DATE DUE

MAY 1 3 2014			

Demco, Inc. 38-293

SALEM HEALTH

MAGILL'S
MEDICAL
GUIDE

SALEM HEALTH

MAGILL'S MEDICAL GUIDE

Sixth Edition

Volume VI

Substance abuse — Zoonoses
Appendixes
Indexes

Medical Editors

Brandon P. Brown, M.D.
Indiana University School of Medicine

H. Bradford Hawley, M.D.
Wright State University

Margaret Trexler Hessen, M.D.
Drexel University College of Medicine

Clair Kaplan, A.P.R.N./M.S.N.
Yale University School of Nursing

Paul Moglia, Ph.D.
South Nassau Communities Hospital

Judy Mouchawar, M.D., M.S.P.H.
University of Colorado Health Sciences Center

Nancy A. Piotrowski, Ph.D.
*Capella University and
University of California, Berkeley*

Claire L. Standen, Ph.D.
University of Massachusetts Medical School

SALEM PRESS
Pasadena, California   Hackensack, New Jersey

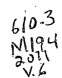

Editor in Chief: Dawn P. Dawson	*Photo Editor:* Cynthia Breslin Beres
Editorial Director: Christina J. Moose	*Production Editor:* Andrea E. Miller
Project Editor: Tracy Irons-Georges	*Acquisitions Editor:* Mark Rehn
Copy Editors: Desiree Dreeuws, Connie Pollock	*Page Design and Layout:* James Hutson
Editorial Assistant: Brett S. Weisberg	*Additional Layout:* William Zimmerman

Illustrations: Hans & Cassidy, Inc., Westerville, Ohio

Magill's Medical Guide: Health and Illness, 1995
Supplement, 1996
Magill's Medical Guide, revised edition, 1998
Second revised edition, 2002
Third revised edition, 2005
Fourth revised edition, 2008
Sixth edition, 2011

∞ The paper used in these volumes conforms to the American National Standard for Permanence of Paper for Printed Library Materials, Z39.48-1992 (R1997).

Note to Readers

The material presented in *Magill's Medical Guide* is intended for broad informational and educational purposes. Readers who suspect that they suffer from any of the physical or psychological disorders, diseases, or conditions described in this set should contact a physician without delay; this work should not be used as a substitute for professional medical diagnosis or treatment. This set is not to be considered definitive on the covered topics, and readers should remember that the field of health care is characterized by a diversity of medical opinions and constant expansion in knowledge and understanding.

Library of Congress Cataloging-in-Publication Data

Magill's medical guide / Brandon P. Brown ... [et al.]. — 6th ed.
    p. cm. — (Salem health)
    Includes bibliographical references and index.
    ISBN 978-1-58765-677-4 (set : alk. paper) — ISBN 978-1-58765-683-5 (v. 6 : alk. paper) —
1. Medicine—Encyclopedias. I. Brown, Brandon P. II. Title: Medical guide.
    RC41.M34 2011
    610.3—dc22
                                                                                    2010031862

First Printing

CONTENTS

COMPLETE LIST OF CONTENTS

VOLUME 1

VOLUME 2

VOLUME 3

Contents lxxiii
Complete List of Contents. lxxvii

VOLUME 4

VOLUME 5

VOLUME 6

Contents clvii

SALEM HEALTH

MAGILL'S
MEDICAL
GUIDE

SUBSTANCE ABUSE

DISEASE/DISORDER

ALSO KNOWN AS: Substance-related disorders

ANATOMY OR SYSTEM AFFECTED: All

SPECIALTIES AND RELATED FIELDS: All

DEFINITION: A pattern of social, psychological, and/or biological problems caused by the way in which a person uses drugs such as alcohol, nicotine, and prescription or illegal drugs.

KEY TERMS:

abuse: a pattern of substance use observed in a twelve-month period resulting in occupational, safety-related, legal, and/or social problems as a consequence of the substance use

addiction: a condition in which an individual is compelled to use a drug, such as alcohol, despite the fact that it is causing significant problems

co-occurring disorders: a situation in which a person has more than one diagnosable problem

dependence: a pattern of substance use problems in a twelve-month period that demonstrates physiological or psychological reliance on a specific substance that results in conditions such as tolerance, withdrawal, inability to regulate one's use, and desire to control or reduce one's use

psychotropic drugs: substances that affect the mind through their influence on the central nervous system

substance of abuse: a drug that affects the mind and body in a reinforcing manner, causing a person to want to repeat use of the drug for its positive effects

tolerance: using a drug and getting less and less effect from the same amount of the drug, or needing more of the drug to get the same effect

withdrawal: symptoms that result when a person ceases or abstains from using a drug; vary from substance to substance and may range from mild irritability to hallucinations and seizures

CAUSES AND SYMPTOMS

There are many substances of abuse. They include drugs such as alcohol and nicotine, the two drugs whose misuse costs society the most in terms of the problems they cause, as well as drugs such as caffeine. They also include illegal and regulated drugs such as marijuana, cocaine, amphetamines, heroin, and hallucinogens. What most people do not realize, however, is that they also include medicinal drugs, such as one might get via a pre-

scription from a doctor, and even substances such as inhalants, including glue and paint.

Problems related to substance use come in several forms. Commonly called substance abuse, the medical description for the group of problems caused by drugs is actually known as substance-related disorders. Substance-related disorders include substance use disorders and substance-induced disorders. Substance use disorders are long-standing problems formally known as abuse and dependence. Substance-induced disorders are slightly different in that they can be very short-lived. Examples of these disorders are intoxication, withdrawal, substance-induced anxiety, substance-induced sleep disorders, and substance-induced sexual disorders. When diagnoses are given for these problems, they are specific to the type of drug(s) the person is using. So a person using marijuana, alcohol, and amphetamines might have diagnoses of marijuana abuse, alcohol dependence, and an amphetamine-induced sleep disorder. The specific diagnoses are made for each drug and will depend on the symptoms that each drug causes on its own.

Problems with substance use may result from many different causes. For conditions such as substance dependence, there can sometimes be a biological component related to genetics. Individuals who have a family history of these problems may carry a genetic

---

INFORMATION ON SUBSTANCE ABUSE

CAUSES: Exposure to addictive substances, repetitive use, genetic risks, other biological risk factors such as other diseases and disorders, social risk factors such as peer and family use, stress, poverty

SYMPTOMS: For abuse, impaired occupational functioning, using in unsafe situations, legal problems, social problems; for dependence, sometimes tolerance, withdrawal, loss of control of use, desire to control use, excessive time spent related to use, reduction of other activities, use despite psychological or physical problems caused or made worse

DURATION: Repeated pattern of problems established within any twelve-month period and time-limited, intermittently repeating, or continuing lifelong

TREATMENTS: Medications, psychotropic drugs, cognitive and behavioral treatments, motivational treatments, family-based treatment, harm reduction treatments, self-help treatments, group-based support, integrated treatments with co-occurring disorders

risk. It is not a guarantee that they will have a problem, but they can have increased risk of developing one. In the same way, even if a person does not have a family history of a problem, it does not mean that they are risk-free. Using substances repetitively, particularly in large doses or very frequently, can also cause problems such as dependence. Patterns of use and frequent use can develop because an individual regularly has access to the drugs through family and/or friends. Also, people may learn how to use the drugs in ways that are not adaptive through these same individuals. This is why having peers who use can be a risk factor for teenagers.

Family history of other problems or characteristics can also contribute to having a greater risk for substance use problems. For instance, a family history of other mental health problems, such as depression, can be a risk factor for developing a substance use problem. Even social characteristics, such as a high amount of family stress, can be a risk factor because individuals may use substances to cope with stress and other life difficulties. Additionally, some individuals may never learn of the risks and consequences associated with substance use because of lack of education or prior exposure to the problems, and so they may use unwittingly and develop problems.

TREATMENT AND THERAPY

Treatments for substance-related disorders vary by the substance involved and the specific type of problem. For instance, if one is experiencing withdrawal from alcohol as compared to another drug such as heroin, different medications are given for treatment. This is the case because the different drugs affect different neurotransmitters in the brain. Also, depending on the severity of the problems or presence of other problems, more than one drug treatment may be used. So someone who has a sleep problem associated with withdrawal from alcohol might be given a sleep medication. If another person withdrawing from alcohol was also showing signs of depression, that individual might be given an additional psychotropic drug to address the depression. In fact, many clients have co-occurring problems, so integrating treatment of the varied problems is important.

It is also important to note that while some treatments focus on reducing symptoms such as withdrawal or sleep problems that are biological in nature, others focus on the more social and behavioral aspects of the problem. Treatments may also vary in their goal. Some

treatments may focus on having an individual achieve abstinence from the problem drug(s), while other treatments may focus on reducing the amount or frequency of drug use, or even reducing other harm from the substance use. Approaches focusing on reducing frequency and amount of use are often focused on moderation as a goal. Approaches focusing on reducing harm are usually known as harm reduction treatments and may focus on reducing associated problems. An example of harm reduction is having individuals who use drugs avoid doing dangerous things such as driving after they have used (thereby reducing risks related to driving while under the influence) or having individuals who inject drugs not share needles (thereby reducing risks related to blood-borne problems such as hepatitis or human immunodeficiency virus, or HIV).

Treatments not including medication may provide therapies that focus on changing specific behaviors or thoughts of the drug user that are related to the problem use. They may also include treatments focusing on helping address the motivation of the individual to change. More specifically, not all people with substance use problems are ready to change immediately. Therefore, sometimes the first treatment needed may be to work on the motivation to change. In fact, sometimes individuals work on their problem on their own, using self-help materials before seeking out treatment professionals. Additionally, it is not uncommon for individuals to seek help for substance use problems through support groups, such as twelve-step groups such as Alcoholics Anonymous.

PERSPECTIVE AND PROSPECTS

Problems related to substances of abuse have been affecting human behavior for all of human existence. Exposure to substances tried as foods or medicines that may have had psychotropic effects, such as fermented berries or mushrooms and plants, are probably some of the first experiences leading to both positive and negative consequences related to substance use. As such, it is a long-standing problem that is likely to stay with human society and require management as time goes on because such substances are available and serve specific needs in human society and/or are ubiquitous in the flora and fauna of the world.

While the formal diagnosis known as substance abuse is likely to change in terms of how it is recognized, the problems related to the condition as currently defined will remain a target of intervention and concern. For example, the parameters defining legal consequences may adjust with new laws as legislation evolves and even new substances of abuse are identified. Similarly, the type and scope of social and safety problems may increase as substances are used in new contexts and with new behaviors. Problems related to role functioning, legal issues, use in unsafe situations, and use resulting in consequences that disturb social relationships remain significant problems and will need continued attention by treatment providers and prevention specialists to address the problem of substance use whether it stands as a condition on its own or as part of a larger spectrum of substance dependence problems and formally diagnosable conditions.

The future is likely to bring continued fine tuning of diagnoses to isolate and identify genetic and physiological aspects of these problems so as to refine prevention and treatment of drug problems involving more biological causes. The balance of the work to refine prevention and treatment will focus on the behavioral and social causes of these conditions which, on their own, may cause problems and also may interact with biological risk factors. Continued understanding of how substance-related conditions interact with other mental health problems, physical conditions, and even cultural differences are also efforts that will improve treatment and prevention.

—*Nancy A. Piotrowski, Ph.D.*

See also Addiction; Alcoholism; Antidepressants; Caffeine; Club drugs; Geriatrics and gerontology; Herbal medicine; Homeopathy; Metabolism; Narcotics; Nicotine; Over-the-counter medications; Pain; Pain management; Pharmacology; Pharmacy; Polypharmacy; Prescription drug abuse; Psychiatry; Psychiatry, child and adolescent; Psychiatry, geriatric; Self-medication; Smoking; Toxicology.

FOR FURTHER INFORMATION:

Bellinir, Karen, ed. *Tobacco Information for Teens: Health Tips About the Hazards of Using Cigarettes, Smokeless Tobacco, and Other Nicotine Products.* Detroit: Omnigraphics, 2007. This resource focuses on one of the most abused drugs in society, nicotine, and provides basic descriptions of key health problems related to its use in varied forms.

DiClemente, Carlo C. *Addiction and Change: How Addictions Develop and How People Change.* New York: Guilford Press, 2006. Provides an easy-to-understand description of problems with addictions, along with useful concepts for thinking about how these problems develop for many people, as well as practical strategies for thinking about how to change.

Julien, Robert M. *A Primer of Drug Action.* 11th ed. New York: Worth, 2007. This is a more technical work that presents a more academic description of what different drugs are, how drugs are processed by the body, their safety issues, and their other effects on the body and brain.

McNeece, C. Aaron, and Diana M. DiNitto. *Chemical Dependency: A Systems Approach.* 3d ed. New York: Pearson, 2005. This textbook provides an integrated way of thinking about substance use problems and their treatment, starting with definitions, epidemiology, etiology, and the biological aspects and other consequences of these problems, while also addressing more advanced topics related to treatment of different types of individuals, such as adolescents, adults, elders, and whole families.

Rosen, Winifred, and Andrew T. Weil. *From Chocolate to Morphine: Everything You Need to Know About Mind-Altering Drugs.* Rev. ed. Boston: Houghton Mifflin, 2004. Source for varying ages provides insight into the broad range of substances that affect the mind.

SUDDEN INFANT DEATH SYNDROME (SIDS)

DISEASE/DISORDER

ANATOMY OR SYSTEM AFFECTED: All

SPECIALTIES AND RELATED FIELDS: Neonatology, pediatrics, psychiatry, psychology

DEFINITION: The abrupt and inexplicable death of any infant or young child, and the most common cause of infant death between the ages of two weeks and one year; postmortem examination fails to demonstrate a definitive cause of death.

KEY TERMS:

apnea: absence of breathing

bradycardia: slowness of the heartbeat

hyperthermia: environmentally influenced elevated body temperature

hypothermia: environmentally influenced lower-than-normal body temperature

hypoxemia: subnormal oxygenation of arterial blood

neonatal: the period of time succeeding birth and continuing through the first twenty-eight days of life

prone: lying face-downward

supine: lying face-upward

tachycardia: rapid beating of the heart

thermolabile: unstable when heated

CAUSES AND SYMPTOMS

The distribution of sudden infant death syndrome (SIDS) is worldwide. Incidence rates vary from 0.12 to 3.0 for every thousand live births. In the United States, rates range from 1.6 to 2.3 for every thousand live births, with considerable ethnic variation: 0.5 among Asians, 1.3 among whites, 1.7 among Latinos, 2.9 among African Americans (5.0 for those of low socioeconomic status), and 5.9 among American Indians.

Cultural practices may make the incidence rate vary. In England, a Birmingham study found that 22 percent of Asian babies were put to sleep on their backs, compared with 3 percent of white babies. Sleeping prone is significantly more common in infants dying of SIDS than in controls. In the same study, 98 percent of Asian babies slept in the same room as their parents for the first year, 34 percent in the same bed. Only 65 percent of white infants slept in the same room as their parents. Perhaps the risk of sudden infant death increases in proportion to the amount of time an infant spends asleep out of parental earshot. In Zimbabwe, SIDS practically does not exist. According to English pediatrician Duncan Keeley, who served in that country for two years, black Zimbabwean infants almost invariably sleep with their mothers, at least until they are six months old and often until they are a year old.

The cause of sudden infant death syndrome is unknown, but a variety of genetic, environmental, and social factors have been associated with an increased risk of SIDS. Besides sleeping in the prone position, other associations include cold weather, overheating, the hours of the day from midnight to 9:00 A.M., and poor socioeconomic conditions, including overcrowding. The young, unmarried mother, especially if she has had no prenatal care, is more likely to have an infant with SIDS; so is the mother who smokes (either before or after the birth), is anemic, or ingests narcotics. Prematurity, especially with a history of apnea or damage to the immature lungs from elevated levels of inspired oxygen while on a respirator, also increases the risk.

Males are at a higher risk for SIDS than are females; so are the brothers and sisters of infants with SIDS. Likewise, a previously aborted episode of SIDS (that is, a "near miss") increases risk. On average, Apgar scores (a measure of infant health immediately after birth) are lower in infants with SIDS than they are in surviving peers. In a family that has lost an infant to SIDS, the risk for the next or subsequent child is about five times the usual risk. Most risk factors, however, are associated with only a twofold or threefold elevation of incidence. Therefore, predicting which infants will die unexpectedly is extremely difficult. Recent immunization is not a risk factor. Breast-feeding is not associated with a decreased risk, as was originally thought. Although the peak incidence of SIDS is around three months of age and coincides with normally low levels of circulating immunoglobulins, the syndrome is not associated with any known pathogen.

Pathologists report a wide variety of findings in their postmortem reports—especially changes in the brain and other parts of the body that suggest chronic or intermittent hypoxemia. Yet pathologists also fail to find an increase in the number of cells in tissue of the carotid bodies, a chemoreceptor that responds to decreases in blood oxygen tension; such a finding weighs against the presence of chronic hypoxia.

Like many other aspects of this disease, the mechanism or mechanisms of death in SIDS are unknown. Does the infant stop breathing, or does some cardiac irregularity occur? An immature cardiorespiratory control mechanism involving the nervous system is the most common hypothesis.

D. P. Davies and Madeleine Gantley of the University of Wales College of Medicine believe that an important mechanism underlying SIDS is failure of respiratory control at a vulnerable stage of development—more a physiological syndrome than a disease in the accepted sense. These doctors hypothesize that the disturbance to this delicate equilibrium might upset the regulation of breathing, sometimes leading to death. Epidemiological risk factors, such as an upper respiratory infection (which is not uncommon), are somehow linked with destabilizing influences to breathing. By avoiding or modulating these factors, the risk of death can be reduced.

INFORMATION ON SUDDEN INFANT DEATH SYNDROME (SIDS)

CAUSES: Unknown; may involve interrelated genetic, environmental, and social factors (sleep disorders, sleep position, cold weather, overheating, poor socioeconomic conditions, premature birth)

SYMPTOMS: Varies and often has no warning signs or symptoms; may include sleep apnea, slow heart rate, low body temperature

DURATION: Acute, with little warning

TREATMENTS: Parent education, placing infants to sleep on their backs

Although the pathogenesis of SIDS remains unclear, Anne-Louise Ponsonby and her colleagues at the University of Tasmania in Australia propose that SIDS be considered as a biphasic event, with the first set of factors operating to predispose the infant and the second set of factors acting as loading factors that operate at a critical stage of the infant's development. The Australian doctors believe that a warm environment could lead to sudden infant death through direct hyperthermia; a thermolabile, sudden fall in blood pressure leading to a diminished oxygen supply to the brain; impaired respiratory control; altered sleep state; or depressed arousal. An asphyxial mode of death would also be more likely, particularly in heavily dressed infants found prone (face down).

Concern for the confusion of SIDS with child abuse should not be ignored, nor should the efforts of the National Sudden Infant Death Syndrome Foundation to provide information about psychosocial support groups and counseling for families of SIDS victims.

TREATMENT AND THERAPY

Since the causes and mechanisms of death from SIDS may continue to be unknown, strategies that might reduce the incidence of this syndrome seem imperative. Cold weather and the hours of midnight to 9:00 A.M. bring increased risks for SIDS. A closer look explains that other risk factors are involved. Overheating as a response to cold weather and leaving the infant alone at night (particularly in Western countries) may be more important. Babies sleeping alone might lose external sensory stimulation that may help stabilize breathing patterns. Davies and Gantley, citing experimental work with mothers and infants co-sleeping in sleep laboratories, have shown how patterns of breathing may interact. They say that the alertness of the babies' caregivers to early symptoms of illness might also be important.

French doctors studied the seasonal variation of death from SIDS in their country for a two-year period in the early 1980's. They concluded that for babies born in the spring, the third month of age was not necessarily associated with the highest SIDS risk. Babies born during other seasons, however, exhibited a normal pattern of increasing risk between the first and third months. Age was an especially critical factor among babies who reached three months of age during the winter months. If they reach this age in July or August, they are less susceptible to SIDS.

This finding, then, leads to a consideration of the risk of overheating. Explanations for the association be-

tween cold weather and SIDS include hypothermia, increased viral illness, and indirect hyperthermia. New Zealand doctors looked at the role of thermal balance in SIDS by investigating the death scene. They found that infants who died of SIDS were significantly more likely to be overdressed for the room temperature at the death scene and in the prone position, when compared to control infants. They also suggest that parents may have responded to infections in their babies by increasing the amount of clothing and bedding or by otherwise warming the infant.

The government of New Zealand initiated a program of education for parents recommending that the prone sleeping position be avoided, that mothers not smoke, and that breast-feeding be encouraged. (Most experts believe that breast-feeding itself does not reduce risks for SIDS. Rather, closer and more frequent contact with mothers is the operative factor.)

A similar education program for parents in Avon, England, was initiated, but it omitted advice on breast-feeding and included suggestions to avoid overheating after a retrospective case-control study that suggested a nearly ninefold relative risk for SIDS from infants sleeping prone. New Zealand and Avon both reported fewer deaths from SIDS after their parental education programs were introduced. The Department of Health extended Avon's campaign nationally.

In an editorial note in 1986, the National Center for Health Statistics acknowledged that "the rapid decline of infant mortality rates in the 1970's has been attributed largely to the advent of medical technology in the area of premature and other clinically ill newborns." Yet, "in the 1980's, this decline has slowed considerably—partly because of a lack of progress in primary prevention of conditions which lead to infant death." Undoubtedly, the United States would benefit from a massive, national program of education for parents. For example, cigarette packages carry a warning of the harmful effects of smoking on the fetus; perhaps they should also include a warning about the dangers to infants of maternal smoking. Another possibility for intervention exists in the area of infections: Pertussis (whooping cough) could be prevented by the immunization of infants under six months of age. In the long term, all nations should work toward improving the socioeconomic status and health care of the poor.

Finally, improved medical technology will be less important over the long haul than will efforts to educate parents in infant care practices. The ability of parents and other members of the household to monitor infants

2868 • Sudden infant death syndrome (SIDS)

and respond appropriately to both true and false alarms is crucial, as is appropriate training in infant CPR (cardiopulmonary resuscitation) and the proper use of monitory equipment. Even if all SIDS is eliminated in at-risk children, there will continue to be cases among children not known to have been at risk.

PERSPECTIVE AND PROSPECTS

The term "sudden infant death syndrome" was popularized by Abraham Berman's book on SIDS in 1969, which grew out of a conference on that subject. Since then, recognition of the syndrome has led to the creation of organizations dealing with it. The Sudden Infant Death Foundation merged, on January 1, 1991, with the National Center for the Prevention of SIDS to form one organization, the Sudden Infant Death Alliance.

In dealing with SIDS, one factor looms most important: Education of parents makes all the difference. In 1991, for example, England's Scarborough district reported a 50 percent fall in the SIDS death rate after parents were advised not to overwarm their small infants. That same year, four other districts in England reported a similar reduction after parents were advised not to let their infants sleep in a prone position. The Foundation for the Study of Infant Deaths and the Department of Health recommend both procedures: a supine sleeping position and prevention of overwarming.

These successes raise two issues: the overall decline in rates of SIDS worldwide in industrial countries and parental guilt. For a number of years, the incidence of SIDS was generally falling. This decline slowed considerably in the 1980's. How much, then, did the parental education programs actually lower the incidence rate in these English districts? No one can say with certainty, but one thing is clear: If doctors make recommendations regarding sleeping positions and warming, they run the risk of inducing guilt in parents who have not followed their recommendations—or, alternatively, who have followed the recommendations but have still lost an infant to SIDS. Parents who have lost a child to SIDS are grief-stricken. They are not prepared for such a tragedy, and their grief is compounded by guilt, because no definitive cause for SIDS has been identified and, as a result, parental behavior seems to be implicated. Investigations conducted by police, social workers, or others who become involved only add to this guilt. Parents may be confronted by questions of whether they positioned their infant correctly or overdressed the child. Regardless of these behaviors, how-

ever, the factors causing the death may not have been under the parents' control.

SIDS will continue to occur until the exact etiologies of the syndrome, its mechanisms, and its correct treatment—based on fact, not simply risks alone—are identified. Until that time, it is expected that incidence rates will continue to go down, based on what is now known of the risk factors and recommendations against prone sleeping positions and overwarming.

—*Wayne R. McKinny, M.D.*

See also Apnea; Death and dying; Grief and guilt; Hyperthermia and hypothermia; Neonatology; Premature birth; Respiration.

FOR FURTHER INFORMATION:

Beers, Mark H., et al., eds. *The Merck Manual of Diagnosis and Therapy.* 18th ed. Whitehouse Station, N.J.: Merck Research Laboratories, 2006. Published since 1899, this classic medical book covers SIDS thoroughly and is easy to read.

Behrman, Richard E., Robert M. Kliegman, and Hal B. Jenson, eds. *Nelson Textbook of Pediatrics.* 18th ed. Philadelphia: Saunders/Elsevier, 2007. This standard pediatric textbook has been around for years and deservedly so. Its excellent chapter on sudden infant death syndrome is a thorough review of the disease.

Byard, R. W., and H. F. Krous. "Sudden Infant Death Syndrome: Overview and Update." *Pediatric and Developmental Pathology* 6, no. 2 (March/April, 2003): 112-127. Details the research advances in the understanding of SIDS since 1990 and discusses historical background, epidemiology, pathology, and pathogenesis.

Samuels, M. "Viruses and Sudden Infant Death." *Pediatric Respiratory Reviews* 4, no. 3 (September, 2003): 178-183. Examines the role of viral respiratory tract inflammation in SIDS, as well as a preceding history of symptoms of minor illness.

SIDS Network. http://sids-network.org. Provides news about current research, frequently asked questions about SIDS, and fact sheets on such topics as sleep, smoking, and apnea.

Southall, D. P., and M. P. Samuels. "Reducing Risks in the Sudden Infant Death Syndrome." *British Medical Journal* 304 (February 1, 1992): 265-266. These acknowledged experts in SIDS have written a thoughtful, thorough review on reducing the risks of SIDS. They strongly suggest that current interventions and socioeconomic factors need monitoring.

SUFFOCATION. *See* **ASPHYXIATION.**

SUICIDE
DISEASE/DISORDER
ANATOMY OR SYSTEM AFFECTED: Psychic-emotional system, all bodily systems
SPECIALTIES AND RELATED FIELDS: Geriatrics and gerontology, psychiatry, psychology
DEFINITION: The deliberate taking of one's own life, usually the result of a mental disorder although sometimes deliberated in the face of life-threatening physical illness, significant interpersonal stress, or when under the influence of one or more substances of abuse.
KEY TERMS:
"no suicide" contract: an agreement, verbally or in writing, that a suicidal person will not act on his or her urges to commit suicide and instead will take other more adaptive action
psychosomatic: referring to physical symptoms interacting with psychological problems
rational suicide: suicide to avoid suffering when there is no underlying cognitive or psychiatric disorder
ritual suicide: a formal, ceremonial, and proscribed form of suicide performed for social reasons in Japanese history
serotonin: an abundant neurotransmitter in the brain that affects many emotional states
suicide cluster: the occurrence of several suicides immediately following a much-publicized suicide
suicide gesture: a superficial suicidal action in which the intention is not to die but to solicit help

CAUSES AND SYMPTOMS
Suicide is the deliberate taking of one's own life. Most often, suicidal individuals are trying to avoid emotional or physical pain that they believe they cannot bear; sometimes, they are very angry and take their lives to lash out at others. Suicide is seen as a solution to an otherwise insoluble problem. Each year, there are about 500,000 self-inflicted injuries and 30,000 completed suicides, with 200,000 family survivors in the United States. In 2006, there were 33,000 suicides, and estimates suggest there were between twelve and twenty-five times as many attempted suicides the same year. Women attempt suicide more often than men, but men complete suicide more often than women because men tend to use more lethal means, such as a gun. It should also be noted that adolescents and the elderly are two high-risk groups.

When an individual contemplates suicide to avoid the physical pain of a terminal illness and does not have a mental disorder, that form of suicidal thought is often called "rational" suicide. This does not imply that this form of suicide is appropriate, moral, or legal but merely that the suicidal thoughts do not arise from a mental disorder (nonrational). Social views on rational suicide vary by culture. For example, many Dutch people consider rational suicide to be acceptable, whereas most Americans do not.

Most suicidal people encountered by physicians, psychologists, social workers, and other mental health professionals experience suicidal thoughts as a result of a mental disorder. The suicidal thoughts and impulses are seen as symptoms of the underlying disorder and require treatment just as any other symptom. The treatment may involve protecting the person against his or her suicidal actions, even to the point of involuntary commitment to a mental hospital.

The rationale behind society's willingness temporarily to deny suicidal individuals' usual civil rights by involuntary commitment is that they are considered to be not "acting in their right mind" by virtue of their mental illness. Thus, they deserve the protection of society until their illness is treated. In fact, suicidal thoughts usually do abate when suicidal patients are treated. The vast majority of these individuals are appreciative afterward; they are glad that they were prevented from killing themselves, as they no longer wish to do so.

The most common mental illness that causes suicidal thoughts is depression. In fact, suicidal thoughts are considered to be a symptom of clinical depression. Other mental disorders associated with suicidal ideation include anxiety disorders such as panic disorder, psychotic disorders such as schizophrenia, substance

INFORMATION ON SUICIDE

CAUSES: Psychological and emotional factors, depression, mental disorders, substance abuse
SYMPTOMS: Depressed and/or anxious mood, hopelessness, loss of normal pleasure in life activities, diminished problem-solving skills, borderline personality disorder, unstable relationships
DURATION: Temporary or recurrent
TREATMENTS: Psychotherapy, counseling, drug therapy

use disorders such as alcohol dependence, and certain personality disorders such as borderline personality disorder.

Although suicide may occur at any time of the year, there is a seasonal variation in its peak incidence. Suicides are most common in both men and women in May; women have a second peak around October and November. This seasonal variation may be attributable to seasonal differences in the incidence of depression.

Suicide appears to have multiple factors involved in its etiology. There are biological, psychological, social, and contextual factors that interact in a complex way to contribute to the causes of suicide in any given individual. The biological factors include genetic contributions to the development of mental disorders such as clinical depression. This may be attributable in part to problems in the neurotransmitter systems in the brain, such as those that control levels of serotonin and dopamine.

Alcohol and other substances of abuse may also cause suicidal ideation. Suicidal thoughts may occur while the individual is using, intoxicated, or in withdrawal. Paradoxically, suicidal thoughts may also arise while the patient is taking antidepressant medications. Fortunately, this side effect is uncommon. and most antidepressant medications do not have such effects. The fact that suicidal thoughts may occur even when on medication, however, underscores the need for individuals taking medications to stay in regular contact with the prescribing physician and to never discontinue their medication without medical consultation. If family members observe a depressed individual taking medication become more depressed, hostile or angry, or suddenly happy or relieved, or if the individual has no apparent response to the medication, then it would be wise to consult with the prescribing physician. This is especially true for family members of children or elders on antidepressant medication.

Psychological factors contributing to suicide include a depressed and/or anxious mood, hopelessness, and a loss of normal pleasure in life activities. Chronically depressed people often have diminished problem-solving skills during periods of depression and can see no way out of their difficulties; suicide is seen as the only solution. There are also personality characteristics that contribute to suicide. In women, borderline personality disorder is often associated with suicide attempts. This disorder is characterized by widely fluctuating moods, rages, feelings of emptiness or boredom, and unstable relationships.

The social factors involved in suicide include cultural acceptance or rejection of suicide. Historically, Japanese people have accepted ritual suicide within their culture and somewhat sanction suicide as a response to a severe loss of face or social esteem. This does not mean that they embrace it, but rather that the history contributes to cultural norms where this is thought of as an option for dealing with shame. Similarly, the Dutch government has legalized rational suicide as an option for dying. In contrast, most Americans have a more negative view of the suicide act. Other social factors that increase the likelihood of suicide include social instability, divorce, unemployment, immigration, and exposure to violence as a child. In the United States, European Americans commit suicide more often than African Americans. Native Americans have a high incidence of suicide. In general, good social support reduces the risk of suicide.

Some patients engage in suicidal gestures; that is, they say they want to kill themselves and take actions such as swallowing some pills or superficially cutting their wrists, but there is no real intention to die. They act this way as a cry for help. For some, this may be the only way to receive attention for what troubles them. Unfortunately, the suicide gesture may go awry and unintended death may occur. Anyone who speaks of suicide or engages in what may appear to be a gesture should be taken seriously.

Most people who are suicidal have ambivalent feelings: Part of them wants to die, part does not. This is one of the reasons that the majority of suicidal people tell others of their intention in advance of their attempts. Most have visited their personal physician in the months prior to the suicide. Adolescents sometimes hint at their wish to die by giving away their prized possessions just prior to an attempt.

Contextual factors, or the circumstances in which people find themselves, can also contribute to individuals attempting suicide. Access to means of self-harm, such as weapons or drugs, can increase the likelihood of a suicide attempt. Similarly, physical isolation from others can also increase the odds, as there is no one to readily intervene. Even painful emotional or physical states, such as exhaustion or those that might be brought on by substance use, can set the stage for impulsive behavior to increase the likelihood of suicide attempts. In contrast, simply talking to someone about suicidal thoughts will not cause someone to commit suicide and instead may be a way to get help from a professional.

Anyone experiencing suicidal thoughts should be thoroughly evaluated by a professional trained in the assessment of suicidal patients. If the risk of suicide is considered to be high enough, the patient will have to be protected. This may require hospitalization, either voluntary or involuntary. It may mean removing suicidal means from that person's environment, such as removing guns from the home. Having someone stay with the patient at all times may be required. These steps should be individualized, taking into account the patient's situation.

Treatment of the underlying cause of the suicidal ideation is very important. Depression and anxiety can be treated with medications and/or psychotherapy. There are treatment programs for alcoholism and drug abuse. Usually, successful treatment of the underlying mental disorder results in the suicidal thoughts going away.

While they await the resolution of the suicidal ideation, patients need to be offered support and hope. Sometimes, a "no suicide" contract is helpful. This is simply a commitment on the part of the patient not to act on any suicidal thoughts and to contact the health professional if the urges become worse. While this contract may be written down, it is usually verbal.

Suicide prevention includes the early detection and management of the mental disorders associated with suicide. Because social isolation increases the risk of suicide, patients should be encouraged to develop and actively maintain strong social supports such as family, friends, and other social groups (church, clubs, and sports teams).

It may also be helpful to provide counseling to teenagers after an acquaintance has committed suicide, as this may prevent social contagion and suicide clusters. A suicide cluster is when several individuals (often teenagers) commit suicide after learning of the suicide of an acquaintance or a person who is attractive to them, such as a music or film star. Suicide clusters have increased among the young.

Family members of a suicide victim often go through a grieving process which is more severe than that which occurs after death from other causes. The stigma of suicide and mental illness is strong, and surviving family members often have greater feelings of both guilt and abandonment. Family survivors also have increased psychosomatic complaints, behavioral and emotional problems, and risk of suicide themselves. Referral to a suicide survivor group may be helpful.

TREATMENT AND THERAPY

An understanding of the causes, detection, and treatment of suicide has led to the development of a number of suicide hotlines and suicide prevention centers. There is evidence that, after these support groups are introduced into a community, the suicide rate for young women decreases. It is not yet known if they have any effect on other groups, such as young men or the elderly.

Most people who contemplate suicide do not seek professional treatment even if they tell people around them of their suicidal ideas. Thus, it is important for physicians, clergy, teachers, parents, and mental health workers to remain alert to the possibility of suicidal thoughts in those in their care. Someone who is depressed or very anxious should be asked about suicidal thoughts. Such a question will not plant the idea in his or her head, and the person may feel relieved after being asked. Once someone with suicidal ideation is identified, evaluation and treatment should proceed quickly. The following sample composite cases illustrate the application of the concepts described in the overview.

Mary is a seventeen-year-old senior in high school. She is from a broken home and was severely abused by her father prior to her parents' divorce ten years ago. Her teachers think that she is a bright underachiever who has a rather dramatic personality. Her friends see her as moody and easily angered. Her relationships with boyfriends are intense and always end with deep feelings of hurt and abandonment. Her mother is best described as cold, aloof, and preoccupied with herself.

Mary is brought to the school counselor by one of her friends when Mary threatens to kill herself and superficially scratches her wrists with a safety pin. The counselor learns that Mary has just broken up with her boyfriend, a young man at a local junior college. She is devastated. When she tried to tell her mother about it, her mother seemed uninterested and said that Mary always makes too much of such little things. It was the next morning that she scratched herself in front of her friend.

While more information is needed, this case illustrates a suicide gesture. In this case, Mary does not want to die but instead wants someone to realize how distressed she is. She feels rejected by her boyfriend and then by her mother. One can suspect a gesture rather than a serious suicide attempt by the superficial, nonlethal means (scratching with a safety pin) and by the likelihood of discovery (done in front of a friend).

Here is a second case. Tom is a forty-eight-year-old accountant. He is separated from his wife and three children and lives alone in an apartment. He has no real friends, only drinking buddies. Like his father and two uncles, Tom is an alcoholic. Each day after work, he stops at his favorite bar and drinks between eight and twelve beers.

He is brought to the emergency room of the local hospital by the police, who found him sitting on the steps of a church sobbing. He threatened to kill himself if his wife did not take him back. The emergency room doctor noted the strong odor of alcohol on his breath and ordered a blood alcohol test, which showed that he was legally intoxicated. Tom insisted that he would kill himself by running in front of a moving bus if he could not be with his family. The emergency room doctor had Tom's belt, pocketknife, and other potentially dangerous items taken from him and arranged for a staff member to sit with him until he was sober. Six hours later, his blood alcohol had returned to near zero. Tom no longer felt despondent and had no more suicidal thoughts. He was embarrassed by his statements a few hours before. An alcoholism counselor was called, and outpatient treatment for his alcoholism was arranged.

This case illustrates suicidal ideation caused by alcohol intoxication. As often happens, the suicidal ideation resolves when the patient becomes sober. The primary treatment is for the underlying addictive disorder.

Here is a third case. Sally is a fifty-three-year-old married mother of two. She is a part-time hairdresser and normally a very active, happy person. For the past three weeks, however, she has gradually lost all interest in her job, her children, her home, and her hobbies. She feels irritable and sad most of the time. Although she is tired, she does not sleep well at night, waking up very early each morning, unable to return to sleep. She is worried by the fact that she is having intrusive thoughts of killing herself. Sally imagines she could end all this dreariness by overdosing on sleeping pills and never waking up. She is a strict Catholic and knows it is against her religion to commit suicide. She calls her parish priest.

After a brief conversation, her priest meets her at the office of a psychiatrist who acts as a consultant for the diocese. The psychiatrist diagnoses major depression as the cause of Sally's suicidal ideation. She has a good social support network, so the psychiatrist decides to treat her as an outpatient and has her agree to a "no suicide" contract. Sally is also started on antidepressant medication, which gradually lifts her depression over a

period of two to three weeks. Simultaneously, her suicidal thoughts leave her.

This case illustrates suicidal thoughts caused by depression. If Sally had been more depressed or her suicidal urges stronger, she would probably have needed hospitalization. If she had required hospitalization and had refused to go voluntarily, the psychiatrist could have had her committed according to the laws of the state where he practiced. Most states require a signed statement by two physicians or one physician and a licensed clinical psychologist. They must attest that the patient is a danger to himself or herself and that no less restrictive form of treatment would suffice.

Finally, here is a fourth case. Harry is a sixty-seven-year-old resident of a hospital, where he has been for the past two years. He has a serious neurological disorder called amyotrophic lateral sclerosis (also called Lou Gehrig's disease). It has caused progressive weakness such that he cannot even breathe on his own. Harry is permanently connected to a respirator attached to a tracheotomy tube in his throat. He has few visitors and mostly stares off and thinks.

Harry tells his nurse that he is "sick of it all" and wants his doctors to disconnect him from the respirator and let him die. His neurologist requests a psychiatric evaluation. The psychiatrist confirms the patient's wish to die. There is no evidence of dementia or other cognitive disorder, nor is the patient showing any evidence of a mental illness. Subsequently, a meeting is called of the hospital ethics committee to make recommendations. Membership on the committee includes physicians, nurses, an ethicist, a local minister, and the hospital attorney.

This case illustrates a difficult example of rational suicide request. The patient has a desire to die and is not suffering from any mental disorder. In this case, he is requesting not to take his own life actively but to be allowed to die passively by removal of the respirator. Some people do not consider this to be suicide at all. They make a distinction between passively allowing a natural process of dying to occur and actively taking one's own life. If this patient requested a lethal overdose of potassium to be injected into his intravenous tubes, such action would be considered suicide and ethically different. In either event, these matters are more ethical, social, and legal than psychiatric.

Perspective and Prospects
Throughout history, there have been numerous examples of suicide. In Western culture, early views on the

subject were mainly from a moral perspective and suicide was viewed as a sin. Mental illness in general was poorly understood and often thought of as weakness of character, possession by evil spirits, or willful bad behavior. Thus, mental illness was stigmatized. Even though society now has a better medical understanding of mental illness, there is still a stigma attached to mental illness and to suicide. This stigma contributes to underdiagnosis and undertreatment of suicidal individuals, as many sufferers are reluctant to come forth with their symptoms.

Suicide remains an important public health problem. In 2006, it was the eleventh most common cause of death in the United States (although it was third for adolescents and second for young adults). Each year, there are about thirty thousand known suicides in the United States. The actual incidence may be higher because an unknown number of accidental deaths or untreated illnesses may actually be undiagnosed suicides. For every suicide death, between eight and twenty-five other individuals attempt suicide.

Unfortunately, most cases of suicidal ideation never come to the attention of health professionals. Therefore, when someone talks of suicide, a high index of suspicion should be maintained. Those people who express suicidal thoughts should be taken seriously and thoroughly evaluated. Increased levels of awareness of suicide may help to improve detection and treatment of this potentially preventable cause of death. Research in this area continues to focus on prevention and early identification and treatment for individuals who are distressed.

—Peter M. Hartmann, M.D.;
updated by Nancy A. Piotrowski, Ph.D.

See also Addiction; Alcoholism; Antidepressants; Anxiety; Death and dying; Dementias; Depression; Euthanasia; Grief and guilt; Hypochondriasis; Midlife crisis; Neurosis; Panic attacks; Phobias; Postpartum depression; Post-traumatic stress disorder; Psychiatric disorders; Psychiatry; Psychiatry, child and adolescent; Psychiatry, geriatric; Psychoanalysis; Psychosomatic disorders; Puberty and adolescence; Schizophrenia; Stress; Terminally ill: Extended care.

For Further Information:

DePaulo, J. Raymond, Jr., and Leslie Alan Horvitz. *Understanding Depression: What We Know and What You Can Do About It.* New York: Wiley, 2003.

A leading expert on depression examines the disease's nature, causes, effects, and treatments.

Hafen, Brent Q., and Kathryn J. Frandsen. *Youth Suicide: Depression and Loneliness.* 2d ed. Evergreen, Colo.: Cordillera Press, 1986. An excellent review of all aspects of teenage suicide, with practical suggestions for helping the suicidal young person.

Jamison, Kay Redfield. *Night Falls Fast: Understanding Suicide.* New York: Alfred A. Knopf, 2000. Jamison, a distinguished psychologist and academic, brings a rare combination of personal and academic experience to bear in this monumental work on suicide.

Kolf, June Cerza. *Standing in the Shadow: Help and Encouragement for Suicide Survivors.* New York: Baker Books, 2002. The author, a veteran of hospice work, addresses the impact of suicide on family members and friends, and explores such emotions as forgiveness and depression, as well as the search for answers.

Koplewicz, Harold S. *More than Moody: Recognizing and Treating Adolescent Depression.* New York: Penguin, 2003. A leading clinician and researcher helps parents distinguish between normal teenage angst and depression, examining the warning signs, risk factors, and key behaviors, as well as treatment options.

Lester, David. *Making Sense of Suicide: An In-Depth Look at Why People Kill Themselves.* Philadelphia: Charles Press, 1997. This book may be helpful for beginning counselors and family members or friends interested in learning more about suicidal behavior.

Peck, M. Scott. *Denial of the Soul: Spiritual and Medical Perspectives on Euthanasia and Mortality.* New York: Random House, 1998. This book discusses controversial issues related to euthanasia and suicide.

Roesch, Roberta. *The Encyclopedia of Depression.* 2d ed. New York: Facts On File, 2001. This volume was written for both laypersons and professionals. Covers all aspects of depression, including bereavement, grief, and mourning. The appendixes include references, self-help groups, national associations, and institutes.

Suicide Awareness Voices of Education. http://www .save.org. Offers resources for suicide prevention, suicide survivors, and for families coping with a suicide loss.

SUNBURN
DISEASE/DISORDER
ANATOMY OR SYSTEM AFFECTED: Skin
SPECIALTIES AND RELATED FIELDS: Dermatology, emergency medicine, family medicine, oncology
DEFINITION: An inflammation of the skin produced by excessive exposure to the sun, sunlamps, or occupational light sources.

CAUSES AND SYMPTOMS
Sunburn is caused by overexposure to ultraviolet light coming directly from the sun or from artificial lighting sources, as well as from reflected sunlight from snow, water, sand, and sidewalks. Scattered rays may also produce sunburn, even in the presence of clouds, haze, or thin fog. Symptoms include red, swollen, painful, and sometimes blistered skin; chills; and fever. In severe cases, nausea, vomiting, and even delirium may be present. Depending on the severity of the burn, tanning and peeling may occur during recovery.

TREATMENT AND THERAPY
To reduce the heat and pain of sunburn, towels or gauze dipped in cool water can be carefully laid on the burned areas. Once the skin swelling subsides, cold cream or baby lotion can be applied to the affected areas. If the skin is blistered, a light application of petroleum jelly prevents anything from sticking to the blisters. Nonprescription drugs, such as acetaminophen, can be used to relieve pain and reduce fever. If necessary, a medical doctor can prescribe other pain relievers or cortisone drugs to relieve itching and aid healing.

PERSPECTIVE AND PROSPECTS
A number of risk factors can greatly intensify the effects of sunburn, including such genetic factors as fair skin, blue eyes, and red or blond hair; the use of

---

INFORMATION ON SUNBURN

CAUSES: Prolonged exposure to sun, sunlamps, or occupational light sources
SYMPTOMS: Red, swollen, painful, and sometimes blistered skin; chills; fever; in severe cases, nausea, vomiting, and possible delirium
DURATION: Acute
TREATMENTS: Prevention through repeated application of sunscreen or sunblock; alleviation of symptoms

---

certain drugs, particularly sulfa drugs, tetracyclines, amoxicillin, or oral contraceptives; and exposure to industrial light sources, such as arc welders. For outdoor activities, a sunscreen or sunblock preparation should be applied to exposed areas of the body. Baby oil, mineral oil, or cocoa butter offer no protection from the sun. Brilliant colored and white clothing that reflect the sun into the face should be avoided. If tanning is a must, sun exposure should be limited to five to ten minutes on each side the first day, adding five minutes per side each additional day. Severe sunburn in childhood can lead to skin cancer later in life.

—*Alvin K. Benson, Ph.D.*

See also Blisters; Cancer; Carcinogens; Dermatology; Dermatology, pediatric; Skin; Skin cancer; Skin disorders.

FOR FURTHER INFORMATION:
Grob, J. J., et al., eds. *Epidemiology, Causes, and Prevention of Skin Diseases.* Cambridge, Mass.: Blackwell Science, 1997.
Kenet, Barney, and Patricia Lawler. *Saving Your Skin: Prevention, Early Detection, and Treatment of Melanoma and Other Skin Cancers.* 2d ed. Chicago: Four Walls Eight Windows, 1998.
Litin, Scott C., ed. *Mayo Clinic Family Health Book.* 4th ed. New York: HarperResource, 2009.
Siegel, Mary-Ellen. *Safe in the Sun.* New York: Walker, 1995.

SUPPLEMENTS
TREATMENT
ANATOMY OR SYSTEM AFFECTED: All
SPECIALTIES AND RELATED FIELDS: Alternative medicine, family medicine, internal medicine, nutrition
DEFINITION: Chemical compounds, concentrated into pills, powders, and capsules, that are taken to prevent or treat diseases.

THE ROLE OF SUPPLEMENTS
Adequate nutrition is the foundation of good health. Everyone needs the four basic nutrients: water, carbohydrates, proteins, and fats. It is important to choose the proper foods to deliver these nutrients and, as necessary, to complement the diet with supplements.
Health-conscious adults have heard the message repeatedly that they can get the vitamins they need from the foods they eat, but surveys have shown that peo-

ple in many countries fail to eat adequate amounts of fruit, vegetables, whole grains, and low-fat dairy foods. Should public health officials or registered dieticians recommend that people take supplements to compensate for poor eating habits? The answer to this question can be found in a discussion of vitamin supplements.

The 1990's brought to light much new information about human nutrition, its effects on the body, and the role that it plays in disease. The fuel for the body's engine comes directly from the food that one eats, which contains many vital nutrients. Nutrients come in the form of vitamins, minerals, enzymes, water, amino acids, carbohydrates, and lipids (fats). These nutrients provide people with the basic materials that human bodies need to sustain life.

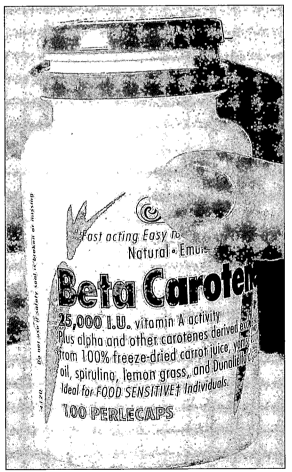

Dietary supplements such as these beta carotene pills have become increasingly popular in the United States, despite a lack of government regulation regarding safety and claims. (SIU School of Medicine)

One of the latest types of dietary supplements are nutraceuticals. These supplements are obtained from naturally derived chemicals in plants, called photonutrients, that make the plants biologically active. They are not nutrients in the classic sense. They are what determine a plant's color, ability to resist disease, and flavor.

Nutritionists have discovered that fruits and vegetables, grains, and legumes contain other healthful nutrients called phytochemicals. Researchers have identified thousands of phytochemicals and have the ability to remove these chemical compounds and concentrate them into pills, powders, and capsules. Phytochemicals are believed to be powerful ammunition in the war against cancer and other cellular mutations. In simple terms, cancer is a mutation of body cells through a multistep process. Phytochemicals are hypothesized to fight that disease by stopping one or more of the steps that lead to cancer. For example, a cancer process can be kindled when a carcinogenic molecule invades a cell, possibly from foods eaten or from air breathed. Sulforaphane, a phytochemical commonly found in broccoli, is then hypothesized to activate an enzyme process that removes the carcinogen from the cell before harm is done.

Researchers and pharmaceutical companies sell concentrated forms of various phytochemicals found in such vegetables as broccoli, brussels sprouts, cauliflower, and cabbage. Because no single supplement can possibly compete with nature, some nutritionists recommend a shopping basket full of fruits and vegetables, as opposed to using expensive bottled supplements. Tomatoes, for example, are believed to contain an estimated ten thousand different phytochemicals.

Natural food supplements can be high in certain nutrients. Examples are aloe vera, bee pollen, fish oils, flaxseed, primrose oil, ginseng, ginkgo biloba, garlic, and oat bran. In general, natural food supplements are composed of by-products of foods that can provide a multitude of health benefits. One caution, however, is that supplements of this type may not have the same kind of quality control or oversight as medications prescribed by a doctor and bought from a pharmacy. As such, the effects of supplements may vary from pill to pill and bottle to bottle.

THE PROMISE OF ANTIOXIDANTS

No discussion of supplements would be complete without mention of antioxidants. They are a group of vitamins, minerals, and enzymes that help to protect the

IN THE NEWS: DIETARY SUPPLEMENT CRACKDOWNS BY THE FDA

In the past, the dietary supplement industry has been loosely regulated. Even though the Food and Drug Administration (FDA) required all the ingredients to be label-listed, there were no rules that limited the manufacturers' recommendations regarding serving sizes or the actual content amount of the nutrients. Moreover, no proof was required to guarantee product safety. However, as a result of the increasing problem of cross-contamination and misleading labeling of dietary supplements, coupled with adverse health outcomes, in March, 2003, the FDA proposed new labeling and manufacturing standards. A final rule was announced in June, 2007, indicating that the current Good Manufacturing Practices (cGMPS) would apply to the dietary supplement business. These standards were already in effect for the pharmaceutical and veterinary industries. The new rulings will establish industry-wide standards to guarantee consistent manufacturing standards in order to assure the public that the dietary supplement industry is safe and provides pure products with known strengths and compositions.

The FDA had been averaging about 550 supplement-related adverse event reports yearly since 1993; however, that figure doubled in 2002. For instance, dietary supplements had to be recalled by one manufacturer because of excessive lead contamination. Another manufacturer of niacin supplements mistakenly marketed a product that contained ten times the safe limit of niacin, which was not reflected on the label. The product was recalled after health reports of nausea, vomiting, and liver damage were received. Dietary supplements containing ephedra, used for weight loss, increased energy, and athletic performance enhancement, have been linked to several deaths, resulting in the banning of ephedra-enhanced products. A sports supplement abuse case involved the use of vitamins by a world-class athlete who failed a drug doping test; the results were later reversed when the product was tested and found to be cross-contaminated by an anabolic steroid compound that was also manufactured at the same laboratory where the vitamins were packaged.

Under the cGMPS ruling, manufacturers are required to document the identity, composition, purity, quality, and strength of the ingredients in dietary supplements. If the product is found to deviate from what the manufacturer has claimed to be the ingredients, the FDA considers the product adulterated. The minimum standards require physical plants to be constructed to ensure proper manufacturing operations, facility maintenance and cleaning, the establishment of quality control procedures, final product testing before going to market, and better methods for handling and resolving consumer complaints. These rulings do not limit consumer's access to dietary supplements but rather ensure a safer product.

—*Bonita L. Marks, Ph.D.*

body from the formation of free radicals. Free radicals are groups of atoms that can cause damage to cells and thus impair the immune system. This damage is also thought to be the basis for the aging process. Free radicals are believed to be formed through exposure to radiation and toxic chemicals such as cigarette smoke, as well as overexposure to the sun's rays.

Some common antioxidants are vitamin A and its precursor, beta carotene; vitamin C; and vitamin E. Zinc and the trace mineral selenium are thought to play an important role in neutralizing free radicals. Each vitamin or mineral has a recommended daily allowance (RDA).

Some in the field of nutrition have recommended higher supplementation doses of antioxidants and specific use of four antioxidant supplements—vitamins C and E, selenium, and mixed carotenes—to protect the

immune system even further. Recommendations such as this are numerous and related to different kinds of supplement use, and they must be weighed carefully against data obtained from controlled clinical trials. While many of the substances touted as beneficial to health may have some benefits, supplements can be harmful in the wrong person; at the wrong dose; if taken in combination with the wrong medications or diet; or if taken in the presence of certain health conditions. For example, it is possible to overdose on vitamins such as A, B, and E, or on iron supplements. Some supplements, like St. John's wort, may create a side effect of light sensitivity, and discontinuing drugs such as valerian root can lead to heart problems. Also, it is easy to succumb to the temptation to seek "health in a bottle" instead of engaging in proven preventive practices. For these reasons, careful consideration and consultation with one's doctor should occur before embarking on any regimen of supplements.

PERSPECTIVE AND PROSPECTS

Use of supplements is based both on modern research and development and on discoveries by mainstream scientists about the benefits of various substances. Substances such as garlic and aloe vera are examples of home remedies that have shown some promise for different kinds of ailments. Natural supplements have been used for centuries in many parts of the world as alternative medicines.

Considered and careful examination of supplement regimens in controlled clinical trials will serve as the ultimate test on the utility of these substances for health purposes. Simultaneously, consumers must remain aware that personal use of these supplements may, at times, be somewhat experimental. Quality control concerns and interactions between supplements and prescribed medications are an important consideration. Additionally, knowledge of the supplements found in pills or popular beverages and how they may interact with street drugs of different types is also important in order to avoid unnecessary harm. This is especially true for children and elders.

—Lisa Levin Sobczak, R.N.C.;
updated by Nancy A. Piotrowski, Ph.D.

See also Aging; Alternative medicine; Antioxidants; Digestion; Ergogenic aids; Food biochemistry; Herbal medicine; Macronutrients; Malnutrition; Nutrition; Osteoporosis; Over-the-counter medications; Phytochemicals; Self-medication; Vitamins and minerals.

FOR FURTHER INFORMATION:

Balch, James F., and Phyllis A. Balch. *Prescription for Nutritional Healing: A Practical A to Z Reference to Drug-Free Remedies Using Vitamins, Minerals, Herbs, and Food Supplements.* 4th rev. ed. Garden City Park, N.Y.: Avery, 2008.

Hendler, Sheldon Saul. *The Doctors' Vitamin and Mineral Encyclopedia.* New York: Simon & Schuster, 1990.

Murray, Michael. *The Pill Book Guide to Natural Medicines: Vitamins, Minerals, Nutritional Supplements, Herbs, and Other Natural Products.* New York: Bantam, 2002.

The PDR Family Guide to Nutritional Supplements: An Authoritative A-to-Z Resource on the One Hundred Most Popular Nutritional Therapies and Nutraceuticals. New York: Ballantine Books, 2001.

Weil, Andrew. *Eight Weeks to Optimum Health: A Proven Program for Taking Full Advantage of Your Body's Natural Healing Power.* Rev. ed. New York: Ballantine Books, 2007.

SURGERY, GENERAL

SPECIALTY

ANATOMY OR SYSTEM AFFECTED: All

SPECIALTIES AND RELATED FIELDS: Anesthesiology, radiology

DEFINITION: A field of medicine that involves a wide range of surgical procedures, from the simple removal of warts and bunions in the doctor's office to complex organ transplantation requiring a large staff in the operating room.

KEY TERMS:

aseptic techniques: procedures that allow surgeons to operate in a germ-free environment

excision: the surgical removal of an organ or tissue

SCIENCE AND PROFESSION

In all probability, surgery has been practiced as long as humans have had cutting tools. Ample reports of battlefield amputations exist almost from the beginning of reported time. Historians tell of rough field surgery, the hacking off of wounded limbs and the sealing of the wounds by searing the lacerated flesh. There are even suggestions that ancient civilizations, such as that of the Egyptians, practiced trepanning, cutting into the skull to operate on the brain.

Until the latter half of the nineteenth century, surgery was a brutal, dirty, and dangerous practice. About this time, the relationship between microorganisms and diseases was first enunciated, a relationship which explained why so many surgery patients sickened and died. It was also at this time that anesthetics were developed, which for the first time allowed the surgeon to deaden the patient's pain.

Surgery today is one of the most respected medical specialties, requiring full training in the disciplines of medicine, as well as years of extensive work in surgical procedures. After becoming physicians, candidates for surgery spend years working under established surgeons learning the techniques that they will use in practice. They are subjected to intensive examination and receive certification only when their peers are convinced that they can perform their duties capably.

The tools and techniques of surgery that the surgical candidate must master present multiple challenges. In their training phase, surgeons learn to become skilled

A Typical Operating Room

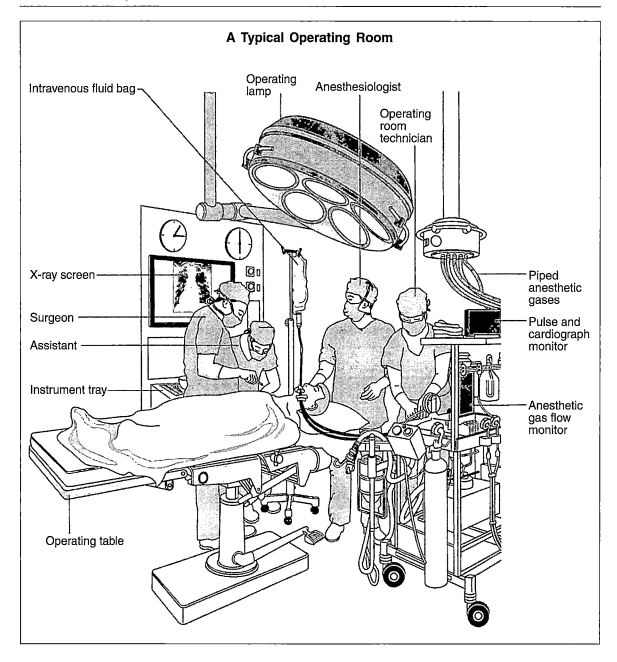

Intravenous fluid bag
Operating lamp
Anesthesiologist
Operating room technician
X-ray screen
Surgeon
Assistant
Instrument tray
Operating table
Piped anesthetic gases
Pulse and cardiograph monitor
Anesthetic gas flow monitor

in the manipulation of all the basic instruments used in surgery, such as the various designs of scalpels, scissors, retractors, forceps, and sutures. The training surgeon learns a wide variety of stitching techniques and the materials used in suturing. Most challenging perhaps is mastery of the many new techniques and instruments that modern surgeons use.

After training and certification, some surgeons elect to practice general surgery. As the term implies, this field covers such diverse areas of the body as the stomach, gallbladder, liver, intestines, appendix, breasts, thyroid gland, salivary glands, main arteries and veins, lumps under the skin, hernias, and hemorrhoids. Other surgeons choose to specialize in disciplines that require still more training, such as heart surgery, bone (or orthopedic) surgery, and eye (or ophthalmic) surgery, to name some of the more prevalent specialties.

Modern surgery is a far-ranging practice involving all body structures and systems. It is also a practice that sees constant advancements and improvements in operating techniques, in instrumentation and tools, and in high-tech equipment. Microsurgery, in which the surgeon uses a microscope to view the operating field and manipulates tiny instruments to repair or excise tissue, was virtually unheard of at the middle of the twentieth century. It is now common practice in virtually every surgical facility in the United States. At one time, a severed limb could never be reconnected, largely because it was impossible to repair severed nerves. Now, because of microsurgery, arms, legs, hands, digits, and other severed body parts can be stitched back on to the body, often with much of their mobility restored.

Much minor surgery takes place in the physician's office or clinic. These procedures are generally simple, involving the excision of skin growths such as warts or cancers, hemorrhoids, and other surface conditions. Emergency surgery in the office, clinic, or emergency room may be necessary to open an airway for a patient whose breathing is impaired or to remove obstructions.

Major surgery usually requires a hospital stay, and its main characteristics are anesthesia and aseptic technique. Anesthesia may be local, regional, or general. For local anesthesia, anesthetic is injected into the site of the operation. The patient is usually fully awake during the surgery but feels no pain in the affected area. In regional anesthesia, a whole part of the body is anesthetized, such as a leg or an arm. As with local anesthesia, the patient is awake during the procedure but may be sedated for comfort. In general anesthesia, the patient is put to sleep and immobilized, usually by injections, and inhaled anesthetics are administered throughout the course of the operation.

To create an aseptic, germ-free environment, the operating room and everything in it are subjected to rigorous sterilization. Surgeons and all operating room staff scrub with antiseptic soaps. They don complete uniforms of sterilized cloth or paper: caps, masks, gowns, gloves, and foot coverings. Avoiding transmission of disease in the operating room can be said to be as important as the operation itself. It is vital that the patient be made safe from infection by the staff and from pathogenic organisms in the ambient atmosphere of the hospital.

It is equally important that staff be protected from infection by the patient. Operating room personnel are particularly vulnerable to blood-borne infections, such as hepatitis B and human immunodeficiency virus (HIV). Surgery can be a bloody procedure. In some operations, copious blood spurts are common, and the likelihood of staff being spattered is high, as is the pos-

sibility of disease transmission. It is possible that there will be a cut or tear in the staff's protective clothing and that the patient's blood or other body fluids can make contact with an abrasion on the body or even land on mucous membranes of the mouth, nose, and throat, where they can infect the caregiver. This has happened so often that the U.S. government has issued rigorous guidelines to high-risk health care personnel—particularly operating room staff—detailing specific procedures to follow to avoid disease transmission.

DIAGNOSTIC AND TREATMENT TECHNIQUES

The surgeon is rarely the first physician whom the patient sees. Usually, a primary care physician makes a diagnosis and may confer with or send the patient to a specialist for confirmation of the diagnosis. When surgery is recommended, the surgeon confers with the primary care physician and/or the consulting specialist and is fully apprised of the patient's condition. He or she reviews the patient's history and inspects all relevant documents and diagnostic reports, such as X rays, computed tomography (CT) scans, and other information that he or she needs to plan and perform the procedure.

For the most part, surgeons deal with their patients only in the immediate context of the operation. They meet before the operation, and surgeons look in on patients afterward to check their progress and recovery. In some cases, follow-up visits to the surgeon are required.

In the operating room, the surgeon assembles the staff needed for the particular procedure. There will be an anesthesiologist, perhaps other specialized surgeons, and various general and specialized operating room nurses. The surgeon or the staff will also order everything needed for the procedure. There is an enormous range of specialized equipment that surgeons can use in their procedures. Cardiac surgeons use heart-lung machines, which take over the task of circulating the patient's blood and allow the surgeon to open and enter the heart itself. The neurosurgeon may operate through specialized microscopic instruments.

A catalog of specialized endoscopes is now available to surgeons, many of which allow them to operate through a tiny hole in the patient's skin, rather than having to make massive cuts with a scalpel. Pulmonary surgeons use a bronchoscope to look down into the patient's bronchial tubes, where they can perform such surgical operations as removing obstructions and excising cancerous tissue. Gastrointestinal surgeons use a gastroscope both to investigate conditions in the stomach and to take small tissue samples for biopsy. Colon and rectal surgeons use a colonoscope to remove polyps from the colon and rectum, a major step in the prevention and treatment of colon cancer. Major surgery, however, still involves cutting the patient open to repair what has gone wrong inside the body. Fortunately, this procedure is now safer and more specialized than it has ever been before.

Management of disease in the United States has reached the point where there are surgical specialties to cover virtually all parts of the body individually. Some surgeons specialize in individual organs, such as the heart, lungs, brain, eyes, and ears. Some surgeons specialize in body systems such as bones or circulation. Furthermore, many surgeons hone their skills in certain specialized surgical techniques and become so adept that they are recognized as experts in highly complex and critical procedures, such as repairing detached retinas, performing heart transplants, correcting slipped disks, or sealing brain aneurysms.

Surgeons are major inventors and designers. Much of the instrumentation and many of the surgical tools that are used in the operating room were invented by surgeons. They often direct the fabrication of specialized tools and instruments to help them in their work. Most of the metal and plastic prostheses implanted to replace damaged internal structures were designed by surgeons. Orthopedic surgeons design prosthetic hips, knees, and other implants. Ophthalmic surgeons design corneal implants. The specialized surgeon knows his or her area of the body better than anyone else does and can visualize what sort of equipment or device is needed to improve the patient's condition.

Surgeons are also at the forefront of major technical innovations that reach across the entire surgical field. They are adept at recognizing potential applications for new technology and adapting it to surgery. For example, fiber-optic science has been applied in surgical endoscopes. Cryosurgery, a technique of freezing tissue, is used in a wide range of procedures, from the removal of hemorrhoids to the reattachment of retinas.

Laser technology is employed in hundreds of surgical procedures. The laser is used for making incisions, for repairing tissue, and for excising diseased tissue, among other applications. One of the major areas that can benefit from the unique advantages of laser use is eye surgery. Ophthalmic surgeons use lasers to relieve diabetic retinopathy, glaucoma, macular degeneration, cataracts, and certain tumors, as well as to reattach torn retinas.

One of the critical qualities of the competent surgeon is judgment. No matter how thoroughly a surgeon may prepare for a procedure, there may be some surprises on the operating table. The surgeon learns the patient's history and status and also reviews all the appropriate diagnostic documents, X rays, and other visualizations, but unforeseen complications may arise during the operation. The surgeon must have the experience and competence to deal with the unexpected.

PERSPECTIVE AND PROSPECTS
Up to the mid-nineteenth century, surgical procedures were probably responsible for as many deaths as cures. Today, surgery extends the lives of millions: heart disease victims, cancer patients, and victims of infection and accidents. Surgery helps improve the quality of life for patients with arthritis and rheumatism, gastrointestinal problems, lung disorders, and circulation problems.

Furthermore, surgery is entering new areas of medicine. For example, operations can now be performed in the uterus to correct anomalies in unborn fetuses. Many more such procedures are predicted for the future.

New areas of surgical expertise are opening constantly; new techniques, instrumentation, and equipment are making many old procedures obsolete. Practicing surgeons face a constant challenge in keeping abreast of what is happening all over the world and deciding what avenues to explore for the benefit of their patients.

—C. Richard Falcon

See also Abscess drainage; Adrenalectomy; Amputation; Anesthesia; Anesthesiology; Aneurysmectomy; Appendectomy; Biopsy; Bladder removal; Bone marrow transplantation; Breast biopsy; Breast surgery; Bunions; Bypass surgery; Cardiac surgery; Cataract surgery; Catheterization; Cervical procedures; Cesarean section; Cholecystectomy; Cleft lip and palate repair; Colorectal polyp removal; Colorectal surgery; Corneal transplantation; Craniotomy; Cryosurgery; Cyst removal; Disk removal; Ear surgery; Electrocauterization; Endarterectomy; Endometrial biopsy; Eye surgery; Face lift and blepharoplasty; Facial transplantation; Fistula repair; Ganglion removal; Gender reassignment surgery; Gastrectomy; Grafts and grafting; Hair transplantation; Hammertoe correction; Heart transplantation; Heart valve replacement; Heel spur removal; Hemorrhoid banding and removal; Hernia repair; Hypospadias repair and urethroplasty; Hysterectomy; Kidney transplantation; Kneecap removal; Laceration repair; Laminectomy and spinal fusion;

Laparoscopy; Laryngectomy; Laser use in surgery; Liposuction; Liver transplantation; Lung surgery; Mastectomy and lumpectomy; Myomectomy; Nail removal; Nasal polyp removal; Nephrectomy; Neurosurgery; Ophthalmology; Oral and maxillofacial surgery; Orthopedic surgery; Parathyroidectomy; Penile implant surgery; Periodontal surgery; Phlebitis; Plastic surgery; Prostate gland removal; Refractive eye surgery; Rhinoplasty and submucous resection; Shunts; Skin lesion removal; Sphincterectomy; Splenectomy; Sterilization; Stone removal; Surgery, pediatric; Surgical procedures; Surgical technologists; Sympathectomy; Tattoo removal; Tendon repair; Testicular surgery; Thoracic surgery; Thyroidectomy; Tonsillectomy and adenoid removal; Tracheostomy; Transfusion; Transplantation; Tumor removal; Ulcer surgery; Vagotomy; Varicose vein removal; Vasectomy.

FOR FURTHER INFORMATION:

Brunicardi, F. Charles, et al., eds. *Schwartz's Principles of Surgery.* 9th ed. New York: McGraw-Hill, 2010. A standard textbook on the topic. Intended for practicing surgeons, but valuable to general readers for its details.

Griffith, H. Winter. *Complete Guide to Symptoms, Illness, and Surgery.* Revised and updated by Stephen Moore and Kenneth Yoder. 5th ed. New York: Perigee, 2006. Covers more than five hundred diseases and disorders and includes information about causes and risk factors, preventive techniques, diagnostic tests, and surgical treatment.

Litin, Scott C., ed. *Mayo Clinic Family Health Book.* 4th ed. New York: HarperResource, 2009. This book covers the surgical aspects of medicine admirably, with clear and concise descriptions of surgical procedures.

Mulholland, Michael W., et al., eds. *Greenfield's Surgery: Scientific Principles and Practice.* 4th ed. Philadelphia: Lippincott Williams & Wilkins, 2006. Covers scientific reviews of wound biology, inflammatory mediators, immunology, and the management of trauma and transplantation in the first part and an overview of surgical practice according to anatomic region and specialty in the second part.

Zollinger, Robert M., Jr., and Robert M. Zollinger, Sr. *Zollinger's Atlas of Surgical Operations.* 8th ed. New York: McGraw-Hill, 2003. A comprehensive examination of surgery. Covers basic surgical anatomy and vascular, gynecologic, gastrointestinal, and miscellaneous abdominal procedures.

SURGERY, PEDIATRIC

SPECIALTY

ANATOMY OR SYSTEM AFFECTED: All

SPECIALTIES AND RELATED FIELDS: Anesthesiology, general surgery, neonatology, pediatrics

DEFINITION: The surgical correction of medical conditions of infants and children.

KEY TERM:

congenital defect: an anatomic defect present at birth; it is not necessarily hereditary

SCIENCE AND PROFESSION

A pediatric surgeon is a general surgeon who has received additional training in operating on infants and children. The full course of training includes four years of medical school, followed by five years of general surgery residency and two years of pediatric surgery residency. Pediatric surgeons generally practice in large referral hospitals or children's hospitals. The relatively small number of American training programs in this specialty are all located at major teaching hospitals.

Children are not simply small adults. They experience some different surgical disorders than adults, especially congenital defects. Their ability to withstand the stress of surgery is less than that of an older person. Also, many of their surgical problems require years of follow-up care by a surgeon who understands child growth and development.

In the first half of the twentieth century, when pediatric surgery was developing as a specialty, the pediatric surgeon was trained to operate on all parts of the child's body. As the specialty matured, however, the pediatric surgeon came to perform only general surgical procedures on infants and children. This trend was made possible by the development of pediatric subspecialties in the other surgical fields, such as neurosurgery and cardiac surgery. In addition, pediatric surgeons work closely with pediatricians. As a team, they share in evaluating the patient and in providing preoperative and postoperative care.

To a degree, pediatric surgeons differ from general surgeons in their point of view. Infants and children change constantly as they grow, and common surgical diagnoses also change with the age of the patient. Additionally, the ability of a child's body to cope with disease and with surgery alters with age. It is therefore necessary for the pediatric surgeon to understand child growth and development.

Although a disorder may be surgically corrected in

infancy, the child may continue to have postoperative difficulty for many years. An example is the removal of a large amount of intestines, which must sometimes be done with premature infants. It takes considerable patience and expertise to follow this sort of patient for years, adjusting the child's diet and treatment to achieve as nearly normal growth as possible. The pediatric surgeon is specially trained to provide this care.

The organs and tissues of an infant or child are much smaller than those of an adult. The pediatric surgeon must develop expert skills to perform surgery on these small structures. Also, the pediatric surgeon is trained to work rapidly when performing surgery. It is important to complete procedures quickly to minimize stress on the pediatric patient.

Congenital defects are, fortunately, relatively uncommon. The pediatric surgeon treats relatively more of these conditions than a general surgeon would and therefore has greater experience in caring for them. Examples of congenital defects treated by pediatric surgeons include defects of the abdominal wall and diaphragm and the obstruction or absence of a part of the intestinal tract.

Because the patient is a child, the pediatric surgeon must also deal with the patient's family. This specialist is trained to build a supportive relationship with parents and to teach them about their child's disorder so that they can be informed participants in decisions regarding the patient's care. Especially with chronic diseases, the parents must be kept aware of their child's progress and changing needs so that they can participate fully in the child's recovery.

DIAGNOSTIC AND TREATMENT TECHNIQUES

The pediatric surgeon's day is split between the operating room and the clinic. This specialist spends relatively more time in the clinic than does a general surgeon. Surgical correction is only one step in pediatric surgery: Careful evaluation and planning must precede any procedure. Afterward, extended follow-up care is often necessary, sometimes for years. This type of care requires patience and an interest in long-range planning on the surgeon's part.

The pediatric surgeon relies heavily on history taking and physical examination of the patient. This information, plus knowledge of the incidence of specific disorders at different ages, leads the surgeon to the most likely diagnosis. Specific laboratory and radiographic tests are ordered to aid in the diagnostic process.

The pediatric surgeon works very closely with the anesthesiologist, the physician responsible for keeping the patient anesthetized and his or her vital functions stable during surgery. The needs of a child are different from those of an adult during surgery. Many hospitals with pediatric surgeons are also staffed with pediatric anesthesiologists.

Like other surgeons, the pediatric surgeon also performs minor surgery on children, often in the clinic. Examples of minor procedures are the suturing of lacerations, the drainage of small abscesses, and the excision of small benign growths under the skin.

PERSPECTIVE AND PROSPECTS

Pediatric surgery began in the United States as an offshoot of general surgery in the first half of the twentieth century. For decades, the specialty met resistance from general surgeons. The American Academy of Pediatrics was first to recognize the value of pediatric surgeons and, following a meeting by the academy in 1948, established a surgical section. C. Everett Koop, the surgeon general under President Ronald Reagan, was a vigorous advocate of pediatric surgical education and a developer of new surgical techniques for children from 1946 through the 1990's. He was an important proponent in the eventual recognition of pediatric surgery as a surgical specialty. It was not until 1973, however, that the Board of Pediatric Surgery certified the first specialists in the field.

In 1995, there were twenty-eight training programs for pediatric surgeons in the United States. Because of the limited number of graduates of these programs, pediatric surgeons will continue to be in great demand.

—*Thomas C. Jefferson, M.D.*

See also Abscess drainage; Adrenalectomy; Amputation; Anesthesia; Anesthesiology; Aneurysmectomy; Appendectomy; Biopsy; Bone marrow transplantation; Cardiac surgery; Cardiology, pediatric; Catheterization; Cleft lip and palate repair; Craniotomy; Cryosurgery; Ear surgery; Electrocauterization; Endocrinology, pediatric; Eye surgery; Fistula repair; Gastroenterology, pediatric; Genetic diseases; Genetics and inheritance; Grafts and grafting; Heart transplantation; Heart valve replacement; Hernia repair; Hypospadias repair and urethroplasty; Kidney transplantation; Laceration repair; Laparoscopy; Laser use in surgery; Lung surgery; Nasal polyp removal; Nephrectomy; Nephrology, pediatric; Neurology, pediatric; Neurosurgery; Ophthalmology; Oral and maxillofacial surgery; Orthopedic surgery; Orthopedics, pediatric; Parathyroidectomy;

Pediatrics; Plastic surgery; Pulmonary medicine, pediatric; Shunts; Splenectomy; Surgery, general; Surgical procedures; Surgical technologists; Sympathectomy; Tattoo removal; Tendon repair; Thoracic surgery; Thyroidectomy; Tonsillectomy and adenoid removal; Tracheostomy; Transfusion; Transplantation; Urology, pediatric.

FOR FURTHER INFORMATION:

Cockburn, Forrester, et al. *Children's Medicine and Surgery*. New York: Oxford University Press, 1996. This volume discusses the basics of pediatrics and features illustrations and an index.

Glick, Philip L., et al. *Pediatric Surgery Secrets*. New York: Hanley & Belfus, 2001. An accessible question-and-answer format addresses general and critical care, thoracic surgery, cardiovascular surgery, gastroenterology, hepatobiliary and spleen surgery, head and neck surgery, genitourinary surgery, trauma, tumors and oncology, and special topics.

Koop, C. Everett. "Pediatric Surgery: The Long Road to Recognition." *Pediatrics* 92 (October, 1993): 618-621. The history of pediatric surgery is discussed. Some believe that pediatric surgery would never have gotten off the ground without the development of pediatric anesthesiology.

O'Neill, James A., Jr., et al., eds. *Principles of Pediatric Surgery*. 2d ed. St. Louis, Mo.: Mosby, 2004. This is a new edition of a classic textbook of pediatric surgery. It is the most comprehensive text available on the subject, a must for all practicing and aspiring pediatric surgeons. Perhaps a bit too comprehensive for nonpediatric surgeons looking for a simple reference book to keep on their shelf.

SURGICAL PROCEDURES

PROCEDURES

ANATOMY OR SYSTEM AFFECTED: All

SPECIALTIES AND RELATED FIELDS: Anesthesiology, general surgery, nursing, plastic surgery

DEFINITION: The treatment of diseases or disorders by physical intervention, which usually involves cutting into the skin and other tissues.

KEY TERMS:

anesthesia: the use of drugs to inhibit pain and other sensations

hemostasis: the control of bleeding

incision: a cut made with a scalpel

suture: a thread used to unite parts of the body

INDICATIONS AND PROCEDURES

Surgery has progressed as rapidly as other areas of medicine. Early surgeries consisted of gross excision (the cutting out of abnormal or diseased tissue). Today, surgery has been transformed by scientific advances so that surgeons commonly use microscopes, lasers, and endoscopes that allow the surgeon to make small incisions in order to gain access to the surgical site. Modern operations are much more precise and emphasize repair or replacement rather than excision.

When a patient requires surgery, several preoperative procedures are performed to increase the chances of a successful outcome. First, the patient is asked to abstain from eating for at least eight hours prior to surgery. This action reduces the chances of the individual vomiting during surgery and aspirating the gastric contents into the trachea (windpipe). After arriving at the hospital or clinic, the patient removes his or her clothes and puts on a gown, allowing the medical staff easy access to the patient for catheter insertion, intravenous line insertion, monitor placement, and preparation of the surgical site. Next, an intravenous (IV) line is placed in a vein of the hand or arm and connected to a bottle or bag of solution, which is suspended above the level of the patient's arm. The intravenous line gives the physician rapid vascular access for sampling blood and injecting drugs. Just before the actual surgery, the patient is usually given a sedative by an anesthesiologist, and electrocardiogram (ECG or EKG) leads and a blood pressure cuff are applied to the patient to monitor heart rate, heart rhythm, and blood pressure. The anesthesiologist will then anesthetize the patient further while the surgical team begins to prepare the site for the operation. Preoperative antibiotics may be given if there is a significant risk of infection.

The surgery may require either general anesthesia, in which the patient is unconscious, or local anesthesia, in which a specific region of the body is anesthetized. For general anesthesia, the patient will be injected with an intravenous anesthetic and quickly intubated, a procedure in which a tube is inserted into the trachea and attached to a ventilator. This arrangement gives the anesthesiologist the ability to administer gaseous drugs such as nitrous oxide and halothane as well as to control the patient's breathing. Surgical assistants prepare the operative site by cleansing the skin with a disinfectant. A sterile drape is used to cover all areas of the body except the surgical site. Surgeons and assistants must mask themselves and prepare for surgery by thoroughly washing their hands and arms. They then carefully put on a sterile gown and gloves. At this point, they must not come into contact with anything nonsterile.

The surgeon uses a scalpel to make an incision through the skin and any underlying structures in order to gain access to the area of the body needing attention. When blood vessels are cut, bleeding must be controlled by cauterizing, clamping, tying off with sutures, or applying direct pressure to the vessel; this process is known as hemostasis.

After the surgery, the incision sites are closed with sutures, and the anesthetic is reversed. The patient is then taken to a recovery room to be monitored closely. Routine care of the patient recovering from anesthesia includes repeated evaluation of body temperature, pulse, blood pressure, and respiration. Postoperative pain medication (such as meperidine, morphine, or fentanyl) is given as needed.

USES AND COMPLICATIONS

Complications from surgery can result from surgical errors, infections, and abnormal patient reactions to the procedure or medications (idiosyncratic reactions). Occasionally, surgery involves damage to healthy tissues, including nerves and blood vessels. Significant intraoperative blood loss may also occur, requiring transfusion. An incision into any part of the body provides an opportunity for bacteria to enter and infect the surgical wound; prophylactic antibiotics help reduce the chance of surgical infection. Rarely, a patient may have an unexpected response to the procedure or drugs, which could result in permanent disability or death. These very infrequent reactions may include a blood clot causing a stroke or heart attack, an abnormal heart rhythm, or severe allergic reactions to medication.

PERSPECTIVE AND PROSPECTS

Modern surgery includes the use of surgical implants, microsurgery, laser surgery, endoscopic surgery, and transplant surgery. Surgery implants are used to replace a part of the body with an artificial implant. These implants include joints, heart valves, eye lenses, and sections of blood vessels or of the skull. During microsurgery, the surgeon uses specially designed instruments and a microscope to perform an operation on minute

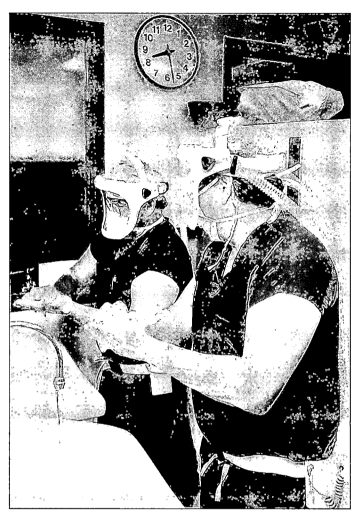

Surgeons scrub their hands and arms before performing an operation. Such procedures are essential to the maintenance of an antiseptic environment. (Digital Stock)

structures such as blood vessels, nerves, and parts of the eyes or ears. Microsurgery is also being used to reattach severed fingers and toes. Laser surgery utilizes a high-energy, narrow beam that can cut through tissues like a scalpel but that also cauterizes blood vessels during the incision. Lasers can be used on the retina, skin blemishes, and even tumors. Recovery from endoscopic surgery, in which a fiber-optic tube is inserted into the body to view the surgical site, is generally faster than from conventional operations because a smaller incision is made and less tissue damage results. Endoscopes are used to remove stones from the urinary tract and gallbladder and to remove or repair damaged cartilage in joints. With the availability of drugs that suppress tissue rejection, damaged organs can now be surgically replaced by donated organs. The most common examples are the heart, lungs, liver, kidneys, and bone marrow.

—Matthew Berria, Ph.D.,
and Douglas Reinhart, M.D.

See also Anesthesia; Anesthesiology; Biopsy; Bypass surgery; Catheterization; Cervical procedures; Colon and rectal surgery; Craniotomy; Cryosurgery; Cyst removal; Electrocauterization; Eye surgery; Fistula repair; Ganglion removal; Grafts and grafting; Hernia repair; Laparoscopy; Laser use in surgery; Lung surgery; Neurosurgery; Orthopedic surgery; Periodontal surgery; Plastic surgery; Shunts; Surgery, general; Surgery, pediatric; Surgical technologists; Thoracic surgery; Tracheostomy; Transfusion; Transplantation; Tumor removal.

FOR FURTHER INFORMATION:

Brunicardi, F. Charles, et al., eds. *Schwartz's Principles of Surgery.* 9th ed. New York: McGraw-Hill, 2010. A standard textbook on the topic. Intended for practicing surgeons, but valuable to general readers for its details.

Leikin, Jerrold B., and Martin S. Lipsky, eds. *American Medical Association Complete Medical Encyclopedia.* New York: Random House Reference, 2003. A concise presentation of numerous medical terms and illnesses. A good general reference.

Mulholland, Michael W., et al., eds. *Greenfield's Surgery: Scientific Principles and Practice.* 4th ed. Philadelphia: Lippincott Williams & Wilkins, 2006. Covers the scope and practice of surgery and includes reviews of wound biology, immunology, the management of trauma and transplantation, surgical practice according to anatomic region and specialty, and musculoskeletal, neurologic, genitourinary, and reconstructive surgery.

Zollinger, Robert M., Jr., and Robert M. Zollinger, Sr. *Zollinger's Atlas of Surgical Operations.* 8th ed. New York: McGraw-Hill, 2003. A comprehensive examination of surgery. Covers basic surgical anatomy and vascular, gynecologic, gastrointestinal, and miscellaneous abdominal procedures.

SURGICAL TECHNOLOGISTS

SPECIALTY

ANATOMY OR SYSTEM AFFECTED: All

SPECIALTIES AND RELATED FIELDS: Anesthesiology, emergency medicine, general surgery, nursing

DEFINITION: Surgical team members whose primary functions are to prepare surgical instruments and hand them to the surgeon as needed and to prevent infection by maintaining a sterile field in the operating room.

KEY TERMS:

analgesia: the absence of pain

anesthesia: the absence of sensation; anesthesia may be achieved systemically (general anesthesia) or in a specific region of the body (regional or local anesthesia)

aseptic techniques: the standard procedures that help prevent wound contamination during the performance of surgical procedures; contamination may be followed by infection or death

circulator: the worker in the operating room whose responsibility is to keep records and to open sterile supplies for the team members wearing gowns and gloves

inpatient procedure: a surgical procedure performed on a patient who comes from a room in the hospital and who will return to a room in the hospital

operating room: a room in which surgical procedures are performed

outpatient procedure: a surgical procedure performed on a patient who comes from outside the hospital and who will most likely leave the hospital after a short stay in the recovery room

prep: a short form of the word "prepare"; to prep means to wash and shave the surgical area and to clean the skin surface immediately before a surgical procedure

recovery room: the room where a patient returns to full consciousness after a surgical procedure; in an outpatient facility, patients can change clothes in the recovery room, which may serve double duty as the preoperative waiting room

scrub: to wash one's hands and forearms in preparation for donning gown and gloves, which protect the patient from the surgical technologist and protect the surgical technologist from the patient

sterile field: an area where only sterile supplies may be placed and that only those wearing sterile gowns and gloves may touch; includes the surgical wound, the surgical drapes, and the extra tables

surgical team: the people working together in the operating room during a surgical procedure, including the surgeon, first assistant, surgical technologist, anesthesiologist and/or anesthetist, and circulator

SCIENCE AND PROFESSION

Surgical technologists work as part of the surgical team in an operating room, so they must be familiar with many aspects of patient care. The surgical team typically includes at least one of each of the following: a surgeon, a first assistant, a surgical technologist, an anesthesiologist and/or anesthetist, and a circulator. As a member of the surgical team, a surgical technologist anticipates the needs of the surgeon, prepares the instruments to be used for surgery, hands instruments to the surgeon, promotes efficiency, and at the same time helps prevent infection by maintaining the sterile field. A surgical technologist may also be referred to as a scrub nurse, a surgical assistant, a private scrub, or simply a scrub.

Surgical technologists work in many types of operating rooms, so their training must be fairly extensive. Courses may be taken at community colleges in one-year or two-year programs. Some of the two-year programs are accredited by the Association of Surgical Technologists. In 2001, the Commission on Accreditation of Allied Health Education Programs (CAAHEP) recognized 350 accredited programs. The courses taken include medical terminology, anatomy, and physiology. Classes specifically focused on surgical technology may include surgical conscience and ethics, the organization of an operating room, principles of microbiology, sterilization and disinfection, aseptic techniques, preoperative preparation and care of the patient, anesthesia, medications used during surgery, proper positioning of a surgical patient, preparation of the surgical site, methods of closing the surgical wound, surgical routines, the supplies found in the operating room, and the legal aspects of surgery.

A surgical technologist may work in one or all of many surgical services, so coursework must provide information about general surgery; obstetrical and gynecological surgery; plastic and reconstructive surgery; ear, nose, and throat procedures; surgery on the mouth and face; orthopedic surgery; neurosurgery; open-heart surgery; lung surgery; pediatric surgery; and surgery on blood vessels not located in the chest.

Students are required to gain experience in an operating room, which is usually done under supervision at a local teaching hospital. At such a hospital, a student gains experience in appropriate operating room procedures and learns the universal precautions against the transmission of infectious diseases.

Although the surgical technologist may work in any of the available medical services, some hospitals require their surgical technologists to specialize—that is, to rotate through different services so that they will gain familiarity with many operative procedures. At other facilities, the surgical technologist will work primarily in one area. For example, if the facility is a plastic surgeon's clinic, only these types of procedures will be performed.

A surgical technologist who has gained some experience may gain a specific area of interest within a broader field and decide to become a specialist. Common areas in which to specialize include eye surgery, neurosurgery, orthopedics, and plastic surgery. If this is the case, the technologist might be invited to work for a certain doctor or may find a number of (perhaps unaffiliated) doctors with whom to work. Working as a private scrub offers a different way to practice in the field. The surgical technologist works directly for the surgeon, instead of working for the hospital or surgical facility, and can usually expect to charge and earn more. There is also the possibility of greater camaraderie with the physician and more trust of the surgical technologist by the physician. Concentrating in a specific area may offer greater remuneration to the surgical technologist, greater rapport with a familiar surgeon, and a more regular schedule, with no requirement for working on the weekends.

DUTIES AND PROCEDURES

Surgical technologists typically work in many areas, both inside and outside the operating room. Within the operating room, they may be either scrubbed or not scrubbed. After washing his or her hands, the surgical technologist dons a gown and gloves, which provides a sterile surface to reduce the possibility of transmission of infection, either from the patient to the surgical technologist or from the surgical technologist to the patient. When scrubbed, surgical technologists perform many duties. They assist surgeons during surgical procedures by handing them instruments, following routine procedures. They promote efficiency by keeping the instrument tables neat and organized. They must anticipate the needs of surgeons, so it is necessary that they know the steps of a procedure and monitor its progress. A surgical technologist places instruments in the surgeon's hands so that the surgeon does not have to look away from the wound in search of an instrument. Surgical technologists also help prevent injuries to the patient.

When necessary, the scrubbed surgical technologist may be asked to act as a first assistant for a procedure. In this capacity, it may be necessary for the surgical technologist to hold tissue out of the way (retract it), so that the surgeon can reach deeper tissues. Surgical technologists may also be required to sponge blood out of the wound or to rinse the surgical site to promote visibility of the tissues. They may also cut sutures. Surgical technologists help count sponges, needles, and instruments when such counts are required; items must be counted so that none are left behind in the patient. These items are counted before, during, and after the surgical procedure, in a specified and orderly manner. It is also the responsibility of the scrubbed surgical technologist to keep track of surgical specimens, pieces of tissue removed from the patient that will be sent to the laboratory for analysis. Many specimens may be taken from a particular procedure, so the surgical technologist must hand them off the sterile field to the circulator and make sure that the circulator labels the specimens properly. Specimens must also be handled and treated properly. Some are sent to the laboratory in preserving solutions, some are sent in salt water, and some are sent dry. It is important to keep track of specimens, to identify them, and to put them in the proper container for transportation to the laboratory.

When the surgical technologist is working in the operating room and is not scrubbed, a registered nurse must be immediately available in case there is an emergency. A registered nurse must also be present if medications are needed on the sterile field. A surgical technologist who is not scrubbed may function as a circulator. The circulator opens sterile supplies onto the operative field. Supplies are wrapped in many different ways, and the circulator must be able to pass the contents of a sterile package to the scrubbed surgical technologist without dropping them. Expiration dates must be checked on all supplies opened. Once the patient for a particular procedure is brought into the operating room, the circulator will help position the patient on the surgical table. The surgical technologist knows the position necessary for the particular procedure. Safe positioning methods prevent injury to patients. Once the patient is on the surgical table, the circulator washes the area with specified soaps and solutions and, if necessary, will shave the area around the surgical wound so that the area can be cleaned for the incision. The circulator ties the gowns of the scrubbed surgical tech-

nologist as well as the surgeon and other scrubbed assistants. If the anesthesiologist or anesthetist asks for help, the circulator provides that help, which may include holding, informing, or reassuring the patient.

It is the function of the circulator to connect tubings and electrical wires from instruments that may be needed on the sterile field, including power cords for cautery units, special lights, and drills, as well as fluid lines and suction cords. The circulator may need to focus or aim the surgical lights. With the scrubbed surgical technologist, the circulator performs the count of the items that need to be counted, including the sutures, sponges, and instruments. The circulator keeps the official legal record of the procedure, the operative report. On this document, the circulator records the particulars of the procedure, including the counts, what was done, and the medications that were given. It is the responsibility of the circulator to receive surgical specimens from the surgical technologist, and to record properly where they came from, before they are sent to the laboratory. It might be necessary for the circulator to wipe the brow of any of the scrubbed personnel, so that sweat will not fall onto the sterile field; however, this is a rare event. The circulator handles all the nonsterile equipment present in the operating room during the surgical procedure. This could involve moving or connecting equipment. In addition, the circulator helps to move the patient from the operating room to the recovery room after the procedure is over.

When not scrubbed for a procedure or functioning as a circulator, a surgical technologist may be asked to perform other duties in the surgery department. Surgical technologists need to be familiar with the protocols for receiving patients in the department. They may be asked to take patients to and from the surgical area or within the surgery department. Surgical technologists may help to order supplies for a department and, when they arrive, may help transport the supplies to the appropriate storage cupboard. Supplies need to be ordered from the central supply department or directly from manufacturers. In the operating room, not only must supplies be restocked but the expiration dates on sterile items must be inspected as well, to ensure that no outdated supplies are present in the operating room and given inadvertently to the patient. Surgical technologists may assist in cleaning instruments and supplies after a surgical procedure and preparing them for sterilization and subsequent reuse. They must be familiar with ways to sterilize instruments and supplies and must know which methods to use for which items. If equipment is working improperly, it is the responsibility of the surgical technologist to make sure that the equipment is repaired or replaced.

Working in an operating room is a very demanding occupation. It requires first of all personal integrity. As with any professional, the surgical technologist must be willing to admit mistakes. Often mistakes can be corrected if they are detected early. For example, the surgical technologist might have to say, "I forgot to sterilize the instruments, so we'll have to wait another fifteen minutes," rather than rush ahead to meet a particular deadline. In addition, a surgical technologist has to be able to handle stress—from providing fast and accurate care to a very sick patient, to having a patient die on the operating room table, to working with individuals with whom one does not get along on a personal level, to changing schedules for emergency procedures, to not being able to take a break to go to the restroom, to standing in one position for a whole day or a whole procedure.

No discussion of surgical technology would be complete without some mention of its legal aspects. As of the early twenty-first century in the United States, no state had licensed or defined the practice of surgical technology, although several states, including Texas, Oregon, and Georgia, were working on licensing initiatives. Therefore, the surgical technologist has only the common rights of a citizen on the street. Although no special license is required for surgical technologists, most hospitals prefer, and others require, certification. Surgical technologists can become certified surgical technologists by completing an approved program of at least one year and passing an examination given by the Association of Surgical Technologists (AST). One thing is certain: The surgical technologist is not allowed to practice medicine or nursing.

Since surgical technologists are not physicians, they may not diagnose or treat disease, inject medicine into the human body, or pronounce death. These actions are limited to physicians, and in some states, a physician may not delegate certain actions (such as suturing, cutting or penetrating the human body, and clamping) to a surgical technologist. Similarly, since the surgical technologists are not nurses, they may not administer medications, which is a practice relegated to the field of nursing. At one time, only registered nurses were permitted to act as circulators. Many hospitals now allow surgical technologists to circulate, with a registered nurse standing by for emergencies. When circulating, however, a surgical technologist must remember that only nurses

may select and measure medications, a right that cannot be delegated to someone without a license.

Surgical technologists must obey the laws in the performance of their duties. They can be prosecuted for breaking a law or for failing to perform a proper job. Surgical technologists must pay attention to laws involving the respecting of property rights, both of patients and of hospitals. In addition to not exceeding the scope of practice, there is another area of concern for surgical technologists: negligence. Any act of carelessness is called negligence, which is legally defined as "the failure to exercise the care that a reasonably prudent person would exercise under similar circumstances." Although negligence itself is not a crime, surgical technologists must remember that carelessness could endanger the safety of the patient.

The most common areas of negligence (and subsequent malpractice lawsuits) that affect surgical technologists involve the following: proper positioning of side rails and patient supports, abandonment of the patient, surgical consent, patient identification, loss of items inside the patient, specimen collections, burns, and explosions. Carelessness involving side rails could result in an anesthetized patient falling on the floor. Abandonment refers to the careless act of leaving an incompetent patient alone. The patient must sign a consent, in which he or she agrees to the surgical procedure; this detailed legal document must be present before the procedure is begun, and the procedure may not wander from the permission given. Sponges, instruments, and needles are counted many times before, during, and after the surgical procedure, which helps to reduce the possibility of leaving anything inside the patient. Burns could be caused by the improper grounding of electrical devices used in the operating room, by the application of the wrong soap to the wrong area, or by the use of recently sterilized instruments, which may be too hot to be placed directly in contact with the patient. Explosions are less likely now than they used to be, because explosive medications are no longer used for general anesthesia. Nevertheless, the presence of oxygen in tanks and tubing increases the possibility of explosion and fire. In summary, there are many things about which the surgical technologist must be careful in order to avoid legal complications and injuries to patients.

PERSPECTIVE AND PROSPECTS

Historically, surgical technology began during World War II, when medical and nursing personnel in the armed forces trained men and women to assist in surgery in order to increase the availability of surgical procedures for the wounded. At that time, workers in this area were called operating room technicians. The name has gradually evolved to reflect the many areas where surgical procedures now take place—not only in hospitals but also in outpatient clinics, delivery rooms, and doctors' offices. In the beginning, surgical technologists had to work directly under the supervision of a registered nurse, who was legally required to be present in the operating room at all times.

The Association of Surgical Technologists began as a wing within the Association of Operating Room Nurses, but it later broke away to become the Association of Operating Room Technicians before later changing its name to the current one. Its headquarters are located in Littleton, Colorado. The AST provides many services for its members. It is a private organization that provides a certificate to those surgical technologists who pass a national examination. Certification, however, has little legal significance. States may not delegate their power to provide licenses to a private organization. The certified surgical technologist has demonstrated a level of skills and knowledge; however, one does not have to be certified in order to work as a surgical technologist. The AST also provides continuing education credits, insurance programs, and a magazine, as well as other services.

As the baby boom generation ages, the numbers of surgical procedures are expected to increase. Technological advances, such as fiber optics and laser technology, also allow new surgical procedures to be performed. For these reasons, the U.S. Bureau of Labor projects that employment opportunities for surgical technicians will grow by approximately 35 to 40 percent through the year 2010.

Working as a surgical technologist can be very demanding, but satisfaction, as in any profession, comes from working with a team in a complex situation in order to achieve a goal. There is satisfaction in a job well done, in being able to work well in stressful situations. There is great satisfaction in seeing the human body in all its complexity and in helping restore it to health. There is satisfaction in knowing in advance what the surgeon is going to use and having it ready at the moment it is needed. It is the excellent surgical technologist who can give the surgeon what is needed and not merely what is asked for.

—*William F. Taylor*

See also Allied health; Anesthesia; Anesthesiology; Education, medical; Malpractice; Nursing; Surgery, general; Surgery, pediatric; Surgical procedures.

FOR FURTHER INFORMATION:
Caruthers, Bob, et al., eds. *Surgical Technology for the Surgical Technologist: A Positive Care Approach.* Florence, Ky.: Cengage Learning, 2009. Includes bibliographical references and an index.
Fuller, Joanna Kotcher. *Surgical Technology: Principles and Practice.* 4th ed. St. Louis, Mo.: Saunders/Elsevier, 2005. An accessible work that functions as a textbook for surgical technologists. Fuller has assembled a wealth of practical clinical information about caring for patients in surgery.
Miller, Benjamin F., Claire Brackman Keane, and Marie T. O'Toole. *Miller-Keane Encyclopedia and Dictionary of Medicine, Nursing, and Allied Health.* Rev. 7th ed. Philadelphia: Saunders/Elsevier, 2005. A comprehensive work which contains much information about the full spectrum of allied health.
Phillips, Nancymarie Fortunato. *Berry and Kohn's Operating Room Technique.* 11th ed. St. Louis, Mo.: Mosby/Elsevier, 2007. Another accessible textbook. This one contains much practical information about what goes on in the operating room.
Rothrock, Jane C., ed. *Alexander's Care of the Patient in Surgery.* 13th ed. St. Louis, Mo.: Mosby/Elsevier, 2007. The bible of surgical techniques and practices. A detailed reference work of the most common surgical procedures.

SWEATING
BIOLOGY
ALSO KNOWN AS: Perspiration
ANATOMY OR SYSTEM AFFECTED: Glands, skin
SPECIALTIES AND RELATED FIELDS: Dermatology, exercise physiology
DEFINITION: The excretion of fluid from the sweat glands in order to cool the body.

STRUCTURE AND FUNCTIONS
Sweat glands are exocrine glands, which secrete products that are passed outside the body. There are two major types. Eccrine sweat glands excrete sweat that contains water and several salts. They are located in the skin throughout the body but are found in greater concentrations in the palms of the hands, soles of the feet, and forehead. Apocrine sweat glands excrete sweat that contains water and fatty substances. They are primarily

found in the armpits and genital area. When bacteria break down the fatty materials, distinctive sweat odors develop.

The primary function of sweating in humans is to regulate body temperature. When the body temperature rises, the blood flow to the skin increases by opening more capillaries in the skin. Since blood can hold heat and circulates throughout the body, the blood can transport heat from the inner core of the body, where the temperatures are higher and the heat is more insulated, to the surface, where the heat is less insulated. In the skin, the warm blood will transfer the heat to the surface, where sweat glands release sweat. When the sweat evaporates, changing its physical state from a liquid to a gas, significant amounts of heat are removed from the body.

DISORDERS AND DISEASES

Sweating is a normal process that is important for the temperature regulation (thermoregulation) of the body, but complications can arise. The most critical result of excess sweating is dehydration. The biggest risk for dehydration occurs when people exercise in hot, humid environments. Therefore, it is important to drink plenty of water. Additionally, when sweating a lot for a period of days, additional salts may be beneficial. Most sports drinks supply adequate salts. In extreme conditions, the excess loss of water in sweat can lead to heatstroke and death. When the body loses too much water, the sweating mechanism shuts down. Without the advantage of sweat evaporation to cool the body, the temperature will continue to rise until death ensues. Anyone who has symptoms of heat stress—such as a body temperature over 105 degrees Fahrenheit, cessation of sweating, or altered mental state—should get immediate medical attention. The intravenous administration of fluids by medical personnel will rehydrate the body quickly.

A less concerning disorder of sweating is hyperhidrosis. People with this condition sweat frequently and in excess of what is required to regulate body temperature. About 1 percent of people have this condition; it is often linked to obesity. There are numerous treatments but no cure. Typical treatments include surgery, medications, biofeedback, relaxation, hypnosis, and weight loss.

—*Bradley R. A. Wilson, Ph.D.*

See also Dehydration; Dermatology; Exercise physiology; Fever; Glands; Heat exhaustion and heatstroke; Host-defense mechanisms; Hyperhidrosis; Physiology; Signs and symptoms; Skin; Sympathectomy.

FOR FURTHER INFORMATION:

Brooks, George A., Thomas D. Fahey, and Kenneth M. Baldwin. *Exercise Physiology: Human Bioenergetics and Its Applications*. 4th ed. Boston: McGraw-Hill, 2007.

McArdle, William, Frank I. Katch, and Victor L. Katch. *Exercise Physiology: Energy, Nutrition, and Human Performance*. 7th ed. Boston: Lippincott Williams & Wilkins, 2010.

Powers, Scott K., and Edward T. Howley. *Exercise Physiology: Theory and Application to Fitness and Performance*. 7th ed. New York: McGraw-Hill, 2009.

SYMPATHECTOMY

PROCEDURE

ANATOMY OR SYSTEM AFFECTED: Back, neck, nerves, nervous system, spine

SPECIALTIES AND RELATED FIELDS: General surgery, neurology

DEFINITION: The surgical interruption of part of the sympathetic nerve pathway.

INDICATIONS AND PROCEDURES

The autonomic nervous system controls the involuntary internal environment of humans, and the sympathetic nerves increase energy expenditures by accelerating the heart rate, increasing the metabolic rate, and constricting and dilating blood vessels, among other actions. Occasionally, the proper regulation of vasoconstriction or vasodilation goes awry, and the sympathetic nervous system causes prolonged and inappropriate constriction of the blood vessels to a specific area. In Raynaud's phenomenon, there is intermittent constricting of blood vessels when the fingers, toes, ears, or nose is exposed to cold. The affected areas change color from white to blue to red, and the condition can be associated with numbness, tingling, burning, and pain. Symptoms of long-term blood vessel constriction associated with decreased blood flow include cold and clammy skin, areas of gangrene, and painful fibrous growths and infections. In other cases, excessive sweating and facial blushing may be candidates for correction with sympathectomy.

After the specific nerves are located, the patient is prepared for surgery and opened in the location of the nerves, typically the neck or back area. Organs are moved or adjusted as needed. The offending region of nerve is clipped from the remainder and removed. The organs are replaced or repaired, and the incisions are closed. Normal vascular dilation will return rapidly and with it warmth to the area and healing of the infections, fibrous tissue, and areas of gangrene.

In the treatment of excessive sweating, often sympathectomy can be performed as an outpatient procedure under local anesthesia. A small incision is made under the armpit and air is introduced into the chest cavity. The surgeon inserts a fiber-optic tube, or endoscope, which projects an image onto a screen. Lasers are used to destroy the ganglia involved in the excessive sweating.

USES AND COMPLICATIONS
To determine if sympathectomy is an appropriate treatment, the nerve in question is injected with a steroid and anesthetic to block the nerve function temporarily. If the condition in question is relieved, then the patient will likely benefit from sympathectomy. After surgery is completed, Doppler ultrasonography, which uses sound waves to measure blood flow, can be used to determine whether the procedure has succeeded in increasing circulation.

Potential complications include those common to all major surgeries. Depending on the type of sympathectomy performed, side effects may involve a decrease in blood pressure when standing, which can lead to fainting spells. About 30 percent of cases of sympathectomy for treatment of excessive sweating result in an increase in sweating of the chest, but the procedure is 90 percent effective in alleviating excessive sweating of the face, hands, and feet.

—*Karen E. Kalumuck, Ph.D.*

See also Circulation; Nervous system; Neuralgia, neuritis, and neuropathy; Neuroimaging; Neurology; Neurosurgery; Sweating; Vascular medicine; Vascular system.

FOR FURTHER INFORMATION:
Ernst, Calvin B., and James C. Stanley, eds. *Current Therapy in Vascular Surgery.* 4th ed. St. Louis, Mo.: Mosby, 2001.

Ganong, William F. *Review of Medical Physiology.* 23d ed. New York: Lange Medical Books/McGraw-Hill Medical, 2009.

Griffith, H. Winter. *Complete Guide to Symptoms, Illness, and Surgery.* Revised and updated by Stephen Moore and Kenneth Yoder. 5th ed. New York: Perigee, 2006.

Rutherford, Robert B., ed. *Vascular Surgery.* 6th ed. Philadelphia: Saunders/Elsevier, 2005.

SYNDROME
DISEASE/DISORDER
ALSO KNOWN AS: Condition, disease, disorder
ANATOMY OR SYSTEM AFFECTED: All
SPECIALTIES AND RELATED FIELDS: All
DEFINITION: A group or pattern of recognizable symptoms or conditions that occur together and indicate a specific disease, psychological disorder, or other abnormal condition.
KEY TERMS:
disorder: abnormal physical or mental condition
symptom: indication of a disorder

CAUSES AND SYMPTOMS
A syndrome is a collection of symptoms that characterize a disorder. For example, metabolic syndrome is the name given to a group of symptoms that warn of potential heart disease, stroke, or diabetes. The symptoms of metabolic syndrome are obesity, high blood pressure, low levels of insulin, and high cholesterol.

Syndromes can be grouped into roughly fourteen categories: environmental (caused by the environment); congenital (existing at birth); gastrointestinal (affecting the stomach and intestines); cardiovascular (involving the heart and blood vessels); iatrogenic (induced by a treatment or procedure); neoplastic (caused by a malignant or benign tumor); endocrine (affecting glands, including sex glands); pulmonary (involving the lung); infectious (caused by a virus, bacterium, or fungus); renal (involving the kidneys); reticuloendothelial (affecting cells, including blood cells); neurological (affecting the nervous system); psychopathological (affecting the mind and behavior); and medically unexplained (cause uncertain).

The causes of syndromes vary. Some come from a single, clear source. For example, toxic shock syndrome is caused by the bacterium *Staphylococcus aureus.* The bacterium enters the body through wounds from injuries or surgery incisions. It also breeds in superabsorbent tampons and contraceptive sponges. Symptoms of this syndrome include fever, headache, vomiting, diarrhea, and muscle aches.

Chinese restaurant syndrome is caused by monosodium glutamate (MSG), a chemical compound widely used to enhance the flavor of foods. MSG can induce headache, dizziness, giddiness, a feeling of facial pressure, tingling sensations over parts of the body, and chest pain.

Some syndromes result from any one of an array of causes. Fanconi syndrome, for instance, activates the release of certain substances from the kidney into the urine instead of the bloodstream. It can be caused by genetic defects, inherited diseases, exposure to heavy metals, a kidney transplant, or any number of medicines or diseases that damage the kidneys.

Other syndromes, such as carpal tunnel syndrome, arise from a combination of causes. This syndrome stems from increased pressure on certain nerves and tendons in the carpal tunnel in the wrist. Most people prone to carpal tunnel syndrome are born with a comparatively small carpal tunnel. This condition is complicated by injury to the wrist, an overactive pituitary gland, an underactive thyroid, rheumatoid arthritis, or repeated use of vibrating hand tools.

The causes of some syndromes remain uncertain. For example, Reye's syndrome is a rapidly appearing, deadly disorder that affects all body organs, most seriously the brain and liver. It attacks adults but is primarily a children's disease. Symptoms include personality changes, seizures, and loss of consciousness. There is no cure. The cause is unknown, but there seems to be a link to the use of aspirin taken for a previous viral disease.

Restless legs syndrome is the nighttime twitching of the legs that often leads to insomnia. The cause is unknown, but there seems to be some connection to a family history of the disorder. Also associated with this syndrome are anemia, diabetes, kidney failure, and certain prescription and nonprescription medicines.

Just as the causes vary, so too do the number and severity of symptoms, depending on the syndrome. Barrett's esophagus, for example, is a condition in which the esophagus (the tube that carries food to the stomach) develops new cells similar to those found in the intestines. Symptoms are nonexistent, and the cause is unknown. It can, however, lead to a deadly type of esophageal cancer.

The symptoms of premenstrual syndrome (PMS) vary widely in number and severity from woman to woman. Some women experience few symptoms; others need several days of bed rest. Symptoms include irritability, headache, backache, weight gain, swelling or tenderness of the breasts, depression, fatigue, and loss of sex drive.

Some fifty different symptoms, or characteristics, are associated with Down syndrome. Characteristics include mental retardation; short stature; slow physical growth; weak muscles; short, stocky arms and legs; a wide space between the big toe and second toe; small, low-set ears; a narrow roof of the mouth; crooked teeth

and other dental problems; heart defects; an underactive thyroid; and hearing problems. So many symptoms require a lifetime of care.

Asperger's syndrome produces no symptoms that require medical attention, but people with this disorder display abnormal behaviors and have limited social skills that can bring on unwanted consequences, such as being shunned by others. Some people with this disorder seem "normal" most of the time. Others just seem odd or different from other people, quieter and disinterested. Still others exhibit somewhat bizarre, or at least socially unacceptable, behaviors, such as inflexible routines, a narrow but intense focus of interests, an inability to empathize with other people, and difficulty understanding some types of humor, especially teasing and sarcasm. Yet they are often above average in intelligence and do no more harm than so-called normal people. The odd behaviors lead people to think that Asperger's syndrome is a mental disorder. In fact, it is a type of autism, a developmental disorder that affects how the brain processes information. The cause is unknown.

TREATMENT AND THERAPY
Treatment of a syndrome depends on the underlying causes and the severity and number of symptoms. Because syndromes run the full range of medical problems, treatments run the full range as well. Drugs, surgery, physical therapy, diet and lifestyle changes, alternative medicine, and psychotherapy are all used to treat syndromes.

PERSPECTIVE AND PROSPECTS
Both Western and Eastern medical practitioners have long recognized that a set of symptoms can describe an abnormal condition. Syndromes are researched, diagnosed, and treated no differently than individual diseases are.

—*Wendell Anderson*

See also Acquired immunodeficiency syndrome (AIDS); Acute respiratory distress syndrome (ARDS); Asperger's syndrome; Blue baby syndrome; Carpal tunnel syndrome; Chronic fatigue syndrome; Cornelia de Lange syndrome; Cushing's syndrome; Diagnosis; DiGeorge syndrome; Disease; Down syndrome; Fetal alcohol syndrome; Fragile X syndrome; Guillain-Barré syndrome; Gulf War syndrome; Hemolytic uremic syndrome; Irritable bowel syndrome (IBS); Klinefelter syndrome; Klippel-Trenaunay syndrome; Kluver-Bucy syndrome; Marfan syndrome; Metabolic syndrome; Multiple chemical sensitivity syndrome; Münchausen syndrome by proxy; Overtraining syndrome; Poly-cystic ovary syndrome; Prader-Willi syndrome; Pre-menstrual syndrome (PMS); Reiter's syndrome; Respiratory distress syndrome; Restless legs syndrome; Reye's syndrome; Rubinstein-Taybi syndrome; Severe acute respiratory syndrome (SARS); Severe combined immunodeficiency syndrome (SCID); Signs and symptoms; Sjögren's syndrome; Stevens-Johnson syndrome; Sturge-Weber syndrome; Sudden infant death syndrome (SIDS); Temporomandibular joint (TMJ) syndrome; Tourette's syndrome; Toxic shock syndrome; Turner syndrome; Wiskott-Aldrich syndrome.

FOR FURTHER INFORMATION:

Kirmayer, Laurence, et al. "Explaining Medically Un-explained Symptoms." *Canadian Journal of Psychiatry* 49, no. 10 (October, 2004): 663-672.

McConnaughy, Rozalynd. "Asperger Syndrome: Living Outside the Bell Curve." *Journal of the Medical Library Association* 93, no. 1 (January, 2005): 139-140.

Pease, Roger, Jr., ed. *Merriam-Webster's Medical Desk Dictionary.* Rev. ed. Springfield, Mass.: Merriam-Webster, 2002.

Rice, Shirley. "Reye's Syndrome Isn't Just Child's Play." *Nursing* 33, no. 9 (September, 2003): 32hn1-32hn4.

Wallis, Claudia. "The Down Syndrome Dilemma." *Time* 166, no. 20 (November 14, 2005).

SYNESTHESIA
DISEASE/DISORDER
ANATOMY OR SYSTEM AFFECTED: Brain, nervous system, psychic-emotional system
SPECIALTIES AND RELATED FIELDS: Genetics, neurology, psychiatry, psychology
DEFINITION: A phenomenon wherein one sensory stimulus—a word or a musical note, for example—automatically induces a second, unstimulated sensory perception, typically a color.
KEY TERMS:
functional magnetic resonance imaging (fMRI): a radiologic technique that shows regional oxygen uptake, indicating brain activity
grapheme: a written character or element—letter, word, or number
photism: in synesthesia, a vivid light or color sensation induced by a different sensory stimulus
positron emission tomography (PET): a technique that creates three-dimensional computer images from

particles emitted after radioactively tagged substances are incorporated into body tissues; particle concentrations identify areas of increased energy metabolism
synesthete: a person who experiences synesthesia by virtue of having a second sensation evoked by a single stimulus

CAUSES AND SYMPTOMS
The term "synesthesia" derives from the Greek *syn-* (union/together) and *aisthesis* (sensation/perception). Regarded as an intriguing but perhaps bogus curiosity, synesthesia was once disparaged as a subjective experience unworthy of scientific interest. Since the 1980's, however, neuroimaging techniques have established the synesthetic experience as a genuine sensorineural phenomenon and a legitimate subject for scientific research. Described as rare by some and as common by others, synesthesia gives rise to widely divergent estimates of its prevalence: from 1 in 20,000 people to 1 in 23.

Various combinations of synesthetic experiences have been documented, but color is the most common concurrent perception. Of the many different types, none has been more intensively studied than grapheme-color synesthesia; specific characters written in black print induce the experience of a specific color. The induced color experiences, termed "photisms," are vivid and consistent; a specific grapheme always induces the same color in the same synesthete. A spoken word or musical note can act as the stimulus, and days of the week or months of the year also trigger colors—for some, Friday will always be chartreuse. Rarer synesthetic experiences involve touch or taste. Mirror-touch synesthesia activates a tactile sensation in the synesthete's body when someone within sight is

---

INFORMATION ON SYNESTHESIA

CAUSES: Unknown; probably increased connectivity and cross-wiring in contiguous brain regions
SYMPTOMS: Subjective manifestations involve two or more concurrent sensory perceptions when only one has been stimulated
DURATION: Generally lifelong
TREATMENTS: Primarily occurs in neurologically and psychologically normal people, does not warrant medical treatment

touched. In tactile-emotion synesthesia, textures induce distinct emotions. Some synesthetes experience a specific taste on hearing a word or piece of music.

Synesthesia has a strong genetic component, although the mode of inheritance is unclear. Familial aggregation in synesthesia was first noted by Sir Francis Galton in 1880. One study found a greater than 40 percent prevalence of synesthesia among first-degree relatives of synesthetes. A report of monozygotic (identical) male twins discordant for grapheme-color synesthesia casts doubt on what was initially believed to be X-linked dominant inheritance; documented male-to-male transmission also argues against it. Genetic linkage studies suggest a complex pattern of inheritance, perhaps with multiple gene loci. Different types commonly coexist in the same family, and heterogeneity is characteristic. Within one type, the same word or letter evokes different colors in different individuals, and the subjective experience differs as well.

DIAGNOSIS AND DETECTION

Recognition begins with a self-report. Various psychological tests can distinguish between synesthetes and nonsynesthetes; neuroimaging is generally limited to research. Some diagnostic criteria have been generally accepted: synesthetic sensory experience is involuntary, automatic, and durable—synesthetes typically report their sensory associations as consistent over years.

Considerable evidence supports the neural basis of synesthesia. Neurologic injury can evoke synesthetic associations, and drugs such as mescaline can induce them. Brain imaging, however, identifies synesthesia as a neural phenomenon. The pattern of cerebral blood flow during a synesthetic experience, first recorded in the 1980's, was described as abnormal. Subsequent studies have used positron emission tomography (PET) and functional magnetic resonance imaging (fMRI) to show differences in brain structure and activity between synesthetes and nonsynesthetes.

Grapheme-color synesthesia has been the main focus of fMRI studies. According to posited models, increased connectivity between contiguous brain areas in the cerebral cortex facilitates cross-activation. The fusiform gyrus, involved both in color and grapheme processing, has shown increased activation in addition to increased cortical thickness, volume, and surface area. Increased white matter volume and connectivity has been observed in brains of some synesthetes compared with those of nonsynesthetic counterparts.

Can developmental mechanisms explain synesthesia? Some investigators suggest that incoming sensory information in infants is normally jumbled together, and pruning of comingled neural and synaptic connections comes with development. According to this hypothesis, sensorineural connections in synesthetic adults somehow escaped the pruning process, perhaps via mutation.

PERSPECTIVE AND PROSPECTS

Synesthesia has a long and distinguished history. Around 1710, an English ophthalmologist reported a blind patient who experienced color visions that were induced by sound. Jonathan Swift's title character in *Gulliver's Travels* (1726) encountered a group of blind apprentices taught by their blind master to mix colors by touch and smell. Swift's source was believed to be the Royal Society scientists of his day, notably Robert Boyle. Francis Galton established synesthesia as a scientific entity in 1880.

The idea that the various senses are fused could be found in literature much before it resonated in neurology. Mary Shelley described the creature in *Frankenstein* (1818) as having a difficult time separating his various sensations because he simultaneously saw, felt, heard, and smelled. Later in the nineteenth century, psychologist William James expressed his view that incoming information from different senses is fused in a child before it is later untangled.

The renaissance of scientific research into synesthesia is prompted by the recognition that synesthesia can be a window into the nature of perception. Among the remaining questions is its true prevalence, which is of more than theoretical interest. Some evidence suggests that synesthetic cross-modal mechanisms are universal, even if below the level of consciousness in most adults. Human sensory experiences and their interconnections will undoubtedly continue to intrigue scientists and artists alike well into the future.

—*Judith Weinblatt, M.A., M.S.*

See also Hearing; Nervous system; Neurology; Neurology, pediatric; Sense organs; Smell; Taste; Touch; Vision.

FOR FURTHER INFORMATION:

American Synesthesia Association. http://synesthesia .info. Raises awareness of synesthesia and sponsors periodic conferences that provide a forum and information source for researchers and synesthetes.

Beeli, Gian, et al. "Synaesthesia: When Coloured Sounds Taste Sweet." *Nature* 434 (March 3, 2005): 38.

Mass, Wendy. *A Mango-Shaped Space*. Boston: Little, Brown, 2003.

Ramachandran, Vilayanur, and Edward Hubbard. "Hearing Colors, Tasting Shapes." *Scientific American* 288, no. 5 (May, 2003): 42-49.

Van Campen, Cretien. *The Hidden Sense: Synesthesia in Art and Science*. Cambridge, Mass.: MIT Press, 2007.

SYPHILIS

DISEASE/DISORDER

ALSO KNOWN AS: "Bad blood," bejel (endemic syphilis)

ANATOMY OR SYSTEM AFFECTED: Anus, bones, brain, eyes, genitals, heart, joints, kidneys, nervous system, reproductive system

SPECIALTIES AND RELATED FIELDS: Bacteriology, embryology, epidemiology, gynecology, internal medicine, microbiology, neonatology, neurology, pediatrics, public health, rheumatology

DEFINITION: A sexually transmitted disease caused by the spirochete bacterium *Treponema palladum* that can progress from a genital lesion to a systemic disorder involving multiple organs.

CAUSES AND SYMPTOMS

Syphilis is a sexually transmitted disease (STD) resulting from infection by *Treponema palladum*. The history of the disease is unclear. Evidence exists that its origin may have been linked with a disease, yaws, found in the Western Hemisphere at the time of explorer Christopher Columbus (1451-1506). Yaws is a relatively mild disease generally transmitted through contaminated objects or open skin lesions, but not generally through sexual transmission; it results from infection by a subspecies of *Treponema* called *T. palladum ssp. pertenue*. The theory suggests that this may have been the form of the disease brought back to Europe on one of Columbus's ships. Mutation and sexual transmission in the population of Europe may have produced the more serious form of the disease.

The disease is characterized by several distinct stages. Initial exposure to the organism during sexual intercourse results in formation of a painless skin lesion called a chancre at the site of infection (primary syphilis), developing anywhere from a week to months after infection. Spirochete bacteria may be isolated from the lesion, as well as being found live inside white blood cells (macrophages and neutrophils) that infil-

trate the area. The white cells may be a mechanism for systemic spread of the organism. The lesion generally heals spontaneously, leaving the impression that the disease has been eliminated.

During the weeks after formation of the chancre, the spirochetes multiply to large numbers and become disseminated throughout the body. A second stage (secondary syphilis) often appears within two months following regression of the chancre. Symptoms are often described as flulike, with malaise, headache, fever, and joint aches. A skin rash often appears, covering most of the body. Sores may develop in the mouth and throat and on many of the mucous membranes in the body. The organism is highly transmissible during this period. The rash and other symptoms generally fade over a period of weeks.

Approximately 10 percent of untreated cases develop a third, or tertiary, stage of syphilis. The organism can infiltrate any organ or system in the body, resulting in soft tumors (gummas) in the eyes, lungs, bone, brain, or other organs. Symptoms are characteristic of the organ infected. For example, infection of the brain or other areas of the central nervous system are described as neurosyphilis or syphilitic dementia, characterized by memory loss, personality changes, and neurodegeneration. Even if tertiary syphilis is treated, prognosis for the patient at this stage is often poor.

Treponema has the ability to cross the placenta, and the infection of a pregnant woman may result in congenital syphilis, or infection of her unborn child. Infection may kill the fetus or cause it to be born with obvious deformities such as blindness or physical abnormalities. The infant may also be asymptomatic. An undiagnosed infection will likely progress, with symptoms appearing within weeks after birth. It is common

---

INFORMATION ON SYPHILIS

CAUSES: Bacterial infection transmitted through sexual contact or congenitally

SYMPTOMS: In sexually transmitted form, painless skin lesion (chancre), malaise, headache, fever, joint aches, rash, sores in mouth and throat, and soft tumors in eyes, lungs, bone, or brain if untreated; in congenital form, stillbirth, blindness, physical abnormalities

DURATION: Progressive, fatal if untreated

TREATMENTS: Antibiotics (penicillin; also erythromycin, tetracyclines, chloramphenicol)

for a rash to appear, with evidence of tertiary stage neurosyphilis or cardiovascular syphilis.

A diagnosis of syphilis can be made through microscopic examination of lesion exudates, noting the presence of spirochetes. However, *Treponema* is notoriously unstable, and the test must be made shortly after obtaining the specimen. More commonly, diagnosis is based upon serological testing for serum antibodies against the organism or tissue lipids released from infected or damaged cells.

TREATMENT AND THERAPY

Penicillin is the preferred method of treatment for both primary and secondary syphilis. If the disease has progressed to the tertiary stage, then antibiotic treatment will still eliminate the organism, but it will not reverse organ damage that may have occurred. Treatment for related organ involvement is symptomatic.

Alternative antibiotics include erythromycin, tetracyclines, and chloramphenicol, if necessary. However, only penicillin is effective during the tertiary stage or for use in pregnant women.

PERSPECTIVE AND PROSPECTS

Despite the long-time existence of effective therapy, penicillin or alternative antibiotics, and the absence of any reservoir for *T. palladum* other than humans, syphilis remains the third most common sexually transmitted bacterial disease in the West. Only gonorrhea and chlamydia are more common.

. As a result of effective therapy and the generally obvious symptoms of the disease, tertiary syphilis has largely disappeared. However, sexual practices continue to sustain spread of the disease, with approximately fifty thousand cases reported each year in the United States. Three factors are primary contributors to the resurgence of the disease: prostitution, the increase in riskier sexual practices among homosexual men, and general apathy toward a disease that is relatively easy to treat in its early stages. An increase in congenital syphilis also reflects the presence of the disease in women of childbearing years. In the absence of condom use, both unwanted pregnancy and the spread of STDs such as syphilis may result.

No vaccine currently exists for syphilis. The inability to culture the organism in the laboratory has made research related to *Treponema* difficult, and the organism does not infect animals other than humans to act as a method of vaccine production. However, genetic engineering has resulted in the cloning of several bacterial gene products related to surface proteins and virulence factors, allowing the possibility for a vaccine in the future. For now, the best means of controlling syphilis remains the prevention of its spread through education and safer-sex practices, as well as early treatment of those infected.

—*Richard Adler, Ph.D.*

See also Antibiotics; Bacterial infections; Birth defects; Chlamydia; Genital disorders, female; Genital disorders, male; Gonorrhea; Lesions; Neonatology; Pregnancy and gestation; Rashes; Sexually transmitted diseases (STDs).

FOR FURTHER INFORMATION:

Centers for Disease Control and Prevention. *The National Plan to Eliminate Syphilis from the United States*. Atlanta: U.S. Department of Health and Human Services, 2006.

Mandell, Gerald L., John E. Bennett, and Raphael Dolin, eds. *Mandell, Douglas, and Bennett's Principles and Practice of Infectious Diseases*. 7th ed. New York: Churchill Livingstone/Elsevier, 2010.

Murray, Patrick R., Ken S. Rosenthal, and Michael A. Pfaller. *Medical Microbiology*. 6th ed. Philadelphia: Mosby/Elsevier, 2009.

Parker, James N., and Philip M. Parker, eds. *The Official Patient's Sourcebook on Syphilis*. San Diego, Calif.: Icon Health, 2002.

Quetel, Claude. *The History of Syphilis*. Baltimore: Johns Hopkins University Press, 1990.

Sutton, Amy L., ed. *Sexually Transmitted Diseases Sourcebook*. 3d ed. Detroit, Mich.: Omnigraphics, 2006.

SYSTEMIC LUPUS ERYTHEMATOSUS (SLE)

DISEASE/DISORDER

ALSO KNOWN AS: Lupus

ANATOMY OR SYSTEM AFFECTED: All

SPECIALTIES AND RELATED FIELDS: Cardiology, dermatology, endocrinology, family medicine, gastroenterology, histology, immunology, internal medicine, nephrology, nutrition, orthopedics, pharmacology, physical therapy, psychiatry, psychology, pulmonary medicine, rheumatology, vascular medicine

DEFINITION: A chronic, inflammatory autoimmune disease in which the immune system attacks the body's own structures. SLE can affect any organ or body system, especially the skin, joints, blood vessels, and kidneys. It is distinguished from two other forms of lupus: drug-induced lupus, which is caused by certain prescription medications, and discoid lupus, which primarily affects the skin.

KEY TERMS:

antibodies: proteins manufactured by the body to attack and neutralize foreign substances, such as bacteria

antinuclear antibody (ANA): an unusual antibody that is directed against structures within the nucleus of cells

autoantibodies: antibodies that attack the body's own cells and tissues

autoimmune: a term describing a disease in which the body produces antibodies against its own cells

connective tissue: the substance holding the body and organs together

cytotoxic: having a damaging effect on cells

discoid rash: raised red patches

erythematosus: characterized by redness of the skin

hyperlipidemia: an excess of lipids (for example, cholesterol and triglycerides) in the blood

malar rash: a redness or rash on the face covering the cheeks and the bridge of the nose; also called butterfly rash

photosensitivity: a sensitivity to light or sunlight

Raynaud's phenomenon: discoloration and pain in the fingertips induced by cold

serositis: inflammation of the lining of the lung or heart

CAUSES AND SYMPTOMS

The cause of lupus is unknown, but scientists believe that both genetic and environmental factors are involved. Although there is a genetic predisposition to lupus, and researchers have identified an associated gene in some cases, only 10 percent of lupus patients have a familial connection and only 5 percent of children born to individuals with lupus will develop the disease. People of African, American Indian, Asian, and Hispanic origin seem to develop the disease more frequently than do non-Hispanic Caucasians. Lupus affects both men and women, but the incidence is ten to fifteen times higher in women and between 85 and 90 percent of patients are women. The majority of lupus diagnoses occur in young women in their late teens to thirties. It is possible that hormonal factors play a role in this disparity, because it is known that symptoms in women increase before menstrual cycles and during pregnancy. Environmental triggers include infections, exposure to ultraviolet light, and extreme

---

INFORMATION ON SYSTEMIC LUPUS ERYTHEMATOSUS (SLE)

CAUSES: Unclear; possibly related to paramyxoviral infection
SYMPTOMS: Red or purple facial lesions, joint pain and swelling, fatigue, low-grade fever
DURATION: Chronic
TREATMENTS: None; alleviation of symptoms

---

stress, as well as antibiotic usage (particularly penicillin and those in the sulfa group). Certain other drugs, particularly hydralazine, procainamide, and isoniazid, can also cause lupus, but this type of drug-induced lupus usually disappears after the offending drug is discontinued.

Symptoms may begin suddenly with fever or may develop gradually over the course of months or years. The clinical course is usually marked by remissions, periods when symptoms are minimal or absent, and relapses (called flare-ups), when the patient experiences an aggravation of symptoms and general malaise.

SLE can affect all organ systems of the body. The production of autoantibodies is the underlying physiologic problem in lupus. These autoantibodies can appear in a great number and variety, differing from patient to patient, thus causing their varying symptoms. General symptoms include fatigue, fever, anemia, weight loss, Raynaud's phenomenon, and headaches. Joint inflammation and pain (arthritis) occurs in about 90 percent of patients and is often the earliest manifestation of the disease. It usually occurs intermittently and generally does not cause permanent joint damage or deformity. Skin manifestations are present in most patients and include malar (butterfly) and/or discoid skin rashes; redness on the hands, fingertips, and nails; mucous membrane ulcers in the mouth and nose; and photosensitivity. Inflammation of the sac around the lungs (pleurisy) or heart (pericarditis) is a frequent occurrence, resulting in pain upon deep breathing or chest pain. On rare occasions, there may be severe complications, such as bleeding into the lungs, which is life-threatening, or cardiac failure. Neurologic complications may also occur, including headaches, thinking impairment, personality changes, seizures, strokes, depression, dementia and psychosis. Kidney involvement may be either minor or progressive, leading to severe nephritis that can be fatal. Ocular changes sometimes occur, causing conjunctivitis or blurred vision. In rare cases, retinitis, inflammation of the blood vessels at the back of the eye, can occur, leading to blindness if not treated quickly.

SLE is difficult to diagnose, due to its variety of symptoms and similarity to many other diseases. The constellation of symptoms appears and progresses differently for each patient and initially may seem vague and unrelated. Usually, patients will first see their family doctors. Upon diagnosis or the discovery of particular body system involvement, the family doctor may refer the patient on to one or more specialists. There is no single test for lupus. A physician will perform several laboratory tests as part of the differential diagnostic process, including various blood and urine tests and biopsies of the skin and kidney. For a positive diagnosis of SLE, a patient must have at least four of the eleven criteria established by the American College of Rheumatology: malar rash, discoid rash, photosensitivity, oral ulcers, arthritis, serositis, renal disorder, neurologic disorder, hematologic disorder, immunologic disorder, and the presence of antinuclear antibodies (ANA).

TREATMENT AND THERAPY

There is no cure for lupus. Treatment is aimed at minimizing symptoms, reducing inflammation, and maintaining normal bodily functions. The treatment approach will vary according to the specific symptoms and organ involvement of the individual patient.

Preventive therapy involves lifestyle strategies aimed at reducing the risk of flare-up episodes. Patients are advised to follow a healthy diet, get adequate rest, and participate in moderate weight-bearing exercise in order to combat fatigue and muscle weakness. Counseling, support groups, and patient education help reduce stress and protect emotional well-being. Other recommendations include smoking cessation, limited alcohol intake, and adequate intake of vitamin D and calcium. Avoidance of excessive sun exposure through the use of protective clothing and sunscreens can reduce the occurrence of skin rashes and possibly systemic disease flares. Patients can learn to recognize the warning signs of an impending flare-up, such as increased fatigue, headaches, dizziness, stomach upset, fever, or the appearance of a rash. Regular laboratory tests can also detect an imminent flare-up. Early treatment of flare-ups can make them easier to control, can prevent tissue damage, and may reduce the length of time that the patient is given high doses of drugs.

Medications are an integral part of the treatment of

lupus, and fall into four main categories: nonsteroidal anti-inflammatory drugs (NSAIDs), corticosteroids, antimalarial drugs, and cytotoxic and immunosuppressive agents.

NSAIDs are used to control symptoms and reduce muscle and joint pain and inflammation. Commonly used NSAIDs include acetylsalicylic acid (aspirin), ibuprofen, naproxen, indomethacin, sulindac, nabumetone, tolmetin, and ketoprofen. Since these drugs can cause stomach upset, patients are usually advised to take them with meals or to take antacids or prostaglandins as well. Some NSAIDs have a prostaglandin added to the capsule. Patients taking NSAIDs must be monitored because of the potential adverse effects to the liver, kidney, and central nervous system.

Corticosteriods are synthetic hormones that have excellent anti-inflammatory and immunoregulatory effects and reduce symptoms promptly. They are used to treat a spectrum of lupus manifestations, especially in cases when organs are threatened. Prednisone is the most commonly used, followed by hydrocortisone, methylprednisolone, and others. Topical formulations are used for skin rashes, and oral doses are given for systemic involvement. Dosages are monitored carefully and tapered after initial inflammation reduction is achieved in order to reduce possible side effects. Corticosteroids may also be administered by injection into the skin or joint. For severe cases, intravenous administration of large doses of methylprednisolone (called pulse steroids) for three days is given. Unfortunately, high doses of corticosteroids over long periods of time can produce unpleasant side effects, such as weight gain, rounded face, acne, emotional lability, hypertension, hyperlipidemia, increased risk of infection, diabetes, and osteoporosis.

Antimalarial drugs are frequently used in the management of skin rashes, joint inflammation, and serositis, though it may take months before their beneficial effects become apparent. They also help protect against the damaging effects of ultraviolet light. The most common agents are hydroxychloroquine (Plaquenil), chloroquine (Aralen), and quinicrine (Atabrine). These medications can be taken in combination with NSAIDs and other drugs to increase their effectiveness. They are particularly helpful when used with corticosteroids in order to decrease the amount of steroid needed. Damage to the retina is a potential side effect and is dose-related. Patients must be evaluated by an ophthalmologist twice a year.

Cytotoxic and immunosuppressive agents are potent

drugs utilized in cases requiring aggressive therapy to protect major organs. They are used in conjunction with, or in place of, corticosteroids in order to spare the patient the side effects of the corticosteroids. Cytotoxics are not approved by the Food and Drug Administration (FDA) for use in the treatment of SLE; however, they are considered part of standard practice. These drugs target autoantibodies, thus suppressing the overactive immune response of lupus patients. Cyclophosphamide (Cytoxin) and azathioprine (Imuran) are both used in the treatment of lupus nephritis and are also effective in combating blood cell deficiencies, pulmonary bleeding, vasculitis, and central nervous system disease. Imuran is less potent but causes fewer side effects than does Cytoxin. Methotrexate, mycophenolate mofetil (CellCept), cyclosporine, chlorambucil, and nitrogen mustard are other cytotoxic agents that have been used in the management of lupus. Intravenous immunoglobulin injections are given to some patients to increase the production of blood platelets. Side effects of cytotoxic drugs include nausea, hair loss, increased risk of certain cancers, increased risk of infection, sterility, and bone marrow suppression.

Pregnancy in a lupus patient requires special care. Even though more than 50 percent of lupus pregnancies follow a normal course, all lupus pregnancies are considered high risk. Doctors recommend planning pregnancy during times of remission. Recent studies contradict the traditional belief that pregnancy increases the chance of flare-ups and also suggest that most flare-ups during pregnancy are mild, consisting only of rashes, fatigue, and arthritis. Frequent doctor visits are a necessity in order to detect and treat any problems early. The obstetrician will regularly check the baby's growth and heartbeat in order to detect any abnormalities that might signal problems. Some lupus medications, such as prednisone, are safe to take during pregnancy because they do not cross the placenta. Others, such as cyclophosphamide, need to be used with caution or discontinued during the pregnancy.

About 20 percent of women with lupus experience preeclampsia during their pregnancy. This is a serious condition in which there is a sudden increase in blood pressure and/or protein in the urine requiring immediate treatment of the patient and delivery of the baby.

About one-third of women with lupus have antiphospholipid antibodies. These antibodies cause blood clots, which puts the patient at risk for developing them in the placenta, interfering with the nourishment of the baby. Since these blood clots usually form in the placenta in the second trimester, often the baby has developed enough to be delivered prematurely. The mother can be treated with heparin, which reduces the chance of clots and miscarriage.

About 50 percent of lupus pregnancies result in birth before full term. The majority of babies born between thirty and thirty-six weeks will grow normally with no problems. Those born before thirty-six weeks are considered premature. Approximately 3 percent of women with lupus will have a baby with a syndrome called neonatal lupus. This syndrome consists of a transient rash and blood count abnormalities and disappears by three to six months of age. Sometimes, a permanent abnormality in the heartbeat also occurs, but it is treatable and the baby is able to grow normally.

PERSPECTIVE AND PROSPECTS

The identification of lupus as a distinct medical entity dates back to the twelfth century, when the term "lupus" (Latin for "wolf") was used to describe ulcerative facial lesions, because they looked similar to either a wolf's bite or a wolf's facial markings. Other descriptions of the various dermatologic manifestations of lupus were noted by physicians over the next several centuries; the first medical textbook illustration occurred in 1856. The Viennese physician Moriz Kaposi, in 1872, was the first physician to recognize and describe the systemic manifestations of lupus, as well as the fact that there seemed to be two distinct forms of lupus, discoid and systemic. This was soon expanded upon by Canadian physician Sir William Osler, who detailed the major organ manifestations. In the late nineteenth century, the usefulness of quinine and salicylates in the treatment of lupus was reported. In the mid-twentieth century, the discovery of the immunologic aspects of lupus were discovered, when the presence of antinuclear antibodies were identified. Around this same time, the first animal models were used for the study of lupus, and the genetic component of lupus was also recognized. A major advance was the discovery of the effectiveness of cortisone in the treatment of systemic lupus. Corticosteroids remain the primary treatment modality, complemented by antimalarials (for skin and joint involvement) and cytotoxic agents (for severe kidney manifestations and other life-threatening complications).

The prognosis for lupus patients has improved dramatically as a result of earlier diagnosis and better treatment. The long-term prognosis for a given patient is still variable, however, and is often related to the severity and the controllability of the initial inflammation. Also, the morbidity patterns of lupus patients have changed because of the increased usage of corticosteroids and cytotoxic drugs. Infections, accelerated atherosclerosis, and osteoporosis have become significant risk factors. Overall, however, the outlook for survival and quality of life has greatly improved. As of 2005, more than 90 percent of lupus patients lived more than ten years postdiagnosis. Those with organ-threatening disease had a lower rate, with only 60 percent surviving fifteen to twenty years.

A proliferation of research into the treatment of lupus that began in the 1950's continues and brings much promise for additional insight into the pathogenesis of lupus as well as new treatment modalities and agents. Some focus areas of current research include investigations into patterns of gene activity, the role of the protein interferon-alpha in the progression of lupus, environmental factors, immune ablation, stem cell transplantation, and the targeting of destructive white blood cells. An intensified effort by the federal government, private industry, and nonprofit organizations, such as the Alliance for Lupus Research and the Lupus Foundation of America, fuels the hope that better treatments, prevention, and ultimately a cure for lupus will be found.

—*Barbara C. Beattie*

See also Arthritis; Autoimmune disorders; Fatigue; Joints; Kidney disorders; Light therapy; Rashes; Skin disorders; Stress; Tuberculosis; Vision disorders.

FOR FURTHER INFORMATION:

Hanger, Nancy C. *Lupus—The First Year: An Essential Guide for the Newly Diagnosed*. New York: Marlowe, 2003. A "patient-expert" guides the reader step-by-step through the first year after diagnosis.

Kasitanon, Nuntana, Laurence S. Magder, and Michelle Petri. "Predictors of Survival in Systemic Lupus Erythematosus." *Medicine* 85, no. 3 (May, 2006): 147-156. This large study correlates various factors, such as demographics, clinical manifestations, and disease activity, to overall survival rates.

Lahita, Robert G., and Robert H. Phillips. *Lupus Q & A: Everything You Need to Know*. Rev. ed. New York: Avery, 2004. Written jointly by an expert on lupus and a psychologist, this book provides straightforward information about all aspects of lupus in an easy-to-read, question-and-answer format.

Lupus Foundation of America. http://www.lupus.org. An organization dedicated to improving the diagnosis and treatment of lupus, supporting individuals and families affected by the disease, increasing awareness of lupus among health professionals and the public, and finding a cure.

Meadows, Michelle. "Battling Lupus." *FDA Consumer* 39, no. 4 (July/August, 2005): 28-34. A complete overview of lupus written for the patient. Includes symptoms, diagnosis, treatment, and future prospects.

Phillips, Robert H. *Coping With Lupus: A Practical Guide to Alleviating the Challenges of Systemic Lupus Erythematosus*. 3d ed. New York: Avery, 2001. Written by an eminent psychologist, this book provides valuable assistance to patients and families on coping with the medical and psychological problems caused by lupus.

Seppa, N. "Self-Help: Stem Cells Rescue Lupus Patients." *Science News* 169, no. 5 (February 4, 2006): 67-68. A description of a promising new therapy procedure for patients with severe forms of lupus.

Wallace, Daniel J. *The Lupus Book: A Guide for Patients and Their Families*. 3d ed. New York: Oxford University Press, 2005. A complete compendium of information from a leading authority, this book provides thorough coverage of the pathogenesis and management of lupus as well as a discussion of standard, alternative, and promising new therapies. Includes references and sources of additional information.

Zonali, M. "Taming Lupus." *Scientific American* 292, no. 3 (March, 2005): 70-77. Authoritative coverage on the complexities of managing the various manifestations and complications of lupus.

SYSTEMS AND ORGANS

ANATOMY

ANATOMY OR SYSTEM AFFECTED: All
SPECIALTIES AND RELATED FIELDS: All
DEFINITION: Groups of tissues and organs dedicated to particular functions, all of which must work together to perform efficiently.

KEY TERMS:

atrium: the chamber of the heart where veins terminate; the atrium receives blood returning to the heart and delivers it to the ventricle

bronchi: the airways conducting air from the mouth to the depths of the lungs

carbon dioxide: the gas produced by the body from the use of oxygen; carbon dioxide and the hydrogen ions it can create may become toxic if not excreted by the body

foodstuffs: the basic components of food that the body can use—carbohydrates (which break down to sugars, primarily to glucose), proteins (which break down to amino acids), and fat

hormone: a chemical released by a tissue to signal another tissue to modify its function

ions: small chemical substances that have a positive or negative charge; the most important ions with a positive charge are sodium, potassium, hydrogen, and calcium, while the most important negative ion is chloride

ventricles: the large chambers of the heart that pump blood into the arteries; the left ventricle pumps blood into the aorta, and the right ventricle pumps blood into the lung's arteries

STRUCTURE AND FUNCTIONS

There are essentially nine systems in the human body: the nervous, cardiovascular, respiratory, gastrointestinal, renal, endocrine, reproductive, thermoregulatory, and skeletomuscular systems. All these systems are essential to sustain life, and many work together to perform their functions efficiently. All the other systems need the nervous system to operate or to coordinate their functions. The first six of these systems will be discussed in this article.

The nervous system is composed of the central nervous system (the brain) and the peripheral nervous system (the spinal cord and nerves extending to every part of the body). The brain receives information from the body by way of the sensory nerves. It then evaluates all the information and sends out the appropriate signals to respond. For example, the ears send information to the brain that there are noises coming from behind; the brain tells the head to turn in the direction of the sounds. The eyes send the signals that the noises are coming from, for example, a gorilla. The brain must decide to run, fight, or stand and try to reason with the gorilla. Meanwhile, the brain tells the heart to beat faster and harder. It also tells the stomach and intestines to stop digestion and reduce its blood flow because blood may be needed by the muscles for running. This is called the "fight or flight" response to stress, which the nervous system controls.

Sensory information can come from any of the five senses—sight, smell, hearing, touch, or taste—but it can also come from other sensors. Sensory nerves send the brain information on pain, temperature, blood pressure, and what is going on in the stomach and intestines (hunger or a full feeling). The brain receives millions of signals each second from every part of the body and must constantly decide how to respond. Humans can choose not to respond instinctively as animals do. For example, humans often eat when they are not hungry.

Different areas of the brain are dedicated to specific functions. The upper portion of the spinal cord and lower portion of the brain (the brain stem) are dedicated to controlling involuntary functions such as breathing, the maintenance of blood pressure and heart rate, and the responses to hot and cold. The middle portion of the brain coordinates movement. The middle brain also coordinates information from upper portions of the brain and generates emotions. The uppermost and outermost portions of the brain (the cerebrum) process the information from the senses and generate responses, such as telling the body to move. The cerebrum also performs such intellectual functions as reasoning.

The cardiovascular system is composed of the heart and blood vessels. Its job is to pump blood containing oxygen and foodstuffs (sugars, proteins, and fat) to every part of the body. Blood is composed of red and white blood cells suspended in plasma, a pale yellow fluid which flows through the cardiovascular system. Red blood cells are the carriers of oxygen, the main source of energy for the body. White blood cells help fight disease and are delivered to parts of the body that are hurt or diseased. The plasma contains platelets that help blood to clot when necessary. Blood also transports wastes produced by the body from tissues to organs that can dispose of them. For example, carbon dioxide is produced by the tissues when oxygen is used for energy. Blood carries carbon dioxide back to the lungs to be removed from the body in exhaled air.

Blood is pumped by the heart in a circuit in the cardiovascular system (also called the circulatory system). The heart has four chambers, two atria and two ventricles. Blood enters the heart through the left atrium, a small pocket of muscles that help pump blood into the left ventricle. The ventricle is a larger chamber with a thick wall of muscle that can pump very hard; it pushes blood into the arteries. The left ventricle pumps blood into the main artery of the body, the aorta. The aorta branches many times into smaller arteries, which in turn branch into capillaries. Every part of the body has millions of tiny capillaries just big enough for a blood cell to pass through them; in fact, blood cells must fold to get through some capillaries. In capillaries, oxygen and foodstuffs leave the blood, and then carbon dioxide and other waste products enter the blood to be taken away. Blood flows from the capillaries into small veins, which join to make larger and larger veins. The largest veins, the venae cavae, empty into the heart, in the right atrium. The blood is pumped from the right atrium to the right ventricle. Blood is then pumped by the right ventricle through the lung and back into the left atrium to start its journey again.

The lungs are the major organ of the respiratory system. The function of the respiratory system is to bring fresh air into the lungs, getting it very close to the blood, and to expel used air. Air enters the respiratory system through the nose and mouth, which connect to the main windpipe, the trachea. The trachea branches into smaller airways called bronchi. Bronchi in turn branch into smaller airways, bronchioles. The ends of bronchioles form many rounded sacs (alveoli) that resemble a bunch of grapes. These sacs of air have very thin walls that are shared with the walls of the lung's capillaries. This close arrangement of air and blood provides a minimal distance for oxygen to travel into the blood and for carbon dioxide to leave the blood.

Air is moved into the lungs when the muscles of respiration contract and expand the lungs. The diaphragm is a large sheet of muscle which separates the chest from the abdomen. When the diaphragm contracts, it pulls the lungs down. At the same time, muscles on the chest wall contract, pulling the lungs up and out. This expansion of the lungs causes air to be sucked into and fill the air sacs. During exhalation, the respiratory muscles are relaxed, the lung collapses somewhat, and air rushes out, carrying carbon dioxide with it.

Blood, specifically red blood cells, is specialized to carry large amounts of oxygen and carbon dioxide. Red blood cells contain hemoglobin, a special substance that attaches to these gases. When the amounts of oxygen and carbon dioxide in the plasma increase, they tend to leak back into the air sacs or tissues, respectively. These gases are effectively removed from the fluid by hemoglobin, allowing more gases to enter the blood without leaking back out. Hemoglobin also coordinates the release of these gases—oxygen to the tissues and carbon dioxide to the lungs—at the correct time.

The gastrointestinal system is a multiorgan system that breaks down food to be absorbed into the blood. Initially, food is broken down by chewing and by mixing with saliva. Then it is swallowed into the esophagus, a tube which travels through the chest to empty into the stomach. The stomach adds acid and other chemicals to the food, which breaks it down even more. The food, now called chyme, passes into the upper small intestine (the duodenum). The pancreas adds enzymes; a chemical called bicarbonate, which neutralizes the acid added by the stomach; and the hormones insulin and glucagon. Insulin is the major hormone secreted by the pancreas. It is absorbed into the blood by the intestine and signals the body to get ready to receive the products of digestion, primarily sugar (glucose). Bile is also added to the contents of the upper duodenum by the liver. Bile helps to break down fat to be absorbed into the blood. As the intestinal contents move along the small intestine, from the jejunum to the ileum, water and mucus are added to help move it along, and carbohydrates are absorbed in their smallest form, glucose. Enzymes attached to the wall of the intestine break up proteins to be absorbed as their component parts, amino acids. Water in chyme is constantly being reabsorbed. Finally the colon, or large intestine, absorbs most of the remaining water. The remaining solids are excreted through the rectum.

Food is moved through the gastrointestinal system by a special type of muscle called smooth muscle. The walls of the gastrointestinal tract are composed of muscle arranged in circular fashion around the tube and along its length. Initially, a circular group of muscles contracts, narrowing a short segment of intestine. This process is called segmentation. The contraction spreads down the muscles arranged lengthwise, squeezing the contents down the length of intestine. Movement of chyme is aided by relaxation of the muscles ahead of the contraction. This motion is called peristalsis. Peristalsis is coordinated by the nervous system, but the intestines have their own set of nerves. These intestinal nerves can control the motion of the intestine without help from the central nervous system.

The kidneys are the primary organs of the renal system. It is the function of the kidneys to regulate both the amount and the composition of the fluid in the body, in spite of wide variations in the human environment and in an organism's intake of food and water. Since blood circulates everywhere in the body, the kidneys can change the composition and amount of plasma, and the other fluids of the body then equalize with it. Therefore, the kidneys can regulate all body fluids. The body has sensors for both the amount of fluid in the blood and the concentration of the important elements in the blood, such as sodium, hydrogen, and potassium.

The kidneys regulate plasma volume and composition by filtering the plasma and returning only the appropriate amounts of fluid and substances back to the blood. Arteries entering the kidneys rapidly branch into capillaries. Approximately 20 percent of all plasma flowing into the kidneys leaves the capillaries and is collected in the capsules that surround them. This fluid is funneled into specialized tubes.

Substances are taken out and put into the fluid in the tubes in order to regulate fluid volume and composition. In the beginning of the tube (the proximal tubule), most of the salt, water, glucose, and amino acids are taken back into the blood. The next sections (the loop of Henle, distal tubule, and collecting ducts) help to regulate the final amount of water excreted in urine. The collecting ducts join to form the ureter, which carries the remaining fluid, urine, to the bladder, where it is stored. From the bladder, the urine is expelled through the urethra.

The endocrine system is another multiorgan system that helps to control and modify the function of almost all other systems. Endocrine glands produce chemicals and release them into the blood to direct the functions of cells and tissues elsewhere in the body. There are three classes of hormones: amines, peptides and proteins, and steroids. Adrenaline is an example of the amine group, insulin is a protein hormone, and estrogen is a steroid hormone. Each of these is produced by a different gland.

The adrenal glands, small glands located near the kidneys, make several hormones. The outer portion, the cortex, produces three types of steroid hormones referred to as corticosteroids: glucocorticoids, mineralocorticoids, and small amounts of androgenic hormones. The major glucocorticoid, cortisol, regulates the production and use of glucose, fats, and amino acids by many cells and tissues. It also plays a helper role for other hormonal actions, such as making them more potent during stress, and it helps prevent inflammation and swelling. The major mineralocorticoid, aldosterone, can modify the kidneys' excretion of sodium, potassium, and hydrogen. A person unable to produce mineralocorticoids will die in a few days without treatment but can be saved by aldosterone therapy. Therefore, these steroids are said to be lifesaving. The androgenic steroids can cause the development of adult male sexual characteristics, the same effect as the male sex hormone, testosterone.

The interior portion, or medulla, of the adrenal glands makes catecholamines, such as adrenaline (epinephrine). Adrenaline helps the cardiovascular system during exercise and stress. It is the hormone that stimulates

much of the "fight or flight" response, making the heart beat faster and harder. Adrenaline also helps to increase blood flow to muscles, in case flight is the action of choice.

The pituitary gland, also known as the hypophysis, is located at the base of the brain and produces many hormones with a variety of actions. The pituitary is divided into two areas: the anterior lobe (also known as the adenohypophysis) and the posterior lobe (also known as the neurohypophysis). The anterior pituitary produces growth hormone, a protein that has a major influence on all metabolic activity. It causes the body to store carbohydrates, to make proteins for growth, and to use fat for energy. The other anterior pituitary hormones cause other glands to increase their production of hormones. The glands stimulated by distinct pituitary hormones are the thyroid, adrenal cortex, ovaries, testicles, and mammary glands. The posterior pituitary produces the peptide hormones antidiuretic hormone (also known as vasopressin) and oxytocin. Antidiuretic hormone (ADH) decreases the amount of water that the kidneys can excrete, which keeps the body from dehydrating. ADH can also cause the blood pressure to rise, which helps if fluid is lost as a result of bleeding. Oxytocin causes the uterus to contract during the birthing process, and it also stimulates the production of milk in new mothers. The pituitary has direct regulating control over many glands and tissues, and it regulates nearly all tissues and organs indirectly by way of its stimulating hormones. This gland is regulated in a similar fashion by the hypothalamus, a small part of the brain just above the pituitary.

The thyroid gland is located in the neck around the voice box, or larynx. The parathyroid glands are located next to the thyroid gland. Thyroid hormones (peptides) cause almost all tissues in the body to increase the use of foodstuffs for the production of proteins, aiding in growth. In addition, the thyroid gland produces calcitonin. Calcitonin and the parathyroid hormones regulate the amount of calcium in the blood. Parathyroid hormone acts by freeing calcium from bone when more calcium is needed in the blood, while calcitonin causes the opposite action. Therefore, when the level of one of these hormones goes up, the other must go down.

The sex organs are also endocrine glands. The ovaries make estrogen and progesterone, while the testes produce testosterone. These steroid hormones cause the body to develop primary and secondary sexual characteristics. When a woman is pregnant, the placenta (the part of a woman's uterus that nourishes the fetus) produces hormones that prepare her body for childbirth and breast-feeding.

DISORDERS AND DISEASES

The body has control mechanisms to ensure that its systems function properly. Many systems use what is called negative feedback to fine-tune their functioning. An example of negative feedback is the control of blood pressure. Sensors in the arteries allow the brain to monitor the body's blood pressure level. When pressure is too high, the brain tells the cardiovascular system to decrease pressure by slowing the heart and opening the blood vessels and tells the kidneys to excrete fluid. Thus, when blood pressure is high, the feedback that the brain provides is negative, because it causes a response that is opposite to the unwanted change from the normal state.

The endocrine system uses negative feedback to regulate many hormones. The simplest endocrine feedback system involves insulin and glucose. When blood glucose increases, insulin secretion increases, which in turn decreases blood glucose. A decrease in blood glucose tells the pancreas to slow down the secretion of insulin. The failure of this system results in diabetes mellitus, a disease in which the ability to regulate blood sugar is lost. When this control is lost, other systems are damaged as a result, such as the renal and cardiovascular systems.

There are also much more complex feedback control systems. The regulation of the adrenal hormone cortisol serves as an example of such a system. Cortisol secretion is controlled by secretion of the pituitary hormone adrenocorticotropic hormone (ACTH), also called corticotropin. The secretion of ACTH is controlled by a hypothalamic hormone called corticotropin-releasing factor (CRF). Stress causes CRF to be released, which causes the release of ACTH and in turn stimulates the secretion of cortisol. In general, when the level of any of these hormones becomes too high, the release of one of the others can be shut down. High levels of cortisol turn off CRF and ACTH secretion. High levels of ACTH can turn off the secretion of the hormone that triggers its secretion, CRF. It is also thought that CRF can provide feedback to its organ of origin, the hypothalamus, and halt its own secretion. Thus, if one of the control systems fails to function, a backup system guards against total malfunction.

The systems and organs of the body are dedicated to specific functions, but each needs the others to function

properly. In addition, each system requires the coordination from the central nervous system to perform efficiently. The lungs bring vital oxygen to the cardiovascular system, and all systems need the nutrients brought to them by the cardiovascular system. Some organs of the endocrine system, such as the adrenal glands, are essential to life. The kidneys keep the blood clean and maintain the body's fluid volume. The reproductive system is essential to maintaining the existence of a species. All these systems must perform their functions for the body to work well. If one system malfunctions, frequently other systems become involved and may malfunction as well.

An example of one system malfunction that causes the failure of many others is renal failure. Kidney failure can be caused by a malfunction of the cardiovascular system such as clogging of the capillaries, which prohibits the kidneys from doing their job. As a result, hydrogen and potassium ions will accumulate. The effects of high levels of hydrogen and potassium ions on the cardiovascular system are a weakened heart and lower blood pressure. The nervous system can sense the increase in hydrogen ions and will tell the respiratory system to breathe faster and deeper to rid the body of carbon dioxide and its hydrogen ions. The increase in breathing helps to lower the hydrogen ion levels in the blood but cannot completely compensate for the kidney malfunction; in fact, the increase in work by the respiratory muscles can produce more hydrogen ions. When levels of hydrogen become too high, the brain begins to malfunction. The patient may experience dizziness, have seizures, or lose consciousness. If these symptoms are not reversed, the malfunction of each system will aid in the deterioration of other systems. The brain will be irreversibly damaged, and the heart will stop.

There are several ways to treat renal failure to avoid multiple-organ sickness. Treatment of infections with antibiotics before they become severe can help to avoid early and mild kidney failure. In severe, long-term kidney failure, kidney transplantation may become necessary. The damaged kidney (or kidneys) is removed and replaced with an organ from a deceased donor or from a living donor (a person can live a normal life with only one functioning kidney). Kidneys, even from deceased donors, are rare, and many people in need of a transplant must wait for years to receive one that will not be rejected by the body's immune system. For such patients, dialysis is necessary for survival. Dialysis is the use of a machine to perform some of the functions of the kidneys. Patients with total kidney failure must be hooked up to an artificial kidney machine for several hours several times per week. Even with this treatment, they will still be very sick because the machine cannot perform all functions of the kidneys.

PERSPECTIVE AND PROSPECTS

In the Middle Ages, it was believed that "spirits" were the essence of life or "vitality"; thus, the treatment for many ailments was bloodletting, the application of leeches to remove the "evil spirit" causing the sickness. It was not until the seventeenth century that William Harvey discovered that blood circulated from arteries to veins in both the lungs and the rest of the body. Oxygen was discovered at the end of the eighteenth century by Joseph Priestley. Knowledge of chemistry, biochemistry, and physiology grew in the nineteenth century, but most of the information about systems and organs contained in this article was revealed in the twentieth century.

Many discoveries have been in the area of how the body's systems and organs interact with and influence one another. New anatomical techniques of investigation have revealed the minute structures of many organs and tissues. As a result, the presence of previously unknown nervous and other tissue parts has been recognized; their functions are under investigation. Chemical techniques have revealed many new hormone and hormonelike substances through which one tissue or organ can influence another. Research into the molecular structure of some of these biochemical signals is helping to explain how they work.

In addition, the events that occur inside a cell or group of cells have been described in greater detail. How a group of cells produces unified organ function and how this function is altered is currently under investigation. Studies into how a cell can change its function in conjunction with surrounding cells have added to the knowledge of how systems and organs can fine-tune their functions. This research involves information regarding how the genes inside cells carry messages and how these messages in turn are expressed in unified physiological functions.

—*J. Timothy O'Neill, Ph.D.*

See also Adrenal glands; Anatomy; Brain; Circulation; Colon; Ears; Endocrine glands; Endocrine system; Eyes; Gallbladder; Gastrointestinal system; Glands; Heart; Immune system; Kidneys; Liver; Lungs; Lymphatic system; Nervous system; Pancreas; Pituitary gland; Reproductive system; Sense organs; Skin; Small intestine; Thyroid gland; Urinary system; Vascular system.

FOR FURTHER INFORMATION:

Asimov, Isaac. *The Human Body: Its Structure and Operation.* Rev. ed. New York: Penguin Books, 1992. Asimov offers an easy-to-understand overview of all the body's organ functions.

Guyton, Arthur C., and John E. Hall. *Human Physiology and Mechanisms of Disease.* 6th ed. Philadelphia: W. B. Saunders, 1997. This physiology text deals with the function of the body in considerable detail. Excellent advanced reading for the physiology student.

Kittredge, Mary. *The Human Body: An Overview.* Reprint. Philadelphia: Chelsea House, 2003. This text explains the general workings of the human body. Provides background to the historical development of medical knowledge and addresses many of the pathologies that can arise in the body.

Page, Martyn, ed. *Human Body: An Illustrated Guide to Every Part of the Human Body and How It Works.* New York: DK, 2009. The first part of the book covers basic human anatomy with full color illustrations, explaining how each individual body system functions. The second part covers diseases and disorders.

Parsons, Jayne, ed. *Encyclopedia of the Human Body.* New York: DK, 2004. A beautifully illustrated and accessible guide to the human body designed for children and teens, covering anatomical concepts, disease mechanisms, and the history of medicine and its pioneers.

Thibodeau, Gary A., and Kevin T. Patton. *The Human Body in Health and Disease.* 4th ed. St. Louis, Mo.: Mosby/Elsevier, 2005. Examines the mechanisms of the human body by examining each system in detail.

TAPEWORMS
DISEASE/DISORDER

ANATOMY OR SYSTEM AFFECTED: Gastrointestinal system, intestines

SPECIALTIES AND RELATED FIELDS: Gastroenterology, public health

DEFINITION: Flatworms of the phylum Platyhelminthes and class Cestoda that are parasitic in the digestive tract of humans and other animals.

CAUSES AND SYMPTOMS

Humans are the definitive hosts for several tapeworm species. Infection is usually caused by ingestion of undercooked muscle tissue with encysted larvae. The larvae attach to the upper part of the small intestine and mature into adults. Adult tapeworms are hermaphrodites, having both male and female reproductive organs, and a single tapeworm can produce millions of eggs during its normal life span of up to twenty-five years. The eggs pass out through the feces and are ingested by intermediate hosts. Larvae emerge from the eggs, invade the muscle tissue of the intermediate host, and form cystlike structures called cysticerci. When an intermediate host's muscle tissue containing cysticerci is eaten by humans, the life cycle continues. Most tapeworm infestations are asymptomatic or cause only minor gastric distress.

The beef tapeworm, *Taenia saginata*, infects humans when undercooked beef containing cysticerci is eaten; it is the most common human tapeworm worldwide. *T. solium*, the pork tapeworm, although less common, is more serious. When humans ingest the cysticerci, an infection much like the one caused by the beef tapeworm usually occurs. However, when humans ingest *T. solium* eggs, larvae emerge that can burrow into human muscle and connective tissue and form cysticerci. They can cause major problems, especially when the cysticerci form in the brain or eyes. Seizures, severe headaches, and loss of consciousness can result from neurocysticercosis, while ocular cysticercosis can lead to many visual problems.

Diphyllobothrium latum is a tapeworm with two intermediate hosts. Eggs hatch into larvae that are ingested by copepods, which are themselves eaten by fish that may in turn be eaten by larger fish. The larvae become encysted in the fish muscle. Humans are infected when they ingest the undercooked fish. In this infection, vitamin B_{12} deficiency and associated me-

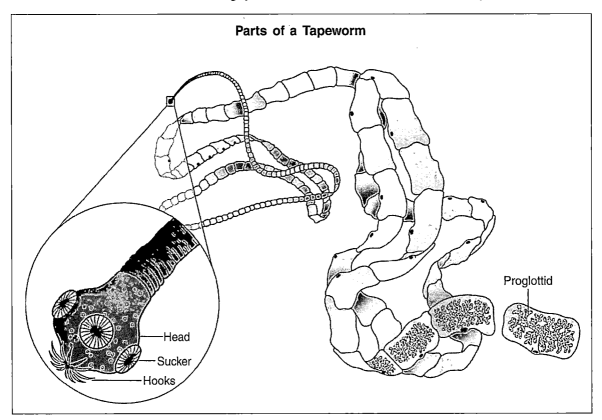

Parts of a Tapeworm

Head
Sucker
Hooks

Proglottid

galoblastic anemia can occur as the worm competes with the host for vitamin B_{12}.

The dwarf tapeworm, *Hymenolepis nana*, normally uses mice as the definitive host and grain beetles as the intermediate host. Unlike all other tapeworms, however, it can go through its entire life cycle in a single host. Humans, especially children, ingest *H. nana* eggs from contaminated soil. The eggs mature into larvae, which then mature into adults that attach to the intestinal wall.

TREATMENT AND THERAPY

T. saginata, *T. solium*, and *D. latum* are usually treated by a single 5 to 10 milligram per kilogram dose of praziquantel. Alternatively, niclosamide and albendazole can be used. The preferred treatment for *H. nana* is a single 25 milligram per kilogram dose of praziquantel. Good personal hygiene, proper waste handling, and effective sewage treatment can break the cycle of infection. In addition, meat and fish from areas where these tapeworms are endemic should be cooked thoroughly.

—*Richard W. Cheney, Jr., Ph.D.*

See also Food poisoning; Insect-borne diseases; Intestinal disorders; Intestines; Parasitic diseases; Worms; Zoonoses.

FOR FURTHER INFORMATION:

Icon Health. *Tapeworms: A Medical Dictionary, Bibliography, and Annotated Research Guide to Internet References*. San Diego, Calif.: Author, 2004.

Kearn, G. C. *Parasitism and the Platyhelminths*. New York: Springer, 1997.

Roberts, Larry S., and John Janovy, Jr., eds. *Gerald D. Schmidt and Larry S. Roberts' Foundations of Parasitology*. 7th ed. Boston: McGraw-Hill Higher Education, 2005.

TASTE
BIOLOGY

ANATOMY OR SYSTEM AFFECTED: Gastrointestinal system, mouth, nervous system, nose

SPECIALTIES AND RELATED FIELDS: Gastroenterology, neurology, nutrition, otorhinolaryngology

DEFINITION: One of the five special senses; chemicals interact with receptor sites in specialized structures of the tongue, and the resulting nerve impulses are classified as certain kinds of taste.

KEY TERMS:

chemoreceptors: specific structures upon which tastant molecules (chemicals that cause a taste sensation on the tongue) adhere; it is presumed that taste receptors have some structural uniqueness because sweet, salty, sour, and bitter can be distinguished there

facial nerve: the seventh cranial nerve pair, which relays signals from the face and the front region of the tongue up to the pons of the brain stem; conducts impulses related to taste, salivation, and facial expression

filiform papillae: the small, rounded projections that form the tough, yet velvetlike, texture of the tongue surface; lacking any chemoreceptors, these papillae do not function in taste

foliate papillae: the folded papillae found on the soft edges of the rear of the tongue and just ahead of the V shape formed by the vallate papillae; although found in the regions that detect bitter or sour tastes, foliate papillae are not specific receptors for bitter or sour tastes

fungiform papillae: the papillae scattered about the tongue surface, in no specific array, that are responsive to tastant molecules; these do not exhibit specificity for a particular type of taste

glossopharyngeal nerve: the ninth cranial nerve, which relays signals pertaining to or controlling salivation; sends neurological information to and from the posterior region of the tongue to the medulla oblongata of the brain stem

gustation: the ability to taste, which is independent of smell (olfaction) or textural and temperature enhancements; ageusia, or apogeusia, is the loss of taste sensation

gustatory stimulation threshold: the minimal quantity of tastant molecules that must be present in a water or saliva solution for a neural response at the taste cell to be initiated and the correct taste perceived; below this threshold, taste is either absent or identified incorrectly

taste bud: a special sensing structure for taste found on taste-responsive papillae; taste buds are made of three cell types—gustatory or taste cells, supporting cells, and basal cells

taste cell: the cellular compartment of a taste bud that contains chemoreceptors; taste hairs, one type of chemoreceptor, are found at the taste pore, or entry point, of a taste cell

vagus nerve: the tenth cranial nerve, which carries taste messages from the limited number of taste buds located in obscure sites such as the palate, epiglottis, uvula, and other structures at the entrance of the esophagus; also sends important information from the thoracic and abdominal viscera to the brain

vallate papillae: the seven to ten papillae mounds, arranged in a V shape, which can be seen when the tongue is fully extended; these taste sensors lack taste specificity

STRUCTURE AND FUNCTIONS

For many people, the thought of biting into a lemon causes a puckering or a tingling sensation in the mouth. A real taste sensation is evoked even though the actual taste stimulus, a lemon, is absent. This kind of response indicates the power of the sense of taste. Taste is also called the gustatory sense, a term derived from the Latin word *gustatus*, meaning taste. This sense evolved to aid animals in the selection of safe, nontoxic foods. Although loss of the ability to experience taste (apogeusia) is not a life-threatening condition, it may indicate the presence of other maladies, some of which are life-threatening. A diminished or absent ability to taste may account for loss of appetite or weight loss in some ill persons; for these persons, sufficient and proper nutrition can become a critical issue.

There are five special senses of the human body: gustation, olfaction (smell), vision, hearing, and equilibrium. The organs associated with the special senses take in information from the environment in the form of chemical, light, sound, or mechanical energy and convert that energy into nerve impulses. Nerve impulses are tiny electrical signals that are carried by the peripheral and central nervous systems to the brain, where the information is integrated in order to assess how dangerous or secure an individual may be in any given environment. Taste is a primitive sense, meaning that it need not be taught; it evokes instinctual responses or reactions.

Although taste is not as essential to survival as the sense of vision, it is an important sense for a variety of organisms. Taste preferences can be observed in humans, elephants, monkeys, fish, and even some microorganisms. Yet not all organisms respond equally to the same tastant; one example is sugar. Cats lack taste receptors for sugar; therefore, if a cat eats a sweet food, it does so for other flavors. Just as a cat does not taste sweetness, however, a human might not notice a tastant that a cat recognizes. A tastant is any food or chemical (such as soap) that causes a taste sensation.

Taste is a nerve impulse that is interpreted by the brain. (In organisms lacking a brain, taste is interpreted by some other structure that serves as the center of integration and coordination.) For humans, and for many of the larger land animals, taste sensations begin upon the intake of food or other substances into the mouth. This signal is prompted by the interaction of tastant molecules or ions and chemoreceptors located in specialized regions within taste buds.

Composed mostly of muscle fiber, the tongue not only serves as a receptor site for taste stimuli but also is responsible for the refined and coordinated movements that produce speech—an important form of communication in the human species. Different sections of the tongue are in contact with specific nerves that allow coordinated and specialized movements of the tongue. The palatine section of the tongue is easily seen when the tongue is fully extended from the mouth; it constitutes the front two-thirds of the tongue. The back one-third is the pharyngeal section; the palatine and pharyngeal sections are visibly, but subtly, separated by a transverse groove.

The surface of the palatine section of the tongue is coated with small, closely spaced projections called papillae. These structures give the tongue the dual properties of being rough and textured while remaining velvety smooth. Papillae are arranged, from the tongue's tip to the back, in more or less parallel rows that run along the medial groove of the tongue. The medial groove divides the tongue lengthwise into equal halves that are independently coordinated by nerves and muscle working together.

Most papillae covering the tongue are of the filiform type. Unlike the other three papillae forms, filiform papillae do not contain taste buds and thus are not responsive to tastants. Instead, filiform papillae aid in the tearing and grating of food particles. Although filiform papillae are not barbed, they do have a rasping mechanical action that aids in cleansing the body through licking (as observed in cats) and moving food particles about in the mouth.

All other papillae—the fungiform, the foliate, and the vallate—are actively involved in tasting, even though they are not present in great abundance or distributed uniformly over the tongue surface. Fungiform papillae, whose projections are shaped like a mushroom cap, are widely scattered on the tip and lateral sides of the tongue. Foliate papillae mimic the texture and appearance of smooth, folded leaves; they are located on both sides of the tongue, flanking the vallate papillae. The vallate papillae make a semicircular pattern (or a V shape) at the back of the tongue. Located on the palatine region just before the pharyngeal segment of the mouth, vallate papillae resemble rounded, soft cushions. Humans have between seven and twelve of these projections, making the vallate papillae the least abundant form of papillae.

Four tastes have commonly been recognized by humans: sweet, salty, sour, and bitter. These tastes are strongly registered in specific zones of the tongue. Much to the frustration of scientists, however, the recognition of taste is not specific to any particular type of taste-responsive papillae (fungiform, foliate, or vallate). Sweet receptors are plentiful at the tip of the tongue, while salty receptors are grouped together on

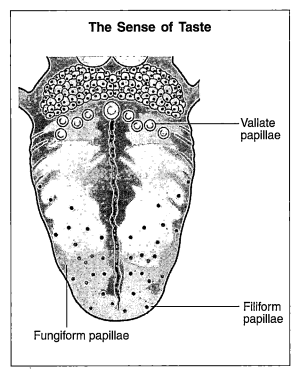

The Sense of Taste

Vallate papillae

Filiform papillae

Fungiform papillae

Special receptors on the tongue send nerve impulses to the brain that are registered as various tastes, such as bitter, sweet, salty, and sour.

either side just beyond the tip. Sour sensations are detected more strongly along the middle sides of the tongue, and bitter sensations are detected at the rear.

Since the vallate papillae are located in the region where only bitterness is tasted and the fungiform papillae are located in the regions sensitive to sweetness, one may assume that a match between papillae structure and taste type exists. Scientific studies, however, prove this to be a false correlation. A simple relationship between kind of taste and type of papillae does not exist, nor is there a complete explanation of the anatomy and physiology of the gustatory sense.

Taste-responsive papillae seem to respond to all tastants that enter their taste buds, whether they are classified as sweet, salty, sour, or bitter. The distinguishing factor seems to be a variation in the intensity of the neural message that a tastant induces. The variable levels of nervous impulses caused by a tastant constitute what is called a taste profile. Taste profiles are mixed neural codes that a taste bud receives from certain tastants.

A tastant molecule causes a nervous impulse to be sent to the brain for interpretation. It has been learned that all three taste-sensitive papillae are fired, to a greater or lesser extent, by all tastant molecules. A neural response is triggered when tastant molecules arrive at specialized sites on the taste buds. Then there is a certain ratio, or firing pattern, that is interpreted as sweet, salty, sour, or bitter. Oddly, this kind of mixed signal can be misread in the brain. For example, if a sweet solution of table sugar and water (tasted and properly identified as sweet) is greatly diluted with very pure water, the sugar solution may be erroneously classified in the brain as salty. The taste sensation is simply able to recognize when something has interacted with a taste chemoreceptor; a weak stimulus may cause a misinterpretation to occur.

For decades, researchers have been on the trail of an elusive fifth taste. While salty, bitter, sour, and sweet were all well-defined tastes, scientists have long suspected the presence of a fifth taste, called umami. Umami is known more familiarly as the flavor enhancer monosodium glutamate (MSG). In the late 1990's, scientists at the University of Miami School of Medicine found compelling evidence of umami. Molecular biologists there demonstrated that a modified form of a brain glutamate, mGluR4, is a taste receptor for umami. Because its receptor was identified, many researchers now recognize umami as the fifth taste. Umami is difficult to describe, but foods such as Parmesan cheese, steak, seafood, mushrooms, and tomato juice have an umami component to them, though it is generally mixed in with other tastes as well.

Taste buds are relatively large, bulbous-shaped structures located on the tips of fungiform papillae and in the grooves of the foliate and vallate papillae. It is within the taste bud structure that sweet, salty, sour, or bitter begin the journey of becoming distinguished taste sensations. A taste bud is not a wholly sensing bundle; it can be divided into at least three distinct parts—taste (or sensing) cells, support cells, and basal cells.

The number of taste buds in humans ranges from two thousand to nine thousand. About half of these are located in the grooved edges of the vallate papillae, making this a very sensitive taste area of the tongue. Taste buds are abundant in infants and children, but a continuous decline is observed from adolescence throughout adulthood. This explains why adults often like to add rich sauces, gravies, and seasonings to foods; adults need to enhance food so that a greater range of taste sensations is triggered in each mouthful. Children tend to shun sauces and spices because they may experience almost overwhelming taste sensations when they consume adult-prepared foods. In the elderly, low numbers of taste cells can contribute to poor eating habits or food selection, putting them at risk during the most vulnerable stage in adult life. It is often recommended that foods be made readily available and prepared in colorful and aromatically pleasing ways to entice the elderly to eat properly.

Tastant particles must dissolve in saliva in order to cause a taste response that can be identified properly. The minimum amount of tastant that must be present for it to be identified correctly is called the gustatory stimulation threshold. The requirement that a tastant be soluble in saliva is particularly true of sweet molecules (sugars and carbohydrates) or sour and some salty ions (salts and acids can release charged groups of atoms called ions when dissolved in saliva). Bitter substances seem to adhere to lipid sites on the papillae, and thus could be thought of as fat-soluble molecules. Sweet, salty, and sour chemicals are generally hydrophilic (water-loving), while bitter chemicals tend to be hydrophobic (water-hating).

Whether hydrophilic or hydrophobic, tastant molecules or ions must get through the entry point on at least some taste cells located on taste buds. At the entry point of a taste cell, a tiny pore has small taste hair projections that are believed to be the true sensors of taste.

The basic premise, according to current theory, is that the ions or molecules of the tastant substance enter the pore and then physically or chemically interact with specialized regions of the taste hairs. This interaction causes an action potential (a nerve impulse) to occur as the permeability of the nerve fibers innervating the taste cell is altered. An action potential will cause a wave of permeability changes all the way up the nerve fibers and into the brain. The medulla oblongata is the first site of the brain to receive the action potentials that will be registered as taste.

The exposure of taste cells to the environment renders them at risk to potential damage. Fortunately, new taste cells are regenerated every seven to ten days; regeneration occurs within the basal cells of the taste buds. It is important to note, however, that this is a regeneration of the taste cells, not of the nerves that innervate them. Olfactory nerves are the only nerve cells in the human body that can regenerate.

DISORDERS AND DISEASES

In the medical sciences, gustatory problems are generally not a cause but an effect. A diminished sense of taste (hypogeusia), an alteration of taste (dysgeusia), or the complete absence of the sense of taste (ageusia, or apogeusia) is generally a symptom of an underlying pathology. It is rare for true apogeusia to be an isolated symptom of a malady; it is even rarer for true apogeusia to exist as an isolated physical malady. Yet apogeusia does, in fact, exist in human populations. Among some descendants of the Ashkenazi Jews, for example, a double recessive genetic code mandates that taste papillae will not develop, resulting in congenital apogeusia.

In discussing when or how noncongenital apogeusia, hypogeusia, or dysgeusia can become a problem, it is important to review the critical components of a taste message. Three discrete structures are involved: taste cells, which contain taste hairs at their pores; nerve fibers, which connect the chemoreceptors (taste hairs) to the brain; and the brain itself. Alterations in the ability to taste can originate in any or all three of these discrete steps along the path.

Some pathologies that can cause a miscommunication at the receptor sites include actual physical or chemical damage to the taste buds, such as a burn that covers the tongue's surface or the ingestion of lye; accidental or therapeutic exposure to radiation; lingual (tongue) or palatal (palate) carcinomas; tumors or lesions of the tongue surface; or a leukemic infiltrate of the tongue surface.

The ability to taste may be altered or lost if damage occurs to certain cranial nerves. Specifically, damage to any of these cranial nerves may be responsible for taste disorders: the facial nerve (the seventh cranial nerve), which carries sweet and salty messages from the front of the tongue; the glossopharyngeal nerve (the ninth cranial nerve), which carries bitter and sour signals; and the large vagus nerve (the tenth cranial nerve), which carries taste sensations from the throat and epiglottis. Damage to these nerves may occur if they are crushed, severed, or pinched or if tumors, lesions, or neural disease interferes with normal function.

Finally, a head injury or malady can account for apogeusia, hypogeusia, or dysgeusia. Regions of particular concern include damage to the medulla oblongata, the thalamus, or the gustatory cortex, which is located in the parietal lobe of the brain. Lesions, tumors, or head injuries resulting from sudden or severe impact can give rise to true taste pathology. In these cases, the brain can either no longer identify tastes properly or no longer receive or interpret taste impulses.

Indirect impairment of taste may occur as a result of an imbalance in body chemistry. Such imbalances may result from exposure to or ingestion of trace metal poisons or other toxins, insufficient dietary intake to allow for cellular repair or development, incomplete intake of essential vitamins or minerals, or metabolic imbalances, such as hypothyroidism (an underactive thyroid gland). In addition, taste-modifying pathologies, whose origins are not directly associated at the chemoreceptor sites, can involve allergic or drug reactions.

Other taste disorders that can be clinically assessed include cacogeusia, the alteration of once-pleasant tastes to ones that are repulsive (for example, the perception that all foods taste rotten); phantogeusia, the presence of a taste sensation in the absence of any tastant; heterogeusia, a distortion of tastes for all foods (for example, sweets may taste salty, salts may taste bitter, and so on); and parageusia, an unusual taste distortion of one taste type that does not cause a repulsive taste response (for example, bitter foods may taste salty).

In diagnosing a taste disorder, the physician must first obtain a full medical history from the patient and perform a physical examination. Because of the anatomy involved in taste function, special attention will be given to the head and neck area. General laboratory analysis of kidney, liver, and endocrine function must be performed, as well as a complete blood study. Also, tests may be administered to determine the possible role of allergies in a given pathology.

The issue of taste disorder is often complicated by the common use of terms that have specific meaning in a clinical setting. Three of these troublesome terms are "taste," "flavor," and "palatability." Taste means, quite literally, the chemoreceptor response of taste cells embedded in taste buds (located on the papillae), which is caused by tastant molecules. The interaction between the tastant and the chemoreceptors produces a nerve signal that travels from the taste receptor site to the brain. In stringent use of the term "taste," other factors, such as aroma, texture, or color, should not be considered in the assessment of this sense.

Flavor generally means the response of the olfactory and gustatory systems, working in unison, to assess the pleasure or displeasure prompted by a tastant. Smell is fundamentally integrated with taste to the point that people generally salivate more when exposed to an appealing odor, especially if the aroma is associated with a particularly pleasing food, such as freshly baked bread. A common exercise used to demonstrate the close connection between the olfactory and gustatory systems is a blind study in which the subjects close their eyes, pinch their noses shut, and sample uniformly sized cubes of solid foods kept at room temperature. Under such circumstances, most humans cannot distinguish among raw potato, raw onion, white cheese, and peeled fresh apple. Taste-testers may be shocked to discover that raw onions seem much the same as raw apples without visual or aromatic cues. This exercise speaks strongly to the significance of how humans integrate all of their senses in gathering data from the environment.

A loss or a decrease in the ability to smell greatly alters one's sense of flavor, even though there is no true loss of the ability to experience taste. A common example of this interrelationship between ability to smell foods or beverages and the connected ability to enjoy flavor has been experienced at first hand by anyone who has ever suffered from a severe head cold. When the nasal passages are coated with thick mucus, as generally occurs during a viral cold, eating is no longer pleasurable; foods are generally described as tasting flat or bland. The cold virus does not in any way interrupt the mechanics of the taste cells, nor does it disrupt the neurons associated with the taste cells. What is disrupted during a cold is the ability to smell and, therefore, enjoy the flavor of foods and beverages. Thus, a head cold alters the ability to experience fully all the sensory aspects of the foods or beverages that create a complete food sensation.

Palatability describes the association of taste with texture, temperature, and feeling. If a slice of bread is expected to be warm, soft, and sweet but what is ingested is cold, hard, and salty, then palatability is greatly diminished. If a person is truly hungry, however, then the lack of palatability, or even flavor, may be overruled by the greater need for nourishment. In the absence of the ability to see or to smell food (as in blindness or anosmia, respectively), texture and temperature take on heightened importance in the consumption of foods and beverages.

Taste disorders can be quantitatively assessed through various stimuli tests to measure the extent and type of taste disorder present. In addition, magnetic resonance imaging (MRI) and computed tomography (CT) scanning can be used to identify problems that may originate in the central nervous system. Positron emission tomography (PET) scanning can also be used to determine if brain lesions are responsible for a taste disorder. Treatments are as highly varied as the pathologies that cause taste disorders. Those disorders that arise from tumors may be treated by the surgical removal of the tumor. For certain metabolic imbalances, supplements rich in zinc ions may be administered. Some cases require simply restoring the patient to a healthy and balanced diet, while some rare disorders are untreatable.

PERSPECTIVE AND PROSPECTS

Tasting is an inborn sense; it requires no training or skills. So-called acquired tastes are attained by adults mainly as a result of the declining population of taste cells, a natural aspect of the aging process. Because adults cannot sense food as fully as children, they may seek out heightened taste sensations, consuming salty foods such as caviar, drinking strong beverages such as whiskey, or enjoying spicy foods such as curry or hot peppers. Given their divergent taste responsiveness, it is reasonable to expect children to have natural aversions to certain foods, as compared to adults. A child is simply more aware of the mixed flavors of a given food, some of which may be bitter or sour relative to the way in which an adult senses the same food.

Like their primitive ancestors, modern humans let the tip of the tongue sample a new food before actually ingesting it. It is believed, therefore, that sweet receptors evolved to occupy the tip of the tongue to help humans seek out and consume safe foods in nature. Sweet foods, such as carbohydrate-rich vegetables, fruits, and (to some extent) proteins, are generally safe and nour-

ishing. Therefore, humans tend to seek sweet flavors, especially in the infant stages, over salty, sour, or bitter ones. This instinctual drive may account for the powerful attraction many people have for sweet desserts and candies.

Bitterness is detected in the mouth nearer the esophagus. This location seems to prevent humans from naturally seeking bitter foods. Furthermore, it allows for the rejection of a bitter food before it enters the esophagus, where the food would be well on its way to digestion and absorption. This adaptation to the environment aids in human survival. Many naturally bitter substances are poisons or potential toxins. Included in the list of bitter taste sources are caffeine-containing tea leaves and coffee beans, cocaine, nicotine, almond bitters, and lye (sodium hydroxide). At the turn of the twenty-first century, scientists identified a new family of genes that encode proteins that function as bitter taste receptors. The discovery opens the way for the identification of additional receptors that detect bitter and sweet tastes and also gives researchers new probes with which to trace the wiring of the taste perception pathways into the brain itself.

In 2002, scientists reported the discovery of a new taste receptor that recognizes most of the twenty naturally occurring amino acids. They theorize that this receptor was evolutionary important because it helps humans select foods rich in these essential nutrients.

Taste is a special sense that facilitates the ability of an organism to survive in or interact with an environment. More than this, however, taste provides the body with great sensory pleasure. Serving as both a tool to survive and as a pleasure-seeking sensor, taste is a unique and enriching sense.

—*Mary C. Fields, M.D.*

See also Aging; Appetite loss; Digestion; Food biochemistry; Food poisoning; Malnutrition; Nervous system; Nutrition; Otorhinolaryngology; Poisoning; Sense organs; Smell; Toxicology.

FOR FURTHER INFORMATION:

Atkins, Peter. *Atkins' Molecules.* 2d ed. New York: Cambridge University Press, 2003. A truly entertaining book supported by pleasing photographs and sketches of some of nature's most intriguing molecules.

Møller, Aage R. *Sensory Systems: Anatomy, Physiology, and Pathophysiology.* Boston: Academic Press, 2003. An excellent text that describes how human sensory systems function, with comparisons of the five senses and detailed descriptions of the functions of each of them. Also covers how sensory information is processed in the brain to provide the basis for communication and for the perception of one's surroundings.

Schmidt, Robert F., ed. *Fundamentals of Sensory Physiology.* Translated by Marguerite A. Biedermann-Thorson. Rev. 3d ed. Berlin: Springer, 1986. A succinct treatment of the anatomy and physiology of taste is provided in chapter 8, "Physiology of Taste."

Shier, David N., Jackie L. Butler, and Ricki Lewis. *Hole's Essentials of Human Anatomy and Physiology.* 10th ed. Boston: McGraw-Hill, 2009. An academic textbook that goes into greater detail about the human body than an introductory biology book. One chapter covers the somatic and special senses and has a section devoted exclusively to the sense of taste.

Tortora, Gerard J., and Bryan Derrickson. *Principles of Anatomy and Physiology.* 12th ed. Hoboken, N.J.: John Wiley & Sons, 2009. This text offers a brief treatment of the structure of taste cells and the stimulation of receptors.

Wolfe, Jeremy M., et al. *Sensation and Perception.* 2d ed. Sunderland, Mass.: Sinauer, 2009. Addresses all five senses. Includes a detailed section on taste.

TATTOO REMOVAL

PROCEDURE

ANATOMY OR SYSTEM AFFECTED: Skin

SPECIALTIES AND RELATED FIELDS: Dermatology, general surgery

DEFINITION: The use of lasers to break up tattoo ink under the skin.

INDICATIONS AND PROCEDURES

Application of a tattoo is relatively easy, although the process is painful. A design is drawn on the skin. Needles are used to push the ink down into the skin. When the skin heals from the multiple punctures, the design remains permanently in place. Attempts have been made to remove tattoos since the first one was applied. Scrubbing with sandpaper or table salt has been tried to scour the surface of the skin and remove the tattoo. The results have usually been disfigurement or scarring.

Currently, light therapy is the most effective way of removing unwanted tattoos. The Food and Drug Administration (FDA) has approved two uses of light to remove tattoos. The first is the use of laser light. The laser emits a brief pulse of light at a specific wavelength—for example, the ruby laser emits red light—covering an area of skin roughly the size of a pencil eraser. The tattoo ink embedded in the skin absorbs the pulse of energy. The laser energy causes the tattoo ink to break up into fragments that can be removed by cells of the body's immune system. The treatment feels like a rubber band snapping against the skin, and local anesthetics may be necessary when attempting to remove large tattoos. Immediately after the laser treatment, the treated area turns white and might swell slightly; over the next few days, blisters and scabs may form. Within seven to ten days, the skin will look normal.

A second, newer, technique that uses light therapy to remove tattoos is called intense pulsed light (IPL), which works in the same manner as the laser. However, whereas lasers use only one wavelength of light, ISL uses a broad spectrum of wavelengths for each pulse, leading to more efficient tattoo removal; light is shone through a prism that is placed on the skin. Also, IPL is less painful than laser treatment, and it usually does not lead to blisters or scabbing.

USES AND COMPLICATIONS

The number of treatments required to remove a tattoo depends on several factors: the color of ink, the amount of ink, the depth of the tattoo, and the location of the tattoo.

Dark colors of ink—such as black, green, red, and blue—are the easiest to remove with laser and IPL therapies because they absorb the energy well. Yellow and fluorescent inks are the hardest to remove. Professional tattoos may require more treatments to remove than those applied by amateurs because professionals tend to use more ink and to apply the ink deeper into the skin. Ideally, treatments are spaced several weeks apart to allow the body's immune system to remove the maximum amount of ink between sessions; this time is also necessary to allow the skin to recover fully before the next treatment.

It is more problematic to remove tattoos from areas of the body with thin skin, such as the face, genitals, and ankles. In the case of tattoo removal, both laser and IPL treatments are designed to remove the unwanted buildup of abnormal pigment (ink) in the skin; however, people with dark skin have high amounts of natural pigment (melanin) in their skin. Sometimes, IPL and lasers cannot distinguish between tattoo ink pigment and normal skin pigment. As a result, both types of pigment are destroyed, leaving pale patches on the skin; these patches can fade with time. Conversely, an increase in pigmentation can be seen after treatment, causing dark patches on the skin; these patches can also fade with time. It is recommended that patients stay out of the sun before and after treatment for tattoo removal. Tattoo removal can lead to scarring, but with the modern laser and IPL methods, this is becoming rarer. The most striking side effect of laser and IPL tattoo removal is the cost, at least five to ten times higher than the cost of the original tattoo.

—*L. Fleming Fallon, Jr., M.D., Ph.D., M.P.H.*

See also Blisters; Dermatology; Healing; Laser use in surgery; Pigmentation; Skin; Skin disorders; Tattoos and body piercing.

FOR FURTHER INFORMATION:

Ahluwalia, Gurpreet S., ed. *Cosmetic Applications of Laser and Light-Based Systems*. Norwich, N.Y.: William Andrew, 2009.

Camphausen, Rufus C. *Return of the Tribal: A Celebration of Body Adornment—Piercing, Tattooing, Scarification, Body Painting*. Rochester, Vt.: Park Street Press, 1997.

Graves, Bonnie B. *Tattooing and Body Piercing*. Mankato, Minn.: LifeMatters, 2000.

Hewitt, Kim. *Mutilating the Body: Identity in Blood and Ink*. Bowling Green, Ohio: Bowling Green State University Popular Press, 1997.

Miller, Jean-Chris. *The Body Art Book: A Complete, Illustrated Guide to Tattoos, Piercings, and Other Body Modifications*. Rev. ed. New York: Berkley, 2004.

Wilkinson, Beth. *Coping with the Dangers of Tattooing, Body Piercing, and Branding*. New York: Rosen, 1998.

TATTOOS AND BODY PIERCING

PROCEDURE

ANATOMY OR SYSTEM AFFECTED: Muscles, skin

SPECIALTIES AND RELATED FIELDS: Dermatology, plastic surgery, public health

DEFINITION: Piercing of the skin to implant devices or make designs.

KEY TERMS:

dermis: the deepest skin layer

epidermis: the outer skin layer

mortification: self-induced physical pain

proof of ordeal: a painful surgical procedure that leaves a scar, design, or skin mutilation

tattooing: piercing of the skin with pigments or dyes

INDICATIONS AND PROCEDURES

Tattooing is accomplished by a variety of techniques, usually by persons who are specialists. Traditionally, a shaman or other religious practitioner would create a tattoo by piercing the skin with a sharpened object (such as a bone splinter or a piece of metal) or with a bundle of porcupine quills or ponderosa pine needles, or by passing a colored string on a needle through the skin. The colors were from mineral salts, charcoal, certain plant juices, and even the feces of dogs that had been fed charcoal.

Coloring inks were available from the end of the nineteenth century and are now supplied in liquid forms. They can be applied in either the so-called European fashion, in which the coloring ink is applied over a small surface and an electric vibrating needle impregnates the epidermis and the dermis, or the American procedure, in which the needle contains the desired pigment.

The skin is prepared in a variety of ways, usually by smearing a thin layer of petroleum jelly over the site to minimize the seepage of blood and tissue fluids that would otherwise obscure the artist's view. When the tattoo is completed, the area is washed and then covered with an antiseptic ointment. Tattoos assume various geometric or curvilinear designs and can be executed over all of a person's body or simply within a restricted area. Extensive tattooing may take several years to complete.

The most obvious forms of body piercing, by both males and females, are performed in the ears, nose, nasal septum, tongue, navel, lips, scalp, eyelids, or cheeks. In some cultures, the lips or ears may be grossly distorted by inserting over time increasingly larger objects, such as pieces of horn, bone, wood, and even metal. Some modern piercing use plastics as a temporary or permanent material. In some cases, the particular style of body piercing may indicate a person's marital status, group membership, or religious affiliation, or it may simply be cosmetic mutilation. Body piercing may also be performed on male or female genitals. The breasts, particularly the nipples, are a common site for the insertion of either closed or threaded rings. The Prince Albert penile ring, which is inserted into the top or either side of the glans, has become fashionable in Western cultures.

USES AND COMPLICATIONS

Tattoos and body piercing of the human body have been practiced by all cultures throughout the world to serve different functions: for religious purposes, as an indication of certain status changes or the accomplishment of culturally significant tasks, as a proof of ordeal, for medical reasons, as body art, as identification marks, to signify membership in either sacred or profane organizations, or to attain visions through mortification of the flesh. Depending on the culture or specific group, men, women, and children may undergo these frequently painful rituals. Various cultures believe that the soul's transition to a life hereafter is facilitated by having certain tattoos and body piercing. Often, the degree of pain experienced during the rituals of tattooing and body piercing, and from the subsequent wounds, not only is a proof of ordeal but also may serve as a physical and spiritual atonement for a person's moral transgressions. Certain groups, such as the Newar of Bhaktapur in Nepal, believe that they may gain a higher incarnation when they sell their tattoos in heaven.

In the United States during the early twentieth century, it became popular for women to be tattooed for eyeliner, cheek blush, and even colored lips. Although tattooing and body piercing were once associated with motorcycle gang members, prisoners, and military personnel, these surgical procedures have become more popular with the general public. Tattooing and self-mutilation by body piercing are gaining popularity as forms of personal expression, particularly with women, who make up approximately 70 percent of the new business.

A concern, however, is the increasing frequency of adolescents engaging in tattooing and body piercing. Today, body piercing in Western cultures is often viewed by teenagers and young adults as a rite of passage, sometimes symbolically in defiance of the established social order. When self-practiced, tattooing and body piercing can lead to infection and even septicemia, particularly when people use instruments and inks that are not sterile. In addition, there has been an increase in the incidence of blood-borne infections such as human immunodeficiency virus (HIV) and hepatitis B and C being transmitted through contaminated needles.

PERSPECTIVE AND PROSPECTS

Some anthropologists believe that the first documented examples of tattooing were practiced in Egypt approximately four thousand years ago. These conclusions are supported by tattooed female mummies and by clay figurines that have puncture "tattoos." Although there is not agreement among scholars, some believe that the practice of tattooing may have diffused from Egypt to other parts of the world.

Perhaps the most artistic and dramatic full-body tattooing was done by the Japanese as early as the fifth century B.C.E. and the Maori of New Zealand; even today, many young male Maori follow this traditional custom. The Maori were noted for facial tattoos, called *moko*, that served to frighten and intimidate their enemies. The word "tattoo," however, comes from the Tahitian word *ta-tau*; it was acquired by eighteenth and nineteenth century European explorers in Polynesia, who introduced tattoos to Europe and America.

A dramatic historical example of body piercing for religious purposes was part of the Sun Dance ritual of many Plains Indian tribes, in which male participants had hard wooden shafts surgically inserted in the pectoral or back muscles. Long thongs were attached to these poles. The participant would then drag heavy bison skulls or would pull away from a pole, causing tearing in the muscles.

—John Alan Ross, Ph.D.

See also Acquired immunodeficiency syndrome (AIDS); Dermatology; Dermatology, pediatric; Hepatitis; Plastic surgery; Puberty and adolescence; Skin; Skin disorders; Tattoo removal.

FOR FURTHER INFORMATION:

Brown, Kelli McCormack, Paula Perlmutter, and Robert J. McDermott. "Youth and Tattoos: What School Health Personnel Should Know." *Journal of School Health* 70, no. 9 (November, 2000): 355-360. Though tattooing has been practiced by various cultures for centuries, this art form has undergone dramatic changes in the past few decades. Today tattoos appeal to diverse populations and mainstream culture.

DeMello, Margo. *Bodies of Inscription: A Cultural History of the Modern Tattoo Community.* Durham, N.C.: Duke University Press, 2000. Although academic, this book has much to recommend it for general collections. DeMello's major interest is in describing the new community of tattooed people, both men and women, for whom new meanings are being forged from the meeting of skin and ink.

Gard, Carolyn. "Think Before You Ink: The Risks of Body Piercing and Tattooing." *Current Health* 25, no. 6 (February, 1999): 24-25. Tattoos and body piercing are popular, but teens should consider the risks associated with these trends. Tattoo dyes can cause allergic reactions.

Gay, Kathlyn, and Christine Whittington. *Body Marks: Tattooing, Piercing, and Scarification.* Brookfield, Conn.: Millbrook Press, 2002. A book for young adults that traces the history of body marking and discusses issues to consider before getting a tattoo or body piercing.

Gilbert, Steve. *The Tattoo History: A Source Book.* New York: Juno Books, 2000. Traces the history of tattooing from diverse eras and cultures from ancient Polynesia to the modern-day punk music scene.

Shields, Sherice L. "Popular Piercing Opens Possibility of Serious Illness." *USA Today,* July, 19, 2000, p. D9. Experts may worry about the health risks associated with body piercing, but lawmakers have focused on the age of consent. The National Conference of State Legislatures says few states enforce health regulations, but twenty-three states have laws regarding piercing minors.

"Support for Body Piercing Checks." *Nursing Standard* 14, no. 30 (April 12-18, 2000): 8. Body piercing outlets should be strictly regulated because piercing can cause blood poisoning, hepatitis, and even death, according to a congress of professional nurses.

TAY-SACHS DISEASE
DISEASE/DISORDER
ANATOMY OR SYSTEM AFFECTED: Nervous system
SPECIALTIES AND RELATED FIELDS: Genetics, neonatology, neurology, pediatrics
DEFINITION: An inherited disorder in which products of fat metabolism (gangliosides) accumulate in and destroy the brain and spinal cord.

CAUSES AND SYMPTOMS
Tay-Sachs disease is a genetic disorder of lipid (fat) metabolism resulting from a missing enzyme. This enzyme normally breaks down special nerve lipids known as gangliosides, which are present in the brain and spinal cord. These substances accumulate and destroy the cells, killing the child by age three or four years.

INFORMATION ON TAY-SACHS DISEASE

CAUSES: Genetic disorder
SYMPTOMS: Initially, cherry-red spots on retina; in later stages, deafness, blindness, muscle paralysis, mental retardation, vegetative state
DURATION: Three or four years, until death
TREATMENTS: Supportive therapy only

Several features at birth may raise the possibility of early detection, particularly cherry-red spots on the retina of the eye. Most newborns with Tay-Sachs disease, however, appear normal at birth. Between the ages of three months and six months, the progressive neurologic damage becomes apparent: deafness, blindness, muscle paralysis, and mental retardation develop. By eighteen months, the infant is usually already in a vegetative state, requiring complete care. The child may survive until three or four years of age, dying from complications associated with comatose and bedridden patients, usually infections.

TREATMENT AND THERAPY
Tay-Sachs disease has no cure, and only supportive measures can be used. Feeding tubes for nutrition and fluids, suctioning of throat secretions, meticulous skin care for bed sores, and oxygen to assist breathing are among the types of support needed. Full-time skilled nursing care at home or at a facility is often necessary.

PERSPECTIVES AND PROSPECTS
While Tay-Sachs disease is the most common lipid (or lysosomal) storage disease, it is rare in the general population. It is nearly one hundred times more common, however, in people of Eastern European Jewish ancestry, occurring in one per 3,600 births. One person in thirty Ashkenazi (Eastern European) Jews is a carrier of the genetic defect. If two such carriers have children, they have a 25 percent chance of having a child with Tay-Sachs disease. Prenatal testing using amniocentesis or chorionic villus sampling can detect affected fetuses. More important is genetic counseling and screening of couples with a family history. A blood test can identify carriers.

Ongoing research is attempting to correct the disease in the developing fetus through the insertion of the missing gene.

—Connie Rizzo, M.D., Ph.D.

See also Amniocentesis; Chorionic villus sampling; Coma; Embryology; Enzymes; Gaucher's disease; Gene therapy; Genetic counseling; Genetic diseases; Genetics and inheritance; Lipids; Metabolic disorders; Metabolism; Neonatology; Niemann-Pick disease; Pediatrics; Screening.

FOR FURTHER INFORMATION:
Behrman, Richard E., Robert M. Kliegman, and Hal B. Jenson, eds. *Nelson Textbook of Pediatrics.* 18th ed. Philadelphia: Saunders/Elsevier, 2007.

Bellenir, Karen, ed. *Genetic Disorders Sourcebook: Basic Consumer Information About Hereditary Diseases and Disorders.* 3d ed. Detroit, Mich.: Omnigraphics, 2004.

Gormley, Myra Vanderpool. *Family Diseases: Are You at Risk?* Baltimore: Genealogical Publishing, 2002.

Harper, Peter S. *Practical Genetic Counselling.* 6th ed. New York: Oxford University Press, 2004.

McCance, Kathryn L., and Sue M. Huether. *Pathophysiology: The Biologic Basis for Disease in Adults and Children.* 6th ed. St. Louis, Mo.: Mosby/Elsevier, 2010.

Milunsky, Aubrey, ed. *Genetic Disorders of the Fetus: Diagnosis, Prevention, and Treatment.* 6th ed. Hoboken, N.J.: Wiley-Blackwell, 2009.

National Tay-Sachs and Allied Diseases Association. http://www.ntsad.org.

Parker, James N., and Philip M. Parker, eds. *The Official Parent's Sourcebook on Tay-Sachs Disease.* San Diego, Calif.: Icon Health, 2002.

Tears and tear ducts
Anatomy

Also known as: Lacrimal ducts, nasolacrimal ducts, tear film

Anatomy or system affected: Eyes, head, nose

Specialties and related fields: Ophthalmology, optometry

Definition: Fluid produced by the eye and the channel that carries it from the eye to the nasal cavity.

Key terms:

canaliculus: a small canal linking the upper and lower puncta to the lacrimal sac

cornea: the transparent front portion of the eye

fluorescein: a brightly colored dye used for diagnostic purposes

instill: to slowly put a liquid into the eye, drop by drop

lacrimal: pertaining to the secretion and conduction of tears

lysosyme: an enzyme found in body secretions that destroys bacteria by breaking down their walls

ophthalmologist: a medical doctor who specializes in the treatment of disorders of the eye

Structure and Functions

The lacrimal gland is located beneath the upper eyelid, on the outer edge of each eye, and its key function is to produce tears. Tears flow constantly across the conjunctiva, which is the front surface of the eye, in order to keep it clean and lubricated. Blinking spreads tears across the eye. This constant flushing of the eye surface also supplies oxygen and nutrients to the cornea. Tears provide an important barrier to infection as they contain the antibacterial enzyme lysosyme, which destroys microorganisms on the eye surface. As new tears are produced, old tears drain from the eye at its inner edge, called the canthus, by being drawn into two small holes, the upper and lower puncta, through capillary action. Tears flow through the canaliculus, entering the lacrimal sac, then to the tear duct, called the nasolacrimal duct, and at last into the nasal cavity. This is the reason that a surplus of tears results in a runny nose.

Tears or tear film is made up of three distinct layers: an outer oily layer to prevent drying, which is produced by the meibomion glands; a watery middle layer, which contains the oxygen and nutrients; and an inner mucous layer, produced by the conjunctival goblet cells, reducing the surface tension of the tears and allowing them to be spread evenly on the surface of the eye.

The body naturally produces tears in order to maintain and protect the eye, but in humans, tears are also produced in response to emotion in the form of crying. During a normal twenty-four-hour day, 0.75 to 1.1 grams of tears are secreted; however, this rate declines with age. Also, approximately 25 percent of tear secretion is lost to evaporation, dependent on the environment.

Disorders and Diseases

The most common disorder associated with tears is excessive tearing. This can occur for many reasons and may require evaluation by an ophthalmologist. An excessive amount of tears can be caused by infection, environmental irritants, glaucoma, certain medications, allergic reaction, eyestrain, dry eyes, foreign material in the eye, scratch on the surface of the eye, or other eyelid or eyelash disorders.

Dry eye, also described as "scratchy eye," can occur when too few tears are being produced or they are draining from the eye too rapidly or evaporating too quickly. Dry eye affects more than twelve million people in the United States. Often the treatment is to instill drops of artificial tears or lubricating gel and avoid excessively dry or warm rooms to prevent evaporation. If the cause of dry eye is that tears are draining too quickly, then a surgeon may modify the tear duct to slow or limit tear drainage.

Another common disorder associated with tear ducts is obstruction. If there is an obstruction of the tear duct (nasolacrimal duct), then tears are not able to drain easily into the nasal cavity. Blockage of the tear duct can occur in early childhood as a congenital blockage or later in life as a result of chronic infection or irritation. In order to test the tear duct for obstruction, a drop of fluorescein dye will be instilled into the lower lid and then the patient will be observed at regular intervals to determine if the dye has traveled through to the nasal cavity.

A congenital blockage occurs in 6 to 20 percent of infants when a membrane remains between the tear duct and nasal cavity. This results in the inability for the eye to drain, and the eye appears excessively watery or filled with mucus. Often the membrane will rupture spontaneously before one year of age, thus resolving the obstruction, but sometimes a probe will need to be inserted by an ophthalmologist.

Tear duct obstruction may cause an acute infection of the lacrimal sac, located at the upper, wider end of the nasolacrimal duct. This form of infection is called dacrocystitis, and patients normally have an overflowing of tears (epiphora) and a swollen painful mass over the area of the lacrimal sac. Dacrocystitis requires systemic antibiotics and sometimes drainage of the mass.

PERSPECTIVE AND PROSPECTS

Research is being conducted to determine if tears not only provide nutrients and moisture to the eye but also have diagnostic uses. Tears are created from blood that has been filtered; therefore, tears can provide medical clues as to things happening in the blood. Studies are being done to determine if biological changes in the eye and eye health can be measured through small variations in the level of inflammatory proteins found in tears. Also, in 2000, a group of contact lens researchers in Australia found that tears contain protein markers that may be used to detect certain types of cancer. Research is continuing in this area in the hope that tears may provide useful information in future diagnoses.

—*April D. Ingram*

See also Eye infections and disorders; Eyes; Glands; Host-defense mechanisms; Ophthalmology; Sense organs; Sjögren's syndrome; Vision; Vision disorders.

FOR FURTHER INFORMATION:

Cohen, Adam, Michael Mercandetti, and Brian Brazzo, eds. *The Lacrimal System: Diagnosis, Management, and Surgery.* New York: Springer, 2006. This book explores the anatomy, diagnosis, and management of a wide range of lacrimal disorders. It includes basic examination skills and an overview of the anatomy.

Sullivan, David, Darlene Dartt, and Michele Meneray, eds. *Lacrimal Gland, Tear Film, and Dry Eye Syndromes 2: Basic Science and Clinical Relevance.* New York: Plenum Press, 1998. This book contains proceedings, abstracts, and papers from the Second International Conference on the Lacrimal Gland, Tear Film, and Dry Eye Syndromes.

Van Haeringen, N. J. "Aging and the Lacrimal System." *British Journal of Ophthalmology* 81 (1997): 824-826. This article explains changes observed in tear production with age and how these changes are associated with medications, eye structure, and other morphology.

TEETH

ANATOMY

ANATOMY OR SYSTEM AFFECTED: Bones, brain, gastrointestinal system, gums, heart, musculoskeletal system, nervous system

SPECIALTIES AND RELATED FIELDS: Dentistry, orthodontics

DEFINITION: Structures that aid animals in processing food prior to swallowing, bringing food into the mouth and grinding; they may also be used for defense, the killing of prey, and displays of either hostility or pleasure.

KEY TERMS:

cementum: the outer covering of the root of a tooth

crown: the portion of the tooth, normally covered with enamel, that is exposed in the oral cavity above the gingiva (gums)

cusp: the conical projection of the chewing surface of the tooth

cuspid: the longest anterior tooth; also called the canine tooth or the eyetooth

dentin: the substance that composes the major portion of the tooth internally

enamel: the tissue that covers the crown of the tooth; the hardest tissue in the body

gingiva: the gum tissue surrounding the neck of the tooth

incisor: one of the front teeth, used primarily to cut or shear food with a scissoring motion

molars: the back teeth used to grind food into smaller portions prior to swallowing

periodontium: those tissues supporting the tooth in the jaws, including the gingiva, the jawbone, and the periodontal ligament that attaches the root of the tooth into the jaw

premolars: the teeth between the cuspids and the molars, used in crushing and grinding food; also called bicuspids

pulp: the internal, living tissue of the tooth, consisting of nerves, blood vessels, and dental cells

root: the portion of the tooth that is below the crown and is embedded in a bony socket of the jaw

STRUCTURE AND FUNCTIONS

Teeth are functional portions of the mouths of animals that assist them in processing food prior to swallowing. This process is called chewing, or mastication. Teeth are also primary offensive and defensive weapons for most animals. Many animals have no hands to grasp or capture food, and their teeth become the principal means of grabbing and killing prey. In humans, teeth not only process food but also have a sociological significance in displaying anger, friendliness, and desirability.

A tooth is composed of three basic parts: the crown, the dental pulp, and the root. The crown of the tooth is that portion exposed above the gingiva, commonly called the gums. The outer surface of the crown is covered by a hard, crystalline substance called enamel. Enamel is an almost completely inorganic material, calcium hydroxyapatite, and it is the hardest tissue in the human body. Underneath the enamel, the bulk of the crown is made up of a substance known as dentin. It, too, is quite hard, but it has more organic material, ground substance and nerve fibers, within it. The dentin is honeycombed by small tubules radiating from the dental pulp chamber at the center of the tooth. These tubules carry nerve fibers from the central nerve within the pulp to the junction of the enamel and dentin.

In the center of the crown is the pulp chamber. The pulp contains nerves and blood vessels that give sensations to and nourish the tooth. These nerves and blood vessels enter at the tip of the root, the apex, and arise from nerve trunks and blood vessels that run through the jawbone.

The root is the portion of the tooth joining the crown to the jawbone. The outer surface of the root is covered by a thin layer of bonelike substance called cementum, and it runs from the junction of the enamel of the crown to the apex of the root. Under the cementum, dentin composes the bulk of the root, continuing from the crown to the apex. The root is attached from the cementum to the bony socket in the jaw by the periodontal ligament. This ligament is composed of elastic connective tissue fibers that act not only as part of the attachment apparatus for the tooth but also as a shock absorber

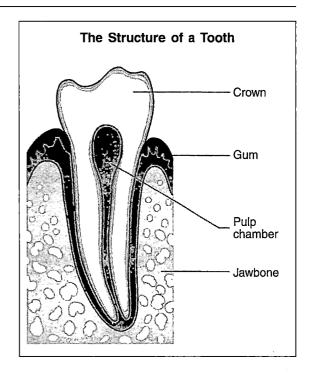

The Structure of a Tooth

Crown

Gum

Pulp chamber

Jawbone

from chewing forces. The pulp chamber narrows into a thin, constricted channel from the pulp chamber to the apex; this is known as the root canal. In some animals, such as rodents, the root canal of incisors remains relatively large throughout life and is called "evergrowing." In most animals, including humans, the root canal constricts to prevent further growth while still providing sufficient blood flow for proper tooth nourishment. These teeth are termed "rooted" (although all teeth are actually rooted). The tooth is surrounded by the tissues of the attachment apparatus called the periodontium, consisting of the gingiva, the periodontal ligament, and the alveolar bone of the jaws.

In humans, there are normally thirty-two adult teeth and twenty deciduous (or baby) teeth. Deciduous teeth start calcifying in the embryo at about five to six weeks of development. Teeth start to form from two types of cells at an interface in the tooth bud, which becomes the dentoenamel junction. The enamel is formed by a cell called an ameloblast, and the dentin is formed by a cell known as an odontoblast. The enamel grows outward and the dentin inward from the interface. The pulp is formed from nerves and blood vessels in the developing jawbone. While the crown is growing, the root starts to form, lengthening as the tooth develops. After the crown is formed, the ameloblast cells rest on the outer surface of the enamel, while the odontoblasts line the internal cavity of the pulp chamber.

When the tooth erupts through the gum tissue, the ameloblasts are compressed and destroyed. Enamel is one of the two tissues in the human body that cannot repair itself (the other being the cornea of the eye). The odontoblasts can be activated inside the pulp chamber to form a secondary or reparative dentin. This formation of insulating dentin is in response to aging, advancing tooth decay, or trauma to the tooth or in reaction to the placement of restorative materials into a tooth.

The deciduous teeth begin to erupt through the gums in infancy and continue to do so until the full complement of primary dentition has erupted. Most of the adult teeth develop below the baby teeth, and as they push on the roots of the primary teeth, these roots are resorbed from the pressure of erupting permanent crowns. The primary teeth are shed throughout childhood and into adolescence. Other animals have both primary and permanent teeth. Sharks continually develop full sets of teeth, sometimes as many as seven or eight at a time; as their teeth loosen or break off, new teeth replace them. Humans, however, possess only one set of permanent teeth, and they are not naturally replaced if they are lost through trauma or disease.

Mammals differ from all other animals in having teeth set in sockets (thecodont) and in having several different kinds of teeth (heterodont), compared to the homodont teeth of animals such as sharks and reptiles.

The shape and size of teeth are closely related to their functions. The four front incisor teeth, both upper and lower, are used to shear and cut food. The movement of the mobile lower jaw, the mandible, against the static upper jaw, the maxilla, causes these teeth to work as scissors on food. Horses crop grasses with their large incisors. Cusps are conical projections of the cuspids and posterior teeth. They act as crushing and grinding segments of the posterior teeth, reducing the food into smaller portions that may be swallowed and digested efficiently. The four cuspids, or canines, are conical and pointed. Their primary function is to grasp and tear food. The fangs of a tiger are cuspids, as are those of lions. The eight premolars have two conical cusps and are called bicuspid teeth. They too are used for tearing, but working against the opposing teeth, they also function as a mill, crushing and grinding the food.

The twelve molars are multicusped teeth that grind food into smaller portions; mixed with saliva, the food is then readied for swallowing. The grooves of the occlusal (chewing) surfaces act as sluiceways to channel the food in the oral cavity. The tongue folds the food back onto the surfaces of the grinding teeth until it is chewed sufficiently.

The third molars are commonly called wisdom teeth. These teeth are the last to develop and are more prone to irregular calcification and morphology. In the course of human evolution, the jaws have shortened, and the third molars often do not have enough room in the jaw to erupt in a normal, perpendicular mode. The result is an irregular angle of eruption. When the third molars lock and push against the second molars and are unable to erupt normally, the condition is called impaction. Thus, in many cases, the wisdom teeth must be removed.

Teeth and their supporting tissues are susceptible to disease. The primary disease of the tooth is dental caries, or tooth decay. Caries (cavities) begin with the decalcification of the enamel crystals by acids. These acids are products of bacteria caught in a sticky film that forms on the teeth called plaque. These bacteria use refined hydrocarbons, principally sugars, for their food. If the plaque is not removed from the surface of the teeth, the acids are kept close to the enamel. Over a period of time, the decalcification of the enamel reaches the internal dentin, and the acid begins to decay the less calcified enamel at a more rapid rate. The acids also can touch the nerve fibers within the dental tubules, causing sensitivity and pain. If this process is not stopped, the decay can penetrate into the pulp and cause infection.

When the pulp becomes infected, it invariably dies. The dead tissues gradually seep through the apex, and bacteria feed on the necrotic material. Inflammatory cells from the blood vessels in the bone try to fight the infection, which can cause swelling, pain, and pus. The result is a periapical abscess.

The periodontium is also susceptible to disease, and again, the bacterial plaque is the chief cause. Surrounding the neck of the tooth is a cuff of gum tissue. The bacteria in the plaque release their waste products into the cuff and irritate the lining. Inflammatory white cells, known as lymphocytes or chronic inflammatory cells, are brought from the blood vessels in the gum tissue to the point of irritation in order to attack the bacteria and their by-products. This disease is called gingivitis, which can be reversed by removing the dental plaque.

If the plaque is allowed to remain on the surface of the tooth, it may calcify into a hard, rough, and porous substance called dental calculus or, more commonly, tartar. This material attracts and entraps more bacteria, and it is abrasive to the soft lining of the gingiva. The gums become further inflamed, bringing more lymphocytes into the area. These cells try to attack the bacteria and dissolve the dead and dying cells of the diseased gingiva.

Over a period of time, the inflammatory cells move deeper into the periodontium, dissolving and detaching the elastic fibers of the periodontal ligament and eroding the crest of the bony socket. This inflammation of the periodontium is called periodontitis. With the destruction of the fibers attaching the gingiva and bone to the root, the cuff of gum tissue deepens into a pocket around the neck of the tooth. The depth of the pocket facilitates the further entrapment of bacteria and makes it more difficult to clean.

If the condition is not corrected, eventually there is enough destruction of the periodontium that the tooth becomes loose. Often, the chronic inflammatory cells at the bottom of a deep pocket are joined by acute inflammatory cells, producing painful swelling and pus. This condition is known as a periodontal abscess. Most extractions of adult teeth are the result of periodontitis.

DISORDERS AND DISEASES

The principal scientific professions requiring knowledge of teeth and their surrounding structures are those of dentistry and dental hygiene. Dentists need to have thorough knowledge of the anatomy and physiology of the teeth and their surrounding structures in the mouth. They must be able to detect and treat diseases of the mouth and all its tissues. Dental caries, infected pulp, diseases of the periodontium, and tooth loss are treated by dentists. Dental hygienists aid dentists by treating and identifying diseases of the mouth. Their principal duty is to remove harmful deposits on the teeth, but hygienists also identify diseases of the teeth and periodontium. Using their anatomical and physiological knowledge of the teeth and surrounding structures, hygienists teach patients preventative techniques that can help prevent or halt the spread of dental disease.

Since the teeth and oral tissues are only a part of the body, knowledge of general human anatomy, physiology, and pathology is a must for dentists. Oral symptomatology discovered by dentists is often the first sign of a serious systemic disease. For example, a certain fruity odor on the breath is a sign of ketosis, which is a symptom of diabetes. Kaposi's sarcoma, a rare type of skin cancer, is often manifested as lesions of the oral tissues; the presence of such lesions may be a strong in-

dication that the patient has acquired immunodeficiency syndrome (AIDS).

The successful treatment of diseases of the teeth and periodontium must be based on a thorough understanding of the anatomy and physiology of these tissues. To restore a decayed tooth, the dentist must know how deep to cut into the tooth, the probable location of the pulp, the irritating factors of the restorative material, the possible traumatic chewing forces on the new restoration, and the compatibility between the restoration and the tissues of the periodontium.

The treatment of tooth loss is literally as old as the pharaohs. An X ray of the skull of an Egyptian mummy displayed an attempt to construct a dental bridge using gold wire to secure a tooth between two natural teeth. At present, there are several ways to restore lost teeth. Cemented fixed bridges constructed of metal and porcelain are often the treatment of choice when there are sound teeth to support them. In the case of a partial or total loss of the teeth, removable dentures constructed of plastic or porcelain teeth fixed in an acrylic plastic base are used.

Introduction of newer materials and techniques for the restoration of teeth is a constant challenge for the dental scientist. While the theory of implanting restorations into the jaw to replace teeth is not new, some of the materials are. The recent use of titanium implants into the jaw reinforces the dentist's need to know the anatomy and physiology of the surrounding tissues. It is known that the bone of the jaw attaches to the surface of titanium, a process called osseointegration. Great care must be used, however, in placing correct chewing forces on the supporting bone, and nonirritating restorations must be placed near the periodontal tissues for the implants to be successful.

Special acrylic plastics called composites are sometimes used in restoring lost tooth structure by chemically bonding to the enamel and dentin. Thin films of these materials are placed in the grooves of the newly erupted posterior teeth. This treatment has been shown to prevent decay in the chewing surfaces of the teeth. Laser technology is being explored by scientists to see if the enamel surface might be fused to withstand decay.

While the bone lost as a result of periodontal disease cannot be regenerated, new techniques of grafting the patient's own bone, freeze-dried sterile bone, and other materials show some promise in strengthening the weakened tooth.

A number of recent studies clearly demonstrate a

close connection between oral health and disease of other body systems. Patients with serious gum disease or tooth decay are at increased risk of cardiac arrhythmias, stroke, and kidney disease. Several studies reveal that older patients are especially susceptible. The American Geriatric Society, for example, published a study showing that patients over the age of eighty with three or more active root caries were twice as susceptible to cardiac arrhythmias when compared to individuals with disease-free teeth and gums.

Increased risk of heart attack and stroke may come from acute and or chronic inflammation caused by bacterial infection originating from bacterial pockets in gums and rotting teeth. Such inflammation leads to platelet activation and elevated levels of clotting factors in the blood, which increases the risk of cryptogenic stroke and cardioembolism.

Periodontal disease has been linked to another heart health problem called subacute bacterial endocarditis, a severe bacterial infection of the lining of the heart that can cause heart irregularities and heart attacks. This disease is also caused by bacterial infections that originate and reside in periodontal pockets known as gingival crevices. These bacteria eventually spread via the blood to all parts of the body and lodge in the tissues that line the heart, causing subacute bacterial endocarditis. Links between heart disease, stroke, and gum diseases are elevated in individuals who have lost teeth because the bacteria colonize the residual periodontal pockets, from which they leach into the bloodstream. Both periodontal disease and the secondary but important inflammations of the heart, brain, and other body systems that result are treatable and preventable conditions for many patients. Periodic cleaning and prompt attention to dental caries, along with complete removal of old amalgam fillings and other metals, have proven very helpful.

PERSPECTIVE AND PROSPECTS

Recorded history and archaeological findings show that humans have tried to treat the teeth and their related diseases probably since the Stone Age. There has been speculation among archaeologists that the practice of trepanning, the surgical opening of the skull, could have been in response to severe toothaches as well as other pain in the head. Mutilation of the teeth by the Incas and Mayans was common in noble families; skulls have been discovered in burial sites of both nations showing the insertion of jade disks in slots filed into the front teeth.

In ancient Greece, Hippocrates wrote of treating a severe tumor of the jaw of a young man. After lancing the lesion, he wrote that the condition was morbid and that the young man would surely die. The Greeks also supposed that tooth decay was caused by small worms that bored into the tooth and ate it from within.

In medieval Japan, dentists were trained to extract teeth with their thumb and forefingers. They practiced on tapered wooden pegs pounded into a board. A soft wood was used at first for easier removal, then successively harder boards and pegs were introduced until the dentist could then remove a tooth from the jaw.

Most of the dentistry in the past was surgical removal of painful teeth. From the Middle Ages to the mid-nineteenth century, barbers performed extractions. Without the benefit of anesthetic, this practice was quite painful. Horace Welles found in 1894 that a patient could be put to sleep with ethyl ether, allowing painless tooth extraction. With the introduction of local anesthetics in the 1920's and later of intravenous drugs, pain during the extraction of a tooth has been virtually eliminated.

In modern practice, the study of the teeth has found new applications. For example, dental forensics contributes to the identification of abusers and criminals who bite their victims. The dental arch and the relationship of the teeth within it are unique, and bite marks are like fingerprints: No two are alike. The forensic scientist can take impressions of the bite marks on the victim's body with an accurate impression material. Plaster casts are formed in the impressions and compared to a cast of the suspect's dental arch. The evidence may either confirm or rule out the suspect's participation in the crime. In addition, dental forensics is used to identify the remains of people who are burned beyond recognition or whose bodies are badly decomposed. The teeth and their dental restorations are often the only way that a deceased person may be identified, especially in a major disaster such as an airplane crash.

The restoration and replacement of diseased teeth is an ongoing challenge, but with the new materials and technology available, humans should have healthier teeth in the future.

—*William D. Stark, D.D.S.;*
updated by Dwight G. Smith, Ph.D.

See also Braces, orthodontic; Cavities; Crowns and bridges; Dental diseases; Dentistry; Dentistry, pediatric; Dentures; Endodontic disease; Fluoride treatments; Forensic pathology; Fracture repair; Gastrointestinal system; Gingivitis; Gum disease; Jaw wiring; Nutrition; Orthodontics; Periodontal surgery; Periodontitis; Plaque, dental; Root canal treatment; Teething; Tooth extraction; Toothache; Veterinary medicine; Wisdom teeth.

FOR FURTHER INFORMATION:

Cook, Allan R., ed. *Oral Health Sourcebook: Basic Information About Diseases and Conditions Affecting Oral Health*. Detroit, Mich.: Omnigraphics, 1998. This handy reference source, which covers all aspects of dental health, includes helpful statistics on dental disease.

Ferracane, Jack L. "Using Posterior Composites Appropriately." *Journal of the American Dental Association* 123 (July, 1992): 53-58. A discussion of the mechanical properties of acrylic composites, including resistance to wear and the use of bonded seals with this restorative material.

Foster, Malcolm S. *Protecting Our Children's Teeth: A Guide to Quality Dental Care from Infancy Through Age Twelve*. New York: Insight Books, 1992. This book, meant for parents, is clear and easy to understand. A good starting point.

Langlais, Robert P., and Craig S. Miller. *Color Atlas of Common Oral Diseases*. 4th ed. Philadelphia: Lippincott Williams & Wilkins, 2009. Provides six hundred color photographs of the most commonly seen oral problems accompanied by descriptive text for each condition.

Parker, James N., and Philip M. Parker, eds. *The Official Patient Sourcebook on Tooth Decay*. San Diego, Calif.: Icon Health, 2002. Self-described as a reference manual for self-directed patient research, this book describes in clear detail relationships among types of tooth decay and relationships between dental problems and overall health. Includes lists of Web links for many topics treated within.

Standring, Susan, et al., eds. *Gray's Anatomy*. 40th ed. New York: Churchill Livingstone/Elsevier, 2008. The definitive book on human anatomy. With 780 illustrations in the text, the interrelationship of nerves, blood vessels, bones, and other anatomical structures of the human body is displayed in a practical manner as a fascinating biological machine.

Zablotsky, Mark H. "The Periodontal Approach to Implant Dentistry." *Journal of the California Dental Association* 19, no. 12 (1991): 39. An excellent article outlining the important relationships between dental implants and the restorations attached to them and the periodontal tissues.

TEETHING
BIOLOGY

ALSO KNOWN AS: Deciduous dentition, tooth eruption

ANATOMY OR SYSTEM AFFECTED: Mouth, gums, teeth

SPECIALTIES AND RELATED FIELDS: Dentistry, orthodontics, pediatrics

DEFINITION: The eruption of the primary, or deciduous, teeth in infancy.

KEY TERMS:

central incisors: the two center top and two center bottom teeth

cuspids: the teeth on either side of the lateral incisors; also known as the canines or eyeteeth

deciduous teeth: a child's first set of teeth, which will be replaced by the child's permanent teeth; also known as the primary or baby teeth

lateral incisors: the teeth on either side of the central incisors

molars: the grinding teeth located at the back of the mouth

STRUCTURE AND FUNCTIONS

A child's teeth begin to develop about the second month of pregnancy. The first tooth does not usually appear above the gum line, however, until the sixth or seventh month after birth. The tooth is pushed upward through the gum by growth at the base of the tooth. At the same time, the root sheath grows downward toward the jaw. Studies indicate that dental development does not seem to be affected by nutrition, illness, or climate. In addition, there seems to be little difference between girls and boys in their dental development.

Dental development follows a typical pattern. The teeth generally emerge in pairs. Usually, the lower central incisors are the first teeth to erupt, between five and seven months after birth, followed by the upper central incisors at six to eight months. The upper lateral incisors make their appearances between nine and eleven months, followed by the lower lateral incisors at ten to twelve months. The first molars, two upper and two lower, usually emerge between twelve and sixteen months. The cuspids follow next, at about sixteen to twenty months. The final deciduous teeth to emerge are the second molars, at twenty to thirty months. Most children will have twenty teeth, ten on the top and ten on the bottom, by their third birthday. By the time that they are six, most children begin to lose their primary teeth as the permanent teeth emerge.

While this is the typical pattern, there is much individual variation in both the time frame and the order of tooth eruption. Some children do not get the first tooth until their first birthday. On the other hand, children are sometimes born with teeth or have their first teeth erupt in the first month after birth. Those teeth present at birth are called natal teeth, and those that emerge soon after birth are called neonatal. Natal and neonatal teeth have been associated with other oral abnormalities, including cleft palate and cleft lip, although many children with these teeth have no abnormalities. Natal and neonatal teeth can present problems for babies, who may cut their tongues on the teeth, and for nursing mothers, who may experience lacerated nipples.

Although not permanent, a child's primary teeth are important. The primary teeth are necessary for the child to chew solid food. In addition, they are important as space holders and guides for the permanent teeth.

DISORDERS AND DISEASES

Some children have a more difficult time teething than do others. Common symptoms of teething in an infant include wakefulness, excessive drooling, fussiness, refusal to nurse, and finger chewing. An infant's gums may also be swollen and tender. These symptoms have also been observed in animals as their teeth erupt.

Some debate exists over other commonly held beliefs concerning symptoms associated with teething. Historically, fever, diarrhea, and ear pulling have been attributed to teething; however, there is no scientific evidence to suggest that teething causes any of these symptoms. In a 1992 article, "Teething," in the *Journal of Pediatric Health Care*, Patricia T. Castiglia suggests that parents often attribute behaviors such as wakefulness to teething because it alleviates parental worry. She further argues that wakefulness at six to nine months is caused by separation anxiety, not teething.

Those researchers who have attempted to associate teething with disease have found it difficult to do so. The teething period is also the period when babies are no longer fully protected by the mother's antibodies but have not yet built up antibodies of their own, thus rendering them susceptible to disease. Consequently, while diseases may coincide with the teething period, it is difficult to associate teething with disease.

Nevertheless, most pediatricians agree that babies experience some discomfort from teething. Many believe that allowing the child to chew on a cold rubber teething ring or damp washcloth will relieve the pain. While some experts suggest offering frozen teething

rings and/or frozen bagels or bread, others argue that neither should be given. They contend that the frozen teething ring can damage the baby's gums, while bits of the frozen bagel can break off, potentially choking the baby. Likewise, there is little agreement about whether acetaminophen should be used.

Most experts discourage using breast-feeding or a bottle to help a teething baby fall asleep. The milk pools around the new teeth, potentially causing decay. Indeed, many pediatricians suggest that a baby's gums and new teeth should be wiped with a clean, damp gauze pad several times a day to remove traces of milk or juice from the mouth.

PERSPECTIVE AND PROSPECTS

Teething has been a concern for doctors and parents for many years. Theorists as early as Hippocrates attributed fever, convulsions, and diarrhea to teething. During the eighteenth and nineteenth centuries, many writers considered teething to be the leading cause of death among infants.

During the last quarter of the twentieth century, however, the use of teething as a diagnosis for diarrhea, fever, and other childhood illnesses diminished among pediatricians, although studies indicated that some pediatricians continued to connect teething with diarrhea.

—*Diane Andrews Henningfeld, Ph.D.*

See also Cleft lip and palate; Cleft lip and palate repair; Dental diseases; Dentistry; Dentistry, pediatric; Neonatology; Pain; Pain management; Pediatrics; Teeth.

FOR FURTHER INFORMATION:

Gorfinkle, Kenneth. *Soothing Your Child's Pain: From Teething and Tummy Aches to Acute Illnesses and Injuries—How to Understand the Causes and Ease the Hurt*. Lincolnwood, Ill.: Contemporary Books, 1998. Aimed at the parents of young patients, this guide includes bibliographical references and an index.

Josephson, Laura. *A Homeopathic Handbook of Natural Remedies: Safe and Effective Treatment of Common Ailments and Injuries*. New York: Villard Books, 2002. Gives an overview of the healing principles and history of homeopathy, guidelines for identifying and treating symptoms, and instructions for preparing and stocking your home kit. Includes an entire section on childhood conditions, including teething.

Kemper, Kathi J. *The Holistic Pediatrician: A Pediatrician's Comprehensive Guide to Safe and Effective*

Therapies for the Twenty-five Most Common Ailments of Infants, Children, and Adolescents. Rev. ed. New York: Quill, 2002. Integrates mainstream and alternative medicine to aid parents in dealing with the most common childhood health problems, such as fever, diaper rash, teething, ear infections, and allergies.

Kump, Theresa. "The Facts About Baby Teeth: From Teething Pain to First Cleanings, Here's What You Do." *Parents* 70, no. 6 (June, 1995): 65-66. Facts surrounding the teething process in babies ages six to twelve months are discussed. Parents can alleviate the pain of teething by offering them teething rings or giving them pain relievers.

Rogoznica, June. "Teething Time." *Parents* 74, no. 3 (March, 1999): 139-140. Babies between the age of one month and one year often become suddenly fussy, finicky, and even slightly feverish because it is teething time.

Shelov, Steven P., et al. *Caring for Your Baby and Young Child: Birth to Age Five.* 5th ed. New York: Bantam Books, 2009. Offers a comprehensive discussion of the developmental stages of young children.

Woolf, Alan D., et al., eds. *The Children's Hospital Guide to Your Child's Health and Development.* Cambridge, Mass.: Perseus, 2002. An authoritative and comprehensive guide to children's health, providing a guide to every common illness or condition that affects children and a carefully designed emergency section.

TELEMEDICINE

OVERVIEW

DEFINITION: The incorporation and use of modern electronic communications systems to exchange medical information from one site to another to deliver health care from a distance.

KEY TERMS:

e-health or eHealth: an umbrella term that encompasses telehealth, telemedicine, storage of medical records, and other types of health-related information and technology

health information technology (HIT): the various initiatives and interdependency of technological innovations as applied to telehealth and telemedicine

telehealth: a broader definition of telemedicine that refers to the transmission of additional nonclinical information such as videoconferencing, transference of still images and data, continuing educational programs for medical personnel, administrative needs, and research

DEVELOPMENT AND APPLICATIONS

With the development of health information technology (HIT), U.S. telemedicine has expanded rapidly and is being used in some form in all states. Most applications of telemedicine fall under the categories of "real time," such as when face-to-face consultations are necessary, or "store and forward," which is the most widely used technology at present. Electronic transmissions of computed tomography (CT) scans, X rays, and test results can be stored and sent to another department, another city, or anywhere in the world. Videoconferencing in real time, on the other hand, allows all parties involved—doctor, patient, specialist, and others—to consult together as if they were in the same room. These applications have been found useful to most medical specialties and particularly in the delivery of services in remote areas. The prefix "tele-" is generally applied to specialties using the technology (telecardiology, teleradiology, telepediatrics).

Services are generally delivered through high-speed lines and the Internet, linking various sites. Other modes of delivery include private networks for specialty needs, used directly or contracted out to private agencies. Home connections for clinical consultation may use single-line phone/video systems and the Web.

Some major advantages of telemedicine include lower costs, greater efficiency, remote delivery of care, better clinical outcomes, immediate returns on investment for agencies, minimization of health care disparities in populations, and easier and more efficient billing procedures.

USE IN TREATMENT AND THERAPY

Since the mid-1990's, tens of thousands of patients have been served by various forms of telemedicine. Physicians may consult with specialists, and patients can be monitored at a distance for better diagnosis and treatment. Vital signs can be taken and instantly transmitted to another site for analysis. Wireless technology is now used in ambulances to transmit vital information en route to the hospital.

Doctors and patients can communicate through telemedicine programs, as well as through the Internet. Consumers can access specialized health information and engage in online discussions with groups providing peer support. Telemedicine has been used primarily for patient care services, although it is also being used for administration and continuing education. There are also a number of developing and innovative potential applications.

The Department of Veterans Affairs is studying the use of telemedicine for the treatment of post-traumatic stress disorder (PTSD), giving veterans broader access to services and group treatment interventions. Such telemental health programs have broad applications for mental health patients and can offer more immediate access, security, and reassurance.

Teletrauma programs allow doctors, especially in rural areas, to talk to trauma specialists through live video hookups. Such programs have already saved a number of lives and have tremendous potential. Teletrauma technology is projected eventually to link most hospitals with top trauma centers.

Health e-stations are off-hour clinics where patients with minor ailments can be treated by a doctor over a plasmá television hookup. Patients can also be monitored at home through home telehealth applications adopted by home health agencies. Such services can empower patients, increase access, and reduce costs and time and can result in less burden on physicians and on emergency room care. Telehospice programs are relatively new, and in the process of development. They may provide pain control, anxiety relief, and comfort measures.

The use of telemedicine in screening can also be extremely valuable in preventing more serious illness or future problems in a population. Dental screening, especially in underserved populations for early childhood conditions, for example, can detect possible serious future problems from infection, malnutrition, and loss of teeth. Retinal screening of diabetics can also provide early detection of loss of sight, allowing early intervention.

PERSPECTIVE AND PROSPECTS

The early roots of telemedicine date from the late 1920's with the development of television and of telephones with visual capabilities. Since then, technological development has culminated in capacities for highly advanced interactive communications enhanced by improved data compression and available bandwidths, setting the stage for future expansion, deployment, and application.

New applications for telemedicine and telehealth are constantly being proposed, researched, and developed. In the case of natural disaster or terrorist attack, for example, a broad telehealth system could provide a rapid and effective response through linking existing networks to form a national medical response grid. The U.S. military is doing research on the extended use of telemedicine to deliver care on the battlefield involving robotic telesurgery, which enables a surgeon in one location to perform surgery remotely through control of a robotic arm in another location.

Some of the barriers faced in developing e-health systems include exploring ways to institute billing and incorporate insurance payments. Information must also be secure and protected. Medicare and Medicaid reimbursement has a number of restrictions. There is also a lack of appropriate technology and infrastructure. A question of licensure of physicians involved in out-of-state consultations, as well as fears of malpractice, makes some physicians hesitant to participate. There are also considerable initial costs for training and equipment. Federal funding is provided through grant programs, reimbursement under Medicare, and services for the military, veterans, American Indians, and correctional populations. A number of companies and health care organizations are interested or involved in research and development in the corporate sector, and telemedicine is expected to have a significant impact on how health care is delivered in the future.

—*Martha Oehmke Loustaunau, Ph.D.*

See also Allied health; Education, medical; Emergency medicine; Emergency medicine, pediatric; Internet medicine; Physical examination; Screening; Self-medication.

FOR FURTHER INFORMATION:

Darkins, Adam William, and Margaret Ann Cary. *Telemedicine and Telehealth: Principles, Policies, Performance, and Pitfalls.* New York: Springer, 2000.

Norris, A. C. *Essentials of Telemedicine and Telecare.* New York: John Wiley & Sons, 2002.

Wootton, Richard, John Craig, and Victor Patterson, eds. *Introduction to Telemedicine.* 2d ed. London: Royal Society of Medicine Press, 2006.

TEMPOROMANDIBULAR JOINT (TMJ) SYNDROME

DISEASE/DISORDER

ANATOMY OR SYSTEM AFFECTED: Bones, head, joints, mouth, muscles, teeth

SPECIALTIES AND RELATED FIELDS: Dentistry, family medicine, psychology

DEFINITION: A disorder that produces pain and stiffness in the joint between the lower jawbone (mandible) and the temporal bone of the skull.

CAUSES AND SYMPTOMS

The exact cause of temporomandibular joint (TMJ) syndrome, or myofacial pain-dysfunction syndrome, is not known. Possible causes include arthritis, bad bite (malocclusion), grinding or clenching of the teeth (bruxism), muscle tension, and psychological stress. X rays and laboratory tests carried out on people with this disorder usually reveal no abnormalities. Another cause of pain and stiffness in the temporomandibular joints at either side of the jaw is rheumatoid arthritis. With rheumatoid arthritis, however, the symptoms are most severe the first thing in the morning, which is not typically the case with TMJ syndrome.

TMJ syndrome affects the temporomandibular joints, producing mild to severe spasms and pain in the jaw muscles that sometimes make it difficult to open the jaw fully. Other symptoms can include blurred vision, sinus problems, and pain that extends into the head, neck, ears, and even as far as the shoulders.

TREATMENT AND THERAPY

If spasmodic pain exists in the jaw muscles, a physician should be consulted. Some type of treatment will usually be arranged to ease the symptoms. Treatment to provide relief varies according to the underlying cause but typically includes local heat therapy, injections or sprays of local anesthetics, and simple analgesics, such as aspirin, ibuprofen, or acetaminophen. Prescribed jaw exercises are also often helpful. Some cases may require dental procedures, and, in the most severe cases, surgery may be necessary to correct the problem.

PERSPECTIVE AND PROSPECTS

TMJ syndrome is fairly common; most people who have spasmodic pain in the jaw muscles have this condition. It is estimated that nearly 25 percent of the population in the United States suffers from some form of TMJ syndrome, ranging from mild to very severe. The majority of cases, however, go untreated.

—*Alvin K. Benson, Ph.D.*

See also Arthritis; Dental diseases; Head and neck disorders; Joints; Muscle sprains, spasms, and disorders; Muscles; Orthopedic surgery; Orthopedics; Orthopedics, pediatric; Pain management; Rheumatoid arthritis; Stress; Stress reduction.

FOR FURTHER INFORMATION:

Bumann, Axel, and Ulrich Lotzmann. *TMJ Disorders and Orofacial Pain: The Role of Dentistry in a Multidisciplinary Diagnostic Approach.* Translated by Richard Jacobi. New York: Thieme, 2002.
Gremillion, Henry A., ed. *Temporomandibular Disorders and Orofacial Pain.* Philadelphia: Saunders/Elsevier, 2007.
Mitchell, David A. *An Introduction to Oral and Maxillofacial Surgery.* New York: Oxford University Press, 2006.
Okeson, Jeffrey P. *Management of Temporomandibular Disorders and Occlusion.* 6th ed. Philadelphia: Mosby/Elsevier, 2008.
Sarnat, Bernard G., and Daniel M. Laskin, eds. *The Temporomandibular Joint: A Biological Basis for Clinical Practice.* Philadelphia: W. B. Saunders, 1992.

TENDINITIS

DISEASE/DISORDER

ALSO KNOWN AS: Epicondylitis, tendinosis, tendon overuse syndrome, tendonitis
ANATOMY OR SYSTEM AFFECTED: Arms, feet, hands, joints, knees, legs, musculoskeletal system, tendons
SPECIALTIES AND RELATED FIELDS: Exercise physiology, family medicine, occupational health, orthopedics, physical therapy, preventive medicine, sports medicine
DEFINITION: An inflammation of a tendon or tendon sheath.
KEY TERMS:
collagen: strengthening protein in tendon tissue
ergonomics: the science of the relationship between the human form and its biomechanical environment
extracorporeal: pertaining to something occurring outside the body, such as therapy
inflammation: a condition of tenderness and disturbed function of an area of the body, caused by a reaction of tissue to injury or infection
tendinopathy: a general term referring to any type of tendon disorder

CAUSES AND SYMPTOMS

Tendons are fibrous cords that attach muscles to bones. Their function is to transmit force and coordinate the activity between muscles and bones. When too much stress is placed upon the tendons, they may become inflamed (tendinitis), or damaged, or both, from the chronic degeneration of tendon collagen (tendinosis). The cause of such stress is usually poor technique, overuse, or repetitive movements in sports, recreational, and occupational activities. The injury usually follows the progression of multiple microscopic tears in the tendon tissue, eventually leading to acute inflammation and pain. The areas most commonly affected are the rotator cuff of the shoulder, the elbow ("tennis elbow" or "golfer's elbow"), the wrist/thumb (de Quervain's disease), the knee ("jumper's knee"), and the ankle (Achilles tendinitis).

Many athletic activities, such as racquet sports, baseball, running, and weight training, involve repetitive movements that may put excessive stress on the tendons. Many occupations also pose a risk; examples include performing assembly line work, playing a musical instrument, and using a keyboard. Tendinitis may also be caused by infection or by a buildup of calcium deposits (calcific tendinitis) or other materials in a joint as a result of a chronic illness such as diabetes or arthritis.

Pain is the usual complaint. It occurs when the patient moves the affected joint but may sometimes persist when the joint is at rest. In severe cases, simple activities such as raising a coffee cup or brushing teeth may cause pain. There may also be swelling, warmth, and redness in the affected area.

TREATMENT AND THERAPY

The term "tendinitis" has traditionally been used as a blanket term for all tendinopathies. However, medical professionals emphasize that tendinitis and tendinosis, while often occurring hand-in-hand, are separate conditions and must be treated accordingly. Tendon overuse conditions have been generally considered inflammatory processes (tendinitis), and therapy has been administered based on that conception. However, it is important to recognize that overuse tendon conditions are frequently caused by collagen damage and degeneration of tendon tissue (tendinosis), eventually leading to an acute inflammatory condition. Tendinosis requires a different approach to therapy once the initial inflammation is treated.

True tendinitis conditions are treated with therapy

INFORMATION ON TENDINITIS

CAUSES: Stress on tendons resulting from poor technique, overuse, or repetitive movements in sports, recreational, or occupational activities; buildup of calcium deposits from chronic illness such as diabetes or arthritis

SYMPTOMS: Pain, swelling, warmth, and redness in affected area

DURATION: A few to several weeks; sometimes recurrent

TREATMENTS: Rest, avoidance of causative activity, alternative application of ice and heat, compression and elevation of affected extremity, immobilization with slings and splints, anti-inflammatory drugs (ibuprofen, corticosteroid injections), antibiotics, sometimes surgery

---

aimed at reducing inflammation. Rest and avoidance of the causative activity, alternative application of ice and heat, compression and elevation of the affected extremity, and immobilization with slings and splints are all helpful measures. Over-the-counter anti-inflammatory medications such as ibuprofen may be suggested. A new method exists for delivering medication to inflamed tissue: iontophoresis, whereby a small electrical current delivers anti-inflammatory medication, such as dexamethasone, through the skin to the inflamed tissue. More severe cases may require corticosteroid injections. Tendinitis caused by infection is treated with antibiotics and sometimes surgery if first-course therapy is not effective. Recovery from tendinitis varies from a few to several weeks.

Tendinosis therapy is aimed at allowing the injured tendon tissue to heal. Rest and avoidance of the offending activity is most important. Icing, ultrasound, and electrical stimulation may enhance collagen production. Once the initial inflammation has been treated, anti-inflammatory medications and corticosteroid injections are not indicated and may actually impede healing. Ergonomic changes in the workplace and the correction of improper technique in sports activities are important. Physical therapy and strengthening exercises play key rehabilitative roles by helping to prevent future injury, and they may also improve collagen formation and thus speed healing. Surgery to remove damaged tissue is used only as a last resort when conservative management has failed. Recovery from tendinosis may take up to several months.

Perspective and Prospects

Tendinopathies have been regarded as conditions that are often recalcitrant to therapy, becoming chronic or frequently reoccurring. It is possible that this difficulty is in part attributable to the lack of distinction between tendinitis and tendinosis. It has been postulated that some of the therapies for tendinitis, when used on tendinosis, may cause further tissue deterioration and thus contribute to the chronic nature of the disorder. Additionally, once the initial inflammation is treated and pain is no longer felt, the injured individual will often begin the offending activity before healing is complete. This leads to further damage and weakened tissue, creating a frustrating cycle. It is therefore crucial that a proper diagnosis is made before treatment begins and that the injured individual follow the full course of therapy and rest to ensure optimal healing.

The investigation of new treatment modalities is ongoing. Extracorporeal shock wave therapy has been shown to have some positive benefits for both tendinosis and calcific tendinitis. The use of ultrasound and electrical stimulation has gained acceptance with some professionals.

Preventive measures can greatly reduce the risk of developing overuse tendinopathies. This approach is becoming more evident in the workplace, where proper ergonomic environments help to decrease employee injury, increase productivity, and reduce injury and absences. Conditioning and emphasis on correct technique in sports and recreational activities will greatly reduce the incidence of tendon overuse disorders.

—*Barbara C. Beattie*

See also Arthritis; Braces, orthopedic; Collagen; Inflammation; Joints; Muscle sprains, spasms, and disorders; Muscles; Orthopedic surgery; Orthopedics; Orthopedics, pediatric; Physical rehabilitation; Rotator cuff surgery; Sports medicine; Tendon disorders; Tendon repair.

For Further Information:

Khan, Karim M., et al. "Overuse Tendinosis, Not Tendinitis: A New Paradigm for a Difficult Clinical Problem." *Physician and Sports Medicine* 28, no. 5 (May, 2000): 38-45.

_____. "Time to Abandon the 'Tendinitis' Myth: Painful, Overuse Tendon Conditions Have a Noninflammatory Pathology." *British Medical Journal* 324, no. 7338 (March 16, 2002): 626-627.

Porter, Robert S., et al., eds. *The Merck Manual Home Health Handbook.* Whitehouse Station, N.J.: Merck Research Laboratories, 2009.

Standish, William D., Sandra Curwin, and Scott Mandell. *Tendinitis: Its Etiology and Treatment.* New York: Oxford University Press, 2000.

Tendon Disorders
Disease/disorder
Anatomy or system affected: Back, bones, legs, ligaments, muscles, musculoskeletal system, tendons
Specialties and related fields: Occupational health, orthopedics, physical therapy, podiatry, sports medicine
Definition: Inflammation or tearing of the tendons.

Tendons are the tough, white, fibrous cords that connect muscles to movable structures such as bone or cartilage. The presence of tendons allows muscles to act at a distance and concentrates the force of the muscle into a small area. Sometimes tendons can change the direction of a muscle's pull, thus allowing the muscle to act around a joint. The structure of a tendon consists of parallel bundles of collagen fibrils, which makes it extraordinarily strong. A sheath, or vagina fibrosa, surrounds the tendon and is responsible for holding it in place. Between the fibrils and the sheath lie a lymphatic network and a fluid that allow tendon movement without excessive friction. Because of the vital functions of tendons, diseases and injuries to them can be debilitating as well as painful. Damaged tendons tend to heal slower than epithelial tissue, for example, because tendons have a lower blood supply than other soft tissues.

Trauma to tendons usually occurs in conjunction with impact, twisting, overstretching, or the simple overuse of a joint. These actions commonly result in partial or complete tears of the fibrous cord. Only if a

---

Information on Tendon Disorders

Causes: Disease, trauma, injury, overuse
Symptoms: Inflammation, pain, abnormal motion
Duration: Acute or recurrent episodes
Treatments: Rest, appropriate stretching, icing, heat, ultrasound, braces, surgery, anti-inflammatory drugs

tendon has not been stretched more than 4 percent of its original length will it return unchanged to its normal state once the force is released. When it is stretched from 4 to 8 percent of its normal length, the molecular bonds between individual collagen fibers begin to fail and the fibers slide past one another. At 8 to 10 percent strain, the tendon itself is in danger of tearing because individual fibers rupture, placing even more force on the fibers that remain intact. Although Golgi tendon organs send signals to the brain regarding excessive strain on tendons, such tearing usually occurs quickly during physical activities. Pain, swelling, and abnormal motion at the joint follow the damage. Tendinitis is the name given to the inflammation of a tendon.

Tendon disorders of the upper body. Tennis elbow, or lateral epicondylitis, involves the elbow joint and can be attributed to excessive extensor movements in the wrist joint and a sustained gripping of objects such as a tennis racket. There is great diversity in opinion as to the development of this disorder, as well as to its treatment. The latter includes methods such as rest, stretching, icing, heat, ultrasound, bracing, and surgery. Golfer's elbow is less often seen but is a similar tendinitis of the common flexor tendon.

Supraspinatus tendinitis, or swimmer's shoulder, is seen in athletes participating in swimming, tennis, and other activities involving overhead arm movement. Repeated overhead arm swings impinge and sometimes tear the supraspinatus tendon located between the acromion and the proximal end of the humerus. The disorder has also been termed impingement syndrome. Treatments include icing, stretching, modifying stroke technique in swimmers, anti-inflammatory drugs, and surgery.

Bicipital tendinitis usually stems from sports that require throwing or paddling. This type of tendon disorder is similar to the supraspinatus type in that pinching of a tendon is involved. The narrow tendon connecting the long head of the bicep muscle to the scapula lies in a groove and is restrained by a ligament therein. Pain occurring while a physician applies pressure to this groove and moves the patient's arm is diagnostic for this particular tendinitis. Treatments are the same as for supraspinatus tendinitis and are almost always successful.

Vigorous throwing can produce triceps tendinitis. Other tendons prone to injury are those attaching the infraspinatus, teres minor, and teres major muscles. Indeed, any tendon may incur damage depending on the specific activities that an individual undertakes.

Synovitis of the wrist extensor tendons is the result of friction between the tendon, its surrounding sheath, and bone processes. Tenosynovitis brings about a thickening of the tendon sheath, and at times a rubbing sound can even be heard during movement. An aching pain develops and may be relieved by methods applied in tendinitis cases. In addition, ultrasound therapy in water is highly successful. The abductor pollicis longus and the extensor pollicis brevis muscles are most often affected.

Tendon disorders of the lower body. Tendons of the lower body undergo greater stress than tendons of the torso because a greater weight is moved and a more continuous motion is involved. Achilles tendinitis often occurs in people participating in sports involving running and jumping. This type of inflammation has become the most common athletic injury. When great tensile strength is needed, the tendon tends to be long compared with the muscle to which it attaches. The Achilles tendon is long and durable but twists as it descends down the lower leg, making certain areas of the tendon vulnerable to the concentration of stress. Quality footwear with slight heel elevation and heel padding can reduce the tearing effect on this tendon. Stretching the gastrocnemius and soleus muscles before athletic exertion ensures that these muscles will absorb a greater portion of the force that would otherwise be transferred to the tendon.

Jumper's knee, or patellar tendinitis, is fairly common in basketball and volleyball players; it is often mistaken for arthritis of the knee. Repetitive extending of the leg at the knee causes microtearing in the kneecap tendon; thus, the torn fibers fray and eventually begin to degenerate. More stress than before is then placed on the remaining intact fibers, resulting in the likelihood of their failing as well.

Many other lower body injuries may involve tendons. Groin pull is most frequent in soccer players because of the sudden stresses involved in kicking and changing direction by planting cleats firmly into the ground and jolting the body into a new configuration. Hamstring pull occurs during bursts of sprinting because the hamstring functions in the forward movement of a leg after a stride is completed. During extremely fast running, the hamstring requires great force to keep pace; thus, damage to the connecting tendon and to the muscle itself is likely to occur if attention is not given to proper stretching techniques before the exertion.

The term "shin splints" refers to several painful injuries to the lower leg. Indicative of shin splints are pain and tenderness along the tibia, or shinbone, and the middle one-third of the leg. The condition develops in athletes who do not use sufficient padding in their shoes or who run and play on hard surfaces. Genuine shin splints do not involve tendons directly; fortunately, tendinitis of the tibial muscles can be differentiated from true shin splints because the pain of tendinitis is located higher up on the leg.

Compartment syndrome is most frequently seen in runners. The leg is divided into three compartments, each encompassed by a tight fascial sheath. When injury occurs to muscles or tendons of a certain compartment, swelling accompanied by a cutting off of the blood supply can cause further problems. Even the sudden growth of muscles as a result of physical activity can impair the function of muscles and nerves deeper in the leg.

—*Ryan C. Horst and Roman J. Miller, Ph.D.*

See also Arthritis; Braces, orthopedic; Collagen; Inflammation; Joints; Muscle sprains, spasms, and disorders; Muscles; Orthopedic surgery; Orthopedics; Orthopedics, pediatric; Osgood-Schlatter disease; Physical rehabilitation; Rotator cuff surgery; Sports medicine; Tendinitis; Tendon repair.

FOR FURTHER INFORMATION:

Delforge, Gary. *Musculoskeletal Trauma: Implications for Sport Injury Management.* Champaign, Ill.: Human Kinetics, 2002.

Józsa, László, and Pekka Kannus. *Human Tendons: Anatomy, Physiology, and Pathology.* Champaign, Ill.: Human Kinetics, 1997.

Stanish, William D., Sandra Curwin, and Scott Mandell. *Tendinitis: Its Etiology and Treatment.* New York: Oxford University Press, 2000.

Weintraub, William. *Tendon and Ligament Healing: A New Approach to Sports and Overuse Injury.* Rev. ed. Brookline, Mass.: Paradigm, 2003.

TENDON REPAIR
PROCEDURE

ANATOMY OR SYSTEM AFFECTED: Bones, feet, hands, joints, knees, legs, ligaments, muscles, musculoskeletal system, tendons

SPECIALTIES AND RELATED FIELDS: General surgery, occupational health, orthopedics, podiatry, sports medicine

DEFINITION: The surgical repair of tendons, the bands of tissue that attach muscle to bone.

INDICATIONS AND PROCEDURES

Tendons are straps of collagenous tissue that attach muscles to bone. They are strong and flexible; a tendon approximately 1.3 centimeters (0.5 inch) thick can support a ton. Tendons are most prominently observed in the hand, where they are associated with the muscles that move the fingers and thumbs, and in the heel, where the Achilles tendon joins the muscles and bones of the foot. The Achilles tendon is the longest and thickest tendon in the body.

Tendon injuries can be of several types. If the hand or foot is badly cut, the slice may enter or sever the tendon, resulting in an inability to move the fingers or toes. Tendons have also ruptured during physical activity; the Achilles tendon is at particular risk during certain running or jumping exercises. The sensation that the patient experiences with initial tear has been likened to a kick. Severance of the Achilles tendon is indicated by an inability to stand on tiptoe.

More often, the Achilles tendon may become inflamed by activity. Such inflammation is usually indicated by pain that develops at the beginning and end of a run but that seems to improve during the exercise. Often, the pain becomes worse at night. Treatment of minor inflammation generally involves rest or cessation of the activity. Corticosteroids may be administered to relieve the inflammation.

If a tendon has been cut or severed, surgery is often required for proper repair. Since tendons are under great tension, they may snap or regress from the site of the injury. The surgeon makes an incision through the affected area, whether hand or foot, and sutures the ends of the tendon together.

USES AND COMPLICATIONS

If carried out properly and quickly, tendon repair is generally satisfactory. The patient may be immobilized for weeks, and some permanent stiffness is common. Because the blood supply to tendons is poor, healing may be a problem. One new method for repairing tendons is platelet-rich plasma therapy. Platelets produce growth factors, proteins that take part in the healing process. Blood is drawn from the patient being treated. The blood is spun down using a centrifuge to separate the plasma, which contains platelets, from the red and white blood cells. The resulting platelet-rich plasma is injected into the site of tendon damage, supplying the tendon with healing growth factors. These healing growth factors had been lacking because of the poor blood supply.

—*Richard Adler, Ph.D.*

See also Collagen; Cysts; Exercise physiology; Ganglion removal; Joints; Muscle sprains, spasms, and disorders; Muscles; Orthopedic surgery; Orthopedics; Orthopedics, pediatric; Physical rehabilitation; Rotator cuff surgery; Sports medicine; Tendinitis; Tendon disorders.

FOR FURTHER INFORMATION:

Garrick, James G., and David R. Webb. *Sports Injuries: Diagnosis and Management.* 2d ed. Philadelphia: W. B. Saunders, 1999.

Irvin, Richard, Duane Iversen, and Steven Roy. *Sports Medicine: Prevention, Evaluation, Management, and Rehabilitation of Athletic Injuries.* 2d ed. Boston: Allyn & Bacon, 1998.

Scuderi, Giles R., and Peter D. McCann, eds. *Sports Medicine: A Comprehensive Approach.* 2d ed. Philadelphia: Mosby/Elsevier, 2005.

Small, Eric, et al. *Kids and Sports: Everything You and Your Child Need to Know About Sports, Physical Activity, and Good Health.* New York: Newmarket Press, 2002.

Weintraub, William. *Tendon and Ligament Healing: A New Approach to Sports and Overuse Injury.* Rev. ed. Brookline, Mass.: Paradigm, 2003.

TERATOGENS

DISEASE/DISORDER

ANATOMY OR SYSTEM AFFECTED: All

SPECIALTIES AND RELATED FIELDS: Embryology, obstetrics

DEFINITION: Agents that alter normal fetal development during pregnancy and cause birth defects.

TYPES AND EFFECTS

Teratogens are agents that cause fetal injury and result in birth defects. Agents such as drugs, chemicals, infections, and environmental contaminants can cause birth defects when a woman is exposed to them during pregnancy. Teratogens can be found at home, in the workplace, or in the environment. The severity of fetal injury and subsequent birth defects that occur are the result of the amount and timing of exposure to a particular agent and the genetic susceptibility of the embryo and mother. At low doses of teratogen, there may be no effect; at intermediate doses, a characteristic pattern of malformations will result; and at high doses, severe malformations will occur that usually result in death of the baby. The first trimester of pregnancy is the most vulnerable time.

Teratogens produce specific abnormalities at specific times during pregnancy. Thalidomide, sold in the late 1950's to help pregnant women with morning sickness, results in babies with phocomelia (lack of long bones and flipperlike hands and feet), while valproic acid and carbamazepine produce spinal cord and brain defects. Other teratogens are also associated with recognizable patterns of birth defects. For example, the antiepileptic drug dilantin/phenytoin results in craniofacial malformations, whereas coumarin anticoagulants, such as warfarin, result in neurological complications.

Teratogenic specificity also applies to individual species. For example, aspirin has been found to be teratogenic in mice and rats but appears to be safe in humans. Thalidomide, on the other hand, was shown not to be teratogenic in rats, cats, dogs, or rabbits but is highly teratogenic in humans, a fact that resulted in approximately ten thousand children born with severe birth defects before it was recognized. The most devastating effects of thalidomide occur when the woman is exposed within the first thirty days of pregnancy.

CLASSIFICATION AND REDUCING RISK

Known teratogens can be classified as infectious agents, environmental agents, and pharmaceutical drugs. Infectious agents include rubella (German measles), cytomegalovirus (CMV), varicella, herpes simplex, toxoplasmosis, and syphilis. Environmental agents include ionizing agents, radiation therapy, X rays, organic mercury compounds, herbicides, polychlorinated biphenyls (PCBs), and industrial solvents. Pharmaceutical drugs include retinoic acid (isotretinoin, Accutane), aminopterin, steroid hormones, busulfan, angiotensin-converting enzyme (ACE) inhibitors (captopril, enalapril), cyclophosphamide, diethylstilbestrol, diphenylhydantoin (Phenytoin, Dilantin, Epanutin), etretinate, lithium, methimazole, penicillamine, tetracyclines, thalidomide, trimethadione, warfarin, and valproic acid.

Public awareness is essential for the prevention of teratogen exposure during pregnancy. Information about fetal malformations that can be caused by exposure to drugs or environmental agents is important because they are potentially preventable. Women who may become pregnant should be aware of any medications and environmental conditions that might be teratogenic, as severe fetal malformations occur very early before the pregnancy might be discovered.

Awareness of teratogenic agents and potential exposure during pregnancy has led to the development of teratogen information databases in many areas of the country. National databases, such as ReproTox and TERIS, and teratology society organizations, such as the Organization of Teratogen Information Specialists (OTIS), have been established to provide detailed information on numerous potential teratogenic agents.

—*Thomas L. Brown, Ph.D.*

See also Addiction; Alcoholism; Birth defects; Carcinogens; Chickenpox; Childbirth; Childbirth complications; Cytomegalovirus (CMV); DNA and RNA; Embryology; Environmental diseases; Environmental health; Fetal alcohol syndrome; Herpes; Imaging and radiology; Mental retardation; Mercury poisoning; Mutation; Obstetrics; Occupational health; Over-the-counter medications; Pharmacology; Pregnancy and gestation; Premature birth; Radiation therapy; Rubella; Self-medication; Sexually transmitted diseases (STDs); Syphilis; Thalidomide; Toxoplasmosis; Viral infections.

FOR FURTHER INFORMATION:

Organization of Teratogen Information Specialists. http://otispregnancy.org.

REPROTOX. http://www.reprotox.org.

Shepard, Thomas H., and Ronald J. Lemire. *Catalog of Teratogenic Agents.* 11th ed. Baltimore: Johns Hopkins University Press, 2004.

Silverman, William A. "The Schizophrenic Career of a 'Monster Drug.'" *Pediatrics* 110, no. 2 (August, 2002): 404-406.

Wilson, James G., and F. Clarke Fraser, eds. *Handbook of Teratology.* 4 vols. New York: Plenum Press, 1977-1978.

TERMINALLY ILL: EXTENDED CARE

SPECIALTY

ANATOMY OR SYSTEM AFFECTED: All

SPECIALTIES AND RELATED FIELDS: All

DEFINITION: The medical, social, and psychological care of patients who are suffering from a terminal illness, the goal of which is to maintain as high a quality of life as possible for the remainder of a patient's life.

KEY TERMS:

adult day care facility: a facility that offers a temporary daytime setting based on either social, maintenance, or rehabilitative services; often used to give the home care provider some time off

extended care facility: a facility that can be found in several settings outside the home, where specialized medical care can be rendered under a physician's orders

home care: the provision of outside services to a person living in a home setting

hospice: a program designed to ease the suffering and grief for terminally ill patients and their families; care can be rendered in the home or in a special hospice setting with special emphasis on the relief of pain

nursing home: a type of extended care facility that can be classified as either skilled or intermediate, depending on the type of care; physicians oversee medical care that is rendered around the clock by a nursing staff

ASSESSING PATIENT NEEDS

Difficult decisions await those trying to care for a patient with a terminal condition. Many families are faced with these decisions soon after the patient leaves the hospital, unable to function alone at home. Physicians and family members are able to choose among several options, depending on the needs and desires of the patient.

The decision process should start when the patient is still in the traditional hospital setting. The decision process should explore all alternatives, based on many factors. The degree of physician involvement is important, since not all doctors make monthly trips to visit patients at other facilities. The possibility of rapid deterioration of health or mental status is a vital concern, and nursing needs and other nonphysician services are also of utmost importance. The patient's desires and the wishes of the family can be addressed through the patient's legal rights to have a living will or durable power of attorney for health care decisions. Both can document, either through the patient's own written directions or through the appointment of a relative as a legal representative, where the patient stands on the issue of being kept alive by artificial means. Specific requests regarding the use of cardiopulmonary resuscitation (CPR) should be made to the physician. These wishes are best discussed long before the patient is near death.

When the terminally ill patient also has a mental illness, such as dementia, the desires of the family members are weighed along with their willingness and ability to care for the person in the home. The problems of mobility, financial constraints, and quality-of-life concerns also enter the picture.

This is a picture that is not clear or easy to visualize. Many questions need to be answered before a suitable arrangement can be made regarding the continued care for a terminally ill person, especially an elderly one. These questions will lead to wiser long-term care decisions.

Extended care includes a wide range of social and support services and can be divided into three categories: in-home services, community-based services, and institutional care. The availability of these long-term care services may vary widely, with differences in eligibility requirements and costs. The choices to be reviewed must fit the family's financial resources. Long-term care should also be based on the medical, personal, and social needs of the patient. Special attention should be paid to the patient's cognitive, psychological/emotional, functional, and economic status. The value system, perspective, beliefs, and goals of the patient are extremely important.

For a terminally ill person, an assessment of the patient's current and potential needs may have to be completed more than once as the illness progresses. A timeline showing the patient's current needs and needs within the next year, or even the next five years, should be made. This long-term planning must address physician involvement; nursing coverage; physical, speech, and occupational therapies; social worker and nutrition consultations; dental care; and the need for medical supplies and equipment. Other services that may be necessary include personal care, preparation of meals, transportation, housekeeping and home maintenance, and assistance with daily living skills. The amount of time for which these services must be available and the necessary financial resources may influence early decisions. Unfortunately, financial considerations often dictate the answer before all options can be explored.

The patient's concerns regarding housing are influenced by such things as the amount of importance that is placed on staying in the present home and questions about living with or near family, friends, and church and about the availability of social activities. When the terminally ill person is elderly, this issue is even more sensitive. Because of the traumatic aspects of moving an elderly person from the home environment, the easiest transition for the patient should be sought. The choices are having a terminally ill patient remain at home or moving the patient to an extended care facility or a hospice center.

Before family members convene a meeting with the physician to discuss the options, all of them should speak with the patient. The terminal patient should not be given the impression that family members are making decisions for him or her. Such meetings allow patients to inform family members of their wishes, allowing the patients optimum input and providing information that the family may not have. Competent adults, even if they are elderly, have legal rights and privileges that must be honored. Some of these rights present ethical issues to family members trying to decide about long-term care. Unfortunately, such discussions often take place immediately after an older person has an emergency or a patient hears the diagnosis of a terminal illness.

When a patient is in an acute care hospital, the decision process should start before discharge. Many persons within an acute care hospital setting are qualified to assist in these decisions. An attending physician has available many tools to evaluate the patient's needs, especially if the patient is elderly and the doctor has specialized in geriatric care. Questionnaires can determine the daily living needs as well as collect psychological data pertaining to cognitive, emotional, and perceptive functions. The family physician, during the discharge planning, can arrange for the family to speak to the social services area within the hospital.

The family and the patient would be wise to make a checklist to determine the areas of most concern, ranking them by importance so that all persons concerned are able to look at the options more objectively. Although each of the alternative living settings is unique, every person involved in these decisions should visit the actual setting, allowing the patient active involvement to make the transition easier.

OPTIONS FOR LONG-TERM CARE

One of the first options available for a terminally ill patient is to return to his or her own home or to live with relatives. This decision of home health care must be based on the support available from the family: who will help provide care, when, and how. The need for home modifications to make the patient more independent or more comfortable may be a concern. If outside services are needed, such as therapy, family members must determine how they can be obtained. Another difficult question is identifying responsibility for the financial costs of special care.

These questions are difficult to ask and even more difficult to answer. Families may underestimate the additional stress involved in caring for a terminally ill person in the home. Fortunately, services are available to help relieve the additional stresses encountered, such as respite care. Having someone come into the home or having the patient placed in a day care facility can relieve some of the stresses temporarily. One of the first types of stress encountered is one of a physical nature, especially fatigue arising from the additional house-keeping activities of cleaning, laundering, shopping, and cooking. Additional emotional stress results from trying to balance time, responsibilities, and pressures. Financial worries may also cause stress, even though the costs of home care are often much less than for care in a hospital or other facility.

Home health care does not mean that the family or the patient is alone. Outside professional care, such as part-time nursing or supportive services, can be rendered when a terminal patient is in the home setting. These types of services fall under two headings: skilled care and supportive care. Skilled care involves physicians, nurses, and therapists. Supportive services are those that enable a patient to continue to live independently in the home. These services may meet personal needs (such as bathing and dressing) or involve the performance of chores (such as shopping, meal preparation, and housekeeping). Supportive services may be obtained as often as necessary, but they are not without cost. Moreover, the absence of one needed service may mean that home care is not the best option for this patient, at least at this point in time. Every patient and family member is entitled to make an objective evaluation of which agency is best suited for the homebound patient. An ongoing evaluation should be conducted to ensure that this option remains the best choice. Especially in the case of a terminally ill elder, home care may not remain a viable option for long: As the patient's physical needs change, his or her environment may need to change as well.

One step beyond living independently in the home or with family members would be for the terminally ill patient to arrange for special housing, often called supportive housing arrangements. This option may include continuing care retirement villages, board-and-care homes, domiciliary care, foster homes, personal care homes, group homes, and congregate care facilities. Board-and-care homes provide regular housekeeping and personal care services. This type of care is called assisted living, or even residential care, because the services vary widely, as do the costs. Another possibility is congregate housing, the environment of which is more like an updated version of an old resort hotel, with costs and services greatly variable. Continuing care communities offer independent living arrangements along with twenty-four-hour nursing care. These communities offer what is referred to as life care, with a wide range of services available, a large entrance fee, monthly charges for services, and a lifetime com-

mitment. They usually cost more than board and care homes or congregate housing.

Adult day care, which lies between home care and institutional care, emphasizes either social or medical needs. The three main types of adult day care are social, maintenance, and restorative, with each specializing in addressing the specific needs of the patient. The social model of adult day care emphasizes socialization while also giving families or caregivers some free time. The maintenance model, a mix of social and remedial components, differs from the restorative model, which offers extensive rehabilitation services. These settings may be alternatives to a nursing home. Some specialized adult day care centers, connected to hospitals, teach patients to live independently after discharge, with a special emphasis on daily living skills and the use of community resources.

If extensive care becomes necessary, especially for elderly patients, yet another option would be a nursing home facility, either an intermediate care or a skilled nursing care facility. The skilled nursing home is for the person needing intensive care, twenty-four-hour supervision under a physician's supervision with treatment by a registered nurse. Intermediate care is suitable for those not needing round-the-clock supervision but unable to live alone. This option is expensive, and the costs generally are not reimbursed, placing all the financial responsibility on the patient or on family members. Although nursing homes in the United States are inspected and controlled by the government, the certification status and quality among homes differ greatly. Attention must be given to ensure good medical coverage, provisions for maintaining the patient's individuality and dignity, available activities, nutritious meals, social and recreational activities, and intellectual stimulation.

The hospice setting offers intense medical supervision in comfortable and peaceful surroundings. The philosophy of hospice emphasizes the concept of supportive care and services for the terminally ill and their families in the home or a special center. Although hospices assist in some home health care services and inpatient care, they are designed for terminally ill patients who are no longer being treated for their diseases, with a life expectancy of only weeks or months. Specialized teams composed of a physician, nursing staff, volunteers, social workers, and clergy administer to the physical, spiritual, and emotional needs of each patient through the management of medical symptoms and the control of pain. If the patient is not placed into a hospice center, specialized care from the hospice team is available in the home to meet the needs of terminally ill patients and their families.

PERSPECTIVE AND PROSPECTS

Caring for a terminally ill family member can be a rewarding experience as well as an exhausting one. The location where this care is traditionally given has changed over time and will continue to change in the future. Care in the patient's home or with relatives is the least restrictive and one of the less expensive of the many options available. In fact, care in the home is often the only option because outside care is too expensive. Some family members are motivated to select home care because of a sense of obligation or a fear that no one else can care for the patient as well.

More supplemental resources are available than ever before, allowing home care to be a viable option for some. For many others, however, the additional stresses of responsibility for a terminally ill relative, especially an elderly one, are too high. At this point, tough decisions must be made about where the patient should live. Family members may not be prepared to care for the patient at the home. Despite the high costs of extended care facilities, this option is sometimes the only choice available. An emphasis on quality of life makes placement in the least restrictive environment a common choice. Concerns about pain management and the need for a caring staff may change this choice, however, when the terminally ill face the end of life.

In the United States, the high cost of health care makes such decisions even more difficult. Until some form of national health care reform allows for extensive coverage to assist these families, the financial burden will often dictate placement for the terminally ill. Although many placement options exist, more will be developed in the future because of the increase in the number of older adults. Some will be suitable and some will not, making this decision process a problem for generations to come. While the final decision about where to live remains with the competent patient, the input of physicians and family members and the influence of financial questions will become larger concerns. Societal influences may also come to the surface as the number of elderly people grows. With improving medical technology, the elderly population will have a greater impact on governmental policy makers and will influence national health care provisions. Advances in medicine may also dictate where and how terminally ill patients are cared for.

Resources for this care are available, but they have specific requirements. Possible benefit providers include the federal government through Medicare and the Social Security Administration's supplemental security income (SSI) program. Qualified persons should contact the Veterans Administration. State programs include Medicaid, the Department of Human Resources, and state supplemental programs. In addition to private insurance coverage, financial help could be sought through community agencies, such as municipal or other local support groups. Several health-related organizations offer some assistance for specific groups of patients, such as the American Cancer Society. Many private agencies, both nonprofit and for profit, offer services. The first and best approach for information when seeking care for a terminally ill patient is through family physicians, hospitals, and local health departments.

—*Maxine M. Urton, Ph.D.*

See also Acquired immunodeficiency syndrome (AIDS); Aging: Extended care; Allied health; Assisted living facilities; Cancer; Critical care; Critical care, pediatric; Death and dying; Emergency medicine; Ethics; Euthanasia; Geriatrics and gerontology; Home care; Hospice; Hospitals; Law and medicine; Living will; Nursing; Oncology; Palliative medicine; Pediatrics; Pharmacology; Psychiatry; Psychiatry, child and adolescent; Psychiatry, geriatric; Resuscitation.

FOR FURTHER INFORMATION:

Appleton, Michael, and Todd Henschell. *At Home with Terminal Illness: A Family Guide to Hospice in the Home.* Englewood Cliffs, N.J.: Prentice Hall Career & Technology, 1995. This popular work examines hospice care and home nursing for the terminally ill.

Beerman, Susan, and Judith Rappaport-Musson. *Eldercare 911: The Caregiver's Complete Handbook for Making Decisions.* Rev. ed. Amherst, N.Y.: Prometheus Books, 2008. A practical guide for elder care. Includes topics such as locating services, managing medications, understanding benefits, choosing a nursing home, coping with memory loss, hiring and handling in-home help, helping a parent who refuses help, and recognizing signs of elder abuse.

Corr, Charles A., Clyde M. Nabe, and Donna M. Corr. *Death and Dying, Life and Living.* 6th ed. Belmont, Calif.: Wadsworth/Cengage Learning, 2009. This book provides perspective on common issues associated with death and dying for family members and others affected by life-threatening circumstances.

Forman, Walter B., et al., eds. *Hospice and Palliative Care: Concepts and Practice*. 2d ed. Sudbury, Mass.: Jones and Bartlett, 2003. A text that examines the theoretical perspectives and practical information about hospice care. Other topics include community medical care, geriatric care, nursing care, pain management, research, counseling, and hospice management.

Levy, Michael T. *Parenting Mom and Dad: A Guide for the Grown-Up Children of Aging Parents*. New York: Prentice Hall, 1991. Discusses common problems, guidelines for financial planning and legal decisions, and health insurance. Outlines how to secure optimal medical care. Special sections cover psychiatric illnesses, dementias, and the deterioration of the body.

Lieberman, Trudy. *Consumer Reports Complete Guide to Health Services for Seniors*. New York: Crown, 2000. Helps consumers navigate Medicare, assisted living, nursing home selection, adult day care, and HMOs and their policies, among many other topics.

Lynn, Joanne, and Joan Harrold. *Handbook for Mortals: Guidance for People Facing Serious Illness*. New York: Oxford University Press, 2001. A handbook for caregivers, patients, and family members designed to guide individuals faced with serious illness and death through the experience. Compassionately covers all facets of end-of-life care, including topics such as how to talk with one's physician, planning ahead for special circumstances, and modern medical technology and the choices it offers.

_____. "Preparing for the Inevitable." *The Washington Post*, May 30, 1999, p. X03. Lynn, Harrold, and their colleagues at the Center to Improve the Care of the Dying reveal why the philosophy of palliative care is so important to the debate about the care of the dying.

Matthews, Joseph L. *Choose the Right Long-Term Care: Home Care, Assisted Living, and Nursing Homes*. 4th ed. Berkeley, Calif.: Nolo, 2002. A comprehensive reference for consumers that guides decisions about protecting assets, arranging home health care, finding nonnursing home residences, choosing a nursing facility, rating nursing homes, insurance, and understanding Medicare, Medicaid, and other benefit programs.

Portnow, Jay, and Martha Houtmann. *Home Care for the Elderly: A Complete Guide*. New York: Pocket Books, 1989. A comprehensive guide covering nutrition, exercise, bathing, grooming, proper environment, bowel and bladder care, and signs of illnesses.

TESTICLES, UNDESCENDED
DISEASE/DISORDER
ALSO KNOWN AS: Cryptorchidism
ANATOMY OR SYSTEM AFFECTED: Genitals, reproductive system
SPECIALTIES AND RELATED FIELDS: Endocrinology, general surgery, pediatrics, urology
DEFINITION: Testicles that neither reside in nor can be manipulated into the scrotum.

CAUSES AND SYMPTOMS
The testicles, or testes, appear in males by seven weeks of gestation; by eight weeks, they are hormonally active. At eleven weeks, they produce testosterone, which is suppressed by maternal estrogens later in the pregnancy. These estrogens decrease before birth, causing a surge in testosterone production that is indispensable for the descent of the testes at about thirty-six weeks of gestation and for future sperm production.

About 3.4 percent of all male infants born after a full-term pregnancy will have undescended testes, or cryptorchidism. Risk factors include being first born or a twin, having a low birth weight, and/or being born prematurely, as well as being delivered by cesarean section. By three months of age, 1 percent of male infants still have undescended testes, a percentage unchanged by one year of age. In premature infants, most testes will descend by three months after the expected date at which the child should have been born (term).

The tissues of descended and undescended testes are the same for the first year. Thereafter, an undescended testis deteriorates and the chance of infertility increases. Rarely will testes descend spontaneously after six months of age.

Cryptorchidism may be isolated or be part of other conditions such as hermaphroditic, genetic, and endocrine disorders. Infertility affects 50 percent of patients

> **INFORMATION ON UNDESCENDED TESTICLES**
>
> **CAUSES:** Genetic, hermaphroditic, and endocrine disorders
> **SYMPTOMS:** Testicles that neither reside in nor can be manipulated into scrotum, increased occurrence of cancer, possible infertility
> **DURATION:** Typically one to twelve months
> **TREATMENTS:** Surgery, prosthesis for cosmetic purposes, hormonal therapy

with unilateral cryptorchidism. Testicular malignancy is twenty-two times as common in these patients as in the general population; malignancy is six times as common in intra-abdominal testes as in other cryptorchid testes. One-fourth of all cancers occur in the contralateral descended testicle.

TREATMENT AND THERAPY

The American Academy of Pediatric Surgery recommends correction of this condition by the first birthday, thereby decreasing the incidence of infertility and tumors and making the testicle accessible for regular examination. If the testicle is absent, a prosthesis may be inserted for cosmetic purposes. Hormonal treatment is also available, with a success rate of 33 to 90 percent but a 10 to 20 percent chance of recurrence. A pediatric surgeon or a pediatric urologist will evaluate the child and decide what is best for the individual patient.

—*Frances García, M.D.*

See also Endocrine system; Endocrinology; Endocrinology, pediatric; Genetic diseases; Genital disorders, male; Glands; Hermaphroditism and pseudohermaphroditism; Hormones; Hydroceles; Men's health; Orchitis; Premature birth; Reproductive system; Sexual differentiation; Sexuality; Surgery, pediatric; Testicular cancer; Testicular surgery; Testicular torsion; Urology; Urology, pediatric.

FOR FURTHER INFORMATION:

Behrman, Richard E., Robert M. Kliegman, and Hal B. Jenson, eds. *Nelson Textbook of Pediatrics.* 18th ed. Philadelphia: Saunders/Elsevier, 2007.

Montague, Drogo K. *Disorders of Male Sexual Function.* Chicago: Year Book Medical, 1988.

Rajfer, Jacob, ed. *Urologic Endocrinology.* Philadelphia: W. B. Saunders, 1986.

Rifkin, Matthew D., and Dennis L. Cochlin. *Imaging of the Scrotum and Penis.* Florence, Ky.: Taylor & Francis, 2002.

Swanson, Janice M., and Katherine A. Forrest. *Men's Reproductive Health.* New York: Springer, 1984.

TESTICULAR CANCER

DISEASE/DISORDER

ANATOMY OR SYSTEM AFFECTED: Endocrine system, genitals, glands, urinary system

SPECIALTIES AND RELATED FIELDS: Endocrinology, general surgery, oncology, radiology, urology

DEFINITION: A tumor that appears as a hard lump, often painless, on one or both testicles.

KEY TERMS:

biopsy: the removal and examination of a tissue sample from a living body

hematocele: a swelling of the scrotum that contains blood and may result from an injury to the testes

hydrocele: a collection of fluid in the scrotum

metastasis: the spread of cancer cells from one part of the body to another

orchiectomy: the surgical removal of a testis

orchitis: inflammation of the testis

seminomas: cancers developing from a single cell type, often from the cells that produce sperm

teratomas: cancers developing from multiple cell types

testis: a male sex organ that produces sperm and manufactures the male sex hormone testosterone

CAUSES AND SYMPTOMS

Testicular cancer occurs infrequently and is most often found in Caucasian males between the ages of fifteen and thirty-five. The disorder is virtually unknown among African American males, among boys who have not yet reached puberty, and in men over fifty. The cause of this type of cancer is still unknown, although it has been observed to be more frequent among males with an undescended testicle than it is among the general population.

The most common symptom is a swelling of one testis. This swelling occasionally is accompanied by pain and inflammation, although more frequently than not it will be painless. Many causes trigger swelling in the scrotum, and most such situations prove to be harmless. Among these is a hydrocele, a collection of fluid in the scrotum that typically disappears over a period of several days. Also, injuries to the scrotum, often sustained by young men who are engaged in athletics, may result in a hematocele, a swelling that contains fluid and blood.

Although most swelling in the genital area is not serious, it is wise, especially for those in the fifteen to thirty-five age group, to have such swelling checked by a physician immediately to verify that no malignancy is present. Where orchitis, an inflammation of the testis, is present, it may be accompanied by severe pain, but it usually does not presage cancer, nor is it likely to persist.

Males are encouraged to make periodical digital examinations of the testes to check for any abnormalities. If a hard lump is detected, even though it may not be tender or painful when it is palpated, immediate medical intervention is indicated.

The most common testicular cancers are seminomas, composed of a single cell type, usually sperm-

INFORMATION ON TESTICULAR CANCER

CAUSES: Unknown; more frequent among males with undescended testicle

SYMPTOMS: Swelling of one testis, occasionally pain and inflammation

DURATION: Chronic

TREATMENTS: Removal of affected testis and adjacent lymph nodes, radiation therapy, sometimes chemotherapy

producing cells, or teratomas, which consist of a combination of different cell types. A handful of testicular cancers result from the growth of testicular tissue or lymph tissue within the testis, but these are extremely rare.

TREATMENT AND THERAPY

If men regularly examine their testes, any abnormalities should be detected in their earliest stages. If a malignant growth is present, then it is likely to grow quite quickly. Where a malignancy is detected, ultrasound examination can dependably determine the parameters of the growth. This procedure is usually followed by a needle biopsy to check testicular tissue for malignant cells.

Physicians attempt to treat such growths before they have had an opportunity to spread to other parts of the body. The most common treatment is orchiectomy, or removal of the affected testis and the adjacent lymph nodes. Such surgery, while drastic, usually does not limit a man's sexual activity, nor does it typically result in infertility.

Following an orchiectomy, the testis that has been removed is examined closely under magnification to detect malignant cells. The surgery is usually followed by a course of radiation therapy on the remaining testis and the nearby lymph nodes. Such treatment is indicated even if there is no evidence that the malignancy has spread.

Where there is any suggestion that the cancer has spread, however, chemotherapy is usually indicated as well. In such cases, cancerous tissue may also have to be excised from the patient's abdomen and from other nearby areas to limit the spread of the malignancy.

PERSPECTIVE AND PROSPECTS

Testicular cancer is among the easiest cancers to detect, simply by examining the testes digitally at least once

every two or three weeks. Digital palpation of both testes will quickly reveal pronounced irregularities. Because the detection process is simpler for this type of cancer than in many other types, early detection is typical. Once an abnormality has been discovered, immediate treatment and follow-up radiation therapy and/or chemotherapy will usually result in a favorable outcome.

In most cases, one of the patient's testes is not affected, so that patients are able to achieve erections and resume a normal sex life. The viability of their sperm usually is not adversely affected by an orchiectomy. The recovery period following surgery is seldom more than a few days, although subsequent radiation therapy and chemotherapy may disable patients for short periods of time following their application.

The cure rate for testicular cancers that are detected early is between 95 and 97 percent. Even in more advanced cases, the cure rate is 80 to 85 percent because of the specificity of treating this disorder surgically and with radiation, especially if the malignancy has not metastasized.

—*R. Baird Shuman, Ph.D.*

See also Cancer; Chemotherapy; Endocrine system; Endocrinology; Endocrinology, pediatric; Genital disorders, male; Glands; Hormones; Men's health; Oncology; Orchiectomy; Orchitis; Radiation therapy; Reproductive system; Testicles, undescended; Testicular surgery; Testicular torsion; Urology; Urology, pediatric.

FOR FURTHER INFORMATION:

Berenberg, Jeffrey L. "Testicular Cancer." In *Oncological Nursing Secrets*, edited by Rose A. Gates and Regina M. Fink. Philadelphia: Hanley & Belfus, 2001.

Gardner, David G., and Dolores Shoback. eds. *Greenspan's Basic and Clinical Endocrinology*. 8th ed. New York: McGraw-Hill, 2007.

LeMone, Priscilla, and Karen M. Burke. *Clinical Handbook for Medical-Surgical Nursing: Critical Thinking in Client Care*. 3d ed. Upper Saddle River, N.J.: Pearson/Prentice Hall, 2004.

Reinhart, M. "Testicular Cancer." In *PET in Clinical Oncology*, edited by Helmut J. Wieler and R. Edward Coleman. Berlin: Springer, 2000.

Tamimi, Rulla, and Hans-Olov Adami. "Testicular Cancer." In *Textbook of Cancer Epidemiology*, edited by Adami, David Hunter, and Dimitrios Trichopoulos. 2d ed. New York: Oxford University Press, 2008.

TESTICULAR SURGERY

PROCEDURE

ANATOMY OR SYSTEM AFFECTED: Endocrine system, genitals, glands, reproductive system

SPECIALTIES AND RELATED FIELDS: General surgery, urology

DEFINITION: The fixation of a testicle to the scrotum or the removal of a testicle or the veins surrounding a testicle.

KEY TERMS:

orchiectomy: surgical removal of the testicle for benign or malignant conditions

orchiopexy: fixation of the testicle to the internal lining of the scrotum to eliminate the possibility of testicular torsion

testicular torsion: twisting of the testicle in the scrotum, with compromise of the blood supply to the testicle, as a result of spermatic cord rotation

varicocele: an enlarged vein surrounding the testicle as a result of incompetent venous valves; most commonly found surrounding the left testicle

INDICATIONS AND PROCEDURES

Fixation of a testicle may be performed as treatment for torsion (twisting) of the testicle and undescended testicle (cryptorchidism). Removal of a testicle may be required because of infection, traumatic rupture, pain, necrosis (death of the testicle), or the presence of a testicular tumor.

Testicular torsion occurs most commonly in males under twenty-five years of age. Torsion is usually associated with acute testicular pain that is intense enough to produce nausea, vomiting, and severe discomfort. The testicle is usually firm, tender, and displaced upward in the scrotum. It is frequently difficult to examine the gland because of the severe pain. Manual elevation of the testicle may relieve discomfort in some patients with infections of the epididymis, but it has no effect on patients with torsion. Testicular torsion is considered a surgical emergency. Information regarding this condition can be obtained using scrotal ultrasound or radionucleotide scans, but most patients require surgical exploration to identify this condition. It is important to relieve the torsion as quickly as possible to restore blood supply to the testicle. Prolonged delay before surgical intervention can result in a nonviable, necrotic testicle.

Treatment of testicular torsion is by a surgical procedure called orchiopexy. After an incision in the scrotum, the testicle is untwisted under direct vision. If more than six hours have elapsed before surgery, a necrotic testicle may result and orchiectomy may be required. If the testicle appears viable, orchiopexy is carried out. In orchiopexy, the testis is anchored in the scrotum with a row of three or more absorbable sutures through the lining of the testicle and the dartos muscle layer of the scrotal wall. These sutures fix the testicle to the scrotum to eliminate further torsion. A small plastic drain may be placed to limit swelling and enhance drainage during recovery. The skin is closed with absorbable sutures. Because testicular torsion frequently occurs on both sides, the opposite testicle is similarly fixed with orchiopexy.

Undescended testes are located outside the scrotum, usually in the inguinal canal, but they may also be found in the abdomen. Orchiopexy should be performed at one to two years of age to preserve future testicular function. While rare cases require microsurgery, most orchiopexies are performed using a scrotal incision with testicular fixation similar to that described for torsion.

Varicoceles occur in approximately 15 percent of adult males, usually following puberty. Their importance is the association with infertility in some men with low sperm counts. Varicoceles occur primarily on the left side and result from abnormalities in the veins draining the left testicle. While tying off the veins of the varicocele is important in adolescent males with an associated decrease in testicular size, most varicoceles do not require surgery. If low sperm count, persistent infertility, decreased testicular volume, or prolonged pain occurs from the varicocele, surgical intervention may be appropriate.

Varicocele surgery can be performed through the abdomen, groin, or scrotum. Most surgeons prefer a high ligation, which involves a small incision just above the groin (internal inguinal ring). The vein draining the testicle is identified beneath the abdominal muscles. It is separated from the vas deferens (sperm tube) and arteries supplying the testicle, is ligated with several sutures, and is divided. This method of treatment is the most direct, least complicated, and most effective for varicocele ligation. The procedure is performed on an outpatient basis. Most patients are able to return to normal activity within seven days. Under certain circumstances, with previous failed high ligations, or with very large scrotal varices, a scrotal incision may be selected by the surgeon to remove all dilated veins from around the testicle. This technique is most useful in patients with decreased testicular volume or pain caused by a varicocele.

Orchiectomy, or removal of a testicle, is used to treat an abscess, infection, traumatic rupture, loss of testicular function, prostate cancer, and testicular tumors. Removal of the testicle for testicular tumors is especially important since these tumors are curable if identified and treated early. This procedure is carried out through an incision in the groin and not in the scrotum, a technique that decreases the chance of testicular tumor spread to the scrotum. A small incision in the groin above the scrotum is made, the spermatic cord is clamped, and the testicle is delivered into the incision and inspected. If a testicular tumor is identified, the spermatic cord is tied and the testis removed. The incision is then closed using standard suture techniques. If a testicle is to be removed for other indications, such as infection, prostate cancer, pain, or trauma, a scrotal incision is appropriate. The incision, which is similar to that described for testicular torsion, exposes the testicle and spermatic cord and allows for clamping and ligation of the spermatic cord prior to testicular removal. A drain is not usually necessary for orchiectomy.

Uses and Complications

Rapid identification of testicular torsion is paramount, before compromise of the blood supply results in the death of the testicle. Diagnosis of testicular torsion should be within six to eight hours of onset. Episodic torsion can also occur and is associated with preservation of testicular function and anatomy. Varicocele ligation is carried out for associated decreased testicular volume, pain, and most commonly infertility with diminished sperm count or sperm activity.

The complications associated with testicular surgery include infection in the scrotum, bleeding into the scrotum, and scrotal swelling. Pain, which is usually short-lived and localized, may occur with the inguinal incisions used for the removal of testicular tumors. Bleeding is the most common significant complication of testicular surgery and results in enlargement of the scrotum, significant discoloration, and pain. Bleeding is most often identified within six to twelve hours after testicular surgery. Testicular surgery is usually performed using absorbable sutures in the scrotal skin, and suture removal after surgery is unnecessary.

Perspective and Prospects

Surgical procedures for scrotal abnormalities have been common urologic procedures for centuries. New technologies such as radiographic embolization of testicular veins for varicoceles have been tried, but they are not generally accepted as superior to simple surgical procedures. These procedures, which are expensive and have unique complications, are less likely to be effective than more common, simple surgical intervention. Laparoscopy has been widely used for varicocele ligation, but it has little advantage over high ligation and is more expensive and time-consuming. Orchiopexy for abdominal or other high-lying testes can now be performed using microsurgical techniques. The testis can be removed and transplanted to a scrotal location, or the spermatic cord rerouted to permit scrotal placement and to avoid orchiectomy.

—*Culley C. Carson III, M.D.*

See also Circulation; Genital disorders, male; Glands; Hydroceles; Men's health; Orchiectomy; Orchitis; Reproductive system; Surgery, pediatric; Testicles, undescended; Testicular cancer; Testicular torsion; Urology; Urology, pediatric; Vascular system.

For Further Information:

Cockett, Abraham T. K., and Ken Koshiba. *Color Atlas of Urologic Surgery.* Baltimore: Williams & Wilkins, 1996. Examines both routine and complex procedures, including open, minimally invasive, and endoscopic techniques.

Graham, Sam D., Jr., et al., eds. *Glenn's Urologic Surgery.* 7th ed. Philadelphia: Lippincott Williams & Wilkins, 2009. Topics include the adrenal gland, kidney, ureter and pelvis, bladder, prostate, urethra, vas deferens and seminal vesicle, testes, penis, and scrotum. Also addresses urinary diversion, pediatric urology, endoscopy, laparoscopy, and frontiers in surgery.

Milsten, Richard, and Julian Slowinski. *The Sexual Male: Problems and Solutions.* New York: W. W. Norton, 2001. Accessible discussion of impotence and its causes, effects, and treatments.

Parker, James N., and Philip M. Parker, eds. *The Official Patient's Sourcebook on Testicular Cancer.* San Diego, Calif.: Icon Health, 2002. A wide-ranging handbook on testicular cancer.

Taguchi, Yosh, and Merrily Weisbord, eds. *Private Parts: An Owner's Guide to the Male Anatomy.* 3d ed. Toronto, Ont.: McClelland & Stewart, 2003. A guide to male genital health.

TESTICULAR TORSION

DISEASE/DISORDER

ANATOMY OR SYSTEM AFFECTED: Circulatory system, genitals, reproductive system

SPECIALTIES AND RELATED FIELDS: Family medicine, pediatrics, urology

DEFINITION: A twisting or rotation of the testicle (testis) or spermatic cord on its long axis, causing acute pain and swelling.

CAUSES AND SYMPTOMS

Testicular torsion is most commonly found in infants, adolescents, or young adult males. Roughly half of the cases occur in the early hours of the morning, and cases usually occur on the left side rather than the right. The condition can occur during sleep, rest, game playing, or hard physical activity, but it is more likely to be caused by direct injury. Testicular torsion may also result if the testicle is unusually mobile within its covering in the scrotum because of inadequate connective tissue.

Testicular torsion makes itself known by pain of varying degrees either in the lower part of the abdomen or in the scrotum itself. The pain intensifies rapidly and is occasionally accompanied by nausea as the testicle becomes swollen and very tender and the scrotal skin becomes discolored. A diagnosis can be made by physical examination.

TREATMENT AND THERAPY

Immediate treatment of testicular torsion is necessary. The testicle must be untwisted immediately and blood flow restored to the testicle, the epididymis, and other structures. Otherwise, complete blockage of the blood supply (ischemia) for six hours or more may result in gangrene (tissue death) of the testicle. Even a partial loss of circulation can produce atrophy.

Manual untwisting should be followed by surgery within six hours of the onset of symptoms to ensure that the torsion has been undone successfully and that there is no recurrence. An incision is made in the scrotal skin, and the testicle is secured to the scrotum by small stitches. If irreversible damage exists, removal of the testicle must be performed. The other testicle, which usually remains capable of producing active sperm, is also anchored to prevent torsion on that side. Prompt surgery ensures a complete recovery.

—*Keith Garebian, Ph.D.*

See also Genital disorders, male; Glands; Hydroceles; Laparoscopy; Men's health; Orchiectomy; Orchitis; Penile implant surgery; Reproductive system; Testicles, undescended; Testicular cancer; Testicular surgery; Urology; Urology, pediatric; Vasectomy.

FOR FURTHER INFORMATION:

Behrman, Richard E., Robert M. Kliegman, and Hal B. Jenson, eds. *Nelson Textbook of Pediatrics*. 18th ed. Philadelphia: Saunders/Elsevier, 2007.

Montague, Drogo K. *Disorders of Male Sexual Function*. Chicago: Year Book Medical, 1988.

Rajfer, Jacob, ed. *Urologic Endocrinology*. Philadelphia: W. B. Saunders, 1986.

Rifkin, Matthew D., and Dennis L. Cochlin. *Imaging of the Scrotum and Penis*. Florence, Ky.: Taylor & Francis, 2002.

Swanson, Janice M., and Katherine A. Forrest. *Men's Reproductive Health*. New York: Springer, 1984.

Taguchi, Yosh, and Merrily Weisbord, eds. *Private Parts: An Owner's Guide to the Male Anatomy*. 3d ed. Toronto, Ont.: McClelland & Stewart, 2003.

TESTS. *See* INVASIVE TESTS; LABORATORY TESTS; NONINVASIVE TESTS.

TETANUS

DISEASE/DISORDER

ALSO KNOWN AS: Lockjaw

ANATOMY OR SYSTEM AFFECTED: Brain, muscles, musculoskeletal system, nervous system

SPECIALTIES AND RELATED FIELDS: Bacteriology, family medicine, internal medicine, neurology, public health

DEFINITION: An often fatal disease of the nervous system characterized by painful, sustained, and violent muscle spasms; it is almost completely preventable through vaccination.

KEY TERMS:

anaerobic: without oxygen; anaerobic organisms grow in an atmosphere free of oxygen

---

INFORMATION ON TESTICULAR TORSION

CAUSES: Injury, hard physical activity, inadequate connective tissue within scrotum

SYMPTOMS: Acute pain and swelling, discolored scrotal skin

DURATION: Acute

TREATMENTS: Manual untwisting, followed by surgery

antibody: a protein found in the blood and produced by the immune system in response to contact of the body with an antigen

antigen: a foreign substance (such as a bacteria, toxin, or virus) to which the body makes an immune response

antitoxin: an antibody against a specific toxin; antitoxins can bind toxins and neutralize them

bacterium: a microscopic single-celled organism that multiplies by means of simple division; bacteria are found everywhere; most are beneficial, but a few species cause disease

endospore: a resistant, dormant structure, formed inside bacteria such as *Bacillus* and *Clostridium*, that can survive adverse conditions

immunity: a capacity to resist a disease caused by an infectious agent

lockjaw: a popular name for tetanus, derived from a symptom associated with the disease

toxin: a poisonous substance produced by some bacteria that cause certain diseases

toxoid: a form of a toxin that can no longer cause the symptoms of a disease but can cause the body to make antibodies against it

vaccination: inoculation with a specific vaccine in order to prevent or lessen the effect of some disease

CAUSES AND SYMPTOMS

Tetanus is a disease of the nervous system caused by the bacterium *Clostridium tetani* (*C. tetani*). Humans and most species of warm-blooded animals are susceptible to tetanus. This disease is not contagious, meaning it cannot be transmitted from one individual to another. It results from the contamination of a natural or surgical wound by spores (endospores) of *C. tetani*. The bacteria grow in the wound and produce a toxin that spreads throughout the body and causes the symptoms of the disease. Neonatal tetanus is the appearance of tetanus in a child less than one month old; it is usually contracted by the infant directly following birth.

C. tetani is an anaerobic, endospore-forming bacterium. Anaerobic bacteria can grow only in an oxygen-free environment. In harsh environments or at times when oxygen is present, all species of Clostridia have the unique ability to form dormant (nongrowing) structures called endospores. These structures develop inside the bacterial cell and serve to protect the genetic material of the cell from harsh environmental stresses that would destroy an actively growing cell. Endospores are very resistant to disinfectants and tempera-

---

INFORMATION ON TETANUS

CAUSES: Bacterial infection through wound or abrasion

SYMPTOMS: Restlessness; irritability; stiff neck; difficulty swallowing; stiffness or spasms of jaw muscles (lockjaw); painful, sustained, and violent muscle spasms

DURATION: Typically three to twenty-one days

TREATMENTS: Antitoxins; antibiotics; cleaning wound of any dead tissue; control of muscle spasms (barbiturates, Valium, D tubocurarine); positive-pressure breathing apparatus to maintain respiration; possible tracheotomy; dark room to reduce auditory and visual stimuli

---

ture changes; thus, the bacteria can remain dormant until the surrounding environment becomes better suited for growth. *C. tetani* spores are found throughout the world in soil, human and animal intestines, and especially in soil fertilized with human or animal feces.

A person can get tetanus only if spores from the soil or elsewhere in the environment enter that person under the proper conditions to become living, growing bacteria. The bacteria will grow only if they enter a wound that is free from oxygen, such as a deep puncture wound or a wound that has considerable dead or crushed tissue. There are always a few cases of tetanus, however, that follow no apparent injury. Typical causes of wounds that could be susceptible to tetanus are compound fractures; gunshots; dog bites; punctures caused by glass, thorns, needles, splinters, or rusty nails; "skin popping" by drug addicts; bedsores; outer ear infections; and dental extractions. The most feared form of tetanus, neonatal tetanus, is usually caused by the cutting of the umbilical cord with an unsterile instrument or by improper care of the umbilical stump. In the United States, most cases of neonatal tetanus are found in home deliveries not attended by a health professional.

Spores of *C. tetani* enter the body through a wound or abrasion. In the absence of oxygen, they will germinate (revert from the dormant endospore state to become living, growing cells). The bacteria will grow and multiply but not spread from the initial site of infection. In many cases, the wound hardly appears to be infected at all. As it grows, *C. tetani* produces a toxin called tetanospasmin that can filter through the body. Once the toxin reaches the central nervous system, it binds to

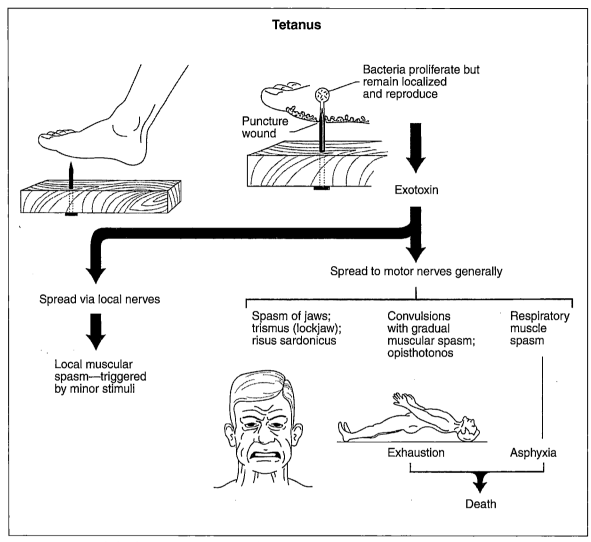

Tetanus is contracted when bacteria enter a wound and produce a toxin, tetanospasmin, that spreads through the body, most often causing death. A program of immunization is nearly 100 percent effective against tetanus.

nerve cells, causing the beginning stages of symptoms to be seen. Symptoms can appear from one day to several months after infection, with the average incubation period (the time during which symptoms appear after infection) being three to twenty-one days. The wide range of incubation time depends on the amount of time needed for anaerobic conditions to develop and the time required for the toxin to reach the central nervous system.

The tetanus toxin, tetanospasmin, is a simple protein. No one knows why *C. tetani* makes this protein. It has no apparent role in the life of the bacterium, and it is unknown whether this toxin gives the bacterium any selective advantage for survival in the environment. It is

unlikely that the bacterium makes this toxin merely to kill people and animals, yet the fact that it does kill them is all that is known about the toxin. Animals vary in their susceptibility to the effects of tetanospasmin; humans and horses are the most susceptible, while birds and cold-blooded animals are resistant. Tetanospasmin is the second most dangerous known toxin, and it is so powerful that an amount of toxin the size of one period on this page could kill thirty people. One milligram of toxin could kill 200 million laboratory mice.

To understand how tetanospasmin works to cause the symptoms of tetanus, one must first understand how muscles function. Most muscles in the body occur in pairs; one muscle in the pair, when contracted, causes that part of the body to move in one direction, and the opposing muscle in the pair, when contracted, causes that part of the body to move in the opposite direction. Normally, the nerves that control the muscle pairs stimulate one muscle in a pair to contract and signal the opposing muscle to relax. In this way, that part of the body is able to move. For example, in using an arm to lift an object, the nerves send a signal to the muscle in the front of the arm to contract and at the same time send a signal to the back of the arm to relax, so that the arm can bend upward at the elbow and lift the object. If the nerves did not signal the opposing muscle to relax, the contraction of the first muscle would cause the opposing muscle to stretch and trigger the "stretch reflex" in that muscle, causing that muscle to contract and counteract the stretch. Tetanus toxin works by binding to the nerve cells at nerve-muscle junctions and somehow blocking the signal of relaxation to the opposing muscle; therefore, when one muscle in a pair of muscles contracts, both muscles contract. The final effect is called spastic paralysis, in which the muscles are in a state of continuous contraction, pulling against each other, causing rigidity in a normally movable part of the body.

The initial symptoms of tetanus include restlessness, irritability, a stiff neck, and difficulty swallowing. In about half of all cases, the initial symptoms include stiffness or spasms of the jaw muscles, known as lockjaw. Gradually, the skeletal muscles (muscles of the arms, legs, back, and stomach) become involved. Muscles move through stages of contractions, from merely twitching to rigid spasms that are brief but may be frequent, painful, and exhausting. Severe stages of the disease are characterized by tetanic spasms (sustained contractions) of some or all of the muscle groups. The slightest disturbance of the victim may cause spasms, generalized seizures, or both. A typical tetanic seizure is characterized by a sudden burst of tetanic spasm of all muscle groups, causing clenching of the jaw to produce a grimace, arching of the back with the neck back, flexion of arms, clenching of fists on the chest, and extension of the lower extremities. The patient is completely conscious during such episodes and experiences intense pain. Some spasms may be severe enough to cause bones to break. Eventually, the muscles of the cardiac and respiratory systems can be affected. Spasms of the throat muscles and respiratory muscles may lead to suffocation or respiratory arrest. The toxin may affect the circulatory system and heart in such a way as to increase the heart rate, increase blood pressure, and cause constriction of blood vessels. Death caused by tetanus is usually a result of circulatory collapse or respiratory failure.

TREATMENT AND THERAPY

Tetanus is diagnosed mainly on the basis of the symptoms present and the case history of the patient—the vaccination record and the type of injury sustained. A patient with no recent history of tetanus vaccination who receives a puncture or trauma wound is often treated for tetanus with an injection of antitoxin even before any symptoms appear. Antitoxin is quite effective when given to prevent the symptoms from appearing, but less so when given after the symptoms have already appeared. While other diseases are diagnosed after the organism that causes the disease is isolated from the site of the infection, it is very difficult to diagnose tetanus based on the ability to isolate the C. tetani bacteria from the wound, for several reasons. First, Clostridia are present in almost every wound, but they do not always cause disease, so finding them does not necessarily mean that the bacteria are active. Second, there are many other contaminating bacteria in wounds, which makes it difficult to tell which may be causing disease or whether Clostridia are there at all. In addition, the number of C. tetani bacteria needed to cause disease is quite small, which makes them harder to isolate. Finally, Clostridia, because of their anaerobic nature, are difficult to grow.

Tetanus may take from a few days to several weeks to run its course. Patients who exhibit certain patterns in the course of the disease usually have a poor chance of recovery. These include patients with a short incubation period between the time of the injury and the onset of seizures, patients who exhibit a rapid development from mild muscle spasms to tetanic spasms, patients with injuries close to the head, patients with a high frequency or strong severity of seizures, and patients who are very young or very old. Patients who do recover usually return to a completely normal state after a variable period of stiffness; except for possible damage to the lungs from pulmonary complications or bone fractures, tetanus leaves no permanent damage. Unfortunately, recovery from the disease does not make the patient immune to future attacks, as with other diseases. The amount of toxin needed to kill a person is not even close to enough toxin to stimulate the patient's immune response to make the patient immune to the disease. Only vaccination with a large dose of inactive toxin can give a person immunity to tetanus.

Tetanus is difficult to treat because no one knows exactly what the toxin does. Doctors know only what kinds of symptoms the toxin causes, so the treatment is mainly symptomatic and is directed at preventing the production of more toxin. Antitoxin is given to block the attachment to the nerve cells of any free toxin that might be circulating in the body. Antitoxin has absolutely no effect on toxin that is already fixed to nerve tissue, but it can fully neutralize any free toxin. Originally, doctors used serum from immunized horses as a source of antitoxin, but this caused serious side effects (namely, serum sickness) in patients, so it is recommended that only pooled hyperimmune human globin (purified serum from immunized humans) be used as a source of antitoxin. Second, large doses of an antibiotic such as penicillin are given to kill any remaining bacteria, in order to prevent the bacteria from producing more toxin. If the patient is allergic to penicillin, tetracycline or clindamycin can be given instead. In addition, the wound may need to be cleansed of any dead tissue, to remove the anaerobic environment necessary for growth of the bacteria. Third, the muscle spasms need to be controlled. Mild muscle spasms are controlled with barbiturates and diazepam (Valium); severe spasms need a curarelike agent (D tubocurarine is used to poison the paralyzed muscles so that they do not contract) that completely paralyzes the patient. These various muscle relaxants are used to ease the contractions until the toxin already present at the nerve sites wears out. The patient can be put on a positive-pressure breathing apparatus to maintain respiration. A tracheostomy (an operation in which an opening into the trachea, or windpipe, is made) may be necessary to minimize respiratory complications. Also, patients are often kept in quiet dark rooms that reduce auditory and visual stimuli, in order to minimize the frequency and severity of the tetanic spasms. Even with all these treatment measures, three out of five persons who contract tetanus will die.

The best means of controlling tetanus is prevention. In fact, tetanus is nearly 100 percent preventable with active or passive immunization. Active immunization involves stimulating a person's immune system to produce its own antibody to fight off the disease. An injection of tetanus toxoid is given to immunize actively against tetanus. Tetanus toxoid is purified tetanus toxin that has been treated with formaldehyde to be rendered nontoxic (meaning that it will not cause any symptoms of tetanus) but is still capable of stimulating the immune system to produce antitoxin antibody. Active immunization usually lasts a long time, because the cells that make the antibody can keep making more antibody when the first batch runs out or whenever the person comes in contact with tetanus toxin in the future. The tetanus toxoid is usually administered as part of the DPT vaccine. This vaccine protects against diphtheria (D), pertussis (P), and tetanus (T). In the United States, it is recommended that persons be immunized against tetanus at two, four, six, and eighteen months of age, with a booster at four to six years of age and one every ten years after that. Surveys indicate, however, that more than 50 percent of adults over sixty years of age are not protected against tetanus. It is as dangerous to receive too many booster shots for tetanus as it is to receive too few. With too few shots, a person runs the risk of succumbing to the disease and dying. With too many shots, a person runs the risk of developing a potentially fatal allergic reaction to the vaccine. It is best to keep careful records of all vaccinations and to be certain that one receives a tetanus booster every ten years.

Passive immunization involves giving a person antibodies (made in an outside source) that will protect that person from a disease, instead of stimulating the individual to make antibodies. Patients thought to be at risk for tetanus can be given an injection of antitoxin for protection. This type of protection works only for a short period of time, because once the antibody in the injection is used up, the patient cannot make more. The way to immunize infants passively against neonatal tetanus is to immunize their mothers actively. A pregnant patient immunized with tetanus toxoid will produce antitoxin that is passed on to the baby's blood through the placenta. The baby is then born carrying some antitoxin antibodies in its blood that can protect it from neonatal tetanus.

PERSPECTIVE AND PROSPECTS

As early as the fourth century B.C.E., Hippocrates described tetanus as a common killer of women in childbirth, wounded soldiers, and infants. It was not until 1889, however, that the cause of tetanus, *C. tetani*, was first isolated by Shibasaburo Kitasato. In the early twentieth century, W. T. Glenny and Gaston Ramon paved the way for the development of a tetanus vaccine by discovering tetanus toxoid. War-related cases of tetanus were virtually eliminated by vaccinating soldiers. During World War II, only 12 cases of tetanus were recorded among 2,735,000 hospital admissions for wounds and injuries in soldiers previously immunized. This result led most state legislatures in America to pass laws requiring adequate immunization for tetanus before entering school.

Despite advances in treatment, the mortality rate for tetanus is quite high. The United States has about one hundred cases per year, mostly in the very young, who are in frequent contact with the soil, or in the very old, who have weakened immune systems. Many cases in the United States arise from trivial but fairly deep injuries that are thought to be too minor to bring to a physician. Sporadic cases are most frequently seen in the South, the Southeast, and the Midwest.

Tetanus is relatively rare in developed countries, where routine immunizations are available; it is, however, a common and uncontrolled disease in the developing world. Tetanus is a health problem in developing countries because of the lack of immunization, unsanitary living conditions, and the performance of common wound-causing procedures (such as ear piercing, tattooing, circumcision, and abortion) in an unsanitary manner. Neonatal tetanus is often caused by mothers or midwives who cut the umbilical cord with an unsanitary instrument. In addition, it is a tradition in many developing nations to apply soil, clay, or cow dung to the cut umbilical cord, which can inoculate tetanus spores right into the wound. Throughout the world, nearly 3.5 million children (mostly under five years of age) die yearly of three infectious diseases for which immunization is available. Two million die of measles, 800,000 die of tetanus, and 600,000 die of whooping cough; another 4 million die of various kinds of diarrhea. In parts of some developing nations, 10 percent of deaths within a month of birth are caused by neonatal tetanus. The World Health Organization is making a concerted effort to reduce the incidence of tetanus—especially neonatal tetanus—in developing nations by providing the personnel and resources needed for vaccination. Strategies for reducing the incidence of neonatal tetanus include providing passive immunity to newborns through the immunization of the mothers. Also important are promotion of safe practices, such as clean deliveries and clean cord cutting, and ensuring that unsanitary substances are not applied to cord wounds.
—*Vicki J. Isola, Ph.D.*

See also Asphyxiation; Bacterial infections; Childhood infectious diseases; Gangrene; Immunization and vaccination; Muscle sprains, spasms, and disorders; Muscles; Paralysis; Seizures; Toxicology; Wounds.

FOR FURTHER INFORMATION:
"CDC Report Finds Tetanus Reaching Younger Adults." *Vaccine Weekly,* July 16, 2003, 21-22. Surveys the types of injuries that can lead to tetanus and gives in-

sight into an upswing in cases occurring in younger people.

Joklik, Wolfgang K., et al. *Zinsser Microbiology.* 20th ed. Norwalk, Conn.: Appleton and Lange, 1997. An excellent textbook describing all infectious diseases. Chapter 46, "Clostridium," discusses all diseases caused by species of *Clostridium,* including tetanus, botulism, and gangrene.

Pan American Health Organization. World Health Organization. *Control of Diphtheria, Pertussis, Tetanus, "Haemophilus influenzae" Type B, and Hepatitis B Field Guide.* Washington, D.C.: Author, 2005. Provides updated information on the prevention of tetanus.

Pascual, F. B., et al. "Tetanus Surveillance: United States, 1998-2000." *Morbidity and Mortality Weekly Report: Surveillance Summaries* 52, no. 3 (June 20, 2003): 1-8. Reviews the incidences, demographics, and causes of tetanus in the United States.

Traverso, H. P., et al. "A Reassessment of Risk Factors for Neonatal Tetanus." *Bulletin of the World Health Organization* 69, no. 5 (1991): 573-579. A controlled study on the factors associated with the risk of neonatal tetanus in Pakistan. Gives a good introduction to the problem of neonatal tetanus in developing countries.

Worf, Neil. "Tetanus—Still a Problem." *RN* 63, no. 6 (June, 2000): 44-49. Nurses need to recognize the symptoms of tetanus and how to treat it. Despite widespread availability of an effective vaccine, the disease still occurs today and kills a third of reported cases. Provides a continuing education test for nurses on this topic.

THALASSEMIA
DISEASE/DISORDER
ALSO KNOWN AS: Cooley's anemia, hydrops fetalis
ANATOMY OR SYSTEM AFFECTED: Blood
SPECIALTIES AND RELATED FIELDS: Family medicine, genetic counseling, hematology, pediatrics
DEFINITION: A group of diverse genetic blood disorders affecting either β or α globin and resulting in decreased amounts of normal hemoglobin.

CAUSES AND SYMPTOMS
Mutations in one or more of the four genes coding for β globin or one or both of the two genes coding for α globin are the causes of thalassemia. The deletions lead to an underproduction of normal hemoglobin, a tetramer of two β and two α globins.

The most severe form of thalassemia is β thalassemia (hydrops fetalis or β thalassemia major), in which all four β globin genes are mutant or deleted and no β globin is produced. Death occurs at or before birth. Milder forms (β thalassemia minor or trait) occur when only two of the β globin genes are nonfunctional or deleted. The mild forms may exhibit mild anemia, but usually no health effects occur. When three β globin genes are deleted or are nonfunctional, the resulting thalassemia is called hemoglobin H disease. Enough β globin is missing in hemoglobin H disease to cause moderate to severe anemia, an enlarged spleen, bone deformities, and fatigue.

In the most severe form of α thalassemia (α thalassemia major or Cooley's anemia), both α globin genes are nonfunctional or deleted and no normal hemoglobin is produced, resulting in severe anemia. Hemoglobin molecules consisting of four β globin chains rather than two β and two α chains are produced, leading to red blood cell aggregates and inclusions that cause red blood cell membrane damage. In milder forms (α thalassemia minor or trait), in which only one α globin gene is nonfunctional or deleted, hemoglobin production is 50 percent of normal, resulting in mild anemia.

TREATMENT AND THERAPY
There is no effective treatment for β thalassemia major. Treatment for α thalassemia major involves red blood cell transfusion every two to three weeks. Transfusion therapy results in an iron overload that is controlled using chelators such as Desferal (desferrioxamine).

PERSPECTIVE AND PROSPECTS
The thalassemias constitute the most common single-gene inherited disease in the world. People with mild forms of the disease (thalassemia minor or trait) are usually heterozygotes or carriers. When two carriers have children, there is a one in four chance that the

---

INFORMATION ON THALASSEMIA

CAUSES: Genetic mutation
SYMPTOMS: Depends on type; ranges from mild or no anemia to moderate or severe anemia, spleen enlargement, bone deformities, and fatigue to death at or before birth
DURATION: Chronic
TREATMENTS: Blood transfusions every two to three weeks

---

child will have the severe form of the disease (thalassemia major). The frequency of the several forms of thalassemia varies geographically, with β thalassemia most common in Africa, the Middle East, India, Southeast Asia, southern China, and around the Mediterranean, and α thalassemia most common in Italy, Greece, the Arabian Peninsula, Iran, Africa, Southeast Asia, and southern China. It has been estimated that two million people in the United States carry one of the genes for thalassemia. The National Institutes of Health recommends testing for the trait.

—*Charles L. Vigue, Ph.D.*

See also Anemia; Blood and blood disorders; Genetic diseases; Hematology; Hematology, pediatric; Sickle cell disease; Transfusion.

FOR FURTHER INFORMATION:
Cooley's Anemia Foundation. http://www.cooleys anemia.org.

Jorde, Lynn B., et al. *Medical Genetics.* 3d ed. St. Louis, Mo.: Mosby/Elsevier, 2006.

Nora, James J., and F. Clarke Fraser. *Nora and Fraser Medical Genetics: Principles and Practice.* 4th ed. Philadelphia: Lea & Febiger, 1994.

Northern California Comprehensive Thalassemia Center. http://www.thalassemia.com.

Pritchard, Dorian J., and Bruce R. Korf. *Medical Genetics at a Glance.* 2d ed. Malden, Mass.: Blackwell Science, 2008.

THALIDOMIDE
TREATMENT

ANATOMY OR SYSTEM AFFECTED: Arms, blood vessels, feet, hands, immune system, legs
SPECIALTIES AND RELATED FIELDS: Immunology, oncology
DEFINITION: A drug that previously had been used as a sedative and then was banned for many years because of its severe effects on the developing fetus, but is now finding application in the treatment of leprosy and different cancers.

INDICATIONS AND PROCEDURES
In 1961, a link was established between the use of thalidomide, a mild sedative, and an increase in the frequency of severe defects in newborn babies in Germany, Great Britain, and other countries around the world where the drug had been in use. The "thalidomide babies" had minor defects of the fingers or toes but had major malformations of the limbs, resulting in

incomplete or even missing arms and legs. The defects resembled those of a rare genetic disorder known as phocomelia ("seal limb"). Following the tragic discovery that thalidomide is a potent teratogen (a substance that causes a birth defect), use of the drug was discontinued.

In recent years, however, it has been discovered that thalidomide may be a useful therapeutic agent in a number of conditions, including leprosy, several other dermatologic disorders, different types of cancer, and acquired immunodeficiency syndrome (AIDS). The Food and Drug Administration (FDA) in the United States has approved thalidomide for use in the treatment of leprosy. Studies have demonstrated that thalidomide can inhibit in vitro angiogenesis, the process of formation of new blood vessels. Since many types of cancers require development of new blood vessels for their continued growth, thalidomide may be especially useful in cases where conventional treatments have ceased to be effective. Its use may be indicated in patients either relapsing after high-dose chemotherapy or who are developing serious side effects and are not able to tolerate additional chemotherapy.

USES AND COMPLICATIONS

Since thalidomide is such a powerful angiogenesis inhibitor, it is being used in disorders requiring antiangiogenic therapy. Successful treatments have been made in cases of ovarian cancer, breast cancer, gastrointestinal carcinoma, renal melanoma, chronic graft-versus-host disease, and multiple myeloma. In some cases, the effectiveness of thalidomide increased when accompanied by other treatments, including immunotherapy, chemotherapy, and surgery.

Thalidomide appears to have few side effects in its new applications, but its return to medical respectability has raised again the specter of "thalidomide babies." Adverse effects noted in a few patients have included lethargy, constipation, and peripheral neuropathy. The potential problems associated with thalidomide causing a new round of severe birth defects may be a more serious consequence.

PERSPECTIVE AND PROSPECTS

The outbreak of thalidomide-related birth defects in the 1950's and 1960's led to the creation of birth defect surveillance programs in many countries. Unfortunately, medical standards and safeguards are not uniformly good, and there already appears to be an increase in birth defects associated with the new applications of thalidomide in South America. It will be necessary to regulate and to monitor closely the prescription, dispensing, and use of the drug. Counseling of patients of childbearing age will be an especially critical component if the tragedy of thalidomide's history is not to be repeated.

—*Donald J. Nash, Ph.D.*

See also Birth defects; Cancer; Leprosy; Pharmacology; Pregnancy and gestation; Teratogens.

FOR FURTHER INFORMATION:

Brynner, Rock, and Trent Stephens. *Dark Remedy: The Impact of Thalidomide and Its Revival as a Vital Medicine.* Cambridge, Mass.: Perseus, 2001.

Fanelli, M., et al. "Thalidomide: A New Anticancer Drug?" *Expert Opinion on Investigational Drugs* 12, no. 7 (July 2003): 1211-1225.

Patrias, Karen, Ronald L. Gordner, and Stephen C. Groft. *Thalidomide: Potential Benefits and Risks— January, 1963, Through July, 1997.* Bethesda, Md.: Department of Health and Human Services, 1998.

Perri, A. J., and S. Hsu. "A Review of Thalidomide's History and Current Dermatological Applications." *Dermatology Online Journal* 9, no. 3 (August, 2003): 5.

THORACIC SURGERY

SPECIALTY

ANATOMY OR SYSTEM AFFECTED: Chest, heart, lungs, respiratory system

SPECIALTIES AND RELATED FIELDS: Cardiology, general surgery, pulmonary medicine

DEFINITION: The branch of surgery that treats diseases of the chest cavity, especially the heart.

KEY TERMS:

aneurysm: a weakened segment of a heart or blood vessel

balloon catheterization: the use of a balloonlike device on the tip of a catheter to widen blood vessels

cardiac catheterization: the guidance of a catheter into the heart or great blood vessels to measure function, assess problems, and identify solutions

computed tomography (CT) scanning: the use of X-ray computer technology to identify diseases of hard and soft tissues, such as bone and the heart

echocardiography: the use of sound waves to examine heart structures

mitral valve: the valve between the heart's left auricle and ventricle

stenosis: the narrowing of heart valves or blood vessels

SCIENCE AND PROFESSION

The chest, or thorax, lies between the neck and the abdomen, from which it is separated by the diaphragm. Its side boundaries are the ribs and the muscle that surrounds them, which are attached to the spine and breastbone (sternum) in the back and front of the body, respectively. Overall, the thorax is cone-shaped, with its small and large ends bounded by the neck and diaphragm. Inside this airtight cavity, the lungs are suspended on the right and left sides, covered by the membranous pleura. Between the lungs is the heart, with its covering, the pericardium.

Also located in the chest cavity are the trachea (windpipe), which leads to the lungs; the esophagus, which connects the mouth and stomach; the major blood vessels that enter and leave the heart; and nerves. The chest cavity inflates and deflates as a result of diaphragm and rib muscle movement. This action provides the entry of oxygen to the blood that is circulated around the body through the cardiovascular system.

Thoracic surgeons, sometimes called cardiothoracic/cardiovascular and thoracic surgeons, handle a wide variety of surgery associated with these organs. Preeminent in many cases is surgery of the heart and major blood vessels. This precise, exacting surgery requires residency training of six years in general surgery and three years in thoracic surgery. In the United States, thoracic surgeons are certified by the American Board of Surgery and the American Board of Thoracic Surgery. Much of the time of thoracic surgeons is spent in hospitals working with critically ill patients whose lives depend on the prompt use of technical and demanding surgical techniques. Most patients are aged fifty-five to sixty-five.

DIAGNOSTIC AND TREATMENT TECHNIQUES

The diagnostic techniques associated with thoracic surgery are highly refined. They include careful patient histories, laboratory tests, and noninvasive techniques such as echocardiography, computed tomography (CT) scanning, electrocardiography (ECG or EKG), and other types of electrophysiology. Invasive procedures include cardiac catheterization and cineangiography of the heart and surrounding blood vessels with fiberoptic devices. Hence, cardiothoracic surgeons require extensive technical backup and wide expertise. After quick, careful assessment of all information obtained, surgery is carried out. Thoracic surgeons are noted for great surgical dexterity, scientific expertise, and logical, stepwise development of a complete picture that enables them to arrive rapidly at sensible decisions before and during surgery.

Entering the chest cavity, thoracotomy, is required for all thoracic surgery. Patients are given a general anesthetic and concurrently have heart and lung function replaced by a heart-lung machine, which oxygenates the blood and pumps it through the cardiovascular system.

Anterior thoracotomy is used to gain access to the heart and its coronary arteries. First, a vertical incision is made from between the collarbone to the lower end of the sternum, to which the ribs are attached. The sternum is divided with a bone saw and pried apart to expose the surgical area. After surgery, a drain is inserted into the chest, the sternum is wired together, and the muscle and skin are closed.

Lateral thoracotomy uses curved incisions made from between the shoulder blades and around the side of the trunk to just below a nipple. It provides access to the lungs and the great blood vessels. This technique is used by thoracic surgeons, general surgeons, and other specialists who perform lung surgery. After the incision is complete, the ribs are spread apart and surgery is performed. Closure is as with the anterior procedure.

Many different thoracic surgery procedures are carried out on heart and great blood vessels when medical and dietary treatments fail or in cases of congenital and traumatic problems. They can be divided into valve replacement, artery surgery, and heart transplantation. Once, bypass surgery was a major aspect of cardiothoracic surgery. Today, it has been largely replaced by balloon catheterization and related techniques carried out by other specialists.

Three types of important cardiothoracic surgery are heart valve replacement, aneurysm resection, and heart transplantation. Heart valve replacement may be necessitated by severe mitral valve damage, which causes mitral insufficiency or stenosis that can lead to heart failure and death. Aneurysms are weakened portions of the heart or great blood vessels. Heart aneurysms are caused by myocardial infarction (the death of parts of the heart muscle), yielding areas of weak, noncontractile scar tissue. Vessel aneurysms are caused by atherosclerosis or infectious disease. In extreme cases, aneurysms can rupture, and they are always painful and/or life-threatening. They are repaired by resection and replacement with graft materials such as Dacron or Teflon appliances. In the most severe cardiac problems, whole heart transplantation is needed using cadaver hearts. When this is not possible but the heart must be aided, ventricular assist pumps and artificial hearts can be connected temporarily.

PERSPECTIVE AND PROSPECTS

Thoracic surgery was first successful in the United States in the early twentieth century. Development of the New York Thoracic Surgical Society in 1917 began its acceptance as a medical specialty. In the 1930's, the *Journal of Thoracic Surgery* started to describe the area, and treatment methods evolved rapidly. Much impetus came from thoracic injuries that occurred during World War II. By the late 1940's, a Board of Thoracic Surgery was affiliated with the American Board of Surgery. In 1971, it became the independent American Board of Thoracic Surgery, which certifies thoracic surgeons. There are several thousand board-certified thoracic surgeons.

Some firsts in this field were the relief of mitral stenosis, by Elliott Cutler (1923); surgical intervention for cardiac aneurysm, by Ernst Sauerbruch (1931); the successful ligation of an arterial duct, by Robert Gross (1939); the development of a heart-lung machine for humans, by John Gibbon (1954); and the relief of congenital pulmonary defects, by Alfred Blalock (1954).

In current thoracic surgery, the treatment of coronary artery disease, once restricted to surgical bypass, has largely been replaced by techniques performed by cardiologists. Nevertheless, thoracic surgical procedures continue to improve, and the development of ever-better diagnostic tools and appliances is expected, such as a satisfactory artificial heart.

—Sanford S. Singer, Ph.D.

See also Aneurysmectomy; Aneurysms; Bypass surgery; Cardiac surgery; Cardiology; Cardiology, pediatric; Chest; Congenital heart disease; Heart; Heart disease; Heart transplantation; Heart valve replacement; Lung surgery; Lungs; Mitral valve prolapse; Pulmonary medicine; Pulmonary medicine, pediatric.

FOR FURTHER INFORMATION:

Beers, Mark H., et al., eds. *The Merck Manual of Diagnosis and Therapy.* 18th ed. Whitehouse Station, N.J.: Merck Research Laboratories, 2006. This is a reference work for physicians, and the nomenclature can be daunting. It is best consulted after more general introductory reading.

Crawford, Michael, ed. *Current Diagnosis and Treatment—Cardiology.* 3d ed. New York: McGraw-Hill

Medical, 2009. Discusses advances in cardiac diagnostics, treatments, and prognostic indicators and includes extensive information on prevention techniques.

Doherty, Gerard M., and Lawrence W. Way, eds. *Current Surgical Diagnosis and Treatment.* 12th ed. New York: Lange Medical Books/McGraw-Hill, 2006. A reference work on general surgery for physicians, this tome is nevertheless comprehensible to laypersons familiar with medical terminology. Presents succinct overviews of procedures and their potential complications; contains finely detailed illustrations.

Eagle, Kim A., and Ragavendra R. Baliga, eds. *Practical Cardiology: Evaluation and Treatment of Common Cardiovascular Disorders.* 2d ed. Philadelphia: Lippincott Williams & Wilkins, 2008. Details advances in cardiac medicine.

Gersh, Bernard J., ed. *The Mayo Clinic Heart Book.* 2d ed. New York: William Morrow, 2000. One of the most respected texts for laypeople on heart disease. Covers all aspects of anatomy, physiology, diagnosis, treatment, and prevention.

Pearson, F. Griffith, et al., eds. *Thoracic Surgery.* 2d ed. New York: Churchill Livingstone, 2002. Discusses diagnostic tests, surgical techniques, and research advances.

Taylor, Anita D. *How to Choose a Medical Specialty.* 4th ed. New York: Elsevier, 1999. Gives a useful description of many medical specialties. Included are information on residency and certification and on the economics of various types of practice, a personal suitability self-examination, and references.

THROAT. *See* ESOPHAGUS; PHARYNX.

THROAT, SORE. *See* SORE THROAT.

THROMBOCYTOPENIA

DISEASE/DISORDER

ANATOMY OR SYSTEM AFFECTED: Blood, circulatory system, liver, spleen

SPECIALTIES AND RELATED FIELDS: Hematology

DEFINITION: A bleeding disorder in which the blood contains an abnormally low count of functional platelets (thrombocytes).

KEY TERMS:

corticosteroids: a family of adrenal cortex steroids used medically as anti-inflammatory agents

hemorrhage: profuse blood loss from the vessels

megakaryocytes: cells that produce platelets in the bone marrow

petechiae: a skin rash of pinpoint purplish-red spots

platelets: small, disk-shaped cells that circulate in the blood and whose function is to take part in the clotting process; platelets store many molecules inside and on their surface that cause them to stick to one another and to the walls of injured blood vessels

CAUSES AND SYMPTOMS

Thrombocytopenia occurs when platelets are lost from the circulation faster than they can be replaced by the bone marrow where they are produced. It may result from either a deficiency in platelet production or an increased clearance rate from the blood. Clinically, thrombocytopenia is defined as a platelet count less than the normal levels of 150,000 to 350,000 per microliter of blood.

There are several specific causes of thrombocytopenia. In artefactual thrombocytopenia, antibodies in a person's blood cause platelets to stick together and cause a falsely low platelet count. In congenital thrombocytopenia, one of several rare genetic diseases causes low platelet counts. Another cause of thrombocytopenia is impaired platelet production, such as in leukemia or lymphoma, where the number of some other cell type in the bone marrow is increased, leaving fewer megakaryocytes for platelet production. Alternatively, the rate of platelet destruction can be increased as in disseminated intravascular coagulation (DIC), in which the blood clotting process is inappropriately activated. Antibodies in the blood, produced because of infections such as human immunodeficiency virus (HIV) or rheumatoid arthritis, can cause platelet removal. Idiopathic or immunologic thrombocytopenic purpura (ITP) causes thrombocytopenia through destruction of platelets by the patient's immune system. Thrombocytopenia can also be attributable to an abnormal distribution of platelets, as when platelets are sequestered in a patient's enlarged spleen. Thrombotic thrombocytopenic purpura (TTP) is a disease resulting in thrombocytopenia. Platelets clump together in areas of clots to the extent that there are fewer platelets in other parts of the body. Finally, a massive transfusion of red blood cells can dilute platelets to thrombocytopenic levels.

Thrombocytopenia can cause excess bleeding and thus has several notable symptoms. Petechiae, rashes, and frequent bruising can appear on the skin, provoked by minor injury or pressure. Bleeding from wounds or body cavities may occur. At extremely low platelet

---

INFORMATION ON THROMBOCYTOPENIA

CAUSES: Platelet deficiency or increased clearance from blood; may result from autoimmune response, genetic defect, infection, diseases such as leukemia, lymphoma, disseminated intravascular coagulation

SYMPTOMS: Petechiae; rashes; frequent bruising; bleeding from wounds or body cavities; spontaneous bleeding; spleen and liver enlargement; blood in stool, urine, vomit, or sputum; anemia, fatigue; elevated heart rate

DURATION: Chronic

TREATMENTS: Depends on cause; may include red blood cell or platelet transfusion, platelet growth factor

---

counts, those below 20,000 per microliter, spontaneous bleeding occurs. The spleen and liver may be enlarged and sensitive to the touch if the thrombocytopenia is caused by splenic activity. Impaired clotting may cause blood to appear in the stool, urine, vomit, or sputum. Thrombocytopenic patients may also experience anemia, feel fatigued, or exhibit an elevated heart rate.

Low platelet counts increase the risk of bleeding, which becomes particularly dangerous when the count falls below 10,000 per microliter. Bleeding from the nose and gums is quite common. Serious hemorrhage can occur at the retina in the back of the eye, threatening vision. The most critical bleeding complication posing a risk to life is spontaneous bleeding in the head or in the lining of the gut.

TREATMENT AND THERAPY

The primary treatment for thrombocytopenia is to address the underlying cause of the deficiency. This is not always possible. If significant blood loss has occurred, then red blood cell or platelet transfusion may be necessary. However, in the condition of thrombotic thrombocytopenia purpura, the use of platelet concentrates is quite hazardous. Platelet growth factor can be used to stimulate increased platelet production in the bone marrow. Additionally, certain drugs such as aspirin and ibuprofen are to be avoided since they are known to cause antiplatelet activity.

If an infection is suspected as the cause of thrombocytopenia, then treatment such as antibiotics for the specific infection is often initiated. Some viral infections such as glandular fever caused by Epstein-Barr virus have no specific treatment, and only close monitoring is applied. If the thrombocytopenia is caused by the presence of cancer cells in the bone marrow, then treatment such as chemotherapy or radiotherapy is directed at the abnormal cells. In such cases, the bone marrow may become damaged and blood platelet counts further lowered. Platelet transfusions are then given to prevent bleeding, until either the platelet count reaches acceptable levels or the bone marrow recovers its ability to produce sufficient numbers of platelets.

PERSPECTIVE AND PROSPECTS

Prior to the development of plasma exchange as an effective treatment in the 1970's, the mortality from thrombotic thrombocytopenic purpura-hemolytic uremic syndrome (TTP-HUS) was 90 percent. During those times, diagnosis was made using five clinical observations, including thrombocytopenia and fever. The availability of effective plasma exchange treatment has lowered the mortality rate to 20 percent. Early diagnosis is important, with thrombocytopenia and one other criterion the only requirements for initiation of treatment since 1991.

At the start of the twenty-first century, the treatment of children with idiopathic or immunologic thrombocytopenic purpura remained controversial. Platelet counts can be increased by treatment with corticosteroids, but clinical outcomes may not improve. Because most children spontaneously recover from severe thrombocytopenia in several days to weeks, only supportive care is sometimes recommended in this case.

—*Michael R. King, Ph.D.*

See also Bleeding; Blood and blood disorders; Bone marrow transplantation; Hematology; Hematology, pediatric; Plasma; Transfusion; Wiskott-Aldrich syndrome.

FOR FURTHER INFORMATION:

Cattaneo, M. "Inherited Platelet-Based Bleeding Disorders." *Journal of Thrombosis and Haemostasis* 1, no. 7 (July, 2003): 1628-1636.
Chong, B. H. "Heparin-Induced Thrombocytopenia." *Journal of Thrombosis and Haemostasis* 1, no. 7 (July, 2003): 1471-1478.
George, J. N. "Platelets." *The Lancet* 355, no. 9214 (April 29, 2000): 1531-1539.
Goldstein, K. H., et al. "Efficient Diagnosis of Thrombocytopenia." *American Family Physician* 53, no. 3 (February 15, 1996): 915-920.
McCrae, Keith R., ed. *Thrombocytopenia.* New York: Taylor & Francis, 2006.
Reid, T. J., et al. "Platelet Substitutes in the Management of Thrombocytopenia." *Current Hematology Reports* 2, no. 2 (March, 2003): 165-170.
Warkentin, Theodore E., and Andreas Greinacher, eds. *Heparin-Induced Thrombocytopenia.* 4th rev. ed. New York: Marcel Dekker, 2007.

THROMBOLYTIC THERAPY AND TPA
TREATMENT

ANATOMY OR SYSTEM AFFECTED: Blood, blood vessels, circulatory system, heart, lungs, nervous system, respiratory system

SPECIALTIES AND RELATED FIELDS: Cardiology, critical care, emergency medicine, hematology, pharmacology, pulmonary medicine, vascular medicine

DEFINITION: The use of drugs to dissolve blood clots blocking an artery or vein (often in the heart, lungs, or brain); TPA is one of the best thrombolytic agents and is frequently administered to patients experiencing heart attacks.

KEY TERMS:

embolism: the blockage of an artery by matter (such as a blood clot) that has broken off from another area

fibrinolysis: the breakdown of fibrin, a major component of blood clots, that occurs after the broken vessel wall has healed; fibrinolytic agents are used to dissolve unwanted clots

hemostasis: a physiological response that arrests bleeding; involves the constriction of the injured blood vessel, the clumping of platelets to form a plug, and the activation of blood-clotting elements such as fibrin

occlusion: the blockage of any vessel in the body, which may be caused by a thrombus or other embolus

plasmin: an enzyme present in the blood that can dissolve clots; plasmin is normally found in its inactive form, plasminogen, until needed

platelets: specialized blood-clotting particles that travel in the blood and become sticky when they come in contact with a damaged blood vessel

thromboembolism: the blockage of a blood vessel by a fragment that has broken off from a thrombus in another blood vessel

thrombolytic drugs: a group of drugs that dissolve blood clots by increasing the level of plasmin in the blood

thrombus: a blood clot that has formed inside an intact blood vessel; a thrombus can be life-threatening if it occludes a vessel that supplies the heart or brain

tissue plasminogen activator (TPA or tPA): a substance produced by the body to prevent abnormal blood clots by stimulating the formation of plasmin from plasminogen; can also be administered to dissolve blood clots

PHYSIOLOGY OF BLOOD CLOT FORMATION

In an undamaged, healthy blood vessel, blood flows smoothly past the lining of the vessel wall. If a blood vessel wall breaks or there is damage to its lining, however, a complex series of biochemical reactions occurs to stop the flow of blood. The blood vessel spasms (vascular spasm), platelets in the bloodstream clump together to form a plug, and proteins form to cause the blood to clot (coagulate). This process is rapid, localized to the area of injury, and carefully controlled. It involves many clotting factors normally present in blood, as well as specialized clotting particles called platelets and some substances that are released by the injured tissues.

The most immediate response to a blood vessel injury is vasoconstriction, a narrowing of a blood vessel. Vasoconstriction decreases the diameter of a vessel, resulting in a decreased flow of blood at the site of damage. Some factors that cause vascular spasm include direct injury, chemicals released by the cells that line a vessel wall, platelets, and nervous reflexes. When the cells that line the interior wall of a blood vessel are damaged, platelets are attracted to the site. They then swell and become sticky. The platelets adhere to the damaged area and release chemicals called prostaglandins, which attract more platelets to the area. Aspirin, in relatively low doses, is an effective inhibitor of prostaglandin synthesis and therefore an excellent therapy for some individuals who are susceptible to inappropriate blood clotting. The vascular spasm and platelet plug help to stop the bleeding at the injury site. Blood-clotting proteins must be activated, however, in order to seal the damaged area of the blood vessel completely.

Once the platelet plug is formed, coagulation is triggered. Several clotting proteins are produced by the liver and released in their inactive form to the blood. Bacteria within the intestinal tract are responsible for synthesizing vitamin K, which is essential for normal production of the clotting proteins by the liver. Vitamin K is absorbed by intestinal blood vessels and transported to the liver.

The mechanism by which clotting proteins are activated is called a cascade. First, a substance called prothrombin activator is formed. Prothrombin activator converts a protein in the plasma called prothrombin into thrombin, which in turn converts another plasma protein, fibrinogen, into fibrin. Fibrin molecules then combine to form a loose meshwork that fills in the gaps between the cells of the platelet plug, preventing blood loss at the site of injury.

A clot is not meant to be a permanent solution. If the clot completely occludes, or stops the flow of blood to, a tissue, the tissue may die. A process called fibrinolysis removes clots that are no longer needed. Because small clots are continually formed in vessels throughout the body, clot dissolution is essential to reestablishing normal blood flow. Without fibrinolysis, blood vessels would gradually become completely occluded.

One essential component of this natural clot-reducing process is the enzyme plasmin, which is produced when the blood protein plasminogen is activated. A large amount of plasminogen, which binds to fibrin, is incorporated into a blood clot. The plasminogen remains inactive until it receives appropriate signals. Healing of the blood vessel and surrounding tissues will cause the release of a substance called tissue plasminogen activator (TPA or tPA). TPA then converts the plasminogen in the clot to plasmin. It is plasmin that breaks down the fibrin, and thus the clot, through fibrinolysis. Enzymes will quickly destroy any plasmin that escapes into the general circulation. Therefore, most of the fibrinolytic effect of plasmin occurs within the clot itself.

It is important to note that once a clot begins to form, something must limit its growth. A clot that is allowed to grow uncontrollably would eventually fill up all the vessels in the body. Several factors regulate the extent of clot formation. Any tendency toward clot formation in rapidly moving blood is usually unsuccessful because the activated coagulation factors are diluted and washed away, preventing them from accumulating to a concentration necessary for clotting. The second mechanism restricting clot formation is that as a clot forms, almost all the thrombin produced is absorbed into the fibrin. Therefore, fibrin effectively acts as an anticoagulant to prevent enlargement of the clot by holding onto thrombin so that it cannot act elsewhere. Any thrombin that escapes is bound by a substance in the blood called antithrombin III. Antithrombin III can be activated by a substance called heparin, a natural anticoagulant produced by some white blood cells and other undamaged cells that line blood vessels. Heparin acts to inhibit thrombin activity, and thus clotting, by stimulating antithrombin III.

Additional factors prevent clotting in undamaged blood vessels. The factors that normally ward off unnecessary clotting include both structural and chemical characteristics of the lining of blood vessels. As long as the cells lining the vessels remain undamaged, there is no vasospasm, no platelet plug forms, and no clot results. The cells on the wall lining can repel platelets using specialized chemicals on their surfaces. They also secrete heparin and a substance known as prostacyclin, both of which prevent platelet activation.

Despite the body's protective mechanisms to prevent inappropriate blood clots, clotting sometimes does occur. A clot that forms in an undamaged vessel is called a thrombus. If the thrombus is large, it may block blood flow to the tissue beyond the occlusion and starve the tissue to death. This starvation process is called ischemia, and the result is infarction, or cell death. A relatively common site for a thrombus to occlude a vessel is in the heart..If the blockage occurs in a coronary artery, a vessel that supplies the heart with blood, the consequences may be death of this tissue and even death of the affected individual.

A thrombus (or any other type of matter, such as lipids) that breaks away from a vessel and floats freely in the bloodstream is called an embolus. An embolus becomes a problem if it enters a blood vessel that is too narrow for it to pass through. For example, emboli that become trapped in a blood vessel going to the lungs can significantly alter an individual's ability to obtain oxygen. An embolus that occludes a vessel feeding the brain will cause a stroke.

What would cause a clot to form in the body when there is no trauma to a vessel? Several factors are known to cause clot formation even when there is no bleeding. Anything that causes the lining of a blood vessel to become roughened or irregular will allow platelets to gain a foothold and cling to the vessel wall, starting the clotting process.

Arteriosclerosis, in which there is an abnormal accumulation of fatty plaques in the wall of an artery, and blood vessel inflammation are the most common causes of irregularities in the lining of blood vessels. Anything that causes the flow of blood to slow and pool enhances clot formation. In this case, clotting factors are not washed away and diluted, so they tend to accumulate until their concentrations are high enough to initiate clotting. Conditions in which this may occur include atrial fibrillation, aneurysms, and varicose veins. Atrial fibrillation is the abnormally rapid beating of the upper chambers (atria) of the heart. Because the contractions that normally force blood into the lower chambers (ventricles) are inefficient, blood pools and clots may form. Aneurysms occur when there is a weakening of an artery wall. This causes the blood vessel wall to bulge out and form a pocket where blood can pool. Thus, aneurysms provide a potential site for inappropriate clotting. Varicose veins are relatively common and usually occur in the veins returning blood from the legs. When the valves in a vein weaken, the flow of returning blood slows and the vein swells. As a result, clotting factors may accumulate in the vein and be returned to the heart or forced into the lungs.

INDICATIONS AND PROCEDURES

If inappropriate clotting occurs in blood vessels supplying critical tissues, such as the brain, heart, lungs, or kidneys, the resulting tissue damage can be debilitating or even life-threatening. Fortunately, physicians have a few options in treating patients with clotting problems.

A blood clot in the arteries supplying oxygen and nutrients to the heart can cause numerous symptoms. Sudden pain, pressure, squeezing, and fullness in the chest that last longer than fifteen minutes may indicate a heart attack. The pain may be excruciating; it may also be mild, resembling heartburn or indigestion. In general, the elderly tend to have less pain during a heart attack. Heart attack pain does not go away with rest and may radiate across the chest to the shoulders (usually on the left side), neck, arms, jaw, or even the middle of the back. Because the pumping mechanism and efficiency of the heart have been impaired, patients often feel dizzy or light-headed. They may even faint, become nauseated or vomit, have difficulty breathing, or begin to sweat.

A number of drugs are used to prevent undesirable clotting in persons at risk for a heart attack. Aspirin is a common drug whose action blocks the production of chemicals called prostaglandins, which cause platelets to adhere to one another. Heparin helps to prevent clot formation. Warfarin is a drug that interferes with the action of vitamin K in the formation of clotting proteins. If a clot has already formed, some drugs are available that will dissolve clots, including TPA, streptokinase, and urokinase. These drugs are known as thrombolytic agents and are often administered in an emergency room to people experiencing heart attacks.

In 2003, researchers announced a breakthrough in

the treatment of persons prone to blood clots. Since the 1950's, warfarin has been given to patients for a period of three to six months. Studies showed an increased risk of severe bleeding with longer use of warfarin, thus preempting its use after six months. However, without warfarin, nearly one-third of patients will form another blood clot within eight years. The 2003 findings showed that after several months of full doses of warfarin, moderate doses of the medicine can follow and can reduce the risk of further clots without introducing the risk of hemorrhage.

The time period for which thrombolytic agents are effective is relatively brief; the sooner these drugs are given, the greater is the benefit. To be effective, these potent drugs must be given before irreversible damage occurs. For heart attack victims, this means within six hours after the onset of symptoms. Most studies indicate that thrombolytic therapy can be given safely and effectively before heart attack victims reach the emergency room and that early treatment reduces the likelihood of death. Therefore, it is important for individuals to contact a physician or emergency medical team promptly after experiencing suspicious symptoms that may indicate a heart attack.

USES AND COMPLICATIONS

Most patients who are thought to be experiencing a heart attack are given TPA or streptokinase intravenously to reverse or at least halt damage. Like all drugs, however, the thrombolytic agents have potentially adverse effects. Because these medications can increase bleeding, patients are not given thrombolytic therapy if they are at high risk for hemorrhage (abnormal bleeding). Some of the factors that may increase the risk of bleeding include surgery within the past six weeks, severe hypertension, diabetic eye disease, recent head trauma, recent stroke, stomach or duodenal ulcers, or recent cardiopulmonary resuscitation.

If the thrombolytic drug is administered and bleeding becomes a significant problem, a drug called aminocaproic acid can be used to help correct the problem. Aminocaproic acid inhibits the thrombolytic effects of TPA, streptokinase, and urokinase by preventing their action and inhibiting plasmin. In lifethreatening situations, the physician may have to give the patient blood transfusions or fibrinogen infusions to reverse the effects of thrombolysis. The adverse effects of thrombolytic agents are relatively rare, however, and should not discourage physicians from the appropriate use of these agents.

Thrombolytic therapy is used in nearly 300,000 patients in the United States each year. Tissue plasminogen activator is the fastest-acting thrombolytic agent. It is produced naturally in the body but can be manufactured in large amounts using genetic engineering techniques. Streptokinase, on the other hand, is produced by bacteria and at about one-tenth the cost of TPA. When these two thrombolytic agents were compared in 41,000 heart attack patients, TPA showed a slightly better effectiveness. In a one-month follow-up study, researchers found that there were 14 percent fewer deaths among heart attack patients given TPA and intravenous heparin (to help keep blood clots from reforming) than among heart attack patients treated with streptokinase and heparin.

In addition to their use as therapeutic agents for heart attacks, thrombolytic drugs are also used to treat abnormal blood clots in the blood vessels of the lungs. These clots, known as pulmonary emboli, usually originate in a leg vein, a condition called venous thrombosis. Part or all of the thrombus breaks away, forms an embolus, and travels to the heart, which then pumps it into the pulmonary arteries. If the embolus is large enough to block the main pulmonary artery leading from the heart to the lungs, or if there are many clots, the condition can be life-threatening. Pulmonary embolism is responsible for more than 50,000 deaths in the United States each year.

The symptoms that a patient may experience depend on the size of the obstructing clot. If an embolus is so large that it blocks the main pulmonary artery, an affected individual will die. Smaller emboli may cause severe shortness of breath, rapid heart rate, dizziness, sharp chest pains when breathing, and coughing up of blood.

Physicians treat pulmonary emboli with similar medical therapy as that used for heart attacks. Anticoagulant drugs such as heparin and warfarin are usually administered to reduce the clotting ability of the blood and to reduce the chance of more clots occurring. Thrombolytic agents, including urokinase and streptokinase, can also be used to destroy the clot in much the same way that they are used in heart attack victims.

The third major use of thrombolytic agents is to clear intravenous catheters of blood clots. A catheter may be placed into a person's vein if health care workers need to draw frequent blood samples or administer drugs at frequent intervals. Because the catheter is in direct contact with the blood, it is a site for potential clot formation. Urokinase can be used to reopen an occluded catheter.

PERSPECTIVE AND PROSPECTS

Each year 1.2 million Americans experience a heart attack. An attack lasts longer than most people realize. It is actually a four to six-hour process that starts when one of the arteries supplying the heart muscle becomes blocked, usually by a blood clot. The pain that one experiences is partially attributable to a cramping of the heart muscle from lack of oxygen and an accumulation of waste products. As a result, heart muscle is destroyed, which interferes with the heart's function. If the amount of muscle destruction is severe, it can lead to the patient's death.

Studies show that individuals treated within one to two hours of the onset of heart attack symptoms have significantly less heart damage than those treated later. Yet, half of all heart attack patients wait more than two hours before getting medical attention. The American Heart Association estimates that 300,000 Americans die of heart attacks each year before reaching a hospital. This number could be greatly reduced if people responded more quickly to the symptoms of a heart attack.

Recent studies have shown that women are even less likely to receive initial medical care within the required four to six-hour time interval. Women frequently see to other responsibilities such as child or elder care before seeking medical help. Many women believe the myth that they are not likely to have a heart attack. This is true before the menopause, but, within five years of the menopause, women have the same risk of heart attacks as men. In addition, physicians are more likely to misdiagnose heart attack symptoms in women, attributing them to anxiety or stress.

The goal in treating a heart attack is to stop it and, if possible, reverse the clotting process. Treatment with thrombolytic agents helps to minimize or even reverse the damage to heart tissue. As with most diseases, however, it is better to prevent heart attacks entirely. Individuals who exercise regularly, who eat a diet relatively low in fat, and who do not smoke have a low incidence of heart attacks and may never need drug therapy to unclog their arteries. Yet, it is comforting to know that these agents are available if the need ever arises.

Because of the success of thrombolytic agents in the treatment of coronary artery disease, these agents are also being tried in patients showing early symptoms of stroke. Strokes and heart attacks occur for similar reasons. In a stroke, blood clots in the arteries that supply the brain prevent the delivery of oxygen and nutrients to the sensitive nerve cells and cause an accumulation of waste products. As a result, these sensitive brain cells die. As in heart attack treatment, timing is critical. In heart attack patients, agents that dissolve clots work best when given within six hours after the onset of symptoms. For stroke patients, it appears that treatment with a thrombolytic drug must begin within three hours to have maximal effectiveness. Therefore, awareness of the early symptoms of stroke is even more important. These symptoms develop rapidly and depend on the region of the brain that is damaged. Some common symptoms include muscle weakness, loss of touch sensations, speech disturbances, and visual disturbances.

If thrombolytic agents are found to be effective in treating strokes, up to 80 percent of all stroke victims may be helped. As with heart attack patients, these drugs cannot be used in stroke patients with hemorrhagic (bleeding) strokes or other disorders in which the risk of bleeding is greater than the potential benefits from such therapy.

—Matthew Berria, Ph.D.;
L. Fleming Fallon, Jr., M.D., Ph.D., M.P.H.;
updated by Bradley R. A. Wilson, Ph.D.

See also Angiography; Angioplasty; Arteriosclerosis; Bleeding; Blood and blood disorders; Blood vessels; Brain; Bypass surgery; Cardiac arrest; Cardiology; Catheterization; Circulation; Echocardiography; Embolism; Emergency medicine; Endarterectomy; Enzymes; Heart; Heart attack; Heart disease; Heart valve replacement; Hematology; Ischemia; Lungs; Pharmacology; Pulmonary medicine; Strokes; Thrombosis and thrombus; Transient ischemic attacks (TIAs); Varicosis; Vascular medicine; Vascular system.

FOR FURTHER INFORMATION:

American Medical Association. *American Medical Association Family Medical Guide.* 4th rev. ed. Hoboken, N.J.: John Wiley & Sons, 2004. Updated, understandable medical information about various diseases including stroke.

Bick, Roger L. *Disorders of Thrombosis and Hemostasis: Clinical and Laboratory Practice.* 3d ed. Philadelphia: Lippincott Williams & Wilkins, 2002. An excellent introduction to the diagnosis and management of clotting and bleeding disorders.

Hales, Dianne. *An Invitation to Health Brief.* Updated ed. Belmont, Calif.: Wadsworth/Cengage Learning, 2010. This book is recommended for anyone who wishes an overview of health topics. Several chapters deal with the function of the heart and how lifestyles influence its health. Covers cardiovascular disease and includes a description of thrombolytic and surgical therapy modalities for helping heart attack patients.

Katzung, Bertram G., et al., eds. *Basic and Clinical Pharmacology.* 11th ed. New York: McGraw-Hill, 2009. This well-written text provides detailed information about thrombolytic and anticoagulant agents. It discusses usage of these drugs, as well as their adverse effects and contraindications.

Loscalzo, Joseph, and Andrew I. Schafer, eds. *Thrombosis and Hemorrhage.* 3d ed. Philadelphia: Lippincott Williams & Wilkins, 2003. Covers an array of relevant topics including the basic elements of hemostasis, the normal function and response of platelets, and specific clinical disorders and laboratory approaches, thrombotic disorders, and management of patients with hemorrhagic and thrombotic conditions.

McCance, Kathryn L., and Sue M. Huether. *Pathophysiology: The Biologic Basis for Disease in Adults and Children.* 6th ed. St. Louis, Mo.: Mosby/Elsevier, 2010. This book contains a comprehensive presentation of diseases, symptoms, and treatments. The authors have done an excellent job of tying together basic physiological principles with the pathology of various organ systems.

THROMBOSIS AND THROMBUS
DISEASE/DISORDER

ANATOMY OR SYSTEM AFFECTED: Blood, blood vessels, brain, circulatory system, head, heart, lungs, respiratory system

SPECIALTIES AND RELATED FIELDS: Cardiology, hematology, internal medicine, vascular medicine

DEFINITION: Thrombosis is an abnormal blood condition in which blood cells called thrombocytes (platelets) produce clots that move through the bloodstream and eventually clog blood vessels; a thrombus is such a clot.

KEY TERMS:

artery: a blood vessel that transports blood away from the heart to the cells and tissues of the body

clot: a clumping of platelets, blood, fibrin, and clotting factors that normally accumulates in damaged tissue as part of the body's healing process

embolus: an object, air bubble, or other material moving through the bloodstream that is capable of creating a blockage to circulation

fibrin: a critical protein produced by platelets during the clotting process in bleeding, damaged tissue; the fibrin seals openings in damaged blood vessels

myocardial infarction: a condition in which the blood and oxygen supply to the cells of the heart muscle is cut off, thereby causing heart cell death; commonly called a heart attack

shock: a situation in which the body or a region of the body is not receiving an adequate supply of blood and oxygen, thereby leading to collapse of the organism

thrombocytes: white blood cells that secrete the proteins thrombin and fibrin in response to chemical signals from damaged tissue in the body; also called platelets

thrombus: an abnormal clumping of platelets and platelet proteins that moves through the bloodstream and may act as an embolus to block circulation through key arteries

vein: a blood vessel which returns blood to the heart from various regions of the body

CAUSES AND SYMPTOMS

Clotting is a critical process in the maintenance of damaged bodily tissue and the prevention of blood loss leading to conditions of shock within the organism. Shock involves the disorientation and collapse of major organ systems within the body when excessive blood has been lost; it can be fatal if it is not treated immediately.

When the body is damaged from a cut or other breach of the body's epithelial and connective tissue defense layers in the skin, chemical signals called chemoattractants stimulate a white blood cell type called a thrombocyte to secrete proteins, leading to the sealing of the damaged tissue region. Thrombocytes, also called platelets, are versatile cells floating in the approximately 10 to 12 liters of blood flowing through roughly 100,000 kilometers of blood vessels within the average human body. There are roughly 500,000 thrombocytes per cubic millimeter of blood. Their clotting response to tissue damage is rapid and efficient, although very intricate in the chemical signaling between cells.

Once activated by alarmones, emergency chemical-signaling hormones released from the damaged tissue, the thrombocytes are activated to respond at the site of tissue damage. Each thrombocyte releases the proteins thrombin and fibrinogen. The thrombin modifies the fibrinogen to produce fibrin, the principal sealant protein for the damaged region. The fibrin is secreted massively from thousands of thrombocytes within only a few minutes of the initial tissue damage. Fibrin protein is put down by the cells in intricately connected layers from the outer edges of the tissue damage progressively inward, eventually forming a plug.

Following the sealing of the damaged tissue by the clotting thrombocytes, other white blood cells of the immune system, called leukocytes, move into the region to immobilize and destroy contaminating bacteria and viruses, as well as to break down damaged cells. Surrounding healthy cells initiate mitotic cell divisions to grow into the damaged region, thereby regenerating the missing tissue. White blood cells such as leukocytes and thrombocytes are termed "white" because they do not produce hemoglobin and hence are not "red." The two white blood cell types work intricately in the maintenance of body tissue primary defense layers.

When the clotting process of thrombocytes and other related cells does not occur properly, problems can arise. Normally, a clot will form at a breach in a blood vessel, whether that vessel is an artery carrying blood away from the heart to the body or a vein returning blood to the heart from the body. Abnormal clotting of thrombocytes and fibrin proteins, however, can form masses that break off from a blood clot and float through the bloodstream. Such a floating blood clot is called a thrombus.

A thrombus is a type of embolism, an object that floats through the bloodstream and can cause a blockage in small arteries, veins, and capillaries. Emboli can be pockets of air or solid clots such as thrombi. Both air emboli and thrombus emboli can cause serious blockages of important vessels supplying blood to particular body regions. As a thrombus or other embolus flows along with blood, it will eventually float through a vessel that becomes progressively smaller in diameter. The

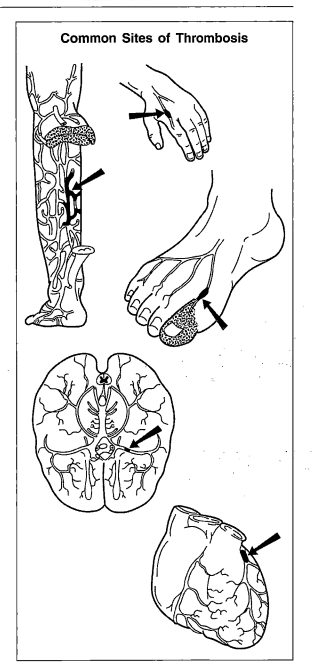

Common Sites of Thrombosis

INFORMATION ON THROMBOSIS AND THROMBUS

CAUSES: Heart attacks, strokes, blood-clotting abnormalities, compromised immune system, bone marrow abnormalities, phlebitis (from surgery or prolonged confinement)

SYMPTOMS: Sudden pain or tenderness along course of vein, skin discoloration, swelling and edema below obstruction, rapid pulse, mild fever

DURATION: Acute

TREATMENTS: Anticoagulants, compression stockings

---

thrombus blocks the vessel so that nothing can pass any farther through it—not the thrombus, not blood, and not the oxygen and nutrients within the blood.

As a result, cells downstream from the blockage will be starved for essential oxygen, sugar, and other nutrients necessary for carrying out the cellular chemical reactions of life. Most cells have only about a ten-minute supply of chemical and oxygen reserves needed for life. These cells depend on a continuous supply of blood to provide oxygen, sugar, and other nutrients and to carry away carbon dioxide and other waste products. The blood clot occludes the artery going to a cell region, thereby preventing blood flow and causing the death of these cells. In many parts of the body, these dead cells cannot be replaced, particularly within the heart, brain, and spinal cord.

The existence of thrombi within the circulatory system is a serious medical condition known as thrombosis. The five principal types of thrombi are agonal, ball, hyaline, laminated, and white thrombi. An agonal thrombus is a type of blood clot that forms from clumping blood cells when a person is dying. A ball thrombus is a spherically shaped blood clot composed of platelets, red blood cells, and fibrin. A hyaline thrombus is a mass of depigmented, hemoglobinless, clumped red blood cells. A laminated thrombus is an array of clumped cell types accumulated at differing times, creating a snowball effect. A white thrombus is a clump of leukocytes of varying types. Regardless of type, all thrombi can seriously impede efficient blood flow and thereby contribute to localized cellular and tissue death, damage that is often irreparable.

Two of the most serious cases of localized cellular and tissue death brought about by thrombi are myocardial infarctions and strokes. A myocardial infarction, also called a heart attack, occurs when the muscular layer of cells within the heart (the myocardium) is starved for oxygen and nutrients, and dies, because of a blockage to one of the branches of the coronary arteries supplying blood to the heart. If only a small branch of the coronary artery is blocked by a thrombus or other occlusion, then only a few hundred myocardial cells will die and the heart attack will be mild.

If the thrombus blockage is to a major coronary artery, however, then many thousands of cells in the myocardium will die, and a major heart attack will occur. It should be emphasized that the death of myocardial cells is permanent; they cannot be replaced. Therefore, a thrombus-induced heart attack causes permanent death of a region of heart muscle, whether large or small. In many cases, the heart attack is so severe that the normal, rhythmic contraction of the heart is disrupted, thereby leading to cardiac arrest and death.

In the same manner, a stroke, also called a cerebrovascular accident, occurs when an artery transporting blood to a region of brain cells is blocked by a thrombus or other embolus. Brain cells downstream from the blockage are starved for oxygen and nutrients; they die within minutes. If a small artery or capillary is blocked,

only a few brain cells will die and the stroke will be minimal, perhaps not even noticeable to the individual. It is possible that many people have such "microstrokes" repeatedly during the course of their lives, although the effects of these small strokes are cumulative over time. Decreased and impaired neurological and motor functioning throughout the body ensue from damaged brain regions in stroke victims.

If the thrombus-induced blockage is to an artery supplying blood to a large brain cell region, however, then millions of brain cells will die. The stroke is severe, perhaps deadly, if the affected brain region is essential for certain bodily life processes. If the severe stroke victim survives, then the effects will be noticeable as sluggish neuromuscular motor activity on the opposite side of the body from the affected brain region. Heart attacks and strokes are manifestations of the same problem: arteries occluded by thrombi and other emboli.

TREATMENT AND THERAPY

Thrombosis is a problem of major concern for the physician facing patients with certain types of medical conditions and patients who recently have had major internal surgery. Furthermore, individuals with blood-clotting abnormalities, compromised immune systems, and bone marrow abnormalities also are prone to forming thrombi and other solid emboli. Phlebitis is an inflammation of a vein brought about by surgery, prolonged confinement to bed, or prolonged sitting, in which blood clots form in deep veins, a condition called deep vein thrombosis (DVT). These blood clots can break off and flow through the general blood circulation, eventually clogging an artery or vein leading to a critical bodily region.

Consequently, thrombi and thrombosis are of major concern to medical doctors because they represent potential complications and side effects from other medical conditions and certain needed surgical treatments. People who have had abdominal or pelvic surgery (such as the removal of certain organs such as the spleen and portions of the stomach because of cancer) or individuals who have been bedridden with leg fractures are prone to forming thrombi and emboli.

The elderly are particularly prone to thrombi because of the gradual decline of the immune system and the breakdown of bone development that accompany the aging process. Moreover, the natural chemical substances in the blood that dissolve floating blood clots are not as prevalent in the elderly. As a result, more cases of thrombi are seen in elderly patients, particularly individuals above the age of seventy.

Once thrombi and other solid emboli have formed, they may float for a long time through an individual's blood vessels. They usually can pass through the heart unimpeded without causing any serious disruptions of cardiac rhythm. Occasionally, large thrombi can become lodged in one of the four valves of the heart, creating an occlusion and triggering a heart attack, but this is very rare. More commonly, the thrombi become trapped in the general circulation in progressively smaller arteries and capillaries going to a localized tissue region.

Within the body, oxygenated blood leaves the left ventricle of the heart through the largest artery in the body, the aorta, and subsequently branches and subbranches through thousands of successively smaller arteries, arterioles, and capillaries until reaching each of the quadrillion cells of the body. These cells extract oxygen and nutrients from the blood and deposit carbon dioxide and waste products into the bloodstream. Small capillaries combine to produce small venules that combine to produce small veins, which in turn combine into larger veins. These veins eventually come together into the inferior and superior vena cavae, returning blood to the right atrium of the heart for eventual delivery to the lungs. Once in the heart, blood flows from the right atrium to the right ventricle and then through the pulmonary arteries branching to the tissues of the lungs, where the blood is oxygenated through breathing. Oxygenated blood returns to the left atrium of the heart via the pulmonary veins and then flows through the left ventricle to the aorta to make another trip through the body.

Thrombi can flow through this system repeatedly. They usually become caught, however, in the progressively smaller arteries and capillaries transporting blood to the tissues. The resulting blockage and starvation of cells downstream from the blockage leads to the death and decay of the affected tissue region, resulting in a localized tissue infarction. The two most serious types of infarctions are the myocardial infarction and the stroke, but both of these infarctions can be caused by other types of blockages, including arterial rupture and fatty clogging of arteries from the conditions atherosclerosis and arteriosclerosis. Nevertheless, thrombi are a major contributory factor to the occurrences of strokes and heart attacks, two leading killers in the United States and other stressful, technological Western nations. In both strokes and heart attacks, thrombal blockages to key cellular regions lead to localized cellular death. Heart cells and brain cells cannot be regenerated. The tissue death is permanent, and the resulting physiological effects will remain with the victims for the rest of their lives if they survive the stroke or heart attack.

Another serious thrombal blockage can occur in the pulmonary arteries and arterioles transporting blood to lung tissue for oxygenation. Such blockages lead to the localized death of lung tissue and sudden shortness of breath in affected individuals. About 10 percent of cases of pulmonary thrombosis and embolism end in death, resulting in a fatality figure much smaller than the hundreds of thousands of deaths from heart attacks and strokes in the United States each year.

Scuba divers who spend excessive periods of time at great depths and then ascend rapidly are prone to decompression sickness, or "the bends," in which nitrogen bubbles form emboli that create the same blockages as thrombi in localized tissue spaces. Nitrogen bubble emboli can accumulate in the heart, lung, and brain tissue and are fatal if not immediately treated in a decompression chamber.

PERSPECTIVE AND PROSPECTS

Thrombi and thrombosis are serious problems that can arise in any individual, although the likelihood increases with age and the corresponding decline in individuals' immune systems. Care must be taken with various surgical procedures, particularly abdominal and pelvic surgery and the treatment of leg fractures, to reduce the chances of thrombi forming. Any severe cut has the potential to form thrombi, but the status of an individual's immune system is an important factor in determining whether these thrombi are captured and dissipated.

In many surgical procedures, including open heart surgery, physicians and surgeons will administer anticlotting agents to minimize the risk of thrombi forming during and following the surgery and in the recovery phase of the operation. These anticlotting agents are administered intravenously and diffuse throughout the patient's circulatory system so that any thrombi and other blood clots dissolve before they can occlude various tissue regions. Medical doctors are versed in the science of thrombi and thrombosis because these conditions often are associated with other medical conditions. Physicians are aware of contributory factors to thrombosis and can take action to guard against thrombal occurrence early in the medical treatment process.

In 2003, researchers announced a breakthrough in

the treatment of persons prone to blood clots. Since the 1950's, the drug warfarin has been given to patients for a period of three to six months. Studies showed an increased risk of severe bleeding with longer use of warfarin, thus preempting its use after six months. However, without warfarin, nearly one-third of patients will form another blood clot within eight years. The 2003 findings showed that after several months of full doses of warfarin, moderate doses of the medicine can follow and can reduce the risk of further clots without introducing the risk of hemorrhage.

—*David Wason Hollar, Jr., Ph.D.*

See also Arteriosclerosis; Behçet's disease; Blood and blood disorders; Blood vessels; Cardiac arrest; Cardiology; Cholesterol; Deep vein thrombosis; Disseminated intravascular coagulation (DIC); Echocardiography; Embolism; Heart; Heart attack; Heart disease; Hyperlipidemia; Hypertension; Infarction; Ischemia; Phlebitis; Plaque, arterial; Strokes; Transient ischemic attacks (TIAs); Varicosis; Vascular medicine; Vascular system; Venous insufficiency.

FOR FURTHER INFORMATION:

Bick, Roger L. *Disorders of Thrombosis and Hemostasis: Clinical and Laboratory Practice.* 3d ed. Philadelphia: Lippincott Williams & Wilkins, 2002. An excellent introduction to the diagnosis and management of clotting and bleeding disorders.

Cohen, Barbara J. *Memmler's The Human Body in Health and Disease.* 11th ed. Philadelphia: Wolters Kluwer Health/Lippincott Williams & Wilkins, 2009. This brief book is an excellent introduction to human anatomy and physiology for the layperson. Excellent definitions, descriptions of processes, and illustrations highlight each short chapter. Chapter 14, "The Heart and Heart Disease," discusses the formation of thrombi, their contribution to heart attacks, and anticlotting thrombolytic drugs.

Lichtman, Marshall A., et al., eds. *Williams Hematology.* 7th ed. New York: McGraw-Hill, 2006. An accessible handbook that covers the pathogenetic, diagnostic, and therapeutic essentials of blood cell and coagulation protein disorders.

Limmer, Daniel, et al. *Emergency Care.* 11th ed. Upper Saddle River, N.J.: Pearson/Prentice Hall Health, 2009. A primer in emergency care for the emergency medical technician (EMT) and paramedic. Offers useful information and illustrated procedures for handling various types of life-threatening emergencies, including strokes and heart attacks.

Loscalzo, Joseph, and Andrew I. Schafer, eds. *Thrombosis and Hemorrhage.* 3d ed. Philadelphia: Lippincott Williams & Wilkins, 2003. Covers an array of relevant topics including the basic elements of hemostasis, the normal function and response of platelets, and specific clinical disorders and laboratory approaches, thrombotic disorders, and management of patients with hemorrhagic and thrombotic conditions.

Wistreich, George A., and Max D. Lechtman. *Microbiology.* 5th ed. New York: Macmillan, 1988. This very detailed work is an outstanding introduction to the sciences of microbiology and immunology. Chapter 17, "Introduction to Immune Responses," discusses the role of thrombocytes and thrombin in the normal immune response.

THUMB SUCKING

DEVELOPMENT

ANATOMY OR SYSTEM AFFECTED: Mouth, teeth

SPECIALTIES AND RELATED FIELDS: Dentistry, pediatrics, speech pathology

DEFINITION: A common oral behavior among young children that may cause physical, psychological, and social problems if it is continued past a certain age.

PHYSICAL AND PSYCHOLOGICAL FACTORS

It has been estimated that 45 percent of all two-year-olds, 36 percent of four-year-olds, 21 percent of six-year-olds, and 5 percent of eleven-year-olds suck their thumbs. As children grow older, by age five, the occurrence of thumb sucking generally begins to fade during the daytime. If children continue to suck their thumbs, it is generally limited to nighttime.

Thumb sucking seems to be reinforcing to children because of its soothing property. For example, it is often observed among children when they are tired, frustrated, hungry, or uncomfortable, such as when teething causes discomfort. Furthermore, thumb sucking tends to increase the level of independence in infants. This becomes evident when observing an infant who is occupied by this self-stimulating behavior.

DISORDERS AND EFFECTS

Although thumb sucking is relatively harmless among children younger than three years of age, problems can develop if the behavior persists. Negative consequences may consist of dental problems, inhibited speech development, and critical peer and negative parental reactions.

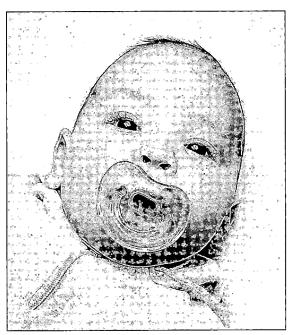

A thumb or pacifier fulfills some infants' strong need for sucking in the early months of life but can become a difficult habit to break. (PhotoDisc)

One of the main problems associated with thumb sucking is dental problems, especially if this behavior persists after the age of four. Thumb sucking can also inhibit speech development in formal and informal settings at school or day care. For example, when children are sucking their thumbs during formal group activities, they are less likely to respond to adult questions. Also, during free-play time, children who are sucking their thumbs are less likely to speak spontaneously.

In addition to causing problems for speech and physical development, thumb sucking can create social difficulties for children. According to the *Pediatrics* article "Influence of Thumb Sucking on Peer Social Acceptance in First-Grade Children," by P. C. Friman and colleagues, "Social acceptance is lower among children who suck their thumb, and they are viewed by their peers as being less intelligent, happy, attractive, likable, or fun, and less desirable as a friend, playmate, seatmate, classmate, or neighbor." Furthermore, thumb sucking can create negative interactions between the parents and children. Because parents are often troubled by thumb sucking, children are routinely asked to stop. These requests can be positively reinforcing to the child and can increase the frequency of the behavior.

Given the problems associated with thumb sucking, many parents wonder at what point in time a child should be treated for this behavior. In their 1989 article "Thumb Sucking: Pediatricians' Guidelines" in *Clinical Pediatrics*, Friman and B. D. Schmitt provide some guidelines to answer this question. As a simple rule, thumb sucking should not be treated until the potential negative consequences outweigh the benefits, which is seldom before the age of four. When children do suck their thumbs, often it is not frequent enough to warrant treatment. They also point out that at times the potential benefits may outweigh the risks, such as when a child uses thumb sucking as a means of coping with fear, pain, or a significant loss. As suggested by these authors, another indication for treatment is chronic thumb sucking, which they define as occurring "across two or more settings (e.g., home and school) and when it occurs day and night."

PERSPECTIVE AND PROSPECTS

Attitudes toward oral behavior in children have fluctuated over the years. It has been viewed as both indulgent and detrimental. There have been high and low attempts to prohibit the activity. Sigmund Freud and his colleagues did much to draw attention to the oral drive in the first year of life, and over the years many writers have made observations about oral habits and psychological health.

The advent and wide use of pacifiers has done much to neutralize concern over oral behaviors. Pacifiers are generally seen as preferable to the thumb, from a dental perspective. Thumb sucking tends to arouse more anxiety for both parents and medical specialists than does the use of the pacifier.

—*Jay D. Schvaneveldt, Ph.D.*

See also Anxiety; Cognitive development; Dental diseases; Dentistry; Dentistry, pediatric; Developmental stages; Phobias; Psychiatry, child and adolescent; Reflexes, primitive; Separation anxiety; Teeth; Teething; Weaning.

FOR FURTHER INFORMATION:

Berk, Laura E. *Child Development.* 8th ed. Boston: Pearson/Allyn & Bacon, 2009. A text that reviews theory and research in child development, cognitive and language development, personality and social development, and the foundations and contexts of development.

Friman, P. C., K. M. McPherson, W. J. Warzak, and J. Evans. "Influence of Thumb Sucking on Peer Social Acceptance in First-Grade Children." *Pediatrics* 91, no. 4 (April, 1993): 784-786. The influence of thumb sucking on social acceptance was assessed among forty first-grade children.

Nathanson, Laura Walther. *The Portable Pediatrician: A Practicing Pediatrician's Guide to Your Child's Growth, Development, Health, and Behavior from Birth to Age Five.* 2d ed. New York: HarperCollins, 2002. An engaging, easy-to-read guide for parents to assess their child's development, medical symptoms, and behavioral problems.

"Thumb Sucking and Teeth." *Pediatrics for Parents* 19, no. 12 (2002): 1-2. Discusses findings of a study from the University of Iowa School of Dentistry that showed that thumb sucking past two years of age adversely affects children's bites.

Van Norman, Rosemary. *Helping the Thumb-Sucking Child.* Garden City Park, N.Y.: Avery, 1999. A step-by-step guide for families.

Walker, C. Eugene, and Michael C. Roberts, eds. *Handbook of Clinical Child Psychology.* 3d ed. New York: John Wiley & Sons, 2001. Covers normal and abnormal development, assessment and diagnosis, psychopathology (in three sections encompassing infancy, childhood, and adolescence), and intervention strategies.

THYMUS GLAND

ANATOMY

ANATOMY OR SYSTEM AFFECTED: Blood, cells, endocrine system, glands, immune system, lymphatic system

SPECIALTIES AND RELATED FIELDS: Biochemistry, endocrinology, immunology, oncology

DEFINITION: A gland that produces types of white blood cells for maintaining the immune system.

STRUCTURE AND FUNCTIONS

The thymus gland is a pinkish-gray organ that lies in front of the ascending aorta, beneath the top of the sternum. It consists of two lobes that are divided into lobules by a septum, or wall. Each thymic lobule is made of connective tissue, which consists of a densely packed outer cortex and less-dense center (medulla). The thymus is relatively large in infants and typically grows to its maximum size around the age of two. After puberty, it gradually decreases in size until it blends in with surrounding tissue.

The major cells of the thymus are morphologically indistinguishable from small, circulating lymphocytes. Lymphocytes (white blood cells) divide, differentiate, and mature in the thymic cortex to become T cells, a heterogeneous group of cells that are essential in protecting the body against infections that can be produced by invading foreign organisms. Once T cells mature, they migrate into the thymic medulla and eventually enter the bloodstream and travel to other lymphatic organs, where they bolster the immune system against disease. The thymus also produces a hormone, thymosin, which stimulates the maturation of lymphocytes in other lymphatic organs.

DISORDERS AND DISEASES

The thymus is critical in developing the immune system in children. If it malfunctions or is surgically removed, then a child has little to no ability to fight off disease. Signs and symptoms of thymus dysfunction include shortness of breath, facial swelling, muscle weakness, blurred vision, double vision, flushing, diarrhea, and neck pain and swelling. Myasthenia gravis, a neuromuscular disease that causes fluctuating muscle weakness, has been linked to thymus dysfunction. Proper diagnosis is critical so that appropriate treatment can be administered.

Although uncommon, thymic cancer can occur. Thymomas are generally slow-growing tumors that are most often found in middle-aged people. A much rarer condition is thymic carcinoma, which develops more quickly than thymoma and is more likely to spread to other parts of the body. If a thymic tumor is found from images produced by chest X rays, computed tomography (CT) scanning, or magnetic resonance imaging (MRI), then the tumor may be surgically removed or treated with radiation.

PERSPECTIVE AND PROSPECTS

The first description of the thymus gland was reported in the early sixteenth century by Italian anatomist Giacomo da Capri. The functions of the thymus were not well understood until the 1960's, when its role in the immune system was discovered. In 2007, it was reported that natural killer T (NKT) cells, a type of regulatory T cells that mature in the thymus, help regulate insulin-dependent diabetes mellitus. Research is focused on the development of NKT cell-based approaches for immunotherapeutic treatment of this disease.

—Alvin K. Benson, Ph.D.

See also Blood and blood disorders; Connective tissue; Diabetes mellitus; Glands; Immune system; Immunology; Immunology, pediatric; Lymphatic system; Myasthenia gravis.

FOR FURTHER INFORMATION:

Anastasiadis, Kyriakos, and Chandi Ratnatunga, eds. *The Thymus Gland: Diagnosis and Surgical Management*. New York: Springer, 2007.

Dabrowski, Marek P., and Barbara Dabrowska-Bernstein. *Immunoregulatory Role of Thymus*. Boca Raton, Fla.: CRC Press, 1989.

Lavini, Corrado, et al., eds. *Thymus Gland Pathology: Clinical, Diagnostic, and Therapeutic Features*. New York: Springer, 2008.

THYROID DISORDERS

DISEASE/DISORDER

ANATOMY OR SYSTEM AFFECTED: Endocrine system, glands, neck

SPECIALTIES AND RELATED FIELDS: Endocrinology

DEFINITION: Underactivity (hypothyroidism) or overactivity (hyperthyroidism) of the thyroid gland.

CAUSES AND SYMPTOMS

The thyroid gland normally weighs about 20 to 35 grams and is located in the neck just below the larynx, or voice box. The gland is named for the shield-shaped "thyroid" cartilage that forms the front of the larynx. The thyroid has two lateral lobes that are connected by an isthmus that crosses in front of the trachea. By placing a finger on the trachea below the larynx it is possible to feel the ridgelike isthmus pass under the finger after swallowing. The bilobed (two-lobed) shape of the rest of the gland can be felt just under the skin of the neck on either side of the midline, although its boundaries are normally indistinct except to a trained examiner.

The thyroid produces two major hormones. Thyroxine, a product of the follicular cells, is the major hormone produced by the thyroid that helps regulate metabolism. Within the thyroid are also parafollicular cells that produce calcitonin, an essential hormone involved in calcium metabolism. In the tissue of the thyroid are also embedded two pairs of parathyroid glands. The parathyroid glands produce parathyroid hormone, which is required to maintain normal levels of blood calcium. In the case of thyroid surgery, it is important that the parathyroid glands are not damaged or removed; otherwise, there may be life-threatening tetanus—the sustained contraction of muscles, including those needed for breathing.

The normal functioning of the thyroid results from an elaborate physiological control system involving the hypothalamus of the brain, the anterior lobe of the pituitary gland, and the thyroid gland. The hypothalamus produces thyrotropic-releasing hormone (TRH), which is passed by special blood vessels to the anterior lobe of the pituitary, the adenohypophysis. The TRH-stimulated cells in the adenohypophysis produce thyroid-stimulating hormone (TSH), which is released into the general circulation. When it reaches the thyroid gland, it stimulates the gland to produce thyroxine. Normally, thyroxine has a negative feedback effect on its own production; that is, thyroxine can inhibit the activity of the hypothalamus and the pituitary to maintain its concentration in the blood. Various thyroid disorders, which are more common in women than in men, can develop from tumors that either increase or decrease the hormones produced in these three interdependent structures.

The normal thyroid (or euthyroid state) produces mainly thyroxine, which is converted into triiodothyronine in the tissues of the body before it has its effects, which are generally to increase the metabolic rate of the body. Some triiodothyronine is directly produced by the thyroid. The thyroxine molecule contains iodide, the negative ion of iodine; iodine is therefore an essential component of one's diet. If iodine is not available in the diet—as in the case of vegetables grown in geographical areas glaciated in the past, such as mountainous terrain and the American Midwest—then the body cannot produce thyroxine. Industrialized countries have iodine added to table salt to ensure an adequate

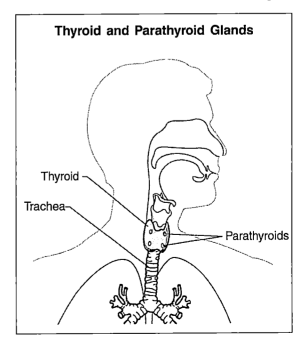

Thyroid and Parathyroid Glands

Thyroid

Trachea

Parathyroids

supply of this element in the diet. A lack of iodine, and therefore a lack of thyroxine, prevents the functioning of the negative feedback effect of thyroxine on the hypothalamus and pituitary, resulting in very low thyroxine levels and high TSH levels in the blood. High levels of TSH cause substantial growth of the thyroid, which will bulge from the neck as a goiter. A person with such a condition would be hypothyroid (that is, have lower-than-normal thyroxine levels in the blood) and may become a cretin (mentally impaired and of short stature) if this condition occurs early in childhood.

Hypothyroidism can arise in other ways as well. Hashimoto's thyroiditis is a common type of hypothyroidism that is caused by an autoimmune reaction whereby white blood cells known as lymphocytes infiltrate the thyroid and gradually destroy its tissue. The presence of antibodies against normal thyroid proteins can be detected with this condition. The usual signs of hypothyroidism are an intolerance of cold, a low body temperature, a lower rate of metabolism, a tendency to sleep longer, a general lack of energy, infrequent bowel movements, constipation, possible weight gain, a puffy face and hands, a slow heart rate, cold and scaly skin, a lack of perspiration, and possible emotional withdrawal and depression.

Graves' disease, the most common type of hyperthyroidism, is an autoimmune disorder in which antibodies mimic the action of TSH and therefore stimulate the thyroid to produce excessive thyroxine. Sometimes, nodules develop in the thyroid that may produce the excessive thyroxine. Although the presence of a nodule in the thyroid may cause a person to suspect cancer, the nodules are usually benign. Hyperthyroidism may be associated with bulging eyes, but this orbitopathy does not always occur. Generally, there is an intolerance of heat, a loss of body weight, a high degree of nervousness, increased or decreased skin pigmentation, more frequent bowel movements, loss of hair, and a very rapid heart rate.

Treatment and Therapy

Patients suspected of having hypothyroidism or hyperthyroidism will have their blood tested for levels of TSH and thyroxine. Ultrasonography can be used to detect tumors and serve as an anatomical guide for potential surgery. Hypothyroidism patients are prescribed a small oral dose (less than 1 milligram per day) of thyroxine, which is adjusted until a euthyroid state is obtained within a few months. Then the patient is maintained on thyroxine, with perhaps yearly checkups by a physician. For hyperthyroidism patients, several modes of treatment are possible. Antithyroid drugs, such as propylthiouracil (PTU) or methimazole, can be given to inhibit thyroxine synthesis. Radioactive iodine is commonly given to destroy part of the thyroid gland and thus reduce its thyroxine output. Second or even third doses of radioactive iodine may be given if the blood thyroxine levels remain high. Radioactive iodine is not used during pregnancy because damage to the fetal thyroid is likely. Additionally, surgery can be performed to remove enough thyroid tissue to restore normal thyroxine levels. Following any of the treatments, a hypothyroidism may be induced that will require that the patient receive thyroxine supplements. Finally, surgery can be used to reduce the bulging of the eyes caused by hyperthyroidism.

—John T. Burns, Ph.D.;
updated by Matthew Berria, Ph.D.

See also Congenital hypothyroidism; Endocrine disorders; Endocrine glands; Endocrinology; Endocrinology, pediatric; Glands; Goiter; Hashimoto's thyroiditis; Hormones; Hyperparathyroidism and hypoparathyroidism; Metabolic disorders; Metabolism; Parathyroidectomy; Thyroid gland; Thyroidectomy; Vitamins and minerals.

INFORMATION ON THYROID DISORDERS

Causes: Tumors, iodine deficiency, autoimmune disorders

Symptoms: In hypothyroidism, intolerance of cold, low body temperature, tendency to sleep longer, lack of energy, infrequent bowel movements, constipation, possible weight gain, puffy face and hands; in hyperthyroidism, bulging eyes, intolerance of heat, weight loss, nervousness, increased or decreased skin pigmentation, more frequent bowel movements, hair loss, rapid heart rate

Duration: Several months to chronic

Treatments: Thyroxine, antithyroid drugs (propylthiouracil, methimazole), radioactive iodine, surgery

---

For Further Information:

Braverman, Lewis E., ed. *Diseases of the Thyroid.* 2d ed. Totowa, N.J.: Humana Press, 2003. A clinical text that covers major topics in the pathophysiology, diagnosis, or management of clinical thyroid disorders.

Brooks, S. J., and Robert S. Bar. *Early Diagnosis and Treatment of Endocrine Disorders.* Totowa, N.J.: Humana Press, 2003. Reviews the early signs and symptoms of common endocrine diseases, surveys the clinical testing needed for a diagnosis, and presents recommendations for therapy.

Griffin, James E., and Sergio R. Ojeda, eds. *Textbook of Endocrine Physiology.* 5th ed. New York: Oxford University Press, 2004. This textbook of basic endocrinology is used widely in medical schools as well as graduate and undergraduate programs.

Hershman, Jerome M., ed. *Endocrine Pathophysiology: A Patient-Oriented Approach.* 3d ed. Philadelphia: Lea & Febiger, 1988. Discusses diseases of the endocrine glands. Includes bibliographical references and an index.

Kronenberg, Henry M., et al., eds. *Williams Textbook of Endocrinology.* 11th ed. Philadelphia: Saunders/ Elsevier, 2008. Text that covers the spectrum of information related to the endocrine system, including thyroid disorders.

Ruggieri, Paul, and Scott Isaacs. *A Simple Guide to Thyroid Disorders: From Diagnosis to Treatment.* Omaha, Nebr.: Addicus Books, 2004. A user-friendly guide that covers how the thyroid gland works and explains common disorders, including hypothyroidism and hyperthyroidism. Special attention is given to how thyroid diseases affect specific populations such as women, children, and the elderly.

Surks, Martin I. *The Thyroid Book.* Yonkers, N.Y.: Consumer Reports Books, 1993. This concise volume discusses diseases of the thyroid gland. Includes an index.

THYROID GLAND

ANATOMY

ANATOMY OR SYSTEM AFFECTED: Endocrine system, glands, neck

SPECIALTIES AND RELATED FIELDS: Endocrinology

DEFINITION: A gland found in the neck that secretes the hormones responsible for the synthesis and breakdown of proteins and the metabolism of carbohydrates.

KEY TERMS:

cretinism: a severe hypothyroidism in which infants are born with insufficiently developed thyroid tissue

endocrine system: a series of ductless glands that de-

liver hormones to target cells directly through the bloodstream

Graves' disease: a common type of hyperthyroidism in which the thyroid gland produces an oversupply of hormone

hormones: chemicals, usually proteins or steroids, that carry messages regulating the body's chemical balance, responses to stimuli, and development

hypothyroidism: a condition in which the thyroid gland produces an insufficient supply of hormone

parathyroid: one of four small endocrine glands physically close to the thyroid that control the calcium balance of the body

pituitary: the endocrine gland responsible for the functioning of the thyroid, along with many other central control activities

thyroxine: the chief hormone of the thyroid gland, an iodine-containing derivative of the amino acid tyrosine

STRUCTURE AND FUNCTIONS

The human body is, to an extraordinary extent, under the metabolic control of chemical secretions called hormones. These molecules are produced by the ductless, or endocrine, glands and carry messages that regulate the rate of production of necessary substances in remote parts of the organism. The endocrine glands in turn are largely controlled by the nervous system, which also uses chemical messengers to manage the multiple and interrelated systems of the body.

The thyroid gland was one of the earliest glands to be studied in detail. It synthesizes, stores, and secretes two principal hormones, thyroxine and triiodothyronine. These substances stimulate carbohydrate metabolism and protein synthesis or breakdown.

The first description of the thyroid that has been accepted as definite was given by Thomas Wharton in 1656; he also named the gland. In his studies of all the glands, he performed animal dissections and human autopsies. Although his written accounts were widely reprinted, it was more than two hundred years later before any serious further work was undertaken.

Nineteenth century clinical studies of goiter (swelling of the thyroid) and hyperthyroidism (the gland's overproduction of hormones) contributed little to an understanding of the thyroid. An exception is found in the study of the insufficient production of hormone by the thyroid, called hypothyroidism. English and Swiss physicians made discoveries that are considered by some medical historians to be as important as the dem-

The Thyroid Gland

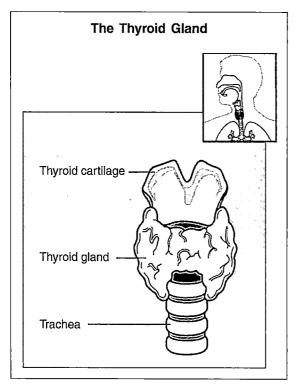

Thyroid cartilage

Thyroid gland

Trachea

The thyroid is an important gland that produces thyroid hormone, the proper level of which is crucial to health; the inset shows the location of the thyroid gland.

onstration that the element iodine is associated with thyroid action.

In the 1870's, the Swiss surgeon Emil Theodor Kocher began to describe the significance of the thyroid gland and its role in goiter formation. He was awarded the 1909 Nobel Prize in Physiology or Medicine for providing a fuller appreciation of the thyroid and associated glands. Kocher was neither a physiologist nor a pathologist by training or disposition, but he recognized that to be an effective surgeon it was essential to understand well the function of the thyroid and its role in the goiters so common in Bern. In this region, 80 to 90 percent of schoolchildren had a malfunctioning thyroid gland and the often-associated goiter. Kocher's drawings in books and papers show that such enlargements are extremely disfiguring and often interfere with normal breathing and speech.

In Kocher's day, little was known about any of the endocrine glands, of which the thyroid is the first to have been studied surgically. Such glands deposit chemical regulatory substances called hormones directly into the bloodstream, which carries them to the sites of their activity.

Later clinical observations provided evidence that the thyroid gland produces some material essential for good health. In 1896, Eugen Baumann made the key discovery that the thyroid contains an unusual amount of iodine. He also showed that this excess iodine is present in a protein that he could decompose with water to yield a new substance. During the next twenty-five years, technical progress was made to the point that the hormone thyroxine could be produced in a pure, crystalline form.

With the new tool of radioactive iodine, a powerful method for the study of thyroid functions and malfunctions became available. For example, overactive and underactive thyroid glands can be easily determined through the ingestion of a tiny amount of one of the radioactive isotopes of iodine and the later determination of the amount of the tracer present in the thyroid.

DISORDERS AND DISEASES

It is possible for the thyroid to produce either too much (hyperthyroidism) or too little (hypothyroidism) of the hormone thyroxine, which plays a role in controlling metabolism and body growth. If an insufficient quantity of it is produced, the condition called Gull's disease results. In children, this condition limits both physical and mental growth and is known as congenital hypothyroidism or cretinism. In Graves' disease and related conditions, the overactive thyroid gland produces too much hormone. Either of these conditions can produce an enlarged thyroid gland, or goiter. This imbalance existed in many different countries, but physicians designated it by various names, thus causing much misunderstanding and confusion. Emil Kocher's studies presented the first organization of the field in the form of these basic definitions.

In his first 101 operations carried out between 1872 and 1883, Kocher completely removed the thyroid gland in 34 cases. After a report by his colleague Jacques Louis Reverdin indicating that removal of the thyroid was a causal factor in cretinism, Kocher made as detailed a follow-up of these patients as possible. His conclusion was that if the entire gland was removed, cretinlike symptoms almost always appeared. If at least some of the gland was left, it appeared to regenerate itself and supply the required hormone. He vowed never to remove a thyroid completely again except in the case of malignancy.

Only in the twentieth century did reliable diagnoses and treatments become available for thyroid disorders. Because of the variety of these conditions and their causes, accurate diagnosis is indispensable. Modern approaches that supplement radioactive iodine include ultrasound and the needle biopsy.

The principal difficulty in the treatment of a malfunctioning thyroid gland is the several variations often displayed. Hyperthyroidism can occur in forms that appear quite unrelated to the most common form, Graves' disease. For example, there may not be a heredity basis, the condition may not spread over the entire gland, the production of antibodies may not be involved, and there may be no progressive failure of the thyroid.

The causes of hypothyroidism are also less than uniform. The age at which the disorder begins is significantly related to its cause. Newborn children with this condition may have never developed the required amount of thyroid tissue. Others may have inherited a defect that prevents the thyroid from producing sufficient hormone. In developing countries, iodine deficiency remains a problem (although an overabundance of that element in the diet of expectant mothers can lead to infants with hypothyroidism and a goiter). Later in life, infection can be the cause of Hashimoto's disease and the loss of thyroid tissue. Finally, the treatment of an overactive thyroid places a person at risk of later underproduction of hormone.

The most common symptoms associated with thyroid problems are a too rapid or too slow heartbeat, nervousness or a tired and run-down feeling, frequent bowel movements or constipation, and weight loss or weight gain. An excess of the hormones that direct the use of food and the production of energy might reasonably be expected to produce the first of each pair of contrasting observations, while a deficiency would lead to the opposite effects.

The treatment of Graves' disease falls into three distinct classes, and in modified application these techniques are employed with the other forms of hyperthyroidism. Since the early 1940's, a series of antithyroid drugs have been synthesized. They function by preventing the gland from making hormone, and the symptoms lessen in a short time. Unfortunately, only about 30 percent of patients remain well when the medication is stopped after six to twelve months.

If antithyroid drugs fail to control the overactive thyroid, a radioactive isotope of iodine is often successful. Since the iodine goes directly to the thyroid and remains there for a period of time, it is able to irradiate and destroy a portion of the tissue. It is a demanding task to calculate the proper amount of iodine to administer, but a surprising 80 percent of patients find their condition under control after a single treatment.

Surgical treatment of Graves' disease and related hyperthyroid conditions became practical with Kocher's efforts, and it remains the method of choice in many cases. Kocher began his Nobel Prize lecture by describing the crucial importance of the work of Louis Pasteur, Joseph Lister, and others in making surgery on internal organs possible, and he suggested the future of thyroid research when he examined the effective use of extracts and the search for chemical means of providing substitutes for the gland's secretions.

The standard treatment of hypothyroidism is oral thyroid hormone tablets. Typically, a synthetic form of thyroxine, called Levothyroxine, is given to compensate for low thyroid hormone levels. As is the case with Graves' disease, good follow-up is essential because the prescribed dosage will likely change with the patient's age. The administration of too much thyroxine can lead to hyperthyroidism.

Two notes should be made in concluding this discussion of malfunctions of the thyroid. First, there is a tendency to believe that iodine prevents and cures goiter. Statements to that effect, found in many general reference books, are both misleading and dangerous. Second, publications for laypersons tend to minimize the importance of thyroid blood tests, which is a serious disservice. Regular and complete physical examinations are essential in maintaining good health.

PERSPECTIVE AND PROSPECTS

Historians of medical history have attributed knowledge of the thyroid gland and the treatment of goiter to many significant figures. The works of Galen, Paracelsus, ancient Chinese writers, and other classical Roman and Greek authors, as well as medieval manuscripts, have been studied. In the twentieth century, the study of the thyroid and goiter illustrates central themes in the evolution of medical practice; these are shown clearly in the career of Emil Kocher. His being chosen as an early Nobel laureate is prophetic—first for his role in creating modern surgery, with its total reliance on a germ-free environment and its demand for detail, and second for successful synthesis of the roles of clinician and research scientist. He both possessed the necessary surgical skill to develop such a delicate procedure as thyroidectomy (removal of the thyroid gland) and appreciated the importance of understanding the role played by the thyroid in controlling distant and seemingly unrelated functions. Finally, Kocher kept abreast of any new discovery that might, in any way, be of significance to his surgical goals.

The study of the thyroid in many ways unlocked the secrets of other endocrine glands. As in many areas of scientific research, new medical knowledge follows quickly after the discovery of materials and techniques. At the same time, the search for knowledge provides both motivation and information driving the discovery of materials and techniques.

The identification of iodine as an elemental substance by the French chemist Bernard Courtois in 1811 rapidly led to its indiscriminate use as a treatment for goiter, along with a wide variety of related conditions. Important work in the mid-nineteenth century by A. Chatin demonstrated the high correlation between goiter and low levels of iodine in the food and water supplies throughout central Europe. In the 1930's, with the creation of radioactive isotopes, including those of iodine, a vital and productive new phase of thyroid research began.

A similar pattern is seen during World War II, when four independent research groups showed that sulfa drugs were capable of exerting a strong influence on the behavior of the thyroid. All these studies were conducted within a two-year period, and it was less than a year later that the therapeutic use of sulfa drugs was demonstrated.

While much knowledge and technical skill concerning the thyroid has been gained, the number of conferences and publications devoted to endocrinology attests to the continued importance of that general field of study. For example, while malignant tumors are rare in the thyroid, benign lumps or nodules are common. The reasons for this pattern and the role of endocrine glands in the development and spread of cancerous cells warrant detailed and continuing study.

—*K. Thomas Finley, Ph.D.*

See also Congenital hypothyroidism; Endocrine disorders; Endocrinology; Endocrinology, pediatric; Glands; Goiter; Growth; Hashimoto's thyroiditis; Hormone therapy; Hormones; Metabolic disorders; Metabolism; Systems and organs; Thyroid disorders; Thyroidectomy.

FOR FURTHER INFORMATION:

Bayliss, R. I. S., and W. M. Tunbridge. *Thyroid Disease: The Facts*. 4th ed. New York: Oxford University Press, 2008. Well written and researched. Provides a wealth of information on thyroid disease in a not-too-technical fashion.

Burman, Kenneth D., and Derek LeRoith, eds. *Thyroid Function and Disease*. Philadelphia: Saunders/ Elsevier, 2007. A textbook that offers a detailed understanding of the entire range of the gland and its medical interest to all readers.

DeGroot, Leslie J., P. Reed Larsen, and Georg Hennemann. *The Thyroid and Its Diseases*. 6th ed. New York: Churchill Livingstone, 1996. Much technical material can be found in this standard textbook, but there are also valuable details to give the reader a greater appreciation of the subject.

Holt, Richard I. G., and Neil A. Hanley. *Essential Endocrinology and Diabetes*. 5th ed. Malden, Mass.: Blackwell, 2007. This text addresses the field of endocrinology, describing the physiology of the endocrine glands and the hormones that they produce. Includes an index.

Marieb, Elaine N. *Essentials of Human Anatomy and Physiology*. 9th ed. San Francisco: Pearson/Benjamin Cummings, 2009. This introductory anatomy and physiology textbook, easily accessible to those with little science background, is richly illustrated with diagrams and photographs, which help to illuminate body systems and processes.

Melmed, Schlomo, et al. *The Pituitary*. 2d ed. Boston: Blackwell Science, 2002. Text covering the biochemistry, molecular biology, physiology, pathophysiology, and clinical aspects of the pituitary. Sections include hypothalamic-pituitary function, hypothalamic-pituitary dysfunction, pituitary tumors, pituitary disease in systemic disorders, and diagnostic procedures.

Moore, Elaine A., and Lisa Moore. *Graves' Disease: A Practical Guide*. Jefferson, N.C.: McFarland, 2001. Discusses both typical and special concerns of patients with Graves' disease, its association with related autoimmune disorders, and the patient's role in the healing process.

Rosenthal, M. Sara. *The Thyroid Sourcebook*. 5th ed. New York: McGraw-Hill, 2009. Wide-ranging examination of thyroid disorders from hyperthyroidism to cancer.

Ruggieri, Paul, and Scott Isaacs. *A Simple Guide to Thyroid Disorders: From Diagnosis to Treatment*. Omaha, Nebr.: Addicus Books, 2004. A user-friendly guide that covers how the thyroid gland works and explains common disorders, including hypothyroidism and hyperthyroidism. Special attention is given to how thyroid diseases affect specific populations such as women, children, and the elderly.

Wood, Lawrence C., David S. Cooper, and E. Chester

Ridgway. *Your Thyroid: A Home Reference.* 4th rev. ed. New York: Ballantine Books, 2005. An excellent description of the entire field, with much wise advice for all, including those suffering with thyroid problems. Includes important supplemental information for those seeking further assistance.

THYROIDECTOMY
PROCEDURE

ANATOMY OR SYSTEM AFFECTED: Endocrine system, glands, neck

SPECIALTIES AND RELATED FIELDS: Endocrinology, general surgery

DEFINITION: The surgical removal of all or a portion of the thyroid gland.

INDICATIONS AND PROCEDURES

A thyroidectomy is performed to remove thyroid tumors, to treat thyrotoxicosis (whereby the thyroid gland excretes very large amounts of thyroid hormone), to evaluate a mass, or to excise an enlarged thyroid that is causing problems with breathing, swallowing, or speaking.

The thyroid gland is located at the base of the neck. It is composed of two lobes that straddle the trachea (throat) and a third lobe that is in the middle of the neck. Surgery on the thyroid is usually performed under general anesthesia. The patient's neck is extended, and an incision along a natural fold or crease is made through the skin, platysma muscle, and fascia that lie over the thyroid. The muscle is cut high up to minimize damage to the nerve that controls it.

The thyroid is next carefully freed from surrounding structures (blood vessels, nerves, and the trachea). One at a time, the upper portion of each lobe is freed to allow identification of the veins that take blood from the thyroid. The veins are ligated (tied) in two places and cut between the ties. The ligaments that suspend the thyroid are cut next. It is important for the surgeon to avoid damaging the superior laryngeal nerve. Once the nerve has been protected, other blood vessels are clamped, tied, and cut. A similar procedure is followed for the lower lobes: ligating and cutting veins, protecting the inferior and recurrent laryngeal nerves, and freeing the remainder of the thyroid lobes.

Four parathyroid glands, each about the size of a pea, are imbedded in the thyroid gland. At least one of these must be preserved, as they play a vital role in regulating calcium. Once these glands are identified, the tissue of the thyroid is cut away, leaving the parathyroids intact.

The remnants of the thyroid gland are folded in and sutured to the trachea to control bleeding. A final inspection for bleeding is made. The fascia is sutured closed over the thyroid; any muscles that were cut are sewn back together. Finally, the edges of skin are carefully brought together and sutured with very fine material; occasionally, clips are used. The instruments needed for a tracheostomy are left nearby to cope with any emergency that might occur during the next twenty-four hours.

USES AND COMPLICATIONS

Approximately one week after a thyroidectomy, the patient returns for a postoperative checkup, and sutures or clips are removed. Many, but not all, individuals having this procedure must take a synthetic thyroid hormone to make up for the tissue removed during the thyroidectomy.

Thyroid surgery is not uncommon. In the past, radiation was used to shrink the thyroid, but this procedure led to many cancers and has been discontinued. Laser techniques may reduce the size of the incision, thus reducing the size of the resulting scar in the neck.

Complications that may occur as a result of a thyroidectomy include bleeding into the neck, causing difficulty breathing; a surge of thyroid hormones into the blood, called thyroid storm or thyrotoxic crisis; and injury to the vocal cords, which can result in changes in voice pitch.

—*L. Fleming Fallon, Jr., M.D., Ph.D., M.P.H.; updated by Sharon W. Stark, R.N., A.P.R.N., D.N.Sc.*

See also Endocrine disorders; Endocrinology; Endocrinology, pediatric; Glands; Goiter; Hashimoto's thyroiditis; Hormone therapy; Hormones; Parathyroidectomy; Thyroid disorders; Thyroid gland.

FOR FURTHER INFORMATION:

Bayliss, R. I. S., and W. M. Tunbridge. *Thyroid Disease: The Facts.* 4th ed. New York: Oxford University Press, 2008.

Burman, Kenneth D., and Derek LeRoith, eds. *Thyroid Function and Disease.* Philadelphia: Saunders/Elsevier, 2007.

Doherty, Gerard M., and Lawrence W. Way, eds. *Current Surgical Diagnosis and Treatment.* 12th ed. New York: Lange Medical Books/McGraw-Hill, 2006.

Kronenberg, Henry M., et al., eds. *Williams Textbook of Endocrinology.* 11th ed. Philadelphia: Saunders/Elsevier, 2008.

MedlinePlus. "Thyroid Gland Removal." http://www
.nlm.nih.gov/medlineplus/ency/article/002933.htm.

Rosenthal, M. Sara. *The Thyroid Sourcebook*. 5th ed.
New York: McGraw-Hill, 2009.

Ruggieri, Paul, and Scott Isaacs. *A Simple Guide to Thyroid Disorders: From Diagnosis to Treatment*.
Omaha, Nebr.: Addicus Books, 2004.

Wood, Lawrence C., David S. Cooper, and E. Chester
Ridgway. *Your Thyroid: A Home Reference*. 4th rev.
ed. New York: Ballantine Books, 2005.

TIAs. *See* TRANSIENT ISCHEMIC ATTACKS (TIAs).

TICKS. *See* LICE, MITES, AND TICKS.

TICS
DISEASE/DISORDER

ALSO KNOWN AS: Habit spasm

ANATOMY OR SYSTEM AFFECTED: Brain, muscles, musculoskeletal system, nerves, nervous system, psychic-emotional system

SPECIALTIES AND RELATED FIELDS: Neurology, psychology

DEFINITION: Small, brief, recurrent, inappropriate, compulsive jerking movements or twitches, sometimes called habit spasms, often set off by stressful events and including tic douloureux, involving the trigeminal nerve, and Tourette's syndrome, a lifelong disorder associated with a large variety of tics.

KEY TERMS:

neuralgia: pain in one of the peripheral nerves

paroxysm: an uncontrolled spasm or convulsion that may sometimes be violent

psychogenic: psychological in origin; set off by psychologically stressful events

stereotyped: performed exactly the same way from one occasion to the next, or from one individual performer to the next

tic douloureux (trigeminal neuralgia): painful tics of the fifth cranial nerve (trigeminal nerve)

Tourette's syndrome: a neurological disorder characterized by bizarre or unusual tics, compulsive swearing, strange facial gestures, and animal-like noises

CAUSES AND SYMPTOMS

Tics are small, inappropriate, involuntary, compulsive jerking or twitching movements that recur uncontrollably and appear to be nonrhythmic (erratic) in pattern. Tics are stereotyped movements of small portions of the body that last only briefly but may be repeated often. They are often set off by psychologically stressful events. In many cases, tics can be voluntary and temporarily suppressed, but often with the result that the same movements occur more forcefully afterward. The term "habit spasm" is often used for tics that occur among children. A tic is a symptom rather than a disease. Many tics are believed to be of psychogenic origin, and certain others seem to be related to epilepsy, encephalitis, or diseases of unknown origin.

Motor tics commonly involve coarse muscle movements of small magnitude, including movements of the face (such as eye blinks, grimaces, or sniffing movements), shruggings of the shoulders, jerks of the neck, or twitches of the body parts. Many motor tics (and also vocal tics) are easily imitated by others but are performed involuntarily and uncontrollably by the patient. Distracting the patient's attention may stop certain tics. In most cases, the tic does not interfere with the patient's use of the hands or feet, even in delicate movements. Several neurologists distinguish simple motor tics (eye winking, head twitching, shoulder shrugs, or facial grimaces) from complex motor tics using more muscles and requiring coordination. Complex motor tics may include touching oneself or other people, jumping, hitting, or throwing things.

Vocal or phonic tics include the making of sounds, which may include grunts, coughs, sniffs, clearings of the throat, animal noises (especially barking and yelping), or understandable words. The words may simply be repeated utterances of the patient's own words (palilalia), repetition of words spoken to the patient (echolalia), or obscene and offensive words (coprolalia). Although coprolalia is one of the more striking symptoms of Tourette's syndrome and has been vividly portrayed in many popular accounts of this disorder, it is usually a mild or transient symptom and appears in only a minority of cases.

Sensory tics are unusual sensations of pressure, cold, warmth, tickling, or other common sensations that are generally brief in duration. Some otherwise inexplicable movements may be interpreted as actions taken by the patient to alleviate these sensory tics. Sensory tics are reported to be present in about 40 percent of patients with Tourette's syndrome.

Tic disorders can be classified into four types: tic douloureux, transient tic disorder of childhood, chronic tic disorder, and Tourette's syndrome. One of the most common forms of tic is trigeminal neuralgia, also called tic douloureux, a disorder that affects about fif-

INFORMATION ON TICS

CAUSES: Stressful events, disease (e.g., epilepsy, encephalitis), tumors, psychological disorders, Tourette's syndrome

SYMPTOMS: Small, brief, recurrent, and compulsive jerking movements or twitches; unusual vocalizations (grunting, coughing, throat clearing, animal noises) or word repetition

DURATION: Acute to chronic with recurrent episodes

TREATMENTS: Surgery, drug therapy, injection of ethyl alcohol into trigeminal nerve ganglion, vitamin supplements, psychotherapy

teen thousand individuals annually in the United States. Tic douloureux is a disorder of the trigeminal or fifth cranial nerve, the nerve that supplies motor stimulation to the jaw muscles and sensory innervation to much of the skin of the face. Tic douloureux usually begins with a very brief but very intense, sharp pain, often described as feeling like an electric shock or a stabbing, swiftly spreading in many cases along the course of the affected nerve. The pain is usually accompanied by uncontrolled spasms or paroxysms that last less than a second but continue to recur for several minutes. These episodes may be separated from one another by tic-free periods lasting from weeks to more than a year. The pain and twitching are generally confined to one side of the face, often to one of the three divisions of the trigeminal nerve, usually the maxillary or mandibular division, or, much less often, the ophthalmic division. In addition to the uncontrollable tics, patients suffering from tic douloureux often wince visibly from the pain; this habit is responsible for the term "tic douloureux," meaning "painful tic."

The immediate event precipitating an attack of tic douloureux is usually a mild stimulation or irritation of a "trigger zone" on or about the face, lips, tongue, or gums. The trigger zone is often a small area that is constant for a particular patient; some patients can trigger an episode by stimulating the trigger zone themselves. The most common locations for the trigger zone are along the cheek or the attached parts of the lips; less common locations include the gums or the floor of the mouth beside the tongue. Some patients suffering an attack of tic douloureux will apply pressure to their faces, but the pain usually goes away by itself. Attacks generally occur during the day rather than at night, and they typically increase in intensity and become more frequent and exhausting to the patient until treatment is sought.

The stimulus that normally evokes an attack of tic douloureux may be an exposure to touch or pressure, to cold, to food in the mouth, or even to a puff of air. Because an attack can be precipitated by touching or otherwise stimulating the trigger zone, many victims of tic douloureux avoid touching the region in which the trigger zone is located. When the trigger zone is on the outside of the face, patients may become very fearful of touching the affected part, and men may avoid shaving. Some patients avoid brushing their teeth and remain unwashed for weeks or even months in the vicinity of their trigger area, with social consequences that often contribute to pessimistic feelings and even depression.

When tongue or cheek movements precipitate attacks, patients suffering from tic douloureux may develop the habit of holding the affected side of their face motionless, which sometimes restricts talking, eating, or similar everyday movements. In some cases, certain chewing movements or the presence of food in certain locations in the mouth may precipitate an attack; in these cases, patients are often very careful to avoid eating or chewing on the affected side, and in extreme cases they may so often avoid eating or drinking that they become dehydrated and emaciated. Some physicians advise such patients to modify their diet and drink only liquids, fortified with vitamins, that can be consumed without chewing. Malnutrition and physical inactivity are in many cases reinforced by the social consequences of facial uncleanliness and lack of hygiene, or by the fear of such consequences. The lack of social contact may result in pessimistic or negative feelings, feelings of inadequacy or lack of worth, preoccupation with loss and with past events, feelings of rejection or powerlessness, and other symptoms of clinical depression in many patients.

Dental disease or trauma may sometimes be associated with tic douloureux, but in most cases the tic has no apparent cause. Tic douloureux is more common after the age of forty and is slightly more common in women than in men. Some researchers believe that infection with a herpesvirus (especially herpes simplex) may be causally related to trigeminal neuralgia, but other researchers doubt this connection. Tumors of the trigeminal (Gasserian) ganglion, brain-stem tumors, multiple sclerosis, or localized damage to the brain stem tissue can sometimes give rise to conditions that closely resemble tic douloureux, but the majority of tics occur among patients having none of these conditions.

The remaining forms of tic disorder are considered by at least some researchers to be related to one another, or to form a spectrum of conditions from mild or imperceptible to severe. The mildest types are the tics or "habit spasms" of children. These tics are usually considered psychogenic in origin because they occur more often under conditions of stress or tension. Tics of this kind are more common in boys than in girls. Common types of childhood tics include eye blinks or other facial movements, as well as occasional vocal tics such as throat-clearing noises. In some children—perhaps many—tics of this kind may disappear (or be "outgrown") spontaneously if no attention is drawn to them.

Chronic tics can be of either the motor or the vocal type. Chronic motor tics are uncommon tics in which three or more muscle groups are usually involved at the same time. Chronic vocal tics are also uncommon and consist of uncontrolled sounds that are more often animal sounds than words of articulate speech. Either kind of chronic tic can originate either in children or in adults, even beyond the age of forty. In either case, they usually last for the remainder of the patient's life. The disorder is equally prevalent in both sexes. Some researchers think that these chronic tics, and possibly also the transient habit spasms of childhood, may result from the same (as yet unidentified) cause as Tourette's syndrome, but in much milder form.

Tourette's syndrome is a neurological disorder characterized by bizarre or unusual tics, compulsive swearing or cursing, strange facial gestures, and sudden barking or other animal-like sounds. The spectrum of these tics and other symptoms is broad, which has complicated earlier attempts to describe the disease or to find its cause. The disease usually first appears in children between five and ten years of age and continues throughout life.

The variability of symptoms is one of the characteristic features or highlights of Tourette's syndrome. According to the American Psychiatric Association's *Diagnostic and Statistical Manual of Mental Disorders: DSM-IV-TR* (4th ed., 2000), among the diagnostic criteria for Tourette's syndrome are that both motor and vocal tics must occur and that the number, frequency, complexity, severity, and anatomical location of these tics must change over time. The tics must occur many times a day, usually in bouts, and they must recur "nearly every day or intermittently throughout a period

of more than one year." The disease must appear before the age of twenty-one to be considered Tourette's syndrome (although in many cases symptoms are so mild as to escape attention).

Associated with Tourette's syndrome are a number of other conditions, including obsessive-compulsive behaviors, attention-deficit disorder, hyperactivity, school phobias, test anxiety, conduct disorders, depression, dyslexia, poor socialization skills, and low self-esteem, though many of these symptoms can also appear by themselves. Several experts consider Tourette's syndrome and attention-deficit disorder to be variable manifestations of a common underlying disorder that may relate to a chemical imbalance in the brain. About half of Tourette's patients also show symptoms of attention-deficit disorder, such as frequent inattention, impulsiveness, and hyperactivity.

The association between Tourette's syndrome and attention-deficit disorder should be regarded as provisional. The two disorders may have an underlying cause in common, such as a common genetic basis. In many cases, however, the motor and vocal tics are made worse by the administration of stimulants such as methylphenidate, which is commonly used for the treatment of the hyperactivity that so often accompanies attention-deficit disorder. Thus it is possible that the presence of Tourette's syndrome in such cases may be attributable not to the attention-deficit disorder, but to the drugs used to treat the disorder. In certain cases, these drugs may have caused a transient or chronic tic disorder to progress to the more severe Tourette's syndrome. Clearly, more research is needed to clarify the exact nature of the relationship between Tourette's syndrome and attention-deficit disorder, both in the presence and in the absence of various drugs.

There are several other aspects of Tourette's syndrome that are being examined. For example, a number of researchers now suspect that the factors that predispose a patient to develop Tourette's syndrome may also predispose male patients to one form of alcoholism. Other researchers believe that the brain disorder responsible for Tourette's syndrome is related to the endorphins, the brain's natural opiates.

Some promising research involves the connection between this disorder and the neurotransmitter dopamine. Neurologists suspect that Tourette's syndrome results from increased sensitivity of certain parts of the brain to dopamine. Some of the evidence for the hypersensitivity of dopamine receptors derives from the observation that drugs such as haloperidol, which is known to inhibit the dopamine receptors, are effective in reducing the symptoms of Tourette's syndrome, while amphetamines and other drugs that enhance dopamine neurotransmission make the symptoms worse. Also, the cerebrospinal fluid of patients with Tourette's syndrome contains reduced levels of homovanillic acid, a breakdown product of dopamine. The corpus striatum in the brain is considered to be the most likely location for the supersensitive dopamine receptors. One researcher has found a total absence of a brain peptide called dynorphin in fibers of the corpus striatum, where this peptide normally occurs. The fibers in question project to the globus pallidus at the base of the cerebral hemispheres.

One theory that attempts to explain the relationship of the several symptoms in Tourette's syndrome is that they all stem from a loss of the inhibition that normally controls involuntary movements. The obscene or offensive words, normally inhibited, are expressed more often than other types of words because the inhibition has been removed. This theory supposes that children who find that they have expressed "bad" words that should not have been said out loud become obsessed with these words and thus (in the absence of inhibitions) say them more often, making the problem worse.

Studies of the families of Tourette's syndrome patients show that there are familial inheritance patterns, with many family members having at least some symptoms of tic disorders, attention-deficit disorders, or both. In many or most cases, the tic disorders of affected family members are so mild that they never caused any problems and were never mentioned to any physician. This finding leads many researchers to conclude that the underlying disorder is variable in the extent of its expression and that it is much more common than medical records show. One expert has even estimated that nearly 1 percent of the population has some form of tic disorder.

If all forms of tic disorder are included, it becomes clear that tics run in families and that Tourette's syndrome is simply one end of a spectrum of variable expression. Studies on identical twins confirm that the trait has a genetic basis. Additional studies of family histories suggest that everyone with the gene experiences symptoms of the disorder. The penetrance of the gene is somewhat greater in males than in females, meaning that more males have symptoms while females are more often symptom-free. Among those family members who have symptoms, the expression of those symptoms is highly variable.

Mimicking some of the symptoms of Tourette's syndrome are the so-called tardive tics that appear during adolescence or adult life. Tardive tics are considered by many researchers to be iatrogenic (drug-induced), arising from the prolonged use of neuroleptic drugs (tranquilizers) such as phenothiazines (Thorazine, Compazine, and Mellaril). Symptoms include isolated, short, quick, uncoordinated jerking movements. The mechanism by which tardive tics appear is unclear, but the same dopamine pathways may be involved as in genuine cases of Tourette's syndrome.

TREATMENT AND THERAPY

Various treatments are available for tic douloureux, both medical and surgical. Partial relief may be afforded by medical treatments, which include carbamazepine (tegretol), trichloroethylene, anticonvulsants such as phenytoin or phenylhydatoin (Dilantin), vasodilators such as tolazoline (Priscoline), analgesic (painkilling) drugs, vitamin B_{12}, or the repeated injection of 95 percent ethyl alcohol directly into the trigeminal nerve ganglion.

None of these treatments is successful in all cases, however, and some, such as trichloroethylene, have toxic side effects. Surgical treatments include neurotomy (cutting of the affected branch of the trigeminal nerve), decompression of the posterior nerve root, or the cutting of one or more of the trigeminal tracts in the brain stem, either in the midbrain or in the medulla. The most frequently performed surgical procedures include destruction, or partial destruction, of the trigeminal ganglion, either by electrocoagulation, by radio frequency therapy, or by mechanical means. The facial paralysis or partial paralysis that follows nerve destruction often resembles Bell's palsy except that the damage is usually permanent, with minimal possibility of recovery.

Treatment of childhood transient tic disorders usually consists of psychological intervention to control or reduce the level of stress. Many cases of transient or chronic tic disorder are so mild that they do not require any treatment.

For Tourette's syndrome, haloperidol (Haldol) is most often prescribed, and it is said to be effective in 50 to 90 percent of the cases, depending on the authority consulted. Other drugs occasionally prescribed include clonidine, penfluridol, and pimozide. These drugs can reduce the severity and frequency of tics and may reduce impulsive or aggressive behavior. They also have side effects, however, causing sedation, depression, and weight gain in many patients.

PERSPECTIVE AND PROSPECTS

Because tics are highly noticeable, suggestions regarding their cause have been made throughout history. It was not until the eighteenth century, however, that scientific studies were conducted on patients exhibiting these movements. Thus, while there are indications that tic douloureux was known and recognized in ancient times, James Fothergill (1712-1780) is usually credited with the first modern description of the disorder in 1773.

Georges Gilles de la Tourette (1857-1904) was a French physician who, in 1885, first described the medical syndrome that bears his name. Tourette described the disorder, which he considered to be heritable, on the basis of eight patients whose symptoms included jerking movements, noises, coprolalia, and echolalia. Tourette was shot three times by one of his patients in 1893; he never recovered from the resulting brain injury. Tourette's syndrome was usually ignored in medical literature or described as a rare disorder until the 1980's, when several researchers studying the families of Tourette's syndrome patients began to notice that many of the family members had mild forms of the same disorder that had previously escaped attention. When they looked more closely for tic symptoms, they discovered that such disorders were much more common than had previously been thought. Connections with obsessive-compulsive disorders and with alcoholism were first noticed from the discovery of these conditions among the relatives of Tourette's syndrome patients.

—Eli C. Minkoff, Ph.D.

See also Anxiety; Attention-deficit disorder; Encephalitis; Epilepsy; Huntington's disease; Motor neuron diseases; Muscle sprains, spasms, and disorders; Muscles; Nervous system; Neuralgia, neuritis, and neuropathy; Neurology; Neurology, pediatric; Palsy; Seizures; Speech disorder; Stress; Tourette's syndrome.

FOR FURTHER INFORMATION:

American Psychiatric Association. *Diagnostic and Statistical Manual of Mental Disorders: DSM-IV-TR.* 4th ed. Arlington, Va.: Author, 2000. The standard work in the field of psychiatry. Lists the criteria for the presence of Tourette's syndrome in a given patient.

Behrman, Richard E., Robert M. Kliegman, and Hal B. Jenson, eds. *Nelson Textbook of Pediatrics.* 18th ed. Philadelphia: Saunders/Elsevier, 2007. Includes a brief and very readable summary of tic disorders, emphasizing Tourette's syndrome. A bibliography is included.

Bloom, Floyd E., M. Flint Beal, and David J. Kupfer, eds. *The Dana Guide to Brain Health.* New York: Dana Press, 2006. An easy-to-understand health guide to the brain from neuroscience, neurology, and psychiatry perspectives. More than seventy psychiatric and neurological disorders, their diagnoses, and their treatments are covered.

Brill, Marlene Targ. *Tourette Syndrome.* Brookfield, Conn.: Millbrook Press, 2002. Uses vignettes of children at all ages to discuss Tourette's syndrome and its symptoms and manifestations, how it can be controlled and treated, and living with the disorder at home, at school, and in society.

Chipps, Esther M., Norma J. Clanin, and Victor G. Campbell. *Neurologic Disorders.* St. Louis, Mo.: Mosby Year Book, 1992. A good, simple reference written for nurses, using everyday language and frequent illustrations. Includes a section on tic douloureux.

Nicholls, John G., A. Robert Martin, and Bruce G. Wallace. *From Neuron to Brain.* 4th ed. Sunderland, Mass.: Sinauer, 2007. An excellent and detailed undergraduate neurobiology text that describes how nerve cells transmit signals, how signals are put together, and how higher functions emerge from this integration.

Victor, Maurice, and Allan H. Ropper. *Adams and Victor's Principles of Neurology.* 9th ed. New York: McGraw-Hill, 2009. A good but somewhat technical source on neurology. Contains a lengthy discussion of Tourette's syndrome.

Waxman, Stephen G. *Correlative Neuroanatomy.* 25th ed. New York: Lange Medical Books/McGraw-Hill, 2002. A very readable treatment, balancing basic information with clinical discussions.

Woods, Douglas W., and Raymond G. Miltenberger, eds. *Tic Disorders, Trichotillomania, and Other Repetitive Behavior Disorders: Behavioral Approaches to Analysis and Treatment.* New York: Springer, 2006. Provides an introductory chapter followed by fourteen chapters that cover assessment; physical and social impairment; and the characteristics, behavioral interventions, and treatment for tic disorders.

TINGLING. *See* NUMBNESS AND TINGLING.

TINNITUS

DISEASE/DISORDER

ANATOMY OR SYSTEM AFFECTED: Brain, ears, head, nerves, nervous system, psychic-emotional system

SPECIALTIES AND RELATED FIELDS: Audiology, family medicine, neurology, otorhinolaryngology, psychiatry

DEFINITION: An auditory sensation originating in the head without external stimulation. This common disorder (often considered a symptom) affects up to 10 percent of the general population in the United States, with the highest prevalence in persons between forty and seventy years old.

KEY TERMS:

acoustic neuroma: a benign tumor of the auditory nerve

auditory cortex: an area of the cerebral surface gray matter where auditory information is ultimately processed

auditory nerve: a sensory nerve (eighth cranial) that conducts hearing and equilibrium impulses

brain stem: a part of the brain that connects the cerebral hemispheres with the spinal cord

cerumen: earwax; secreted by glands at the outer third of the ear canal

cochlea: the coiled part of the inner ear containing the hearing receptors (hair cells with fine cilia)

Eustachian tube: an auditory tube extending from the middle ear to the nasopharynx

Ménière's disease: an inner-ear fluid imbalance resulting in recurrent episodes of hearing loss, tinnitus, severe dizziness, and ear pressure

oto-: a combining form indicating "ear"

otosclerosis: an abnormal bone growth in the middle ear

CAUSES AND SYMPTOMS

One proposed classification of tinnitus distinguishes two main categories. Subjective tinnitus, the most common type, is perceived only by the patient, usually as a continuous "phantom" sensation. Objective tinnitus, the second type, can be heard through a stethoscope placed over head and neck structures and is frequently perceived as a pulsatile sound.

Continuous subjective tinnitus occurs in a multitude of ear conditions. It is most often encountered in the context of hearing loss due to aging, excessive noise exposure, or ototoxic medication (such as salycilates, aminoglycoside antibiotics, chemotherapeutics, and diuretics). The auditory sensation can be induced or worsened by ear infections or excess of cerumen.

Other otologic causes are Ménière's disease, otosclerosis, and acoustic neuroma. Neurologic conditions (multiple sclerosis, stroke, head injury), temporomandibular joint (TMJ) disorder, and metabolic and psychogenic factors can also lead to tinnitus.

The causes of continuous tinnitus are often difficult to pinpoint, and the pathophysiology is still poorly understood. Prominent theories include repetitive discharge from injured cochlear hair cells that generate continuous impulses in the auditory nerve, spontaneous auditory nerve activity, hyperactive brain stem auditory nuclei, and decreased suppression of peripheral nerve impulses by the auditory cortex. A neurobiological model that has gained acceptance includes two essential events: initial damage to peripheral auditory structures, which triggers the tinnitus, and subsequent (maladaptive) plastic changes in the central auditory pathway, with increased activity in brain stem and cortical areas.

Pulsatile tinnitus is caused by blood flow perturbations (through either normal or abnormal blood vessels near ear structures) and mechanical factors. Atherosclerosis, vascular tumors, arteriovenous malformations, aneurysms, and vascular loops often lead to unilateral tinnitus and can be identified using imaging techniques. Vascular inflammation and thrombosis are additional causes of pulsatile tinnitus. Conditions associated with high cardiac output, such as pregnancy, anemia, or an overactive thyroid, can result in tinnitus. Mechanical causes of pulsatile tinnitus are represented by open Eustachian tubes and middle-ear muscle spasms.

Patients with tinnitus report a disturbing noise localized in one or both ears and sometimes in the head. They describe it as ringing, whistling, hissing, swishing, roaring, buzzing, or clicking. Ear fullness or pain can be present. The severity ranges from an occasional

---

INFORMATION ON TINNITUS

CAUSES: Various otologic, neurologic, vascular, and metabolic conditions

SYMPTOMS: Sound sensations without external physical stimulus

DURATION: Acute (days to weeks) or chronic (more than six months)

TREATMENTS: Pharmacotherapy, surgical intervention, hearing support, cognitive and behavioral therapy

awareness of the noise to a frustrating, even unbearable sound. Epidemiologic studies indicate that 25 percent of patients with tinnitus experience a pronounced discomfort, while the rest do not report significant distress. Sensations perceived as severe can result in attention deficit, anxiety, and depression. In general, pulsatile tinnitus, unilateral tinnitus, and tinnitus associated with additional ear symptoms should be investigated carefully because they can signal a potentially serious underlying disorder.

TREATMENT AND THERAPY

The assessment of a patient with tinnitus includes physical examination, blood pressure measurements, audiometric profile, complete blood chemistry, hematocrit and lipid levels, thyroid studies, and brain imaging. Most cases of tinnitus should be evaluated by an ear, nose, and throat (ENT) specialist.

Therapeutic steps vary according to the type of tinnitus diagnosed and how the symptoms affect a patient's life. Specific treatment should be provided for any underlying illness. Inflammatory ear disease is treated with antibiotic and anti-inflammatory medication. Conditions such as tumors, vascular abnormalities, otosclerosis, and Ménière's disease may warrant surgical intervention. If the tinnitus is caused by hearing damage, then reassurance is often sufficient. Hearing aids, noise-masking devices, and cognitive and behavioral therapy are sometimes recommended. Patients should avoid ototoxic medication, loud noise, and stress.

Many treatments are still in the experimental phase or have variable efficacy. Proposed pharmacologic therapies for severe cases include antianxiety and antidepressant agents, lidocaine, and carbamazepine. Drugs that improve brain metabolism (nootropics) and neurotransmitter-directed agents might prove beneficial. Additional approaches focus on neck exercises, sound therapy, acupuncture, and electrical brain stimulation.

PERSPECTIVE AND PROSPECTS

Tinnitus has been considered a disease entity for centuries. It was only in the second half of the twentieth century that physicians were able to discriminate between various types of tinnitus and their underlying pathology. Tinnitus remains a perplexing disorder, both for the sufferer and for the physician. No single treatment is truly efficacious, especially in subjective tinnitus. Many variables are associated with this "phantom" sensation, and a multitude of biological mechanisms

can cause it. Nevertheless, the neurobiology of tinnitus has become less mysterious. A growing body of research continues to unveil striking neural changes. Animal models are employed to elucidate brain activity patterns in tinnitus and to explore therapeutic avenues. As a result of this complexity, it is likely that successful therapeutic strategies will have to target multiple factors simultaneously.

—*Mihaela Avramut, M.D., Ph.D.*

See also Audiology; Ear infections and disorders; Ears; Hearing; Hearing loss; Ménière's disease; Nervous system; Neurology; Otorhinolaryngology; Sense organs; Signs and symptoms.

FOR FURTHER INFORMATION:

Claussen, Claus F. "Tinnitus." In *Conn's Current Therapy 2008*, edited by Robert E. Rakel and T. Edward Bope. Philadelphia: Saunders/Elsevier, 2009.

Crummer, Richard W., and Ghinwa A. Hassan. "Diagnostic Approach to Tinnitus." *American Family Physician* 69, no. 1 (January 1, 2004): 120.

Tyler, Richard S., ed. *The Consumer Handbook on Tinnitus*. Sedona, Ariz.: Auricle Ink, 2008.

TIREDNESS. *See* FATIGUE.

TOENAIL REMOVAL. *See* NAIL REMOVAL.

TOILET TRAINING
DEVELOPMENT

ANATOMY OR SYSTEM AFFECTED: Bladder, gastrointestinal system, genitals, intestines, kidneys, psychic-emotional system, urinary system

SPECIALTIES AND RELATED FIELDS: Family medicine, gastroenterology, pediatrics, psychiatry, psychology, urology

DEFINITION: Toilet use is a complex skill that children usually master within the first four years of life.

KEY TERMS:

encopresis: defecating outside the toilet

enuresis: urinating outside the toilet

PHYSICAL AND PSYCHOLOGICAL FACTORS

Toilet use may seem simple, but it is a complex skill. Children must learn to produce both urine and bowel movements on the toilet, stay dry when not on the toilet, clean themselves, dress and undress, initiate going to the toilet without being reminded, and stay dry while asleep. Most children are fully toilet trained—dry all day and night with complete independence in cleaning and dressing—by the age of four. All successful toilet training methods have three things in common: timing, consistency, and a positive approach.

Two kinds of timing are important. First, training should begin when the child is ready. The child is physically ready when voluntary control over the urethral and anal sphincters is established, usually between twelve and twenty-four months of age. Behavioral signs of physical readiness include a reduction in the frequency of urination. Another sign of readiness is seeking out privacy, often under or behind furniture, before defecating.

The child may indicate psychological readiness by showing awareness of being wet, revulsion or irritation when soiled, or interest in watching parents and older children in the bathroom. Some children show these signs of readiness as early as twelve months of age; others never do. Nearly all children can begin toilet training successfully by twenty-four months of age.

The second type of timing is in visiting the toilet. Children need to use the toilet after meals, every two or three hours between meals, and before bedtime or long car trips, just as adults do. Encouraging the child to sit on the toilet at these times for a few minutes each visit usually produces results.

Consistency is also important. A consistent schedule for meals and visits to the toilet is helpful, as is a consistent place for the child to use the toilet, such as a child-sized toilet, or potty, in the bathroom. Training pants help children to recognize when they are wet and should be worn every day once toilet training starts—although diapers can still be used at night. Finally, parents should respond consistently, showing pleasure every time that the child is successful and remaining calm when accidents occur.

A positive approach includes providing small treats or special activities to celebrate successes, giving children encouragement and affection whether or not they succeed, and discussing toilet use with the child in a calm and encouraging manner. Picture books for toddlers can provide an easy way for parents to talk to their child about toilet use.

DISORDERS AND EFFECTS

Children who have developmental delays or physical disabilities may have difficulty with toilet use. Sometimes, mild developmental delays or health problems are first discovered because of problems with toilet training. Special training methods for these children include positive reinforcement; liquid, food intake, and bathroom trips scheduled to maximize the chance of success; timers to remind children to use the bathroom; and sensors in clothing that trigger an alarm when wet. In some cases of physical malformation or disease, biofeedback, medication, or surgery may be attempted. Even children with very severe disabilities can learn to use the toilet, although they may continue to need reminders or physical assistance.

Toilet use problems of typically developing children include enuresis; fear of the toilet, urine, or feces; encopresis and hiding or playing with feces; retention of feces or urine; and frequent tantrums and accidents. It is normal for children under the age of four occasionally to have any of these problems, stressful as they are for parents. For older children, medical causes should be ruled out. Family therapy directed at both toilet use and discipline problems is often helpful. Nighttime enuresis, or bed-wetting, is the most common toilet use problem experienced by older children and adults. The cause of most cases of bed-wetting is probably developmental immaturity and may be inherited; it is rarely caused by mental illness, as many once believed. Effective treatments are available for this common problem.

PERSPECTIVE AND PROSPECTS

In European history, toilet training recommendations have ranged from sitting the child on the toilet at three months to giving no training at all. Punitive methods such as tying the child on the toilet, forcing food or drink, or hitting the child were common. By the early twentieth century, two schools of thought on toilet training had developed. Sigmund Freud, the founder of psychoanalysis, believed toilet training that was too early, punitive, indulgent, or sexualized would cause lifelong personality problems. The behaviorist school of thought held that with the right technique, children could be toilet trained quickly at any age in as little as a day. Neither camp had any direct evidence in support of its position.

Freudian ideas dominated popular advice on child care in the United States from the 1940's through the 1960's, leaving many parents anxious about ruining their children's lives with the wrong toilet training methods. During the 1960's, researchers discovered the variety of actual toilet training practices around the world. They found that toilet training before thirteen months was not effective and that training after thirteen months through age three was typical and rarely led to problems. Often, children who were punished during toilet training not only developed toilet use problems but also had nightmares, tantrums, and discipline problems throughout childhood. In addition, they found that children and adults with disabilities—previously thought to be untrainable—could be toilet trained using positive methods. By the early 1980's, developmental psychologists concluded that consistency, encouragement, and patience produce the best long-term results.

—Kathleen Zanolli, Ph.D.

See also Anxiety; Bed-wetting; Developmental stages; Emotions: Biomedical causes and effects; Motor skill development; Phobias; Psychiatry, child and adolescent; Soiling; Stress.

FOR FURTHER INFORMATION:

Berk, Laura E. *Child Development.* 8th ed. Boston: Pearson/Allyn & Bacon, 2009. A text that reviews theory and research in child development, cognitive and language development, personality and social development, and the foundations and contexts of development.

Faull, Jan. *Mommy, I Have to Go Potty! A Parents' Guide to Toilet Training.* Seattle: Parenting Press, 1996. Faull's overall tone is one of guiding and teaching, not rigid "training," and is therefore easier on both parent and child. A section entitled "Stories from the Bathroom," which details parents' experiences, will be helpful to any parent attempting toilet training.

Frankel, Alona. *Once upon a Potty.* Woodbury, N.Y.: Barron's, 1994. With millions of books sold, this resource is widely recognized as a premier picture book about toilet training. Published in different versions for girls and boys.

Rogers, June. "Child Centered Approach to Bed-Wetting." *Community Practitioner* 76, no. 5 (May, 2003): 163-165. A pediatric continence adviser explores the role that nurse-led community enuresis services play in effectively diagnosing and treating the underlying causes of childhood bed-wetting.

Schaefer, Charles, and Theresa Foy DiGeronimo. *Ages and Stages: A Parent's Guide to Normal Childhood Development.* New York: Wiley, 2000. An excellent resource that helps set expectations for children's growth and development. Includes numerous examples, stories, and activities parents can use to positively influence their child's development.

"Toilet Training: Is Your Child Ready?" *Health News* 18, no. 3 (June/July, 2000): 8. Most child development experts advocate a child-centered approach to toilet training. Signs that a child is ready to begin toi-

let training and steps parents can take to encourage their child to become potty-trained are discussed.

Warner, Penny, and Paula Kelly. *Toilet Training Without Tears or Trauma.* Minnetonka, Minn.: Meadowbrook Press, 2003. The authors, a pediatrician and a child development expert, provide advice for a stress-free toilet training experience for parents and children using research advances and "quick tips" from experienced parents.

TONSILLECTOMY AND ADENOID REMOVAL

PROCEDURES

ANATOMY OR SYSTEM AFFECTED: Lymphatic system, respiratory system, throat

SPECIALTIES AND RELATED FIELDS: General surgery, otorhinolaryngology, pediatrics

DEFINITION: The removal of the palatine tonsils (tonsillectomy) or the palatine tonsils and the adenoids (pharyngeal tonsils), in adenotonsillectomy.

KEY TERMS:

abscess: a painful, localized collection of pus in any part of the body; caused by tissue infection and deterioration

antibody: a blood protein that provides immunity against a disease-causing microorganism

crypt: a pit or cavity in the surface of a body organ (such as a tonsil)

lymphocyte: a white blood cell that produces antibodies

lymphoid tissue: tissue that can make lymphocytes; any portion of the lymphatic system

pharynx: the throat

INDICATIONS AND PROCEDURES

In common use, the term "tonsils" indicates two pinkish palatine tonsils, almond-shaped masses of soft lymphatic tissue located on either side of the back of the mouth. There are two other tonsil types: the lingual tonsils, positioned at the back of the tongue, and the pharyngeal tonsils (adenoids), found in the pharynx and near the nasal passages. Together, the three types of tonsils constitute an irregular band of lymphatic tissue that roughly encircles the throat at the back of the mouth. This tissue band is called Waldeyer's ring. The surface of each tonsil is composed of many deep crypts that, in the case of the palatine tonsils, often become the sites where food debris lodges or sites of bacterial and viral infections. The resulting inflammation of the tonsils is called tonsillitis.

In many cases, acute tonsillitis causes severe throat

pain that is easily cured by antibiotic treatment, without recurrence. In others, it returns repeatedly, leading to chronically infected palatine tonsils. Infection of the pharyngeal tonsils (adenoids) causes nasal congestion, and it sometimes produces hearing loss as a result of the obstruction of the Eustachian tubes, which lead from the ear to the throat. This obstruction of the Eustachian tubes may also predispose a person to ear infections.

Severe, chronic tonsillitis is most often treated by surgery to remove the palatine tonsils. When such surgery is carried out, physicians often elect to remove the infected adenoids as well. This double surgery is called adenotonsillectomy. The lingual tonsils are rarely removed because they do not often become infected. While the exact function of the components of Waldeyer's ring is not clear, they are seen as important to the production of bacteria-killing lymphocytes and antibodies, which protect the throat and digestive system from infection. For this reason, unlike in the past, the tonsils are removed only when absolutely necessary, and tonsillitis (or adenoid infection) is most often treated with antibiotics; penicillins and cephalosporins are the drugs of choice.

Usually, the onset of acute tonsillitis is signaled by sudden and severe throat pain, high fever, headache, chills, and diffuse pain in the lymph glands of the neck. These symptoms will normally clear up in five to seven days. The most dangerous form of tonsillitis is caused by streptococcal bacteria, usually the *Streptococcus pyogenes* species. Associated complications increase with the severity of the infection.

Especially severe cases of tonsillitis may lead to a deep infection of the throat involving peritonsillar abscess (quinsy). Many cases of quinsy must be treated by lancing the infected region, causing it to drain. The most severe complications of inappropriately or incompletely treated streptococcal tonsillitis are acute nephritis (kidney disease) and rheumatic fever, which may lead to serious heart problems. Both glomerulonephritis and rheumatic fever are due to autoimmune processes triggered by the infection.

When tonsillectomy is carried out, the adenoids are not removed unless they too cause frequently recurring health problems. The removal of the adenoids alone (adenoidectomy) is sometimes deemed necessary in children when repeated blockages of the nasal passages have caused excessive breathing through the mouth. Prolonged mouth breathing in children can lead to facial deformities because of stress on the developing facial bones.

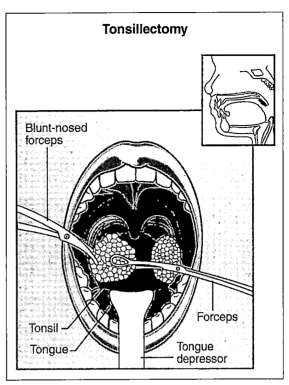

Tonsillectomy

Blunt-nosed forceps

Tonsil

Tongue

Forceps

Tongue depressor

Although this procedure is performed less often than in the past, the removal of the tonsils may still be required by chronic or severe infections; the inset shows the location of the tonsils.

The tonsils of children are removed under general anesthesia. With adults, local anesthesia is used whenever possible. Tonsillitis in children is much more severe and frequent than in adults because the tonsils decrease in size as one gets older. Similarly, the surgery is more difficult and severe in children because of larger tonsil size.

Uses and Complications

In most cases, tonsillectomy, adenotonsillectomy, and adenoidectomy are simple surgeries with few complications. The entire recovery period from such a procedure is usually several weeks. Most patients experience severe throat pain during the first few days of the recovery period, but this pain diminishes rapidly with time. It is important for the patient to eat soft food during recovery in order to prevent bleeding, which can become dangerous in some cases. Palatine tonsils do not grow back after surgery, although adenoids may sometimes reappear. The secondary adenoids, however, rarely become troublesome. Tonsillectomy, adenotonsillectomy, and adenoidectomy do not lead to freedom from sore throats. They do usually result, however, in a decreased frequency and severity of throat infections.

—*Sanford S. Singer, Ph.D.*

See also Abscesses; Adenoids; Antibiotics; Bacterial infections; Ear infections and disorders; Hearing loss; Lymphatic system; Otorhinolaryngology; Pediatrics; Pharynx; Quinsy; Sore throat; Strep throat; Streptococcal infections; Tonsillitis; Tonsils.

FOR FURTHER INFORMATION:

Beers, Mark H., et al., eds. *The Merck Manual of Diagnosis and Therapy.* 18th ed. Whitehouse Station, N.J.: Merck Research Laboratories, 2006. This is a reference work for physicians, and the nomenclature can be daunting. It is best consulted after more general introductory reading.

Ferrari, Mario. *PDxMD Ear, Nose, and Throat Disorders.* Philadelphia: PDxMD, 2003. A clinical yet accessible reference text that provides a comprehensive list of disorders, with a summary of the condition, background, diagnosis, treatment, outcomes, prevention, and resources.

Icon Health. *Tonsillectomy: A Medical Dictionary, Bibliography, and Annotated Research Guide to Internet References.* San Diego, Calif.: Author, 2004. Designed for physicians, medical students, researchers, and patients.

Tierney, Lawrence M., Stephen J. McPhee, and Maxine A. Papadakis, eds. *Current Medical Diagnosis and Treatment 2007.* New York: McGraw-Hill Medical, 2006. This text, updated yearly, is the point of reference for physicians and other health care practitioners. It incorporates each year's biomedical research discoveries that have immediate, relevant, and applicable use for the patient.

Townsend, Courtney M., Jr., et al., eds. *Sabiston Textbook of Surgery.* 18th ed. Philadelphia: Saunders/ Elsevier, 2008. A standard textbook of surgery.

TONSILLITIS
DISEASE/DISORDER

ANATOMY OR SYSTEM AFFECTED: Ears, lymphatic system, throat

SPECIALTIES AND RELATED FIELDS: Family medicine, general surgery, otorhinolaryngology, pediatrics

DEFINITION: Inflammation, infection, and enlargement of the palatine tonsils, two small masses of lymphoid tissue located on either side of the back of the throat, and frequently of the pharyngeal tonsils, or adenoids, which are located high in the throat above the soft palate.

CAUSES AND SYMPTOMS

Four small pairs of lymphatic tissue called tonsils together form a ring that circles the nasal cavity and mouth. In children, these tonsils help filter and protect the respiratory and alimentary tracts from infection. As children grow, however, this function dwindles and the tonsils shrink. Tonsillitis, or an infection of these tissues, can be either viral or bacterial in origin. Viral infections are more common in children under three, while older children usually suffer from bacterial infections. A throat culture can determine whether bacteria are present, thus indicating antibiotic treatment.

The two pairs of tonsils most often infected and inflamed are the palatine tonsils, which are those removed in a tonsillectomy, and the adenoids. Symptoms of infected and enlarged tonsils include a sore throat, difficulty swallowing, fever, chills, bad breath, and breathing exclusively through the mouth.

TREATMENT AND THERAPY

Viral tonsillitis is self-limiting and typically lasts for five days or less. In these cases, treatment should be symptomatic and includes a soft or liquid diet, warm saltwater or mild antiseptic gargles, throat lozenges, rest, and an analgesic drug such as acetaminophen. If a throat culture indicates bacterial causes, treatment should also include a ten-day course of penicillin or other appropriate drug and a second culture to determine the effectiveness of the treatment.

Occasionally, tonsillectomy (removal of the palatine tonsils) and adenoidectomy (removal of the adenoids) may also be indicated. Because the tonsils play an important role in the development of the immune system, children under three should not be surgically treated.

INFORMATION ON TONSILLITIS

CAUSES: Bacterial or viral infection

SYMPTOMS: Sore throat, difficulty swallowing, fever, chills, bad breath

DURATION: Acute

TREATMENTS: Alleviation of symptoms (soft or liquid diet, warm saltwater or mild antiseptic gargles, throat lozenges, rest, analgesics); antibiotics; tonsillectomy if needed

Before the discovery of penicillin and other antibiotics, a tonsillectomy was the treatment of choice for children who suffered recurrent tonsillitis. Because of the inherent risks of even minor surgery, however, tonsillectomies are now performed only if infected and enlarged tonsils are so problematic that they threaten to obstruct breathing.

—*Jane Marie Smith, M.S.L.S.*

See also Abscess drainage; Abscesses; Adenoids; Antibiotics; Bacterial infections; Immune system; Inflammation; Nasopharyngeal disorders; Otorhinolaryngology; Pharyngitis; Quinsy; Sore throat; Strep throat; Streptococcal infections; Tonsillectomy and adenoid removal; Tonsils; Viral infections.

For Further Information:

Beers, Mark H., et al., eds. *The Merck Manual of Diagnosis and Therapy.* 18th ed. Whitehouse Station, N.J.: Merck Research Laboratories, 2006.

Icon Health. *Tonsillitis: A Medical Dictionary, Bibliography, and Annotated Research Guide to Internet References.* San Diego, Calif.: Author, 2004.

Kemper, Kathi J. *The Holistic Pediatrician: A Pediatrician's Comprehensive Guide to Safe and Effective Therapies for the Twenty-five Most Common Ailments of Infants, Children, and Adolescents.* Rev. ed. New York: Quill, 2002.

Litin, Scott C., ed. *Mayo Clinic Family Health Book.* 4th ed. New York: HarperResource, 2009.

Silverstein, Alvin, Virginia B. Silverstein, and Laura Silverstein Nunn. *Sore Throats and Tonsillitis.* New York: Franklin Watts, 2000.

Woolf, Alan D., et al., eds. *The Children's Hospital Guide to Your Child's Health and Development.* Cambridge, Mass.: Perseus, 2002.

Tonsils
Anatomy

Anatomy or system affected: Immune system, lymphatic system

Specialties and related fields: Family medicine, oncology, otorhinolaryngology, pediatrics

Definition: The palatine tonsils are two compact bodies of lymphoid tissue located laterally between the opening of the mouth and the pharynx.

Key terms:

B lymphocytes: immunologically active lymphocytes predominantly found in tonsil tissue

group A streptococcus: the most common bacterial infection of the tonsils

human papillomavirus (HPV): a common virus affecting skin and mucosal surfaces

tonsillar fossa: the bed in which the tonsil sits

tonsillectomy: the common operative procedure used to remove diseased or hypertrophic tonsils

tonsilloliths: small white plugs or stones that form within the crypts of tonsil tissue

Waldeyer's ring: the ring of lymphoid tissue at the upper end of the pharynx consisting of the palatine tonsils laterally, the adenoids superiorly, and the lingual tonsils at the back of the tongue

Structure and Functions

The palatine tonsils are the largest bodies of lymphoid tissue in Waldeyer's ring. In contrast to the adenoid and lingual tonsil tissues, which are diffuse and adherent to the nasopharynx and the base of the tongue, the palatine tonsils are encapsulated by a specialized fascia and are easily dissected from their muscle beds. The tonsil tissues have ten to thirty deep crypts that extend into each tonsil and are lined by stratified squamous epithelium. Each tonsil sits in a tonsillar fossa in the lateral wall of the opening between the mouth and the pharynx. This tonsil bed is composed of three muscles that hold the tonsil in place. The anterior pillar of the tonsil is formed by the palatoglossus muscle, the posterior pillar is formed by the palatopharyngeal muscle, and the floor of the tonsil bed is formed by the superior constrictor muscle of the pharynx. The tonsils get their blood supply primarily at their lower pole from branches of the dorsal lingual and facial arteries. The tonsils' main nerve supply is from the tonsillar branches of the glossopharyngeal nerve.

The tonsils are immunologically active lymphatic organs. The lymphocytes of tonsil tissues are approximately composed of 60 percent B lymphocytes and 40 percent T lymphocytes. The location of the tonsils in the upper part of the aerodigestive tract exposes them to many airborne allergens. Tonsil crypts are able to trap foreign material and transport it to lymphoid follicles. When stimulated by antigens, B cells can proliferate in the germinal centers of the tonsils and produce all five major antibody classes. It has been shown that the immunologic activity of the tonsils and the adenoids in Waldeyer's ring helps protect the entire upper aerodigestive tract. Tonsils are most immunologically active between the ages of four and ten. Although it has been a point of controversy over the years, there is no evidence that removing the tonsils results in any immunologic deficiency.

DISORDERS AND DISEASES

Acute tonsillitis is commonly caused by both virus and bacteria. Enlargement of the tonsils without exudates is common with the common cold virus. Epstein-Barr virus may cause mononucleosis with high fever, dysphagia, and tonsillitis characterized by thick gray exudates. The most common bacterial infection of the tonsils is group A streptococcus, which is most commonly seen in children at age five to six years. Before antibiotics, acute streptococcal tonsillitis was a frequent precursor of rheumatic fever.

Recurrent tonsillitis and chronic tonsil hypertrophy are the most common reason for performing tonsillectomy in children. Enlarged tonsils can contribute to airway obstruction and sleep apnea. A peritonsillar abscess is more likely to be seen in young adults. The abscess usually forms between the tonsil and the anterior pillar, causing pain, dysphagia, and drooling, and requires drainage. The combination of exudates and bacteria in the crypts of the tonsils can lead to the formation of plugs or stones called tonsilloliths that can cause pain and bad breath. In severe cases, this condition may also be an indication for tonsillectomy.

Cancer of the palatine tonsil accounts for less than 1 percent of all cancers. Men are affected four times more frequently than women, with an age range between fifty and seventy. More than 70 percent of malignancies are squamous cell carcinomas, with lymphoma accounting for most other tonsil malignancies. Risk factors for squamous cell carcinoma include smoking, drinking alcohol, and infection from HPV.

PERSPECTIVE AND PROSPECTS

Tonsillectomy is one of the oldest recorded surgical procedures, with the first removal of tonsils being described by the Roman surgeon Aulus Cornelius Celsus in 30 C.E. Between 1911 and 1917, Samuel J. Crowe, professor of otolaryngology at Johns Hopkins, reviewed one thousand tonsillectomies performed. His description of sharp dissection with low incidence of complications opened the way to common use of this procedure. By the middle part of the twentieth century, there were more than two million tonsillectomies being performed every year in the United States. Between 1915 and 1960, tonsillectomy and adenoidectomy was the most frequently performed surgery in the United States. Today that number has dropped to about 700,000 cases per year. The introduction of new techniques such as electrocautery, laser surgery, and high-

frequency ablation have further contributed to lowering the complication rate associated with tonsillectomy to the point that about 80 percent of procedures are now done as outpatient surgery.

Recent research regarding cancers of the oral cavity including squamous cell tonsillar cancers has centered on the emerging role of HPV. HPV is one of the most common viruses in the world. In most cases, these viruses are relatively harmless. However, sexually transmitted types HPV 16 and 18 have been strongly linked to cervical cancer, and they are increasingly being recognized as a cause of oral cancer as well. Smoking and drinking alcohol may promote the invasive ability of these viruses in the oral cavity. Recent studies suggest that as many as 25 percent of oral cancers may be positive for HPV. Some studies suggest that HPV-positive oral cancers have a better prognosis than HPV-negative cancers. Another recent study suggests that HPV-positive tumors are more likely to begin within the tonsillar crypts. Understanding the relationship and effect of HPV on tonsil cancer may lead to novel approaches for prevention, targeted therapy, and improved ability to predict the prognosis of these tumors.

—Chris Iliades, M.D.

See also Abscess drainage; Abscesses; Antibiotics; Bacterial infections; Head and neck disorders; Immune system; Inflammation; Nasopharyngeal disorders; Otorhinolaryngology; Pharyngitis; Quinsy; Sore throat; Strep throat; Streptococcal infections; Tonsillectomy and adenoid removal; Tonsillitis; Viral infections.

FOR FURTHER INFORMATION:
Cummings, W. Charles, et al. *Cummings Otolaryngology: Head and Neck Surgery.* 4th ed. Philadelphia: Mosby/Elsevier, 2005.
Lalwani, K. Anil. *Current Diagnosis and Treatment in Otolaryngology—Head and Neck Surgery.* 2d ed. New York: McGraw-Hill, 2008.
Luginbuhl, A., et al. "Prevalence, Morphology, and Prognosis of Human Papilloma Virus in Tonsillar Cancer." *Annals of Otology, Rhinology, and Laryngology* 118, no. 10 (October, 2009): 742-749.
Pasha, Raza. *Otolaryngology: Head and Neck Surgery—A Clinical and Reference Guide.* 2d ed. San Diego, Calif.: Plural, 2005.

TOOTH DECAY. *See* **CAVITIES.**

TOOTH EXTRACTION

PROCEDURE

ANATOMY OR SYSTEM AFFECTED: Gums, mouth, teeth

SPECIALTIES AND RELATED FIELDS: Dentistry, orthodontics

DEFINITION: The surgical removal of a tooth because it is damaged by decay, disease, or trauma; threatening the health of other teeth; or near the site of significant disease.

INDICATIONS AND PROCEDURES

A tooth may have to be extracted for one of several reasons. Impaction is a condition in which a developing tooth is forced into an adjacent tooth, blocking its progress; the impacted tooth can threaten the health and proper alignment of nearby teeth if it is not extracted. The occurrence of crooked or misaligned teeth may also require surgical removal. In tooth decay, dental tissue weakens in a gradual process and can eventually be destroyed. Decay usually begins in the outer layer of the tooth, penetrates to the underlying dentin, and kills the innermost tissue (pulp) of the tooth. Tooth extraction is necessary if this process of decay cannot be halted.

The extraction of teeth is one of the most common procedures in dentistry. Dentists usually perform simple extractions, but they often refer patients needing more complicated procedures to oral surgeons.

In simple extractions, the dentist first applies a local anesthetic to deaden the area surrounding the tooth that is to be pulled. Then, the dentist uses forceps and short levers to loosen the tooth in its socket. The tooth is removed in one piece by breaking the ligaments that hold the tooth in place. Once the tooth has been extracted, the dentist cleans the empty socket and ensures that the blood flowing from the socket is clotting properly. The socket is dressed to protect it and help it heal.

The oral surgeon may use a general anesthetic with a patient needing a complex extraction. The surgeon may need to cut through gum and bone to gain access to the tooth requiring extraction. The tooth may be cut into small pieces before it can be removed. Sutures may be required to close the wound.

The pain caused by extraction usually peaks a few hours after the procedure. Patients are given analgesics (painkillers) and are encouraged to keep the head elevated and to use an ice pack.

—Russell Williams, M.S.W.

See also Braces, orthodontic; Cavities; Dental diseases; Dentistry; Endodontic disease; Gum disease; Oral and maxillofacial surgery; Orthodontics; Periodontal surgery; Periodontitis; Root canal treatment; Teeth; Toothache.

FOR FURTHER INFORMATION:

Christensen, Gordon J. "When It Is Best to Remove a Tooth." *Journal of the American Dental Association* 128, no. 5 (May, 1997): 635-636. Christensen describes situations in which removing teeth might be more acceptable than retaining them.

Connecticut Consumer Health Information Network. *Your Dental Health: A Guide for Patients and Families.* http://library.uchc.edu/departm/hnet/dental health.html. This is a user-friendly, practical Web resource for patients and the parents of younger patients, covering a wide range of information sources, including books and Web-based and printed pamphlets.

Diamond, Richard. *Dental First Aid for Families.* Ravensdale, Wash.: Idyll Arbor, 2000. Retired dentist Diamond discusses what to do when a dental problem arises and an immediate visit to the dentist is impossible. His practical advice is built on just enough basic science to put dental problems in context.

Klatell, Jack, Andrew Kaplan, and Gray Williams, Jr., eds. *The Mount Sinai Medical Center Family Guide to Dental Health.* New York: Macmillan, 1991. Designed for the lay reader, this handbook covers oral hygiene and dental care. Includes an index.

Langlais, Robert P., and Craig S. Miller. *Color Atlas of Common Oral Diseases.* 4th ed. Philadelphia: Lippincott Williams & Wilkins, 2009. Provides six hundred color photographs of the most commonly seen oral problems accompanied by descriptive text for each condition.

Morant, Helen. "NICE Issues Guidelines on Wisdom Teeth." *British Medical Journal* 320, no. 7239 (April 1, 2000): 890. The routine practice of prophylactic removal of disease-free, impacted third molars should be discontinued, according to the National Institute for Clinical Excellence.

Smith, Rebecca W. *The Columbia University School of Dental and Oral Surgery's Guide to Family Dental Care.* New York: W. W. Norton, 1997. This classic text provides easy-to-understand explanations of all common dental problems and procedures and many less common procedures. The text is written for the general reader.

Toothache
Disease/disorder
Anatomy or system affected: Gums, mouth, teeth
Specialties and related fields: Dentistry
Definition: Pain around a tooth or in the jaw.

Causes and Symptoms
Toothache is most commonly due to a cavity, which is decay that produces a hole in a tooth. Another frequent cause is inflammation of the gums, the soft tissue around the teeth. Cavities and gum disease are both caused by bacteria that accumulate, along with saliva and food particles, in deposits, called plaque, on the teeth. Cold, heat, or chewing may intensify toothache.

Initially, a decaying tooth is not painful. Pain may arise after the bacterial assault progresses through the tooth's hard, outermost layer of enamel and reaches the dentin. When the disease advances to the pulp, the blood vessels and nerves of this soft, innermost tooth tissue may die. At this stage, known as endodontic disease, severe pain and swelling may arise, especially if an abscess develops.

The early stages of gum inflammation—called gingivitis—also are not painful. Pain develops during the next stage, known as periodontal disease, when bacterial toxins erode the jawbone and weaken the attachments of the teeth to it. An abscess may form.

Other causes of toothache include exposure of the tooth roots, fracture of a tooth, and clenching or grinding of teeth. Toothache occasionally results from a problem not originating in the teeth or jaw, as in sinus congestion, heart disease, or ear infection.

Treatment and Therapy
A dentist will most commonly treat a cavity by placing a filling in the tooth. An advanced cavity, however, may require a crown, or cap, for the tooth. For decay that has reached the pulp, the dentist may refer the patient to an endodontist for a root canal procedure, in which the dying pulp tissue is removed. In extreme cases, the tooth may be extracted.

If a toothache is caused by gum disease, then the dentist will clean the teeth to remove plaque or, in severe cases, refer the patient to a periodontist for more elaborate treatment. Antibiotics may be administered.

Toothache caused by the exposed root of a tooth is often treated with a topical fluoride gel, special toothpaste, or protective filling. If a dentist cannot determine

---

Information on Toothache

Causes: Cavities, gum disease, exposure of roots, tooth fracture, clenching or grinding of teeth; may be worsened by cold, heat, or chewing
Symptoms: Pain, sometimes with swelling and abscess development
Duration: Chronic, progressive if untreated
Treatments: Depends on cause; may include fillings, crowns, root canal treatment, tooth extraction, plaque removal, antibiotics, topical fluoride gels, special toothpastes

---

the cause of a toothache, then the patient may need to consult with a physician to determine whether there is other underlying illness.

Perspective and Prospects
Toothache is mentioned in the writings of ancient civilizations of the Middle East and Far East. Remedies included filling or extracting decayed teeth and splinting loose ones.

Since the mid-twentieth century, dental research has increased greatly, resulting in a decreased prevalence of toothache. Research areas that may one day reduce the incidence even further include genetically engineered bacteria. Dental research is conducted both at dental schools and at the National Institute of Dental and Cranio-Facial Research.

—*Jane F. Hill, Ph.D.*

See also Cavities; Dental diseases; Dentistry; Dentistry, pediatric; Endodontic disease; Gingivitis; Gum disease; Periodontal surgery; Periodontitis; Root canal treatment; Sinusitis; Teeth; Tooth extraction.

For Further information:
Christensen, Gordon J. *A Consumer's Guide to Dentistry.* 2d ed. St. Louis, Mo.: Mosby, 2002.
Connecticut Consumer Health Information Network. *Your Dental Health: A Guide for Patients and Families.* http://library.uchc.edu/departm/hnet/dental health.html.
Porter, Robert S., et al., eds. *The Merck Manual Home Health Handbook.* Whitehouse Station, N.J.: Merck Research Laboratories, 2009.
Smith, Rebecca W. *The Columbia University School of Dental and Oral Surgery's Guide to Family Dental Care.* New York: W. W. Norton, 1997.

TORTICOLLIS
DISEASE/DISORDER
ALSO KNOWN AS: Spasmodic torticollis
ANATOMY OR SYSTEM AFFECTED: Muscles, neck
SPECIALTIES AND RELATED FIELDS: Neurology, physical therapy
DEFINITION: A form of dystonia (muscle rigidity) in which the neck muscles contract involuntarily, causing spasms, abnormal movements, and posture of the neck and head backward (retrocollis), forward (antercollis), or sideways (torticollis).

CAUSES AND SYMPTOMS
Torticollis occurs equally in the sexes and may develop in childhood or adulthood. Its causes are unknown, but some cases seem to be genetic, while others are acquired from secondary damage to the nerves affecting the head or neck muscles. Congenital torticollis may be caused at birth by malpositioning of the head in the uterus or by prenatal injury of the muscles or blood supply in the neck. Torticollis results from abnormal functioning of the basal ganglia, situated at the base of the brain, which control all coordinated movements.

The first symptoms may appear gradually as the head tends to rotate or turn to one side involuntarily. Other symptoms may involve asymmetry of an infant's head from sleeping on the affected side, enlargement or stiffness of the neck muscles, limited range of head motion, neck pain, and even headaches.

TREATMENT AND THERAPY
Because the cause of torticollis is unknown in most cases, presently no certain cure exists. Drug therapy is frequently employed, but these medications often produce only unpredictable, short-term benefits. Some patients experience relief when treated by physiotherapists, who may use local moist heat, ice, ultrasonography, or a custom-fitted soft collar. Surgery is not recommended as an initial treatment, but it has proven helpful in cases unresponsive to medication.

INFORMATION ON TORTICOLLIS

CAUSES: Unknown; possibly genetic
SYMPTOMS: Muscle spasms, abnormal movements and posture of neck and head, tingling and numbness, headaches
DURATION: Short-term to chronic
TREATMENTS: Drug therapy, physical therapy

PERSPECTIVE AND PROSPECTS
Torticollis is easiest to correct in infants and children and in adults who receive early treatment. With chronic conditions, tingling and numbness may develop as nerve roots in the cervical spine become depressed. Recent innovative surgical procedures are helpful, but they are not a complete cure for chronic spasmodic torticollis. Patients with long-term torticollis will probably retain some degree of head tilt or rotation.

—*John Alan Ross, Ph.D.*

See also Botox; Head and neck disorders; Headaches; Muscle sprains, spasms, and disorders; Muscles; Neurology; Neurology, pediatric; Numbness and tingling.

FOR FURTHER INFORMATION:
American Medical Association. *American Medical Association Family Medical Guide*. 4th rev. ed. Hoboken, N.J.: John Wiley & Sons, 2004.
Litin, Scott C., ed. *Mayo Clinic Family Health Book*. 4th ed. New York: HarperResource, 2009.
Moore, Keith L., and Arthur F. Dalley II. *Clinically Oriented Anatomy*. 6th ed. Philadelphia: Kluwer/Lippincott Williams & Wilkins, 2010.
Nagler, Willibald. "Rehabilitating a Stiff Neck." *Family Practice News* 36, no. 3 (February 1, 2006): 38.
Noback, Charles R., et al. *The Human Nervous System: Structure and Function*. 6th ed. Totowa, N.J.: Humana Press, 2005.
Pathak, Mayank, Karen Frei, and Daniel Truong. *The Spasmodic Torticollis Handbook: A Guide to Treatment and Rehabilitation*. New York: Demos Health, 2003.

TOUCH
BIOLOGY
ANATOMY OR SYSTEM AFFECTED: Nerves, nervous system, skin
SPECIALTIES AND RELATED FIELDS: Dermatology, neurology
DEFINITION: One of the five special senses; nerve endings and specialized structures in the skin and other tissues send the brain data about the organism's environment, both internal and external.
KEY TERMS:
adaptation: a decreased sensitivity to a stimulus, even though the stimulus may still be present, ultimately resulting in an ever-slowing release of nerve impulses until the impulses stop entirely
exteroceptors: sensory receptors generally located on

the skin or body surfaces that supply the brain with information about the external environment in which the body is located

mechanoreceptors: sensory receptors that, when mechanically deformed (such as being pressed on), send nerve impulses causing sensations of pressure and touch

Meissner's corpuscles: receptors at which the sense of a light touch or low-frequency vibrations are detected; also called corpuscles of touch

Merkel's disks: sensory receptors located in deeper layers of epidermal (skin) cells; also called tactile disks

modality: the ability to distinguish one sensation from another; the ability to discriminate light or heavy touch, pain, pressure, vibratory, or hot and cold sensations from one another

Pacinian corpuscles: receptors at which the sensations of heavy touch or deep pressure originate; also called lamellated corpuscles

projection: the process whereby the cerebral cortex determines where the point of a stimulus is located

root hair plexus: a network of sensory receptors located at hair roots that generates an impulse when hairs are moved

Ruffini endings: sensory receptors that respond to heavy and continuous touch and pressure; also called type II cutaneous mechanoreceptors or the end organs of Ruffini

STRUCTURE AND FUNCTIONS

An essential attribute of the survival of a species is the ability to detect both the internal and the external environment. This is necessary so that appropriate and life-sustaining actions can be taken at all times. When changes or modifications of these environments take place, many responses can occur within an individual, ranging from rolling over during sleep to restore blood flow to an arm to avoiding contact with a prickly pear cactus. This kind of monitoring occurs within the general and special sense organs or structures found in humans and many other species.

One way in which the body monitors its internal and external environments is through the general senses. General sensations include temperature, pain, touch, pressure, vibration, tickle, and proprioception (internal sensations relating to how one's body is situated in space). Sensations of touch usually originate at or very near the skin surface; some originate from receptors found in deeper, subcutaneous (below-the-skin) layers. Many of the general senses are collectively called the

tactile senses, notably those of touch, pressure, vibration, and tickle. In addition, the term "somatic senses" refers to the sensory receptors associated with skin, muscles, joints, and visceral organs. Receptors in the muscles or joints are essential for the awareness of body movement. Visceral receptors play important roles in monitoring changes in body pain, as in stomach pain, hunger, and thirst. The somatic senses provide a means by which the internal and external environments are monitored with regard to touch, pressure, stretch, pain, and temperature. While these terms are not precisely interchangeable, there is overlap in the sensations of touch, pressure, vibration, and tickle with all three categories: general, tactile, and somatic sensations.

Another means whereby a human interacts with the environment is controlled by the special senses. Special senses include taste, vision, smell, hearing, and body equilibrium in space (or balance). Special senses involve relatively large and specialized structures of the tongue, eyes, nose, and ear and inner ear, in contrast to the general senses, in which the structures are relatively simple but are more widely dispersed throughout the entire body. The neurological pathways are also simplified relative to the neurological events that occur in the special senses' organs and pathways. Combined, the general and special senses form an intricate and elegant system that allows for an individual's survival.

Sensations occur when a receptor receives a stimulus from the external or internal world. The result is a neural impulse that can be utilized in the brain to provide some awareness of the body and its immediate environment. Perception results from the interpretation of the sensory information at a conscious level. Conscious awareness of sensory stimulation generally occurs only when a sufficiently large, or sometimes abrupt, change in the status quo happens in either the internal or the external environment. At that point, the perception of a sense will be registered and noted in the cerebral cortex.

An untold number of sensory receptors are stimulated at any given second, including receptors that note where each body part is placed—from the tiniest portion of each finger and toe, to the position of the body in a chair. Other receptors respond to inhalation and exhalation pressure changes or feel air brushing past. All receptors work simultaneously and in harmony in a healthy person, but most of this activity is on a subconscious level. Only if a sufficient change in either the internal or the external world occurs will a sensation no

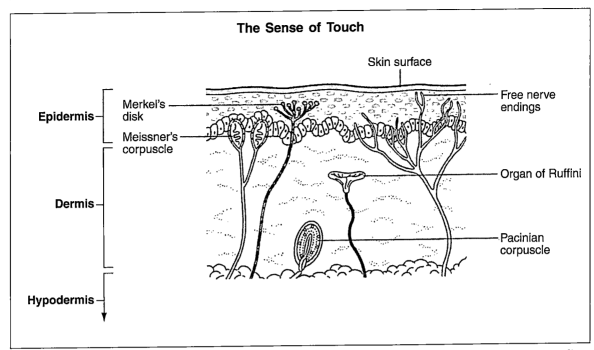

The Sense of Touch

Skin surface

Epidermis
- Merkel's disk
- Meissner's corpuscle

Dermis

Hypodermis

Free nerve endings

Organ of Ruffini

Pacinian corpuscle

The sensation of touch is produced by special receptors in the skin that respond to temperature and pressure stimuli.

longer be simply monitored but instead cause a conscious response. An example is feeling the hard coolness of a bench when being seated: At first, the perception of the hard and cold surface is pronounced, but this perception will decrease over time until one seemingly "forgets" about being seated on an uncomfortable bench. This kind of decreased sensitivity to a stimulus is called adaptation.

It appears that adaptation prevents the conscious mind from being overloaded with "meaningless" data or data that require no particular response. Adaptation may also allow for new, perhaps more important, stimuli to be noted at the receptor sites. Thus, the adaptation mechanism acts as a "reset" button. Consider the bench example again: In spite of one's "forgetfulness" about the bench being beneath the body, the stimulus is not, in fact, gone. Rather, the mind conveniently elects to ignore the stimulus unless a change occurs that reminds the brain of the bench's presence. This new perception of the bench might recur if a shift in body position causes new receptors to receive stimuli from new contact places between the body and the bench. Eventually, these new sensations will undergo the adaptation process and the bench will once again be "forgotten." (Although thermal equilibrium will be reached between the bench and the person, this process is slow and does not account for the quick rate of adaptation.)

There are four necessary components of sensation: a stimulus, which is generally caused by a change in the environment; a receptor, which can experience a stimulus and produce a generator potential to initiate a nerve impulse; an impulse, which carries the signal from the point of stimulation of the receptor to the brain; and a translation of the impulse within the brain, so that a meaningful interpretation of the kind of sensations experienced, such as a tickle or a floral fragrance, can be made.

All sense receptors are very excitable, but only if stimulated by the specific sensation that they are designed to monitor. This means that sensory receptors are highly specialized in their function. Sense receptors have a low threshold of response to the type of stimuli to which they are designed to respond, while having a high threshold of response to other kinds of stimuli. (Pain receptors are an exception to this rule, perhaps because of the variety of stimuli that can include a sense of pain.) An example of specialization of the receptors is seen in the fact that certain regions of the body are more susceptible to sensing a tickle than others. Specialization of receptors is attributed to the unique structures of the receptors, even though all sense receptors contain dendrites from sensory neurons.

At a receptor site, a stimulus may induce a generator potential, which sometimes is called the receptor potential. The generator potential is a localized and graded response that may reach its threshold if enough depolarization of the dendrites occurs. In other words, if threshold potential is achieved at the receptor, then a nerve impulse will ensue. This kind of response is an all-or-none response, the landmark characteristic of nerve cells.

The cerebral cortex is essential in the perception (interpretation) of a sensation. All different impulses arriving at the cerebral cortex are chemically the same; the only difference between an impulse carrying a message of a soft touch or of a heavy pounding is where the impulse arrives within the cerebral cortex. Impulses arriving at different locations of the cortex allow the brain to identify, classify, and locate the origins of a stimulus. The ability to distinguish one sensation from another is called modality; the ability to locate precisely the point at which the stimulus is applied is called projection. Modality and projection are functions of the cerebral cortex. In addition, the cortex can prompt many shifts in body position (such as stretching after reading) or body chemistry (such as the release of epinephrine to increase heart rate and blood flow in a crisis) if a response to the stimulus is deemed necessary.

Receptors can be classified according to the location or type of stimuli that cause the receptors to respond. Touch receptors can be classified as exteroceptors by virtue of the fact that these sensory receptors are externally located, mainly on the skin surface. Other classes of somatic receptors are located internally. Visceroreceptors monitor internal organs for data on hunger, thirst, pressure, and nausea. Proprioceptors monitor the muscles, tendons, joints, and inner ear for exacting knowledge of body position and body movement.

Mechanoreceptors are an alternative classification for touch receptors. This label is based on the type of stimuli—a mechanical displacement or disfiguring, for which touch receptors have a low threshold. Light touch is felt when the skin is very gently touched and no indentation or distortion of the skin results. Touch pressure is felt when a heavy touch causes a distortion of the skin surface, either laterally, as in a tugging sensation, or vertically, as in a depression of the skin surface.

Six types of touch receptors have been identified in the human anatomy: root hair plexuses; free nerve endings; tactile disks, or Merkel's disks; corpuscles of touch, or Meissner's corpuscles; type II cutaneous mechanoreceptors, or end organs of Ruffini; and Pacinian corpuscles, or lamellated corpuscles. At these structures, a mechanical stimulus can be transformed

into a sensation, provided that the stimulus is sufficiently strong to bring about a threshold potential.

Root hair plexuses are located in networks at the hair roots. On the scalp, these generate a sensation of touch when the hair is being pulled, brushed, or stroked. On the body surface, these receptors are sensitive to movement of the hair, as can occur if a small breeze passes over the skin or if a silk scarf is dragged lightly over the skin hairs. Root hair plexuses are not structurally supported, nor are they protected by any surrounding structure.

Free nerve endings are everywhere on the skin surface and seem to be responsive to many kinds of stimulus. These little dendritic processes of sensory neurons are not protected or supported by surrounding structures.

Made of disklike formations of dendrites, Merkel's disks, or tactile disks, are found in the deeper layers of the skin. Merkel's disks are particularly abundant on the fingertips, palms, soles of the feet, eyelids, lips, nipples, clitoris, tip of the penis, and tip of the tongue. Merkel's disks are particularly suited to receiving stimuli of fine touch and pressure.

Meissner's corpuscles, or corpuscles of touch, are egg-shaped dendritic masses that are sensitive to light touch and vibrations of a low frequency. Found in the hairless portions of the skin, these receptors are also used in making judgments about the textures of whatever the skin may contact. Two or more sensory nerve fibers enter each corpuscle of touch; the nerve fibers terminate as tiny knobs within the corpuscle. In addition, Meissner's corpuscles contain dendritic extensions. The entire mass is enclosed in connective tissue, which offers some support and protection to the disks. Corpuscles of touch are found in the external genitalia, tip of the tongue, eyelids, lips, fingertips, palms and soles, and nipples of both sexes.

The end organs of Ruffini, or type II cutaneous mechanoreceptors, are found all over the body but especially in the deep dermis (skin) and deeper tissues below the dermis. These are also called corpuscles of Ruffini and are responsive to heavy and continuous touch and pressure.

Finally, the Pacinian corpuscles are relatively large ellipses that are found in the subcutaneous tissue (below the skin) and deeper subcutaneous tissues. Also known as lamellated corpuscles, these touch receptors are found under tissues that contain mucous membranes, serous membranes, joints and tendons, muscles, mammary glands, and external genitalia. Pacinian receptors are sensitive to deep and heavy pressure and vibrations of low frequency. As such, these receptors detect pulsating, vibrating stimuli. There is an abundance of Pacinian receptors in the penis, vagina, feet and hands, clitoris, urethra, breasts, tendons, and ligaments. Inside each ellipsoid are dendrites from sensory nerves; the bundle itself is wrapped in connective tissue that can serve as a protective support.

DISORDERS AND DISEASES

Loss of tactile senses is a symptom rather than a disease. In general, a lost ability to sense touch, pressure, vibration, or tickle is a result of physical damage to a group of nerves or of a disease of the nervous system. Sensory receptors are not themselves targets of disease, but they can be physically or chemically impaired, especially if the skin is severely damaged.

An example of severe damage to the skin that will cause a loss of tactile sensations is a third-degree burn of the body. Third-degree burns are marked by the total destruction of the full thickness of the skin. This destruction includes the epidermis, the dermis, and any associated skin structures, such as secretion glands, hair, and the general sensory receptors. No pain is sensed when regions of the body that have received a third-degree burn are touched, because the nerve fibers that innervate the touch receptors and the free nerve endings, as well as nerves located in the subcutaneous layers, have been destroyed by the burn. In such cases, total destruction of the nerve fibers and the skin has occurred. Third-degree burns can have a charred, dry appearance or a mahogany or ash-white color. Regeneration of the dermis and the subcutaneous structures is slow and painful as the healing occurs. Although skin grafting can facilitate the regeneration process, it is not uncommon for scarring to result from the rapid contraction of the wounded area as it heals.

The sense of touch is largely lost in scar tissue, since new nerve fibers cannot be formed. (Nerve cells are formed only during gestation and early life and are designed to last a lifetime.) Some tactile senses can return to scarred regions through a process called sprouting. This process involves the branching forth, or the sprouting, of dendritic processes originating in undamaged nerve cells near to, but removed from, the injured site. In this kind of recovery, the healthy nerves assist in restoring tactile senses, to a limited degree, in the damaged regions.

Aside from a total loss of sensation, a sense of numbness can indicate a loss of proper blood circulation to a body region. For example, if one sits or folds oneself into a position so that a leg is receiving pressure from other body parts, the sensation of touch and pressure on the leg will eventually cause a sense of numbness; a form of pain ensues that feels like a tingling sensation that is often described as "pins and needles" all over the leg. The loss of blood circulation to the numbed region actually triggers pain receptors, sending an impulse to the cerebral cortex that warns of an odd feeling. The cerebral cortex will perceive the problem and command responses of the skeletal and muscular systems to change body position. Proprioceptors will sense the new body position and, as blood circulation restores a normal environment, the tingling decreases until it disappears. Numbness can also be a symptom of nerve damage or can result from the use of certain drugs, such as Novocain, that are used in dental and medical applications.

Changing of body position is an important outcome of the touch, pressure, and pain senses. Without the ability to change the position of the body, as can happen in some elderly or quadriplegic persons, damage to the areas on which the whole of the body is resting can occur. Neglect of these persons in home care or in health care facilities will result in bedsores developing at these pressure points. If left unchecked, these bedsores will grow and can lead to gangrene. As a part of their care, such individuals require physical therapy or physical aid in moving body parts and in changing sitting and sleeping positions several times each day.

Damage to the right lobe of the brain may cause abnormalities in the senses of touch and pressure, which in turn can cause a deficit in the ability to locate precisely where a tactile sensation originates on the body surface (the ability to project tactile sensations), making adjustment to and interaction with the external environment challenging. Right lobe damage, therefore, may give rise to a condition called passive touch deficit. Passive touch deficits are revealed by an impaired ability to discriminate touch sensations and by altered thresholds of touch and pressure that cause a sensation to be perceived.

Damage to the right lobe may also lead to deficits in active touch, meaning that such descriptors as size, shape, and texture cannot be readily discerned in touch tests. Generally, right lobe damage also leads to the loss of fine motor control of the fingers, which is especially challenging for piano players, authors, computer operators, painters, surgeons, and others who require exacting motor control of the fingers.

Sometimes, lesions in the right lobe of the cerebral cortex will lead to a condition called tactile agnosia. Tactile agnosia will occur only in the left hand, given the contralateral arrangement of the hands and neurological pathways to the cortex. The symptom of tactile agnosia is the diminished ability, or the inability, to identify common items (such as a key, pencil, or comb) when it is placed in the left hand. Fortunately, this condition is not common.

Another interesting form of loss of touch can occur in an odd behavior called neglect. Again, the problem with this loss of sensation originates from damage to the cerebral cortex, not to the touch receptors of the body. In neglect, lesions of the right parietal lobe are generally present but the contralateral neural pathway results in lost sense on the left side of the body. The ability to perceive a left-side stimulus is lost; patients may not notice anything in the internal or external environments on the left side of the body. In left-side neglect, patients may step into the right leg of a pair of pants but not the left leg and will not know that anything is wrong. Left-side neglect can also result in only right turns being made in walking patterns, and stimuli from the visual, auditory, and tactile sensations are not at all perceived. The sensation is traveling from the point of stimulation, but the cerebral cortex cannot process the sensation.

Finally, the issue of the phantom limb has significance in the medically related aspects of the sense of touch. "Phantom limb" is the term used to describe a sensation that seems to arise from a limb that has been amputated. Patients who have lost body parts to amputation, either surgically or mechanically (as a result of trauma, such as a car accident or an accident while operating a meat-processing machine), often describe sensations of itching, burning, or heat or cold, as well as other general sensations in the limb that is missing.

Although the limb—such as a finger, toe, or part of a leg or arm—may be absent, general sensations seem to arise from these absent body parts because of the neurological pathways that would normally connect the limbs to the cerebral cortex. In addition, a sensation is only as accurate as the cortex's ability to locate and identify the stimulus. This recall is called perception. Perception, however, is not an exact science; it results from experiences and associations that teach the cortex how to sort and analyze sensory data. Much information comes into the brain on common pathways, as if only a few streets led into a special city and all cars wanted to travel those streets to get there. An index fin-

ger may have had priority access to the paths during the training days of a young concert pianist. If, however, the pianist loses that index finger, neurological activity along the pathway to which the finger was once connected has not stopped. In fact, during the adjustment and recovery period immediately following the amputation, neurological activity may be heightened. As these sensory receptors and neurons send impulses along the avenues as before, these impulses will now be dominant in the absence of the index finger. Although the conscious mind is fully aware that the finger is absent, the subconscious mind has not yet acclimated itself to the change. Thus, a false association is made before the conscious mind can "correct" the perception and realize that the stimulus must be originating from a place other than the absent body part.

PERSPECTIVE AND PROSPECTS

Responsiveness to different kinds of touch at different locations on the body reveals a relationship between receptor structures and their subsequent function. Specifically, the hands of the human body are exquisitely sensitive to touch. The calculated innervation (number of nerve connections) for touch alone on the palms of the hands is 17,000 units.

On the palms, the most abundant type of touch receptors are Meissner's corpuscles. Accounting for 43 percent of all the touch receptors of the palms, they are responsible for the sensations of texture, light touches, and low-frequency vibrations and clearly play an important role in the human experience. Meissner's corpuscles are particularly abundant on the tips of all fingers and both thumbs. Although these receptors adapt at a moderately rapid pace, they are not so fast at adapting that the pleasure of stroking a cat or caressing a baby's head is lost.

After Meissner's corpuscles, Merkel's disks are second most abundant on the palms. Constituting 25 percent of the touch innervation density, these cells are suited for fine touch and pressure. Mainly confined to the digits' and thumbs' full length, Merkel's disks are important in tactile pursuits such as painting, drawing, sewing, writing, and dentistry. They are equally important in the expression of loving gestures to other people, animals, and plants via touch. Merkel's disks are slow to adapt; thus, these sensations are somewhat sustained.

Constituting 19 percent of the palms' innervation are the Ruffini endings. These are scattered throughout the palm surface area and are not localized. Ruffini endings are receptive to heavy and continuous touch and are slow adaptors. While a person is carrying a stack of books, for example, these endings are "firing" the nerves that connect to them.

Finally, making up only 13 percent of the palms' innervation to touch are the Pacinian corpuscles. Having a slight clustering in the fingertips, these are very quick at adapting to stimuli. They are receptive to deep and heavy pressure, such as the sensations that can be felt while massaging the hands.

Hairless regions of the skin, such as the palms, soles, penis, and vagina, contain Merkel's disks, Ruffini endings, Meissner's corpuscles, and Pacinian corpuscles. The combinations of receptors within these regions make these body parts acutely aware of and sensitive to light or heavy touch, rough or velvety textures, and pulsating or vibratory stimuli. These areas are also associated with pleasure centers of the body, in part because of their heightened tactile sensitivity.

Hairy skin, such as on the legs, chest, and arms, contains tactile disks, Ruffini endings, root hair plexuses, and Pacinian corpuscles. These body parts are sensitive to vibratory stimuli, breezes and other forms of displacement of body hairs, and pressure and tugging or pulling of the skin.

People are often willing to go to extra lengths to take care of their special sensory organs—the eyes, ears, mouth, and nose—because of their unique and important functions in the human body, but rarely do the general senses receive such attention. In spite of being largely overlooked, the general senses provide humans and other species with something so fundamental to life that it is often forgotten: touch. Offering a means of experiencing the most intimate communication and connection between self and others or between self and the environment, touch is an integral aspect of life.

—*Mary C. Fields, M.D.*

See also Acupressure; Amputation; Burns and scalds; Grafts and grafting; Nervous system; Neuralgia, neuritis, and neuropathy; Neurology; Neurology, pediatric; Numbness and tingling; Physical rehabilitation; Sense organs; Skin.

For Further Information:

Møller, Aage R. *Sensory Systems: Anatomy, Physiology, and Pathophysiology.* Boston: Academic Press, 2003. An excellent text that describes how human sensory systems function, with comparisons of the five senses and detailed descriptions of the functions of each of them. Also covers how sensory informa-

tion is processed in the brain to provide the basis for communication and for the perception of one's surroundings.

Schmidt, Robert F., ed. *Fundamentals of Sensory Physiology.* Translated by Marguerite A. Biederman-Thorson. Rev. 3d ed. Berlin: Springer, 1986. Chapters 1 through 4—"General Sensory Physiology, Psychophysics," "Somatovisceral Sensibility," "Neurophysiology of Sensory Systems," and "Nociception and Pain"—address the topics of touch sensations. Sketches and postreading quizzes assist the reader in comprehension.

Shier, David N., Jackie L. Butler, and Ricki Lewis. *Hole's Essentials of Human Anatomy and Physiology.* 10th ed. Boston: McGraw-Hill, 2009. An academic textbook designed to give more detail about the human body than an introductory biology book. Chapter 12, "The Somatic and Special Senses," has a section devoted exclusively to receptors and sensations. Related topics, such as the anatomy and organization of the brain and nervous system, are described in exquisite detail.

Tortora, Gerard J., and Bryan Derrickson. *Principles of Anatomy and Physiology.* 12th ed. Hoboken, N.J.: John Wiley & Sons, 2009. Provides a treatment of the topic of touch. Covers the sensory, motor, and integrative systems.

Wolfe, Jeremy M., et al. *Sensation and Perception.* 2d ed. Sunderland, Mass.: Sinauer, 2009. Addresses all five senses. Includes a detailed section on touch.

Tourette's syndrome

Disease/disorder

Also known as: Gilles de la Tourette syndrome

Anatomy or system affected: Brain, muscles, musculoskeletal system, nerves, nervous system, psychic-emotional system

Specialties and related fields: Biochemistry, family medicine, genetics, neurology, psychiatry, psychology

Definition: A disorder characterized by recurrent, multiple motor tics and one or more vocal tics that causes stress and impairs social functioning.

Key terms:

coprolalia: involuntary vocalization involving the uttering of obscenities or other socially inappropriate comments

copropraxia: a complex motor tic that involves involuntary, obscene gestures

echolalia: repetition of the words or gestures of others

palilalia: repetition of one's own words
tic: a sudden, rapid, recurrent, irresistible, nonrhythmic, and stereotyped movement; tics may involve motor movements, sudden vocalizations, or a combination of both

CAUSES AND SYMPTOMS

Tourette's syndrome is a disorder marked by multiple motor tics, involuntary vocalizations, and significant impairment of social functioning, often resulting in low self-esteem. For a diagnosis of Tourette's syndrome, the symptoms must persist for a period of at least one year, although they may decrease or subside during that time for brief periods of three months or less. Onset must be prior to eighteen years of age. The motor and vocal tics manifested must not be a consequence of drug use or the result of a previously existing medical condition such as Huntington's chorea.

Definitive causes for Tourette's syndrome remain under investigation. Research in the late 1990's included an exploration of genetic factors that might cause a susceptibility to the disorder and studies of the frequency of the disorder in subsequent generations within families. Studies in brain chemistry were also conducted.

Tourette's syndrome differs from a disease in that sufferers manifest a number of symptoms that occur together. Symptoms may be seen in sequence or in combination. Simple motor or vocal tics are most often first noticed in children between the ages of two and seven, but initial symptoms may be seen in the teenage years. Typically, the first symptoms noticed are simple motor tics such as eye blinking, tongue protrusion, facial grimacing, or other movements in the head area, such as grunting, coughing, throat clearing, or unusual vocalizations.

Complex motor tics include such behaviors as involuntary touching, knee bends, touching of objects in sequence, or other repetitive behaviors. Although many patients first display eye blinks, the anatomical location, severity, and frequency of the tics may change over time. As a youngster matures, the tics may involve other areas of the body, such as the torso or the limbs.

The social implications of this disorder are as important as the physical ones for a child with Tourette's syndrome. Such motor tics as touching inappropriately and involuntary utterances and outbursts can be disastrous to both self-image and social standing. Palilalia, echolalia, coprolalia, copropraxia, and bizarre behaviors brought about by involuntary compulsions cause

affected children much anxiety. That their symptoms may mimic or coexist with other disorders is another concern. Although some children may outgrow the disorder in their twenties, generally Tourette's syndrome is a lifelong disorder. Social difficulties abound for those afflicted and for their families. With concentration and relaxation techniques, tics may be delayed or suppressed for brief periods, but they present ongoing problems for those living with Tourette's syndrome.

TREATMENT AND THERAPY

By the turn of the twenty-first century, physical treatment for Tourette's syndrome involved a combination of relaxation techniques and medication therapy. Counseling has also proven useful, in conjunction with other treatments, in helping to deal with the social and emotional effects of this disorder. Relaxation techniques such as visualization of a calm setting and a variety of related therapies have proven successful in reducing the number and severity of the tics. Touch therapy and related techniques such as stroking and rocking have been helpful in reducing stress, as have some forms of massage.

Music is another effective means of relaxing the mind and the body. Some researchers have recommended that musical selections with a beat close to one's resting heartbeat are the most effective in reducing stress levels. Musical instruments and other forms of creative expression have proved to be effective tools against stress and associated tics. Hobbies, diaries, written expression, and counseling have all been used effectively to treat the physical and emotional symptoms of Tourette's syndrome.

A number of medication therapies are also being used. Catapres has been helpful in the treatment of tics,

---

INFORMATION ON TOURETTE'S SYNDROME

CAUSES: Unknown; possibly genetic
SYMPTOMS: Repetitive eye blinking, tongue protrusion, facial grimacing, or other head movements; unusual vocalizations (grunting, coughing, throat clearing); involuntary touching, knee bends, touching of objects in sequence, or other repetitive behaviors
DURATION: Chronic
TREATMENTS: Relaxation techniques, drug therapy, counseling, touch therapy, music therapy

with some side effects. Drugs such as Haldol and Orap have also had success, but with undesirable side effects. Children also suffering from related disorders such as attention-deficit disorder (ADD) have been treated successfully with Ritalin. Drugs such as Anafinil and Prozac have proven useful in treating obsessive-compulsive disorder and other anxiety disorders sometimes seen in conjunction with Tourette's syndrome.

PERSPECTIVE AND PROSPECTS

Treatment and understanding have evolved substantially since 1885 when Georges Gilles de la Tourette first identified Tourette's syndrome, which was thought to be a psychological disorder influenced by environmental factors. Many significant gains have been made since the 1980's in the clinical and scientific understanding of this complex disorder. Research in the late 1990's explored connections between brain chemistry and Tourette's syndrome. The role of genetics in the transmission and manifestation of the disorder was also studied extensively. Promising new medications continue to be developed as well.

—*Kathleen Schongar, M.S., M.A.*

See also Antianxiety drugs; Anxiety; Attention-deficit disorder (ADD); Learning disabilities; Motor skill development; Nervous system; Neurology; Neurology, pediatric; Obsessive-compulsive disorder; Psychiatric disorders; Psychiatry; Psychiatry, child and adolescent; Tics.

FOR FURTHER INFORMATION:

American Psychiatric Association. *Diagnostic and Statistical Manual of Mental Disorders: DSM-IV-TR*. 4th ed. Arlington, Va.: Author, 2000. The bible of the psychiatric community, this is a compendium of descriptions of disorders and diagnostic criteria widely embraced by clinicians.

Brill, Marlene Targ. *Tourette Syndrome*. Brookfield, Conn.: Millbrook Press, 2002. Uses vignettes of children at all ages to discuss Tourette's syndrome and its symptoms and manifestations, how it can be controlled and treated, and living with the disorder at home, school, and in society.

Cohen, Donald J., Ruth D. Bruun, and James F. Leckman, eds. *Tourette's Syndrome and Tic Disorders*. New York: John Wiley & Sons, 1988. Covers aspects of Tourette's syndrome, tic disorders, and other diseases of the central nervous system.

Koplewicz, Harold S. "Tourette Syndrome." In *It's Nobody's Fault: New Hope and Help for Difficult Chil-*

dren and Their Parents. New York: Three Rivers Press, 1997. Designed for the lay reader, this volume offers helpful advice to parents. Includes an index.

Kushner, Howard I. *A Cursing Brain? The Histories of Tourette Syndrome*. Rev. ed. Cambridge, Mass.: Harvard University Press, 2000. A fascinating exploration of the history of the understanding of Tourette's syndrome, detailing the role of cultural and medical assumptions in mediating its definition in the nineteenth and twentieth centuries.

Parker, James N., and Philip M. Parker, eds. *The Official Parent's Sourcebook on Tourette Syndrome*. San Diego, Calif.: Icon Health, 2002. Guides patients in using the Web to educate themselves about Tourette's syndrome and draws from public, academic, government, and peer-reviewed research to provide comprehensive information on a range of topics related to the condition.

Shimberg, Elaine Fantle. *Living with Tourette Syndrome*. New York: Simon & Schuster, 1995. Designed for sufferers of Tourette syndrome and their families and friends, this practical guide offers detailed information about diagnosing, treating, and dealing with Tourette syndrome at home, school, and work.

Tourette Syndrome Association. http://www.tsa-usa .org. A group supporting advocacy, education, and research related to the disorder.

TOXEMIA
DISEASE/DISORDER
ALSO KNOWN AS: Preeclampsia, eclampsia
ANATOMY OR SYSTEM AFFECTED: Blood vessels, circulatory system, reproductive system
SPECIALTIES AND RELATED FIELDS: Obstetrics
DEFINITION: A common disorder of pregnancy characterized by hypertension and proteinuria (protein in the urine). When severe, toxemia can affect multiple organ systems and even lead to seizures.

CAUSES AND SYMPTOMS
The precise cause of toxemia is unknown. Multiple theories exist, the leading ones pointing to an immunologic or vascular cause. Toxemia occurs after twenty weeks of gestation and is associated with a number of risk factors, including nulliparity, twin gestation, family history of toxemia, diabetes, antiphospholipid syndrome, chronic hypertension, and renal disease.

Symptoms and signs that are required for a diagnosis of toxemia are systolic blood pressure over 140 and di-

---

INFORMATION ON TOXEMIA

CAUSES: Unknown; risk factors include first pregnancy, more than one fetus, family history of toxemia, diabetes, antiphospholipid syndrome, chronic hypertension, renal disease

SYMPTOMS: Elevated blood pressure and facial edema; in severe cases, headache, visual changes, upper abdominal pain, decreased urine output, overactive reflexes, fluid in lungs

DURATION: Chronic during pregnancy

TREATMENTS: Depends on severity and gestational age of fetus; may include blood pressure medications (hydralazine, labetalol), bed rest, delivery of baby

---

astolic blood pressure over 90 across a span of six hours and urine with protein in excess of 300 milligrams over twenty-four hours. Other symptoms may be present, such as facial edema. In severe cases, headache, visual changes, upper abdominal pain, decreased urine output, hyperreflexia (overactive reflexes), or fluid in the lungs may be present. These symptoms may be accompanied by laboratory abnormalities indicating liver, kidney, red blood cell, or platelet disorders. Toxemia may also manifest as seizures, with the risk of concomitant stroke, which is termed eclampsia. In women with prolonged preeclampsia, uteroplacental insufficiency (decreased blood supply to the fetus) may occur, leading to oligohydramnios (too little amniotic fluid) and/or restriction in fetal growth.

TREATMENT AND THERAPY

The treatment of toxemia depends on the severity of the disease and the gestational age of the fetus. High blood pressure can be controlled with medications such as hydralazine or labetalol. The patient is placed on bed rest, and the patient's fluid status is monitored. Delivery of the infant and placenta is curative. While this is the treatment of choice when the infant is full term, the treatment plan in preterm pregnancies is more complex.

In a preterm pregnancy, ultrasonography and fetal heart tone monitoring are carried out to check for any adverse effects of toxemia on the fetus. If toxemia becomes severe or there is evidence of fetal compromise, then the decision for delivery may be made, even if the infant is preterm. If delivery is anticipated, then the patient will receive intravenous magnesium to decrease

the risk of seizures. If the fetus is less than thirty-four weeks of gestation, then the patient also receives steroid injections to facilitate fetal lung maturity. If seizures occur, a bolus of magnesium can be given to stop the seizures, and stabilization measures are taken to maximize maternal and fetal safety.

—*Anne Lynn S. Chang, M.D.*

See also Blood pressure; Childbirth; Childbirth complications; Embryology; Hypertension; Obstetrics; Preeclampsia and eclampsia; Pregnancy and gestation; Premature birth; Seizures; Vascular medicine; Vascular system; Women's health.

FOR FURTHER INFORMATION:

Brewer, Thomas H. *Metabolic Toxemia of Late Pregnancy: A Disease of Malnutrition.* Rev. ed. New Canaan, Conn.: Keats, 1998.

Cunningham, F. Gary, et al., eds. *Williams Obstetrics.* 23d ed. New York: McGraw-Hill, 2010.

Gabbe, Steven G., Jennifer R. Niebyl, and Joe Leigh Simpson, eds. *Obstetrics: Normal and Problem Pregnancies.* 5th ed. Philadelphia: Churchill Livingstone/Elsevier, 2007.

Sibai, Baha M. "Treatment of Hypertension in Pregnant Women." *New England Journal of Medicine* 335, no. 4 (July, 1996): 257-265.

TOXIC SHOCK SYNDROME

DISEASE/DISORDER

ANATOMY OR SYSTEM AFFECTED: All

SPECIALTIES AND RELATED FIELDS: Critical care, emergency medicine, general surgery, gynecology, internal medicine, microbiology

DEFINITION: A potentially fatal infection causing failure of multiple organs of the body, most notably associated with tampon use.

CAUSES AND SYMPTOMS

Toxic shock syndrome, an overwhelming and potentially life-threatening infection, is most commonly known for its association with tampon use in young women. Although this is still the most commonly affected population, toxic shock syndrome can affect nonmenstruating women and men as well.

Two distinct organisms can be responsible for toxic shock syndrome, each associated with a different constellation of symptoms. The bacteria *Staphylococcus aureus* (staph) causes all cases of menstrual toxic shock syndrome, and some nonmenstrual cases as well. Nonmenstrual cases can arise from an infected surgical wound or infections elsewhere in the body. The bacteria *Streptococcus pyogenes* (strep) is responsible for nonmenstrual toxic shock syndrome only.

All patients with staph toxic shock syndrome have high fevers, lightheadedness associated with low blood pressure, and a diffuse rash resembling a sunburn. The

IN THE NEWS: SINUS INFECTIONS LEADING TO TOXIC SHOCK SYNDROME IN CHILDREN

A retrospective study at The Children's Hospital of Denver found that rhinosinusitis (infection of the nose and paranasal sinuses) can be a primary cause of toxic shock syndrome in young children. The study published in the June, 2009, issue of *Archives of Otolaryngology—Head and Neck Surgery* describes data from seventy-six pediatric patients admitted between 1983 and 2000 who were identified through medical records as having toxic shock syndrome. Of these patients, 21 percent had rhinosinusitis. Study authors, including Kenny Chan, chief of Pediatric Otolaryngology at Children's Hospital of Denver and professor of otolaryngology at the University of Colorado, suggest that physicians consider rhinosinusitis a primary cause of toxic shock syndrome when another site of infection cannot be identified. Because toxic shock syndrome can be fatal, quick treatment and identification of the source are critical.

Sinus infections have not been well reported as a potential primary source of toxic shock syndrome. A study published by Paul D. Gittelman from New York University Medical Center and colleagues found an association between toxic shock syndrome and rhinologic surgery and medical devices. The study, published in *Laryngoscope* in 1991, included 140 adult patients. Toxic shock syndrome was linked to circulating exotoxin of a toxogenic strain of *Staphylococcus aureus*. About 30 percent of patients in the study selected for surgery were *S. aureus* carriers, with toxin-capable isolates identified in 40 percent of those tested. The study also found users of cocaine, topical decongestants, and steroid sprays had a statistically higher rate of *S. aureus* compared to nonusers.

—*Sandra Ripley Distelhorst*

eyes, mouth, and vagina can become red and irritated, and several weeks following the initial illness, the skin on the palms and soles begins to slough. Other symptoms may include vomiting, diarrhea, muscle aches, jaundice, kidney failure, and confusion.

Strep toxic shock syndrome typically arises at a site of minor trauma to the skin, either an injury or a recent surgical wound. Severe pain at the site is the most common finding. The patient may have a fever, confusion, and low blood pressure. Severe swelling at the site of infection can lead to major damage to the skin and underlying tissues; this necrotizing fasciitis (so-called flesh-eating bacteria) is a well-known manifestation of strep toxic shock syndrome.

TREATMENT AND THERAPY

Because of the severity of the illness, almost all patients with toxic shock syndrome require hospitalization. Intravenous fluids and other medications are administered to improve the blood pressure, and antibiotics are used to kill the bacteria and to decrease production of the toxins that they release.

In cases of menstrual toxic shock syndrome, removal of the tampon is critical. For infected surgical wounds, removal of bandages and packing is required, as well as occasional removal of infected tissue with further surgery.

INFORMATION ON TOXIC SHOCK SYNDROME

CAUSES: Bacterial infections with staphylococci (menstrual cases, associated with tampon use) or streptococci (nonmenstrual cases, as from injuries, surgical wounds, infections elsewhere in body)

SYMPTOMS: In staph cases, high fever, lightheadedness, low blood pressure, diffuse rash, redness and irritation of eyes, mouth, and vagina, vomiting, diarrhea, muscle aches, jaundice, kidney failure, confusion; in strep cases, severe pain and swelling at injury site, fever, confusion, low blood pressure, tissue death (necrotizing fasciitis)

DURATION: Acute

TREATMENTS: Hospitalization, intravenous fluids, antibiotics, removal of cause (tampon, bandages or packing), sometimes surgery to remove infected tissue

In cases of necrotizing fasciitis, surgical removal of infected tissue is necessary and may involve a loss of a significant amount of skin and underlying muscle.

PERSPECTIVE AND PROSPECTS

The initial association of toxic shock syndrome with highly absorbent tampons in 1980 led to a withdrawal of such products from the market. Consequently, the number of cases of menstrual toxic shock syndrome has declined; however, tampon use remains a risk factor for toxic shock syndrome. Frequent tampon changes and tampon use only on the heaviest days of bleeding should reduce this risk. Women who have had menstrual toxic shock syndrome or other problems with staph infections should avoid tampon use.

—*Gregory B. Seymann, M.D.*

See also Antibiotics; Bacterial infections; Bacteriology; Genital disorders, female; Gynecology; Menstruation; Methicillin-resistant *Staphylococcus aureus* (MRSA) infections; Necrotizing fasciitis; Staphylococcal infections; Streptococcal infections; Wounds; Women's health.

FOR FURTHER INFORMATION:

Beers, Mark H., et al., eds. *The Merck Manual of Diagnosis and Therapy*. 18th ed. Whitehouse Station, N.J.: Merck Research Laboratories, 2006.

Icon Health. *Toxic Shock Syndrome: A Medical Dictionary, Bibliography, and Annotated Research Guide to Internet References*. San Diego, Calif.: Author, 2004.

Mandell, Gerald L., John E. Bennett, and Raphael Dolin, eds. *Mandell, Douglas, and Bennett's Principles and Practice of Infectious Diseases*. 7th ed. New York: Churchill Livingstone/Elsevier, 2010.

Parker, James N., and Philip M. Parker, eds. *The Official Patient's Sourcebook on Toxic Shock Syndrome*. San Diego, Calif.: Icon Health, 2002.

Sheen, Barbara. *Toxic Shock Syndrome*. San Diego, Calif.: Lucent Books, 2006.

TOXICOLOGY

SPECIALTY

ANATOMY OR SYSTEM AFFECTED: All

SPECIALTIES AND RELATED FIELDS: All

DEFINITION: The scientific study of the effects of poisonous substances (also known as toxicants or toxins) on organisms. Poisons interfere with physiological functions and are typically chemicals generated either naturally (such as poisonous plants, venom-

ous snakes, pathogenic microorganisms, and geochemical cycling) or artificially (industrial products such as PCBs, tetraethyl lead, and certain pharmaceutical or personal care products).

KEY TERMS:

acute toxicity: rapid development of disease symptoms following exposure of an organism to toxic agents (ranging from a few minutes to several hours; typically less than fourteen days)

chronic toxicity: slow or cumulative expression of disease symptoms following exposure of organisms to toxic agents (typically more than one year)

poison: a chemical substance that can cause injury, sickness, or death to organisms; may be from natural or artificial sources

toxicant: the preferred term used to denote a poisonous substance strictly from artificial sources that has been introduced into the environment and has a capacity to adversely affect humans, wildlife, and ecosystem processes

toxin: the preferred term used to denote a poisonous substance strictly from biological sources, such as toxic algae or the tetanus toxin from the bacterium *Clostridium tetani*

SCIENCE AND PROFESSION

Since its inception, toxicology has gone through many paradigmatic shifts and now has several subdisciplines, each with their own approaches and techniques, but they are united by the fundamental challenge of understanding and controlling the interaction between toxic agents and physiological processes. The scale of analysis in which toxicological questions are investigated ranges from molecules to ecosystems, and toxicologists study all kinds of organisms, from the smallest viruses to the largest terrestrial and aquatic organisms.

"The dose makes the poison" is a popular expression that is one of the key principles of toxicology. It refers to the fact that adverse physiological effects can be produced by practically any substance if given at a dose large enough to overwhelm the body's natural capacity to process it. Extremely toxic chemicals impart their effects at very small doses. A key measure of toxicity is the lethal dose (LD), which is defined as the amount of a toxic substance that kills an organism. Because the individuals in a group of organisms do not exhibit identical responses, the actual quantitative measure is termed "LD-50," which is the dose that kills 50 percent of the individuals in an exposed population.

There are three major branches of toxicology: descriptive, mechanistic, and regulatory toxicology. All three branches contribute to risk assessment, which is the main societal application of toxicological knowledge. Mechanistic toxicology is concerned with elucidating the biochemical mechanisms underpinning the expression of toxic effects of poisons at the cellular and/or molecular levels. Assessing the potential toxicity risks associated with new chemicals depends largely on the work of mechanistic toxicologists, who are able to determine whether toxic effects observed in laboratory species are relevant to human exposure levels and physiological attributes. Mechanistic toxicologists also study dose-response relationships that are important for establishing safety thresholds of exposure for industrial chemicals used in manufacturing products and for pharmaceuticals used to treat diseases.

Regulatory toxicology involves the study of how best to protect people from toxic chemicals through the formulation of regulatory policies that govern the manufacture of commercial products, the use and disposal of potentially toxic chemicals, and the protection of workers from toxic exposures at occupational settings. The final responsibility for rejecting or approving specific chemicals for use in commerce rests with regulatory toxicologists, who are trained to evaluate data generated by mechanistic and descriptive toxicologists in the light of federal and regional policies designed to protect public and environmental health. Regulatory toxicologists must make judgments following an evaluation of risks associated with short-term exposures and immediate effects (acute toxicity) as well as longer-term exposures and small doses that may result in symptoms long after the initial exposure occurs (chronic toxicity).

Descriptive toxicology forms the bridge between mechanistic and regulatory toxicology. Descriptive toxicologists are responsible for using toxicity testing for comparative risk assessment. For example, the Food and Drug Administration (FDA) is charged with protecting public health through rigorous evaluation of toxicity levels of drugs and food additives, and descriptive toxicologists employed by the FDA are experts in selecting the best toxicity tests for that purpose. Descriptive toxicologists in the service of the U.S. Environmental Protection Agency (EPA) or the U.S. Department of Agriculture (USDA) collaborate in the comparative toxicity assessment of pesticides used on crops or to control disease vectors. Industrial toxicologists perform similar roles for chemicals used in man-

ufacturing, to minimize adverse impacts on people and the environment.

Toxicologists are usually trained at graduate-level institutions that award master's or doctorate degrees following specialization in one or more subdisciplines. Clinical toxicology is typically studied and practiced in the hospital setting to quickly recognize the symptoms of toxic exposure, usually in an uncommunicative patient, and to identify the responsible poison, followed by administration of antidote or other forms of therapy. Environmental toxicology is the study of the sources, transportation, transformation, and sinks of toxicants in the environment, and how humans come into contact with, and suffer from, exposure to these toxicants. Ecotoxicology is a subspecialty of environmental toxicology that deals strictly with the study of the effects of toxicants on wildlife and ecosystems. Forensic toxicology is the study of how poisons kill people and how to measure residual levels of poisons in corpses in order to determine the cause and time of death. Forensic toxicology is essential practice in cases of suicide or homicide involving poisons. Molecular toxicology is the study of the effects and metabolism of toxic materials in the body at the level of molecules, typically involving molecular genetic analysis and biochemical enzymology. Molecular toxicologists also study how variability in individual genetic characteristics affects human sensitivity to toxic agents, just as age, gender, and body size can all influence human exposure and sensitivity to toxic substances. Pharmacotoxicology is the study of the toxic effects of pharmaceutical products intended for human or animal consumption. It is aimed at finding the appropriate dose of a chemical that has a healing effect without overwhelmingly toxic side effects.

Most practicing toxicologists belong to the professional Society of Toxicology, an organization that defines the responsibilities of toxicologists. The first is to develop new and improved ways of determining the potentially harmful effects of chemical and physical agents and the dose that will cause these effects. This responsibility requires a thorough understanding of the molecular, biochemical, and cellular processes responsible for diseases caused by exposure to toxic substances. The second responsibility is to study commercial chemicals and products using carefully designed and controlled empirical analyses and modeling to determine the conditions under which they can be used with minimum or no adverse effects on human health, wildlife, and ecosystems. The third is to conduct toxicological risk assessments, including estimating the probability that specific chemicals or processes pose significant risks to human health and/or the environment. The risk assessments form the basis for establishing rules and regulations that underpin government policies designed to protect public health and the environment.

DIAGNOSTIC AND TREATMENT TECHNIQUES

The diagnostic and treatment techniques used by toxicologists depend largely on the branch of toxicology in which they practice. For example, clinical toxicologists in the hospital setting must be proficient at rapid diagnostic techniques for implementing emergency response to acute exposure to poisons. According to data published by the American Association of Poison Control Centers (AAPCC), which operates a toxic exposure surveillance system (TESS), 2,438,644 cases of human exposure to poisons were reported by sixty-two participating poison centers across the United States during 2004, representing an increase of 1.8 percent compared to 2003. These poison response centers deal with a new poisoning case approximately every fourteen seconds; local poison control centers in the United States can be reached by calling (800) 222-1222.

More than half of all poisoning cases occur in children younger than six years of age, although these incidents are rarely fatal. A major challenge for toxicologists is to quickly diagnose poisoning events in children who typically may not have the vocabulary or level of consciousness to describe the exposure event to their caregivers or to the emergency response staff when they are brought to the hospital. Most poisonings occur in the home from domestic items such as cosmetics and personal care products, cleaning fluids, medications, and pest control chemicals. Therefore, the first step in diagnosis is to identify as precisely as possible the specific chemical(s) that caused the poisoning; this can most easily be achieved through perusing the list of ingredients on the suspected container but is not always possible. It is more difficult if the poison is gaseous with a remote source. Therefore, body fluid samples (saliva, urine, or blood) can be tested using rapid techniques to identify major categories of common poisons, their known physiological effects, or biomarkers of exposure.

Application of first aid techniques is the first line of treatment for poisonings after ensuring that the patient is removed completely from the source of exposure. Follow-up treatment of poisoned patients involves three major steps. The first is facilitating the elimination of ingested or injected poison from the body. Stomach pumping is sometimes effective for ingested poisons if applied within a time frame that occurs before a fatal dose is absorbed in the stomach. Typically, in a gastric lavage process, a siphon tube is inserted into the stomach through the mouth to repeatedly flush and empty the contents. The second step is applying effective antidotes that aid the excretion or inactivation of the poison either through natural liver functions or through specific biochemical reactions. Activated charcoal may be given, preferably to conscious patients through the mouth, for the purpose of absorbing the poison, thereby reducing the biologically available dose. In serious situations in which poisons are injected into the bloodstream or when poisons have been absorbed extensively from the stomach or lungs, hemodialysis may be performed to filter the blood directly through the use of artificial kidneys. Where artificial kidneys are not available, charcoal may be used for blood filtration (hemoperfusion). For poisoned patients exhibiting respiratory distress, breathing support through ventilators is essential treatment strategy. The third step is treating symptoms and aiding recovery. Depending on the nature of the poison, treatment may involve controlling seizures, correction of irregular heartbeat, regulation of blood pressure, and the repair or replacement of damaged organs, including kidney and liver.

Posttreatment counseling is recommended to prevent further poison exposures through educational programs, drug rehabilitation, or mental health referrals in cases of suicide attempts. Poisoning cases may also involve substantial legal proceedings for forensic toxicologists or in cases where homicide is intended.

PERSPECTIVE AND PROSPECTS

Poisons and their effects on human health have been known since antiquity, but the scientific study of poisons and systematic information on their synthesis and mode of action is a relatively recent development. The German scientist Auroleus Phillipus Theostratus Bombastus von Hohenheim (1493-1541), popularly known as Paracelsus, is considered by many to be the world's first authority on and founder of toxicology as a scientific discipline. Among his several notable accomplishments, Paracelsus is credited with introducing the use of mercury and arsenic into medical practice for curative purposes. Furthermore, he is the source of the famously paraphrased anecdote, "The dose makes the poison." His exact statement in German translates as

"All things are poison and nothing is without poison, only the dose makes a thing be poison."

Toxicology is a rapidly evolving specialty, driven by innovations in chemical manufacturing and the growing number of toxic substances accessible to the general population. Progress in toxicology is also driven by discoveries in human genomics and proteomics. The more that is learned about the variability in the nucleotide sequences of individuals in a population, the better understood are the differences in human response to toxic chemicals. Additional work in mechanistic toxicology and descriptive toxicology remains to be done to understand adequately the interactions among genetics, age, gender, body size, and behavioral traits that mediate human exposure and response to poisons. Furthermore, the human body is exposed to a large number of chemicals on a daily bases. Very little is known about how these chemicals interact to make people more or less vulnerable to the toxic effects of poisons.

It is important to create a seamless strategy for translating laboratory data, including those based on animal or microbial model systems, into regulatory policies designed to protect the most vulnerable members of society. It is also important to create a seamless strategy for understanding the interactions of toxic chemicals in ecosystems and how these interactions influence human vulnerability and sensitivity to toxic exposures at the workplace, on the streets, and at home. Finally, toxicology has been neglected for too long by the engineering professions that create the products upon which society relies. Toxicology must be engaged as much as possible in the product design stage, before large-scale manufacturing of consumer products that end up endangering the public and ecosystems through the expression of toxicity at various stages of the product life cycle.

—*Oladele A. Ogunseitan, Ph.D., M.P.H.*

See also Asbestos exposure; Biological and chemical weapons; Bites and stings; Blood testing; Botulism; Carcinogens; Critical care; Critical care, pediatrics; Dermatitis; Eczema; Emergency medicine; Environmental diseases; Environmental health; Enzyme therapy; Food poisoning; Forensic pathology; Hepatitis; Herbal medicine; Homeopathy; Insect-borne diseases; Intoxication; Itching; Laboratory tests; Lead poisoning; Liver; Mercury poisoning; Occupational health; Pathology; Pharmacology; Pharmacy; Poisoning; Poisonous plants; Rashes; Snakebites; Teratogens; Toxoplasmosis; Urinalysis.

FOR FURTHER INFORMATION:

Agency for Toxic Substances and Disease Registry. http://www.atsdr.cdc.gov. ATSDR is a public health agency under the U.S. Department of Health and Human Services. An excellent resource for current information on risks associated with toxic substances for specialists and for the public.

Hodgson, Ernest, and Robert C. Smart, eds. *Introduction to Biochemical Toxicology.* 3d ed. New York: Wiley Interscience, 2001. More than forty experts contributed chapters to this introductory book on molecular and biochemical approach to toxicology.

Hoffman, David J., et al. *Handbook of Ecotoxicology.* Boca Raton, Fla.: CRC Press, 1995. A comprehensive introduction to ecotoxicology, with more than fifty contributors who are experts in their research subject.

Klaassen, Curtis D., ed. *Casarett and Doull's Toxicology.* 7th ed. New York: McGraw-Hill, 2008. With more than seventy authors, this is considered the authoritative source on toxicology. It is more or less the classic text for the discipline, written at a level suitable for senior undergraduate and graduate students. A good reference for researchers.

Landis, Wayne G., and Ming-ho Yu. *Introduction to Environmental Toxicology.* 3d ed. Boca Raton, Fla.: Lewis, 2004. Takes an unusual ecosystems approach to describe environmental toxicology, which makes it overlap somewhat with books explicitly on ecotoxicology.

Malachowski, M. J., and Arleen F. Goldberg. *Health Effects of Toxic Substances.* Rockville, Md.: Government Institutes, 1995. A straightforward, easy-to-read guide on the history of industrial toxicology and a review of how poisons affect human physiology.

TOXOPLASMOSIS

DISEASE/DISORDER

ANATOMY OR SYSTEM AFFECTED: Gastrointestinal system, immune system, nervous system, skin

SPECIALTIES AND RELATED FIELDS: Family medicine, pediatrics

DEFINITION: A widespread, infectious disease caused by a protozoan parasite.

CAUSES AND SYMPTOMS

The parasite *Toxoplasma gondii*, which causes toxoplasmosis, is fairly common and can infect warm-blooded animals as well as reptiles, but the ordinary domestic cat is the only known animal that sheds the toxoplasma parasite in its feces. Humans can also be infected by coming into contact with cat feces in a litter box or by eating raw or undercooked meat from infected animals.

The parasite may be acquired or congenital. Both forms seem to have a wide variety of clinical outcomes, ranging from a mild, asymptomatic state to an infection with fatal results. Congenital infection may manifest itself with jaundice, fever, anemia, convulsions, inflammation of the retina (chorioretinitis), an enlarged liver or spleen, and lymphadenopathy.

Acquired toxoplasmosis infection may be mild or severe. The vast majority of people who contract the disease have no or few symptoms, while others may have swollen glands, headaches, or a sore throat. These symptoms generally appear within ten to fourteen days after infection and subside within two to twelve weeks. Severe toxoplasmosis manifests itself by a possible fever, rash, pneumonia, encephalitis, myocarditis, pericarditis, hepatitis, and muscle inflammation (polymyositis).

When toxoplasmosis is acquired during pregnancy, it may badly harm the fetus, even if the mother did not have any symptoms. The degree to which the infection damages the fetus depends upon the stage of pregnancy. The parasite can be passed to the fetus in 15 percent of women infected during the first trimester, in approximately 25 percent infected during the second trimester, and in up to 65 percent of those infected during the last trimester. It is possible for the pregnant woman to suffer a spontaneous abortion or a stillbirth or to deliver a premature or a full-term child in whom birth defects are present.

Toxoplasmosis can occur when the immune system is impaired. Reactivation of previously acquired toxoplasma organisms has become a serious problem for HIV-infected persons. Improved HIV treatment and prophylaxis for toxoplasmosis with trimethoprim-sulfamethoxazole have reduced the incidence of disease. Similar reactivation of toxoplasma has also occurred in immunologically suppressed solid-organ and bone-marrow transplant patients.

TREATMENT AND THERAPY

Pyrimethamine and sulfa drugs have reduced the complications from toxoplasmosis. When pyrimethamine is given to a pregnant woman during her first trimester, however, birth defects may occur. Physicians will prescribe sulfa drugs alone for infections occurring during pregnancy.

PERSPECTIVE AND PROSPECTS

The sporozoan *Toxoplasma gondii* was first isolated from an African rodent and was eventually described as a new species in 1909. In 1940, it was established as a factor for human disease.

It is possible to prevent toxoplasmosis by feeding cats only well-cooked meat or commercial cat food; keeping cats indoors, so that they cannot hunt and eat birds or mice; staying away from cats and having someone else clean the litter box during pregnancy; washing one's hands after touching uncooked meat; and cooking meat at a minimum of 151 degrees Fahrenheit (66 degrees Celsius).

—*Earl R. Andresen, Ph.D.*

See also Birth defects; Blindness; Brain damage; Encephalitis; Eye infections and disorders; Eyes; Fever; Glands, swollen; Headaches; Hepatitis; Parasitic diseases; Pneumonia; Pregnancy and gestation; Protozoan diseases; Rashes; Sore throat; Vision disorders; Zoonoses.

FOR FURTHER INFORMATION:

Ambroise-Thomas, Pierre, and Eskild Petersen, eds. *Congenital Toxoplasmosis: Scientific Background, Clinical Management, and Control.* New York: Springer, 2000.

Despommier, Dickson D., et al. *Parasitic Diseases.* 5th ed. New York: Apple Tree, 2006.

Joynson, David H. M., and Tim G. Wreghitt, eds. *Toxoplasmosis: A Comprehensive Clinical Guide.* Rev. ed. New York: Cambridge University Press, 2005.

Martin, Richard J., Avroy A. Fanaroff, and Michele C. Walsh, eds. *Fanaroff and Martin's Neonatal-Perinatal Medicine: Diseases of the Fetus and Infant.* 2 vols. 8th ed. Philadelphia: Mosby/Elsevier, 2006.

INFORMATION ON TOXOPLASMOSIS

CAUSES: Parasitic infection; may be acquired or congenital

SYMPTOMS: Often asymptomatic; may include swollen glands, headaches, sore throat, jaundice, fever, anemia, spleen or liver enlargement

DURATION: Two to twelve weeks

TREATMENTS: Pyrimethamine, sulfa drugs

Parker, James N., and Philip M. Parker, eds. *The Official Patient's Sourcebook on Toxoplasmosis*. San Diego, Calif.: Icon Health, 2002.

Roberts, Larry S., and John Janovy, Jr., eds. *Gerald D. Schmidt and Larry S. Roberts' Foundations of Parasitology*. 7th ed. Boston: McGraw-Hill Higher Education, 2005.

TRACHEA

ANATOMY

ALSO KNOWN AS: Windpipe

ANATOMY OR SYSTEM AFFECTED: Chest, neck, respiratory system

SPECIALTIES AND RELATED FIELDS: General surgery, otorhinolaryngology, pulmonary medicine

DEFINITION: The cartilaginous tube that conducts air from the larynx to the bronchi and into the lungs.

KEY TERMS:

bronchi: the right and left branches from the trachea which supply air into the lungs

hyaline cartilage: the most common type of human cartilage

larynx: the organ of voice placed at the upper part of the air passage

respiratory mucosa: the mucous membrane that lines the respiratory tract

tracheal stenosis: a narrowing of the tracheal lumen

tracheomalcia: a weakening of the tracheal lumen that allows collapse during respiration

tracheostomy: a surgical opening into the trachea

STRUCTURE AND FUNCTIONS

The trachea, also commonly referred to as the windpipe, is that part of the airway that connects the larynx to the two main bronchi. The trachea is made up of sixteen to twenty hyaline cartilage rings that maintain the airway lumen width at about 2.5 centimeters. The cartilage rings are incomplete and flattened posteriorly, where they are completed by fibrous tissue and muscle fibers. The first cartilage ring is thicker than the others and connected by the cricotracheal ligament to the lower edge of the cricoid cartilage of the larynx. At its lower end, the trachea bifurcates into the right bronchus, which is wider, shorter, and more vertical, and the left bronchus which is narrower. This explains why aspirated foreign bodies are more likely to lodge in the right bronchus. The length of the trachea from top to bottom in an adult is 10 to 12 centimeters.

The anatomical relations of the trachea include the esophagus posteriorly and the great vessels of the neck laterally. The thyroid gland lies over the anterior surface in the lower neck. As the trachea enters the thorax, it is protected by the bony manubrium sterni. The cartilaginous structure is enclosed by an elastic fibrous membrane, and supported by nonstriated longitudinal muscle externally. Internally, transverse fibers of the trachealis muscle form a connection between the posterior ends of the cartilage rings.

In addition to its function of maintaining a patent (open) airway, the trachea also has the function of trapping foreign particles and of warming and moistening the air that flows to the lungs. It accomplishes this function by virtue of the lining of the tracheal lumen. The ciliated, respiratory mucosa of the tracheal lumen contains goblet cells that produce mucus. In the submucosa are numerous blood vessels that give warmth and seromucous glands that contribute to the lubrication of the airway. Blood supply to the trachea is from the inferior thyroid arteries. Nerve supply is from branches of the vagus and recurrent laryngeal nerves.

DISORDERS AND DISEASES

The most serious disorders of the trachea are those that cause interference with the airway. Tracheal stenosis can develop from trauma, tumors, radiation therapy, autoimmune diseases, and infection. The most common cause is prolonged intubation. Symptoms include shortness of breath, cough, and stridor. Treatment involves correcting any underlying medical condition, laser surgery, reconstructive surgery, dilation, and airway stenting. In 2008, the first tracheal transplant using patient stem cells was reported.

Tracheomalacia occurs when the lumen of the trachea collapses inward, obstructing the airway during breathing or coughing. The most common cause of tracheomalacia is chronic obstructive pulmonary disease (COPD). Other causes include prolonged intubation, recurrent infection, injury from tracheostomy, and tumors or abnormal blood vessels that press against the trachea. A form of congenital tracheomalacia also exists. Symptoms are due to a compromised airway and are similar to tracheal stenosis. Management is also similar, including short- and long-term stenting and reconstructive surgery.

Acute inflammation of the trachea is usually the result of bacterial infection. Symptoms may resemble croup or epiglottitis with cough, fever, and stridor. Bacterial tracheitis has become more common than acute epiglottitis as a cause of airway distress from bacterial infection. It is much less common than croup, occurring in only 0.1 cases per 100,000 children. Bacterial infection may follow trauma during intubation or a viral infection and is more common in pediatric patients. Treatment is usually successful with airway support and appropriate antibiotics, although mortality rates have been reported at 4 to 20 percent.

PERSPECTIVE AND PROSPECTS

Tracheostomy is the most common surgical procedure performed on the trachea. The term "tracheotomy" implies a surgical opening made in the trachea. The term "tracheostomy" refers to an opening into the trachea that is kept open with a cannula or made permanent. In most medical literature, however, the term "tracheostomy" is used to describe both procedures. The purpose of tracheostomy is to gain access to the tracheal airway in order to bypass a respiratory obstruction or to facilitate breathing. This potentially lifesaving procedure has been known since ancient times. There is a description of a healed tracheotomy incision in the Sanskrit hymns of the *Rigveda*, dating to 2000 B.C.E. The physician Chevalier Jackson (1865-1958) of Philadelphia is the founder of the modern tracheostomy, having described the indications, complications, and the basics of the modern surgical procedure. In the nineteenth century, the procedure was commonly done to relieve airway obstruction in diphtheria patients, and in the twentieth century polio was a frequent indication. Today, the most common indication is for prolonged ventilator-assisted breathing.

Tracheal surgery made history in 2008 when the first tracheal transplant using a patient's own stem cells was successfully performed. This milestone was accomplished by a team of doctors in Barcelona, Spain. The patient was a thirty-year-old woman who had scarring of her trachea from tuberculosis. A donor trachea was obtained and stripped of living cells. Stem cells from the woman's bone marrow were then seeded into the trachea prior to transplantation.

—*Chris Iliades, M.D.*

See also Asphyxiation; Bronchi; Cartilage; Choking; Critical care; Critical care, pediatric; Emergency medicine; Paramedics; Pulmonary medicine; Pulmonary medicine, pediatric; Respiration; Resuscitation; Tracheostomy.

FOR FURTHER INFORMATION:

Cummings, W. Charles, et al. *Otolaryngology Head and Neck Surgery.* 4th ed. Philadelphia: Mosby/ Elsevier, 2005.

Drake, L. Richard, et al. *Gray's Anatomy for Students.* 2d ed. New York: Churchill Livingstone/Elsevier, 2009.

Engels, P. T., et al. "Tracheostomy: From Insertion to Decannulation." *Canadian Journal of Surgery* 52, no. 5 (October, 2009): 427-433.

Lalwani, K. Anil. *Current Diagnosis and Treatment: Otolaryngology Head and Neck Surgery.* 2d ed. New York: McGraw-Hill, 2008.

Macchiarini, P., et al. "Clinical Transplantation of a Tissue-Engineered Airway." *The Lancet* 372 (2008): 2023-2030.

TRACHEOSTOMY

PROCEDURE

ANATOMY OR SYSTEM AFFECTED: Neck, respiratory system, throat

SPECIALTIES AND RELATED FIELDS: Critical care, emergency medicine, general surgery

DEFINITION: The creation of a hole in the trachea, thus providing an alternative source for getting air into the lungs.

INDICATIONS AND PROCEDURES

A tracheostomy is the surgical creation of an opening into the trachea through the throat. It is done to relieve upper airway obstruction, decrease the effort of breathing, provide access for mechanical ventilation, and improve patient comfort. It is uncommonly used in an emergency except in the field; the preferred method of establishing an airway is to pass a tube through the trachea via the mouth.

Local anesthesia is used to deaden the skin of the front of the neck. A horizontal incision is made over the space between the second and third tracheal rings. If the thyroid gland is encountered, it is divided. Bleeding must be carefully controlled throughout the procedure. The trachea is entered through an incision that will divide the second and third rings of cartilage. In an adult, a small portion of the third ring may be removed. A previously tested tracheostomy tube with a cuff is inserted within the interior of the trachea. The wound is loosely closed, and a gauze dressing is applied. An X ray is taken after the procedure to ensure that the tube has been correctly placed and that there is no free air in the mediastinum or thorax.

USES AND COMPLICATIONS

Once a tracheostomy has been performed, ambient air in a patient's room must be humidified and warmed.

Tracheostomy

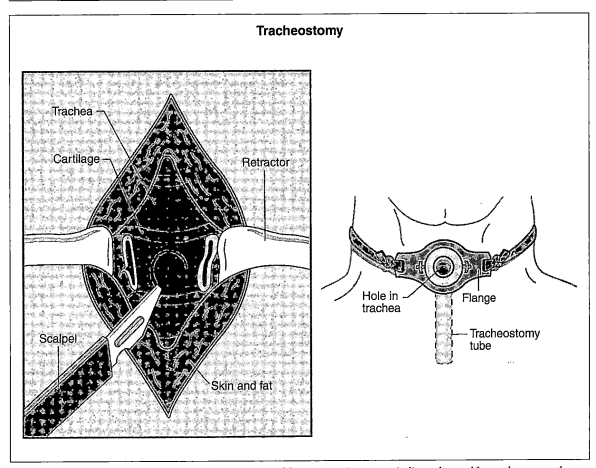

Certain throat disorders and diseases or the emergency need for an open airway may indicate the need for tracheostomy, the creation of a hole in the trachea (windpipe) through which the patient can breathe.

If any secretions develop, the tracheostomy site must be suctioned in a sterile manner. If shortness of breath is observed, the tracheostomy site should be examined for a mucus plug. The tracheostomy tube should be removed and the opening closed at the earliest possible time that is consistent with the condition of the patient.

Some potential problems are associated with a tracheostomy. The most common is bacterial contamination of the lungs or adjacent tissues. Air may enter the space between the lungs and the tissue that lines the cavity containing the lungs, a condition known as pneumothorax. The tube may also become displaced. Attempting to replace the tube blindly can result in obstruction.

PERSPECTIVE AND PROSPECTS

Although dramatic when portrayed on television programs, a tracheostomy is a delicate surgical procedure that requires skill and training. With the invention of modern laryngoscopes, tracheostomies are uncommon, being used primarily in cases of fracture of the anterior neck.

—*L. Fleming Fallon, Jr., M.D., Ph.D., M.P.H.*

See also Asphyxiation; Choking; Critical care; Critical care, pediatric; Emergency medicine; First aid; Paramedics; Pulmonary medicine; Pulmonary medicine, pediatric; Respiration; Resuscitation; Trachea.

FOR FURTHER INFORMATION:

Kertoy, Marilyn. *Children with Tracheostomies: Resource Guide.* Albany, N.Y.: Singular/Thomson Learning, 2002.

Kittredge, Mary. *The Respiratory System.* Edited by Dale C. Garell. Philadelphia: Chelsea House, 2000.

Levitzky, Michael G. *Pulmonary Physiology.* 7th ed. New York: McGraw-Hill Medical, 2007.

Mason, Robert J., et al., eds. *Murray and Nadel's Text-*

book of Respiratory Medicine. 5th ed. Philadelphia: Saunders/Elsevier, 2010.

Myers, Eugene N., and Jonas T. Johnson, eds. *Tracheotomy: Airway Management, Communication, and Swallowing*. 2d ed. San Diego, Calif.: Plural, 2008.

Parker, Steve. *The Lungs and Breathing*. Rev. ed. New York: Franklin Watts, 1991.

TRACHOMA
DISEASE/DISORDER
ANATOMY OR SYSTEM AFFECTED: Eyes
SPECIALTIES AND RELATED FIELDS: Environmental health, family medicine, ophthalmology, pediatrics
DEFINITION: An infectious disease of the eyes that causes blindness.

CAUSES AND SYMPTOMS
Trachoma is caused by the *Chlamydia trachomatia* bacteria. It is carried primarily by children throughout the developing world, where water is scarce and washing is difficult. Combined with a general lack of hygiene, blowing dust and smoke from cooking fires provide a perfect environment for *Chlamydia trachomatia* bacteria to take hold.

Flies from refuse areas crawl on faces of children who sleep in crowded conditions. The insects touch those children with the bacteria, then infect and reinfect others rapidly throughout an entire village. The eyes become red, painful, and sticky, causing irritation to the underside of the eyelid. Infection easily spreads as children touch the faces of their mothers and other children.

Left untreated, the eyelid and eyelashes turn in, damaging the cornea. The disease becomes more painful and injurious to adults as the eyelashes break off. This bristlelike effect lacerates the cornea and opaque scarring builds (a condition called trichiasis). Blindness is inevitable, usually by the age of forty to fifty.

INFORMATION ON TRACHOMA

CAUSES: Bacterial infection
SYMPTOMS: Red, painful, and sticky eyes; irritation to underside of eyelid; turning in of eyelid and eyelashes with corneal damage; eventual blindness
DURATION: Typically six weeks
TREATMENTS: Tetracycline eye ointment, face cleansing, surgery if prolonged

---

TREATMENT AND THERAPY
Tetracycline eye ointment, twice a day for six weeks, gets rid of the infection. Face cleansing, especially for children, is the best way to prevent infection, along with environmental improvement and education. After the disease has advanced, the last hope is a surgical procedure to rotate the eyelid to its original position. The procedure is relatively simple. Nurses, medical assistants, and technicians can be trained to perform it at local clinics. Efforts to eliminate *Musca sorbens*, the aggressive flies in Africa and Asia, are also effective in controlling trachoma.

PERSPECTIVE AND PROSPECTS
The World Health Organization (WHO) estimates trachoma has blinded 6 million of the 38 million blind people in the world. Active infectious trachoma affects 150 million children. Areas most affected are Mexico, Brazil, Burkina Faso, Egypt, Kenya, China, Myanmar, and interior Australia.

In 1997, WHO launched a concerted effort to control trachomatous blindness by forming a consortium, the Global Elimination of Trachoma by 2020 (GET 2020). Strategy for GET 2020 is summarized by the acronym "SAFE," which refers to the four field-tested activities for control of trachoma; *s*urgery, *a*ntibiotics (tetracycline), clean *f*aces, and *e*nvironmental change. Trachoma control is one of the most affordable health interventions.

Education of the peoples involved is difficult. Because the disease is not fatal, they have little concern, accepting the disease as a fact of life. Mothers are being educated to find time to retrieve well water for washing their children's faces even when drought and poverty make feeding their families a trial. Mothers are being taught to understand the relationship between dirt on children's faces and the eye diseases making their own eyes red and sore. As such environmental improvement techniques are taught, villages are motivated to cooperate with worldwide and local agencies in the interest of curing trachoma.

—*Virginiae Blackmon*

See also Bacterial infections; Blindness; Childhood infectious diseases; Epidemiology; Eye infections and disorders; Eyes; Insect-borne diseases; Vision; Vision disorders; World Health Organization; Zoonoses.

FOR FURTHER INFORMATION:
Buettner, Helmut, ed. *Mayo Clinic on Vision and Eye Health: Practical Answers on Glaucoma, Cataracts,*

Macular Degeneration, and Other Conditions. Rochester, Minn.: Mayo Foundation for Medical Education and Research, 2002.

Dawson, Chandler. "Flies and the Elimination of Blinding Trachoma." *The Lancet* 353, no. 9162 (April 24, 1999): 1376.

Hertle, Richard, David B. Schaffer, and Jill A. Foster, eds. *Pediatric Eye Disease: Color Atlas and Synopsis.* New York: McGraw-Hill, 2002.

Johnson, Gordon J., et al., eds. *The Epidemiology of Eye Disease.* 2d ed. New York: Oxford University Press, 2003.

Miller, Stephen J. H. *Parsons' Diseases of the Eye.* 19th ed. New York: Elsevier, 2002.

Schachterm, J., et al. "Azithromycin in Control of Trachoma." *The Lancet* 354, no. 9179 (May, 1999): 630.

Sutton, Amy L., ed. *Eye Care Sourcebook: Basic Consumer Health Information About Eye Care and Eye Disorders.* 3d ed. Detroit, Mich.: Omnigraphics, 2008.

TRANSFUSION
PROCEDURE

ANATOMY OR SYSTEM AFFECTED: Blood, circulatory system, immune system

SPECIALTIES AND RELATED FIELDS: Critical care, emergency medicine, general surgery, hematology, immunology, neonatology, serology, vascular medicine

DEFINITION: The introduction of whole blood or blood components (such as platelets, red blood cells, or fresh-frozen plasma) directly into the bloodstream.

KEY TERMS:

allogeneic: of the same species; in allogeneic blood transfusion, recipients are transfused with blood from another human being

alloimmunization: immunization by means of antibodies that react against substances from another person (such as blood)

apheresis: the removal of whole blood from a donor, followed by its separation into components, the retention of the desired component, and the return of the recombined remaining elements

autologous: self-derived; in autologous blood transfusion, recipients are transfused with their own blood

plasma: the liquid portion of blood in which the particulate components, such as proteins, are suspended; plasma is the origin of the blood components fresh-frozen plasma and cryoprecipitate

platelets: small, disk-shaped structures in blood that play a key role in blood clotting

red blood cells: blood cells that contain hemoglobin; the role of red blood cells is to transport oxygen

white blood cells: blood cells involved in the defense systems of the body; granulocyte components consist of white blood cells and are used to combat infections

whole blood: blood from which none of the elements has been removed

INDICATIONS AND PROCEDURES

Blood transfusion is the introduction of whole blood or blood components directly into the bloodstream. Human blood has been transfused with success since the early nineteenth century. Modern transfusion therapy, however, is largely the result of scientific advances made during the twentieth century and is, therefore, a young discipline. Blood transfusion plays a critical role in modern medical practice by enabling physicians to provide care, both surgical and nonsurgical, which is not feasible in its absence. Until relatively recent times, transfusion options were limited to two items: whole blood and plasma. The introduction of blood component therapy in the 1960's had a major impact on transfusion practice.

Physicians are now able to choose from a large variety of specific blood products. Some products are the result of manufacturing processes that concentrate a portion of blood (blood derivatives), such as factor VIII concentrates for the treatment of hemophilia A. Other products, such as red blood cells or platelet concentrates (blood components), are separated, produced, and distributed by blood collection facilities for transfusion purposes. The cardinal principle of modern transfusion therapy is to administer the specific blood products that patients require. Portions of blood not required by the patient should not be transfused. Therefore, indications for the use of whole blood are very limited and its use is considered, in general, to be wasteful. The two major categories of transfusion are autologous and allogeneic. Autologous transfusion is the infusion of an individual with his or her own blood. Allogeneic transfusion is the infusion of blood collected from a person or people other than the transfusion recipient.

Autologous transfusion. Currently, there are four distinct types of autologous blood transfusion services available; preoperative donation, intraoperative hemodilution, intraoperative blood collection and reinfusion, and postoperative collection and reinfusion.

Patients scheduled for surgical procedures in which blood transfusion is likely are candidates to donate and store their own blood in advance for use at the time of surgery. This is preoperative donation. It may be possible to collect and store multiple units of blood with this technique. Close communication between patient and physician is critical in preoperative donation because the number of autologous units required must be determined and a donation schedule must be established. Usually, the last donation occurs no later than seventy-two hours before the scheduled operation. For surgical procedures in which the likelihood of transfusion is remote, preoperative donation has not proven to be cost-effective.

Intraoperative hemodilution is the removal of one or more units of blood from a patient at the beginning of an operation for reinfusion during or at the end of the procedure. The volume of blood removed is replaced by the infusion of solutions that contain no blood cells and no risk of infection, such as Ringer's lactate or albumin. Intraoperative hemodilution is considered beneficial for a number of reasons. First, this technique lowers blood viscosity (that is, it thins the blood), which may improve blood flow to vital organs. Second, the amount of actual blood loss during the operation is decreased because the patient's blood is diluted at the start of the surgery. Third, a supply of fresh, normal autologous blood for transfusion is available during and at the end of the surgery.

Intraoperative blood collection and reinfusion refers to the collection and return of blood recovered from the operative field or from machines used for the performance of an operation, such as a return of blood from the cardiopulmonary bypass machine used in cardiovascular surgery. Intraoperative autologous transfusion has proven to be an effective form of blood conservation in a number of surgical procedures, including cardiac, vascular, orthopedic, urologic, trauma, gynecologic, and transplantation surgeries.

Postoperative blood collection and reinfusion refers to the collection and return of blood recovered from surgical drains following an operation. This technique has been used predominantly following cardiac or orthopedic surgery. The overall effectiveness of this technique is still being clarified.

The different types of autologous transfusion should not be considered independently of one another. A coordinated approach using multiple techniques offers the greatest opportunity to maximize the value of autol-

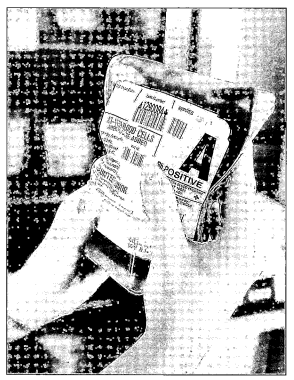

A bag of type A whole blood is stored for transfusion if needed. (Digital Stock)

ogous transfusion and minimize the chance that allogeneic transfusion will be required.

Allogeneic transfusion. This type of therapy begins with blood collection from informed, healthy donors. The allogeneic blood supply in the United States has never been as safe as it is at present. Blood donors are selected according to criteria designed to maximize donor safety and minimize recipient risks. Donor selection criteria are based on a high standard of medical practice and must comply with federal, state, and local regulations concerning blood collection. Facilities that collect and/or process blood and blood components for transfusion must comply with the United States Public Health Service's "Current Good Manufacturing Practice for Blood and Blood Components." These manufacturing practices are defined by the Code of Federal Regulations and are administered by the Food and Drug Administration (FDA). State and local laws often govern blood donor age requirements and the filing of reports, such as to state and county health departments, pertaining to donors whose laboratory tests reveal the presence of infectious diseases.

Blood donor selection starts with education regarding donor qualifications. Prior to every donation, potential blood donors are given information about human immunodeficiency virus (HIV) and acquired immunodeficiency syndrome (AIDS). Information is provided on the potential of HIV transmission to individuals receiving blood and on risk behaviors associated with HIV infection. Potential donors are informed of the absolute necessity of refraining from donation if they are at risk for HIV infection. Honest donor self-exclusion is a critical step in maintaining a safe blood supply.

The next phase of the donation process is the health history interview. Confidential interviews, often consisting of both a self-administered questionnaire and direct questioning, are conducted prior to every blood donation. Prospective donors are also tested for hemoglobin level (to check for the presence of anemia), temperature, pulse, and blood pressure. Some individuals are excluded because it is determined that blood donation poses an unacceptable health risk for the donor. Some exclusions, such as when a donor has a history of infectious disease or risk factors for HIV infection, are designed to protect blood recipients. Prospective donors are allowed to terminate the blood donation process at any time. Prior to the start of the actual blood donation, eligible donors are given the opportunity to ask additional questions and provide additional information. They are then asked to sign an informed consent statement. Some individuals may feel obligated to donate blood despite the realization that they do not qualify as safe donors. In this situation, donors are provided another opportunity to disqualify themselves through confidential unit exclusion (CUE). In CUE, blood donors choose "Transfuse" or "Do Not Transfuse" by marking a form or selecting a bar code label following the blood donation.

Laboratory testing of donor blood is required before whole blood or blood components can be made available for routine transfusion. A blood sample from every donation must pass an FDA-licensed test and be found to be negative for hepatitis B surface antigen (HBsAg) and for antibodies to HIV viruses types 1 and 2 (anti-HIV 1/2), hepatitis B core antigen (anti-HBc), hepatitis C virus (anti-HCV), human T-cell lymphotropic viruses types I and II (anti-HTLV-I/II), and West Nile virus. Other tests routinely performed with every donation include a test for syphilis and a test for liver function called the alanine aminotransferase (ALT) level; these tests must be negative and normal, respectively.

Units of blood collected for "Autologous Use Only"

at blood centers are ordinarily tested for syphilis, anti-HIV 1/2, HBsAg, anti-HCV, and anti-HBc. Blood units remain acceptable for autologous transfusion despite positive results in one or more tests. Some health care facilities collect Autologous Use Only blood components for transfusion within the institution. Such blood components drawn, stored, and infused at one facility may have not been tested for all the above-mentioned infectious diseases. If autologous blood donors have been screened and tested in a manner identical to allogeneic blood donors, unused autologous blood may be used for allogeneic blood transfusions. Most transfusion services, however, opt to destroy unused autologous blood.

The transfusion process begins with a physician's assessment of patient need and a formal order, clearly identifiable in the patient record, specifying the blood product to be transfused, the quantity, and any special administration requirements. This order is then transcribed to a special transfusion request form; computer-transmitted requests are acceptable as long as the required information is present. Forms requesting blood or blood components and forms accompanying blood samples from the patient must contain sufficient information for positive identification of the recipient. The first and last name and unique identification number of the patient are required. With the exception of extreme emergencies, such as patients who will bleed to death if there is any delay in transfusion of blood or blood components, the ABO (A, B, AB, or O) and Rh (positive or negative) types of the intended recipient must be determined before blood or blood components are issued for transfusion.

If the patient is to receive whole blood, red blood cells, granulocytes, or platelet components containing more than 5 milliliters of red cells (red cell-containing components), the recipient's serum (plasma lacking coagulation factors) must also be tested for the presence of clinically significant unexpected antibodies and for compatibility with the donor red blood cells. The only expected antibodies in a patient's serum are those directed at the A and/or B groups. Individuals who are in blood group O have antibodies directed toward the A and B groups, those who are in group A have anti-B antibodies, and group B individuals have anti-A antibodies. People who are in group AB do not have antibodies directed toward the A or B groups. There is no anti-O antibody. If the serum of a prospective transfusion recipient contains a clinically significant unexpected red cell antibody, red cell-containing components chosen for transfusion must lack the corresponding antigen (the determinant to which the antibody is directed).

With the exception of emergencies, the recipient's serum is usually tested with red blood cells from the donor prior to the release of red cell-containing components for transfusion. This procedure is known as the major crossmatch, and if recipient serum does not react with donor red cells, the red cell-containing unit is termed crossmatch compatible. It is now acceptable to use properly functioning computer systems to select compatible red cell units for transfusion in the place of a major crossmatch for recipients who do not have clinically significant unexpected antibodies. Blood components that do not contain 5 milliliters or more of red blood cells, such as fresh-frozen plasma, cryoprecipitate, and most platelet components, do not have to be crossmatched.

Patients should receive blood and blood components of their own ABO group whenever possible. For red cell-containing components, with the exception of whole blood, alternative choices exist when ABO identical components are not available. For red cell-containing components, the donor red cells must be compatible with the recipient's plasma. For example, group A recipients may receive group O red blood cells. When transfusing components that contain plasma (whole blood, fresh-frozen plasma, cryoprecipitate, or platelets), it is best to transfuse blood products that are compatible with the recipient's red blood cells. For example, group A recipients may receive group AB fresh-frozen plasma since the plasma from group AB donors does not contain anti-A. Whole blood transfusion should be ABO identical because donor red cells and plasma must be compatible with the recipient.

For whole blood, red blood cells, platelets, and granulocytes, Rh-identical products should be provided whenever possible. Rh-negative units are acceptable for transfusion into Rh-positive individuals, but Rh-negative units should be reserved for Rh-negative recipients because of the limited supply of Rh-negative blood. The transfusion of Rh-positive blood into Rh-negative recipients will likely result in the formation of antibodies to the Rh antigen and therefore should be avoided in all but emergency situations. Rh type is not a consideration when transfusing fresh-frozen plasma or cryoprecipitate.

When there is a desperate requirement for blood, there may be a need to transfuse uncrossmatched red blood cells. If the recipient ABO group and Rh type are unknown, group O red cells should be transfused, and it is preferable that they be Rh negative. If there has been time to determine the recipient's ABO and Rh types with a current blood sample, then appropriate ABO and Rh type blood can be issued uncrossmatched (that is, uncrossmatched A-positive red cells can be provided to a recipient determined to be A positive). Previous records must not be used to determine which blood group to issue, nor may the recipient's blood type be taken from other records such as credit cards, dog tags, or a driver's license.

Whole blood. A unit of whole blood contains approximately 450 milliliters of blood and 63 milliliters of anticoagulant/preservative solution. All the elements that make up human blood are in whole blood. Whole blood stored for more than twenty-four hours, however, contains few functional platelets or white blood cells. In addition, the levels of two proteins in whole blood necessary for normal blood clotting, known as coagulation factors V and VIII, decrease with storage. Stored whole blood, therefore, cannot be considered a source of functional platelets, functional white cells, or therapeutic levels of coagulation factors V and VIII. Whole blood provides oxygen-carrying capacity and blood volume expansion. Oxygen-carrying capacity is accomplished through the red blood cells present in whole blood. Red blood cells carry oxygen, which they deliver to vital organs and tissues. The approximately 500-milliliter volume of a unit of whole blood may make a significant addition to the total blood volume of a patient. The maintenance of a normal blood volume is vital to maintaining a proper level of pressure within the vascular system to get blood to and from vital organs and tissues. Patients lacking in blood volume may benefit from the volume provided by whole blood. Whole blood transfusions may be used, therefore, when there is a need for blood volume support combined with oxygen-carrying capacity, such as in patients experiencing severe acute hemorrhage.

For patients requiring oxygen-carrying capacity only, such as patients who have a normal blood volume but are anemic, red blood cell transfusion is recommended. When blood volume support is the sole need, such as in the early stages of acute blood loss when oxygen-carrying capacity has not yet become compromised but the blood volume is diminished, blood volume expanders that pose no risk of infectious disease—for example, normal saline (a salt and water solution)—are favored. Whole blood and other red cell components should not be used in patients with anemias that can be treated safely with specific medications such as iron, vitamin B_{12}, recombinant erythropoietin, or folic acid. Coagulation factor deficiencies, such as hemophilia, are more effectively treated with other blood components or derivatives. The storage period for whole blood varies from twenty-one to thirty-five days, based on the type of anticoagulant/preservative solution. As a result of time constraints posed by prerelease testing, whole blood that is less than twenty-four hours old is not routinely available. Whole blood stored less than seven days is often considered a desirable blood product for exchange transfusions in neonates (newborn children).

Red blood cell components. These components are produced when centrifugal or gravitational separation of red cells from plasma in whole blood is followed by the removal of 200 to 250 milliliters of plasma. The storage period of red cells collected and stored in an anticoagulant/preservative solution known as CPDA-1 is thirty-five days. Many red cell components contain a supplemental additive solution in addition to the anticoagulant/preservative. Additive systems in current use extend the storage period for red blood cells to forty-two days. Red cell transfusions increase oxygen-carrying capacity by increasing the circulating red blood cell mass. Increasing oxygen delivery to the body's organs and tissues with red cell transfusions may correct or prevent the manifestations of anemia. Red cell transfusions should be administered to patients with symptomatic anemia when other treatments are unavailable or ineffective and to those patients for whom rapid replacement of red cell mass is of critical importance. A unit of red blood cells contains essentially the same number of red cells as a whole blood unit. The volume of a red cell unit, however, is approximately 50 to 66 percent of whole blood. Thus, the use of red cells allows delivery of more red cells per milliliter transfused than whole blood, and smaller volume transfusions are required to achieve desired increases in oxygen-carrying capacity. When red blood cell components are used for exchange

IN THE NEWS: THE DEVELOPMENT OF BLOOD SUBSTITUTES

Red blood cell (RBC) substitutes were initially developed both to address the needs of the military by providing an improved resuscitation fluid and to avoid concerns about blood safety among the general population. A blood substitute with a long shelf life that is pathogen-free and universal in type would find wide clinical use: Human blood used for transfusions is sensitive to periodic blood shortages and cannot be used on patients with religious convictions against RBC transfusion. Blood substitutes can be classified into two general categories: hemoglobin-based oxygen carriers (HBOCs) and perfluorochemicals (PFCs).

The first HBOC to reach advanced Phase III clinical trials was a tetramer made of four connected hemoglobin molecules called Hemassist. Development of Hemassist was terminated after an interim review of data showed that twenty-four of fifty-two patients receiving the product had died, giving a mortality rate of 46.2 percent; the control group experienced a mortality rate of 17.4 percent. As of 2007, no HBOC had been approved for use in the United States. However, one HBOC based on bovine hemoglobin, Hemopure, had been approved for use in general surgery in the Republic of South Africa. Moreover, by 2003, at least ten HBOCs were under development and were being studied in either preclinical, Phase II, or Phase III clinical trials.

The other category of blood substitutes under development is PFCs. PFCs are synthetic, highly fluorinated, inert organic compounds that can dissolve large volumes of oxygen and other gases. They are unreactive in the body and are excreted as vapor by exhalation. PFCs can be safely injected into the bloodstream as microscopic drops, with one such product, Oxygent, in advanced clinical trials in Europe and China.

—*Michael R. King, Ph.D.*

transfusion, it is common to use units that are less than seven days old. Stored red blood cells do not contain functional platelets or white blood cells.

In adults, a hemoglobin value of 7 grams per deciliter or less is commonly used as a guideline for red cell transfusion. (An example of a normal range for hemoglobin is 13.5 to 16.5 grams per deciliter in adult men and 12.0 to 15.0 grams per deciliter in adult women.) This is a useful guideline; however, the decision to transfuse red cells should be based on patient clinical status. Laboratory data should be utilized as part of overall patient assessment and not as a sole indicator for transfusion therapy. Signs and symptoms reflecting a possible need for red cell transfusion include fainting, shortness of breath, a drop in blood pressure when sitting up or standing up, rapid heart rate, chest pain, and transient neurologic deficits. In rapid acute blood loss, the hemoglobin value may not reflect circulating red cell mass. Red cell transfusion decisions in this setting are based on assessments of blood loss, cardiorespiratory status, and oxygen delivery to tissues. Certain diseases compromise oxygen delivery to tissues or the adequate oxygenation of red blood cells, such as heart disease, lung disease, and disease of the blood vessels supplying the brain. Such patients may need to be transfused at higher hemoglobin levels than other patients in order to maintain adequate organ and tissue oxygenation. In summation, the decision to transfuse red cells should be based on patient symptoms, laboratory data, underlying diseases, and the urgency of need for oxygen-carrying capacity.

In neonates, red cell transfusions are usually small in volume (5 to 10 milliliters per kilogram) and administered frequently. The most common indication for red cell transfusion in neonates is to replace blood drawn for laboratory studies. Blood losses caused by laboratory sampling are proportionately large in neonates because of their small blood volumes. Usually, red cells are transfused following the removal of 5 to 10 percent of the estimated blood volume from sick neonates requiring frequent monitoring. Neonates with severe respiratory disease, particularly those requiring oxygen and/or respiratory support, are usually transfused to maintain a hematocrit level (a laboratory test used as a marker for anemia) above 40 percent. An example of a normal range for hematocrit values in children is 40 to 50 percent. Similar transfusion guidelines have been established for neonates with congenital heart disease. In neonates without severe respiratory or heart disease, it has been recommended that red cell transfusions be given to maintain hematocrit levels above 30 percent for infants with shortness of breath, rapid breathing, episodes of no breathing, rapid heart rate, and abnormal heart rhythms. Some physicians advocate red cell transfusions to maintain hematocrit levels above 30 percent for infants experiencing poor weight gain.

Red cell components may be modified by centrifugation, filtration, washing, sedimentation, or freezing/thawing to remove white blood cells. White cell removal procedures must result in a component that contains fewer than 5×10^8 residual white blood cells while maintaining at least 80 percent of the original red cells.

Many currently available white cell filters achieve much higher levels of white cell removal. White cell-depleted blood components are used to prevent febrile transfusion reactions (fever), to prevent or delay alloimmunization to white blood cell antigens, to prevent poor responses to platelet transfusions as a result of alloimmunization, and to prevent the transmission of white blood cell-associated viruses, such as cytomegalovirus, by cellular blood components.

Automated techniques are available for the washing of red cell units with sterile saline. This is less effective than filtration for white blood cell removal. The washing of red cells, however, does remove as much as 99 percent of the plasma from the red cell unit. Washed red cells may be indicated for patients requiring minimal plasma exposure. Examples include patients with a disease known as paroxysmal nocturnal hemoglobinuria, patients with IgA antibodies, and patients who have experienced recurrent or severe allergic transfusion reactions. Signs and symptoms of allergic reactions include hives, wheezing, low blood pressure, swelling of the throat, and fluid in the lungs.

Frozen red cells are prepared through the addition of glycerol, a cryoprotective (cold-protecting) agent, to red cells that are usually less than six days old, followed by freezing. The storage period for frozen red cells is ten years from the date that the unit was collected. When needed for transfusion, frozen red cells are thawed and washed with a series of saline-glucose solutions to remove glycerol. The unit is resuspended in sterile saline or a saline-glucose mixture. After thawing, washing, and resuspension, the storage period is twenty-four hours at 1 to 6 degrees Celsius. Frozen/thawed red cells are virtually devoid of plasma, anticoagulant, and platelets. The degree of white cell removal with this procedure is comparable to current filtration methods. Freezing is useful for the storage of rare red cell units and for the long-term preservation of autologous red cells. Because frozen/thawed red cells contain minimal amounts of plasma and white blood cells, they may be used when leukocyte-depleted and/or plasma-depleted red cell units are indicated.

Platelets. Platelet concentrates are prepared from whole blood by centrifugation. Most platelet concentrates contain at least 5.5×10^{10} platelets. The usual storage period for platelet concentrates is five days at 20 to 24 degrees Celsius. Platelets are often administered as a pool of concentrates.

Apheresis platelets are the second type of platelet component available. They are collected from a donor through the use of a blood cell separator in a procedure known as plateletpheresis. Most apheresis platelets contain at least $3 \times 10_{11}$ platelets. An apheresis platelet (collected from one donor) is the equivalent of six to eight units of platelet concentrates. Apheresis platelets are sometimes beneficial in patients who are not responding satisfactorily to platelet concentrates because of antiplatelet antibodies (alloimmunization). Antiplatelet antibodies often arise in response to human leukocyte antigens (HLAs) present on donor platelets; these antigens aid the immune system in recognizing "self" or "nonself" material. Donors possessing HLAs that are identical or similar to those of the recipient may be selected to provide platelets for transfusion. Such components are known as HLA-matched platelets. Apheresis platelets can be used to decrease the number of blood donor exposures for a recipient and to reduce or delay the development of alloimmunization.

A low number of platelets (less than 50,000 per cubic millimeter) is known as thrombocytopenia; the normal range for platelets is 150,000 to 400,000 per cubic millimeter of blood. Thrombocytopenia may result from disease processes, such as leukemia or aplastic anemia, or from the medical treatment of diseases, such as the use of chemotherapy for the treatment of cancer. Thrombocytopenia can lead to bleeding problems. Patients with functionally abnormal platelets may experience bleeding and have normal platelet counts. Platelet transfusions may be indicated to treat significant active bleeding or to protect against bleeding prior to invasive procedures, such as major surgery, in patients with platelet dysfunction or thrombocytopenia. Prophylactic platelet transfusions are commonly administered to prevent bleeding in patients with thrombocytopenia caused by decreased platelet production, as with cancer therapy. A commonly accepted threshold for prophylactic platelet transfusion in such patients is a platelet count of less than 20,000 per cubic millimeter. Platelet transfusions are usually not effective in the setting of rapid platelet destruction, such as in a condition known as idiopathic (or autoimmune) thrombocytopenic purpura (ITP). Platelets are also not recommended for routine use in a condition known as thrombotic thrombocytopenic purpura (TTP). In the event of life-threatening hemorrhage in ITP or TTP, however, platelet transfusions may be necessary.

Prophylactic platelet transfusions are recommended for all neonates with a platelet count less than 20,000 per cubic millimeter. In the presence of active bleeding or prior to invasive procedures, platelet transfusions are recommended to keep the platelet count above 50,000 per cubic millimeter. In stable premature neonates, prophylactic platelet transfusions are recommended to maintain a platelet count above 50,000 per cubic millimeter. In sick premature neonates, platelet transfusions are given to maintain a platelet count above 100,000 per cubic millimeter.

Fresh-frozen plasma. The fluid portion of whole blood is called fresh-frozen plasma (FFP). It can be separated and frozen at −18 degrees Celsius or colder within eight hours of whole blood collection. FFP may be stored for up to one year at −18 degrees Celsius or colder. It contains all plasma proteins present in normal blood.

FFP may be used to treat isolated deficiencies of coagulation proteins (factors II, V, VII, IX, X, and XI) when more specific components are not available or appropriate. Patients on oral anticoagulant therapy, such as warfarin, may require FFP to reverse anticoagulant effect rapidly prior to emergency invasive procedures or because of active bleeding. Depletion of multiple coagulation factors may occur in patients who have developed a deficiency of vitamin K, in those patients receiving massive blood replacement, or with a condition known as disseminated intravascular coagulation (DIC). The use of FFP may be necessary to treat such problems. FFP may be required for patients with liver disease who are actively bleeding or who face invasive procedures. FFP contains antithrombin III (AT-III), a naturally occurring anticoagulant, and it may be used in patients requiring AT-III. Plasma components, either through simple transfusion or as part of plasma exchange procedures, have become a vital aspect of therapy for TTP.

Indications for FFP in neonates include liver failure, inherited coagulation factor deficiencies, bleeding caused by vitamin K deficiency, the treatment of DIC, protein C deficiency (another naturally occurring anticoagulant), and AT-III replacement therapy.

FFP is not recommended for coagulation abnormalities that can be treated more effectively or safely with specific therapy such as vitamin K (in less serious situations, vitamin K deficiency is treated with vitamin K replacement instead of FFP), cryoprecipitate, or specific coagulation factor concentrates. FFP should not be used as a volume expander or as a nutritional source.

Cryoprecipitate. A concentrated source of certain plasma proteins, cryoprecipitate is a white precipitate that forms when FFP is thawed at between 1 and 6 degrees Celsius. The cryoprecipitate is removed and refrozen at −18 degrees Celsius or colder. A single bag of cryoprecipitate has a volume of 10 to 15 milliliters. Cryoprecipitate has a storage period of one year when stored at −18 degrees Celsius or colder. Several proteins necessary for normal blood clotting are present in cryoprecipitate, including factor VIIIc, von Willebrand factor (vWF), fibrinogen, and factor XIII.

Cryoprecipitate is used in the treatment of hemophilia A (a deficiency or abnormality of factor VIIIc), von Willebrand's disease (a deficiency or abnormality of vWF), inherited or acquired fibrinogen deficiency or dysfunction, and factor XIII deficiency. Cryoprecipitate has been beneficial in some kidney disease patients with abnormal bleeding. It is used to prepare fibrin glue, a material with adhesive and hemostatic properties that has been shown to be of value as a sealant in many operative procedures.

Granulocytes. Units of white blood cells (granulocytes) may be obtained by apheresis or by removal from units of fresh whole blood. Granulocytes collected by apheresis have a volume of 200 to 300 milliliters and should contain more than $1.0 \times 10_{10}$ granulocytes. To maximize therapeutic effect, granulocytes should be transfused as soon as possible following preparation. If storage is necessary, granulocytes may be stored for twenty-four hours at 20 to 24 degrees Celsius.

Granulocyte transfusions have been used to aid treatment of serious infections in patients with dysfunctional or very low numbers of white blood cells who are not responding to conventional therapies. Neonates with blood infections (sepsis) may receive granulocyte transfusion as a supplement to antibiotic therapy.

USES AND COMPLICATIONS

The use of autologous transfusion has increased markedly since the mid-1980's. This increase is largely the result of concerns of patients and physicians about the transmission of certain diseases, such as AIDS and hepatitis. In addition to minimizing the risk of transmitting such diseases, autologous transfusion provides numerous other advantages. Alloimmunization, the formation of antibodies to substances (alloantigens) present in allogeneic blood, will not occur when autologous blood is used. Some patients requiring blood transfusion are already alloimmunized from previous allogeneic transfusion or pregnancy. The provision of compatible allogeneic blood to such patients can sometimes be difficult. Therefore, the availability of auto-

logous blood in these situations, when possible, is advantageous.

A number of transfusion reactions may result from exposure to allogeneic blood—allergic reactions, fever, hemolytic reactions, graft-versus-host disease (GVHD)—that are prevented with autologous blood. Allogeneic blood appears to suppress the immune systems of transfusion recipients. Although there is still much to be learned about this phenomenon, the effect may adversely influence recurrence rates and mortality following some forms of cancer surgery and may lead to increased susceptibility to viral and bacterial infections. Autologous blood usage avoids these potential immunosuppressive effects. The use of autologous blood also leads to the conservation of vital blood resources. In the absence of the availability of autologous blood, transfusion needs must be met through the use of a volunteer allogeneic blood supply. For practical purposes, transfused autologous blood can be thought of as conserving a like amount of allogeneic blood. The availability of autologous blood may also lessen patient anxiety regarding the need for transfusion.

The overall risk of HIV infection from allogeneic blood transfusion is estimated at one in 225,000 per unit of blood (whole blood and blood components). The transfusion-transmitted infection rates for hepatitis B virus, HTLV-I/II, and HCV are estimated to be one in 200,000, one in 60,000, and one in 3,300 per unit, respectively. Although fear of HIV infection is a primary concern of transfusion recipients, transfusion-transmitted HCV infection is the principal infectious disease risk. The incidence of other transfusion-transmitted infections is very low in the United States. The current estimate of risk is less than one in one million per unit for transfusion-transmitted yersiniosis (*Yersinia enterocolitica* infection), malaria, babesiosis, and Chagas' disease (trypanosomiasis).

Transfusion-associated GVHD is a rare but severe complication of transfusion therapy. While patients with underdeveloped or impaired immune systems are at the greatest risk for developing this disease, it can occur in patients with normal immune systems. The transfusion of blood and blood components donated by blood relatives may put a recipient at risk for transfusion-associated GVHD. Gamma irradiation of whole blood and cellular blood components is the only currently acceptable method to reduce the risk. Fresh-frozen plasma and cryoprecipitate have not been implicated in this disease.

It is an absolute necessity that proper identification

of recipients be obtained prior to any transfusion procedure. Transfusing facilities must have strict policies to guarantee that the appropriate types of blood or blood components are transfused to the correct patients. Blood and blood components are visually inspected prior to their release for transfusion. If their fitness is questioned upon inspection, they will not be released. Visual abnormalities include hemolysis (evidence of red cell breakage), follicular material, cloudy appearance, or a deviation from the usual color of the blood or blood component. Blood and blood components are prepared by techniques designed to safeguard sterility through their expiration date. Once the seal of a blood component has been broken for any reason, the expiration time is four hours if maintained at room temperature (20 to 24 degrees Celsius) or twenty-four hours if refrigerated (1 to 6 degrees Celsius). All transfusions must be administered through a filter. Transfusion recipients should be observed carefully during the first fifteen minutes of a transfusion. If a life-threatening transfusion reaction occurs, such as from the mistaken transfusion of incompatible red blood cells, it usually develops following the infusion of only a small volume of the blood or blood component. Blood transfusion must be completed prior to the expiration time of the component or within four hours, whichever is sooner. All adverse reactions to transfusion, including possible bacterial contamination or suspected disease transmission, must be reported to the transfusion service.

PERSPECTIVE AND PROSPECTS

The first well-documented transfusion of human blood to a patient was administered by James Blundell on September 26, 1818. For most of the first hundred years of human blood transfusion, blood was transfused from donor to recipient by means of a direct surgical communication between the donor and recipient blood supplies. Numerous transfusion-related fatalities resulted, probably from the infusion of incompatible blood. A landmark event in the history of transfusion medicine occurred in 1901 when Karl Landsteiner published his observations that the sera of some individuals caused the red cells of others to agglutinate (clump). This led to the discovery of the ABO blood group system and set the stage for safe transfusion therapy. Reuben Ottenberg and David J. Kaliski subsequently published their key observations on the importance of pre-transfusion compatibility testing in 1913.

Despite these advances, blood transfusion remained

a cumbersome technique until the value of blood anticoagulants was noted by multiple investigators in 1914 and 1915. For the first time, blood donation could be separated, in time and place, from blood transfusion. Blood could be drawn and set aside for use at a later time. This led to the development of blood banks for the storage and distribution of blood. The first hospital blood bank in the United States was established at Cook County Hospital in Chicago in the mid-1930's. Blood was collected in glass bottles that were washed, sterilized, and reused following transfusion. The introduction of plastic containers for blood in 1952 led to the development of disposable plastic systems for the collection, separation, and preservation of blood products. The advent of such plastic systems allowed whole blood to be separated easily into multiple blood components, thus setting the stage for modern blood component therapy.

Transfusion medicine has become a vital aspect of modern medical practice. Patients with cancer may be treated more aggressively because of the support provided by blood products. Organ and tissue transplantation (such as liver, kidney, and bone marrow transplants) and other complex surgical procedures have become possible because of blood and blood component therapy.

The use of blood and components is constantly evolving. Continual efforts are being made to maximize the safety and availability of the blood supply. Indications for blood and blood component transfusions continue to be analyzed and clarified. Alternatives to allogeneic blood transfusion, such as autologous transfusion, the use of blood growth factors (such as recombinant erythropoietin), and manufactured blood substitutes (such as oxygen-carrying perfluorochemical solutions), continue to be explored and are expected to receive more widespread application.

—*James R. Stubbs, M.D.*

See also Anemia; Bleeding; Blood and blood disorders; Blood banks; Blood testing; Catheterization; Circulation; Critical care; Critical care, pediatric; Emergency medicine; Hematology; Hematology, pediatric; Immune system; Immunology; Immunopathology; Phlebotomy; Plasma; Rh factor; Serology; Surgery, general; Surgery, pediatric; Surgical procedures; Transplantation; Vascular medicine; Vascular system.

FOR FURTHER INFORMATION:
American Association of Blood Banks, American Red Cross, and Council of Community Blood Centers.

Circular of Information for the Use of Human Blood and Blood Components. Arlington, Va.: Author, 2002. This small pamphlet is considered an extension of blood component container labels and as such is a standard informational source on the use of blood and blood components.

Brecher, Mark, ed. *Technical Manual.* 15th ed. Bethesda, Md.: American Association of Blood Banks, 2005. This book is the bible of blood banking and transfusion practice. An indispensable source of information that deserves a place in every blood bank. The chapters are filled with easy-to-understand, practical information on blood banking.

Hillyer, Christopher D., et al., eds. *Blood Banking and Transfusion Medicine.* 2d ed. Philadelphia: Churchill Livingstone/Elsevier, 2007. Draws data from basic, transnational, and clinical studies and explores the latest advances in the use of blood products, new methods of disease treatment, and stem cell transplantation, and addresses a range of controversies in practice.

McCullough, Jeffrey. *Transfusion Medicine.* 2d ed. Philadelphia: Churchill Livingstone/Elsevier, 2005. Transfusion medicine, a young science, is continuously growing and changing. The result is a great body of knowledge about the practical aspects of blood collection and transfusion, and an incomparably better understanding of the blood groups and of the unintended effects of transfusion at the molecular level.

Petz, Lawrence D., et al., eds. *Clinical Practice of Transfusion Medicine.* 3d ed. New York: Churchill Livingstone, 1996. Another comprehensive, detailed textbook on virtually all aspects of transfusion medicine.

Schaub Di Lorenzo, Marjorie, and Susan Strasinger. *Blood Collection in Healthcare.* Philadelphia: F. A. Davis, 2002. Details all phlebotomy issues important in collecting a quality blood specimen and includes excellent photographs that clearly demonstrate the preferred techniques, supplies, and collection procedures.

Starr, Douglas P. *Blood: An Epic History of Medicine and Commerce.* New York: Perennial, 2002. Starr reflects on the societal role of blood as it transformed from a mythical enigma to a scientific entity to a product of industry. He examines the past racism of blood banks, the spread of the AIDS epidemic among hemophiliacs, and the role of blood in helping the Allies win World War II.

TRANSIENT ISCHEMIC ATTACKS (TIAs)
DISEASE/DISORDER
ALSO KNOWN AS: Ministrokes
ANATOMY OR SYSTEM AFFECTED: Blood vessels, brain, circulatory system
SPECIALTIES AND RELATED FIELDS: Neurology, vascular medicine
DEFINITION: Temporary interference with blood flow to the brain, resulting in transient strokelike symptoms.

CAUSES AND SYMPTOMS

A transient ischemic attack (TIA) is very similar to a stroke. Most physicians define a TIA as an episode of strokelike symptoms that fully resolves within twenty-four hours. A stroke, on the other hand, is defined as an episode that produces neurological symptoms that are permanent.

Strokes and TIAs are caused when the blood supply to the brain is interrupted. This interruption may occur because of a hemorrhage in an artery in the brain. Other causes of stroke or TIA may include a blood clot or piece of plaque that breaks loose from somewhere else in the body and eventually lodges in an artery that feeds the brain, or from severe narrowing in an artery that feeds the brain. Symptoms from a stroke or TIA that originates in the carotid arteries (the main arteries in the front of the neck) include weakness or numbness on

---

INFORMATION ON TRANSIENT ISCHEMIC ATTACKS (TIAs)

CAUSES: Temporary interruption of blood supply to brain from hemorrhage, embolism, severe narrowing in artery; risk factors include high blood pressure, high cholesterol, smoking, diabetes, advancing age, cardiac disease, stress, lack of physical activity, genetics

SYMPTOMS: In carotid arteries, weakness or numbness on one side, temporary loss of vision in one eye, difficulty speaking; in back of brain, dizziness, difficulty walking, drop attacks

DURATION: Acute episodes that resolve within twenty-four hours

TREATMENTS: Emergency care, sometimes surgery to remove narrowed section, medications (anticoagulants, antiplatelet drugs, clopidogrel, ticlopidine, dipyridamole)

one side of the body, temporary loss of vision in one eye, and difficulty speaking. When the back of the brain is damaged, symptoms such as dizziness, difficulty walking, or a drop attack (sudden loss of leg strength) may occur.

One might think that since the symptoms of a TIA go away, such an attack is not a serious condition. However, a TIA is often a warning signal of an impending stroke. For this reason, anyone suffering a TIA should immediately seek medical attention.

The risk factors for TIA and stroke are similar. They include high blood pressure, high cholesterol, smoking, diabetes mellitus, advancing age, cardiac disease (especially irregular heart rhythm problems), stress, and lack of physical activity. Genetics can make one more likely to have a stroke or a TIA as well.

TREATMENT AND THERAPY

A person experiencing symptoms of a TIA should call paramedics in order to be seen in an emergency room immediately. Doctors can assess the patient's situation and determine whether treatment can be initiated that will limit the amount of time that the brain is starved of oxygen. A stroke has been referred to as "brain attack" to underscore the need to seek prompt medical attention quickly, as one would for a heart attack.

Diagnostic tests will likely include magnetic resonance imaging (MRI) of the brain to check for hemorrhage or damage. Other tests may include magnetic resonance angiography (MRA) of the arteries or an ultrasound of the arteries that serve the brain. If these studies show a narrowing of the carotid arteries, then surgery can be done to remove the narrowed section before it causes more damage.

In some cases, medications will be used to lessen the risk of a full-blown stroke. They may include anticoagulants (blood thinners) and antiplatelet drugs such as aspirin, clopidogrel (Plavix), ticlopidine, and dipyridamole (Aggrenox). Drugs that lower cholesterol may also be prescribed.

—Steven R. Talbot, R.V.T.

See also Angiography; Arteriosclerosis; Brain; Brain damage; Brain disorders; Carotid arteries; Cholesterol; Circulation; Embolism; Hyperlipidemia; Hypertension; Ischemia; Numbness and tingling; Paralysis; Plaque, arterial; Speech disorders; Strokes; Subdural hematoma; Thrombolytic therapy and TPA; Thrombosis and thrombus; Vascular medicine; Vascular system.

FOR FURTHER INFORMATION:

Adams, Harold P., Jr., Vladimir Hachinski, and John W. Norris. *Ischemic Cerebrovascular Disease.* New York: Oxford University Press, 2001.

American Stroke Association. http://www.stroke association.org.

Chaturvedi, Seemant, and Steven R. Levine, eds. *Transient Ischemic Attacks.* Malden, Mass.: Blackwell Futura, 2004.

Kikuchi, H., ed. *Strategic Medical Science Against Brain Attack.* New York: Springer, 2002.

Parker, James N., and Philip M. Parker, eds. *The Official Patient's Sourcebook on Transient Ischemic Attack.* Rev. ed. San Diego, Calif.: Icon Health, 2004.

TRANSPLANTATION

PROCEDURE

ANATOMY OR SYSTEM AFFECTED: Blood, circulatory system, eyes, heart, immune system, kidneys, liver, lungs, pancreas, respiratory system, spleen, urinary system

SPECIALTIES AND RELATED FIELDS: Cardiology, emergency medicine, general surgery, genetics, immunology, nephrology, oncology, urology

DEFINITION: The transfer of tissue or organs from one individual to another, usually from cadavers or living related donors.

KEY TERMS:

acute rejection: the rejection of a transplanted organ by cells of the immune system; acute rejection is common days to weeks after cadaveric organ transplants and can usually be treated successfully with antilymphocytic drugs

allotransplantation: the transplantation of tissue or organs between unrelated individuals

chronic rejection: the rejection of a transplanted organ months or years after the procedure because of mechanisms that are poorly understood; most long-term graft losses are caused by chronic rejection, and no effective therapy exists

distributive justice: allocating transplanted organs to recipients based on need

hematopoietic stem cell transplantation (HSCT): transplantation of the bone marrow cells to a recipient

human leukocyte antigens (HLAs): structures located on the surface of each cell that are unique to an individual; also called transplantation antigens

material justice: allocating transplanted organs to recipients based on who would most benefit

orthotopic: the placement of a transplanted organ in the position occupied by the original organ

tissue typing: the process of identifying a person's transplantation antigens

utilitarianism: an ethical theory in which individuals make moral decisions based on the likelihood of benefitting the maximum number of people

vascularized transplant: transplanted tissue or organs that must have blood vessels reattached in the recipient in order to function (such as a kidney); corneal or bone marrow transplants are examples of nonvascularized transplants

xenotransplantation: the transplantation of tissue or organs between different species (such as baboon to human)

THE IMMUNE SYSTEM AND TRANSPLANTATION

Transplantation antigens are proteins expressed on the surface of an individual's cells. Every individual has a unique set of these proteins, called human leukocyte antigens (HLAs), which are encoded on chromosome 6. Each parent contributes one HLA-containing chromosome, and both chromosomes are expressed in the offspring. The purpose of these antigens is to help the body recognize what is "self" and what is not. In this manner, bacteria and other pathogens harmful to the individual can be sensed as "nonself" and destroyed by the immune system.

When an organ is transplanted between unrelated people (allotransplantation), it will not be recognized as self in the recipient's body, and the immune system will start to attack it in a process called rejection. In the same way, transplants between identical twins, with the same HLA proteins on their cells, will be recognized as self and not be rejected.

White blood cells (lymphocytes) are intimately involved in the body's immune response. They protect the individual from invading bacteria, viruses, and fungi. Lymphocytes can be divided into two subsets: B and T cells. The T cell is the main cell involved in the recognition and destruction of allotransplants. Receptors found on the T lymphocyte cell surface are stimulated by the foreign antigens found on allotransplants. With T-cell stimulation, events are initiated that lead to the allotransplant's destruction.

With the knowledge that T cells are responsible for rejection, methods of modulating T cell activity were developed. One of the first approaches was to destroy them using total-body irradiation. This method had only limited success, and the side effects of the radia-

tion were severe. Attention then turned toward drugs that acted directly on T cells.

Azathiaprine was one of the first drugs to be used successfully. By preventing the biosynthesis of essential components of cell growth, azathiaprine inhibits T cells from replicating. Steroids were next found to have immunosuppressive properties. Azathiaprine and steroids at one time were used in combination to prevent rejection in human kidney allografts. Although these drugs were effective, they were not specific for T cells. Other cells were affected, and both immunosuppressive drugs had serious side effects in high doses. In 1978, a T-cell-specific inhibitory drug was tried clinically for kidney allotransplants. This drug, named cyclosporine, has since become the mainstay of immunosuppressive therapy for all vascularized allotransplants. In most transplant centers, patients who have received allotransplants are given a combination of the above three drugs, since each drug works differently on T-cell function. The harmful side effects of these drugs can be minimized by using all three in smaller amounts, thus preventing the side effects from larger doses.

With the advent of cyclosporine, patients receiving kidneys without matching HLAs do almost as well in the short term (one to five years) as those receiving HLA-matched kidneys. Transplanted kidneys with HLAs in common, however, function significantly longer (ten years). Therefore, physicians try to match HLAs between donor and recipient. Most organs available for transplantation are from cadavers. It takes days to tissue-type the cadaver, find a compatible recipient, and transport the organ to him or her. Kidneys are the only organ that can be stored this long and still function. Therefore, only kidneys are matched for HLAs. With the liver, heart, and pancreas, only blood type is matched between donor and recipient. Currently, kidneys may be stored up to three days. The liver and pancreas must be transplanted within eighteen to twenty hours.

INDICATIONS AND PROCEDURES

With the advent of dialysis in 1960, renal failure is no longer fatal and patients can live by having their blood filtered several times per week. Kidney transplantation, however, offers a significant improvement in the quality of life compared with dialysis. Unfortunately, while more than 9,000 patients in the United States receive kidney transplants each year, another 8,500 patients remain on waiting lists. With only 13 percent of potential donors actually being utilized, there is much room for greater success.

Two donor options are available to the recipient awaiting a kidney transplant: living related and cadaveric. The first option involves removing a kidney from a willing family member and transplanting it into the recipient. Removing one of two donor kidneys does not significantly affect a healthy individual. The second option is for the recipient to be placed on a waiting list for a cadaveric kidney. When a cadaveric kidney that is of a compatible blood type for a particular recipient becomes available, arrangements are made to admit this patient to the hospital for transplant.

Approximately 25 percent of all kidney transplants are living related. The advantages of a living related transplant are twofold. First, the waiting period for a cadaveric kidney is eliminated, as the operation can be scheduled as soon as the recipient has been evaluated. Second, kidneys from living related donors tend to work immediately, with better long-term results. Because of organ shortages, some medical centers will allow unrelated volunteers to donate a kidney to a recipient. Such transplants usually occur between spouses.

A typical kidney transplant operation takes three hours to perform. Usually, the patient's own kidneys are not removed, and the transplanted kidney is placed in the pelvis. The vessels of the new kidney are sewn into the iliac blood vessels of the leg. After the transplant procedure, patients stay in the hospital ten days before returning home. They must take medications every day to prevent rejection but otherwise are independent.

Orthotopic liver transplantation is now considered the optimal form of therapy for end-stage liver disease in adults and children. Since no machine exists to take the place of the liver, transplantation is the only alternative in patients with liver failure. Cadaveric livers are the source for transplants because individuals have only one liver. Because of a shortage in cadaveric organs, many patients die each year waiting for a liver transplant. For this reason, a few medical centers have experimented with living related liver transplants, usually from parent to child. In this operation, one of the two lobes of the donor's liver is removed and transplanted to the recipient. The remaining liver in the donor will grow back to normal size in one week.

A liver transplant is one of the most difficult operations to perform. Unlike heart operations, there is no machine to take the place of the liver during surgery, and speed is vital. The liver is the largest organ in the body, weighing about 5 pounds in an adult. Because the liver is so large, and its blood supply complex, it is nec-

essary to remove the patient's own liver during the transplant. The average time for a liver transplant varies, ranging from five to thirty hours. The worst complication of liver transplant is failure to function after surgery. The only treatment is to find another liver for transplantation before the patient dies.

Pancreas transplants are done exclusively for patients with complications of insulin-dependent diabetes mellitus (IDDM). Around half of the 15,000 new cases of IDDM per year will develop complications such as renal failure and blindness. There is no way to predict which patients will develop these complications. Currently, combined pancreas-kidney transplants are done for diabetics who experience renal failure. The transplanted pancreas prevents damage from recurring in the new kidney and also makes the individual insulin-independent. Pancreas transplants are not performed for diabetics without complications because the risk of immunosuppression is not worth the benefit of insulin independence.

Unlike with liver transplants, short operative time for pancreas-kidney transplantation is not essential to patient survival. Both the pancreas and the kidney are placed into the pelvis, and the pancreas is anastomosed (sewn) to the right iliac vessels and the kidney to the left. Operative time is about ten hours. As with kidney transplants, the patient's own pancreas and kidneys are left in place because there is no advantage to removing them.

The transplantation of bone marrow, sometimes called hematopoietic stem cell transplantation (HSCT), is less demanding than transplantation of vascularized organs. The bone marrow is composed of stem cells that are primarily responsible for developing into red and white blood cells. A stem cell is any cell from which a whole population of different cells may develop. Transplant recipients, who usually have a blood disease such as leukemia, undergo a process of chemoradiotherapy to destroy their own stem cells. Once it is certain that all their own cells are destroyed, the donor cells are injected into the long bone of the leg. Following HSCT, the recipient may be immunologically incompetent for some time. The functioning of the immune system is vital to the success of this type of transplant. The white blood cells begin to reappear in the blood during the second or third week after the transplant. Although many lymphocytes begin functioning as soon as they are generated, the T and B cells do not become active until later. This is primarily due to the suppression of WBC function due to the presence of

IN THE NEWS:
DONOR BONE MARROW
INSTEAD OF REJECTION DRUGS

Transplantation using bone marrow cells has dramatically increased over the past four decades. Bone marrow transplantation is used as treatment for certain types of cancer, including lymphoma and leukemia. Two types of bone marrow transplantation are termed allogenic (nonself) or autologous (self). Allogenic transplant requires blood cells from a donor, while autologous transplant requires only a patients own cells.

In autologous transplant, the bone marrow or blood cells are taken from a patient, frozen, and subsequently given back to that patient (transplanted) after chemotherapy has been given. After the autologous stem cells are given back to a patient, the cells can mature into one of three types: red blood cells, which carry oxygen; white blood cells, which fight infection; or platelets, which help blood clotting.

Despite efforts to match a donor's blood cells to a recipient, complications often occur in allogenic transplants. For instance, a complication known as graft-versus-host disease (GVHD) develops in about 50 percent of patients undergoing allogenic bone marrow transplant with related matched donors. To prevent this complication, the patient may receive medications that suppress the immune system (antirejection drugs). In contrast, autologous transplants have a lower incidence of GVHD, which sometimes allows for less antirejection medication. Despite this benefit, autologous transplants do have a higher incidence of cancer relapse causing death (73 percent in autologous transplants versus 33 percent of allogenic transplants).

Autologous transplants do have other benefits, including better results when used instead of chemotherapy alone in certain advanced brain cancers, such as neuroblastoma. For example, the three-year disease-free survival rate is higher for patients that undergo autologous transplant for advanced stage neuroblastoma; however, the patient survival rate does not exceed 35 percent.
—*Jesse Fishman, Pharm.D.*

immunosuppressive drugs. There is evidence from immunologist Katalin Poloczi that bone marrow recipients have normal immune responses and may be vaccinated against various diseases. However, he has also observed that such patients must get booster shots more often than "normal" individuals to maintain immunity.

Fetal tissue transplantation therapy is related to stem cell therapy in that vascularized organs are not transplanted. Fetal tissue cell lines, sometimes called pleuripotent stem cells, have the ability to develop into any cell types found in the adult human body: brain cells for Alzheimer sufferers, pancreas cells for diabetics, heart cells for cardiac patients, and more. There are four sources for pleuripotent stem cells: preimplanted human embryos from in vitro fertilization (IVF), umbilical cord blood, cadaveric human fetal tissue, and human germ cell tumors. Although potentially very valuable, research in this area has become an ethical firestorm due to the embryonic source of the tissues. There is the worry that to obtain these cells researchers may actively begin aborting human embryos. Despite this controversy, the stem cell treatment holds such therapeutic promise that no one has yet abandoned the concept.

In 2001, researchers at the University of Wisconsin announced that they had successfully coaxed embryonic stem cells to form blood cells, a key step toward one day being able to make an alternative source of blood in a lab dish. This discovery signaled the future possibility of making blood for transfusions that is safe from germs, easing blood shortages, and offering a cure for cancer patients who need bone marrow transplants but lack a suitable donor. Unfortunately, since the sources of cells used in such laboratory research were aborted, preimplanted human embryos, ethical questions of whether this is tainted research are ongoing. The funding for these investigations was chiefly private, since the U.S. government has banned funding for research into development of these human cell lines.

Another controversial process is xenotransplantation, the transplanting of organs from one species to another. Xenotransplantation, if successful, could dramatically increase the supply of organs worldwide. Porcine transplants to replace human hearts and kidneys are being considered. Because of fears of transmitting animal diseases into human populations, some researchers have demanded a worldwide ban on such research. It is not clear whether these fears are justified. For example, a 2000 study from Stellan Welin of Göteborg University reported that patients with porcine transplants displayed no signs of porcine endogenous retrovirus. Even if xenotransplants do not transmit diseases, many ethical problems remain. One such problem is whether researchers should genetically modify source animals to change their immunological profiles. The consequences to altered livestock are still not clear. For example, a transgenic pig making bovine growth hormone may grow faster than normal but may be more susceptible to numerous uncharacterized, pathologic changes.

PERSPECTIVE AND PROSPECTS

There are a number of ethical problems connected to organ transplantation. Primary among these is the problem of donor selection. Cadaverous donors sometimes present the problem of whether sufficient permission was given to donate organs. Without full consent of the donor, it is considered unethical to harvest tissues. In cases where the potential donor died without giving consent, very often relatives who knew of their wish will give consent in their stead. In the case of living donors who are donating kidneys or bone marrow, questions will sometimes arise of their ability to give full consent; for example, whether the donor is fully competent and informed of what consent means. These questions of competence will usually arise with the mentally ill, but often arise when the donor potentially has been coerced by physicians or relatives. Coercion on anyone's part eliminates full consent from the donor.

Another recent ethical dilemma is the use of human newborns or late stage embryos as organ donors. Is it ethically permissible to use a fetus as an "organ farm"? There have been reports in the last several years of parents with a terminally ill child conceiving another child to act only as an organ donor. Although most often these donor infants become family members, they are sometimes aborted because the needed organ can only be obtained in that way. The bioethicist Mary Anne Warren has argued that the mere "potential to become a person"—unaccompanied by awareness, consciousness, and perception—does not entitle one to life compared to that of a person who needs a transplant. Warren finds no ethical objection to killing a fetus, an "entity below the level of personhood," in order to save the life of a grown human being. Whether or not there is abortion involved in the harvesting process, the ethicist Daniel C. Maguire submits that "person" is a relative term and even baby persons are intrinsically related to other persons. Maguire argues that using the uterus as an organ farm or the "objectified" fetus as an organ

bank is intrinsically wrong at the level of consent. What right does anyone have to presume the permission of the baby to donate an organ to a sibling or even a parent? He suggests that the privacy and autonomy of the baby be protected until it grows and can itself consent to an organ donation.

Maguire's argument has also been applied to the harvest and use of embryonic stem cells. When the cells are harvested directly from an embryo, whether that embryo was discarded from IVF or conceived for that specific purpose, the question of consent still remains unanswered.

Finally, allocation of transplanted organs has become increasingly difficult in recent years as the number of available organs has become overwhelmed by the number of potential recipients. A series of ethical questions has arisen in organ transplant allocation. Will the young or old recipient better benefit from a transplant? Should countries limit organ donations from their citizens to non-immigrant aliens? Should organ recipients of particular note, such as film stars and athletes, be moved ahead of "commoners" who are already on the waiting list? Should the location of the recipient affect the decision to provide an organ?

One principle that has been suggested as a guide to allocation is called "distributive justice." Distributive justice suggests that donor organs should go to those most in need. Most countries have now devised rules by which available organs go to those who are the most critically ill. The problem with this selection strategy is that the patients who are in the greatest need are the least likely to survive long term. If the goal is to maximize the overall benefit to society, as the ethical theory of utilitarianism suggests, then this method reduces the overall advantage to society compared to a system that would donate to patients with a better prognosis.

The opposing theory, called "material justice," suggests that patients who are likely to benefit most from transplantation get the organs first. This would maximize the benefit to society, which is risking less on a recipient with a better prognosis. One interpretation of this principle is that children with longer lives ahead of them would get preference for transplantation over adults or the elderly.

These two principles seem at odds with one another. Although the individual will benefit most from distributive justice, society may suffer, and the opposite might be true of material justice where society will benefit, but the individual may suffer. To make allocation as just as possible, the United Network of Organ Sharing (UNOS), the primary body which coordinates organ donors and recipients worldwide, has utilized a point system since August 1995. This point system creates a value for determining the suitability of a recipient for a particular donor based on number of years waiting, rank on the waiting list, HLA tissue mismatches, immune reactivity, and age.

Besides these other factors, very often the geographic profile of the recipient can be problematic. If a potential transplant recipient has come to the United States from the developing world, where organ donors are rare, in the hope of more easily getting a transplant, should he or she be considered a serious candidate? Should that person be placed ahead of native or naturalized citizens on the waiting list? Should an American citizen and potential recipient living in an isolated geographic location be placed lower on a waiting list because of his or her isolation? These questions are difficult to answer because they bring geography and politics into the equation with medicine and human needs. In September, 2000, the U.S. Department of Health and Human Services (DHHS) proposed rules to reduce the importance of geographic and political boundaries on organ allocation. The prime selection criterion—especially in heart and lung transplantation—would be altered by the DHHS primarily to reflect waiting time. Under these criteria, it would not matter where the candidate resided or where they originated. The only basis for selection would be their need and how long they had been waiting for a transplant.

It has been proposed that organ donors be allowed to sell transplanted organs to the highest bidder. This concept has been defended as "allowing the free market economy to flourish" and letting the poor have the right to "do with their bodies as they see fit." One ethical difficulty with the idea of commercializing human organ sales is that those who are richest will tend to receive the "best" organs. Organ allocation would suffer from these sales, and just distribution would become meaningless. No longer would the most needful recipient get an organ, but rather those who could most afford it. Furthermore, the poor would be victimized, become commodities, and be dehumanized as they potentially become organ farms. Legislation was passed by the World Health Organization and the Transplantation Society in 1999 to universally prohibit the sale of organs.

—*Edmund C. Burke, M.D.,*
and Peter N. Bretan, M.D.;
updated by James J. Campanella, Ph.D.

See also Bone marrow transplantation; Cancer; Cirrhosis; Corneal transplantation; Diabetes mellitus; Dialysis; Eye surgery; Eyes; Facial transplantation; Fetal tissue transplantation; Grafts and grafting; Hair loss and baldness; Hair transplantation; Heart; Heart transplantation; Hepatitis; Immune system; Immunology; Kidney transplantation; Kidneys; Leukemia; Liver; Liver transplantation; Renal failure; Systems and organs; Xenotransplantation.

FOR FURTHER INFORMATION:
Brunicardi, F. Charles, et al., eds. *Schwartz's Principles of Surgery.* 9th ed. New York: McGraw-Hill, 2010. A chapter reviewing most aspects of surgical transplantation is provided in this text. The section on transplant immunology is particularly excellent, with most of the important terms clearly defined.
Chopra, Sanjiv. *The Liver Book: A Comprehensive Guide to Diagnosis, Treatment, and Recovery.* New York: Simon & Schuster, 2002. Covers a great deal of information about liver disorders, including how doctors diagnose liver ailments, what to expect from tests and screening, hepatitis B and hepatitis C, liver transplants, and the role of alternative treatments.
Mulholland, Michael W., et al., eds. *Greenfield's Surgery: Scientific Principles and Practice.* 4th ed. Philadelphia: Lippincott Williams & Wilkins, 2006. Covers the scope and practice of surgery and includes reviews of the management of trauma and transplantation, surgical practice according to anatomic region and specialty, and musculoskeletal, neurologic, genitourinary, and reconstructive surgery.
National Research Council. Institute of Medicine. *Stem Cells and the Future of Regenerative Medicine.* Washington, D.C.: National Academy Press, 2002. A lay exploration of the scientific and ethical debate surrounding stem cell research, as well as an overview of medical advances and leading recommendations for the use of stem cells.
OrganDonor.gov. http://www.organdonor.gov. Site provides advice on how to become an organ and tissue donor and answers questions about the many myths and facts surrounding donation.
Stewart, Susan K. *Autologous Stem Cell Transplants: A Handbook for Patients.* Highland Park, Ill.: Blood and Marrow Transplant Information Network, 2000. Explains the procedure with solid medical and pharmaceutical information and tells the stories of people who have gone through the experience.

Toouli, James, et al., eds. *Integrated Basic Surgical Sciences*. New York: Oxford University Press, 2000. Offers a concise, well-written chapter that summarizes the facts and operative details regarding kidney, liver, and pancreas transplantation. Written by leaders in the field of transplantation.

Townsend, Courtney M., Jr., et al., eds. *Sabiston Textbook of Surgery*. 18th ed. Philadelphia: Saunders/Elsevier, 2008. An outstanding textbook that details all aspects of transplantation and immunology. The milestones in transplantation history are well covered. The authors of individual sections are all pioneers in the field of transplantation.

Trzepacz, Paula T., and Andrea F. Dimartini, eds. *The Transplant Patient: Biological, Psychiatric, and Ethical Issues in Organ Transplantation*. New York: Cambridge University Press, 2000. This excellent book addresses many ethical issues dealing with transplant patients, including specialty transplant populations, psychopharmacology, and assessment of the psychiatric characteristics of transplant patients.

TREMORS

DISEASE/DISORDER

ALSO KNOWN AS: Trembling, shaking

ANATOMY OR SYSTEM AFFECTED: Arms, feet, hands, head, legs, muscles, nerves, nervous system, throat

SPECIALTIES AND RELATED FIELDS: Genetics, geriatrics and gerontology, internal medicine, neurology, pharmacology, psychiatry, serology, toxicology

DEFINITION: Rhythmic, oscillating, and involuntary movements that vary with respect to frequency, amplitude, pattern, and anatomical site.

CAUSES AND SYMPTOMS

A very fine physiological tremor is present in the limbs of all people and may be noticeable when the hand is outstretched. This normal tremor is aggravated by fear and anxiety, cold, stress, fatigue, caffeine, alcohol withdrawal, toxin exposure, and a variety of drugs. For example, enhanced physiological tremor is a side effect of antipsychotic drugs that interfere with dopamine uptake in the brain.

The immediate cause of tremor is the repeated contraction and relaxation of muscles. This muscular pattern may be the consequence of neurological damage to the extrapyramidal structures of the brain, including the basal ganglia, or may be an inherited condition.

Two major types are rest and action tremor. The former occurs when a person is resting and typically dis-

appears or is reduced by voluntary movement, whereas the latter occurs when the person is active.

A "pill-rolling" rest tremor in the hand is usually the first noticeable sign of Parkinson's disease; later, the arms and then the legs may become tremulous. If the rest tremor becomes severe enough, then a postural tremor occurs when maintaining a position against gravity. Hence, rest and action tremors may be present at the same time.

Essential tremor is hereditary and is erroneously called senile tremor. It typically affects one hand and then the other, progressing to the arms, and may involve the head and voice. Essential tremor tends to worsen with age and is most visible during slow movements.

Cerebellar tremor is a slow tremor that is visible with targeted, voluntary movements. The probable cause is damage to a cerebellar pathway. This damage may be the result of disease, such as multiple sclerosis, stroke, or trauma to the brain.

Psychogenic tremor is subconsciously controlled by the person. The symptoms and signs point to both rest and action tremors, complicating the diagnosis. The onset may be sudden. The tremor may diminish or disappear when the person is distracted, and there may be a history of somatization disorder. Metabolic disorders and liver or kidney failure resulting in brain damage can also manifest themselves as tremors, known as flapping tremors, which are characterized by oscillations of the hand between dropping and rising positions.

INFORMATION ON TREMORS

CAUSES: Repeated contraction and relaxation of muscles; may result from neurological damage, inherited condition, or Parkinson's disease and be aggravated by fear and anxiety, cold, stress, fatigue, caffeine, alcohol withdrawal, toxin exposure

SYMPTOMS: Involuntary movement, either with rest or with activity

DURATION: Acute or chronic and progressive

TREATMENTS: Depends on type and cause; may include anxiety management with cognitive-behavioral therapy, treatment of alcoholism, reduction of caffeine intake, sleep improvement, medications (dopamine receptor agonists, beta-blockers, anticonvulsants, benzodiazepines), stereotactic brain surgery, deep-brain stimulation

TREATMENT AND THERAPY

The treatment of tremor depends on the type. For example, nondrug interventions are sometimes appropriate for enhanced physiological tremor and may include managing anxiety with cognitive-behavioral therapy, treating alcoholism, reducing caffeine intake, improving sleep, and so on.

A variety of drugs can be used for the treatment of tremor, including dopamine receptor agonists, beta-blockers, anticonvulsants, and benzodiazepines. For example, propanolol, a common beta-blocker, may reduce essential tremor as well as parkinsonian tremors. Drug therapy is less effective for cerebellar tremor. Stereotactic brain surgery (involving spatial coordinates for precision) to destroy part of the thalamus and thus interrupt the circuitry generating tremors or deep-brain stimulation via an electric probe implanted in the thalamus may provide relief.

—*Tanja Bekhuis, Ph.D.;*
updated by W. Michael Zawada, Ph.D.

See also Aging; Alcoholism; Anxiety; Brain; Brain damage; Brain disorders; Caffeine; Fatigue; Multiple sclerosis; Muscle sprains, spasms, and disorders; Muscles; Nervous system; Neurology; Palsy; Parkinson's disease; Psychosomatic disorders; Seizures; Stress; Strokes; Toxicology.

FOR FURTHER INFORMATION:

Beers, Mark H., et al., eds. *The Merck Manual of Diagnosis and Therapy.* 18th ed. Whitehouse Station, N.J.: Merck Research Laboratories, 2006.

International Essential Tremor Foundation. http://www.essentialtremor.org.

Owens, D. G. Cunningham. *A Guide to the Extrapyramidal Side-Effects of Antipsychotic Drugs.* New York: Cambridge University Press, 2000.

Velickovic, Miodrag, and Jean-Michel Gracies. "Movement Disorders: Keys to Identifying and Treating Tremor." *Geriatrics* 57, no. 7 (July, 2002): 32-37.

TRICHINOSIS

DISEASE/DISORDER

ALSO KNOWN AS: Trichinellosis

ANATOMY OR SYSTEM AFFECTED: Gastrointestinal system, intestines, muscles, musculoskeletal system

SPECIALTIES AND RELATED FIELDS: Microbiology, public health

DEFINITION: A parasitic disease of humans caused by nematodes of the *Trichinella* genus and acquired by eating contaminated, undercooked meat.

CAUSES AND SYMPTOMS

Trichinosis is a zoonosis (disease acquired from animals) caused by nematodes (roundworms) belonging to the *Trichinella* genus, most commonly *T. spiralis.* *Trichinella* are parasites of carnivores that show little host specificity, infecting pigs, bears, horses, and humans among other mammals. Undercooked, contaminated pork and bear meat are the most important sources of human infection. While food processing requirements in developed parts of the world have resulted in decreases in trichinosis, other areas, particularly Latin America (Argentina, Mexico, Chile) and Thailand, continue to experience outbreaks of this disease.

The worms are ingested as larvae that are encysted in the muscle of the infected animal. Once ingested, the larvae hatch from the cysts and mature as adults in the upper intestine. There, the worms mate. Gravid female worms penetrate the intestinal mucosa and deposit larvae that migrate in the bloodstream, eventually becoming encapsulated in the muscle of the infected individual.

Ingesting large numbers of larvae results in gastrointestinal symptoms such as nausea, vomiting, diarrhea or dysentery, fever, and sweating that begin seventy-two hours after infection and may last two weeks. As the larvae migrate, edema (swelling) may be observed around the eyes, side of the nose, temples, and hands. Encysted larvae often result in muscle inflammation and pain, and respiratory symptoms such as cough and hoarseness may be observed late in the infection.

Diagnosis is difficult because of the number of body systems affected and the variety of symptoms. Changes in blood, including an increase in the number of eosinophils (eosinophilia), can be monitored. Because the nematodes are highly antigenic, the human immune response is strong, and antibodies in the blood indicate infection. Sensitive tests involving fluorescently labeled antibodies and enzyme-linked immunosorbent assay

---

INFORMATION ON TRICHINOSIS

CAUSES: Parasitic infection transmitted through ingestion

SYMPTOMS: Nausea, vomiting, diarrhea or dysentery, fever, sweating, swelling in face and hands, muscle inflammation and pain, coughing, hoarseness

DURATION: Chronic

TREATMENTS: Antihelminthic agents (e.g., mebendazole), corticosteroids

(ELISA) can be used to detect circulating antigens in blood serum. Definitive diagnosis is made by examining muscle biopsies for the presence of encysted larvae.

Treatment and Therapy

Trichinosis is usually treated using antihelminthic compounds. Early in the infection, mebendazole (Vermox) may be used. Treatment with these compounds is often accompanied by the administration of corticosteroids to prevent hypersensitivity reactions. The effectiveness of treatment depends on a variety of factors, including the stage of infection, the nature of the infected individual's immune response, the species of nematode, and the initial number of larvae ingested.

Control of the disease is primarily through control of feeding and processing of meat food products, especially pork. In Europe, feeding garbage to pigs has been banned, and in the United States, any garbage-fed pigs and hogs must be pretreated. Inspectors examine animals at slaughter, and in the United States freezing, heating, or freeze-drying of meat products is required during processing. Educating the public to cook pork thoroughly to a temperature of 71 degrees Celsius (161 degrees Fahrenheit) is an important thrust of control and prevention efforts.

—Michele Arduengo, Ph.D.

See also Food poisoning; Insect-borne diseases; Intestinal disorders; Intestines; Parasitic diseases; Worms; Zoonoses.

For Further Information:

Centers for Disease Control and Prevention. "Fact Sheet: Trichinellosis." http://www.cdc.gov/ncidod/dpd/parasites/trichinosis/factsht_trichinosis.htm.

Doyle, Michael P., Larry R. Beuchat, and Thomas J. Montville, eds. *Food Microbiology: Fundamentals and Frontiers.* 2d ed. Washington, D.C.: ASM Press, 2001.

Forbes, Betty A., Daniel F. Sahm, and Alice S. Weissfeld. *Bailey and Scott's Diagnostic Microbiology.* 12th ed. St. Louis, Mo.: Mosby/Elsevier, 2007.

Jay, James M., Martin J. Loessner, and David A. Golden. *Modern Food Microbiology.* 7th ed. New York: Springer, 2005.

Moorhead, A., et al. "Trichinellosis in the United States, 1991-1996: Declining but Not Gone." *American Journal of Tropical Medicine and Hygiene* 60 (1999): 66-69.

Ray, Bibek. *Fundamental Food Microbiology.* 4th ed. Boca Raton, Fla.: Taylor & Francis, 2008.

Trichomoniasis

Disease/disorder

Also known as: Trich

Anatomy or system affected: Genitals, reproductive system, urinary system

Specialties and related fields: Epidemiology, gynecology, neonatology, obstetrics, perinatology, public health, urology

Definition: A sexually transmitted disease in which motile *Trichomonas vaginalis* protozoans become established in the genitourinary tract of men and women.

Key terms:

asymptomatic: infected but with no discernable symptoms of disease

carrier: a person infected by an organism who can transmit that organism to other people but who is asymptomatic

Centers for Disease Control and Prevention (CDC): a government facility, located in Atlanta, that coordinates investigations of disease occurrence in the United States

protozoan: a unicellular organism with an organized nucleus

sexually transmitted disease (STD): a disease that is usually transmitted from person to person through contact between the vaginal or urethral discharges from an infected person and the genital mucous membranes of a person susceptible to infection

urethritis: inflammation and infection of the urinary tract

vaginitis: inflammation and infection of the vagina

Causes and Symptoms

Flagellated motile protozoans known as *Trichomonas vaginalis* cause trichomoniasis, one of the most widespread and common of sexually transmitted diseases (STDs). The disease is common among people with multiple sex partners, those who engage in unprotected sex, and those who seek services at STD clinics. Trichomoniasis in pregnant women is a leading cause of premature birth in the United States.

Some estimates suggest that 180 million people a year are infected with trichomoniasis worldwide. The most common population found to be infected is females sixteen to thirty-five years old, which is prime childbearing age. This is an important epidemiological group, as trichomoniasis infections are a leading cause of premature rupture of the placenta, premature birth, and low birth weight.

After infection, there is an incubation period of about seven days, with a range from about four to twenty days. Although up to 70 percent of infected women may remain asymptomatic, *T. vaginalis* infections may sometimes produce a frothy yellow or green vaginal discharge. Women's symptoms may also include urethritis, vaginitis, and itching of the vulva. Sometimes, vaginal inspection shows a distinctive "strawberry cervix" (red patches on the cervix) and red spots on the vaginal walls. Men's symptoms sometimes include urethritis, dysuria, a frothy or purulent urethral discharge, and, in rare cases, scrotal pain as the tube connecting the testicle with the vas deferens becomes inflamed.

The symptoms of infection by *T. vaginalis* are of questionable value in diagnosing the infection. In addition, many infected people remain asymptomatic for many years, and most existing tests, such as microscopic viewing of wet mounts, Pap tests, and polymerase chain reaction (PCR), often fail to show the infectious agent in people with symptoms. Culture of vaginal and urethral smears is considered to be the most effective way of detecting *T. vaginalis* infection. These factors add to the difficulty in reducing infection rates.

TREATMENT AND THERAPY

The CDC's *Sexually Transmitted Diseases Treatment Guidelines 2006*, which includes trichomoniasis, focuses on microbiological cure, alleviation of signs and symptoms, prevention of sequelae, and prevention of transmission.

The infection is treated with a single oral dose of either metronidazole or tinidazole. Any sex partner should be treated simultaneously even if he or she is asymptomatic. Treatment is successful in 90 to 100 percent of cases. Treatment during pregnancy is controversial, but no case of fetal malformation has been attributed to metronidazole. Studies have shown that trichomoniasis is associated with low infant birthweight, premature rupture of the membranes, and preterm births. However, studies of pregnant women with trichomoniasis who are treated failed to show an improvement in preterm deliveries and even trended toward more preterm deliveries; therefore, treatment remains controversial.

PERSPECTIVE AND PROSPECTS

Many men and women infected by the organism remain asymptomatic for years, spreading the disease to other people through sex. Safer sex practices help pre-

---

INFORMATION ON TRICHOMONIASIS

CAUSES: Protozoan infection transmitted via sexual contact or congenitally

SYMPTOMS: In sexually transmitted form, ranges from asymptomatic to frothy yellow or green vaginal discharge, urethritis, vaginitis, itching, red patches on cervix and vaginal walls (in women) and frothy or purulent urethral discharge, urethritis, dysuria, and scrotal pain (in men); in congenital form, placental rupture, premature birth, low birth weight

DURATION: Chronic

TREATMENTS: Metronidazole

---

vent transmission. People with multiple sex partners should use latex or polyurethane condoms to help curtail the spread of this disease. It is crucial that sex education programs emphasize that people with any unusual genital symptoms, including urethritis and vaginal discharge, seek medical treatment.

People infected by *T. vaginalis* may also be infected by other STD organisms, especially the bacterium that causes gonorrhea. Medical professionals believe that infection by the *Trichomonas* protozoan predisposes a person to infection by the human immunodeficiency virus (HIV) upon exposure through unprotected sex with infected partners.

Trichomoniasis in young children may indicate sexual abuse, and health professionals may be obligated to report such infections, if local regulations require it.

—Anita Baker-Blocker, M.P.H., Ph.D.

See also Acquired immunodeficiency syndrome (AIDS); Epidemiology; Genital disorders, female; Genital disorders, male; Gonorrhea; Gynecology; Human immunodeficiency virus (HIV); Men's health; Preventive medicine; Protozoan diseases; Sexually transmitted diseases (STDs); Urethritis; Urinary disorders; Urinary system; Women's health.

FOR FURTHER INFORMATION:

Boston Women's Health Collective. *Our Bodies, Ourselves: A New Edition for a New Era.* 35th anniversary ed. New York: Simon & Schuster, 2005. A popular book dealing with all aspects of women's sexuality, including STDs and safer sex.

Centers for Disease Control and Prevention. *Sexually Transmitted Diseases Treatment Guidelines.* http://www.cdc.gov/std/treatment. The official government recommendations for diagnosing and treating STDs, including trichomoniasis.

Heymann, David L., ed. *Control of Communicable Diseases Manual.* 19th ed. Washington, D.C.: American Public Health Association, 2008. An official report of the American Public Health Association. Includes an index.

Scharbo-DeHaan, Marianne, and Donna G. Anderson. "The CDC 2002 Guidelines for the Treatment of Sexually Transmitted Diseases: Implications for Women's Health Care." *Journal of Midwifery and Women's Health* 48 (February, 2003): 96-104. Reviews the government recommendations for the diagnosis and treatment of trichomoniasis and other STDs.

Sutton, Amy L., ed. *Sexually Transmitted Diseases Sourcebook.* 3d ed. Detroit, Mich.: Omnigraphics, 2006. Offers consumer health information about trichomoniasis and a variety of other sexually transmitted diseases.

TROPICAL MEDICINE
SPECIALTY
ANATOMY OR SYSTEM AFFECTED: All

SPECIALTIES AND RELATED FIELDS: Bacteriology, critical care, environmental health, epidemiology, immunology, microbiology, neonatology, nutrition, pediatrics, pharmacology, preventive medicine, public health, virology

DEFINITION: The prevention, diagnosis, and treatment of diseases that are prevalent in tropical regions, particularly those occurring in poor countries with inadequate health care delivery.

KEY TERMS:

arthropod: a member of the phylum Arthropoda, which includes mites, ticks, spiders, and insects

helminths: a general term for roundworms (nematodes) and flatworms (platyhelminths), many of which are parasites of humans and animals

morbidity: in medical statistics, the occurrence of clinical disease, in contrast to mortality (death) and occurrence (which includes subclinical infections)

parasite: an organism whose principal food source is another living organism; in medicine, the term refers to unicellular and multicellular animals

reservoir: an animal population infected with a disease that can be transmitted either to other animals or to humans; also called alternate hosts

vector: an organism, usually an insect or other arthropod, which transmits a disease from one host to another; the vector may itself be a host in which the pathogen multiplies, or it may merely transmit the pathogen mechanically

SCIENCE AND PROFESSION

Humankind evolved in tropical Africa, and it is presumed that many of the diseases and parasites characteristic of the tropical environment were inherited from nonhuman primate ancestors. Over the centuries, tropical diseases have challenged the limited resources of tribal medical practitioners and the more sophisticated medical learning of Chinese and Arab physicians. Western involvement in tropical medicine developed as a consequence of colonial expansion. The great number and diversity of tropical diseases may be grouped according to the nature of the causative agent, the symptoms involved, their mode of transmission, or their geographical distribution. The causative agent is the focus of this entry.

Viral diseases have become the most important infectious diseases in the temperate zone since the introduction of antibiotics. In the tropics, they are important but not preeminent. The principal tropical viral diseases are yellow fever and dengue fever, which are transmitted by arthropods. The transmitted viruses are called arboviruses. Yellow fever and dengue fever are acute illnesses with mortality (death) rates that exceed 50 percent if left untreated. The diseases occur sporadically when mosquitoes transmit the virus from a primate reservoir. There is potential for devastating epidemics to occur if a breakdown in health care delivery prevents prompt immunization of the population in affected areas. Arboviruses are distributed throughout tropical areas of both the New and Old Worlds. Until a massive eradication campaign orchestrated by the World Health Organization (WHO) eliminated smallpox, they exceeded other viral diseases in mortality and morbidity (illness).

Other viral diseases affect tropical regions. Human immunodeficiency virus (HIV), the agent that causes acquired immunodeficiency syndrome (AIDS), is prevalent and spreading in East and Central Africa, as well as in Haiti and Brazil in the New World. Influenza and measles, although not predominantly tropical, have high mortality rates among poor tropical populations. Hepatitis is endemic throughout the developing world. Until recently, poliomyelitis was virtually universal in the tropics, although paralytic cases were infrequent. Rabies claims a small number of victims. Finally, scientists are constantly encountering new viral diseases. Some (such as filoviruses) are exceedingly virulent. Ebola, Marbourg, and Bolivian hemorrhagic fevers are examples. Their distribution is confined to relatively small areas, probably because of the rapidly fatal nature of these diseases.

Tropical diseases caused by bacteria include some of the diseases most feared by humanity: cholera, bacillary dysentery, typhoid fever, tuberculosis, leprosy, and bubonic plague. As a result of the lack of safe sources of drinking water, there has been a resurgence of epidemic cholera in urban slums in the developing world. Fortunately, the discovery of inexpensive methods of oral rehydration therapy has reduced mortality from cholera and dysentery. Leprosy is surprisingly common and, because of its low infectivity and slow onset of debilitating symptoms, is not always perceived as a major menace. Bubonic plague occurs in isolated outbreaks within and outside the tropics where rodent reservoirs exist. In the southwest United States, approximately one hundred cases of plague are reported each year. Trachoma, an inflammation of the eyelids, affects large numbers of people—as many as a million in Brazil alone—and is a leading cause of blindness. Vaccines and antibiotics exist for the most prevalent bacterial diseases.

Spirochetes of the genus *Treponema* cause syphilis and yaws, which are chronic, endemic, and degenerative illnesses characterized by skin ulcers and neurological involvement. Yaws was the most common major tropical disease reported by WHO in the 1950's, affecting twelve million people in Southeast Asia alone. The disease is rarely fatal. Since then, aggressive wholesale treatment campaigns employing penicillin have reduced the incidence of yaws considerably in Asia and the Americas. Typhus and relapsing fever, arthropod-transmitted rickettsial diseases, can occur in epidemics.

Parasitic diseases caused by protozoa and helminths constitute the classic tropical diseases. These groups of organisms typically have complex life cycles that involve invertebrate vectors (flies, worms, and amoebas). Since many organisms are intolerant of freezing, human parasites are much more common in tropical areas.

A mosquito-transmitted protozoan causes malaria. Schistosomiasis is caused by a flatworm whose alternate hosts are aquatic snails that inhabit rice paddies and irrigation canals. These two diseases are arguably the greatest threats to human health anywhere in the world today. They affect enormous numbers of people throughout the tropics and warm temperature regions. Both cause chronic infections that may persist for decades, undermining the health and vigor of the host. In poorer tropical nations, malaria, schistosomiasis, and ancylostomiasis (hookworm) affect much of the adult population. These victims are chronically malnourished and may harbor other parasites. Trypanosomiasis, African sleeping sickness and its South American counterpart, Chagas' disease, is caused by insect-transmitted protozoa. Both diseases declined in frequency and geographical distribution following aggressive attempts to eliminate vectors.

Kala-azar is a lethal, disseminated form of the disease leishmaniasis. It is comparatively rare; some experts predict a resurgence because of increases in vector populations and drug resistance. Cutaneous leishmaniasis is widespread throughout the tropics. The organism responsible for amebic dysentery is universal in contaminated water in the tropics; infection is extremely common. Carriers are often asymptomatic; unsuspecting tourists and natives with compromised immune systems contract the most serious forms of the disease. Filariasis, called elephantiasis in its extreme

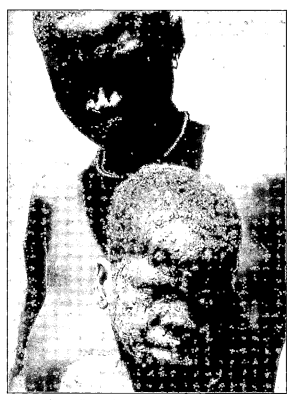

A young boy suffering from yaws. (National Library of Medicine)

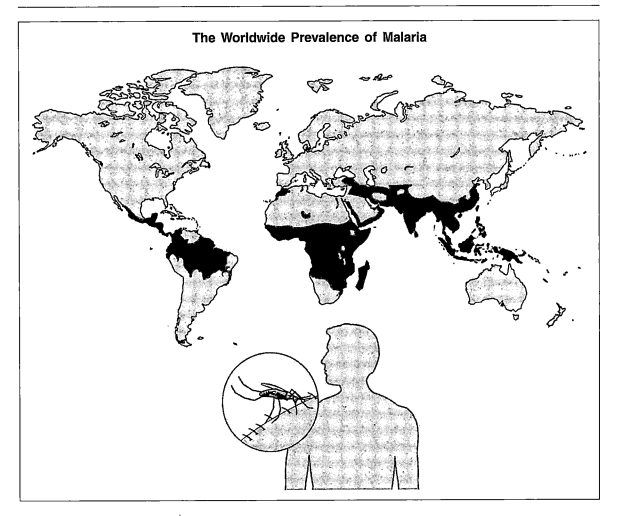

The Worldwide Prevalence of Malaria

form, is caused by a mosquito-transmitted nematode. It is common in Africa and the Indian subcontinent. In 1998, the pharmaceutical company SmithKline Beecham announced that it would donate its anti-parasitic drug albendazole for use by the one billion people at risk for contracting filiarisis until the disease is eliminated completely. Onchocerciasis, also called river blindness, is a parasitic disease found primarily in Africa. It is one of the leading causes of blindness in the world. Approximately one million people become blind each year as a result of this disease. Economic limitations and politics have hampered campaigns to treat onchocerciasis. There are many other parasitic diseases, including guinea worm, that occur locally in the tropics.

Nutritional deficiencies primarily result from extreme poverty and parasitic infection but also from ignorance and poor dietary practices. Characteristic of tropical regions is kwashiorkor, a protein deficiency

disorder affecting primarily very young children and increasing in regions where modernization encourages early weaning. Children with kwashiorkor are fed carbohydrates but inadequate amounts of protein. Marasmus (wasting) is usually caused by a combination of insufficient total calorie intake and very inadequate intake of protein. It is made worse by dysentery or other parasitic infections and the B-complex vitamin deficiencies beriberi and pellagra.

Diseases caused by other factors are not as prevalent in tropical countries. While severe systemic fungal diseases are predominantly tropical, the total number of cases is not high. Sickle cell disease, an inherited disorder, is frequent in central Africa because the mild, heterozygous form confers immunity to malaria. Little is known, however, about other genetic disorders in the tropics as a whole. In South Africa, genetic diseases are more common in white than in black populations. Typical so-called diseases of affluence may also pose a particular threat to people who make an abrupt transition from tribal to urban life in developing countries. The urban black population of South Africa is experiencing high rates of obesity and adult-onset diabetes.

DIAGNOSTIC AND TREATMENT TECHNIQUES

Tropical medicine is a vast field in which progress is slow and sporadic, with gains in one area often offset by losses in another. Tropical medicine, especially in developed countries that are located in temperate climates, is hampered at every stage, from research to clinical practice, by the low proportion of resources devoted to basic research in tropical disease etiology and ecology. Pharmaceutical companies often assign low priorities to the development of medicines and therapeutic agents for tropical diseases because of the potentially low returns on their investments. In affected countries, governmental policies are often established that ignore human health consequences. Extreme poverty among affected populations slows efforts to improve sanitation and general health. Explosive population growth and social and political instability slow efforts to improve infrastructures that, in turn, would improve human health. Persistent customs and attitudes in many tropical regions, which may once have been adaptive, are often harmful in modern settings. Finally, health care facilities and professionals are in short supply and unevenly distributed throughout the world and within countries affected by tropical diseases.

All these factors are important. No tropical country enjoys an average life span as long or an infant mortality rate as low as Western Europe, North America, or Japan. Nevertheless, the overwhelming influence of poverty and lack of health care access is well illustrated by contrasting the health status of the populations of Puerto Rico, Okinawa, or Taiwan with the conditions in Central Africa and the Indian subcontinent. In relatively prosperous, politically stable countries, diseases that can be prevented by immunization (such as polio) or easily cured by chemotherapy (such as yaws) are unimportant. Education, better sanitation, and environmental management have dramatically reduced the incidence of the parasites that cause malaria, schistosomiasis, and hookworm. In developed countries, severe malnutrition is rare.

Existing medical knowledge is constantly being refined, and an increased commitment to tropical medical research is needed. It is worth noting, however, that many typical tropical diseases were prevalent in the southeastern United States before World War I. Furthermore, the medical knowledge and governmental agencies available in the 1920's proved effective in combating malaria, yellow fever, hookworm, and pellagra in the United States.

The development of drugs to combat disease is largely the business of a pharmaceutical industry based in developed countries. These companies have been accused of neglecting tropical diseases because of a low potential for profit. WHO has provided incentives in some cases but has also opposed exclusive licensing of drugs developed under its aegis, a potential disincentive. Less than 5 percent of health research worldwide is devoted to the health problems of developing nations.

The pharmaceutical industry has also been implicated in marketing drugs to developing nations that have been banned as ineffective or dangerous in the United States. This practice underscores a wider and growing health threat: multinational corporations exporting pesticides, industrial chemicals, and manufacturing processes that undermine human health to the developing world. Any process resulting in wholesale environmental disruption produces an increase in disease in ways that are unpredictable.

Drug-resistant strains of pathogens are most likely to evolve when large populations are treated with a single therapeutic agent and when treatment is insufficient to cure patients completely. The risk of this pattern occurring is high in tropical countries. Drug-resistant strains of malaria are already increasing and complicate the task of combating this dangerous disease.

Poverty among individuals leads to malnutrition, overcrowding, poor sanitation, lowered resistance to infection, and an inability to avoid exposure to vectors and contaminated water. In many tropical areas, access to medical care ranges from limited to nonexistent. On a regional and national level, poverty leads to political and social instability and an inability to implement public health programs. Political upheaval facilitates the interregional spread of pathogens.

In much of the tropics, efforts to improve infant health and agricultural productivity backfire because social and economic customs favor large families. The resulting population increase exacerbates poverty-dependent variables responsible for disease. Training skilled medical personnel and maintaining clinics are costly. In the developing world, however, this cost is less because labor costs are low.

If market forces alone dictate the allocation of medical resources, health care providers gravitate toward the most prosperous areas. Medically trained developing world nationals frequently emigrate to Europe or the United States. Paramedic personnel, such as the so-called barefoot doctors of China, are effective only to the extent that their training, supervision, and support services are adequate. The number of doctors relative to the population in many tropical countries is too low to provide adequate medical care even without the additional factors of uneven distribution and higher incidence of serious disease.

PERSPECTIVE AND PROSPECTS

The Old World tropics, especially tropical Africa, were dubbed the "white man's grave" because European military personnel and colonists lacked both inherited resistance and customary methods of avoidance to protect themselves from the ravages of malaria, yellow fever, Asiatic cholera, and scores of other life-threatening diseases. Occasionally, disease resulted in the failure of colonial enterprise. In Hispaniola (Haiti), black slaves were successful in their bid for independence after yellow fever killed all but six thousand of the thirty thousand troops sent by Napoleon to quell the rebellion. In Africa, large areas in which sleeping sickness was endemic were inaccessible to European colonization.

The period of maximum European colonial expansion (from 1830 to 1914) coincided with great strides in the understanding of disease causation and prevention, although effective cures lagged until the beginning of World War II. In 1900, Walter Reed, in the course of investigating a devastating epidemic of yellow fever among workers and soldiers digging the Panama Canal, discovered that the disease was mosquito-borne. In 1898, the Italian researchers Amico Bignami, Giovanni Grassi, and Giuseppe Bastianelli, who were also working with malaria, made a similar discovery. These observations paved the way for effective control through exclusion and eradication of the vectors.

European activities in the tropics have often exacerbated tropical disease problems. The African slave trade introduced a number of tropical diseases into the southern United States, including schistosomiasis, one of the most debilitating and intractable of tropical parasitic infections. Bengalis in India dubbed kala-azar "the British government disease," since road-building and improved communication introduced a previously localized pathogen into large areas, with disastrous results. Dam-building and artificial irrigation dramati-

cally increase the incidence of schistosomiasis in tropical areas. Paradoxically, medical intervention reducing infant mortality and allowing rapid population growth tends to undermine health and increases the incidence of nutritional disorders and parasitic infections. Inadequate sanitation in rural clinics, especially the use of poorly sterilized hypodermic needles, contributes to the spread of disease and has been implicated in the spread of AIDS in Africa.

The examples of Brazil and China, however, illustrate how nationally coordinated efforts within a tropical region of low per capita income can be effective. In China's regimented society, a blanket application of environmental control measures with mobilization of a large rural workforce, mass screening and treatment, education at all levels, and coordinated targeted research have been shown to be feasible. Between 1956 and 1987, the areas in which schistosomiasis occurred and the number of people at risk of exposure were halved. At the same time, the number of infected individuals declined by a factor of ten. In Brazil, the Superintendency for Public Health Campaigns (SUCAM) works in frontier areas where social control is slower and channels for education and communication do not function well. SUCAM relies on the Guarda, a field staff composed of a large number of paraprofessionals trained to recognize symptoms and risk factors in a particular disease and to implement control measures. SUCAM has had notable success against Chagas' disease, which can be controlled by eliminating the insect vector from houses through the use of insecticides and renovation. Egypt, Zimbabwe, and the Philippines have also mounted successful campaigns that have reduced the incidence of parasitic diseases.

Education of women is an important factor in the health of poor populations. Women play a crucial role in maintaining the health of infants and children. They are also more likely to be vulnerable to neglect and ill health than are adult males as a result of cultural attitudes. In the Indian state of Kerala, longevity and infant mortality statistics are now comparable to those of African Americans because the government has devoted a large proportion of resources to universal education and public health. Nearby Bangladesh, which has a comparable climate and per capita income but lacks the commitment to education and health access, has some of the worst statistics on survival and longevity in the developing world.

The net result of improving public health in the developing world has been an increase in average life expectancy of approximately ten years, from fifty to sixty, between 1970 and 1990. Increased longevity results in an increase in diseases of old age and their demands on the health care system. This is most true in China, where life expectancy approaches seventy years and aggressive measures have reduced the birth rate dramatically.

In an age of international travel, virtually any communicable disease has the potential to spread rapidly. The worldwide epidemic of AIDS clearly illustrates this phenomenon. Some medical ecologists view the large AIDS-infected population in Africa as a medical time bomb in which a novel, virulent pathogen, such as the Ebola virus, could gain a foothold. Military incursions and tourism in the tropics expose people from the temperate zone to tropical ailments. These factors should provide an additional impetus for research into tropical diseases and general awareness of them by physicians.

Tropical diseases extract an enormous toll in human productivity that, by perpetuating poverty and hindering all forms of development, contributes to global political instability. The interaction of tropical disease processes and European colonialism was destructive for both Europeans and colonial subjects. Medical science and social policy are a long way from solving the medical problems of the tropics.

—*Martha Sherwood-Pike, Ph.D.; updated by*
L. Fleming Fallon, Jr., M.D., Ph.D., M.P.H.

See also Acquired immunodeficiency syndrome (AIDS); Antibiotics; Bacterial infections; Bacteriology; Beriberi; Chagas' disease; Childhood infectious diseases; Cholera; Dengue fever; Diarrhea and dysentery; Drug resistance; Ebola virus; Elephantiasis; Emerging infectious diseases; Epidemics and pandemics; Epidemiology; Fungal infections; Immunization and vaccination; Insect-borne diseases; Kwashiorkor; Leishmaniasis; Leprosy; Malaria; Malnutrition; Microbiology; Nutrition; Parasitic diseases; Plague; Poliomyelitis; Protozoan diseases; Rabies; Schistosomiasis; Sleeping sickness; Syphilis; Typhoid fever; Typhus; Viral infections; World Health Organization; Worms; Yellow fever; Zoonoses.

FOR FURTHER INFORMATION:

Busvine, James R. *Disease Transmission by Insects: Its Discovery and Ninety Years of Effort to Prevent It.* Amsterdam: Springer, 1993. This interesting history of tropical medicine is complete and relatively easy to read.

Camus, Emmanuel, James House, and Gerrit Uilenberg, eds. *Vector-Borne Pathogens: International Trade and Tropical Animal Diseases.* Rev. ed. New York: New York Academy of Sciences, 1999. This extensive and highly readable work provides a wealth of information concerning the spread of tropical diseases through commerce and rapid world transportation.

Garrett, Laurie. *The Coming Plague: Newly Emerging Diseases in a World out of Balance.* New York: Penguin, 1995. This book contains an excellent discussion of many tropical diseases and the efforts of the World Health Organization to eradicate them. The author has a style that is easy to read. This book is highly recommended.

Jong, Elaine C., and Russell McMullen, eds. *Travel and Tropical Medicine Manual.* 4th ed. Philadelphia: Saunders/Elsevier, 2008. A very useful reference manual with advice on preventing, evaluating, and managing diseases that can be acquired in tropical environments and countries outside the United States. Covers topics such as emerging infectious diseases, travel advice for infants, children, and women, and HIV infection.

Liese, Bernhard H., Paramjit S. Sachdeva, and D. Glynn Cochrane. *Organizing and Managing Tropical Disease Control Programs: Case Studies.* Washington, D.C.: World Bank, 1992. A summary of the organization, financing, and implementation of public health programs in Brazil; schistosomiasis control programs in China, Egypt, the Philippines, and Zimbabwe; and malaria and tuberculosis control in the Philippines.

Peters, Wallace, and Herbert M. Gilles. *Tropical Medicine and Parasitology.* St. Louis, Mo.: Mosby, 1999. This handbook provides illustrations and descriptions of symptoms, pathogens, and vectors, with maps of distribution, for serious tropical diseases. It includes those that are widespread and globally important and some that are rare and local, but of interest from a medical standpoint.

Sandford-Smith, John. *Eye Diseases in Hot Climates.* 4th ed. Boston: Butterworth-Heinemann, 2005. This text devotes an extensive section to onchocerciasis. The disease, attempts to treat it, and problems associated with economic development are discussed.

Sen, Amartya. "The Economics of Life and Death." *Scientific American* 268 (May, 1993): 40-47. This article contrasts the health of nations with the wealth of nations, focusing on areas with low per capita income and comparatively high longevity. The author suggests that longevity and infant mortality are better measures of the well-being of a population than income alone.

Strickland, Thomas, et al., eds. *Hunter's Tropical Medicine and Emerging Infectious Diseases*. 8th ed. Philadelphia: W. B. Saunders, 2000. This is a classic textbook written by internationally known experts in the field. Although it uses some technical words, most readers should find the text understandable.

TUBAL LIGATION
PROCEDURE
ANATOMY OR SYSTEM AFFECTED: Abdomen, reproductive system, uterus

SPECIALTIES AND RELATED FIELDS: Gynecology, obstetrics

DEFINITION: A surgical procedure that closes the Fallopian tubes and causes permanent sterilization.

INDICATIONS AND PROCEDURES
Tubal ligations are performed strictly for sterilization of a female patient. While there has been some success with reversing the procedure, it must be considered permanent. The woman must be well informed and certain that she does not want additional children under any circumstances.

The most common technique for tubal ligation is laparoscopy. As an outpatient, the woman receives local anesthetic and a light sedative. A small incision is made in the navel, and gas is used to inflate the abdomen, allowing easy visibility of the patient's Fallopian tubes.

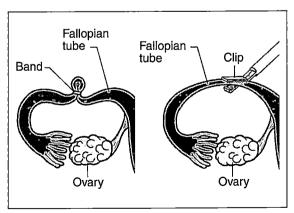

A common means of sterilization for women is tubal ligation, in which the Fallopian tubes through which eggs must pass to reach the uterus are severed or interrupted with clips or bands.

An instrument called an intrauterine cannula is inserted through the vagina, and a clamp called a tenaculum is positioned on the cervix. Both are used to manipulate the tubes into position. A laparoscope, a thin tube containing a camera and light, is inserted through the incision in order to view the tubes. An instrument to block the tubes is inserted through the laparoscope. The tubes may be blocked by burning, cutting, or applying rings or clips. The incision is sewn closed.

In a minilaparatomy, a small incision is made above the woman's pubic bone. The tubes are brought through the incision and are tied and cut. Tubal ligations can also be performed through a woman's vagina (culdoscopy or colpotomy).

Many tubal ligations are done immediately, or within a day, following the delivery of a baby. If a patient has a cesarean section, then tubal ligation is often done as part of the same surgical procedure. Following a vaginal delivery, a woman desiring a tubal ligation is usually brought to the operating room the next day. In cases in which there is a problem with the baby (including extreme prematurity, anomalies, or sepsis), the sterilization procedure is often delayed, pending a good outcome for the infant.

USES AND COMPLICATIONS
The only purpose of tubal ligation is sterilization. It is highly effective (with a 0.2 percent failure rate) and largely irreversible. Depending on the type of blockage used, it is about 30 percent reversible; however, only 10 percent of women become pregnant after undergoing tubal reconstruction. Other forms of birth control are recommended for any patient who is not absolutely certain about the procedure.

Tubal ligations take only thirty minutes to perform, and there is only minor postsurgical pain. A rare complication may be an ectopic pregnancy within the Fallopian tube, which could rupture. Other potential problems are those associated with any abdominal surgery, including unintentional damage to other internal organs, bleeding, and infection. One recent study indicated that there is no change in the level of hormones produced by women prior to or following tubal ligation.

—*Karen E. Kalumuck, Ph.D.; updated by Robin Kamienny Montvilo, R.N., Ph.D.*

See also Contraception; Gynecology; Hysterectomy; Laparoscopy; Pregnancy and gestation; Reproductive system; Sterilization; Women's health.

FOR FURTHER INFORMATION:

Ammer, Christine. *The New A to Z of Women's Health: A Concise Encyclopedia*. 6th ed. New York: Checkmark Books, 2009.

Berek, Jonathan S., ed. *Berek and Novak's Gynecology*. 14th ed. Philadelphia: Lippincott Williams & Wilkins, 2007.

Connell, Elizabeth B. *The Contraception Sourcebook*. Chicago: Contemporary Books, 2002.

Cunningham, F. Gary, et al., eds. *Williams Obstetrics*. 23d ed. New York: McGraw-Hill, 2010.

Gentile, Gwen P., et al. "Hormone Levels Before and After Tubal Sterilization." *Contraception* 73, no. 5 (May, 2006): 507-511.

Manassiev, Nikolai, and Malcolm I. Whitehead. *Female Reproductive Health*. New York: Parthenon, 2004.

Quilligan, Edward J., and Frederick P. Zuspan, eds. *Current Therapy in Obstetrics and Gynecology*. 5th ed. Philadelphia: W. B. Saunders, 2000.

Zite, Nikki, Sara Wuellner, and Melissa Gilliam. "Barriers to Obtaining a Desired Postpartum Tubal Sterilization." *Contraception* 73, no. 4 (April, 2006): 404-407.

Zollinger, Robert M., Jr., and Robert M. Zollinger, Sr. *Zollinger's Atlas of Surgical Operations*. 8th ed. New York: McGraw-Hill, 2003.

TUBERCULOSIS

DISEASE/DISORDER

ANATOMY OR SYSTEM AFFECTED: Chest, lungs, respiratory system

SPECIALTIES AND RELATED FIELDS: Bacteriology, microbiology, public health, pulmonary medicine

DEFINITION: A chronic, highly infectious lung disease that can destroy tissue.

KEY TERMS:

BCG: a weakened version of *Mycobacterium bovis* that is used in vaccines to protect against tuberculosis

PPD (purified protein derivative): proteins from mycobacteria used in the tuberculin test; exposure to tuberculosis will result in the sensitization of the immune system to these proteins

primary tuberculosis: a form of tuberculosis that often does not produce symptoms and that develops after exposure to tuberculosis-causing bacteria

sanatorium: an institution designed for the treatment of chronic illnesses, such as tuberculosis

secondary tuberculosis: the recurrence of tuberculosis in individuals who chronically carry the bacterium; a more severe form of the disease in which the lungs are usually damaged

tuberculin test: a skin test used to detect exposure to tuberculosis; a useful test in countries in which vaccines against tuberculosis are not routinely administered

tuberculosis bacilli: bacteria that belong to the genus and species *Mycobacterium tuberculosis*; sometimes called tubercle bacilli, these organisms are the causative agents of tuberculosis

CAUSES AND SYMPTOMS

Tuberculosis derives its name from the Latin word *tubercle*, which means "little lump." Tubercles, or small nodules of diseased tissue, are often found in the lungs of infected individuals. In humans, bacteria that belong to the genus *Mycobacterium* cause tuberculosis. In the vast majority of cases, *Mycobacterium tuberculosis*, often referred to as the tuberculosis bacillus or the tubercle bacillus, is the responsible organism. Other species within the genus may also cause tuberculosis or tuberculosis-like diseases. For example, *M. avium*, a disease-causing organism, or pathogen, is found in birds and swine; it can cause a tuberculosis-like disease in humans. Before it was common to pasteurize milk, *M. bovis*, a pathogen found in cattle, was responsible for cases of human tuberculosis of the digestive tract. In most cases of tuberculosis in humans, the lungs are the major organs affected, but other tissues and organs such as the bones, skin, and digestive tract may also be sites of infection.

Poverty, overcrowding, unsanitary conditions, poor health, and poor nutrition provide ideal conditions for the spread of tuberculosis. It is found at a high frequency in the developing areas of the world, such as parts of Africa, Asia, and Oceania. Immigrants from these countries present a serious public health concern when they enter the United States and other countries. In the United States, the incidence of tuberculosis is still relatively high in African Americans, Asians, Pacific Islanders, American Indians, Alaskan natives, and Hispanics. Tuberculosis cases among foreign-born persons now living in the United States account for nearly half of the national total of tuberculosis patients. Other individuals who have a greater risk for developing tuberculosis infection are inmates of correctional institutions, alcoholics, intravenous drug users, the homeless, and the elderly.

People at a particularly high risk of developing tuberculosis after exposure are those whose immune systems are compromised or suppressed, such as cancer patients receiving chemotherapy, organ transplant recipients, or people with acquired immunodeficiency syndrome (AIDS). Diabetics and individuals with a lung condition known as silicosis are also at high risk of developing tuberculosis as a result of exposure to the disease. Silicosis is an occupational disease that develops as a result of exposure to silica. Silica is found in sand and is a crystalline material encountered by miners, tunnel diggers, stonecutters, glassmakers, and those involved in sandblasting operations.

Under a microscope, tuberculosis bacilli appear as straight or slightly curved, rod-shaped organisms. Their widths vary from 0.3 to 0.6 of a micrometer, and their lengths vary from 1 to 4 micrometers. Mycobacteria have unique properties that appear to be linked to their abilities to cause tuberculosis. The cell wall, a protective layer that surrounds all bacteria, is unique in mycobacteria because it contains some unusual lipids. These lipids, which include mycolic acid, give the bacteria special staining properties. Mycobacteria are the only bacteria that resist decolorization with a solution of acid and alcohol (hydrochloric acid and ethyl alcohol) and are thus termed acid-fast. Acid-fastness is the most important characteristic of mycobacteria because it can be used to differentiate them from other types of bacteria. The acid-fast staining procedure can be used to identify mycobacteria and to visualize them in clinical specimens such as lung tissue and sputum.

Mycobacteria populations grow very slowly compared to other bacteria. Under optimal conditions, typical mycobacteria will divide every twelve to eighteen hours, while many other bacteria will divide in twenty to thirty minutes. Mycobacteria require oxygen for growth and are very resistant to drying, most likely because of the lipids in their cell walls. Mycobacteria also resist many chemical and physical agents that would normally kill bacteria. This resistance allows them to survive both in the body and in the exterior environment. Cultures of *M. tuberculosis* maintained in a laboratory usually remain viable for many years. These bacteria can also remain viable outside both a laboratory and the human body. They can retain their pathogenic properties in dried sputum for many months. They are sensitive to ultraviolet light, however, and are killed in about two hours after exposure to direct sunlight.

The mycobacteria that cause tuberculosis are found in the droplets released when a person with active tuberculosis coughs, sneezes, or even talks. This mist of tiny droplets can remain aloft for hours. The manner by

---

INFORMATION ON TUBERCULOSIS

CAUSES: Bacterial infection
SYMPTOMS: Ranges with severity; may include low-grade fever, fatigue, chest pain, appetite loss, weight loss
DURATION: Chronic
TREATMENTS: Antituberculosis drugs, antibiotics

---

which a person becomes infected with tuberculosis usually involves the inhalation of these droplets. The tuberculosis bacilli can then be carried to the lungs. It is fortunate that most individuals who are exposed to tuberculosis will not develop the disease. Tuberculosis is less contagious than the common childhood diseases (such as measles, chickenpox, and mumps) and is usually contracted only after long exposure to an infectious individual who has an active case of tuberculosis. Of all newly infected individuals, approximately 5 percent will show symptoms of tuberculosis within a year. The remaining infected individuals continue to have some risk of developing the disease at any time.

When tuberculosis infection does occur, the initial period is referred to as the primary infection. During this period, an infected individual may not experience any symptoms of illness, or the symptoms may be nonspecific, such as low fever and tiredness. Tuberculosis bacilli in the lung become the focus of an attack by the body's immune system. Primary tuberculosis may also involve the lymph nodes and the pleural cavity. This reaction may lead to the accumulation of fluid within the pleural cavity, accompanied by fever or chest pain. As a result of activities of the immune system and the ingestion of tuberculosis bacilli by white blood cells known as macrophages, the primary infection will often spontaneously subside without medical intervention. Yet, although healing occurs, the tuberculosis bacilli can remain in a somewhat dormant state, walled up in the primary lesions. They live within the cells of the immune system but do not divide. The bacilli can remain in this state for years or decades without producing further symptoms of the disease. Untreated individuals will remain infected throughout their lifetimes even though the disease is in remission.

Most individuals recover from primary tuberculosis. In a small percentage of cases, however, the disease progresses and lung destruction occurs. The reactivation of the disease is referred to as secondary tuberculosis and most frequently occurs when the immune system is weakened. Destruction of lung tissue is a hallmark of this phase of the disease. Much of the damage produced in the lung is the result of efforts by the immune system to destroy the tuberculosis bacilli. Parts of the lung suffer tissue death (necrosis) and soften. These lesions can merge, enlarge, liquefy, and discharge their contents of tuberculosis bacteria into the bronchi. The bacteria can spread to other parts of the lung and be coughed up in sputum, where they contaminate the environment and serve as a source of infectious organisms that will spread the disease. Secondary tuberculosis, if untreated, is a chronic condition in which the symptoms worsen progressively to include fever, fatigue, loss of appetite, and weight loss.

If the bacteria spread to other parts of the body, a condition known as miliary tuberculosis results. Multiple small lesions that resemble millet seeds are found throughout the body. The most common sites in which these lesions are found are the bones and joints, the urogenital system, lymph nodes, the meninges (membranes surrounding the brain and spinal cord), and the peritoneum. Individuals with AIDS are at an increased risk for contracting tuberculosis outside the lungs (extrapulmonary tuberculosis).

TREATMENT AND THERAPY

On a global basis, close to ten million new cases of tuberculosis are diagnosed each year, and approximately three million deaths are attributable to this disease. Every minute, ten new people become infected with tuberculosis; of these, three will die from it. Since tuberculosis presents a serious public health concern, many countries have employed strategies to prevent its spread. Control of the spread of tuberculosis could decrease the numbers of new cases seen each year. Improvements in living conditions, sanitation, and general standards of living have, in the past, been associated with the decreased incidence of tuberculosis in populations. These goals cannot easily be met in impoverished regions of the world. The medical approaches designed to inhibit the further transmission of tuberculosis include vaccination, rapid diagnosis, and the development of effective drug treatments.

In the United States after the mid-twentieth century, measures were developed to diagnose tuberculosis and prevent its transmission. This program resulted in a marked decrease in death rates from tuberculosis. Total death rates declined dramatically until the mid-1980's. Believing that the disease was one of the past, New York City officials dismantled the entire public tuberculosis health infrastructure of hospitals, sanatoriums, and diagnosis centers during the 1970's. Only a decade later, the city was forced to rebuild that system at a cost of $1 billion to contain a new tuberculosis outbreak that included deadly drug-resistant strains. Prior to the 1980's, most cases of tuberculosis occurred in Native American Indian reservations. By the 1990's, tuberculosis was once again on the rise, but the distribution pattern of the disease had changed. Tuberculosis began to be seen more in African American and Hispanic patients and in individuals with AIDS. The rate of tuberculosis infection became much higher in patients with AIDS than in any other group in the population. The immunocompromised nature of AIDS patients renders them highly susceptible to tuberculosis. An illustration of the extent of this phenomenon is the fact that all individuals newly diagnosed with tuberculosis are also presumed to have AIDS until laboratory tests prove otherwise.

The tuberculin skin test is a safe and reliable diagnostic test for tuberculosis. When some of the proteins from the tubercle bacilli, in a preparation known as purified protein derivative (PPD), are injected into the skin of an individual who has been exposed to tuberculosis, a characteristic skin reaction will occur. The reaction is characterized by redness and swelling around the injection site, which appears in forty-eight to seventy-two hours. The accumulation and activities of cells of the immune system that recognize the bacterial protein cause this reaction. This type of immune response is referred to as a delayed hypersensitivity reaction and will be seen only in persons who have been previously exposed to these bacterial proteins, usually following infection with tuberculosis bacilli. A positive test does not necessarily mean that a person has an active case of tuberculosis and could therefore be contagious; it merely indicates that at some time, past or present, a tuberculosis infection occurred, even if the individual did not display symptoms of the disease.

The tuberculin skin test is not useful in those parts of the world where many individuals in the population have been vaccinated against tuberculosis with a vaccine composed of Bacillus Calmette-Guérin (BCG). The BCG vaccine contains proteins that sensitize the immune system to PPD. After this occurs, a tuberculin skin test will be positive in an individual who has been vaccinated, even though the individual has never been exposed to live tuberculosis bacilli. In the United States, BCG vaccination is not routinely performed because of the great value in tuberculin skin testing as a public health measure. All individuals who may become exposed to tuberculosis, such as medical personnel, are advised to receive the tuberculin skin test at regular intervals. If an individual should have a positive skin test, it is common practice to begin treatment with antituberculosis drugs.

In 2005, a new blood test for the diagnosis of tuberculosis was approved by the Food and Drug Administration (FDA). The test, QuantiFERON-TB-Gold, is an enzyme-linked immunosorbent assay (ELISA) that can be used in all instances where the PPD skin test is used; no follow-up visit is required for skin-test reading. The test also can be used in individuals who have had prior BCG vaccination.

Other methods for the diagnosis of tuberculosis include the detection of acid-fast mycobacteria in sputum, chest X rays to examine the lungs, and the laboratory culture and examination of mycobacteria grown from clinical specimens. The latter procedure may take from four to six weeks because mycobacteria grow so slowly. The growth and examination of these organisms in the laboratory is necessary, however, to confirm diagnosis when tuberculosis is suspected because of the patient's history and the lung damage seen on X ray but microscopic examination fails to show the presence of mycobacteria.

The treatment of tuberculosis changed drastically in the last half of the twentieth century. In the place of quarantine in a sanatorium, a common practice to prevent the spread of the disease, or surgery to remove portions of the diseased lung tissue, tuberculosis patients are now treated with antituberculosis drugs and antibiotics on an outpatient basis. Once treatment is begun, individuals can no longer transmit the disease and are therefore not contagious.

The most effective antituberculosis drugs include isoniazid, pyrazinamide, ethambutol, and the antibiotics rifampicin and streptomycin. The prescribed antituberculosis medications must be used for a long period, usually about nine months, to ensure the destruction of all live tuberculosis bacilli. An ever-increasing problem in the treatment of tuberculosis is the appearance of tuberculosis bacilli that are resistant to drug therapy. These bacteria develop resistance as a result of genetic mutation, and when such drug-resistant bacteria are present in a patient, the disease will not respond to that particular drug. For this reason, most treatment procedures involve the use of three to four different antituberculosis drugs. The probability of the development

of two or more separate mutations is much less than the development of a single mutation.

Even though tuberculosis bacilli are less likely to be resistant to more than one drug, multiple-drug-resistant bacteria are emerging in populations throughout the world. Combined drug therapy is ineffective because these organisms can withstand exposure to several of the antituberculosis drugs at once. Without an effective means of treatment, patients who harbor these multiple-drug-resistant organisms are a continued source of infection to the community unless they are kept in isolation.

Because of the long treatment period, some tuberculosis patients stop taking their medication before the destruction of all tuberculosis bacilli. Some of these patients discontinue their medication because their symptoms have disappeared and they believe that they are cured. A recurrence of the disease is highly probable when the full course of treatment is not followed.

In some countries, the BCG vaccine is widely used as a preventive measure. This vaccine is prepared from live bacteria that belong to a strain of *M. bovis* that has lost its pathogenic properties. The effectiveness of the vaccine is not absolute; studies show that in countries where the vaccine is employed, there may be a 60 to 80 percent decrease in the incidence of tuberculosis. The BCG vaccine is not used in the United States because the incidence of tuberculosis in the general population is quite low compared to other countries. In addition, if the BCG vaccine were widely used, it would negate the utility of the tuberculin skin test as a reliable and valuable diagnostic tool.

PERSPECTIVE AND PROSPECTS

Throughout the ages, tuberculosis has been a scourge of humankind. Human fossils, excavated from a Neolithic burial ground dated about six thousand years ago, show evidence of tuberculosis of the spine. Egyptian mummies from 1000 B.C.E. with signs of tuberculosis suggest that the disease was widespread in ancient Egypt. Symptoms of tuberculosis such as fever, excessive weight loss, night sweats, breathlessness, pain in the side and chest areas, and coughing up of sputum and blood are described in the writings of ancient Hindu, Greek, and Roman writers. The widespread nature of the disease appears in accounts from early European history, from the fifth to eighteenth centuries, which refer to a "touching" ceremony that was performed by English and French monarchs and believed to cure scrofula (tuberculosis of the lymph glands in the neck region).

One of the greatest causes of disease and death in the world, tuberculosis has been known by many names, including scrofula, phthisis, and consumption. In writings, it has been referred to as "the white plague" and "the captain of all the men of death." During the nineteenth century, tuberculosis was widespread in Europe. The symptoms of tuberculosis were not thought to represent a disease but rather hallmarks of an especially sensitive personality—the ideal for an artist, musician, poet, or writer. At that time, it was somewhat fashionable to be pale and thin, and to have a slight cough.

Although tuberculosis has been a serious health threat for such a long period of human history, the disease and its cause were poorly understood until the 1880's. Robert Koch is credited with discovering the tuberculosis bacillus. His masterful treatise, published in 1882 and translated under the title "The Etiology of Tuberculosis," presented convincing experimental evidence for implicating a bacterium that came to be known as *M. tuberculosis* as the causative agent of tuberculosis. Despite this great breakthrough, a rational effective treatment for the disease could not be found. One type of therapy that became popular was simply rest and fresh air. Edward Livingston Trudeau, an American physician who suffered from tuberculosis, observed that he regained his health when he traveled to Saranac Lake in the Adirondack Mountains in the state of New York. He attributed his recovery to the restful environment and clean air. Trudeau later founded a sanatorium at Lake Saranac that became popular for tuberculosis patients.

It was not until the discovery of the antibiotic streptomycin in 1943 by Selman A. Waksman that a truly potent antituberculosis agent was found. The tuberculosis bacilli, however, proved to be quite resistant to a multitude of other antibiotics and antibacterial drugs. Fortunately, several antibiotics and antibacterial drugs, especially when used in combination and for the full duration of their prescription, can cure many tuberculosis patients.

The disease's spread seemed to slow again by the early 1990's. Over an eight-year period, from 1992 to 2000, the number of new tuberculosis cases decreased an average of 7 percent per year. However, from 2000 to 2001, this rate of decrease slowed to 2 percent, reflecting transmission in foreign-born patients; in crowded shelters and prisons where people are weakened by poor nutrition, drug addiction, and alcoholism; and in long-term care facilities such as nursing homes where residents develop active tuberculosis from infec-

tions with *M. tuberculosis* that occurred much earlier in life because their general health has declined. Thus, in today's world, the major problems presented by tuberculosis are the increasing incidence of the disease, the increasing prevalence of cases that display multiple-drug resistance, and the association with AIDS. These cases of tuberculosis are difficult to treat and further the possibilities for widespread transmission of the disease.

—*Barbara Brennessel, Ph.D.; updated by*
L. Fleming Fallon, Jr., M.D., Ph.D., M.P.H.
See also Acquired immunodeficiency syndrome (AIDS); Antibiotics; Bacillus Calmette-Guérin (BCG); Bacterial infections; Bacteriology; Coughing; Drug resistance; Epidemics and pandemics; Epidemiology; Immunization and vaccination; Lungs; Pulmonary diseases; Pulmonary medicine; Respiration; Wheezing.

FOR FURTHER INFORMATION:

American Lung Association. http://www.lungusa.org. A group initially founded to fight tuberculosis, it now targets its efforts toward asthma, tobacco control, environmental health, and the global rise of tuberculosis. The Web site offers a comprehensive fact sheet about the disease, as well as resources for advocacy, research, and relevant news stories.

Daniel, Thomas M. *Captain of Death: The Story of Tuberculosis*. Rochester, N.Y.: University of Rochester Press, 1997. This book is written for nonprofessional readers. It is interesting and well researched.

Dormandy, Thomas. *The White Death: A History of Tuberculosis*. New York: New York University Press, 2000. Accessible scientific and sociological history are combined by Dormandy, a consulting pathologist in London, in this account of a tenacious disease that has claimed victims since ancient Egypt.

Gandy, Matthew, and Alimuddin Zumla, eds. *Return of the White Plague: Global Poverty and the "New" Tuberculosis*. New York: Verso, 2003. Examines the global rise of tuberculosis from a socioeconomic and medical perspective, arguing that the increase can be blamed on collapsing health care services, shifting patterns of poverty and inequality, the spread of HIV, and the emergence of virulent drug-resistant strains.

Levitzky, Michael G. *Pulmonary Physiology*. 7th ed. New York: McGraw-Hill Medical, 2007. A clinical text that describes the structure and function of the respiratory system. Covers topics such as the physical process of respiration from the interrelationship of basic lung mechanics, the microscopic changes at the alveolar level of gas exchange, the "non-respiratory" functions of the lungs, and how the lungs respond to stress.

Lutwick, Larry I., ed. *Tuberculosis: A Clinical Handbook.* Chicago: Chapman and Hall, 1995. This well-written book, intended for general practitioners and internists, provides an account of the disease, its manifestations, and prevention in children, adults, and HIV-infected patients.

Mazurek, Gerald H., et. al. "Guidelines for Using the QuantiFERON-TB Gold Test for Detecting Mycobacterium Tuberculosis Infection, United States." *Morbidity and Mortality Weekly Report (MMWR)* 54 (December 16, 2005): 49-55.

Rom, William N., and Stuart M. Garay, eds. *Tuberculosis.* 2d ed. Philadelphia: Lippincott Williams & Wilkins, 2004. A group of experts wrote chapters for this book, which can be easily understood by general readers.

Scharer, Lawrence, and John M. McAdam. *Tuberculosis and AIDS: The Relationship Between Mycobacterium TB and the HIV Type 1.* New York: Springer, 1995. This book considers the relationship between tuberculosis and patients with AIDS. It is written for professionals but contains a wealth of information for general readers.

West, John B. *Pulmonary Pathophysiology: The Essentials.* 7th ed. Philadelphia: Wolters Kluwer/Lippincott Williams & Wilkins, 2008. Examines lungs afflicted with obstructive, restrictive, vascular, and environmental diseases. Bronchoactive drugs, the causes of hypoventilation, and the pathogenesis of asthma and pulmonary edema are new topics covered in this edition.

TULAREMIA
DISEASE/DISORDER

ANATOMY OR SYSTEM AFFECTED: Abdomen, joints, lymphatic system, muscles, respiratory system, skin

SPECIALTIES AND RELATED FIELDS: Bacteriology, emergency medicine, environmental health, epidemiology, immunology, public health

DEFINITION: A highly infectious bacterial disease, caused by *Francisella tularensis*, that is of concern as a potential biological weapon.

KEY TERMS:

biological warfare: also called biowarfare; warfare using biological agents or toxins produced by biological agents

biological weapon: also called a bioweapon; a biologi-

cal agent or toxin produced by a biological agent used as a weapon

zoonoses: a disease that can be transmitted from animals to humans and vice versa

CAUSES AND SYMPTOMS

Tularemia is a bacterial disease, caused by *Francisella tularensis*, that is of significant concern as a potential biological weapon because it is easily spread via airborne routes and is highly infectious—inhaling as few as ten bacterial cells is enough to cause disease in humans. If the bacteria were released in a densely populated area, then large numbers of people could fall ill within days.

The bacterium *F. tularensis* was discovered following a plaguelike disease that swept through ground squirrels in Tulare County, California, in 1911. Shortly after its initial discovery, it was demonstrated to cause disease in humans. The organism is common throughout North America and Eurasia. The disease is transmitted via a number of routes: bites of infected insects, contact with the carcasses of infected animals, eating contaminated food or drinking contaminated water, and breathing in the bacteria. The disease is not spread via person-to-person contact.

After infection, symptoms typically appear within two weeks. They include fever, chills, aches, pain, headaches, diarrhea, coughing, and, as the disease progresses, increasing weakness. Some individuals develop skin ulcerations and swollen lymph nodes, as well as pneumonia with accompanying chest pain, bloody sputum, and difficulty breathing—sometimes leading to respiratory failure.

TREATMENT AND THERAPY

Tularemia can be treated with a number of antibiotics, but preventing infections is ideal. Infection may be pre-

---

INFORMATION ON TULAREMIA

CAUSES: Infection with *Francisella tularensis* bacteria through insect bites, contact with infected animals, contaminated food or water, inhalation

SYMPTOMS: Fever, chills, aches, headache, diarrhea, coughing, progressive weakness, skin ulcerations, swollen lymph nodes, pneumonia

DURATION: Acute

TREATMENTS: Antibiotics

vented by controlling exposure to insect and animal carriers of the bacterium, eating thoroughly cooked food, and drinking clean water.

Vaccines may also be used to prevent the disease. Russia has used a tularemia vaccine in areas where the disease naturally occurs since the 1930's. A vaccine has been under review by the Food and Drug Administration (FDA) but is not yet available in the United States.

PERSPECTIVE AND PROSPECTS

Since tularemia is easily contracted via inhalation of a small number of bacterial cells, it has been tested by some countries as a weapon to be released via the air. Japanese germ warfare units researched the use of tularemia as a weapon in Manchuria from 1932 through 1945. Tens of thousands of German and Russian troops were sickened by the disease on the Eastern Front in World War II, and some researchers suspect that the infections were intentional rather than natural. The United States and other countries have continued to research tularemia as a weapon since the war.

—*David M. Lawrence*

See also Bacterial infections; Bacteriology; Biological and chemical weapons; Environmental diseases; Environmental health; Epidemiology; Food poisoning; Insect-borne diseases; Plague; Pulmonary diseases; Zoonoses.

FOR FURTHER INFORMATION:

Farlow, Jason, et al. "*Francisella tularensis* in the United States." *Emerging Infectious Diseases* 11, no. 12 (December, 2005): 1835-1841.

Henderson, Donald A., Thomas V. Inglesby, and Tara Jeanne O'Toole. *Bioterrorism: Guidelines for Medical and Public Health Management.* Chicago: American Medical Association, 2002.

Sidell, Frederick R., and Ernest T. Takafuji. *Medical Aspects of Chemical and Biological Warfare.* Washington, D.C.: Borden Institute, Walter Reed Army Medical Center, 1997.

TUMOR REMOVAL

PROCEDURE

ANATOMY OR SYSTEM AFFECTED: All (primarily brain, breasts, gastrointestinal system, intestines, lungs, respiratory system)

SPECIALTIES AND RELATED FIELDS: General surgery, histology, oncology

DEFINITION: The removal—through surgery, chemotherapy, or radiotherapy—of any neoplasm.

KEY TERMS:

computed tomography (CT) scanning: a medical imaging technique which involves the X-ray observation of cross sections of tissue

magnetic resonance imaging (MRI): a medical imaging technique in which the image is produced by the scanning of a magnetic field

metastasis: the spread of cancer cells from the primary tumor to other sites in the body

neoplasm: an uncontrolled growth of cells which can develop into a tumor; may be malignant (cancerous) or benign

oncogene: a regulatory gene in a cell which, when mutated, may cause that cell to become cancerous

INDICATIONS AND PROCEDURES

The uncontrolled, progressive growth of cells, termed a neoplasm, usually results in a mass or tumor. The tumor may be malignant (cancerous) or benign. Generally, benign tumors remain localized, are often encapsulated, and contain cells that remain well differentiated. Since the cells of a benign tumor do not metastasize, the tumor is usually less of a threat to life. The site of the tumor, however, can be as critical as its malignant or nonmalignant state: Tumors within inoperable portions of the brain may pose a threat regardless of whether they are malignant.

Most tumors are initially observed as localized masses of cells, or lumps. Any symptoms that occur result from tumor growth in this particular tissue. While any tissue or cell is at risk for the development of a tumor, most such forms of uncontrolled growth are found in the female breasts, the colon, and the lungs, the latter a result of the increased use of cigarettes in the twentieth century.

When a tumor is observed, several options exist for its elimination. Surgery remains the method of choice when applicable. This method poses two advantages: Under ideal circumstances, surgery can result in complete removal of the tumor and total cure. In addition, the removal of the tissue allows for proper diagnosis, and subsequent prognosis, of the form of tumor. Surgery may also play a palliative role, allowing for elimination of some of the tumor mass, temporary relief of symptoms, and a greater chance for alternative forms of therapy to effect a cure.

While alternative methods of noninvasive diagnosis were developed during the latter half of the twentieth century, most notably computed tomography (CT) scanning and magnetic resonance imaging (MRI), surgery remains the best method for both tumor diagnosis and cure. The procedure for diagnosis of most tumors is relatively straightforward. When the patient is examined, a complete analysis of symptoms is carried out. The tumor, though not necessarily its prognosis, may be directly observable, such as a lump in the breast. Sometimes, symptoms may be secondary, such as blood in the feces resulting from a tumor in the colon or a cough associated with lung cancer. Biopsy of the material, often in conjunction with surgery, may be necessary to determine whether the tumor is malignant; many tumors are not. If the tumor is determined to be malignant, the material obtained in the biopsy may also be useful in determining the staging of the tumor, a classification system used to identify the extent of the tumor, its degree of spread, and the likely prognosis. Though several methods of staging are used, the most popular is the TNM system. T refers to the size of the tumor (T0 to T4, depending on its size), N refers to the extent of lymph node involvement (N0 to N2), and M indicates whether metastasis has occurred (M0 or M1).

If the tumor is localized, surgical removal remains the best chance for a cure. In general, the patient is anesthetized and the region of the tumor is surgically removed. For a tiny breast tumor, this may involve a lumpectomy (removal of the lump only). For larger tumors, extensive amounts of tissue may have to be excised. Surgery usually involves the use of a knife, though alternative forms such as laser surgery or electrosurgery may be used under specific circumstances. The surgeon will attempt to remove the area of cancer or, when warranted, the entire organ and a margin of adjacent normal-looking tissue, in the event that a few cells have spread beyond the visible tumor. Localized lymph glands may also be removed, both to estimate the chance of metastasis and to improve the chance of removing all the tumor since the local lymph nodes are generally the sites to which cancer cells initially spread.

When the tumor is too large, or if metastasis has occurred, additional forms of treatment to effect tumor removal may be needed. Radiation therapy, the use of beams of high-energy X rays, may be used to reduce the size of a tumor or to eliminate any cancer cells that remain in the vicinity of an excised tumor. Chemotherapy, the use of metabolic poisons, is often employed when the tumor has spread beyond its initial site.

Tumor removal may also be palliative, a procedure employed for the reduction of symptoms or for the restoration of normal organ function. For example, the removal of a tumor on the colon may reduce pain and re-

store function temporarily, even if the tumor has spread and the prognosis is poor. Common benign tumors may also cause discomfort, even if not life-threatening. Nearly one-quarter of women over the age of thirty develop fibroid tumors on the wall of the uterus, a condition which is more of a nuisance than dangerous; surgical removal of such tumors may be necessary to eliminate pain or bleeding.

The decision regarding the methodology of tumor removal often depends on the site and extent of the tumor. The biopsy of the material may be immediately followed by surgical removal of the tumor while the patient remains under anesthesia. This is often the method of choice if the tumor is small or confined to a single organ. After surgery, any additional options can be discussed with the patient. If various options exist for tumor removal, the results of the biopsy may first be discussed with the patient, and a decision on specific forms of treatment may follow.

The most convenient procedure for biopsy during surgery is needle aspiration, the insertion of a small needle into the tumor for the removal of a small number of cells. If more tissue is needed, a larger needle may be used. If the tumor is small enough, the entire tumor may be removed at this stage.

When the tumor has been removed, the entire tissue is given to a pathologist. Analysis of this gross specimen allows for a firmer diagnosis of the form of tumor, its staging, and a possible prognosis.

Uses and Complications

Two strategies are associated with tumor removal: First is the attempt to effect a cure. Ideally, complete elimination of a malignant tumor will result in a cure for the disease. The assumption in this case is that metastasis has not occurred. If the tumor is benign, removal should alleviate any symptoms associated with its growth. As indicated above, fibroid tumors of the uterus, while common in middle-aged women, rarely pose a threat to life; it is their very presence that results in discomfort or other symptoms. Likewise, parotid tumors, growths in the salivary gland, may result in unsightly lumps in the region of the jaw, as well as pain or discomfort; on some occasions, there may be facial paralysis. Removal of the tumor, generally through surgery but with radiation or chemotherapy if the condition warrants, may be indicated.

Colon cancer is one of the more common forms of cancer among adults, with more than 100,000 cases per year in the United States. Symptoms include rectal bleeding, diarrhea, loss of weight, and loss of appetite. If a patient complains of such symptoms, the physician will likely recommend a rectal examination, including the removal of tissue for biopsy, generally as part of a colonoscopy (the visual examination of the colon with a flexible fiber-optic tube).

Treatment for colon cancer depends on the results of the biopsy and the general health of the patient. Surgical removal, however, is the most common treatment. If the tumor is small and confined, as in the form of a polyp, the removal of the polyp (polypectomy) is usually sufficient to effect a cure. If the tumor is relatively large, both the tumor and surrounding tissue must be removed (wedge resection). The extent of tissue removal depends on the size and stage of the tumor. Complete removal often includes supplementary treatments such as chemotherapy or radiation therapy. Since metastasis has often occurred by the time that symptoms appear, the prognosis for colon cancer is often poor.

Surgical procedures for smaller, more accessible tumors in other parts of the body are more straightforward. In the case of a parotid tumor, diagnosis often includes a CT scan or MRI, along with a biopsy. If the tumor is benign, removal of the lump is relatively simple. In rare instances in which the tumor is malignant, radiation therapy may be included as part of the treatment.

Breast cancer is one of the more common forms of cancer in women. In addition to its life-threatening potential, the disease can result in disfigurement as a result of treatment. Nearly 200,000 women per year in the United States are diagnosed with the disease.

Breast cancer often is first observed as a lump in the breast. If the biopsy shows it to be malignant, several courses of action may be considered, usually associated with surgical removal of the tumor along with healthy surrounding tissue. If the tumor is very small, removal of the lump may be sufficient; if the tumor has spread, complete removal of the breast is often the choice (mastectomy). Radical mastectomy, which also involves the removal of surrounding muscle, may be necessary if the cancer has spread into that tissue. Nearby lymph nodes from the armpit (axillary nodes) are often included in order to evaluate whether the cancer has metastasized.

PERSPECTIVE AND PROSPECTS

The first attempts at the surgical removal of tumors date to as early as 1600 B.C.E. in Egypt. These procedures were obviously crude and limited. Modern surgical treatment for tumor removal is credited to the American surgeon Ephraim MacDowell, who in 1809 removed a 22-pound tumor from a patient. (The patient survived and lived another three decades.) Two complications limited such forms of surgery, even for localized, readily accessible tumors: pain and infection. Though extracts from the poppy and the drinking of alcohol were both used to deaden pain in earlier centuries, it was not until the routine use of ether in the mid-nineteenth century that pain could be eliminated from surgery. In 1846, William T. G. Morton demonstrated the use of ether as a general anesthetic, first in the extraction of a tooth and later in a public demonstration in which a vascular tumor of the jaw was removed from a young patient. The pain-free operation lasted nearly thirty minutes and ushered in the era of general surgery.

Though pain during surgery could now be eliminated, there was still the problem of infection. Tumor removal in the mid-nineteenth century was confined to those of the breast or superficial areas of the body. It remained for Joseph Lister in the 1860's and 1870's to develop the antiseptic procedures necessary to reduce the chances for infection and subsequent mortality associated with surgery as a means of tumor removal.

Surgical procedures continued to improve in the twentieth century. Following the discovery of radioactivity by Wilhelm Conrad Röntgen, the use of X rays was added to the repertoire for the elimination of tumors. By damaging the genetic material of cells, radiation was demonstrated to be capable of reducing the size of tumors or of eliminating localized tumors altogether. The discovery in the mid-twentieth century of chemicals that interfere with the growth or metabolism of cancer cells resulted in the development of chemotherapy as a method of treatment.

Technological advances have resulted in better methods both for the diagnosis of tumors and in their elimination. Both CT scanning and MRI have the advantage of being noninvasive, though surgical biopsy remains the method of choice for diagnosis and staging of a tumor. Along with the development of these techniques have come more aggressive forms of treatment. Until the 1970's, tumor removal generally involved surgery, chemotherapy, or radiation therapy, but not often in combination. It became apparent that the elimination of the tumor was more effective when these procedures were used together: Radiation therapy could be used first to shrink the tumor, allowing for more effective surgical removal. As knowledge of the immunology of cancer (and the immune system in general) developed, physicians began to apply the immune system itself as a form of therapy. Interleukins and other chemicals secreted by the body's immune cells were seen to boost the immune response, aiding in the killing of tumor cells.

Many of the future goals in this medical field center on prevention of tumor formation, as well as their elimination. It is known that certain carcinogens such as cigarette ingredients are involved in the induction of tumors. Reduction in the number of persons smoking would have a significant impact on the prevalence of smoking-related tumors of the mouth and respiratory system. In addition, many tumors have been found to have a genetic basis; specific forms of cancer are associated with oncogenes in the cell. Through periodic screening, it is possible to observe whether such genes have undergone mutation and to remove any tumors that occur while they are still small and before they have undergone metastasis.

—*Richard Adler, Ph.D.*

See also Biopsy; Bladder cancer; Brain tumors; Breast biopsy; Breast cancer; Breasts, female; Cancer; Cervical, ovarian, and uterine cancers; Chemotherapy; Colonoscopy and sigmoidoscopy; Colorectal cancer; Colorectal polyp removal; Cryosurgery; Electrocauterization; Gallbladder cancer; Gastroenterology; Gastrointestinal disorders; Gastrointestinal system; Gynecology; Kidney cancer; Lung cancer; Lung surgery; Lungs; Malignancy and metastasis; Mammography; Mastectomy and lumpectomy; Melanoma; Mouth and throat cancer; Myomectomy; National Cancer Institute (NCI); Oncology; Plastic surgery; Prostate cancer; Prostate gland; Prostate gland removal; Pulmonary diseases; Pulmonary medicine; Radiation therapy; Stomach, intestinal, and pancreatic cancers; Testicular cancer; Tumors.

For Further Information:

Brunicardi, F. Charles, et al., eds. *Schwartz's Principles of Surgery.* 9th ed. New York: McGraw-Hill, 2010. A detailed discussion of surgery as a method of tumor removal that requires some knowledge of basic anatomy. A good reference for the reader wanting surgical details.

Doherty, Gerard M., and Lawrence W. Way, eds. *Current Surgical Diagnosis and Treatment.* 12th ed. New York: Lange Medical Books/McGraw-Hill, 2006. A compromise between a dictionary and a comprehensive surgical treatise. Contains extensive discussions and diagrams of surgical treatments such as tumor removal. The depth of coverage is appropriate for a basic reference book.

Dollinger, Malin, et al. *Everyone's Guide to Cancer Therapy.* 5th ed. Kansas City, Mo.: Andrews McMeel, 2008. An excellent resource on types of cancers, terminology, options, and discussions of topics for cancer patients such as questions to ask, methods of payment, and forms of therapy.

Griffith, H. Winter. *Complete Guide to Symptoms, Illness, and Surgery.* Revised and updated by Stephen Moore and Kenneth Yoder. 5th ed. New York: Perigee, 2006. Covers more than five hundred diseases and disorders and includes information about causes and risk factors, preventive techniques, diagnostic tests, and surgical treatment.

Mulholland, Michael W., et al., eds. *Greenfield's Surgery: Scientific Principles and Practice.* 4th ed. Philadelphia: Lippincott Williams & Wilkins, 2006. Covers the scope and practice of surgery and includes reviews of wound biology, immunology, the management of trauma and transplantation, surgical practice according to anatomic region and specialty, and musculoskeletal, neurologic, genitourinary, and reconstructive surgery.

Sarg, Michael J., and Ann D. Gross. *The Cancer Dictionary.* 3d ed. New York: Checkmark Books, 2007. More than simply serving as a dictionary, this book provides an extensive discussion of all major aspects of tumors. Included are descriptions of various forms of tumors, treatments, and terminology. An excellent source for the nonspecialist.

Zollinger, Robert M., Jr., and Robert M. Zollinger, Sr. *Zollinger's Atlas of Surgical Operations.* 8th ed. New York: McGraw-Hill, 2003. A comprehensive examination of surgery. Covers basic surgical anatomy and vascular, gynecologic, gastrointestinal, and miscellaneous abdominal procedures.

Tumors

Disease/disorder

Anatomy or system affected: All

Specialties and related fields: Endocrinology, histology, internal medicine, oncology, pulmonary medicine

Definition: Abnormal growths of bodily tissues caused by genetic changes within normal cells; tumors may be benign (noninvasive) or malignant (invasive).

Key terms:

benign tumor: a tumor that grows rapidly within a localized area without invading other tissue regions; noncancerous *cancer:* a malignant tumor that grows rapidly and uncontrollably, starting with a transformed cell and spreading throughout the affected body, causing organ damage, failure, and death

carcinogen: a mutagenic substance that triggers cellular biochemical events causing normal cells to become cancerous

cellular transformation: the biochemical process by which a normal body cell becomes tumorous, especially cancerous

differentiation: the physiological event in all multicellular organisms by which identical cells with identical genetic information specialize to become different tissue types

gene regulation: the control of whether a gene is active (that is, encoding messenger RNA and protein) or inactive (that is, not encoding RNA or protein), a process often affected by hormones

malignant tumor: a cancerous mass of cells that invades various body regions, contributing to tissue and organ failure as well as to the eventual death of the entire organism

metastasis: the breaking off and movement of cancer cells from one body tissue region to another, with transport being facilitated by the organism's bloodstream

mutagen: a substance (usually chemicals or ionizing radiation) that penetrates body cells and alters the nucleotide sequence of deoxyribonucleic acid (DNA), thus generating a mutation

virus: an obligate intracellular parasite, composed of genetic information protected by protein, that reproduces within living cells

CAUSES AND SYMPTOMS

Tumors, also called neoplasms, are caused by a variety of factors—including mutations, improper hormonal signaling, viruses, and environmental influences—which cause certain normal body cells to deviate from a genetically determined developmental pattern for that particular organism. Tumors arise in all multicellular eukaryotic organisms, such as animals, plants, and fungi, where colonies of cells are intricately connected and are dependent on one another.

A tumor arises when a mistake is made in the cellular expression of a given gene. At a certain point in the cell's development, a gene may be activated when it should not produce protein, or it may be inactivated when it should be producing protein. In either case, a cascade of subsequent developmental changes within the cell may be initiated. The cell may function inefficiently, die, or start to grow and divide at a faster rate than normal. In this latter scenario, the cell has become tumorous.

Many developmental biologists view the tumorous state as a throwback to the early embryonic development of the organism, when cells are undifferentiated and do not reveal the effects of specific hormonal genetic controls. Therefore, tumors reflect a dedifferentiated state of the cell. Tumors may be benign or malignant. A benign tumor grows as an enlarged tissue region without spreading elsewhere; often, it is only an inconvenience or irritant to the organism without harming the individual. A malignant tumor is invasive, spreading rapidly throughout many tissues, draining the organism of various resources, and eventually destroying key tissues and killing the individual. The breaking off and rapid spread of malignant tumors is termed metastasis.

The changes within genes and the subsequent gene expression or cellular dedifferentiation associated with tumors are brought about by mutations, changes within the nucleotide sequence (the genetic code) of the genes. Mutations can be caused by a number of agents called mutagens. Two major classes of mutagens are chemical mutagens (including benzene, carbon tetrachloride, and diethylstilbestrol) and radiation such as ultraviolet light, X radiation, and gamma radiation. Some mutagens also are carcinogens, causing malignant tumors. Not all mutagens, however, are also carcinogens. Caffeine, for example, is mutagenic but not carcinogenic.

Tumors can arise within cells of any of the five principal tissue types: epithelia, endothelia, connective tissue, nerve, and muscle. Epithelial tissue lines the organs outside and inside the body, including the skin, exocrine glands (such as oil and sweat glands), the digestive tract, and the reproductive organs. Endothelial tissue includes blood cells, blood vessels, and lymph

---

INFORMATION ON TUMORS

CAUSES: Genetic and environmental factors, disease, improper hormonal signaling, viruses

SYMPTOMS: Varies with affected region and severity; may include discomfort, pain, swelling, bloating, diarrhea, vomiting, constipation, skin lumps or lesions

DURATION: Short-term to recurrent

TREATMENTS: Removal through surgery, lasers, freezing, chemotherapy, radiation therapy

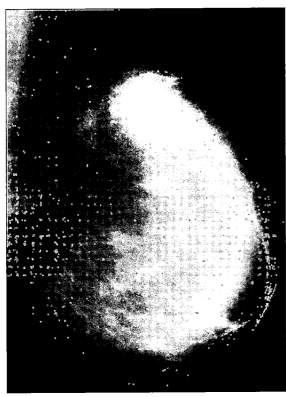

A mammogram showing a tumor in the breast. (SIU School of Medicine)

nodes and glands. Connective tissue includes bone, fat cells, and cartilage. Nerve tissue includes the billions of nerves that compose the brain, spinal cord, and peripheral sensory and motor nerves. Muscle tissue includes the heart, more than six hundred skeletal muscles, and tens of thousands of smooth muscles.

Epithelial tissue cancers collectively are called carcinomas; they include adenocarcinomas, basal cell carcinomas, melanomas, malignant melanomas, squamous cell carcinomas, cervical cancer, uterine cancer, prostate cancer, colorectal cancer, and lung cancer. Whereas benign tumors of the skin such as freckles, moles, and warts are not serious, cancers of the skin and internal organ membranes can be fatal. Adenocarcinomas affect glands. Basal cell carcinomas, melanomas, and squamous cell carcinomas are serious cancers of the skin that can arise from prolonged sun exposure. Malignant melanoma is a rapidly invasive skin cancer which can penetrate other body tissues and cause death within two or three months. Cervical and uterine cancers are serious tumors of the female reproductive tract. Prostate cancer is prevalent among males and is a leading cause of cancer deaths. Colon and rectal cancers,

believed to be triggered by the lack of roughage in diets, are also relatively common in the United States. Lung cancer may result from exposure of lung tissue to cigarette smoke and air pollution.

Endothelial tissue cancers include leukemias, which affect blood cells, and lymphomas, which affect lymphatic tissue. Most leukemias affect the immune system's white blood cells (leukocytes) or the stem cells from which they are derived. Leukemias include acute lymphoblastic leukemia, acute myeloblastic leukemia, acute monoblastic leukemia, chronic lymphocytic leukemia, and chronic granulocytic leukemia. Lymphatic cancers attack the lymph nodes and glands that serve as blood reservoirs for the circulatory system. Lymphatic cancers include lymphosarcomas, Hodgkin's disease, and Burkitt's lymphoma, which is induced by the Epstein-Barr virus.

Connective tissue tumors include benign varieties such as osteomas and osteochondromas affecting bone, chondromas affecting cartilage, and lipomas affecting adipose (fat) tissue. Connective tissue cancers are called sarcomas. Chondrosarcomas are cartilaginous tissue cancers affecting joints. Osteosarcomas are bone cancers. Liposarcomas are fatty tissue cancers that attack a variety of bodily regions. Fibrosarcomas are cancers of the dense, fibrous tissue that holds together many bodily structures, including the skin.

Benign muscle tissue tumors are called myomas, whereas malignant muscle cancers are called myosarcomas. Leiomyosarcoma is a malignancy of smooth, visceral muscle. Rhabdomyosarcoma is a malignancy of cardiac and skeletal muscle.

Benign tumors of the central nervous system are called neuromas and neurofibromas. They include multiple neurofibroma, a condition in which numerous nerve tumors develop throughout the body, thereby causing a severely distorted physical appearance; multiple neurofibroma (or neurofibromatosis) is also known as the "Elephant Man" syndrome after the term used to describe Joseph (or John) Merrick, a nineteenth century Englishman who suffered from this disease. Nervous system cancers include brain cancer and neurogenic sarcoma, glioblastoma, neuroblastoma, and malignant meningioma.

The formation of tumors is probably triggered by many factors. For example, the stress associated with living in a fast-paced technological society causes severe disturbances to the normal homeostatic balance within the body, particularly with reference to the nervous and endocrine systems. The nervous system activates many organ systems and tissues throughout the body. Even more potent in its effects is the endocrine system, which directly controls gene expression in various body cells and tissues via chemical messengers called hormones. When these hormones are hyperactivated by stress, they may activate or inactivate certain genes and their protein products at the wrong time in an individual's development, thereby causing drastic changes in cellular functioning, often accompanied by abnormal growth of tissue into a tumor.

Virus infections may also result in cancer. In 1908, cell-free extracts prepared from leukemia in mice were shown to transmit the disease. In 1910, Peyton Rous discovered that a similar filterable agent would transmit a solid tumor, a sarcoma, in chickens. However, it was felt at the time that cancers in animals represented special circumstances, and that the work was not directly applicable to human cancer. The existence of the Rous sarcoma virus (RSV) was corroborated later by other researchers, culminating in the awarding of the 1966 Nobel Prize in Physiology and Medicine to Rous. Most human cancers are of endogenous (genetic) origin and not associated with viral infection, but there are a number of notable exceptions. Hepatitis B virus infection is associated with a hepatocarcinoma, or cancer of the liver. The Epstein-Barr virus, the etiological agent of infectious mononucleosis, is also the cause of both Burkitt's lymphoma and nasopharyngeal carcinoma.

TREATMENT AND THERAPY

Oncologists and other medical researchers study both benign and malignant tumors. Studies are devoted to the occurrence of these tumors, improved means of diagnosis, and the development of effective treatments. Cancer is the second-leading cause of death in the United States and many Western nations. Stress, viruses, pollution, and an individual's everyday exposure to hazardous materials increase the chance of developing tumors.

Regardless of a tumor's cause, it is important that it be identified and treated. The American Cancer Society's seven warning signs for cancer serve as an important model for tumor and cancer prevention. The warning signs are a sore that does not heal, persistent coughing, a lump anywhere on the body, unusual bleeding, a change in a wart or mole, a change in bladder or bowel movements, and difficulty swallowing.

Tumors may be benign or malignant. Benign tumors are less severe in most cases because they continue to grow within a localized region without invading other tissue regions. Benign tumors may press on critical organs and cause discomfort, however, thereby necessitating their surgical removal or inactivation using lasers, freezing, cytotoxic chemicals, or radiation. Warts represent a good example of a benign tumor. Warts are caused by a papillomavirus which infects skin cells of the dermis and enters a lysogenic phase, where it lays dormant in the host cell DNA but accelerates cell growth into a small tumor. A person can contract a papillomavirus merely by shaking an infected individual's hand; nearly thirty million Americans have this type of tumor. Some warts may become malignant.

Malignant tumors are invasive cancers that multiply rapidly, break off into the bloodstream, and colonize other body regions, where they destroy tissues, organs, and sometimes the entire organism. Malignant cancer cells are immortal in the sense that they reproduce without any developmental barriers. Many malignant colonies can manipulate available blood supplies away from normal tissue, thereby promoting their own growth. Malignant cancers are classified according to tissue type. Any tissue is subject to cancerous growth, given the appropriate stimuli.

Genetic and biochemical research focuses heavily on the study of neoplastic cellular transformation. The prime emphasis is upon gene regulation, the ultimate control point that determines whether a cell will function properly. Mutations in gene regulatory regions, improper hormonal signaling, or viral interference via lysogeny may contribute to abnormalities in cellular growth.

Benign and malignant tumors can be induced and studied in laboratory animals. The application of a chemical mutagen to a localized tissue region in a mouse usually gives rise to a tumor. Female mice infected with the mouse mammary tumor virus pass the virus to their young via milk during suckling; this virus generates grotesquely large tumors that are often as big as the mouse itself. Tumors or sections of tumors removed from humans are studied by biopsy and subsequent biochemical analysis. Human cells are grown in tissue culture in flasks and roller bottles containing fetal calf serum so that medical researchers can study the nature of the neoplastic tumorous cells.

PERSPECTIVE AND PROSPECTS

The study of tumors is of critical importance to medicine because tumor formation is a major cause of illness in millions of people yearly. An understanding of the genetic mechanisms underlying tumor formation is directly applicable to both the study of cancer and the understanding of mechanisms that regulate cell growth in general.

Critical to understanding the genetic basis of cancer was the discovery of retroviruses, RNA viruses that replicate using a DNA intermediate. These viruses were discovered to carry oncogenes, cancer-causing genes that the viruses originally acquired from the cells they infected. It was discovered that oncogenes actually encode a variety of proteins that regulate cell growth, including growth factors and DNA regulatory proteins. The genetic basis behind most human cancers seems to involve mutations in these genes. The study of the mechanism by which these proteins function may eventually lead to a fuller understanding of how cancers develop.

Since most cancers have a genetic origin, the ability to screen for certain genetic patterns allows clinicians to observe patients most at risk for the disease. For example, women who carry certain forms of the genes *BRCA1* and *BRCA2* are at greater risk for developing ovarian or breast cancer.

Developing cancers in certain tissues may also secrete unique forms of proteins, allowing for detection of the disease at an early stage. For example, prostate tumors, the leading form of cancer in men, secrete a prostate specific antigen (PSA); elevated levels of PSA in the blood suggest a possible tumor in the prostate.

Oncofetal proteins, normally found on fetal cells, may also be reexpressed by certain tumors. Elevated levels of alpha-fetoprotein and carcinoembryonic antigen in serum may indicate liver or colorectal cancer. The increasing sensitivity of such screening methods holds out the prospect that the most common forms of cancer may be detected in a "curable" stage.

—David Wason Hollar, Jr., Ph.D.;
updated by Richard Adler, Ph.D.

See also Anal cancer; Biopsy; Bladder cancer; Bone cancer; Brain tumors; Breast biopsy; Breast cancer; Cancer; Carcinoma; Cervical, ovarian, and uterine cancers; Colorectal cancer; Cysts; Endometrial biopsy; Gallbladder cancer; Hodgkin's disease; Kidney cancer; Leukemia; Liver cancer; Lung cancer; Lymphadenopathy and lymphoma; Malignancy and metastasis; Mammography; Mastectomy and lumpectomy; Mouth and throat cancer; Mutation; National Cancer Institute (NCI); Neurofibromatosis; Oncology; Ovarian cysts; Prostate cancer; Sarcoma; Skin cancer; Stomach, intestinal, and pancreatic cancers; Testicular cancer; Tumor removal; Warts.

FOR FURTHER INFORMATION:
Alberts, Bruce, et al. *Molecular Biology of the Cell.* 5th ed. New York: Garland, 2008. This enormous textbook, written by six pioneers of molecular biology, is a presentation of genetics, cellular biochemistry, and developmental biology in a language understandable to the beginning biology student.

American Cancer Society. http://www.cancer.org. A comprehensive Web site dedicated to cancer education, prevention, and advocacy.

Chiras, Daniel D. *Biology: The Web of Life.* St. Paul, Minn.: West, 1993. Chiras's introductory biology textbook is clearly written with numerous examples, detailed sketches and photographs, and guest essays by leading scientists. Chapter 9, "Molecular Genetics," discusses gene regulation and the role of mutation in cellular transformation.

Dollinger, Malin, et al. *Everyone's Guide to Cancer Therapy.* 5th ed. Kansas City, Mo.: Andrews McMeel, 2008. An excellent source of medical information about cancer, written for the general public. Describes various cancer sites in the body. Includes a helpful glossary of medical terminology.

Eyre, Harmon J., Dianne Partie Lange, and Lois B. Morris. *Informed Decisions: The Complete Book of Cancer Diagnosis, Treatment, and Recovery.* 2d ed. Atlanta: American Cancer Society, 2002. This text from the American Cancer Society is intended for the layperson. It is exemplary in its discussion of cancer.

Janes-Hodder, Honna, and Nancy Keene. *Childhood Cancer: A Parent's Guide to Solid Tumor Cancers.* 2d ed. Cambridge, Mass.: O'Reilly, 2002. Covers a range of helpful information for parents with children suffering from cancer, including medical information about solid tumor childhood cancers such as bone sarcomas, liver tumors, and soft tissue sarcomas. Procedures, hospitalization, and school, social, and financial issues are additional topics covered, among others.

Kindt, Thomas J., Richard A. Goldsby, and Barbara A. Osborne. *Kuby Immunology.* 6th ed. New York: W. H. Freeman, 2007. A detailed examination of the field of immunology. Several chapters deal with subjects of cell regulation apropos to tumor development. Included is an update of tumor-specific markers.

Ross, Michael H., and Wojciech Pawlina. *Histology: A Text and Atlas.* 5th ed. Baltimore: Lippincott Williams & Wilkins, 2006. Introductory text on histology that covers a vast array of topics, including methods, the cell, the classification of tissues, epithelial tissue, connective tissue, cartilage, bone, blood, muscle, nerves, cardiovascular tissue, lymphatic tissue, and the esophagus and gastrointestinal tract.

Stark-Vance, Virginia, and M. L. Dubay. *One Hundred Questions and Answers About Brain Tumors.* 2d ed. Sudbury, Mass.: Jones and Bartlett, 2011. A patient-oriented guide that covers a range of topics related to brain tumors, including risk factors and causes; methods of prevention, screening, and diagnosis; available treatments and how to choose among them; and ways of coping with common emotional and physical difficulties associated with the diagnosis and treatment.

Varmus, Harold, and Robert Weinberg. *Genes and the Biology of Cancer.* New York: W. H. Freeman, 1993. Insight into the genetic mechanisms behind tumor formation. Discussions include the roles played by carcinogens, viruses, and oncogenes. Profusely illustrated at a level appropriate for the nonscientist.

TURNER SYNDROME
DISEASE/DISORDER
ALSO KNOWN AS: Gonadal dysgenesis, Bonnevie-Ullrich syndrome, monosomy X
ANATOMY OR SYSTEM AFFECTED: Cells, endocrine system, reproductive system
SPECIALTIES AND RELATED FIELDS: Endocrinology, genetics, gynecology, obstetrics
DEFINITION: A genetic condition in which cells are missing all or part of an X chromosome.

CAUSES AND SYMPTOMS
Turner syndrome affects an estimated one out of every 2,000 to 2,500 girls conceived. The disorder is congenital, which means that it begins at conception. Normal males have one X and one Y chromosome. Normal females have two X chromosomes. Females with Turner syndrome have only one X chromosome (an XO pattern) in each of their cells or two X chromosomes with one being incomplete. Although the exact cause is unknown, scientists believe that the disorder may result from an error during the division of the parent's sex cells.

Shortness is the most common feature of Turner syndrome. The average height of a woman with this condition is 4 feet, 8 inches. Other physical features associated with the syndrome include puffy hands and feet at birth, a webbed neck, prominent ears, a low hairline at the back of the neck, drooping eyelids, flat and broad

---

INFORMATION ON TURNER SYNDROME

CAUSES: Genetic defect
SYMPTOMS: Short stature, puffy hands and feet at birth, webbed neck, prominent ears, soft fingernails that turn up at end, ovarian failure leading to infertility and incomplete sexual development, cardiovascular problems
DURATION: Chronic
TREATMENTS: Hormonal therapy for some symptoms

---

chest, and soft fingernails that turn up at the end.

Most patients experience ovarian failure. Since the ovaries normally produce estrogen, girls and women with Turner syndrome lack this essential hormone, resulting in infertility and incomplete sexual development. Cardiovascular disorders are the single source of increased mortality in patients with Turner syndrome.

TREATMENT AND THERAPY
No treatment is available to correct the chromosome abnormality that causes this condition. Nevertheless, injections of human growth hormones can restore much of the growth deficit. Unless they take hormone therapy, women and girls with Turner syndrome will not menstruate or develop breasts and pubic hair. Although infertility cannot be altered, pregnancy may be possible through in vitro fertilization.

PERSPECTIVE AND PROSPECTS
Turner syndrome was first identified by Henry Turner in 1938. In 1959, C. E. Ford discovered that a chromosomal abnormality involving sex chromosomes causes the syndrome.

Research is under way to assess the best way to administer female sex hormones that provide maximum bone development and growth in adolescents who need this therapy.

—*Fred Buchstein; updated by Sharon W. Stark, R.N., A.P.R.N., D.N.Sc.*

See also Dwarfism; Endocrine system; Endocrinology; Endocrinology, pediatric; Genital disorders, female; Genetic diseases; Genetics and inheritance; Growth; Hormone therapy; Hormones; Infertility, female; Menstruation; Ovaries; Puberty and adolescence; Reproductive system; Sexual differentiation; Women's health.

FOR FURTHER INFORMATION:

Henry, Helen L., and Anthony W. Norman, eds. *Encyclopedia of Hormones*. 3 vols. San Diego, Calif.: Academic Press, 2003.

Kronenberg, Henry M., et al., eds. *Williams Textbook of Endocrinology*. 11th ed. Philadelphia: Saunders/Elsevier, 2008.

Lewis, Ricki. *Human Genetics: Concepts and Applications*. 9th ed. Dubuque, Iowa: McGraw-Hill, 2009.

MedlinePlus. "Turner Syndrome." http://www.nlm.nih.gov/medlineplus/ency/article/000379.htm.

Milunsky, Aubrey, ed. *Genetic Disorders and the Fetus: Diagnosis, Prevention, and Treatment*. 5th ed. Baltimore: Johns Hopkins University Press, 2004.

Money, John. *Sex Errors of the Body and Related Syndromes: A Guide to Counseling Children, Adolescents, and Their Families*. 2d ed. Baltimore: Paul H. Brookes, 1994.

Pinsky, Leonard, Robert P. Erickson, and R. Neil Schimke. *Genetic Disorders of Human Sexual Development*. New York: Oxford University Press, 1999.

Rosenfeld, Ron G., and Melvin M. Grumbach, eds. *Turner Syndrome*. New York: Marcel Dekker, 1990.

Turner Syndrome Society of the United States. http://www.turner-syndrome-us.org.

TWINS. *See* **MULTIPLE BIRTHS.**

TYPHOID FEVER

DISEASE/DISORDER

ANATOMY OR SYSTEM AFFECTED: Circulatory system, gallbladder, gastrointestinal system, intestines, kidneys, liver, skin, spleen

SPECIALTIES AND RELATED FIELDS: Bacteriology, environmental health, epidemiology, internal medicine, public health

DEFINITION: An acute, systemic, febrile disease caused by bacteria that are transmitted through contaminated food or water.

CAUSES AND SYMPTOMS

Typhoid fever, a serious disease with the potential to become epidemic under conditions of poor sanitation, is caused by the bacterium *Salmonella enterica*, serotype Typhi (formerly *Salmonella typhi*). These bacteria are transmitted to humans through the consumption of water or food contaminated with the feces from individuals who carry the serotype Typhi but who most often remain asymptomatic.

An infective dose of bacteria in susceptible individuals is estimated to be quite small, generally less than one thousand cells. The ingested bacteria pass through the stomach to the small intestines, where they establish an initial site of infection. These intestinal lesions usually ulcerate, and the bacteria spread to other body tissues via the bloodstream and lymphatic system. The organs most often affected by these secondary infections include the liver, spleen, kidneys, bone marrow, and especially the gallbladder. Symptoms include

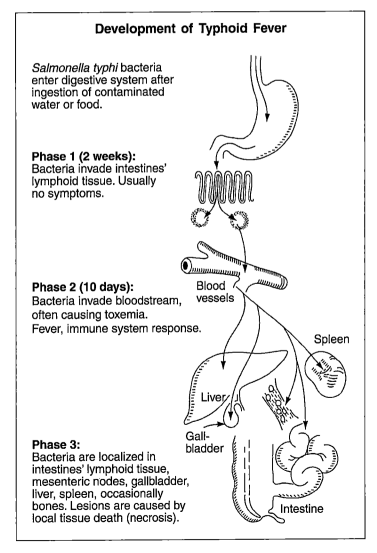

Development of Typhoid Fever

Salmonella typhi bacteria enter digestive system after ingestion of contaminated water or food.

Phase 1 (2 weeks): Bacteria invade intestines' lymphoid tissue. Usually no symptoms.

Phase 2 (10 days): Bacteria invade bloodstream, often causing toxemia. Fever, immune system response.

Phase 3: Bacteria are localized in intestines' lymphoid tissue, mesenteric nodes, gallbladder, liver, spleen, occasionally bones. Lesions are caused by local tissue death (necrosis).

Blood vessels, Spleen, Liver, Gallbladder, Intestine

headache, abdominal pain, general malaise, and a generalized rash with rose-colored spots. If no complications ensue, then the fever will abate after about three weeks, but mortality rates average about 15 percent in untreated cases.

TREATMENT AND THERAPY

The first drug with demonstrable effectiveness in treating typhoid fever was chloramphenicol, which became generally available in 1948. Other antibiotics, notably ampicillin and ciprofloxacin, have largely replaced chloramphenicol as the treatment of choice, and their use has reduced the death rate to approximately 1 percent. Improved sanitation and living conditions since the 1920's have drastically reduced the incidence of this disease in the United States, although worldwide it remains a major public health concern. Each year at least 16 million cases and 600,000 deaths can be attributed to typhoid fever.

A vaccine has been available since the early 1950's, but its effectiveness is suboptimal. Temporary immunity is acquired by about 60 to 70 percent of vaccinated individuals. Individuals who recover from the disease often become healthy carriers of the bacteria, and surgical removal of the gallbladder may be necessary to rid them of their carrier status.

PERSPECTIVE AND PROSPECTS

The most famous case of a healthy carrier of the typhoid fever bacteria was a cook by the name of Mary Mallon, called "Typhoid Mary," who worked in several establishments in New York during the period from 1902 to 1915. In those years, she was linked to several different outbreaks of typhoid fever, resulting in fifty-one cases of illness and three deaths. When she repeatedly refused to cooperate with public health authorities, she was eventually taken into custody and confined in a state hospital. After almost three years, she was released, but she soon skipped parole and disappeared. Four years later, she was apprehended again

---

INFORMATION ON TYPHOID FEVER

CAUSES: Bacteria transmitted through contaminated food or water
SYMPTOMS: Fever, headache, abdominal pain, malaise, rash with rose-colored spots
DURATION: Three weeks
TREATMENTS: Antibiotics

---

as the source of a typhoid fever outbreak that involved twenty-five cases and two deaths. She was returned to the secure hospital in 1915, where she remained until her death in 1938. The important legal issues generated by her case, including incarceration for having an infectious disease and forced surgery, were the driving forces behind the founding of the American Civil Liberties Union (ACLU).

—*Jeffrey A. Knight, Ph.D.*

See also Antibiotics; Bacterial infections; Bacteriology; Epidemics and pandemics; Fever; Food poisoning; Gallbladder diseases; Immunization and vaccination; Microbiology; Salmonella infection.

FOR FURTHER INFORMATION:

Lock, Stephen, John Last, and George M. Dunea, eds. *The Oxford Companion to Medicine.* New York: Oxford University Press, 2005.

Murray, Patrick R., Ken S. Rosenthal, and Michael A. Pfaller. *Medical Microbiology.* 6th ed. Philadelphia: Mosby/Elsevier, 2009.

Tortora, Gerard J., Berdell R. Funke, and Christine L. Case. *Microbiology: An Introduction.* 9th ed. San Francisco: Pearson Benjamin Cummings, 2007.

TYPHUS

DISEASE/DISORDER

ALSO KNOWN AS: Epidemic typhus, rickettsiosis
ANATOMY OR SYSTEM AFFECTED: Circulatory system, kidneys, nervous system, respiratory system, skin
SPECIALTIES AND RELATED FIELDS: Bacteriology, environmental health, epidemiology, internal medicine, public health
DEFINITION: An acute, systemic, febrile disease caused by bacteria that are transmitted through the bite of a body louse.

CAUSES AND SYMPTOMS

The causative agent of epidemic typhus is the bacterium *Rickettsia prowazeckii*, an obligate intracellular parasite. These bacteria are transmitted to humans following the bite from an infected body louse, *Pediculus humanus corporis*. The pathogen is excreted with the louse feces and invades the site of a louse bite when the bitten host scratches the bite. The onset of the disease is marked by a high and prolonged fever with accompanying headache and rash. The bacteria are spread throughout the body through the bloodstream and can cause secondary lesions in many tissues, including the kidneys, heart, and brain. Mortality can be as high as 50 percent in untreated cases.

TREATMENT AND THERAPY

Antibiotic treatment is essential to reduce the severity of the disease, and chloramphenicol, tetracycline, and doxycycline are the antibiotics of choice. Improved sanitation and living conditions since the 1920's has virtually eliminated this disease in the United States. The last epidemic was in 1922, and there have been sporadic recent reports of isolated cases in the United States involving transmission from flying squirrels, indicating a possible animal reservoir. Epidemic typhus still persists in some regions of Africa, Central America, and South America, and an effective vaccine is available for travelers to these regions.

PERSPECTIVE AND PROSPECTS

Epidemic typhus is primarily a disease of crowded, substandard living conditions and poor sanitation. Millions of cases occurred in the trenches of World War I and the concentration camps of World War II. Anne Frank, the noted teenage diarist, died of typhus contracted while at a concentration camp. It has been said that Napoleon's retreat from Russia was started by a louse, and that lice have defeated the most powerful armies of Europe and Asia.

The pioneering investigations of Howard Taylor Ricketts and Stanislas von Prowazeck in the early twentieth century paved the way for the discovery of both the bacteria and the louse vector, although both men died from the disease that they studied. They were honored posthumously when the bacterium was named *Rickettsia prowazeckii*.

—*Jeffrey A. Knight, Ph.D.*

See also Antibiotics; Bacterial infections; Bacteriology; Bites and stings; Epidemics and pandemics; Fever; Insect-borne diseases; Lice, mites, and ticks; Microbiology; Parasitic diseases; Zoonoses.

FOR FURTHER INFORMATION:

Lock, Stephen, John Last, and George M. Dunea, eds. *The Oxford Companion to Medicine.* New York: Oxford University Press, 2005.

Murray, Patrick R., Ken S. Rosenthal, and Michael A. Pfaller. *Medical Microbiology.* 6th ed. Philadelphia: Mosby/Elsevier, 2009.

Tortora, Gerard J., Berdell R. Funke, and Christine L. Case. *Microbiology: An Introduction.* 9th ed. San Francisco: Pearson Benjamin Cummings, 2007.

Zinsser, Hans. *Rats, Lice, and History.* New York: Black Dog & Leventhal, 1996.

ULCER SURGERY

PROCEDURE

ANATOMY OR SYSTEM AFFECTED: Gastrointestinal system, intestines, stomach

SPECIALTIES AND RELATED FIELDS: Gastroenterology, general surgery, nutrition

DEFINITION: The removal of areas of the stomach or duodenum that are ulcerated; a procedure often avoided by nonsurgical treatment.

KEY TERMS:

duodenum: the first part of the small intestine

metastasis: the transfer of disease-producing cells to other parts of a body

partial gastrectomy: the removal of part of the stomach

pepsin: a substance in the stomach that breaks down most proteins

peritonitis: inflammation of the peritoneum or stomach lining

pyloric stenosis: a narrowing of the passageway between the stomach and the duodenum

INDICATIONS AND PROCEDURES

Many people who are host to peptic ulcers have no symptoms. As these ulcers—which may occur as single or multiple eruptions having a diameter between 0.75 centimeter (0.3 inch) and 2.5 centimeters (1 inch) and a depth of about 0.02 centimeter (0.01 inch)—enlarge and multiply, however, symptoms often become apparent. These symptoms include a burning or gnawing pain in the abdominal region, particularly when the stomach is empty. Therefore, people who are asymptomatic during the day, when they are ingesting food at regular intervals, may become symptomatic at night. One way to allay symptoms, particularly those caused by a duodenal ulcer, is to eat, so that the gastric juices feed on the food rather than on the lining of the stomach or duodenum. Symptoms often reappear, however, a few hours after eating.

In some cases, patients experience a loss of appetite. If the ulcer is in the duodenum, however, the opposite may occur, in which case it is best to eat small quantities of food that is not overly spicy. Belching often accompanies ulcer problems, although, in and of itself, this is not categorically indicative of ulcers. People suffering from ulcers sometimes lose weight, largely because they feel bloated and therefore tend to eat less. Nausea and vomiting accompany some ulcer problems.

In extreme cases, an ulcer may start to bleed, in which case the patient may vomit blood. Black, tarry stools are also an indication of bleeding in the stomach, although elements in one's diet, particularly iron, can also produce darkened stools. Where bleeding is profuse, the patient may require a blood transfusion. On rare occasions, an ulcer may eat through the back wall of the digestive tract and involve the pancreas, causing a pain that reaches as far as the patient's back. When ulcers eat through the front of the duodenum, the result may be peritonitis, a life-threatening inflammation of the abdominal lining that requires immediate attention.

If ulcers persist and go untreated, they can cause dangerous scarring of the stomach lining and duodenum. As a result, the passageway between the stomach and duodenum narrows. When this condition, called pyloric stenosis, occurs, patients usually experience vomiting and weight loss.

Some ulcers are malignant (cancerous) and must be removed surgically at once. Follow-up radiation and/or chemotherapy may be indicated in such cases. The surgical removal of ulcers involves making an incision in the abdomen and removing the portion of the stomach or duodenum that is ulcerated. The area affected is then joined and sutured. Large portions of the stomach may be removed if necessary and will, in time, regenerate.

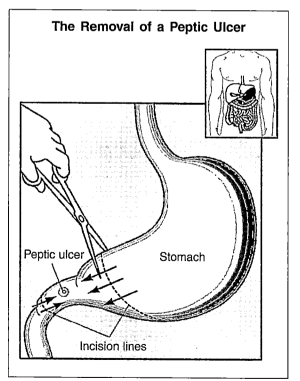

The Removal of a Peptic Ulcer

With a severe peptic ulcer, it may be necessary to remove a section of the stomach and join the remaining ends; the inset shows the location of the stomach.

USES AND COMPLICATIONS

Except where a malignancy is suspected, ulcer surgery is a treatment of last resort. Often, changes in diet can control the situation, as can discontinuing smoking and the drinking of alcoholic beverages or beverages that contain caffeine. Aspirin and nonsteroidal anti-inflammatory drugs (NSAIDs) can irritate the stomach and are usually not advised for people with ulcers. The appearance of ulcers has been linked to stress, so changes in lifestyle can result in considerable improvement.

The most common early treatment is with nonprescription antacids or with similar prescription drugs that coat the stomach lining and neutralize the acids that are causing the problem. Prescription drugs such as H2 blockers and proton pump inhibitors, as well as antimicrobial treatment of the ulcerogenic bacteria *Helicobacter pylori*, can almost invariably cure gastric and duodenal ulcers, leaving surgery for removal of malignancies and control of bleeding that cannot be stopped by endoscopic cautery. Ulcer patients are also generally advised to eat several small meals a day rather than two or three large ones. Doing so helps to keep food in the stomach, and even nibbling through the night produces favorable results in some patients.

Because ulcer surgery is major and is usually done under general anesthesia, it carries the risks associated with any major surgery. The recovery rate after ulcer surgery is good, however, particularly as the areas around the excision begin to return to normal through regeneration. Where a malignancy has been detected early and removed surgically, metastasis can usually be prevented, particularly if follow-up radiation or chemotherapy is employed.

PERSPECTIVE AND PROSPECTS

Ulcers were once treated by bed rest and a bland, boring diet, mostly of such soft foods as boiled eggs, toast, and custards accompanied by plenty of milk, which supposedly lined the stomach and protected it from damage by gastric juices. Such treatment is now generally considered unnecessary. Most ulcer patients can remain active and can eat sensibly but relatively normally. Extremely spicy food, which can irritate an ulcer, should be avoided if ulcer symptoms are present.

In the past, another method of ulcer treatment was to freeze the affected area, which seemed to produce immediate, favorable results. In time, however, many of the ulcers treated in this way returned. This treatment,

although appealing for its short-term results, is now uncommon because its benefits do not appear to be lasting.

In recent years, the management of ulcers has become increasingly conservative, with surgery the least frequent and most extreme treatment of all. In the foreseeable future, it is likely that ulcer surgery will become an increasing rarity.

—*R. Baird Shuman, Ph.D.*

See also Digestion; Endoscopy; Food biochemistry; Gastrectomy; Gastroenterology; Gastrointestinal disorders; Gastrointestinal system; Intestinal disorders; Intestines; Peritonitis; Small intestine; Stress; Stress reduction; Ulcers; Vagotomy.

FOR FURTHER INFORMATION:

Griffith, H. Winter. *Complete Guide to Symptoms, Illness, and Surgery.* Revised and updated by Stephen Moore and Kenneth Yoder. 5th ed. New York: Perigee, 2006. Covers more than five hundred diseases and disorders and includes information about causes and risk factors, preventive techniques, diagnostic tests, and surgical treatment.

Margolis, Simeon, and Sergey Kantsevoy. *Johns Hopkins White Papers 2002: Digestive Disorders.* New York: Rebus, 2002. Covers the diagnosis, treatment, and preventive measures for a range of disorders, including peptic ulcer disease, gastroesophageal reflux disease, gastritis, gallstones, diarrhea, and ulcerative colitis.

Swabb, Edward A., and Sandor Szabo, eds. *Ulcer Disease: Investigation and Basis for Therapy.* New York: Marcel Dekker, 1991. Twenty-four contributed chapters in four sections give medical researchers and practicing clinicians a review of the origins, presentations, therapies, and human investigation of ulcer disease.

Szabo, Sandor, and Carl J. Pfeiffer, eds. *Ulcer Disease: New Aspects of Pathogenesis and Pharmacology.* Boca Raton, Fla.: CRC Press, 1989. Data on the pathogenesis of ulcer disease are presented in this text, with the emphasis that an understanding of the pathogenesis and etiology of ulcer diseases represents the most rational approach to pharmacology.

Tytgat, G. N. J., ed. *Peptic Ulcer Disease.* Orlando, Fla.: W. B. Saunders, 2000. Discusses conceivable mechanisms by which *Helicobacter pylori* provokes duodenal ulcer disease and the management of gastroduodenal ulcers caused by nonsteroidal anti-inflammatory drugs.

Zakim, David, and Andrew J. Dannenberg, eds. *Peptic Ulcer Disease and Other Acid-Related Disorders.* Armonk, N.Y.: Academic Research Associates, 1991. Discusses gastric acid secretion and digestive system diseases generally. Includes bibliographical references and an index.

Zinner, Michael. *Atlas of Gastric Surgery.* New York: Churchill Livingstone, 1992. This text covers stomach surgery, peptic ulcers, and gastrointestinal diseases generally. Includes an index.

Zollinger, Robert M., Jr., and Robert M. Zollinger, Sr. *Zollinger's Atlas of Surgical Operations.* 8th ed. New York: McGraw-Hill, 2003. A comprehensive examination of surgery. Covers basic surgical anatomy and vascular, gynecologic, gastrointestinal, and miscellaneous abdominal procedures.

ULCERS

DISEASE/DISORDER

ANATOMY OR SYSTEM AFFECTED: Gastrointestinal system, mouth, stomach

SPECIALTIES AND RELATED FIELDS: Family medicine, gastroenterology, internal medicine, nutrition

DEFINITION: Ulcers, specifically those referred to as peptic ulcers, are open sores that develop on the mucous membranes that line the gastrointestinal tract and are caused by excessive secretion of gastric juices, particularly from the pancreas into the intestine.

KEY TERMS:

acid pump inhibitors: a group of drugs that block the stomach cells' mechanism for producing hydrochloric acid

histamine II blockers: the general term used to describe various drugs that block the hormonal stimulation of histamine, one inducer of stomach acid

nonulcerous dyspepsia: a condition that exhibits many of the symptoms of peptic ulcers but does not involve actual lesions in the linings of the stomach or intestines

pepsin: the first component of gastric juice to be discovered, in the 1830's; the term "peptic ulcer" derives from the name of this digestive fluid

prostaglandins: chemical substances in the stomach lining that help fight ulceration by increasing blood flow to the lesion area

Zollinger-Ellison syndrome: a rare condition in which secretions of acid are so sudden and excessive that normal gastric defenses cannot prevent the immediate ulceration of stomach membranes

CAUSES AND SYMPTOMS

In the most general of terms, an ulcer is an open sore that does not respond readily to the normal processes of healing. It may occur on the skin itself or on internal mucous membranes. A corneal ulcer, for example, may occur as a result of infections stemming from local injuries of, or foreign objects lodged in, the eye. Circulatory disturbances associated with varicose veins or long periods in bed without sufficient body exercise can also cause skin ulcers. The latter form is sometimes referred to as bedsores.

The most commonly occurring ulcer, however, is the peptic ulcer, which occurs at various points in the gastrointestinal tract. Specifically, such ulcers affect the lower portion of the esophagus, the stomach (in which case the term "gastric" ulcer may be employed), and two locations in the small intestine: the duodenum and the jejunum. Approximately 10 percent of the general population in the United States and Western Europe is thought to suffer from peptic ulcers. A substantially higher percentage of the population may suffer from a condition that resembles ulcers in its symptomatic levels of discomfort and pain but that does not actually involve lesions. This condition is called nonulcerous dyspepsia.

When ulceration of the stomach or intestinal tissue advances past a certain stage, internal bleeding usually occurs. Reaction to this stage of deterioration may involve vomiting, in which case the granular bloody material that is expulsed resembles partially digested food and is brownish rather than red in color. This condition stems from the effect of acidic gastric juices on the blood that has been released. If bleeding from ulcers becomes evident through the presence of blood in the stools, the effect is different: The fecal material is black in color, a condition that was referred to in past generations as "tarry stool."

Although modern medical science has identified the

INFORMATION ON ULCERS

CAUSES: Excessive secretion of gastric juices worsened by alcohol, smoking, and aspirin use; bacterial infection; prolonged stress, nervousness, and hostility

SYMPTOMS: Vomiting, tarry stool

DURATION: Acute or recurrent

TREATMENTS: Antibiotics, stomach acid inhibitors, histamine II blockers, surgery

hydrochloric acid content of the gastric juice as the corrosive agent that causes ulcer sores in all these regions of the digestive system, the term "peptic ulcer" is still commonly used to refer to all ulcers. This label was first applied following the discovery, in 1836, of the enzyme pepsin, one of the first subcomponents of the gastric juice to be isolated in the laboratory.

In the twentieth century, the original contributions of physicians to the understanding of what ulcers are were combined with equally scientific observations of social and psychological factors that can bring about ulcers. Increasingly, many of these causes were associated with environmental and nervous emotional factors.

The likelihood of ulcers forming in the gastrointestinal tract is increased if an imbalance occurs in the normal functioning of a specific phase of the digestive process. That phase begins when, at the time that foods are taken into the mouth and swallowed, the body secretes gastric juice containing both acid and pepsin. The essential acid in gastric juice is hydrochloric acid, which is highly dangerous in its pure state and poisonous if swallowed directly. Pepsin is an enzyme produced in the lining of the stomach that has proteolytic, or protein-degrading, characteristics. Both these components in gastric juices are essential in the first stages of digestion to break down the foodstuffs in the stomach and to facilitate their passage into the small intestine, where other secretions from the liver and pancreas continue the process of digestion. In the case of the enzyme pepsin, it is secreted in an inactive chemical state; it therefore requires the presence of hydrochloric acid (also secreted in the stomach lining) to convert it chemically to an active state and an optimum degree of acidity (pH 1 to 3) for the digestive function it fulfills. If the chemical conversion of pepsin into an active digestive agent does not make use of all the hydrochloric acid that has been secreted, the excess acid is free to do damage to the sensitive tissue of the stomach or intestinal lining.

Ulcers can occur in any of several areas of the gastrointestinal tract when excessive amounts or imbalanced component proportions of gastric juice are secreted. In recent times, doctors established that a continuing state

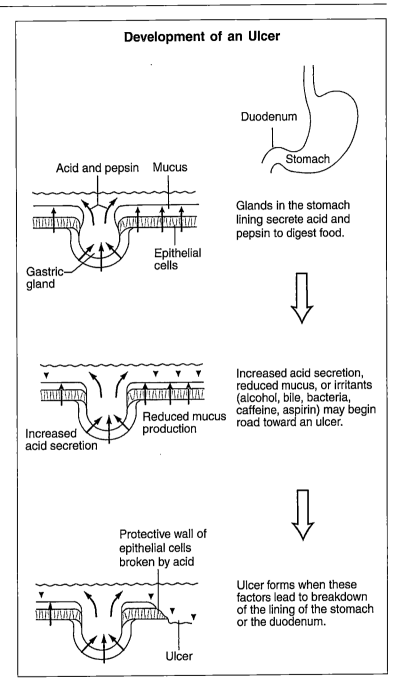

Development of an Ulcer

Duodenum

Stomach

Acid and pepsin Mucus

Epithelial cells

Gastric gland

Glands in the stomach lining secrete acid and pepsin to digest food.

Increased acid secretion

Reduced mucus production

Increased acid secretion, reduced mucus, or irritants (alcohol, bile, bacteria, caffeine, aspirin) may begin road toward an ulcer.

Protective wall of epithelial cells broken by acid

Ulcer

Ulcer forms when these factors lead to breakdown of the lining of the stomach or the duodenum.

of nervousness or hostility can cause gastric juice to flow almost continuously. Such hypersecretion will damage the mucous membranes lining the digestive tract unless a more-or-less constant supply of food is taken in by the organism. Thus, the nervous eater who is constantly consuming foods may be unconsciously trying to control the potential development of ulcers in his or her gastrointestinal tract. The side effects on the body of constant nervous eating may be potentially as harmful as the localized effects associated with ulcers.

In essence, what happens when an ulcer begins to form is that the acid and pepsin in the gastric juice begin to digest membrane tissue in the gastrointestinal tract itself. Normally, the stomach has a series of internal defenses to combat localized attacks by active gastric juice against its own sensitive membranes. In the first place, the mucous lining of the internal organs themselves forms a sort of barrier between membrane tissue and the combined food-gastric juice content of the functioning organ.

The cells of the stomach lining also secrete a natural antacid in the form of bicarbonate of soda. If the normal presence of these two protective agents is insufficient to prevent deterioration of the stomach or intestinal lining, a more active struggle ensues in the area where an ulcer has begun to develop. Surface cells begin to constrict to form a more resistant surface area around the nascent lesion. If the process does not proceed too rapidly, damaged cells may be replaced by healthy cells in the immediate area of the lesion.

Even more specialized reactions in the area of ulceration are associated with prostaglandins, which are chemical agents in the stomach lining that stimulate increased blood flow to nourish besieged cells. Prostaglandins can also bring about higher levels of antacid production and mucus accumulation where they are needed most.

With one notable and fairly rare exception, known as the Zollinger-Ellison syndrome (excessive production of acid), almost all cases of stomach ulcers (gastric ulcers) occur as a result of dysfunction in the defensive systems described above. As for duodenal (upper small intestine) ulcers, it appears that only about a third of all cases stem from higher-than-normal secretions of acid.

Doctors are not in full agreement regarding the way in which certain externally introduced substances may cause, or seriously contribute to, ulcers. Most have concluded, however, that a "big three" of clearly abusive substances—cigarettes, alcohol, and some over-the-counter drugs, especially aspirin—play a significant role. Cigarette smoking has been linked with the slowing down of essential body functions that either provide defenses against ulcers or contribute to their healing. One such function is the rate of blood flow itself, which is vital for the nourishment of cells that may be under attack by ulcers. Other side effects of smoking may include reduced production of prostaglandins, which make important contributions to the defensive reaction of the body against ulcerations.

As for the other potentially abusive agents, alcohol and certain over-the-counter or otherwise common drugs, it is the latter that are almost universally condemned for their negative effects on the proper functioning of the gastrointestinal system.

Alcohol, for its part, apparently does nothing to stimulate excessive acid production in the stomach. It does, however, interfere with the healing processes that are so vital in combating ulcers.

While caffeine is not usually considered to be an over-the-counter drug, it is known to be an important stimulator of acid secretions. Some doctors consider it to be second only to aspirin as a negative "foreign agent" affecting the sensitive mechanism of digestion in the stomach and small intestine.

Another common drug, aspirin, shares a dubious reputation in this respect with a number of other drugs classified as nonsteroidal anti-inflammatory drugs (NSAIDs) that are used to treat arthritis and other muscular or joint inflammations.

There is a widespread consensus that the occurrence of ulcers may be linked to external agents that are taken into the body. The simplest evidence of this hypothesis revolves around associations that have been established between the bacillus *Helicobacter pylori* and ulcerous conditions in the stomach and intestines.

Doctors had observed the presence of this bacillus (along with many others) in the human stomach for at least a century. Studies by the Australian researchers Bernard Marshall and J. R. Warner, however, noted that a very high percentage (nearly 100 percent) of patients diagnosed as having ulcers also had substantial traces of *H. pylori*.

TREATMENT AND THERAPY

As the debate over the role of *H. pylori* in causing ulcers took form in the early 1990's, those researchers who wanted to find proof that medicine was on the verge of a major breakthrough organized a full campaign to prescribe drugs that were known to kill the suspect bacillus.

It is now clear that *H. pylori* is a major contributing factor not only in ulcer development but also in the extremely high recurrence rate of relapse in healed patients. Because of the inflammation that the infecting organism causes in the stomach and duodenal linings, normal protective mechanisms break down. Once these barriers that protect the lining from damage by the acid and enzymes used in digesting food are gone, the process of ulceration begins. Even after the ulcer has healed, very high rates of recurrence are found unless the bacterial infection is eradicated.

Because so many people are infected with these common bacteria but not everyone develops ulcers, other contributing factors are clearly present. In the vulnerable patient, a combination of the well-known risk factors along with infection work together to bring about ulcers. It is now a routine treatment to administer antibiotics and stomach acid inhibitors simultaneously. Cure rate times and relapse rates have improved significantly.

Whatever the ultimate explanation concerning the causes of this surprisingly common ailment may be, the medical world remained, in the late twentieth century, devoted to the necessary use of a number of drugs to control the effects of gastric and peptic ulcers by fighting the flow of gastric juices that do the physical damage of ulceration. On the whole, these drugs, which are called histamine II blockers, aim at one objective: to block the formation of stomach acid. A similar effect is produced by several widely used (and markedly expensive) medicines that are prepared under commercial labels: Tagamet, Zantac, Pepcid, and Axid. Drugs in the class called acid pump inhibitors, such as Prilosec, also block stomach acid, but by a different and nearly complete method: They prevent the stomach cells from actually making the acid, in the final step before it is secreted into the stomach. These drugs are effective even in the most difficult cases of ulceration.

Much more complicated than the problem of treating normal cases of ulcers is the technical question of how to guard against the further deterioration of ulcers into different forms of gastrointestinal cancer. New forms of technology were being tested in the late twentieth century that allowed physicians to examine the inner mucous membranes of the intestines directly. One such device, called the fiber-optic endoscope, consists of a long tube that is passed through the esophagus and stomach to penetrate the upper portions of the small intestine. The fiber-optic endoscope not only views and photographs the surface areas affected by ulcers but also allows the physician to biopsy the tissue at the same time. This and other methods of diagnosis, although not available to all hospitals and clinics, and not mastered by all physicians who were trained in the pre-fiber-optic generation, represent enormous potential advances over the rather basic therapies developed during the previous century.

PERSPECTIVE AND PROSPECTS

Long before modern scientific research techniques provided the medical world with a relatively precise idea of what causes ulcers and how to treat them, an entire literature on the disease had accumulated. It was apparently Hippocrates himself, in the fifth century B.C.E., who first studied the gastric hemorrhaging that can result from a peptic ulcer. Others, including the first century C.E. Roman Celsus, noted the favorable effect of prescribing a nonacid diet to patients suffering from ulcers. It was not until the eighteenth and nineteenth centuries, however, that doctors prepared the first clinical accounts of the effects of ulcers based on pathological studies.

Not much had changed by the early twentieth century regarding the attitude of physicians toward the role of acids in the stage-by-stage degenerative process of ulceration. The American doctor Bertram W. Sippy was often quoted after his famous 1912 statement to medical students that "where there is no acid, there is no ulcer." The question of what caused the presence of excess acid in the intestines aside, medical science would try to come closer to being able to detect the actions of the "culprit at work." To the general public, the advanced process of fiber-optic endoscopy gives the appearance of having been developed overnight in the last decades of the twentieth century. In fact, a number of necessary prestages had been pioneered all over the globe for more than a century.

As early as 1868, nearly thirty years before X rays were discovered, German physician Adolf Kussmaul performed experiments that involved inserting a hollow lighted tube into patients' stomachs. He was actually able to see the interior surface of the stomach with the naked eye. Later, also in Germany, in 1908, a doctor named Hammeter was able to display a gastric ulcer by using barium meal X-ray technology. At a certain point, still well before the advent of fiber-optic endoscopy, a technique called arteriography was employed to explore the extent of ulcer damage when hemorrhaging occurred. This method, which still complemented fiber-optic endoscopy into the 1990's, involves the injection, through a fine tube passing through key arteries, of a dye whose movement in the intestinal tissue is then traced by means of a rapid series of X-ray images.

—*Byron D. Cannon, Ph.D.;*
updated by Connie Rizzo, M.D., Ph.D.

See also Abdomen; Abdominal disorders; Acid reflux disease; Acidosis; Alcoholism; Bacterial infections; Behçet's disease; Canker sores; Cold sores; Endoscopy; Esophagus; Gastrectomy; Gastroenterology; Gastrointestinal disorders; Gastrointestinal system; Heartburn; Indigestion; Intestinal disorders; Intestines; Lesions; Small intestine; Ulcer surgery.

FOR FURTHER INFORMATION:

Goldman, Lee, and Dennis Ausiello, eds. *Cecil Textbook of Medicine.* 23d ed. Philadelphia: Saunders/ Elsevier, 2007. The standard medical reference text. Difficult but complete, it covers the disease process from its inception through diagnosis, treatment, and course.

Janowitz, Henry D. *Indigestion: Living Better with Upper Intestinal Problems, from Heartburn to Ulcers and Gallstones.* New York: Oxford University Press, 1994. A general text exploring various symptoms of digestive ailments and what causes them. Several chapters are devoted to peptic ulcers.

_____. *Your Gut Feelings: A Complete Guide to Living Better with Intestinal Problems.* Rev. ed. New York: Oxford University Press, 1995. An early, scientifically based contribution to general knowledge of the digestive processes and dangers of imbalances that may exist.

Kapadia, Cyrus R., James M. Crawford, and Caroline Taylor. *An Atlas of Gastroenterology: A Guide to Diagnosis and Differential Diagnosis.* Boca Raton, Fla.: Pantheon, 2003. Provides a fully illustrated, nonspecialist understanding of myriad gastrointestinal diseases, including ulcers, heartburn, dyspepsia, diarrhea, irritable bowel syndrome, and pancreatitis. Includes bibliographic references and an index.

Litin, Scott C., ed. *Mayo Clinic Family Health Book.* 4th ed. New York: HarperResource, 2009. An excellent medical text for the layperson, detailing medical disorders, illnesses, and safety and health issues that affect families. Although the information is derived from a wide variety of highly technical sources, the articles are written to be easily understood by a general audience.

Margolis, Simeon, and Sergey Kantsevoy. *Johns Hopkins White Papers 2002: Digestive Disorders.* New York: Rebus, 2002. Covers the diagnosis, treatment, and preventive measures for a range of disorders, including peptic ulcer disease, gastroesophageal reflux disease, gastritis, gallstones, diarrhea, and ulcerative colitis.

Monroe, Judy. *Coping with Ulcers, Heartburn, and Stress-Related Stomach Disorders.* New York: Rosen, 2000. A book for young adults that surveys different types of ulcers, irritable bowel syndrome, food intolerances and allergies of all types, and heartburn and acid reflux. Offers tips for good digestive health through fitness, a slower-paced approach to eating, and stress management.

Parker, James N., and Philip M. Parker, eds. *The 2002 Official Patient's Sourcebook on Peptic Ulcer.* San Diego, Calif.: Icon Health, 2002. Draws from public, academic, government, and peer-reviewed research to provide a wide-ranging handbook for patients with ulcers.

ULTRASONOGRAPHY
PROCEDURE

ANATOMY OR SYSTEM AFFECTED: Abdomen, bladder, blood, gallbladder, heart, kidneys, reproductive system, urinary system, uterus

SPECIALTIES AND RELATED FIELDS: Cardiology, embryology, gynecology, internal medicine, obstetrics, radiology, urology, vascular medicine

DEFINITION: A technique that directs ultrasonic waves into body tissues and uses the reflections to create visual images, making it possible to view the anatomy of organs and blood vessels and to evaluate the dynamics of blood flow.

KEY TERMS:

Doppler effect: the relationship of the apparent frequency of waves, such as sound waves, to the relative motion of the source of the waves and the observer or instrument; the frequency increases as the two approach each other and decreases as they move apart; an effect also known as the Doppler shift

duplex scan: an ultrasound representation of echo images of tissues and blood vessels combined with a Doppler representation of blood flow patterns

frequency: the number of complete cycles, such as sound cycles, produced by an alternating energy source; sound is measured in cycles per second, and one cycle per second is equal to 1 hertz

oscilloscope: an instrument that displays a visual representation of electrical variations on the fluorescent screen of a cathode-ray tube transducer (probe): a device designed to transfer ultrasound waves into the body noninvasively, receive the returning echoes, and transform those echoes into electrical voltages

ultrasonic: referring to any frequency of sound that is higher than the audible range—that is, higher than 20,000 cycles per second (20 kilohertz)

INDICATIONS AND PROCEDURES

Sound waves are mechanical pressure waves that can propagate through liquids, solids, and, to some extent, gases. A sound wave is composed of cyclic variations that occur over time; one cycle per second is called 1 hertz (Hz). Ultrasound waves have a frequency of oscillation that is higher than 20,000 hertz, placing ultrasound above the audible range for humans. The useful frequency range for medical diagnostic ultrasound is between 1 and 10 megahertz (10 million hertz), although surgical instruments often use carrier frequencies greater than 20 megahertz.

The basic ultrasound system has two principal components. The first, and perhaps more important, component is the transducer, or probe. The transducer converts electrical pulses into mechanical pressure (sound) waves that are transmitted into the tissues. It then detects the echoes that are reflected from the tissues and transforms those echoes into electrical voltages. The second component is the audiovisual electronic component, which processes and displays the reflected echoes in the form of an image of internal organs and structures or an image of the movement of red blood cells.

Ultrasound waves are created when the crystalline material within the transducer is excited by an electrical voltage produced by the instrument's oscillator. The application of an electrical charge causes the crystalline particles to expand and contract, producing mechanical waves and pulses. These pulses of sound pass from the face of the transducer into the body, where they strike the organs, bones, and blood vessels. The reflected echoes in turn strike the face of the transducer, again causing the crystalline particles to vibrate and produce an electrical charge. Such crystalline material is said to have piezoelectric (a combination of the Greek word piesis, meaning "pressure," and the word "electric") properties.

Ultrasound systems commonly employ sound in two modalities. The transducer uses sound waves to create an echo image of body structures. The audiovisual component uses the Doppler shift theory to analyze the range of velocities over which red blood cells are moving.

To create an echo image, millions of pulses of sound must be transmitted into the body each second. For each transmitted pulse, one line of echo information is received by the transducer crystal. To build up an image rapidly and depict the real-time motion of body structures, the pulses are sent into the body from many angles as the sound beam is moved over the body surface. The depth of the echoes is displayed as a function of time, and a two-dimensional image is created by relating the sound's direction of propagation to the direction of the echo-image trace that appears on the instrument's oscilloscope.

The time required for a sound pulse to travel from the transducer to its target within the body, reflect, and return to the transducer can be used to measure the distance to the target, as radar does. In body tissues, sound travels at a speed of 1,540 meters per second. It takes approximately thirteen microseconds for a sound pulse to travel 1 centimeter into the body and return to the transducer. The depth and orientation of echoes may be determined by using this information.

As a sound beam travels through tissues, it is attenuated, or reduced in amplitude and intensity. Attenuation occurs as the energy from the beam is absorbed by the tissues and transformed into heat. Additionally, a part of the beam may be reflected into the surrounding tissues at an angle away from the incident angle or backscattered as the long wavelength of the sound beam strikes the smaller red blood cells. Only a small fraction of the returning echoes reach the face of the transducer.

Because the attenuation of the sound beam increases as the depth of penetration increases, the echoes that return from the deepest part of the image field will be reduced in intensity when compared to the echoes that return from the structures nearer the skin surface. The echo intensity is dependent on the degree of change and impedance of each tissue through which the echo passes, the strength of the incident sound beam, and the degree of attenuation of the beam. To equalize the intensity of the echoes from all depths of the image field, the echoes that travel farthest, and therefore take the longest time to reach the transducer, are amplified over time by using time-gain compensation methods.

For medical imaging applications, the returning echoes may be displayed in several ways. The amplitude mode (A-mode) depicts the returning echoes as deflections on the instrument's oscilloscope; the height of the deflection depends on the strength of the returned signal, and the distance between the deflections depends on the depth of the signal. The brightness mode (B-mode) depicts the strength of the echoes as shades of gray, with the strongest echoes appearing the brightest. The B-mode display makes it possible to differentiate tissue texture characteristics. The time-motion mode depicts movement over time by moving the B-mode trace across the face of a high-persistence oscilloscope, showing the depth, orientation, and strength of echoes with respect to time.

The transducer crystal determines the shape and focus of the sound beam and the frequency of the sound waves, features that are important in resolving echo information into complex images. The beam may be divided into three parts: the near field, the focal zone, and the far field. The beam width, close to the face of the transducer, is equal to the width of the transducer. The beam converges as it travels away from the transducer and then diverges at its narrow focal zone. In order for tissue targets to be resolved into discrete image points, both the lateral and the axial planes of the beam must be narrow. The focusing of the beam is facilitated by placing convex acoustic lenses in front of the transducer crystal to shorten the near field to a narrow focal point, thereby increasing the lateral resolution.

Axial resolution is the ability to distinguish targets along the sound beam. If a single pulse is emitted from the transducer, echo sources lying close together in the axial path of the beam may not be separated. Multiple short bursts of sound are used to separate the echo sources; each echo is captured as a discrete burst. Because axial resolution is inversely proportional to the duration of the ultrasound pulse (and the resonant frequency of the crystal is inversely proportional to its diameter), small-diameter, high-frequency crystals are used to obtain maximum axial resolution.

Ultrasound may be used to determine the velocity of blood flow. This velocity is determined in relation to the frequency of the incident sound beam according to

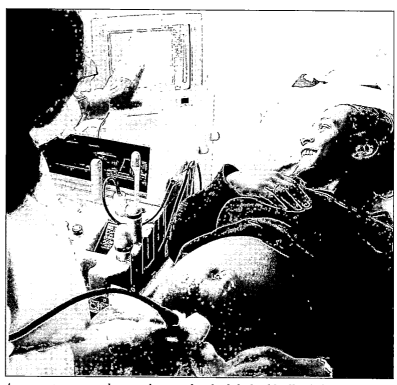

A pregnant woman undergoes ultrasound to check the health of her baby. (PhotoDisc)

the Doppler theory. Several different techniques may be used to process and display the echoes from moving red blood cells. The ultrasound system's computers may be programmed to perform fast Fourier transform analysis, a complex mathematical method for ranking the speed of the echoes returning over time. The signals may be displayed either as spectral tracings of the range of Doppler frequency shifts, represented in the returned echoes recorded throughout the cardiac cycle, or as color-coded Doppler-shifted signals from within the blood vessels, superimposed on a gray-scale image of the surrounding tissues.

USES AND COMPLICATIONS

High-resolution abdominal ultrasonography is a valuable technique for the visualization of intra-abdominal organs and disease processes. For example, liver conditions such as parenchymal abnormalities, abscesses, hematomas, cysts, and cancerous lesions can be identified easily by means of this technique. B-mode and Doppler color-flow imaging are particularly valuable technologies that can be used to evaluate the tissue characteristics and blood flow patterns of transplanted organs. An ultrasound examination of the gallbladder may reveal gallstones, obstruction of the common bile duct, or inflammatory disease. Ultrasound imaging of the pancreas is used to identify pancreatitis, pancreatic pseudocysts, and carcinoma of this organ. An ultrasound examination of the spleen may reveal splenomegaly, or enlargement of the spleen in response to disease or trauma. Additionally, ultrasonography can be used to evaluate splenic volume and to identify hematomas, congenital cysts, infarctions, and tumors within the organ. The technology is particularly well suited for the study of tumors and abscesses within the abdomen. Ascites and other fluid collections may be recognized, and primary tumors and lymph node metastases within the abdominal cavity may be identified by means of pulse-echo imaging.

Ultrasound has certain characteristics that make it particularly valuable for examining the kidneys and the genitourinary tract. The ability to image both native and transplanted kidneys noninvasively from the longitudinal and transverse planes provides additional diagnostic information in uremic patients for whom the injection of contrast agents is undesirable or may fail to provide sufficient information. Urologic ultrasonography may be used to determine renal size and position or to identify cysts and masses, kidney or bladder stones, obstruction of the ureters, and bladder contour.

Transabdominal scanning of the pelvic organs, which is used to determine the presence or absence of suspected lesions, makes possible the precise localization and quantitative mapping of pelvic abdominal masses, facilitating the determination of disease stages and the positioning of radiation ports. The technology is used to differentiate cysts from solid tumors and to determine if pelvic tumors are of uterine, ovarian, or tubal origin.

The sonographic resolution of deep abdominal structures is achieved by internal scanning; endorectal or endovaginal approaches are used to reduce the distance between the transducer and the target organ. During these procedures, the transducer probe either is in direct contact with the genital organs or prostate gland or is separated from them by the thin walls of the bladder or rectum. The information obtained with these techniques is thought to be submacroscopic, observed at approximately twenty to thirty times light magnification.

Ultrasonography plays a major role in the evaluation of obstetrical cases. Ultrasonic imaging is used to study early pregnancy and high-risk cases, as well as to confirm ectopic pregnancy (development of the fetus outside the uterus). In cases of spontaneous abortion, ultrasound procedures are used to indicate whether the fetus and placenta have been retained. Ultrasonography is often used to determine fetal growth rate and placental development and to confirm intrauterine fetal death, threatened abortion, and fetal abnormalities. It is the best method for guiding amniocentesis (the sampling of placental fluids).

Echocardiography, the ultrasound evaluation of the heart, is a reliable and useful tool for the study of patients with congenital and acquired heart disease. The role of cardiac ultrasound in the investigation of cardiac dysfunction, tetralogy of Fallot, transposition of the great vessels, and atrial septal defect has been well defined. Echocardiology is used to detect pericardial effusion; is coupled with Doppler ultrasound to evaluate the pulmonic, mitral, tricuspid, and aortic valves; and is used to investigate primary myocardial disease and atrial tumors. Improved resolution of cardiac structures and patterns of blood flow can be achieved by using endoesophageal (transesophageal) imaging and Doppler color-flow technology.

The vascular system of the body can be studied by combining pulse-echo imaging of the blood vessels and Doppler ultrasound detection of red blood cell movement. This combined technology, known as duplex scanning, not only offers information that is relevant to the anatomy and morphology of blood vessels but also—and this is most important—provides the opportunity to evaluate the dynamics of blood flow and the pathophysiology of vascular disease. Duplex technology is used to demonstrate the presence and characteristics of atherosclerotic disease and to define the severity of vascular compromise resulting from the progression of disease or the presence of blood clots in vessels (thrombosis).

Applications of the technology have been extended to the evaluation of arteries and veins of the extremities, the abdomen, and the brain. Advances in computer technology have made it possible to color-code the Doppler-shifted signals returning from moving red blood cells within the vessels. Doppler color-flow imaging has facilitated the investigation of vascular disorders that result in slow or reduced blood flow (venous thrombosis or preocclusive narrowing of vessels) or that affect the vascularity of organs and tissues (tumors or transplanted organs). Therefore, vascular ultrasonography plays a major role in the evaluation of patients with arterial occlusive disease and those suspected of having thrombosis of the deep or superficial venous systems.

PERSPECTIVE AND PROSPECTS

Ultrasonic techniques have assumed a preferred role in the diagnosis of many diseases and have become an essential component of quality medical care. In contrast to the rapid development and use of X-ray technology in medical diagnosis, the application of diagnostic ultrasound has been relatively slow. Progress depended in large part on the development of high-resolution electronic devices and transducers. Early research into medical applications involved the adaptation of instruments that had been designed for industrial or military purposes.

The first attempts to locate objects with ultrasound probably occurred following the sinking of the *Titanic* in 1912. Improvements in the technology led to the widespread industrial and military use of ultrasound for the detection of flaws in metals, for the determination of range and depth information, and for navigation. The first application of ultrasound to medical diagnosis occurred in 1937, when K. T. Dussik attempted to image the cerebral ventricles by measuring the attenuation of a sound beam transmitted through the head. In 1947, Douglas H. Howry pioneered the ultrasonic imaging of soft tissues and constructed a pulse-echo system that utilized a transducer submerged in water. The system utilized surplus Navy sonar equipment, a high-fidelity recorder power supply, and a metal cattle-watering trough in which the patient and the transducer were immersed.

In the 1960's, Howard Thompson and Kenneth Gottesfeld performed obstetric and gynecologic examinations using the first contact scanner, which had been produced in 1958 by Tom Brown, an engineer, and Ian Donald, a professor of midwifery, at Glasgow University in Scotland. The first commercial scanner marketed in the United States was designed by William L. Wright, an engineer at the University of Colorado.

The two-dimensional scanning system was developed in 1953 by John Reid, an engineer, in cooperation with John Wild, a physician who demonstrated that ultrasound could detect differences between normal tissues, benign tumors, and cancers. The collaboration between medicine and engineering has propelled diagnostic ultrasonography forward at a phenomenal rate of development since that time.

The field of echocardiography was pioneered by Inge Edler, who discovered in the 1950's that echoes from the moving heart could be received and displayed by using a time-motion ultrasonic flow detector. Using this technology, Edler diagnosed mitral stenosis, pericardial effusion, and thrombus in the left atrium.

The use of ultrasound to evaluate blood flow was first described by S. Satomura in 1959. This investigator observed that ultrasound could be transmitted through the skin to derive information about the velocity of blood flow by using the Doppler effect to analyze the reflected signals from the moving blood cells. The first transcutaneous continuous-wave Doppler system was developed at the University of Washington in the 1960's. The instrument was first used to detect fetal life by demonstrating the fetal heartbeat. This application of Doppler ultrasound spurred research under the guidance of Eugene Strandness, Jr., that ultimately led to the development of duplex scanners, instruments that combine pulse-echo imaging with analysis of blood flow patterns derived from the Doppler effect. As a result of the efforts of these early investigators and others, diagnostic medical ultrasonography has evolved into a highly useful tool with diverse clinical applications.

—Marsha M. Neumyer

See also Abdomen; Abdominal disorders; Abscesses; Amniocentesis; Blood vessels; Cholecystitis; Circulation; Echocardiography; Ectopic pregnancy; Embryology; Gallbladder diseases; Heart; Heart disease; Imaging and radiology; Lithotripsy; Noninvasive tests; Obstetrics; Pancreas; Pancreatitis; Pregnancy and gestation; Stone removal; Stones; Tumors; Uterus; Vascular medicine; Vascular system.

FOR FURTHER INFORMATION:

Bates, Jane A. *Abdominal Ultrasound.* 2d ed. New York: Churchill Livingstone/Elsevier, 2004. Offers a wealth of practical clinical information on normal and abnormal anatomy and sonographic techniques.

Bernstein, Eugene F., ed. *Vascular Diagnosis.* 4th ed. St. Louis, Mo.: Mosby, 1993. This bible of noninvasive vascular technology contains chapters written by experts in the field. This important text not only presents updated information on diagnostic vascular ultrasonography but also takes a futuristic look at the clinical applications of this technology.

Griffith, H. Winter. *Complete Guide to Symptoms, Illness, and Surgery.* Revised and updated by Stephen Moore and Kenneth Yoder. 5th ed. New York: Perigee, 2006. Covers more than five hundred diseases and disorders and includes information about causes and risk factors, preventive techniques, diagnostic tests, and surgical treatment.

Hagan, Arthur D., and Anthony N. DeMaria. *Clinical Applications of Two-Dimensional Echocardiography and Cardiac Doppler.* 2d ed. Boston: Little,

Brown, 1989. This exceptional textbook correlates normal and abnormal cardiac anatomy with two-dimensional echocardiography and pathophysiology.

Kremkau, Frederick W. *Diagnostic Ultrasound: Principles and Instruments.* 7th ed. St. Louis, Mo.: Saunders/Elsevier, 2006. A well-organized, programmed text for the student of ultrasound. Each chapter contains easy-to-understand information on the physical principles of ultrasound followed by written, self-assessed review exercises.

Pagana, Kathleen Deska, and Timothy J. Pagana. *Mosby's Diagnostic and Laboratory Test Reference.* 9th ed. St. Louis, Mo.: Mosby/Elsevier, 2009. A clinical handbook that gives alphabetically organized laboratory and diagnostic tests for easy reference. Each listing includes such things as alternate or abbreviated test names, type of test, normal findings, possible critical values, test explanation and related physiology, and potential complications.

UMBILICAL CORD
ANATOMY
ANATOMY OR SYSTEM AFFECTED: Blood vessels, skin
SPECIALTIES AND RELATED FIELDS: Neonatology, perinatology
DEFINITION: The cord connecting the developing fetus to the placenta.

STRUCTURE AND FUNCTIONS
The umbilical cord is composed of a thickened fibrous covering over a gelatinous material that protects three blood vessels. Two umbilical arteries carry blood from the baby to the placenta and coil around the single umbilical vein. Blood containing oxygen and other essential nutrients returns from the placenta through the umbilical cord.

At term, the umbilical cord measures approximately 20 inches. The cord may be short if there is little amniotic fluid and if the baby has a muscular weakness, limiting movement inside the uterus. Umbilical cord lengths of less than 14 inches have a high incidence of traumatic separation and fetal blood loss at the time of a vaginal delivery.

DISORDERS AND DISEASES
Normally, the umbilical cord dries rapidly after birth, with most of its fluid content evaporating in two days. The base of the cord is then colonized by bacteria. An immune system response to the bacteria and chemicals released by white blood cells are required for the final

shedding of the dried cord. The untreated umbilical cord is shed approximately seven to ten days after birth. Any treatment (such as alcohol) used to dry or delay cord bacterial colonization allows the cord to persist for nearly twice as long as in the untreated condition.

Persistence of an umbilical cord beyond three weeks after drying may be caused by a persistent blood supply and may require evaluation by a pediatric surgeon. Conditions that are associated with a persistent cord blood supply include a hemangioma, a connection from an artery in the skin to the vein of the umbilical cord, a small outpouching of the lining of the abdominal cavity, or retained elements of tissue connected to the bladder.

Once the cord has been fully shed, a reactive overgrowth of tissue may occur at the base of the cord. This is termed an umbilical granuloma and is readily managed by the application of silver nitrate, which cauterizes the tissue. There should be no further drainage from the base of the umbilicus beyond six weeks after birth.

During normal embryonic development, the umbilical cord is associated with a portion of two extraembryonic membranes, the yolk sac and the allantois. In late embryonic stages, the umbilical region normally herniates out of the embryo's body wall and is then fully retracted. If part of the herniated bowel is not returned to its normal position, then a connection between the base of the umbilical cord and the small intestine may occur. This is known as a Meckel's diverticulum of the ileum. Similarly, if the allantois does not completely degenerate, then it can leave a connection between the umbilical cord and the top of the bladder, known as a patent urachus. Both conditions are usually easily corrected by surgery.

PERSPECTIVE AND PROSPECTS
Within the last decades, the umbilical cord has taken on new significance as the source of embryonic stem cells. Blood from the umbilical cord taken immediately after the infant has been born can be isolated and cryoprotected for many years. Should the infant (or even individuals who are not perfectly matched immunologically) require new blood stem cells to repopulate the immune system after chemotherapy or radiation therapy, then the cord blood stem cells can be thawed and injected into the recipient. A host of diseases have been successfully treated using cord blood, including many genetic diseases, and thousands of parents have opted to bank their infant's cord blood. The cost of harvesting and maintaining cord blood, however, is a source of controversy. Harvesting and storing cord blood is ex-

pensive, and the chances of an individual spontaneously acquiring a childhood neoplasm or serious genetic disease that would require cord cell therapy is not high. In addition, alternative therapies, such as bone marrow transplants, are sometimes available. On the other hand, parents in which such diseases run in the family may seriously consider cord blood banking.

The hope of stem cell technology in the future lies in the possibility that specific differentiated cell lineages can be stimulated to cure disease and not simply to reconstitute the immune system. For example, diabetic patients might have stem cells in cord blood engineered to produce insulin-secreting cells under appropriate control of circulating glucose concentration. Using the patient's own cord blood to produce such differentiated stem cells would avoid the problem of host-graft rejection.

—*David A. Clark, M.D.;*
updated by Alexander Sandra, M.D.

See also Blood vessels; Childbirth; Childbirth complications; Circulation; Embryology; Hernias; Hypertrophy; Neonatology; Pediatrics; Perinatology; Placenta; Pregnancy and gestation; Stem cells; Uterus; Vascular medicine; Vascular system.

For Further Information:

Cunningham, F. Gary, et al., eds. *Williams Obstetrics.* 23d ed. New York: McGraw-Hill, 2010.

Kurtzberg, J., A. D. Lyerly, and J. Sugarman. "Untying the Gordian Knot: Policies, Practices, and Ethical Issues Related to Banking of Umbilical Cord Blood." *Journal of Clinical Investigation* 115 (October, 2005): 2592-2597.

Moore, Keith L., and T. V. N. Persaud. *The Developing Human.* 8th ed. Philadelphia: Saunders/Elsevier, 2008.

Oppenheimer, Steve B. *Introduction to Embryonic Development.* 4th ed. Upper Saddle River, N.J.: Pearson Education, 2004.

Patten, Bradley M. *Patten's Human Embryology.* Edited by Clark Edward Corliss. Rev. ed. New York: McGraw-Hill, 1982.

Reynolds, Karina, Christoph Lees, and Grainne Mc-Carten. *Pregnancy and Birth: Your Questions Answered.* Rev. ed. New York: DK, 2007.

Simkin, Penny, Janet Whalley, and Ann Keppler. *Pregnancy, Childbirth, and the Newborn: The Complete Guide.* 3d ed. Minnetonka, Minn.: Meadowbrook Press, 2008.

Tsiaras, Alexander, and Barry Werth. *From Conception to Birth: A Life Unfolds.* New York: Doubleday, 2002.

Unconsciousness
Disease/Disorder

Anatomy or system affected: Brain, head, nervous system

Specialties and related fields: Emergency medicine, neurology

Definition: A state in which an individual is unaware of either surroundings or self and lacks response to stimuli.

Causes and Symptoms

Unconsciousness occurs when the mind lacks awareness of that individual's environment and the body does not respond to external stimuli such as light and sound. Sleep can be seen as a common, natural example of such a state, although it can be interrupted easily with sufficient stimuli. Unconsciousness as a medical condition, however, is more profound. It can be caused by a variety of events or situations, including breathing difficulty, shock, drugs, poisons, or electrolyte imbalances. Often, it results from a lack of oxygen to the brain. Other causes include injury, stroke, seizures, brain tumors, or infection. Unconsciousness can range from brief fainting to more prolonged states, such as coma.

Treatment and Therapy

The treatment of unconsciousness depends on the cause. A brief episode may not require medical attention if it was induced by an identifiable external or internal source that no longer presents a danger and the individual did not suffer an injury as a result.

In many cases, however, the cause of a loss of consciousness is not easily diagnosed. In others, any known precipitating factors are clearly dangerous, or such an event may be a symptom of an underlying condition. Therefore, in most cases of unconsciousness, emergency care should be sought. Treatment will depend on cause and duration and may range widely,

---

Information on Unconsciousness

Causes: Trauma, disease, breathing difficulty, shock, drugs, poisons, electrolyte imbalances, stroke, seizures, brain tumors

Symptoms: Lack of awareness of surroundings or self, lack of response to stimuli

Duration: Acute to long-term (coma)

Treatments: Depends on cause; usually emergency care

from cardiopulmonary resuscitation (CPR) at the scene to long-term supportive care in a hospital.

—*Jason Georges and Tracy Irons-Georges*

See also Asphyxiation; Bleeding; Brain; Brain damage; Brain disorders; Choking; Coma; Concussion; Critical care; Critical care, pediatric; Dizziness and fainting; Drowning; Electrical shock; Emergency medicine; Epilepsy; Head and neck disorders; Heart attack; Heat exhaustion and heatstroke; Hypoxia; Intoxication; Resuscitation; Seizures; Shock; Strokes.

FOR FURTHER INFORMATION:

American Academy of Orthopaedic Surgeons. *Emergency Care and Transportation of the Sick and Injured.* Edited by Benjamin Gulli, Les Chatelain, and Chris Stratford. 9th ed. Sudbury, Mass.: Jones and Bartlett, 2005.

American Heart Association. *Heartsaver CPR.* Dallas, Tex.: Author, 2006.

Bledsoe, Bryan E., Robert S. Porter, and Bruce R. Shade. *Brady Paramedic Emergency Care.* 3d ed. Upper Saddle River, N.J.: Brady/Prentice Hall, 1997.

Handal, Kathleen A. *The American Red Cross First Aid and Safety Handbook.* Boston: Little, Brown, 1992.

Krohmer, Jon R., ed. *American College of Emergency Physicians First Aid Manual.* 2d ed. New York: DK, 2004.

Markovchick, Vincent J., and Peter T. Pons, eds. *Emergency Medicine Secrets.* 4th ed. Philadelphia: Mosby/Elsevier, 2006.

UNDESCENDED TESTICLES. *See* TESTICLES, UNDESCENDED.

UPPER EXTREMITIES
ANATOMY

ANATOMY OR SYSTEM AFFECTED: Arms, bones, hands, lymphatic system, muscles, musculoskeletal system, nerves, nervous system, skin

SPECIALTIES AND RELATED FIELDS: Neurology, orthopedics, physical therapy

DEFINITION: The arms (upper arms, forearms, and hands), which are attached to the shoulder blade at the shoulder joint and which consist of muscles, bones, blood vessels, lymph vessels, nerves, skin, and fingernails.

KEY TERMS:

carpus: the wrist

distal: farther away from the base or attached end

elbow: the joint between the upper arm and the forearm

forearm: the region from the elbow joint to the wrist; also called the antebrachium

humerus: the bone that forms the structural beam of the upper arm

proximal: closer to the base or attached end

radial: toward the edge of the forearm and hand containing the radius and thumb

radius: the shorter of the two forearm bones, on the thumb side

ulna: the larger of the two forearm bones, forming the principal part of the elbow joint with the humerus

ulnar: toward the edge of the forearm and hand containing the ulna and little finger

upper arm: the region from the shoulder joint to the elbow joint; also called the brachium

STRUCTURE AND FUNCTIONS

The upper extremities consist of the upper arms, forearms, and hands. Each extremity is attached to the shoulder blade (or scapula) at the shoulder joint. The upper extremity is made mostly of bones and muscles, but it also contains blood vessels, lymphatics, nerves, skin, fingernails, and other associated structures. Important directional terms associated with the upper extremity include proximal (closer to the base or attached end), distal (farther from the base or attached end), radial (on the same side as the radius and the thumb), and ulnar (on the same side as the ulna and the little finger). Along the forearm and hand, the surface bearing the palm is called palmar; the opposite surface is called dorsal.

The bones and muscles of the shoulder provide support structures for the upper extremity. Beyond the shoulder, the major parts of the upper extremity include the upper arm (or brachium), from the shoulder joint to the elbow; the forearm, from the elbow to the wrist; the carpus, or wrist; and the manus, or hand. Beginning with the thumb, the five fingers of the hand are numbered one through five. Digit two is also called the index finger, digit three the middle finger, digit four the ring finger, and digit five the little finger.

Like other parts of the body, the upper extremity is clothed in skin, or integument. The skin covering the armpit (or axilla) has more hair and also more glands (especially the apocrine sweat glands) than most other parts of the body. The palm of the hand is unusual, along with the sole of the foot, in being completely hairless and in having a very thick outermost layer, called the stratum corneum. The ridges on the palm and fingers form individually characteristic patterns called dermatoglyphics, both fingerprints and palm prints.

The Bones of the Hand

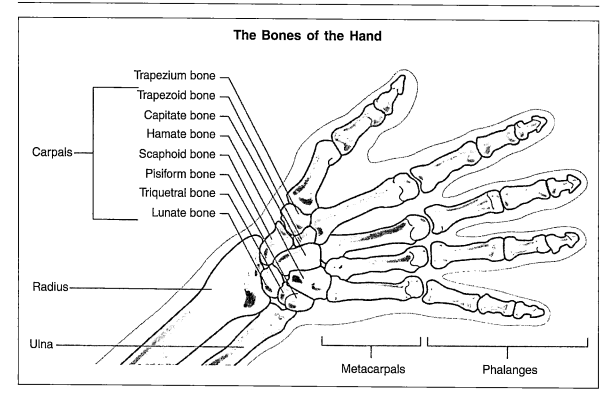

Trapezium bone

Trapezoid bone

Capitate bone

Hamate bone

Carpals

Scaphoid bone

Pisiform bone

Triquetral bone

Lunate bone

Radius

Ulna

Metacarpals

Phalanges

Each finger also has on its dorsal surface a fingernail; the thin crescent of semitransparent skin covering the base of the fingernail is called the eponychium.

The bones of the upper extremity include the scapula, clavicle, humerus, radius, ulna, carpals, metacarpals, and phalanges. The scapula, or shoulder blade, develops as part of the skeleton of the upper extremity and remains more strongly attached to the upper arm than to the trunk of the body. The outer (superficial) surface of the scapula is marked by a ridge called the spine, perpendicular to the scapular blade; the outer tip of this blade is called the acromion. The sculpted area above the spine is called the supraspinous fossa; the larger sculpted area below the spine is called the infraspinous fossa. The flat undersurface of the scapula is the subscapular fossa. The superior border of the scapula is marked by a hooklike coracoid process. At the shoulder joint itself, the scapula has a nearly spherical glenoid cavity into which the head of the humerus fits. The clavicle, or collarbone, runs from the upper end of the sternum (the manubrium) to the edge of the glenoid cavity of the scapula. It strengthens the shoulder region and provides additional support to the upper extremity.

The humerus runs from the shoulder joint to the elbow. At the shoulder joint, it attaches to the scapula by means of a rounded head that fits into the glenoid cavity

of the scapula. The head is flanked by two protruding structures, the greater and lesser tuberosities, to which various muscles attach. At the elbow joint, the humerus attaches to the ulna by means of a pulleylike structure called the trochlea. The humerus also attaches to the radius by a smaller, rounded structure called the capitulum. Areas for muscle attachment on the lower end of the humerus include the lateral epicondyle (on the outer side) and the medial epicondyle (on the inner side).

The forearm contains two bones, the radius and ulna. The ulna is the larger of the two and forms the principal attachment with the humerus by means of a semilunar notch. Part of the ulna extends proximally beyond this semilunar notch to form a projection called the olecranon process (the hard structure on which one rests the elbows). The smaller of the two forearm bones is the radius, which articulates loosely with the humerus and more strongly with the wrist and hand.

The carpus, or wrist, includes two rows of small bones. The proximal row includes (in order from the radial side to the ulnar) the scaphoid, lunate, cuneiform (triquetrum), and pisiform bones. The distal row includes the trapezium, trapezoid, capitate, and hamate bones, also in order from radial to ulnar. The trapezium supports the thumb, the trapezoid supports the index finger, the capitate supports the middle finger, and the hamate supports the two remaining digits. An important ligament called the transverse carpal ligament (or flexor retinaculum) runs across the palmar side of the wrist, forming a tunnel through which the tendons of the flexor muscles run. A similar ligament, the dorsal carpal ligament (or dorsal retinaculum) crosses the back of the wrist, forming a similar tunnel through which the tendons of the extensor muscles run. Beyond the wrist, the palm of the hand is supported by five bones called metacarpals, numbered one through five. The thumb contains two finger bones, or phalanges; each of the remaining fingers contains three phalanges.

The muscles of the upper extremity are divided into extensors (which straighten joints) and flexors (which bend joints). The shoulder muscles attaching the upper extremity to the trunk of the body include the trapezius, pectoralis major, pectoralis minor, deltoideus, coracobrachialis, subscapularis, supraspinatus, infraspinatus, teres major, teres minor, and latissimus dorsi. Of these, the trapezius, deltoideus, and supraspinatus are extensors; the coracobrachialis, latissimus dorsi, and the two pectoralis muscles are flexors; and the remaining muscles are primarily responsible for rotational movements. The trapezius originates from the cervical and thoracic vertebrae, including the adjoining ligaments and the adjacent part of the skull; its fibers converge mostly onto the spine and acromion of the scapula, but some also insert onto the clavicle. The pectoralis major is triangular; it originates from the sternum, costal cartilages, and a portion of the clavicle, from which its fibers converge toward an insertion on the greater tuberosity of the humerus. The pectoralis minor originates from the third through fifth ribs and inserts onto the coracoid process of the scapula. The deltoideus is a triangular muscle that originates from the clavicle and from the spine and acromion of the scapula; its fibers converge to insert by means of a strong tendon onto the shaft of the humerus. The coracobrachialis runs from the coracoid process to an insertion along the shaft of the humerus. The subscapularis originates from the subscapular fossa and inserts onto the lesser tuberosity of the humerus. The supraspinatus originates along the supraspinous fossa and inserts onto the greater tuberosity of the humerus. The infraspinatus originates from the infraspinous fossa and inserts onto the greater tuberosity of the humerus. The teres major and teres minor originate from the lower (inferior) border of the scapula; the teres major inserts onto the lesser tubercle of the humerus, and the teres minor inserts onto the greater tubercle. The latissimus dorsi is a broad, flat muscle that originates from the lower half of the vertebral column (and part of the ilium) by way of a tough tendinous sheet (the lumbar aponeurosis); it inserts high on the humerus.

The major flexors of the upper arm include the biceps brachii and the brachialis. The biceps brachii originates in two heads, one from the coracoid process of the scapula and one from the capsule of the shoulder joint. Both heads insert by means of a strong tendon onto a raised tuberosity of the radius. The brachialis originates from the shaft of the humerus and inserts high on the ulna.

The major extensor of the upper arm is the three-part triceps brachii, but a smaller anconeus and an epitrochlearis are sometimes present as well. The long head of the triceps originates from the scapula just below the armpit; the other two heads originate along the shaft of the humerus. All three heads insert onto the olecranon process by means of a strong tendon. The anconeus (or subanconeus) is not always present; its fibers run directly from the shaft of the humerus to that of the ulna. The epitrochlearis (or dorsoepitrochlearis), also variably present, may be viewed as a connecting band of muscle tissue from the latissimus dorsi onto the triceps brachii.

Flexors of the forearm include the flexor carpi radialis, palmaris longus, flexor carpi ulnaris, pronator teres, flexor digitorum superficialis, flexor digitorum profundus, flexor pollicis longus, and pronator quadratus. Many of these muscles have long, thin tendons that run in the tunnel formed beneath the transverse carpal ligament. The first five of these muscles originate from the medial epicondyle of the humerus. The pronator teres runs at an angle and inserts onto the shaft of the radius. The flexor carpi radialis inserts by a long, thin tendon onto the base of the second metacarpal. The palmaris longus ends in a broad tendon that spreads out over the palm of the hand to form the palmar aponeurosis, a sheet that sends tendinous branches into the fingers. The flexor carpi ulnaris inserts by a tendon onto the pisiform bone; the tendon then continues onto the hamate bone. The flexor digitorum superficialis originates from parts of the radius and ulna as well as the humerus; its strong tendon passes beneath the transverse carpal ligament, then divides into four branches to each of digits two through five. Each of these branches splits and then reunites to allow a tendon of the flexor digitorum to penetrate. The flexor digitorum profundus originates mostly from the shaft of the ulna; it gives rise to four strong tendons that run beneath the transverse carpal ligament, separate from one another over the palm of the hand, run into the second through fifth fingers, penetrate through the openings in the tendons of the flexor digitorum superficialis, and insert onto the base of the terminal phalanx of each finger except the thumb. The flexor pollicis longus arises from the radius alongside the previous muscle; its tendon runs beneath the transverse carpal ligament and inserts onto the base of the distal phalanx of the thumb. The pronator quadratus consists of a muscular sheet running between the distal portions of the radius and ulna.

The more superficial (shallower) extensors of the forearm include the brachioradialis, extensor carpi radialis longus, extensor carpi radialis brevis, extensor carpi ulnaris, extensor digitorum communis, and extensor digiti minimi. The brachioradialis originates from a ridge on the shaft of the humerus and inserts onto the radius at its distal end. The extensor carpi radialis longus originates from the shaft of the humerus; its tendon passes beneath the dorsal carpal ligament to insert near the base of the second metacarpal. The next four muscles originate together from the lateral epicondyle of the humerus. The extensor carpi radialis brevis gives rise to a tendon that passes beneath the dorsal carpal ligament to insert onto the base of the third metacarpal. The extensor carpi ulnaris gives rise to a tendon that passes beneath the dorsal carpal ligament and inserts onto the base of the fifth metacarpal. The extensor digitorum communis gives rise to four tendons that pass beneath the dorsal carpal ligament, then diverge to run into each finger except the thumb, where they each insert onto the base of the second phalanx, the base of the terminal phalanx, and a tendinous sheath covering the first phalanx. The extensor digiti minimi gives rise to a tendon that runs beneath the dorsal carpal ligament and unites over the first phalanx of the fifth finger with the tendon to that digit of the extensor digitorum communis.

The deeper extensors of the forearm include the supinator, abductor pollicis longus, extensor pollicis brevis, extensor pollicis longus, and extensor indicis. The supinator originates mostly from the proximal end of the ulnar shaft, but some of this muscle also originates from the capsule of the elbow joint and from the lateral epicondyle of the humerus. Its fibers spiral toward the midline of the body and insert onto the shaft of the radius. The abductor pollicis longus originates beneath the supinator from the shaft of the radius; it inserts by means of a tendon onto the base of the first metacarpal. The extensor pollicis brevis originates from

the shaft of the radius and inserts by means of a tendon onto the base of the first phalanx of the thumb. The extensor pollicis longus originates from the middle portion of the shaft of the ulna; it gives rise to a tendon which runs beneath the dorsal carpal ligament to insert onto the base of the distal phalanx of the thumb. The extensor indicis arises beside the preceding muscle from the shaft of the ulna; its tendon passes beneath the dorsal carpal ligament and eventually attaches to the tendon going to the index finger from the extensor digitorum communis.

The flexor muscles that are "intrinsic" to the hand— that is, those confined to the hand—include the flexor pollicis brevis, abductor pollicis brevis, adductor pollicis, opponens pollicis, palmaris brevis, flexor digiti minimi, abductor digiti minimi, opponens digiti minimi, the lumbricales, and the interossei. There are no intrinsic extensor muscles in the hand.

The upper extremity can move in various ways. At the shoulder joint, possible movements include extension (or protraction) of the shoulder, which raises the arms; flexion (or retraction) of the shoulder, which lowers the arms; adduction of the arms, bringing them closer together; and abduction of the arms, pulling them farther apart. The two movements possible at the elbow joint are extension (straightening) and flexion (bending). Two special movements are possible within the forearm: Pronation is an inward rotation of the radius upon the ulna in such a way that the palms face downward; supination is an outward rotation of the radius upon the ulna in such a way that the palms face upward. Various movements are possible at the wrist, including flexion (bending), extension (straightening), hyperextension (bending the hand upward), radial abduction (twisting the hand toward the thumb side), and ulnar abduction (twisting the hand toward the little finger side). Movements of the phalanges include flexion (bending), extension (straightening), abduction (spreading the fingers), and adduction (bringing the fingers back together).

Blood vessels of the upper extremity include both arteries and veins. The brachial artery is the major continuation of the subclavian and axillary arteries into the upper arm; as it approaches the elbow, it divides into the radial and ulnar arteries, which supply most of the forearm. Near the wrist, each of these last two arteries divides into a branch that runs closer to the palm and another that runs closer to the back of the hand. The two palmar branches then connect with each other to form a loop called the palmar digital arch; the other two branches also connect, forming a loop called the dorsal digital arch. From these two digital arches arises a secondary digital arch running into each finger, connecting in each case to the palmar arch at one end and to the dorsal arch at the other end. This type of arrangement, called collateral circulation, uses multiple alternate routes to permit blood flow even if one of the routes is temporarily blocked.

There are several important veins draining the upper extremity. Several of these run just beneath the skin: the cephalic vein, running along the radial margin of the forearm and upper arm; the median antebrachial vein, draining the palmar surface of the hand and forearm; and the basilic vein, continuing the median antebrachial vein along the inner side of the upper arm. The deep veins of the arm all drain into the brachial vein. As it flows into the shoulder, the brachial vein joins with the basilic vein to form the axillary vein, which then becomes the subclavian vein when it reaches the rib cage.

The major nerves to the upper extremity arise from a series of complex branchings known as the brachial plexus, originating mostly from the fifth through eighth cervical nerves and the first thoracic nerve. The major nerves of the brachial plexus are a lateral cord (formed from branches of the fifth, sixth, and seventh cervical nerves), a medial cord (formed from branches of the last cervical and first thoracic nerves), and a posterior cord (formed from branches of the sixth, seventh, and eighth cervical nerves). The major nerves of the arm include a musculocutaneous nerve arising from the lateral cord, an axillary nerve and a radial nerve arising from the posterior cord, an ulnar nerve and a medial antebrachial cutaneous nerve arising from the medial cord, and a median nerve arising from both the lateral and the medial cords. The musculocutaneous, ulnar, and median nerves constitute the main nerve supply to the flexor muscles of the arm and hand, while the axillary nerve supplies the deltoid muscle and the radial nerve supplies the remaining extensor muscles. In addition, the radial nerve supplies sensory branches to the skin of the dorsal side of the forearm and hand (except for the fifth finger and part of the fourth), while the musculocutaneous and medial antebrachial cutaneous nerves supply sensory branches to the skin over the palmar or flexor side of the arm and forearm. The median nerve sends sensory branches to the skin over most of the palmar surface of the hand from the thumb up to the middle of the fourth finger, while the ulnar nerve sends sensory branches to the skin on both the palmar and dorsal sides of the fifth finger and the ulnar half of the

fourth. At the elbow, the ulnar nerve passes around the olecranon process just under the skin, where it is easily subject to accidental pressure; the tingling that results from such pressure is the source of the term "funny bone."

Disorders and Diseases

Many types of medical conditions and disorders can affect the upper extremities. For example, many types of contact dermatitis, from poison ivy to "dishpan hands," are first noticed on the surface of the hands and forearms. Other medical problems of the upper extremity include animal bites, injuries, and an assortment of neuromuscular disorders.

Neuromuscular disorders involving the upper extremity include nerve paralyses, uncontrolled shaking (choreic) movements, muscular atrophies, and muscular dystrophies. Nerve paralyses may arise from traumatic injury, but the most common type of paralysis is cerebral palsy. Cerebral palsy is actually a group of paralytic disorders that begin at birth or in early childhood. The extent of the paralysis may vary, often involving large groups of muscles while sparing others. In addition to the lack of muscular control of the limbs, other symptoms may include spasms, athetoid (slow, rhythmic, and wormlike) movements, or muscular rigidity. Some types of cerebral palsy may result from injuries received at birth or in early infancy.

Uncontrolled, purposeless, and irregular shaking movements of the extremities are called choreic movements. These disorders, which involve the upper extremities more often than the lower, include both Sydenham's chorea and Huntington's chorea. Sydenham's chorea (true chorea) typically begins in children and young adults, with maximum disability occurring two to three weeks after symptoms begin. Choreic symptoms typically diminish and disappear in a few months, but they may recur at a later time. The movements can be controlled with drugs. Huntington's chorea, also called Huntington's disease, seldom begins before the age of forty. It typically begins with uncontrolled choreic movements of the hands. The disease progressively worsens and ultimately causes death about fifteen years after onset. The disease is caused by a single dominant gene.

Muscular atrophies are a variety of diseases in which muscle tissues become progressively weaker and smaller, usually beginning between forty and sixty years of age. Spastic movements may sometimes occur. The small muscles of the hands are usually affected sooner and more severely in comparison to the large muscles of the arms and shoulders. Amyotrophic lateral sclerosis (ALS), commonly called Lou Gehrig's disease, is a progressive muscular atrophy that usually begins with weakness and deterioration of the hand muscles. The disease proceeds to affect the rest of the extremities, then other parts of the body; it is usually fatal within three to five years after onset. A more rare type of atrophy, myelopathic muscular atrophy (or Aran-Duchenne atrophy), also begins in the small hand muscles and slowly spreads to the arms, shoulders, and trunk muscles, in that order. A degenerative lesion of the gray matter in the cervical region of the spinal cord is usually responsible. Weakness and wasting of the muscles of the hands and forearms also characterize syringomyelia, a disorder of the glial cells in the cervical region of the spinal cord. Impairment of the cutaneous senses often occurs with this disease and frequently results in burns and other injuries to the hand when the patient, unaware of a threat, fails to withdraw or take other countermeasures.

Muscular dystrophy is an inherited disease—actually several related diseases—that usually begins in early childhood and affects males more often than females. The most common type, Duchenne muscular dystrophy, is believed to be caused by a sex-linked recessive trait. Spastic movements do not occur, and the disease affects the large muscles of the shoulder, arm, and thigh more than the small muscles of the hand. The affected muscles become very weak but remain approximately normal in size or increase as fatty and fibrous tissue replaces muscle. Progressive weakening makes walking impossible, but patients can live for decades with proper care.

Repetitive motion injuries of the upper extremity may occur at the elbow joint (tennis elbow) or in the vicinity of the wrist. Some repetitive wrist movements are capable of producing carpal tunnel syndrome, an injury of the tendons running through the tunnel beneath the transverse carpal ligament.

PERSPECTIVE AND PROSPECTS

The first well-illustrated anatomical texts were produced by Andreas Vesalius (1514-1564); they showed the major muscles and bones of the upper extremities. An accurate medical understanding of the circulatory system began with the studies of the Renaissance physician William Harvey (1578-1657), who examined the veins in the arms of many patients. Harvey noticed the valves in the veins and was able to prove that the blood circulates outward from the heart, throughout the body, and then back again to the heart.

Injuries to the arm are generally treated surgically. Whenever possible, broken bones are set in place, immobilized in a cast, and then allowed to heal. Torn muscles (or tendons) must be sewn together, and nerve endings must be placed in their former positions for them to grow back correctly. If the whole hand is severed at the wrist, many tendons and blood vessels must be reattached; such an operation is very difficult. When a portion of the upper extremity must be amputated, the stump is generally covered with a flap of skin. Sometimes an artificial hand is attached to the muscles that are still usable.

—*Eli C. Minkoff, Ph.D.*

See also Amputation; Arthritis; Arthroplasty; Arthroscopy; Bone disorders; Bone grafting; Bones and the skeleton; Carpal tunnel syndrome; Casts and splints; Fracture and dislocation; Fracture repair; Frostbite; Grafts and grafting; Lower extremities; Marfan syndrome; Muscle sprains, spasms, and disorders; Muscles; Nail removal; Orthopedic surgery; Orthopedics; Orthopedics, pediatric; Osteopathic medicine; Prostheses; Rheumatoid arthritis; Rheumatology; Warts; Wounds.

FOR FURTHER INFORMATION:

Agur, Anne M. R., and Arthur F. Dalley. *Grant's Atlas of Anatomy.* 12th ed. Philadelphia: Wolters Kluwer Health/Lippincott Williams & Wilkins, 2009. Includes excellent, detailed illustrations of the human body.

Marieb, Elaine N. *Essentials of Human Anatomy and Physiology.* 9th ed. San Francisco: Pearson/Benjamin Cummings, 2009. This introductory anatomy and physiology textbook, easily accessible to those with little science background, is richly illustrated with diagrams and photographs, which help to illuminate body systems and processes.

Rosse, Cornelius, and Penelope Gaddum-Rosse. *Hollinshead's Textbook of Anatomy.* 5th ed. Philadelphia: Lippincott-Raven, 1997. A thorough, modern, and detailed reference with good descriptions and illustrations.

Standring, Susan, et al., eds. *Gray's Anatomy.* 40th ed. New York: Churchill Livingstone/Elsevier, 2008. A classic, with the most thorough descriptions of anatomical structures. Most of the excellent color illustrations offer considerable, realistic detail, and others provide well-selected highlights.

Uremia

Disease/disorder

Anatomy or system affected: Bladder, blood, circulatory system, heart, kidneys, urinary system

Specialties and related fields: Cardiology, hematology, nephrology, urology

Definition: A condition that occurs when an excess of urea and other waste elements accumulate in the blood as the result of reduced or inadequate kidney function, or both.

Key terms:

amino acids: any of a number of nitrogen-rich compounds used by the body for the production of protein

antihypertensive drugs: medicines designed to reduce and control elevated blood pressure

diuretics: drugs used to increase urination and eliminate wastes from the bloodstream

edema: an abnormal accumulation of watery fluid in the connective tissues, resulting in swelling

hemolytic uremia: a type of uremia that afflicts mostly young children and infants

renal failure: the failure of the kidneys, making it impossible for them to function efficiently

urea: the waste product when proteins and other nitrogen-rich compounds are broken down

Causes and Symptoms

Uremia is a condition that results when the waste products in the blood, notably urea and creatinine, build up in the bloodstream and are not excreted, as would normally be the case by being transported to the liver and subsequently expelled in the urine. In some patients suffering from uremia, a marked reduction or absence of vitamin B_6 is noted. Often, there is inadequate blood supply to the kidneys, especially in cases where hemorrhaging or shock have occurred.

Congestive heart failure may accompany uremia or may be, at least in part, an initial cause of it. Renal azotemia is a disease affecting the kidneys and may lead to kidney failure. Postrenal azotemia occurs when the flow of urine in the area below the kidneys is blocked. This condition may be attributed to several causes, including kidney stones, pregnancy, compressed ureters, enlargement of the prostate, or bladder stones, often associated with gallbladder problems. When the amino acids that the body uses to produce protein get out of control, uremia may result. In such cases, there is usually no underlying kidney

disease, but a heightened resistance to the flow of urine can result in its backing up into the kidneys, which leads to a condition known as hydronephrosis. This condition can lead to dangerous toxicity and, in extreme cases, may prove fatal.

A unique kind of uremia that is found largely in infants and young children is hemolytic uremia. The origins of this disorder are not fully understood, but it appears to result from damage to the red blood cells in the kidneys. Hemolytic uremia is accompanied by excessively high blood pressure. Many specialists in the field believe that the disorder has viral or bacterial origins.

Treatment and Therapy

Patients suffering from uremia sometimes become disoriented and confused. They lose energy and tire easily. They may become nauseated and lose interest in food and in eating. They may also experience some outward manifestations including eruptions on the skin, sores and/or edema in the mouth, and excessive thirst. Medications to deal with nausea and to help the patient return to more normal eating habits are indicated where nausea is a continuing factor.

In relatively mild cases, therapy with vitamin B_6 may partially or wholly eliminate the condition. Patients may also respond well to changes in their diet, strongly reducing the protein content of what they consume. This solution, however, must be adhered to strenuously and continued throughout one's life span unless such treatment as a kidney transplant is successful and permits the patient to experience better health overall.

Extreme cases may require hemodialysis to cleanse the blood of its impurities or may indicate the removal of uric toxins by modified blood separation and absorp-

---

Information on Uremia

Causes: Excessive levels of nitrogen compounds in blood, resulting in decreased cardiac output

Symptoms: Lethargy, pale skin color, deposits of solid uric compounds resembling frost on skin, rapid pulse, markedly acute thirst, dry mouth, edema in mouth, mental confusion, fluctuations in blood pressure, exhaustion, nausea, vomiting

Duration: Indefinite; extreme cases may result in death

Treatments: Dietary changes, hemodialysis, kidney transplantation, diuretics, antihypertensive medication, vitamin B_6 therapy when deficiency exists

tion therapies. Such treatments can make serious inroads on one's normal life because treatment in sixty- to ninety-minute sessions is often indicated three or more times a week. In cases of renal failure, a kidney transplant may offer the most effective long-term solution.

When uremia elevates the blood pressure to dangerous levels, particularly in hemolytic uremia, treatment with antihypertensive medications is essential and is usually successful. Dialysis may be necessary so that impurities can be removed, giving the kidneys a chance to recover.

In such cases, the patient may find it virtually impossible to urinate and what urine is excreted may be streaked with blood. Despite such disturbing manifestations, most patients suffering from hemolytic uremia make a full recovery, often in as little as two weeks.

PERSPECTIVE AND PROSPECTS

Uremia exists in varying degrees, but much of it can be managed successfully and controlled to the point that it appears to be cured. With adequate care during the acute stages of the disorder, some patients recover in anywhere from seven to fifteen days, although they may incur some kidney damage, either temporary or permanent.

Uremia is most dangerous when it is accompanied by acute pancreatitis, as it often is. In cases involving this complication, the prognosis is not encouraging, although with adequate care, the death rate is substantially reduced.

—*R. Baird Shuman, Ph.D.*

See also Dialysis; Diuretics; Edema; End-stage renal disease; Hemolytic uremic syndrome; Incontinence; Kidney disorders; Kidney transplantation; Kidneys; Lithotripsy; Nephrectomy; Nephritis; Nephrology; Nephrology, pediatric; Polycystic kidney disease; Proteinuria; Pyelonephritis; Renal failure; Stone removal; Stones.

FOR FURTHER INFORMATION:

Brenner, Barry M. *Brenner and Rector's The Kidney.* Philadelphia: Saunders/Elsevier, 2008.
Chen, Shuang. *The Guide to Nutrition and Diet for Dialysis Patients.* Coral Springs, Fla.: Metier Books, 2008.
Gennan, F. John. *Medical Management of Kidney and Electrolyte Disorders.* New York: Dekker, 2001.
Massry, Shaùl G., and Richard J. Glassock, eds. *Massry and Glassock's Textbook on Nephrology.* Philadelphia: Lippincott Williams & Wilkins, 2001.
Nissenson, Allan R., and Richard N. Fine, eds. *Dialysis Therapy.* Philadelphia: Hanley and Belfus, 2002.
Tamparo, Carol D. *Diseases of the Human Body.* Philadelphia: Davis, 2000.

URETHRITIS
DISEASE/DISORDER
ANATOMY OR SYSTEM AFFECTED: Bladder, genitals, urinary system
SPECIALTIES AND RELATED FIELDS: Bacteriology, family medicine, internal medicine, urology
DEFINITION: An infection or inflammation of the urethra, which may be caused by infective organisms, ingested irritants, or trauma.

CAUSES AND SYMPTOMS
Urethritis is most often contracted through intercourse with a partner infected with a sexually transmitted disease (STD), particularly gonorrhea and chlamydia. It will usually appear a few days after sex. Urethritis may also be caused by a variety of other organisms, including *Escherichia coli* (*E. coli*) and *Mycoplasma genitalium* bacteria, *Trichomonas vaginalis* protozoa, and herpes simplex viruses. Another source of the disease is irritation of the urethra produced by soaps, lotions, or spermicides. Trauma produced by medical instruments, such as urinary catheters or cystoscopes, can also generate urethritis. Complicated urethritis may be associated with kidney stones, a weak immune system, or malformations of the urinary tract. There are

---

INFORMATION ON URETHRITIS

CAUSES: Infection with STDs, bacteria, protozoa, or viruses; irritation from soaps, lotions, or spermicides; trauma from catheters or cystoscopes; kidney stones; weakened immune system; urinary tract malformations
SYMPTOMS: Burning or pain with urination, frequent urination, chills or fever; pus-filled and cloudy penile discharge in men and vaginal discharge, rectal discomfort, pain or bleeding during intercourse in women
DURATION: One to two weeks with treatment; sometimes recurrent
TREATMENTS: Antibiotics (doxycycline, azithromycin, erythromycin, roxithromycin, tetracycline); increased fluid intake rate (especially cranberry juice)

cases of nonspecific urethritis that have no known cause.

General symptoms for males and females include burning or pain when urinating, unusually frequent urination, and chills or fever. In males, pus and cloudy discharges may come from the penis, and the opening to the penis may stick together from dried-up secretions and may be red, sore, and itchy. In females, vaginal discharge may be present, as well as discomfort in the rectal area and pain or bleeding during sexual intercourse. In some cases, no accompanying symptoms are associated with urethritis.

TREATMENT AND THERAPY

To assess possible bacterial sources of urethritis, urinalysis and urine culture laboratory tests are performed. Abnormal genital discharges and, in some cases, urethral swabs are also examined. If urethritis is diagnosed, then antibiotics are usually administered. The most common ones used are doxycycline, azithromycin, erythromycin, roxithromycin, and tetracycline. Even for cases of nonspecific urethritis, antibiotics have provided an effective treatment. Drinking copious fluids can help dilute bacteria and flush the urinary system. Acupuncture and homeopathic therapies sometimes help relieve the effects of urethritis.

If symptoms of urethritis are present, then the urethra should be rested by abstaining from sexual intercourse and masturbation until medical treatment has been received. When treated quickly and correctly, the symptoms are usually resolved in one to two weeks. Without proper treatment, serious complications might include infection spreading into the bladder or kidneys, as well as transmission of the causative organism to a sexual partner.

When it is not associated with a general urinary tract infection, urethritis is more common in males than females, probably because males have a longer urethra. In some individuals, nonspecific urethritis can have a high recurrence rate. Burning during urination can be reduced by adding a small amount of baking soda to drinking water to reduce the acidity of urine. Cranberry juice contains a compound that prevents bacteria from sticking to the urethra and growing there.

—*Alvin K. Benson, Ph.D.*

See also Bacterial infections; Chlamydia; Cystitis; *E. coli* infection; Genital disorders, female; Genital disorders, male; Gonorrhea; Men's health; Reproductive system; Sexually transmitted diseases (STDs); Trichomoniasis; Urinalysis; Urinary disorders; Urinary system; Urology; Urology, pediatric; Women's health.

FOR FURTHER INFORMATION:

Beers, Mark H., et al., eds. *The Merck Manual of Diagnosis and Therapy.* 18th ed. Whitehouse Station, N.J.: Merck Research Laboratories, 2006.

Kasper, Dennis L., et al., eds. *Harrison's Principles of Internal Medicine.* 16th ed. New York: McGraw-Hill, 2005.

Schmitt, Barton D. *Your Child's Health: The Parents' One-Stop Reference Guide to Symptoms, Emergencies, Common Illnesses, Behavior Problems, Healthy Development.* Rev. ed. New York: Bantam Books, 2005.

URETHROPLASTY. *See* HYPOSPADIAS REPAIR AND URETHROPLASTY.

URINALYSIS

PROCEDURE

ANATOMY OR SYSTEM AFFECTED: Bladder, kidneys, urinary system

SPECIALTIES AND RELATED FIELDS: Biochemistry, microbiology, nephrology, toxicology, urology

DEFINITION: The chemical, microscopic, and/or physical examination of urine.

KEY TERMS:

dipstick: a chemically treated paper strip used for the chemical analysis of urine

ketones: the by-products of fat metabolism; their presence may be indicative of diabetes mellitus

pH: a value that represents the relative acidity or alkalinity of a solution; values below pH 7 are acidic, while values above pH 7 are basic

specific gravity: the density of a solution relative to that of water; abnormal values can be indicative of elevated sugar or protein levels in urine

INDICATIONS AND PROCEDURES

Urinalysis is one of the oldest and most useful of noninvasive clinical tests. In addition to aiding in the diagnosis of urinary tract or kidney disease, the procedure may be applied to the analysis of most metabolic by-products that pass through the kidneys. Thus it may be applied to observations of kidney or liver abnormalities and metabolic diseases such as diabetes mellitus.

For routine analysis, approximately 10 to 15 milliliters of urine are collected in a clean jar, though larger volumes are preferable. Initial examination involves the physical appearance of the urine sample: color, turbidity, and possible odor. Normal urine is generally pale yellow in appearance, though variation from such color is not necessarily abnormal. Bacteria may cause alterations in this color, as can simple by-products of the diet. Normal urine is generally clear, though as with color, turbidity (cloudiness) may be associated with a variety of causes. Fresh urine also has a characteristically mild odor.

The specific gravity of the urine may be analyzed at this time, though the usefulness of this test is limited to those circumstances in which the water intake of the patient is known. Generally, the only specimen of use for this test is one utilizing the first urine output of the day. The pH is most accurately determined using a pH meter, though dipstick pads impregnated with colored pH indicators can be used when frequent (or inconvenient) monitoring is necessary.

Hematuria, the presence of blood in the urine, is never normal, though its detection need not indicate a significant pathology. Hemoglobin may be detected using a dipstick method, with follow-up necessary to determine the specific cause.

The microscopic examination of urine consists of centrifugation of a volume of urine under specified conditions, followed by resuspension of the sediment in a standard volume of liquid. The presence of any blood cells, bacteria, yeast, or other types of sediment can then be determined.

Chemical analysis can be utilized for determination of the presence of a wide variety of chemicals or drugs. Routinely, chemical procedures are used to detect sugar, protein, or by-products of fat metabolism such as ketones. Dipsticks are available for routine analysis.

USES AND COMPLICATIONS

Diagnosis of urinary or metabolic problems cannot necessarily be made from a single abnormal test result, as a variety of factors have a potential impact on test results. Rather, analysis of a combination of tests is often necessary in diagnosis of a problem.

Urinalysis involves the physical, chemical, and microscopic analysis of urine. Physical examination centers on the color, turbidity, and odor of urine. A pink or red color can be indicative of the presence of blood, though microscopic or chemical examination is needed for confirmation. (For example, a red color may simply indicate that the patient recently ate beets.) An increase in turbidity can result from the presence of yeast or mucus, indicating infection, or from diet by-products

such as lipids. Likewise, abnormal odors can result from urinary tract infection (elevated levels of ammonia) or certain metabolic diseases; however, ingestion of asparagus may also result in unusual odors.

Chemical analysis of urine ranges from the determination of pH to the detection of any of a variety of chemicals. On a routine basis, this usually involves examination for sugar, protein, or ketones. Normal urine is usually acid (pH 6), though the patient's diet will often affect such values as well. A high pH may be indicative of urinary tract infection; microscopic detection of microorganisms may be used to confirm this diagnosis.

Small quantities of protein in the urine are normal. Elevated levels of proteinuria, however, can result from kidney disorders, particularly those associated with glomerular damage, or from urinary tract disease. Likewise, small quantities of sugar in the urine are generally of no clinical significance. In the case of diabetes, however, with resultant high levels of glucose in the bloodstream, significant quantities of glucose may be found in the urine. Persons with severe diabetes are unable to remove and utilize glucose from the blood; metabolism in such individuals will switch to the utilization of fat, with resultant breakdown products such as ketones being secreted in the urine. Such products are volatile and may disappear from urine if the sample is not analyzed within sufficient time. Since fat metabolism is employed as a source of energy in the absence of carbohydrates, severe dieting may also result in the excretion of ketones.

PERSPECTIVE AND PROSPECTS

Analysis of urine for diagnosis of disease was among the earliest of medical procedures. Greek physicians at the time of Hippocrates observed the color of urine and its taste. Pouring urine on the ground to see if insects were attracted to it could be used to test for sugar.

Until the mid-twentieth century, chemical tests on urine utilized a variety of liquid reagents. The introduction of dipsticks significantly improved the efficiency of such analysis, in addition to their convenience. The dipstick consists of a thin strip of plastic with a cellulose pad attached. Impregnated in the pad are the chemicals necessary to carry out the specific test. For example, the dipstick used in the analysis of pH contains an indicator that will change color depending on the degree of acidity or alkalinity.

Instrumentation is becoming available that will allow the analysis of a combination of tests simultaneously, much as a blood sample can be analyzed. Either the dipstick or the urine sample itself may be inserted into a machine for urinalysis. For simple home analysis in which only a single test is necessary, commercial production began in the 1980's of analogous materials for detection of urinary chemicals. For example, home pregnancy kits are available, and, in theory, similar kits could be used for the detection of any substance in urine.

—*Richard Adler, Ph.D.*

See also Bladder cancer; Bladder removal; Cystoscopy; Cytology; Cytopathology; Hematuria; Laboratory tests; Noninvasive tests; Pathology; Pregnancy and gestation; Proteinuria; Urethritis; Urinary disorders; Urinary system; Urology; Urology, pediatric.

FOR FURTHER INFORMATION:

Boston Women's Health Collective. *Our Bodies, Ourselves: A New Edition for a New Era.* 35th anniversary ed. New York: Simon & Schuster, 2005. Contains in-depth discussions of topics covered in this article. This book was written by women for women and is one of the best reference works available on this subject for the general reader.

Griffith, H. Winter. *Complete Guide to Symptoms, Illness, and Surgery.* Revised and updated by Stephen Moore and Kenneth Yoder. 5th ed. New York: Perigee, 2006. Covers more than five hundred diseases and disorders and includes information about causes and risk factors, preventive techniques, diagnostic tests, and surgical treatment.

Humes, H. David, et al., eds. *Kelley's Textbook of Internal Medicine.* 4th ed. Philadelphia: Lippincott Williams & Wilkins, 2000. A medical textbook that is particularly useful, with its inclusion of definitions and descriptions of the clinical presentation of the disease, diagnosis, and treatment.

Pagana, Kathleen Deska, and Timothy J. Pagana. *Mosby's Diagnostic and Laboratory Test Reference.* 9th ed. St. Louis, Mo.: Mosby/Elsevier, 2009. A clinical handbook that gives alphabetically organized laboratory and diagnostic tests for easy reference. Each listing includes such things as alternate or abbreviated test names, type of test, normal findings, possible critical values, test explanation and related physiology, and potential complications.

Simon, Harvey. *Staying Well: Your Complete Guide to Disease Prevention.* Boston: Houghton Mifflin, 1992. A description of various diseases, their causes and symptoms. Much of the book deals with methods of prevention, including the importance of proper nutrition and exercise. A portion of the text covers screening for urinary tract infections.

Strasinger, Susan J., and Marjorie Schaub Di Lorenzo. *Urinalysis and Body Fluids.* 5th ed. Philadelphia: F. A. Davis, 2008. A clinical text that covers all aspects of analysis and interpretation of urine and body fluids. Topics include sharp, radioactive, and chemical hazards; renal function; urine specimen handling; and physical, chemical, and microscopic examination of urine.

URINARY DISORDERS

DISEASE/DISORDER

ANATOMY OR SYSTEM AFFECTED: Abdomen, bladder, kidneys, urinary system

SPECIALTIES AND RELATED FIELDS: Gynecology, nephrology, urology

DEFINITION: Diseases or pathologies associated with any organs of urine production or secretion, such as the kidneys, ureters, urinary bladder, and urethra.

KEY TERMS:

bacteriuria: the presence of bacteria in the urine

cystitis: inflammation of the urinary bladder, often characterized by pain and dysuria

dysuria: painful or difficult urination, often the result of urinary tract infection or obstruction

urethra: the tubular structure that drains the urine from the bladder

urethritis: inflammation of the urethra, often characterized by dysuria

urinary bladder: the muscular organ that stores urine to be discharged through the urethra

urinary tract infection: infection involving any organs associated with the urinary system

CAUSES AND SYMPTOMS

Diseases of the urinary tract represent one of the most common forms of infection by microorganisms. In the United States, the prevalence of urinary tract infections is a reflection of both gender and age. By the age of five, bacteriuria is found in approximately 4 to 5 percent of girls, which is about ten times the rate among boys. Infections are far more common among female adolescents and young women than among men, with a yearly prevalence of approximately 20 percent of American women in the age group of sixteen to thirty-five years accounting for approximately six million reported cases each year. The prevalence of infection among both men and women rises sharply among the elderly, often reflecting problems with aging, including enlargement of the prostate in men. Most infections are self-limiting, particularly among the young. If not treated properly, however, such infections have the potential to be more serious.

Normally, urine is free of microbial contamination. The much higher incidence of urinary tract infections in women reflects, to a large degree, the anatomical differences between males and females. In women, the close proximity of the urethra to the rectum permits relatively easy access of intestinal flora to the urinary tract. Not surprisingly, most urinary infections are caused by enteric bacteria. The most common infectious agent, *Escherichia coli*, represents approximately 80 percent of the acquired infections of the urinary tract. Other bacterial genera of importance include *Enterobacter, Klebsiella*, and *Proteus. Proteus* infections may be of particular significance because colonization by that organism may lead to the deposition of urinary calculi (stones). Less often, *Streptococcus faecalis* or *Pseudomonas aeruginosa* may be involved; the latter can be a particular problem because of its high level of drug resistance.

Urinary tract infections usually begin with entry of the organisms into the distal end of the urethra; the migration of microorganisms into the vagina may occur in a similar manner. Most bladder infections result from ascending movement of the microbial agents along the urethra into the urinary bladder. Inflammation of the urethra (urethritis) or urinary bladder (cystitis) results from a combination of microbial colonization and the host's immune response to the infection. Often, such inflammation may be the first symptom of these infections.

Various factors appear to predispose certain individuals to urinary tract infections. Strains of *E. coli* that colonize the urethra appear to have a greater ability to adhere to the surface tissue. In particular, those strains that frequently ascend into the ureters or kidneys often possess unique types of fimbriae (filamentous structures), which promotes adherence to the epithelial cells that line the surface of the urinary tract; this bacterial structure may be of particular importance to the course of the infection, since the flushing action of urinary flow is a mechanism by which the body maintains the sterility of the urinary tract. Likewise, anything with the potential to interrupt micturition (urination), such as the presence of calculi or tumors, may predispose an individual to a urinary tract infection. Enlargement of the prostate gland in older men is a frequent cause of such problems. Among children, congenital abnormalities at the site of ureter entry into the bladder may result in a vesicoureteral reflux, or urine backflow, which may interfere with normal urine flow. Such abnormalities, which are not uncommon, are found in equal numbers among both young boys and girls; they frequently disappear naturally by the time of puberty. Nevertheless, such problems may contribute to infections among those in this age group.

Certain forms of birth control, in addition to the act of intercourse itself, may contribute to urinary infections. The term "honeymoon cystitis" is often applied, reflecting the bacteriuria often found following intercourse. The colonization of *E. coli* may be associated with the use of diaphragms or spermicides. The reasons for this connection are unclear, but both appear to represent an alteration in the normal flora of the periurethral area and vagina.

Clinical manifestations of urinary tract infections vary with age and are often nonspecific. The infiltration of leukocytes (white blood cells), resulting in inflammation, accounts for many of the symptoms. Among children, abdominal pain is often present, accompanied by fever and sometimes vomiting. Among adults, cystitis and urethritis are often accompanied by difficulty in urination (dysuria), including painful urination and frequent urination, particularly in women. A sensation of abdominal heaviness or lower back pain, in addition to low-grade fever, is often observed. The urine may be bloody or turbid, reflecting a mixture of microbial agents and white blood cells. Bacteriuria is detected by the collection of a sample of voided urine and inoculation of an appropriate culture dish; the presence of at least 100,000 colony-forming units per milliliter of sample constitutes "significant bacteriuria."

INFORMATION ON URINARY DISORDERS

CAUSES: May include bacterial infections, catheters, prostate gland enlargement, stones, tumors, STDs, cancer
SYMPTOMS: Depends on cause; may include abdominal pain, fever, vomiting, painful and frequent urination, abdominal heaviness, lower back pain
DURATION: Typically acute
TREATMENTS: Depends on cause; may include antibiotics, surgery, chemotherapy, radiation therapy

Infection of the urinary tract may also result from a variety of sexually transmitted organisms. Chlamydial infections are common in both males and females, and they represent one of the most commonly observed forms of sexually transmitted disease (STD). *Chlamydia trachomatis* causes urethritis in both males and females; though many chlamydial infections are asymptomatic, they can lead to severe complications. Urethritis may also result from other microbial STDs, both viral and bacterial.

The use of catheters, particularly among hospitalized elderly persons, is a frequent cause of urinary infections. An estimated 40 percent of nosocomial (hospital-acquired) infections result from the use of catheters. Despite attempts to maintain sterility through the use of closed, sterile drainage systems, by two weeks after catheterization 50 percent of both men and women have developed a urinary tract infection, and with longer or permanent catheterizations, nearly all persons will develop some degree of infection. In most cases, these infections are inapparent, but such persons remain predisposed to cystitis or urethritis.

The urinary tract is also subject to other disorders, including cancer. The most common form of neoplasm of the urinary tract is bladder cancer. Such cancers tend to be highly aggressive, often occur as multiple growths, and are difficult to cure once metastasis has begun. Approximately two-thirds of cases of bladder cancer are diagnosed in men, perhaps in part a reflection of risk factors. Exposure to both cigarette smoke and carcinogens, particularly those used in the petrochemical industry, has been linked to an increased incidence of bladder cancers. The symptoms of bladder cancer resemble those of urinary tract infections: dysuria, cystitis, and the frequent need to urinate. If the tumor is diagnosed early enough, electrosurgery or resection may be sufficient to remove the lesion. If the tumor has begun to infiltrate the bladder tissue, complete removal of the bladder may be necessary. Radiation and chemotherapy are also commonly used in the treatment of certain forms of urinary tract cancers.

TREATMENT AND THERAPY

Standard treatment for urinary tract infections consists of a regimen of antimicrobial drugs. Ideally, the antibiotics of choice are secreted in the urine over a prolonged period, rather than achieving high concentrations in the blood serum. In this manner, the drug is directed at the infection itself, with minimal effect on the normal flora elsewhere in the body.

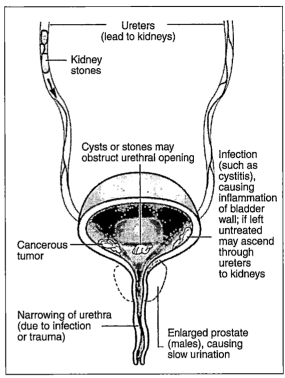

In addition to the variety of infections that may attack the urinary system, urinary disorders may be caused by cancerous tumors, cysts, stones that cause obstruction, reactions to trauma, and in males pressure from an enlarged prostate.

Depending on whether the infection is limited to the lower urinary tract (urethra or bladder) or has spread to the upper tract (ureters or kidneys), the period of regimen may last for several days or up to two weeks. Generally, infections of the upper urinary tract require more prolonged treatment and may be subject to recurrence.

Standard therapy of conventional lower-tract infections routinely consists of a three-day regimen of trimethoprim-sulfamethoxazole (TMP-SMX), or TMP alone. Since most of the drug combination is excreted in the urine, there is a minimum of side effects and little danger to the normal flora within the body. The short duration of treatment also minimizes the chances of encouraging the growth of resistant populations of bacteria. Elderly patients or persons with diabetes mellitus may require longer treatment. If the person shows evidence of upper-tract infection, treatment is generally given over a two-week period.

If there is evidence of kidney involvement or inflammation (pyelonephritis), the patient is often hospitalized in order to monitor treatment, which usually involves a fourteen-day course of TMP-SMX. Severe illness or evidence of spreading may require more intensive therapy with other antibiotics.

Since the flushing action of urine is itself a nonspecific means of removing bacteria from the bladder or urethra, patients are usually advised to drink as much water as possible. In this manner, weakly adherent or nonadherent bacteria may be flushed from the site of infection, reducing the number of bacteria and supplementing the course of antimicrobial therapy. In some cases, this action is sufficient to relieve symptoms or even cure the infection.

In situations in which the infection is asymptomatic, unless the situation warrants treatment (such as impending surgery), antimicrobial therapy may not be necessary, as the infection is self-limiting. Given the large proportion of persons, particularly women, who develop bacteriuria, forgoing therapy may minimize the chances for the artificial selection of resistant strains. In individuals with heart disease, renal failure, or diabetes, however, such therapy may be necessary as a preventive measure for later problems.

Bacteriuria during pregnancy represents a special situation. During early pregnancy, from 4 to 7 percent of women develop bacteriuria, which is probably related to such physiological changes as the dilation of the bladder and uterus, along with vesicoureteral (bladder and urethra) reflux. Even though the infection may be asymptomatic, urinary tract infection is associated with increased risk of both pyelonephritis and loss of the fetus; about one-third of women with untreated bacteriuria during pregnancy develop infections within the upper urinary tract by the third trimester. For this reason, it is generally recommended that pregnant women be screened for such infections and undergo treatment if bacteriuria is present. Pregnant women generally undergo a three-day treatment regimen, though with alternative antibiotics considered safer in the presence of a developing fetus: ampicillin, nitrofurantoin, or cephalexin. Patients should be monitored at intervals during the pregnancy to prevent recurrence. If pyelonephritis should develop, the woman is routinely hospitalized to allow close monitoring of both the mother and the fetus during therapy.

Bacteriuria associated with catheterization is generally treated only when it is symptomatic, since recurrence of the infection is common; long-term treatment presents no advantage and may select for antibiotic-resistant strains. Since the catheter may harbor bacteria, it usually is removed at the start of therapy.

The treatment of sexually transmitted diseases follows much the same pattern. Fortunately, most STDs can be treated or controlled. Both chlamydial infections and gonorrhea are generally treated with doxycycline, a derivative of tetracycline.

PERSPECTIVE AND PROSPECTS

Urinary tract infections are notoriously difficult to prevent. Because in most cases the associated etiological agents are the normal intestinal flora, vaccination or prophylactic use of antibiotics would be impractical. Proper hygiene appears to be the most effective means of prevention among young adults.

STDs can be a source of urinary tract disease. Either a decrease in sexual promiscuity or more effective use of physical barriers (such as condoms) is necessary to reduce the level of such forms of infection. While vaccines against some of the more prevalent forms of STD (gonorrhea, chlamydia) remain a possibility, antibiotic therapy continues to be the most reliable means to treat urinary infections within the individual.

Catheters represent an important source of infection among the elderly, particularly those who are hospitalized. Since a single catheterization results in infection among less than 1 percent of patients, limiting catheterization, or avoiding it entirely, would appear to be the most effective preventive measure. The use of closed drainage systems has also reduced significantly the incidence of such infections. Antiseptic solutions and ointments have had limited success in the prevention of urinary tract infections. The use of antibiotic therapy has been effective in the short term, but over time such therapy may simply select for resistant mutants among the microorganisms. Development of catheters that do not lend themselves to microbial colonization, or that actively inhibit microbial growth (such as silver-impregnated catheters), may reduce the chances of such types of urinary tract infections.

—*Richard Adler, Ph.D.*

See also Abscess drainage; Abscesses; Adrenalectomy; Bed-wetting; Bladder cancer; Bladder removal; Candidiasis; Catheterization; Cystitis; Cystoscopy; Cysts; Dialysis; Diurectics; Endoscopy; Fistula repair; Genital disorders, female; Genital disorders, male; Hematuria; Hemolytic uremic syndrome; Hypertension; Incontinence; Internal medicine; Kidney cancer; Kidney disorders; Kidney transplantation; Kidneys; Laparoscopy; Lithotripsy; Nephrectomy; Nephritis; Nephrology; Nephrology, pediatric; Proteinuria; Pyelonephritis; Renal failure; Reye's syndrome; Sexually transmitted diseases (STDs); Stone removal; Stones;

Ultrasonography; Urethritis; Urinalysis; Urinary system; Urology; Urology, pediatric; Women's health.

FOR FURTHER INFORMATION:

Ammer, Christine. *The New A to Z of Women's Health: A Concise Encyclopedia.* 6th ed. New York: Checkmark Books, 2009. A respected classic that covers the full spectrum of women's health issues, including reproduction, the aging process, methods of contraception, childbearing, herbal medicines, mammography, and advances in infertility research and hormone therapy. Includes helpful charts and illustrations.

Boston Women's Health Collective. *Our Bodies, Ourselves: A New Edition for a New Era.* 35th anniversary ed. New York: Simon & Schuster, 2005. An updated discussion of topics related to women's health. A compendium of material relevant to a wide variety of issues, the book contains a well-written section dealing with urinary tract problems.

Gorbach, Sherwood L., John G. Bartlett, and Neil R. Blacklow, eds. *Infectious Diseases.* 3d ed. Philadelphia: W. B. Saunders, 2004. A textbook dealing with the general topic of infectious disease. The section covering urinary tract infections provides a thorough discussion of the subject. An excellent source for someone interested in such material in depth.

Humes, H. David, et al., eds. *Kelley's Textbook of Internal Medicine.* 4th ed. Philadelphia: Lippincott Williams & Wilkins, 2000. A medical textbook containing a section on urinary tract infections that is thorough in its analysis of the subject. This source is particularly useful, with its inclusion of definitions and descriptions of the clinical presentation of the disease, diagnosis, and treatment.

Parker, James N., and Philip M. Parker, eds. *The Official Patient's Sourcebook on Urinary Tract Infection.* San Diego, Calif.: Icon Health, 2002. Draws from public, academic, government, and peer-reviewed research to provide a wide-ranging handbook for patients with recurring urinary tract infections.

Schrier, Robert W., ed. *Diseases of the Kidney and Urinary Tract.* 8th ed. Philadelphia: Wolters Kluwer Health/Lippincott Williams & Wilkins, 2007. Covers the full range of biochemical, structural, and functional correlations in the kidney, as well as hereditary diseases, urological diseases and neoplasms of the genitourinary tract, and acute renal failure.

Stamm, W. E., and T. M. Hooton. "Current Concepts: Management of Urinary Tract Infections in Adults." *New England Journal of Medicine* 329 (October 28, 1993): 1328-1334. The authors present a moderately detailed overview of the types and management of urinary tract disease. Offers a good synopsis of the most common infectious agents involved. A useful reference for anyone interested in a brief survey of these forms of illness.

URINARY SYSTEM

ANATOMY

ANATOMY OR SYSTEM AFFECTED: Abdomen, bladder, kidneys

SPECIALTIES AND RELATED FIELDS: Nephrology, urology

DEFINITION: A system, composed of the kidneys, ureters, urinary bladder, and urethra, that removes body waste, maintains the proper amount of body water, and regulates the acid-base balance of the blood.

KEY TERMS:

glomerular filtration: the first step in urine formation; passive filtration in which fluids and solids dissolved in the fluid (solutes) are forced through a membrane, resulting in the filtration of the blood

nephron: tiny blood-processing unit located in the kidneys that carries out the processes that form urine; each kidney contains approximately one million nephrons

tubular reabsorption: the process of returning important solutes that were filtered out of the blood back into the blood; these important solutes include glucose, amino acids, vitamins, and most ions

tubular secretion: the process of tubular reabsorption in reverse; important solutes moved from the filtrate to the urine include hydrogen and potassium ions, organic acids, ammonia, and creatine

ureters: slender, expandable tubes that carry urine from the kidney to the urinary bladder

urethra: a muscular tube that transports urine from the urinary bladder out of the body

urinary bladder: a stretchable, muscular sac that functions to store urine

STRUCTURE AND FUNCTIONS

The urinary system consists of two kidneys, two ureters, a urinary bladder, and a urethra. The kidneys function to remove metabolic waste from the blood, maintain proper water balance for the body, and maintain the proper acid-base balance in the blood. The ureters, urinary bladder, and urethra are involved in the moving of the urine formed in the kidneys to the external environment. The kidneys play the major role in the function of the urinary system.

Most people have two kidneys, located at the lower end of the rib cage and lying against the back of the body wall. Typically, the right kidney is positioned a little lower than the left kidney because the right kidney is pushed down by the liver. An adult kidney is about 12.5

The Anatomy of the Urinary System

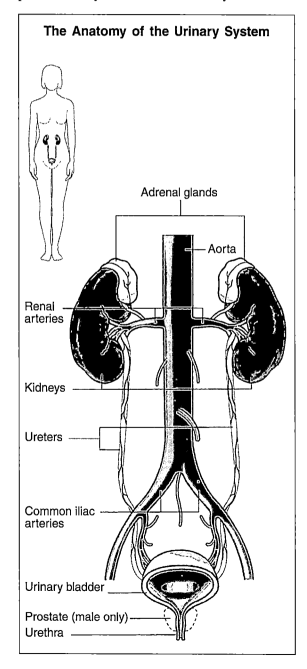

Adrenal glands

Aorta

Renal arteries

Kidneys

Ureters

Common iliac arteries

Urinary bladder

Prostate (male only)

Urethra

centimeters long, 7.5 centimeters wide, and 2.5 centimeters thick and is shaped like a kidney bean. Each kidney is surrounded by a thick layer of fat, which is important for holding the kidneys in their normal body position.

Inside each kidney is a lighter outer region called the renal cortex. Deep in the cortex is a darker layer called the renal medulla. Within the cortex and medulla are found tiny structures called nephrons. Each kidney contains approximately one million nephrons, most of which are in the renal cortex. Nephrons are the functional units of the kidney, carrying out the processes involved in urine formation.

Each nephron consists of two main parts, the glomerulus and the renal tubule. The glomerulus is composed of a knot of capillaries that fit inside the Bowman's capsule, the cup-shaped head of the renal tubule. The rest of the renal tubule is about 2.5 centimeters long. The neck of the renal tubule undergoes a high degree of coiling and twisting just before it makes a hairpin loop. This part of the renal tubule is called the proximal convoluted tubule. The hairpin loop of the renal tubule is termed the loop of Henle. After coming out of this loop, the renal tubule again undergoes a high degree of coiling and twisting and is called the distal convoluted tubule. The distal convoluted tubule then enters another tube, the collecting duct. Surrounding and encasing the renal tubule is the peritubular capillary bed.

Urine formation occurs in the nephron and is the result of three processes: glomerular filtration, tubular reabsorption, and tubular secretion. The glomerulus acts as a filter. This process of glomerular filtration occurs as a result of the capillaries in the glomerulus being somewhat leaky as compared to other capillaries in the body. This process of filtration is a passive process that does not require any metabolic energy. High pressure in the glomerular capillaries causes the formation of a filtrate that consists primarily of blood, except that it lacks the red blood cells and blood proteins. (Both red blood cells and blood proteins are too large to pass through the leaky glomerular capillaries.) The filtrate contains the metabolic waste as well as the many useful substances found in the blood, including glucose, amino acids, vitamins, and water. This filtrate will be continually formed as long as the systemic blood pressure is normal.

The filtrate that is formed is caught in the Bowman's capsule of the renal tubule. From here, the filtrate will pass into the proximal convoluted tubule. Rather than losing the useful substances in the urine, the nephron works to put them back into the blood through the process of tubular reabsorption. Tubular reabsorption begins as soon as the filtrate enters the proximal convoluted tubule. Cells within the tubule take up needed substances from the filtrate and pass them out to the space between the proximal convoluted tubule and the surrounding peritubular capillaries. Once these useful substances are brought into this space, termed the extracellular space, they can be absorbed back into the blood contained within the peritubular capillaries. Some of this reabsorption is passive, not requiring any metabolic energy; water is an example of a substance that is reabsorbed passively. Most substances, however, depend on membrane transporters to carry them out to the extracellular space. These membrane transporters require metabolic energy in the form of adenosine triphosphate (ATP). There are a large number of membrane transporters for those substances that need to be reabsorbed, and few if any transporters for those substances that do not need to be transported. This imbalance helps to explain why substances such as glucose and amino acids are almost completely reabsorbed back into the blood while metabolic waste products such as urea and uric acid are not.

The process of tubular secretion occurs in the loop of Henle and is essentially opposite to that of tubular reabsorption, with substances taken from the blood and put back into the filtrate. Some substances that are secreted from the blood and into the filtrate include hydrogen and potassium ions, ammonium ions, and certain drugs (for example, penicillin). It is the process of tubular secretion that allows the kidneys to remove toxins and drugs from the body, as well as to maintain the acid-base balance of the blood.

The regulation of the volume of urine secreted is controlled by the distal convoluted tubules and the collecting ducts to which they attach. After the filtrate has gone through the proximal convoluted tubules and the loop of Henle, it is fairly concentrated and therefore does not contain a large amount of water. The distal convoluted tubule and collecting duct are impermeable to water when a substance called vasopressin, or antidiuretic hormone (ADH), is present, in which case the filtrate will contain little water and the final urine volume will be small. If ADH is not present, the distal convoluted tubule and collecting ducts become permeable to water and, because the concentration of solutes is higher in the distal convoluted tubule and collecting duct, water enters into these two structures from the

blood. The result is a dilution of the filtrate, with an increased water content and a large volume of urine. The role of ADH in determining urine volume can be seen with the ingestion of alcohol or coffee, both of which inhibit ADH release from the pituitary gland: The distal convoluted tubule and collecting duct become permeable to water, and the urine volume and the frequency of urination increase. It is by this mechanism that the kidneys regulate the body's water balance.

Once the urine is formed in the kidney, it will flow into a tube, the ureter. The ureters, one for each kidney, are passageways that carry urine from the kidney to the urinary bladder. Because the ureters run downward from the kidney, it might seem that the movement of urine to the urinary bladder is created by gravity. In reality, the ureters, which are stretchy and muscular tubes, contract at a rate of one to five times per minute to force the urine toward the bladder, a process termed peristalsis (the same type of contractions that move food through the digestive system). Where the ureters enter the urinary bladder, small, valvelike folds prevent the backflow of urine from the urinary bladder toward the kidneys.

The urinary bladder is a muscular, collapsible sac located in the pelvic cavity. When the bladder is empty, it is only 5.0 to 7.5 centimeters long and its walls are thrown into folds. As urine enters the bladder, it causes the organ to expand. A moderately full bladder is about 12.5 centimeters long and will contain approximately one-half of a liter of urine. A completely full bladder is capable of holding approximately 1 liter of fluid. The kidneys are continually forming urine. Thus, the bladder acts as a temporary storage unit for urine, allowing the individual to empty the bladder when it is convenient.

The urethra is a thin-walled tube that carries urine from the urinary bladder to the exterior of the body. Near where the urethra exits the urinary bladder is a band of smooth muscle that makes up the internal urethral sphincter. This sphincter, which is not under conscious control, acts to keep the urethra shut when urine is not being voided. A second sphincter, the external urethral sphincter, is found farther down the length of the urethra and is composed of skeletal muscle. This sphincter is under voluntary control: When it is not convenient to void the urine, it is this sphincter that is used to prevent urination.

The urge to urinate is brought about by the stretching of the bladder. Ordinarily, the urge to urinate occurs when the bladder contains about 200 milliliters of urine. This amount of urine causes a stretching of the bladder that sends impulses to the spinal cord initiating the contraction of the urinary bladder. The contractions of the urinary bladder force urine past the internal urethral sphincter. It is at this time that a person will feel the need to void the urine, a process termed micturition.

DISORDERS AND DISEASES

Renal and urinary disorders can be categorized based on their mechanism of action and the portion of the urinary system that they affect. These disorders include obstructive disorders that interfere with normal urine flow anywhere within the urinary tract, urinary tract infections, and glomerular disorders, which affect the glomeruli in the kidneys.

Obstructive disorders of the urinary system can be caused by many different factors. Obstruction of the passage of the urine will usually cause a backing up of the urine into the kidney or kidneys. The result is a swelling of the kidney termed hydronephrosis.

Perhaps the most common obstruction is that caused by kidney stones, also referred to as renal calculi. Kidney stones consist of crystallized minerals such as calcium, magnesium, or uric acid salts that form hard stones in the distal end of the collecting ducts. If the stones are small, they will pass through the remainder of the urinary tract. Larger stones, however, get caught in the ureters, thus blocking the passage of urine from the kidneys to the urinary bladder. This blockage usually results in intense pain as the ureters rhythmically contract in an effort to dislodge the stone; this condition is sometimes referred to as renal colic. If the stone does not move from its position of blockage, a buildup of urine in the kidney may occur; if this continues, damage may be done to the kidneys.

Damage to the nerves that innervate the bladder, termed neurogenic bladder, can also result in an obstructive disorder. Damage to these nerves results in the loss of normal control over the voiding of urine from the bladder. Consequently, there is a retention of urine in the bladder since there is no signal telling the bladder to contract.

Tumors of the urinary system may also cause obstruction of urine flow. Another cause of obstruction is the loss of the fat surrounding the kidney. When this occurs, one or both kidneys may drop from their normal position, a condition referred to as renal ptosis. When the kidneys drop, there is a chance that the ureters exiting the kidney may become kinked and prevent the normal flow of urine from the kidneys to the urinary bladder.

Urinary tract infections are usually caused by bacteria and can involve the urethra, ureters, urinary bladder, kidneys, or all the above. Urinary infections in the urethra are termed urethritis and result in the inflammation of the urethra. The two most common bacterial infections involved in urethritis are gonorrhea and chlamydia. Males are more likely than females to have urethritis.

Cystitis refers to any inflammation of the urinary bladder. This condition usually results from bacterial infections, but it may also be caused by tumors or by the presence of stones in the bladder. Cystitis occurs more frequently in women than in men and is characterized by pelvic pain, a frequent urge to urinate, and possibly blood in the urine.

Nephritis is a general term used to describe inflammatory kidney diseases. The inflammation of the nephrons within the kidney is referred to as pyelonephritis. Pyelonephritis is often attributable to bacterial infection but may also be caused by viral infections, tumors, kidney stones, or pregnancy.

Glomerulonephritis is a term that refers to any type of glomerular disorder. It can be further subdivided into two categories: acute glomerulonephritis and chronic glomerulonephritis. Acute glomerulonephritis is the most common form and may be caused by bacterial infection. Chronic glomerulonephritis refers to noninfectious kidney disorders. It commonly occurs when the immune system reacts to and destroys the body's own glomeruli. This type of glomerulonephritis eventually leads to kidney failure. Acute glomerulonephritis, if it is left untreated or it does not respond to treatment, can become chronic glomerulonephritis.

Renal (kidney) failure is simply the inability of the kidneys to form urine. Renal failure can be classified as either acute or chronic. Acute renal failure is the abrupt loss of kidney function, which may result from excessive loss of blood, severe burns, pyelonephritis, glomerulonephritis, or infection or obstruction of the urinary tract. Chronic renal failure is the slow destruction of the nephrons in the kidney. This form of renal failure may result from infections, glomerulonephritis, tumors, obstructive disorders, or autoimmune diseases. Unless the progression of nephron loss is stopped, chronic renal failure will eventually lead to death.

Diabetes insipidus is a disease that does not directly attack the urinary system, but it has a profound effect on the urinary system through its influence on the pituitary gland and the hypothalamus. With diabetes insipidus, the pituitary gland fails to release antidiuretic hormone, as a result of an injury or tumor of the posterior portion of the pituitary gland or hypothalamus. Because of the decreased amount of antidiuretic hormone, large amounts of urine, and thus water, are flushed from the body daily. If left untreated, diabetes insipidus can lead to dehydration and electrolyte imbalances. To offset the loss of water in the urine, individuals with diabetes insipidus must drink large amounts of water.

PERSPECTIVE AND PROSPECTS

The complexity of the human kidney can be characterized by science's inability to build an artificial kidney that is continually functional and can be inserted into the body in the position of the normal kidney. Until the development of tubing that contained miniature holes (dialysis tubing), kidney failure nearly always resulted in death. Dialysis tubing allowed the development of renal dialysis, which cleanses the blood of toxic substances and helps to regulate electrolyte balance. The process of renal dialysis is carried out using a thin membrane that is permeable to only a few select substances. The tubing is immersed in a bathing solution that is very similar to normal blood plasma. As blood circulates through the tubing, toxic substances and some electrolytes move out of the blood and into the bathing solution. This dialysis tubing and the bathing solution are often referred to as an artificial kidney. Dialysis is usually done three times a week, with each session requiring about four to eight hours. Although effective, dialysis is a far cry from the functioning of the human kidney and is no cure for chronic renal failure. When the kidneys are no longer functioning, the only hope is a kidney transplant.

Because the kidneys are so effective at filtering the blood of toxic substances and drugs, the urine formed by the kidney is the principal fluid used for drug testing and drug screening. Furthermore, the kidney also secretes some white blood cells into the urine. As techniques continue to develop, it will be possible to perform genetic tests on these white blood cells to determine genetic traits such as sex and the color of hair and eyes, as well as the possibility of the presence of genetic diseases or personality traits. Such technology could have considerable impact on the future of individual privacy, as many companies and employers require a mandatory analysis of urine, primarily for the presence of drugs in the urine, prior to the possibility of employment. Thus, with a simple urine sample,

the company could know not only the possible drug use of prospective employees but also their genetic makeup.

—*David K. Saunders, Ph.D.*

See also Abdomen; Abdominal disorders; Abscess drainage; Abscesses; Adrenalectomy; Bed-wetting; Bladder cancer; Bladder removal; Candidiasis; Catheterization; Circumcision, male; Cystitis; Cystoscopy; Cysts; Dialysis; Diuretics; *E. coli* infection; Endoscopy; Fistula repair; Fluids and electrolytes; Geriatrics and gerontology; Hematuria; Hemolytic uremic syndrome; Host-defense mechanisms; Hypertension; Incontinence; Internal medicine; Kidney cancer; Kidney disorders; Kidney transplantation; Kidneys; Laparoscopy; Lithotripsy; Nephrectomy; Nephritis; Nephrology; Nephrology, pediatric; Pediatrics; Penile implant surgery; Proteinuria; Pyelonephritis; Renal failure; Reye's syndrome; Schistosomiasis; Stone removal; Stones; Systems and organs; Transplantation; Ultrasonography; Uremia; Urethritis; Urinalysis; Urinary disorders; Urology; Urology, pediatric.

FOR FURTHER INFORMATION:

Greenberg, Arthur, et al., eds. *Primer on Kidney Diseases*. 4th ed. Philadelphia: Saunders/Elsevier, 2005. A publication from the National Kidney Foundation that covers such topics as fluid and electrolyte disorders, hypertension, dialysis, and renal transplantation.

Guyton, Arthur C., and John E. Hall. *Guyton and Hall Textbook of Medical Physiology*. 12th ed. Philadelphia: Saunders/Elsevier, 2011. This textbook gives many examples of diseases and pathological conditions of the urinary system. Does an excellent job of describing how the diseases and pathologies affect the normal function of the urinary system.

Marieb, Elaine N. *Essentials of Human Anatomy and Physiology*. 9th ed. San Francisco: Pearson/Benjamin Cummings, 2009. An excellent book to begin the study of the urinary system. This text is easy to read and understand because it uses little technical jargon and explains the jargon that it does use. Provides good descriptions and drawings of most parts of the urinary system.

Marieb, Elaine N., and Katja Hoehn. *Human Anatomy and Physiology*. 9th ed. San Francisco: Pearson/Benjamin Cummings, 2010. Provides a detailed look at the urinary system and its function. Nevertheless, written in a style that makes the physiology of the urinary system understandable. Also contains illustrations of the urinary system and photographs from described specimens.

O'Callaghan, C. A., and Barry Brenner. *The Kidney at a Glance*. Malden, Mass.: Blackwell Science, 2000. Covers a range of topics related to the kidneys, presenting text on one page and accompanying illustrations on the facing page. Covers basic anatomy and physiology and the pathologies and presentations of renal and urinary tract disease.

Patt, Gail R. *Carola Human Anatomy and Physiology*. 3d ed. New York: McGraw-Hill, 1995. This text provides an easy-to-follow discussion of the urinary system's structure and function. The illustrations are well done, and the book also contains some photographs of parts of the urinary system in cadavers. Uses flowcharts to help explain the physiological functions of the urinary system.

Thibodeau, Gary A., and Kevin T. Patton. *Anatomy and Physiology*. 7th ed. St. Louis, Mo.: Mosby/Elsevier, 2009. Provides understandable and logical descriptions of the functions of the urinary system. Excellent illustrations aid the reader in understanding the discussion in the text.

Urology

Specialty

Anatomy or system affected: Abdomen, bladder, genitals, kidneys, reproductive system, urinary system

Specialties and related fields: Family medicine, gynecology, microbiology, nephrology, obstetrics, proctology

Definition: The branch of medicine that deals with the physiology and disorders of the urinary system (kidneys, ureters, bladder, and urethra) and the male genital tract.

Key terms:

-otomy: combining form meaning an opening or incision in an organ or structure; for example, a ureterotomy is an opening in the ureter

ureter: either of the two tubes that carry urine from the kidneys to the bladder

urethra: the tube that carries urine from the bladder, voiding the liquid from the body

-uria: combining form meaning the presence of a substance in urine; for example, hematuria refers to blood in the urine

urinalysis: the physical, chemical, and microscopic analysis of urine

urinary system assessment: the evaluation of the complete urinary tract, including kidneys, bladder, ureters, and urethra; also includes an analysis of the patient's personal medical history

urine: fluid collected in the kidneys that contains metabolic wastes, including urea and salts

urogram: the injection of a radiopaque substance, followed by X rays of the urinary tract as the substance passes through it

Science and Profession

The urinary system consists of a complex series of structures that includes the kidneys, ureters, urinary bladder, and urethra. Since in males the urinary tract is closely associated with the genital tract, urology properly deals with disorders of the male genitourinary tract and the female urinary tract. Urologists may also study disorders of the adrenal glands, which are closely associated with the kidneys.

Urine production begins in the kidneys, a pair of bean-shaped organs found within the abdomen. Urine is produced through a complex system of units called nephrons; approximately one million nephrons are found within each kidney. Each nephron consists of a ball-shaped capillary network called the glomerulus, which is surrounded by a capsule (Bowman's capsule) through which the actual filtration of blood takes place. Blood enters the glomerulus under high pressure, forcing the liquid and dissolved material through the basement membrane into the renal tubules that extend from the capsule.

The long, convoluted tubule that extends from each capsule follows a circuitous route through the kidney. As it emerges from the capsule, the proximal convoluted tubule is found within the outer region, or cortex, of the kidney. The tubule then passes through the inner portion, or medulla, of the kidney, forming an extended loop called the loop of Henle. The tubule winds its way back to the cortical region as the distal convoluted tubule. Blood circulates completely through the kidneys about twenty times each hour. Approximately 20 percent of the plasma (liquid portion of the blood) is filtered through the Bowman's capsules during this time, the equivalent of some 180 liters of fluid per day. Much of the plasma and nearly all the nutrient material found within the liquid that passes through the tubules are reabsorbed into the capillary network surrounding the tubules. Approximately 80 percent is absorbed within the proximal convoluted tubule, the remainder as it flows through the tubule system. The rest of the fluid, approximately 1 liter per day for the average person, contains nitrogenous material such as urea, salts, and other metabolic wastes, which are voided.

The distal tubules emerge from the cortex of the kidney and again pass into the medulla, where they now merge into increasingly larger collecting ducts. The collecting ducts form clearly visible pyramids, or papillae, within the medulla. The merging of the largest ducts within the renal pelvis, the lowest portion of the kidney, results in the formation of a single tube, the ureter. One ureter emerges from each kidney to empty the urine into the bladder.

The ureters are thick-walled tubes that extend through the pelvic region. They enter the bladder in a slanted manner, which helps prevent backup of the urine from the bladder when it is full. Urine is actually pumped through the ureters by means of peristaltic, or rhythmic, contraction of the smooth muscle that lines the ureters.

The urinary bladder is a membranous organ in the pelvis that serves to store and discharge urine. The bladder is capable of holding approximately one-third to one-half of a liter of liquid in the average individual. When full, it is quite capable of causing the lower abdomen to bulge visibly. Since the structure is adjacent to the uterus in women, conditions such as pregnancy may significantly lower the carrying capacity of the bladder.

The musculature in the lower portion of the bladder is thickened, forming the bladder neck, and serves to retain the liquid within the organ. The muscle, in turn, is continuous with that of the urethra, the tubular structure that drains the urine from the bladder.

In women, the urethra is 3 to 4 centimeters in length and emerges just in front of the vagina. In men, the tube is approximately 20 centimeters long. Emerging from the bladder in the male, it passes through the prostate gland and into the penis, where it serves both for the elimination of urine and as a passage for semen during ejaculation.

Since urine formation begins in the kidney, the branches of medicine that constitute nephrology and urology may overlap each other at times. Strictly speaking, however, nephrology deals with the kidney as a regulatory organ for fluid and salt levels in the body, in addition to its role as an endocrine gland. Urology deals with disorders of the urinary tract, in addition to problems associated with the genitourinary tract in males, since the two systems are so closely associated.

Approximately 20 percent of adult visits to a physi-

cian involve problems associated with the genitourinary tract. Urinalysis—the physical, chemical, and microscopic evaluation of collected urine—thus becomes an important diagnostic tool. The process begins with proper collection of urine into a sterile specimen container. The sample initially undergoes a macroscopic examination in which color and appearance are evaluated. Since recent ingestion of food may result in the discoloration of urine or alteration in its pH, it is best to obtain the sample several hours after the patient has eaten. Generally, the odor is unimportant; for example, by-products of asparagus ingestion may produce a rather characteristic odor in urine that is of no medical significance. Nevertheless, a pungent aroma may signify an infection. Metabolic diseases may also produce by-products that have characteristic smells.

Macroscopic examination of urine also involves a determination of the specific gravity, or density, of the solution, and its pH. Densities outside the normal density range for urine may be indicative of diabetes mellitus or renal dysfunction. The pH is a measurement of hydrogen ion concentration in the fluid. A pH of 7.0 is neutral. Normal levels in urine vary considerably, from an acid level of 4.6 to an alkaline pH of 8.0. Generally, urine samples obtained soon after a meal will be slightly alkaline, but a consistently alkaline level may be indicative of a urinary tract infection. Other macromolecules that may be observed in urine as a result of various pathologies include elevated levels of protein or sugar and the presence of blood (hematuria).

Microscopic analysis of urine is a necessary part of a thorough urinalysis. The urine sample is centrifuged, or spun at high speed, to concentrate material in a smaller volume. The pellet from the centrifugation is stained and observed for bacteria or blood cells. Normally, the number of bacteria and white blood cells in urine is low; indeed, some bacterial contamination of the specimen during collection is common. Large numbers of either, however, may be indicative of an infection. The presence of red blood cells in urine is always considered abnormal and may signify inflammation or bleeding within the urinary system.

DIAGNOSTIC AND TREATMENT TECHNIQUES
A thorough urinary system assessment involving the examination of the kidneys, ureters, bladder, and urethra may be necessary for an accurate diagnosis of certain pathologies. In addition to the normal urinalysis, including the use of a catheter for obtaining a urine sample, the patient's medical history and vital signs are

included in the study. The diagnosis of urinary problems may include procedures for obtaining images of the urinary tract: X rays of the kidneys or urinary tract, as well as excretory or intravenous urography. The latter involves the injection of a radiopaque solution into the system, either of solids containing barium or of gas (such as air), followed by X-ray analysis as the solution passes through the tract. Direct observation through cystoscopy may also be carried out. Methodology developed during the 1980's also includes computed tomography (CT) scanning and magnetic resonance imaging (MRI).

Depending on the problem, treatment may be as simple as the prescription of antibiotics. Urologic surgery becomes necessary if diagnostic procedures reveal a tumor or obstruction. Under these circumstances, direct surgical removal may be necessary. Surgical reconstruction, as well as possible relocations, may be required for certain problems. For example, damage to the urinary system as a result of neurologic or neoplastic (cancerous) conditions may require the diversion of urine through an opening in the abdomen, a ureteroileostomy, instead of through normal channels.

Pathologic conditions of the urinary tract may take a variety of forms, such as obstructions, which interfere with urinary flow, or infections by any of a wide number of bacteria. Either condition may lead to inflammation and subsequent urinary problems. Damage may also result from external forces, such as injuries caused by falling or blunt force.

Urinary obstructions are generally classified on the basis of several characteristics: the etiology or source of the obstruction, the length of time over which the obstruction takes place (acute or chronic), and the site of the obstruction. The source of obstruction may be congenital, often resulting from a stenosis, or narrowing, of the meatus (opening or tunnel) within the urethra. An additional congenital abnormality may result from the inability of the ureterovesical junction, the site at which the ureters enter the bladder, to prevent urine reflux, or backflow, into the ureter. The result of any obstruction is frequently infection, pyelonephritis, within the urinary system. Since any infection may ascend to the kidney, damage can occur at any site in the urinary tract.

Obstructions may result from injury to the urinary tract, from benign or malignant tumors, or from the formation of stones. In addition, in women extension of the uterus during pregnancy may impinge on the ureters, interfering with normal flow.

The obstructions may develop anywhere along the urinary tract. The lower urinary tract consists of the region along the urethra. An obstruction in this region may cause ballooning or dilation of the urethra; in men, this dilation may extend into the prostate gland. The weakening of the urethral wall may result in the formation of diverticula, pouchlike herniations in the muscle wall. If the region becomes infected, a likely possibility, the increased hydrostatic pressure coupled with the weakening of the wall may cause the urethra to rupture.

Midtract obstructions are associated with the bladder. To compensate for increased resistance to urine flow, the muscle of the bladder may initially thicken, sometimes increasing its thickness by a factor of two or three. The increased size in the musculature of the bladder may in turn actually decrease the urine flow from the ureter as a result of the downward pull on these tubes. The resulting backflow may cause damage to the ureters or kidneys.

The increased pressure within the bladder may also force the tissue, or mucosa, between bundles of musculature, resulting in pockets called cellules. Continued pressure may result in larger pockets, or diverticula, being formed within the bladder wall. Since these regions tend to retain urine, infections are common, and surgery may be necessary to remove the diverticula.

Obstructions of the upper urinary tract are associated with the ureters and kidneys. In addition, increased pressure from backflow may cause dilation of the ureter wall, with an increase in muscle development as compensation. This stage is generally followed by one of decompensation, in which the ureters lose their ability to contract and maintain urine flow. Likewise, the kidneys may be subjected to increased pressure. Normally, the pressure from within the urinary tract on the kidneys is very low. When the pressure is increased on the kidney pelvis, the regions in which the collecting ducts form, the pelvis becomes subject to pressure, ultimately having an impact on blood flow. The result is ischemia (lack of oxygen to the region). The kidney itself may atrophy, followed by renal failure.

Generally, obstructions can be visualized through a variety of procedures. Calcified stones within the tract, or tumors, will show on X rays. In addition, an excretory urogram, a technique in which the urinary tract is X-rayed following injection of a radiopaque substance, may reveal the precise site of the obstruction. The urogram is preferred for observation of certain forms of urinary tract stones that may not appear on conventional X rays. The urogram can also be used to observe sites of both dilation and stenosis.

Depending on the source of obstruction, urologic surgery may become necessary for its removal. If kidney function is significantly reduced, temporary or permanent dialysis, even transplantation, may be necessary. On the other hand, temporary urinary diversion may provide relief to the system, allowing natural healing to repair dilated tubes once the obstruction has been removed. For example, ureteroileostomy has been used under such circumstances. With this technique, a portion of the ureter is diverted through an opening, or stoma, in the intestine.

Urinary stones remain the most common cause of obstructions. The formation of stones is related to a variety of causes, including the diet and metabolic state of the patient, genetics, and the anatomic features of the urinary tract. The result is increased deposition of salts such as calcium around an initial foreign body in the urine. Eventual crystallization leads to steady increases in the size of the stone and, unless it is passed naturally within the urine, eventual obstruction. Stones may form anywhere in the tract, but they tend to be less common in the urethra. In general, stones are crystals of either calcium salts or, less often, uric acid.

A variety of techniques exists for the elimination of urinary stones. Stone dissolution, including lithotripsy (the breaking up of the stone with a surgical instrument or shock waves), is preferred, since minimal invasiveness and hospitalization are required. Hemiacidrin, a magnesium-containing solution, has been used successfully in dissolving certain stones. Ultrasonographic lithotripsy, which utilizes ultrasonic vibrations to dissolve the stone, has also been proved successful. Some stones, however, particularly those composed of calcium, may not respond adequately to these forms of treatment. If the obstruction is significant, and particularly if an infection is present, surgical removal may become necessary.

Infections of the urinary tract may be primary (a direct result of contamination) or secondary (the result of other pathological conditions, such as obstructions). Infections may be confined to a single site or may spread to other organs or areas. Since the clinical signs of infection may resemble those of other conditions, recognition of the microbial cause is necessary for proper treatment. In addition, infections that spread to the kidney may cause significant damage or organ failure.

Infections are categorized as being "specific" or "nonspecific." Specific infections are those in which a particular disease is manifested as a result of a particular agent. For example, sexually transmitted diseases (STDs) are specific in the sense that gonorrhea is caused only by *Neisseria gonorrhoeae* and urinary tuberculosis by *Mycobacterium tuberculosis*. Nonspecific infections are diseases in which the pathology or manifestation may be similar but in which the symptoms may be caused by any of a variety of bacteria. For example, common causes of nonspecific urinary infection include *Escherichia coli* (*E. coli*) and members of the genera *Proteus* and *Staphylococcus*.

The most common cause of urinary tract infections is *E. coli*, a natural colon bacillus. Secondary problems may also result from specific agents. For example, members of the genus *Proteus* produce urease, an enzyme capable of splitting urea to form ammonia. The result is a rise in pH, an alkaline condition that may cause precipitation of magnesium or calcium salts and subsequent stone formation.

The specific physical manifestation of the infection is generally related to the site within the urinary tract. Urethritis, accompanied by reduced or painful urination, often results from STDs. Infection may spread as far up as the kidney, with resulting pyelonephritis. Both *E. coli* and STDs are common causes, though other bacteria may also cause similar types of infections. Proper diagnosis of bacterial infections generally requires the isolation and identification of the organism, if possible, and the ruling out of other possible causes of the symptoms (for example, diabetes). The agent may be isolated from pus, from urine, or through the insertion of a needle into the lesion itself. Treatment usually involves antimicrobials (antibiotics) suited to the particular etiological agent. Abscesses, particularly those in the kidney, may require surgical drainage. If the abscess is too large or does not respond to treatment, then nephrectomy (the surgical removal of a kidney) may be necessary.

Damage from external sources may also result in injury to the urinary tract. Depending on the damage, surgical repair or realignment of the urethra, bladder, or ureters may be necessary. Observations through the use of X rays, cystograms, or urethrograms are routinely used for such assessment.

PERSPECTIVE AND PROSPECTS

The understanding of urine formation and excretion had its roots in the work of the Roman physician Galen during the second century C.E. Though observations had been carried out before this period, it remained un-clear whether the source of urine was the kidney or the bladder. Galen settled the issue by tying off the ureters in animals, demonstrating that no urine would be found below the stricture; urine formation began in the kidney.

Urology as a branch of medicine, and indeed clinical interest in urine formation, arguably began in the early decades of the nineteenth century. In 1827, English physician Richard Bright described a form of chronic nephritis, now called Bright's disease, in which pro-gressive kidney failure generally resulted in the death of the individual. Bright demonstrated that as a result of kidney failure, instead of urine being secreted from the body, its constituents are retained in body fluids. It was also in 1827 that German chemist Friedrich Wöhler chemically synthesized urea, the first demonstration of the synthesis of an organic compound from inorganic materials.

Carl Ludwig, beginning in 1844, attempted to ex-plain urine formation on the basis of a purely physical process. Ludwig suggested the hydrostatic pressure of the blood is sufficiently high that a protein-free filtrate is forced through the kidney glomeruli, followed by passage through the tubules, and ultimately into the ureters. The first definitive work on urine secretion was a 1917 monograph, The Secretion of Urine, by Arthur Robertson Cushny. Cushny believed—and he was sub-sequently proved to be essentially correct in this por-tion of his hypothesis—that urine secretion involves both an active and a passive process: mechanical filtra-tion and movement through the urinary tract, and active tubular reabsorption of most nutrients before the liquid leaves the kidney. (The mechanics of Cushny's reab-sorption were less than accurate, however, and were later refined by others.)

The development of noninvasive techniques for the elimination of stones and improved surgical methods for urinary diversion marked much of the progress in urology in the 1970's and 1980's. Extracorporeal shock-wave lithotripsy (ESWL), the use of ultrasonic vibration for the disintegration of stones, eliminated the need for the surgical removal of these obstructions in most cases. The use of ureterosigmoidostomy (im-plantation of the ureter into the intestinal tract) dated to the nineteenth century. It was replaced with alternate methods of bladder augmentation. The ureter itself could be replaced with segments of intestinal ileum, or it could be joined to the other ureter (ureteroureteros-tomy).

—Richard Adler, Ph.D.

See also Abdomen; Bed-wetting; Bladder cancer; Bladder removal; Catheterization; Chlamydia; Circum-cision, male; Cystitis; Cystoscopy; Dialysis; Diuretics; E. coli infection; Endoscopy; Fluids and electrolytes; Gender reassignment surgery; Genital disorders, fe-male; Genital disorders, male; Geriatrics and gerontol-ogy; Gonorrhea; Hematuria; Hemolytic uremic syn-drome; Human papillomavirus (HPV); Hydroceles; Hypospadias repair and urethroplasty; Incontinence; Infertility, male; Kidney cancer; Kidney disorders; Kid-ney transplantation; Kidneys; Laser use in surgery; Lithotripsy; Nephrectomy; Nephritis; Nephrology; Ne-phrology, pediatric; Pediatrics; Pelvic inflammatory disease (PID); Penile implant surgery; Prostate cancer; Prostate gland; Prostate gland removal; Proteinuria; Pyelonephritis; Reproductive system; Schistosomia-sis; Sexual differentiation; Sexual dysfunction; Sexu-ally transmitted diseases (STDs); Sterilization; Stone removal; Stones; Syphilis; Testicular surgery; Trans-plantation; Ultrasonography; Uremia; Urethritis; Uri-nalysis; Urinary disorders; Urinary system; Urology, pediatric; Vasectomy; Warts.

FOR FURTHER INFORMATION:

Chisholm, Geoffrey D., and William R. Fair, eds. Sci-entific Foundations of Urology. 3d ed. Chicago: Year Book Medical, 1990. A detailed description of urol-ogy. Portions of the book are for the specialist, but numerous illustrations make this a useful reference for the layperson.

Gillenwater, Jay Y., et al., eds. Adult and Pediatric Urology. 4th ed. Baltimore: Lippincott Williams & Wilkins, 2002. A clinical set that covers a range of urologic diseases and disorders in adults and chil-dren.

Stamm, W. E., and T. M. Hooton. "Current Concepts: Management of Urinary Tract Infections in Adults." New England Journal of Medicine 329 (October 28, 1993): 1328-1334. This journal article provides a thorough description of the types and management of urinary tract diseases. A clinical review, but much of the material is appropriate for anyone with an in-terest in the subject.

Tanagho, Emil A., and Jack W. McAninich, eds. Smith's General Urology. 17th ed. New York: McGraw-Hill, 2008. An outstanding overview of kidney structure and function.

Wallace, Robert A., Gerald P. Sanders, and Robert J. Ferl. Biology: The Science of Life. 4th ed. New York: HarperCollins, 1996. Contains a nice section on the excretory system. Provides clear illustrations and text that is concise and without clinical details. A good introduction to the subject.

Walsh, Patrick C., et al., eds. *Campbell-Walsh Urology.* 9th ed. 4 vols. Philadelphia: Saunders/Elsevier, 2007. This edition of a classic urology text maintains its encyclopedic approach while following a new organ systems orientation. Halftone illustrations and contributions by multiple authors. Includes a CD-ROM.

UROLOGY, PEDIATRIC
SPECIALTY
ANATOMY OR SYSTEM AFFECTED: Abdomen, bladder, genitals, kidneys, reproductive system, urinary system

SPECIALTIES AND RELATED FIELDS: Microbiology, neonatology, nephrology, pediatrics, urology

DEFINITION: The treatment and/or surgical correction of disorders of the urinary tract and associated sexual organs in infants and children.

KEY TERMS:
congenital defect: an anatomic defect present at birth; it is not necessarily hereditary
renal: pertaining to the kidneys

SCIENCE AND PROFESSION
The pediatric urologist, who is usually a urologic surgeon, has received extra training in urological procedures on infants and children. The full course of training for this type of surgeon requires a medical degree followed by two years of general surgery training. The physician then undergoes four years of urology residency and two additional years of training on pediatric cases.

The urinary system is the group of organs responsible for filtering waste chemicals from the blood and excreting them in the urine. It begins in the back of the mid-abdomen with the two kidneys, left and right. As blood passes through the kidneys, water and chemicals are filtered, concentrated, and collected in the central portion of each kidney. This urine is then transported through the ureters, long, thin tubes that run from each kidney to the bladder in the pelvis. Urine is then eliminated from the body through the urethra, which opens in the female's vulva or at the tip of the male's penis.

The pediatric urologist is particularly skilled in the repair of congenital deformities of the urinary tract and in the long-term management of the urinary disorders of childhood. Defects of the urinary tract may be present congenitally. Rarely, the bladder may develop in a defect of the abdominal wall, appearing inside out at birth. External genitalia that are abnormal in function or appearance may require surgical correction. Males may have an abnormally positioned opening of the urethra. The testes may not be properly positioned in the scrotum. The female urethra may open in an abnormal place, such as the vagina. Such congenital defects may be corrected or improved by urologic surgery.

Many of these abnormalities may lead to frequent urinary tract infections or to backward pressure in the urinary system, eventually damaging the sensitive kidneys. The damage may be severe enough to cause renal failure and the need for dialysis or kidney transplantation.

Urologists are often involved in the evaluation and treatment of recurrent urinary tract infections. Although surgery faded in importance for treating these chronic infections by the 1980's, urologists continue to be important participants in the management of children who have them.

Another pediatric disorder that requires help from the pediatric urologist is neurogenic bladder. The nerves that control bladder sensations and function come from the spinal cord, leaving the spinal canal in its lowest, sacral, region. Spinal cord damage anywhere above this level, because of injury or congenital defects, can result in damage to these nerves. Consequently, the child has no sensation of bladder filling or urination. Also, the muscles of the bladder wall and the sphincter, both of which permit and control urination, develop uncoordinated contractions. As a result, the bladder retains urine between urinations. This urine repeatedly becomes infected, with eventual damage to the bladder, the ureters, and, most important, the kidneys. The pediatric urologist uses a variety of medications and surgical procedures to treat this serious disorder, in an attempt to avoid permanent renal damage.

Family practitioners and pediatricians perform routine circumcisions on newborn males. If routine circumcision is not performed in the first month of life, a pediatric urologist is generally consulted to perform the procedure if it is needed later.

DIAGNOSTIC AND TREATMENT TECHNIQUES
Pediatric urologists usually practice in large cities, often at universities or children's hospitals. Their day typically is divided between the operating room and the clinic. In the clinic, urinary tract disorders are evaluated and treated medically. Surgery is scheduled when it is indicated or when medical treatment fails. The sur-

gical procedures are often quite difficult. Sometimes, multiple procedures are required to remedy a complicated abnormality. The goal is to achieve as near to normal appearance and function of the affected organs as possible.

Common laboratory tests used by the pediatric urologist include complete blood counts, chemistry tests of renal function, and examination of the urine. Urine examination, called urinalysis, involves two steps, which are usually performed by a laboratory technician. First, a plastic strip impregnated with chemicals is dipped in the urine to test for acidity, concentration, sugar, protein, and other compounds. Then, after being concentrated in a centrifuge, the urine specimen is examined microscopically to detect clues of urinary tract disease, such as white and red blood cells, bacteria, and crystals of excreted compounds. If there is suspicion of a urinary tract infection, a small volume of urine is placed on a culture medium to allow the growth of any bacteria that might be present. Normal urine should be sterile. A number of imaging studies, such as renal ultrasonography, bladder X rays, and intravenous pyelography, help assess the urinary tract's anatomy and function.

Pediatric urologists also perform cystoscopy, the examination of the bladder interior with a scope passed through the urethra. Stones of the kidney or bladder, although rare in children, may require removal using the cystoscope or a wire basket passed through it into one of the ureters.

PERSPECTIVE AND PROSPECTS

General urologists have always performed urologic surgery on children. With the increasing technical complexity of many of these procedures, however, the Society for Pediatric Urology was formed in the 1960's to advance the specialty. Pediatric urology fellowships were developed in the 1970's.

A major challenge for the specialty has been to correct congenital anomalies in such a way as to result in normal urinary function and, as an adult, normal sexual function for the patient. Improved techniques, including microsurgery, point to increasing success.

—*Thomas C. Jefferson, M.D.*

See also Abdomen; Bed-wetting; Catheterization; Circumcision, male; Cystitis; Cystoscopy; Dialysis; *E. coli* infection; Endoscopy; Fluids and electrolytes; Hydroceles; Hypospadias repair and urethroplasty; Incontinence; Kidney disorders; Kidney transplantation; Kidneys; Nephrectomy; Nephritis; Nephrology; Nephrology, pediatric; Pediatrics; Pyelonephritis; Re-

productive system; Schistosomiasis; Sexual differentiation; Surgery, pediatric; Testicular surgery; Transplantation; Ultrasonography; Urethritis; Urinalysis; Urinary disorders; Urinary system; Urology.

FOR FURTHER INFORMATION:

Baskin, Laurence S., and Barry A. Kogan, eds. *Handbook of Pediatric Urology.* 2d ed. Philadelphia: Lippincott Williams & Wilkins, 2005. This convenient handbook is an accessible, reliable guide to the diagnosis and treatment of urologic disorders in infants, children, and adolescents. In an outline format that is ideal for quick reference, the book provides complete information on the full range of urologic problems seen in pediatric patients.

Behrman, Richard E., Robert M. Kliegman, and Hal B. Jenson, eds. *Nelson Textbook of Pediatrics.* 18th ed. Philadelphia: Saunders/Elsevier, 2007. Text covering all medical and surgical disorders in children with authoritative information on genetics, endocrinology, etiology, epidemiology, pathology, pathophysiology, clinical manifestations, diagnosis, prevention, treatment, and prognosis.

McMillan, Julia A., et al., eds. *Oski's Pediatrics: Principles and Practice.* 4th ed. Philadelphia: Lippincott Williams & Wilkins, 2006. Contains many good descriptions and illustrations of different stages of development, various disorders common in children, and several treatments for these disorders.

Martin, Richard J., Avroy A. Fanaroff, and Michele C. Walsh, eds. *Fanaroff and Martin's Neonatal-Perinatal Medicine: Diseases of the Fetus and Infant.* 8th ed. 2 vols. Philadelphia: Mosby/Elsevier, 2006. This classic reference work is one of the most comprehensive to date and features discussions on the diverse practice of neonatal-perinatal medicine, pregnancy disorders and their impact on the fetus, delivery room care, provisions for neonatal care, and the development and disorder of organ systems.

Sanghavi, Darshak. *A Map of the Child: A Pediatrician's Tour of the Body.* New York: Henry Holt, 2003. A comprehensive tour of a child's eight vital organs, beginning with the lungs and proceeding through the heart, blood, bones, brain, skin, gonads, and gut. Interspersed with personal stories of children with disorders and afflictions and how medical science was or was not able to intervene.

UTERINE CANCER. *See* CERVICAL, OVARIAN, AND UTERINE CANCERS.

Uterus

ANATOMY

ALSO KNOWN AS: Womb

ANATOMY OR SYSTEM AFFECTED: Genitals, reproductive system

SPECIALTIES AND RELATED FIELDS: Embryology, gynecology, obstetrics, oncology, perinatology

DEFINITION: The organ, located in the pelvis of the female, in which a fetus develops after conception.

STRUCTURE AND FUNCTIONS

The uterus provides a space for a fetus to grow. Situated in the pelvis in front of the rectum and behind the bladder, the uterus is a bulb-shaped pouch about 3 inches (8 centimeters) in length that has heavily muscled walls and is held firmly in place by several ligaments. The uterus has two main parts: the body (corpus) includes the area above the opening to the two Fallopian tubes, while the fundus is the larger area below the Fallopian tubes to the cervix, all positioned at about a ninety-degree angle to the vagina; the cervix is a funnel that connects the body to the vagina. During a woman's reproductive years, the body is about double the size of the cervix, but that proportion reverses after menopause. The thick muscle (myometrium) of the uterus is lined with mucous membrane, the endometrium.

During ovulation, sperm can enter the body through the cervix on its way to fertilize an egg in a Fallopian tube. During menstruation, blood and excess endometrium exit the uterus through the cervix. During gestation, the uterus expands to accommodate the growth of the fetus, and during labor the walls contract to impel the fetus through the cervix and vagina.

DISORDERS AND DISEASES

Among common disorders specific to the uterus are various noncancerous growths. Fibroids are masses of muscle and fibrous tissue, of unknown cause, in the uterine wall that occur in about 20 percent of women more than thirty-five years old. If small, they are seldom noticed, but large fibroids can affect urination and menstruation and cause pain. Adenomyosis involves enlargement of the uterus after glandular tissue obtrudes into the myometrium; it can result in heavy, painful periods, sensations of pressure, and bleeding between periods. Endometriosis occurs when bits of

the endometrium grow outside the uterus, which may produce pain in the lower abdomen or pelvis. The uterus is also subject to abnormal bleeding and vaginitis, inflammation caused by chemical irritants, bacteria, or yeast (candidiasis). Sometimes, because of pregnancy or birth, the uterus sags and protrudes into the vagina, a condition known as prolapsed uterus.

Two cancers in the uterus are among the most common to afflict women. Endometrial cancer grows in the membrane lining the body. It usually develops between the ages of fifty and sixty and has a high cure rate if detected early. Cervical cancer usually develops between the ages of thirty-five and fifty-five, following infection by the human papillomavirus, and is also curable if detected early. Untreated, both penetrate the uterine wall and spread to nearby organs.

—Roger Smith, Ph.D.

See also Abortion; Amenorrhea; Amniocentesis; Assisted reproductive technologies; Cervical, ovarian, and uterine cancers; Cervical procedures; Cesarean section; Childbirth; Childbirth complications; Conception; Culdocentesis; Dysmenorrhea; Ectopic pregnancy; Endometrial biopsy; Endometriosis; Gamete intrafallopian transfer (GIFT); Genital disorders, female; Gynecology; Hysterectomy; In vitro fertilization; Infertility, female; Menopause; Menorrhagia; Menstruation; Miscarriage; Multiple births; Obstetrics; Pap test; Pelvic inflammatory disease (PID); Pregnancy and gestation; Premature birth; Premenstrual syndrome (PMS); Puberty and adolescence; Sexual differentiation; Sexually transmitted diseases (STDs); Sterilization; Stillbirth; Systems and organs; Tubal ligation; Ultrasonography; Women's health.

FOR FURTHER INFORMATION:

Beers, Mark H., ed. *The Merck Manual of Medical Information: Second Home Edition*. Whitehouse Station, N.J.: Merck Research Laboratories, 2003.

Fortner, Kimberley B., ed. *The Johns Hopkins Manual of Gynecology and Obstetrics*. Philadelphia: Lippincott Williams & Wilkins, 2007.

Parker, Steve. *The Human Body Book*. New York: DK Adult, 2001.

Thibodeau, Gary A., and Kevin T. Patton. *Structure and Function of the Human Body*. 13th ed. St. Louis: Mosby/Elsevier, 2008.

VACCINATION. *See* IMMUNIZATION AND VACCINATION.

VAGOTOMY

PROCEDURE

ANATOMY OR SYSTEM AFFECTED: Gastrointestinal system, nerves, nervous system, stomach

SPECIALTIES AND RELATED FIELDS: Gastroenterology, general surgery, neurology, nutrition

DEFINITION: The surgical cutting of the vagus nerve or nerves as part of the treatment for gastric ulcers.

INDICATIONS AND PROCEDURES

The vagus nerves, the longest nerves in the body, pass from the head through the neck, chest, and abdominal regions. They regulate such processes as speech, coughing, swallowing, heart rate, and the hunger sensation. Branches of the vagus nerve also stimulate gastric acid secretions and gastric movements.

Vagotomy is generally carried out in conjunction with treatments for gastric (stomach) and duodenal (intestinal) ulcers. Such peptic ulcers are characterized by the loss of mucous membranes in regions exposed to such stomach secretions as hydrochloric acid and the digestive enzyme pepsin. Mild ulcers may heal on their own, but chronic ulceration may result in significant damage or scarring to the stomach or intestinal wall. In addition to the pain and discomfort associated with an ulcer, under some circumstances the ulcer may become cancerous. While the formation of peptic ulcers is

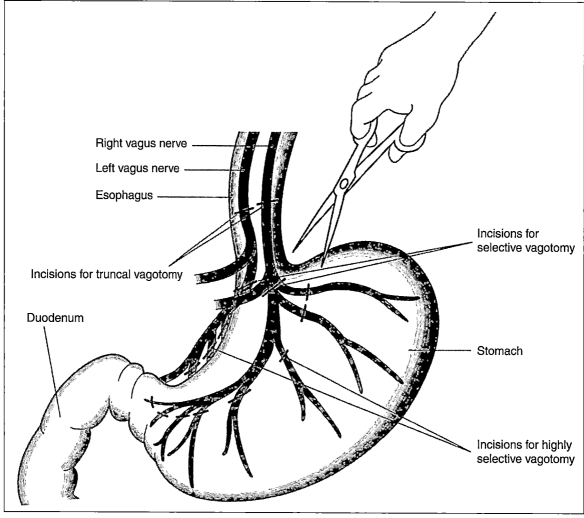

Vagotomy, the severing of the vagus nerve, is a radical treatment for chronic acid reflux, in which gastric juice backs up into the esophagus.

poorly understood, it is known that acid secretion by the stomach can aggravate the condition.

Since the vagus nerve serves to stimulate acid secretions by the parietal cells of the stomach, cutting of the nerve is an effective way to reduce such secretions. Since cutting of the vagus nerve will also reduce or eliminate peristalsis, the rhythmic contraction of muscle that forces food through the stomach, additional procedures are often carried out in combination with vagotomy. For example, an artificial opening between the stomach and small intestine may be created (gastroenterostomy) in order to allow the food to move directly from the stomach to the intestine without the necessity of stomach peristalsis.

The specific region of the vagus nerve on which the vagotomy will be carried out depends on the site of the ulcer. For example, in the case of a duodenal ulcer, the most common form of ulcer, the branch innervating the parietal area of the stomach is severed, reducing the amount of acid produced by the cells in that outer portion of the stomach. Recovery is similar to that for any other general surgical procedure. Medication is provided for pain, and food is reintroduced gradually.

—Richard Adler, Ph.D.

See also Acid reflux disease; Digestion; Enzymes; Gastroenterology; Gastrointestinal disorders; Gastrointestinal system; Nervous system; Neurology; Peristalsis; Sympathectomy; Ulcer surgery; Ulcers; Vagus nerve.

For Further Information:

Abrahams, Peter H., Sandy C. Marks, Jr., and Ralph Hutchings. *McMinn's Color Atlas of Human Anatomy.* 6th ed. St. Louis, Mo.: Mosby/Elsevier, 2008.

Baron, J. H., et al., eds. *Vagotomy in Modern Surgical Practice.* Boston: Butterworths, 1982.

Margolis, Simeon, and Sergey Kantsevoy. *Johns Hopkins White Papers 2002: Digestive Disorders.* New York: Rebus, 2002.

Monroe, Judy. *Coping with Ulcers, Heartburn, and Stress-Related Stomach Disorders.* New York: Rosen, 2000.

Tortora, Gerard J., and Bryan Derrickson. *Principles of Anatomy and Physiology.* 12th ed. Hoboken, N.J.: John Wiley & Sons, 2009.

Zollinger, Robert M., Jr., and Robert M. Zollinger, Sr. *Zollinger's Atlas of Surgical Operations.* 8th ed. New York: McGraw-Hill, 2003.

Vagus nerve

Anatomy

Also known as: Tenth cranial nerve

Anatomy or system affected: Brain, neck, tongue

Specialties and related fields: Gastroenterology, neurology

Definition: The tenth cranial nerve, which starts in the brain stem within the medulla oblongata and sends sensory information about the function or state of the body parts to the central nervous system.

Structure and Function

The vagus nerve is actually two nerves that run from the brain stem and exit from the skull at its base through the jugular foramen and descend the neck through the carotid sheath between the internal carotid artery and the internal jugular vein. The vagus nerve passes not only through the neck and head but also through the chest and abdomen, where it contributes to the innervation of the viscera. The superior laryngeal nerve is the first branch that travels with the superior thyroid artery, whereby this nerve innervates the cricothyroid muscle through its external branch, thus supplying sensation to the supraglottic larynx. The facial nerve, the glossopharyngeal nerve, and the vagus nerve can all recognize flavor. The swallowing reflex is connected to the vagus nerve as well.

Activation of the vagus nerve lowers blood pressure and reduces the heart rate, which typically occurs with gastrointestinal illness (acute cholecystitis or viral gastroenteritis) or in response to other stimuli such as the Valsalva maneuver or pain in having blood drawn.

Disorders and Diseases

The vagus nerve can be tested by a clinician through the gag reflex, usually with a tongue depressor or observing the uvula and the back of the throat when the patient speaks. If anything about these processes is unusual, then further examination of the ninth and tenth cranial nerves is warranted. Some people who suffer from a congenital vagus nerve disorder may have trouble breathing and may need a breathing apparatus or even a pacemaker to keep the heart regular. Fainting can possibly be related to a vagus nerve problem.

A particular disorder related to the vagus nerve is called gastroparesis or delayed gastric emptying, in which the stomach takes a longer time than usual to empty. Basically, the stomach starts its contraction to move food down into the small intestines for the digestion process. This disease occurs when the vagus nerve is damaged whereby the muscles of the intestines and stomach do not function correctly. The food slows down or completely stops in the digestive tract. The most common cause of gastroparesis is diabetes. When the blood sugar is high, a chemical reaction occurs in the nerves that damages blood vessels that carry nutrients and much needed oxygen.

PERSPECTIVE AND PROSPECTS

Vagotomy is the cutting of the vagus nerve to reduce acid buildup to the stomach. Vagotomy is being researched as a less evasive procedure for weight loss than gastric bypass surgery.

—*Marvin Morris, L.Ac., M.P.A.*

See also Blood pressure; Digestion; Dizziness and fainting; Gastroenterology; Gastrointestinal disorders; Gastrointestinal system; Nervous system, Neurology; Otorhinolaryngology; Vagotomy.

FOR FURTHER INFORMATION:

Flint, Paul W., et al., eds. *Cummings Otolaryngology— Head and Neck Surgery.* 5th ed. Philadelphia: Mosby/Elsevier, 2010.

"Motor Speech and Swallowing Disorders." In *Neurology and Clinical Neuroscience,* edited by Anthony H. V. Schapira et al. Philadelphia: Mosby Elsevier, 2007.

"Sarcoidosis of the Nervous System." In *Neurology and General Medicine,* edited by Michael J. Aminoff. 4th ed. Philadelphia: Churchill Livingstone, 2007.

VARICOSE VEIN REMOVAL

PROCEDURE

ANATOMY OR SYSTEM AFFECTED: Blood vessels, circulatory system, legs

SPECIALTIES AND RELATED FIELDS: General surgery, plastic surgery, vascular medicine

DEFINITION: A surgical procedure that is used to rid the body of swollen blood vessels.

INDICATIONS AND PROCEDURES

Varicose veins are caused by an expansion of a superficial vein that is associated with incompetence of the valves within the vein. Conditions such as pregnancy and tumors that increase intra-abdominal pressure contribute to varicose vein formation. Initial treatment involves compression with support stockings.

Sclerotherapy is a more invasive treatment option. In this technique, several injections of a small amount of a solution are made into the affected vessels over an extended period of time. This solution irritates and destroys the inner lining of the blood vessel. The vein subsequently ceases to carry blood, and circulation is improved by the elimination of this diseased blood vessel. Each vessel usually requires one to six treatments at intervals of three to four weeks. Although the procedure is relatively painless, the fading of vessels is a slow process that can take one to six months.

The traditional method of treating varicose veins is surgery, which is usually performed on an outpatient basis. The most common site of varicose veins is in the lower extremities. The varicose veins are marked out on the surface of the leg. The leg is prepared with iodine and draped from the groin to the toes. A local anesthetic is injected in the skin overlying the ends of the varicose veins. A transverse incision is made over each end. The most distant (distal) end is freed, and a suture is tied around the vein. The surgeon must take care to avoid nearby sensory nerves. The near (proximal) end of the vein is similarly located and tied off. The vein is then cut, and a thin wire is passed from the distal to the proximal incision. A bullet-shaped stripper is tied to the wire; the vein is secured to the stripper. The stripper is slowly pulled out, removing the varicose vein. If a branch prevents the vein from moving, an incision is made, a suture is placed around the branch, and the branch is cut.

After the stripper passes through the entire vein, the varicosity has been removed. The path of the vein is then compressed with warm towels for several minutes to stop small branches from bleeding. Other marked branches are removed. The incisions are closed with sutures or tape. Dressings are placed over the path of the vein, and the leg is wrapped from the toe to groin with rolled, soft gauze and elastic bandages. The patient is instructed to walk but not to sit for prolonged periods of time for at least two days.

Several newer and less invasive techniques for treating varicose veins include radio frequency ablation, ambulatory phlebectomy, laser surgery, and intense pulsed light therapy. Radio frequency ablation or closure is a nonsurgical technique that uses heat in the form of radio frequency energy to collapse and seal varicose veins. The problem vein is essentially shut down, and other, healthy veins take over the blood flow. This procedure is much less invasive than vein stripping. In the closure technique, a thin catheter (flexible tube) is inserted into the vein through a small opening. The catheter delivers the radio frequency energy to the

The Stripping of Varicose Veins

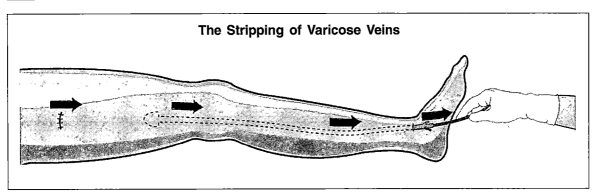

Varicose veins, which are identified by their characteristic swollen appearance, usually occur in the legs; although they are not harmful, many patients wish to have them stripped for cosmetic reasons.

vein wall, causing it to heat up and seal shut. The vein is eliminated by placing the catheter in the lower portion of the vein and then advancing the catheter up the vein using ultrasound guidance. There is no bleeding. After this one-day procedure, patients with little trauma can ambulate more quickly and wear compression dressings for a shorter period of time than in traditional vein stripping.

Ambulatory phlebectomy is a minimally invasive technique in which a varicose vein is removed through small punctures or stab incisions along the path of the vein. Through these tiny holes, the surgeon uses a surgical hook to remove the varicose vein.

In laser surgery, a high intensity laser beam focuses a single wavelength of light at a tiny point on the vein. The light heats the vein but passes through the skin with only minimal surface damage. The underlying vein, however, is damaged by the heat and is then slowly reabsorbed by the body over a period of a few weeks. As opposed to laser surgery, intense pulsed light therapy focuses a broad spectrum of light in a range of wavelengths that are adjustable through the use of filters and computer-guided parameters of energy delivery. This adjustability allows the physician to customize precisely the characteristics of the light energy according to the needs of each patient, thereby minimizing damage to surrounding tissue and reducing recovery time.

USES AND COMPLICATIONS

Nonabsorbable sutures are removed after a week during a postoperative visit to the surgeon; elastic bandages are used for at least two weeks. Medication for pain may be needed for two to four days. The patient is instructed to walk increasing distances over the next few weeks. Patients who walk rarely experience complications.

PERSPECTIVE AND PROSPECTS

The prevention of varicose veins is preferable to surgical removal. Removing excess weight, exercising, and avoiding articles of clothing that constrict the top of the thighs will help. Varicose veins affect men as well as women, although they are more common among the latter.

—*L. Fleming Fallon, Jr., M.D., Ph.D., M.P.H.;*
updated by Genevieve Slomski, Ph.D.

See also Blood vessels; Circulation; Deep vein thrombosis; Laser use in surgery; Lower extremities; Plastic surgery; Varicose veins; Vascular medicine; Vascular system.

FOR FURTHER INFORMATION:

Goldman, Mitchel P., John J. Bergan, and Jean-Jérôme Guex. *Sclerotherapy: Treatment of Varicose and Telangiectatic Leg Veins*. 4th ed. Philadelphia: Mosby/Elsevier, 2007.

Hobbs, J. T. *The Treatment of Venous Disorders: A Comprehensive Review of Current Practice in the Management of Varicose Veins and the Post-thrombotic Syndrome*. Philadelphia: J. B. Lippincott, 1977.

Narins, Rhoda, and Paul Jarrod Frank. *Turn Back the Clock Without Losing Time: Everything You Need to Know About Simple Cosmetic Procedures*. New York: Three Rivers Press, 2002.

Saltin, Bengt, et al., eds. *Exercise and Circulation in Health and Disease*. Champaign, Ill.: Human Kinetics, 2000.

Townsend, Courtney M., Jr., et al., eds. *Sabiston Textbook of Surgery*. 18th ed. Philadelphia: Saunders/Elsevier, 2008.

Weiss, Robert A., Craig Feied, and Margaret A. Weiss, eds. *Vein Diagnosis and Treatment: A Comprehensive Approach*. New York: McGraw-Hill, 2001.

VARICOSE VEINS

DISEASE/DISORDER

ANATOMY OR SYSTEM AFFECTED: Blood vessels, circulatory system

SPECIALTIES AND RELATED FIELDS: Cardiology, plastic surgery, vascular medicine

DEFINITION: The distension of superficial veins, usually affecting the legs and causing the appearance of twisted, swollen, blue veins, especially on the backs of the calves.

CAUSES AND SYMPTOMS

The main task of normal leg veins is to return blood to the heart and lungs. This is difficult because the blood must be pushed upward, against the constant force of gravity. The force that propels the blood up the leg comes from the contraction of the calf muscles surrounding the deep veins that occurs during the act of walking. This forward momentum is quickly lost as gravity pulls the blood back down; however, one-way valves attached to the inside of the vein wall allow blood to pass up the leg freely, then close before the blood can be pulled back down. With each step taken, the column of blood moves up the leg until it eventually reaches the heart.

The system works well until one of the valves fails. Valves may fail because of congenital defect or because of damage from venous thrombosis (blood clots in the veins of the leg). As one ages, long periods of standing or straining eventually cause even normal veins to become stretched out and dilated, causing the valve leaflets to close improperly. When a vein valve does not close correctly, blood leaks backward, placing extra pressure on the valve beneath it. This increased pressure causes the vein to become dilated and twisted. Such veins are said to be "varicose." If this vein is near the skin, it will

---

INFORMATION ON VARICOSE VEINS

CAUSES: Aging process; damage from venous thrombosis; long periods of standing, sitting, or straining; pregnancy; congenital valve or vessel defects; obesity

SYMPTOMS: Twisted, swollen, blue, or bulging veins; achiness or heaviness in legs; swollen feet and legs

DURATION: Short-term to chronic

TREATMENTS: Compression stockings, surgery, sclerotherapy

---

bulge out and become visible. These unsightly veins become more pronounced while standing and disappear or become less noticeable when lying down.

Once damaged, the valve cannot repair itself. The increased pressure continues to damage valve after valve until the small bump eventually becomes a large, bluish rope. Varicose veins are frequently accompanied by an aching sensation or a feeling of heaviness in the legs. These symptoms are aggravated by sitting or standing. People who must be on their feet all day usually experience severe discomfort. As the condition worsens, the legs and feet swell. These symptoms, which are often absent upon arising from bed in the morning, usually become more severe as the day progresses.

Although varicose veins are embarrassing and sometimes painful, they are not always a serious condition. Most people experience only minor inconvenience from them. If allowed to progress, however, varicose veins lead to more serious conditions. One of the most common—and most serious—of these complications is a blood clot within the varicose vein. As long as blood is moving quickly in a vessel, it is very difficult for it to clot. When a vein becomes varicose, the dilated portion of the vein allows blood to pool. If blood stagnates, it can become a solid mass of blood called a thrombus, or a blood clot. This blood clot may continue to grow up the vein. It can fill the entire vein from the foot to the groin and enter the deep veins of the leg.

A clot in a deep vein is a potentially life-threatening condition, as it may break loose, pass through the heart, and lodge in the arteries that take blood to the lungs. This condition is referred to as a pulmonary embolism. If this happens, and the blood clot is small, the patient experiences shortness of breath and chest pain. If the clot that breaks loose is big and lodges in a larger lung artery, it can result in sudden death. Blood clots limited to the superficial veins (near the skin) are far less likely to break loose and result in a major pulmonary embolism. The symptoms of clot in the superficial veins are pain and redness directly over the vein involved. The varicose vein may also become hard. This is called a superficial cord. As the clot grows, the redness, pain, and cord move up the leg. This is a serious condition and requires immediate medical attention.

Other complications associated with varicose veins relate to the impact of having increased venous pressure in the legs over a long period of time. When the valves are working, the pressure in the tissue at the ankle is kept at a low level. When varicose veins are severe, the pressure in the tissue becomes so high that

Varicose Veins

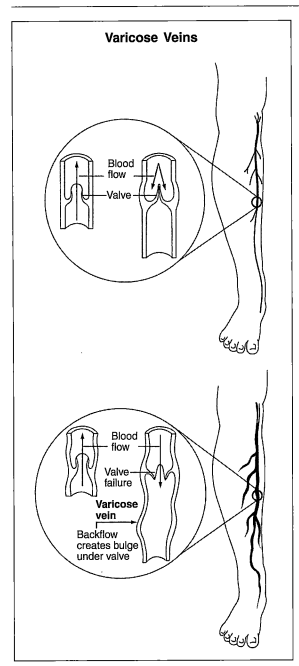

In normal veins, the wings of the valves shut completely, preventing backflow of blood; in varicose veins, backflow creates a bulge in the vein that leads to the characteristic appearance of branched blue veins on the legs.

blood flow to the skin decreases. If this occurs over a long period of time, the skin becomes discolored and hardens. Ultimately, the skin breaks down, and venous ulcers occur. These open, weeping sores can become infected and become a chronic problem.

TREATMENT AND THERAPY

Minor varicose veins are managed quite effectively—if caught early—with well-fitting elastic compression stockings. These place pressure over the superficial veins, giving them support and preventing additional damage to them. This also forces blood into the deep veins. Assuming the deep veins have functioning valves in them, this provides relief and slows progression of the problem. Another popular approach is to surgically remove the damaged vein. This operation, called stripping, removes the veins with damaged valves, forcing blood to go through healthy veins. This can resolve the symptoms of varicose veins altogether. However, other veins may eventually become varicose.

Another intervention to get rid of varicose veins is injection therapy, or sclerotherapy, in which the patient is injected with a material that irritates the varicose vein, causing a clot to form in it. The clot is carefully controlled so that it stays only in the vein being treated. The clot attaches to the vein wall, causing the vein to shrink. This shrinking of the vein makes it seem to disappear. Sclerotherapy is not appropriate in more serious cases of varicose veins.

PERSPECTIVE AND PROSPECTS

Although varicose veins can occur at any time, they are particularly predominant among the elderly; 50 percent of all individuals can expect to develop varicose veins by the age of fifty.

Nothing can be done to change congenital or inherited factors that cause varicose veins. Simple measures, however, can prevent the development of varicose veins before they occur or can slow their progression once they have developed. These preventive measures all have a common theme: avoiding long periods of sitting or standing and keeping the calf muscle active. Doctors advise people who must sit or stand for any length of time to flex and relax their calf muscles by pulling their feet up and pushing them back down. This keeps the blood moving and keeps it from pooling. Other measures include breaking up long periods of inactivity by walking a few minutes every hour, elevating the legs from time to time, and wearing loose clothing that does not restrict blood flow. Some doctors also recommend eating a high-fiber diet since some varicose vein problems result from straining during difficult bowel movements.

—Steven R. Talbot, R.V.T.

See also Blood vessels; Circulation; Deep vein thrombosis; Embolism; Lower extremities; Plastic surgery; Thrombosis and thrombus; Varicose vein removal; Vascular medicine; Vascular system; Venous insufficiency.

FOR FURTHER INFORMATION:
Baron, Howard C., and Barbara A. Ross. *Varicose Veins: A Guide to Prevention and Treatment.* New York: Facts On File, 1997.
Goldman, Lee, and Dennis Ausiello, eds. *Cecil Textbook of Medicine.* 23d ed. Philadelphia: Saunders/Elsevier, 2007.
Kumar, Vinay, et al., eds. *Robbins Basic Pathology.* 8th ed. Philadelphia: Saunders/Elsevier, 2007.
Narins, Rhoda, and Paul Jarrod Frank. *Turn Back the Clock Without Losing Time: Everything You Need to Know About Simple Cosmetic Procedures.* New York: Three Rivers Press, 2002.
Townsend, Courtney M., Jr., et al., eds. *Sabiston Textbook of Surgery.* 18th ed. Philadelphia: Saunders/Elsevier, 2008.
Weiss, Robert A., Craig Feied, and Margaret A. Weiss, eds. *Vein Diagnosis and Treatment: A Comprehensive Approach.* New York: McGraw-Hill, 2001.

VAS DEFERENS

ANATOMY

ALSO KNOWN AS: Ductus deferens

ANATOMY OR SYSTEM AFFECTED: Genitals, reproductive system

SPECIALTIES AND RELATED FIELDS: Urology

DEFINITION: The tube that conveys sperm from the epididymis to the urethra in the male reproductive system.

STRUCTURE AND FUNCTIONS

In the male reproductive system, the testes make sperm, which is then stored in an adjacent structure, the epididymis. The epididymis is connected to the urethra via the vas deferens (plural, vasa deferens), a smooth tube about 18 inches (45 centimeters) in length with thick, muscular walls that forms part of the spermatic cord along with various nerves, muscles, and blood vessels.

A male has two vasa deferens. From the epididymis by each testes a vas deferens leads up into the abdominal cavity through the inguinal canal (a passageway through the groin). It curves around behind the bladder and, via an enlargement called the ampulla, merges with the seminal vesicle near the base of the bladder.

From there it passes through the prostate gland into the urethra.

During sexual intercourse, the walls of the vas deferens contract to move sperm out of the epididymis. The sperm collects seminal fluids from the seminal vesicle, prostate gland, and bulbourethral glands (Cowper's glands). The ampulla and duct of the seminal vesicle together are the ejaculatory duct through which sperm is propelled into the urethra for ejaculation from the penis.

DISORDERS AND DISEASES

Congenital defects of the male reproductive system that cause infertility include malformation or absence of one or both of the vasa deferens. The exact mechanisms behind the defects are unknown, although there is a correlation with the genetic markers for cystic fibrosis. Obstructions in the vas deferens also occur, or an inguinal hernia may pinch it.

A principal means of contraception by sterilizing men involves the vas deferens. This is the vasectomy (also, deferentectomy). The vasa deferens are either cut and sealed, clipped, or injected with a material to block them. Urologists perform the procedure, usually during an office visit, and it takes about twenty minutes. Possible complications include reduced sexual desire, bleeding, inflammation, sperm leakage, and spontaneous reopening. Postvasectomy pain syndrome is a condition of chronic pain in some men because of pressure, inflammation, or physical changes in the vas deferens. In some cases, a vasectomy can be reversed surgically so that the man is again fertile.

—*Roger Smith, Ph.D.*

See also Conception; Contraception; Erectile dysfunction; Genital disorders, male; Glands; Infertility, male; Masturbation; Men's health; Orchitis; Penile implant surgery; Prostate cancer; Prostate enlargement; Prostate gland; Prostate gland removal; Puberty and adolescence; Reproductive system; Semen; Sexual dysfunction; Sexuality; Sexually transmitted diseases (STDs); Sterilization; Testicles, undescended; Testicular cancer; Testicular surgery; Testicular torsion; Vasectomy.

FOR FURTHER INFORMATION:
Beers, Mark H., ed. *The Merck Manual of Medical Information: Second Home Edition.* Whitehouse Station, N.J.: Merck Research Laboratories, 2003.
Denniston, George C. *Vasectomy.* Victoria, B.C.: Trafford, 2002.

Parker, Steve. *The Human Body Book*. New York: DK Adult, 2001.

Thibodeau, Gary A., and Kevin T. Patton. *Structure and Function of the Human Body*. 13th ed. St. Louis: Mosby/Elsevier, 2008.

VASCULAR MEDICINE

SPECIALTY

ANATOMY OR SYSTEM AFFECTED: Blood vessels, circulatory system, lymphatic system

SPECIALTIES AND RELATED FIELDS: Cardiology, family medicine, hematology

DEFINITION: The diagnosis and management of diseases of the arteries, veins, and lymphatic system, exclusive of the heart and lungs.

KEY TERMS:

aneurysm: an abnormal area of an artery (or, less commonly, a vein) that enlarges for a variety of reasons and produces a focal ballooning

atherosclerosis: hardening of the arteries; a nonspecific term for the buildup of fatty material in the wall of any artery; over time, this buildup can obstruct the flow of blood through the artery and lead to adverse consequences in the organ it supplies

bypass graft: a surgical procedure that reroutes blood around an obstruction, usually caused by atherosclerosis; the "new" artery can be either plastic or constructed from an expendable, healthy section of vein in another part of the patient's body

embolus: any particle in the arterial or venous system that travels with the flow of blood and eventually lodges in the lungs, brain, or other organ or blood vessel

endarterectomy: a surgical procedure during which an artery is opened and the atherosclerotic material is manually removed, effectively cleaning out the artery and restoring more normal blood flow

ischemia: a state of blood deprivation of any organ in the body; ischemia may occur as a result of atherosclerosis in the main artery that supplies the organ, decreasing the amount of blood that can reach the organ

plaque: the fatty material composed of cholesterol, degenerating cells, and proteinaceous substances that can build up in the wall of any artery

thrombosis: the act of complete clotting of an artery or vein, through which no blood can then flow

SCIENCE AND PROFESSION

Vascular medicine, especially peripheral vascular surgery, has become an important specialty of general surgery. In the past, general surgeons performed surgery on the arteries and veins, but technical advances have led to the creation of vascular surgery as a field of its own.

Western society has produced an older population because of its high level of primary care, but with this older population come the ravages of atherosclerosis. The modern lifestyle is ideally suited to the formation of atherosclerosis in many arteries as a result of cigarette smoking, stress and high blood pressure, a fatty diet, and a sedentary lifestyle. Peripheral vascular surgeons can contribute in a positive way and help many patients with these diseases. This can be in the form of stroke prevention, the restoration of blood flow to a leg that might otherwise not be saved, and occasionally the saving of a life through repair of a ruptured aortic aneurysm.

One of the most common arteries affected by atherosclerosis is the carotid artery, in the neck. This artery branches high in the neck near the jawline. One branch continues up into the brain, supplying a large part of the area that controls motor and sensory function. For some reason, presently unknown, atherosclerosis tends to occur at areas of branching arteries; the carotid bifurcation is no exception. The buildup of material in this location is especially hazardous, because small pieces of the material, called emboli, can break off the arterial wall, travel up the artery, and lodge in the brain. When an embolus lodges in the small arteries of the brain, it blocks the flow of blood to the area of brain tissue supplied by those arteries. This results in ischemia—less blood flow—and the body functions controlled by that part of the brain may be altered. If the ophthalmic artery is involved, then blindness can ensue. If the middle cerebral artery is involved, then symptoms of motor and sensory dysfunction—such as abnormal sensation, numbness, weakness, or paralysis of one side of the body—can occur. Fortunately, very small emboli often do not cause permanent loss of neurological function, and a complete recovery is possible. They are, however, warning signs that atherosclerotic debris resides in the carotid artery, and if treatment is not begun, a permanent stroke might occur if the brain tissue is irreversibly damaged. If a permanent stroke occurs, there is a loss of some neurologic function and patients may be unable to see to their own daily needs. They also may need extensive and expensive rehabilitation. Strokes can be prevented, however, if the warning signs are properly interpreted and acted upon.

Atherosclerosis also results in blockages, or stenoses, in other arteries. Depending on the location of these blockages, a variety of symptoms can result. If the arteries to the intestines are involved, patients can feel abdominal pain that is very difficult to diagnose, given that there are many other causes of abdominal pain (such as ulcer disease, gallbladder problems, and colitis). Intestinal ischemia is somewhat rare and often is not thought of as a cause of abdominal pain. These patients may have to endure this pain for a long period of time and experience severe eating problems, weight loss, and addictions to painkillers. Many patients can be helped with nonsurgical and surgical techniques, however, resulting in the cessation of pain, the regained ability to eat, and thus the maintenance of proper nourishment.

A particularly interesting form of atherosclerotic arterial disease is called renovascular hypertension. In this syndrome, plaque builds up in the renal arteries (kidney arteries). Patients with renovascular hypertension exhibit a type of high blood pressure (hypertension) that is somewhat different from the kind of high blood pressure that affects most patients. The majority of patients with hypertension have "essential hypertension" for which there is no known cause. For that minority of patients whose hypertension results from pathology in the renal arteries, the blood flow in these arteries is decreased because of atherosclerotic plaques in the arterial walls that severely limit the space through which blood can flow. When this happens, the kidney "senses" this decreased flow and elaborates a variety of chemical hormones that serve to increase the blood flow. These hormones indirectly raise the blood pressure by trying to preserve blood flow to the kidney.

Renovascular hypertension is often difficult to diagnose and to treat medically. Many patients need to take up to five kinds of blood pressure pills to keep their pressure under reasonable control; it is this kind of patient who must be screened for renovascular hypertension. A variety of treatments can be offered to these patients when the diagnosis is made, although the medicines they must take all have significant side effects.

The arteries that supply the muscles and nerves of the extremities also can be affected by atherosclerotic disease. Peculiarly, the upper extremities are usually spared of this disease, whereas the lower extremities are not. The mildest form of lower-extremity disease manifests itself in the form of "claudication" (the term that describes the specific symptoms that develop in an ischemic limb). Most of the time there are no symptoms when a patient is at rest, but when the patient undergoes the physical stress of walking or other exercise, pain develops in the limb in certain areas that correspond to the areas of muscle tissue supplied by the blocked artery. A characteristic pain syndrome develops after a certain amount of exercise and repeats itself regularly. The pain stops after exercise, and this cessation of pain also follows a pattern.

Claudication is the classic example of arterial occlusive disease. If the disease is severe enough, it may cause resting pain. Such patients have profound ischemia of their leg(s), which is limb-threatening and requires intervention. People afflicted with ischemia of the leg have difficulty in healing small scrapes and cuts on the feet, which may turn into large lesions that do not heal. If these lesions become secondarily infected, they can also become limb-threatening and result in amputation. In many patients, however, amputation can be avoided by timely intervention with either surgery or other techniques.

A rather curious phenomenon occurs in some patients whereby there is a focal dilatation of a portion of an artery. The mechanism by which this occurs is largely unknown, but it may be related in some way to the atherosclerotic process. Instead of a buildup of debris in the arterial wall resulting in a blockage in the artery, aneurysms have a thinned-out wall. They enlarge over time and can cause problems. They may clot off entirely or be a source of emboli giving rise to problems farther down the arterial tree. The most devastating complication of an aneurysm, however, is acute rupture. Laplace's law of hemodynamics states that wall tension in a tube of fluid is related to the fourth power of the radius. Accordingly, as an aneurysm enlarges, the wall tension increases in exponential fashion. If rupture does occur, it can lead to rapid blood loss if expert medical and surgical care are not readily available.

Aneurysms can form anywhere in the body, but they most commonly occur in the aorta (the main artery coming out from the heart) directly beneath the umbilicus. Because this location is surgically accessible, repair of these aneurysms is a common operation. In this location, most aneurysms will not cause a problem until they measure approximately 5 centimeters in diameter; at that size, the risk of rupture becomes significant. Smaller aneurysms are usually followed with serial examinations over time, and if they do enlarge, then the appropriate therapy can be instituted. Other, less common areas of aneurysm formation include the splenic, renal, iliac, femoral, and popliteal arteries. Similar complications can ensue with these aneurysms.

The majority of peripheral vascular surgery practice deals with the diseases of the arteries, but venous disease is a very common problem that many physicians in many specialties must address. Patients with simple phlebitis of the superficial veins of the leg usually require no more than supportive care until they feel better, but if the clots are in or extend into the deep veins of the leg, much more aggressive treatment is necessary. A clot in this location has a chance of migrating into the lungs (pulmonary embolus) and can be fatal. Therefore, intensive treatment with intravenous and then oral blood thinners (anticoagulants) is mandatory. There are some patients who then have chronic venous problems because the clots in their legs can damage the valves in the veins. This results in severe pain, swelling, and even ulceration of the legs that can be very difficult to treat.

DIAGNOSTIC AND TREATMENT TECHNIQUES

Many patients who suffer from vascular diseases are not treated with surgery right away. They may ultimately need an operation, but often long periods of time elapse before surgery is undertaken. Nonoperative therapy is often all that is needed to control certain aspects of the patient's symptoms, in the form of cessation of cigarette smoking, lowering of serum cholesterol, or an exercise program. Vascular surgeons provide guidelines for patients who need this sort of therapy.

Atherosclerosis may appear in many ways and affect patients differently. For example, a forty-five-year-old postal carrier complains of pain in the thighs of the legs in the same location whenever he walks more than a few hundred feet. He may have been a heavy smoker for many years, his cholesterol levels may be elevated, and there may be many relatives in his family with "hardening of the arteries." Such a person has a classic case of claudication resulting from atherosclerotic occlusive disease of the arteries that supply the thigh muscles. The patient has several options. Other causes of leg pain must be ruled out, such as nerve problems or back conditions, but when this is accomplished, the field of vascular surgery can help this patient maintain his lifestyle. If the patient would like to investigate options for intervention, an arteriogram is performed next. In this procedure, specially trained radiologists insert a small tube into the arteries and take pictures after dye has been injected. This allows an exact replica of the patient's arterial anatomy to be projected in two dimensions. The arteriogram allows the surgeons and radiologists to determine the best course of action for this patient.

Some atherosclerotic plaques are in particular locations that may allow their treatment with balloon angioplasty rather than open surgery. In this procedure, again performed by trained radiologists or some vascular surgeons, a catheter with a balloon at its end is inserted into the artery and the balloon is inflated in the area of the offending plaque in an effort to open the clogged artery. This procedure is often performed on the arteries of the heart, but it can also be performed on other arteries: those of the kidneys, intestines, and legs. A vascular surgeon usually oversees the care of the patient, as not all the balloon procedures are completely successful and open surgery is sometimes necessary. Open surgery might include a bypass graft with a woven or knitted prosthetic artery or a graft made with an expendable vein in the patient's leg, utilizing the same vein as for heart bypass surgery. The postal worker described above could be a candidate for a balloon procedure or a surgical bypass graft, but in either case he should be restored to almost normal walking capability and be able to return to his job.

Another common scenario might involve a more serious situation. A person may have an open sore on his foot that has been there for more than six months and is getting bigger, perhaps infected. This person may also be a heavy smoker with cholesterol problems and severe diabetes mellitus. He has not walked more than a block in the past few years because his feet hurt when he does. His problem may relate to poor blood flow to his legs and feet, and the diabetes certainly does not help. Before vascular surgery techniques became popular, this patient ultimately would have required an amputation of his leg either below or above the knee. It is physically and emotionally difficult for patients to cope with such a loss: The long, expensive period of rehabilitation includes learning to walk with a prosthetic extremity. This patient would be a good candidate for an arteriogram and would undoubtedly need some surgery. This would most likely be in the form of a bypass graft, which could stretch from the groin all the way to the foot, crossing the knee and the ankle. Ultimately, a successful outcome would be healing of the open sore and control of the infection; the patient would then be able to continue walking with his own leg.

Another situation that might involve vascular surgery is as follows. A patient has a history of deep vein clots following prior major surgery. Treatment consisted of long-term blood thinners, and the patient may have had no major problems since that time. The patient now needs a hip operation, however, and hip operations carry a high risk of blood clot formation in the deep veins of the leg. Because deep-vein thrombosis carries risks of a pulmonary embolus as well as chronic problems in the leg, a vascular surgeon is called upon to help design a program that can prevent these complications from occurring. The usual methods of prophylaxis do not necessarily apply in this patient, and as the patient is labeled "high-risk," it might be most prudent to place a device in the body to catch any pulmonary emboli if they occur. The theory behind this management is that, in the high-risk patient, the formation of blood clots in the legs is almost unavoidable and that the majority of effort should be aimed at preventing the most serious, potentially fatal complication, the pulmonary embolus. In this circumstance, vascular surgeons could place a filter device in the main vein that carries blood to the heart and lungs, which would effectively trap any free-floating emboli that could cause a problem.

PERSPECTIVE AND PROSPECTS
Peripheral vascular surgery has assumed a paramount role in medical practice. By 1900, significant contributions had been made regarding the basic reconstructive techniques needed to sew arteries together. The work of Alexis Carrel in the early twentieth century is considered the most important contribution to the technical art of vascular surgery. He reported the techniques of transplanting organs and sewing arteries together that are still routinely performed. By the 1950's, synthetic materials were introduced as arterial replacements, which became acceptable treatment for many patients.

Nonsurgical techniques for opening blocked arteries and veins to improve blood flow have so far been somewhat disappointing in peripheral vascular surgery, but new techniques are being developed and tested at a rapid pace and may eventually become commonplace. Although technically performing a bypass graft is feasible, the graft cannot approach the durability and performance of a native artery. Research involving the transplantation of human arteries may solve some of these problems and allow more patients to benefit from surgery.

Vascular surgery can benefit large numbers of people simply because of the nature of atherosclerosis. It may be a product of habits, the environment, and/or genetic makeup, but it is widely accepted that as the population ages, more and more people will suffer from diseases that can be helped by vascular surgery, allowing them to maintain lifestyles that are as productive as possible. Basic scientific research of the mechanisms of atherosclerosis may yield important answers and guide new therapies for patients with this disease.

—*Mark Wengrovitz, M.D.*

See also Amputation; Aneurysmectomy; Aneurysms; Angiography; Angioplasty; Arteriosclerosis; Behçet's disease; Biofeedback; Bleeding; Blood and blood disorders; Blood pressure; Blood vessels; Bypass surgery; Carotid arteries; Catheterization; Cholesterol; Circulation; Claudication; Deep vein thrombosis; Diabetes mellitus; Dialysis; Embolism; Endarterectomy; Exercise physiology; Glands; Healing; Hematology; Hematology, pediatric; Hemorrhoid banding and removal; Hemorrhoids; Histology; Hypercholesterolemia; Hyperlipidemia; Ischemia; Klippel-Trenaunay syndrome; Lipids; Lymphatic system; Mitral valve prolapse; Phlebitis; Phlebotomy; Podiatry; Shunts; Stents; Strokes; Sturge-Weber syndrome; Systems and organs; Thrombolytic therapy and TPA; Thrombosis and thrombus; Transfusion; Transient ischemic attacks (TIAs); Varicose vein removal; Varicose veins; Vascular system; Vasculitis; Venous insufficiency.

FOR FURTHER INFORMATION:
Ancowitz, Arthur. *Strokes and Their Prevention: How to Avoid High Blood Pressure and Hardening of the Arteries.* New York: Jove, 1980. Provides useful information on nonpharmacological treatments of vascular disease. Available in most public libraries.

Ernst, Calvin B., and James C. Stanley, eds. *Current Therapy in Vascular Surgery.* 4th ed. St. Louis, Mo.: Mosby, 2001. This advanced textbook is superbly edited and has contributions by the leaders in the vascular surgical field. Discusses treatments for all vascular disorders.

Jaff, Michael, and C. Goldman. *Handbook of Vascular Medicine for the Cardiologist: The Basics of Vascular Diagnosis and Therapy.* Boston: Blackwell, 2003. A clinical text that covers basic vascular medicine and a range of vascular disorders.

Marieb, Elaine N. *Essentials of Human Anatomy and Physiology.* 9th ed. San Francisco: Pearson/Benjamin Cummings, 2009. This introductory anatomy and physiology textbook, easily accessible to those with little science background, is richly illustrated with diagrams and photographs, which help to illuminate body systems and processes.

Rutherford, Robert B., ed. *Vascular Surgery.* 6th ed. Philadelphia: Saunders/Elsevier, 2005. Long considered to be the classic text on vascular surgery by many surgeons, this book provides a wealth of information on all vascular diseases.

Tortora, Gerard J., and Bryan Derrickson. *Principles of Anatomy and Physiology.* 12th ed. Hoboken, N.J.: John Wiley & Sons, 2009. An outstanding textbook of human anatomy and physiology, with good coverage of the vascular system.

Vascular system

Anatomy

Anatomy or system affected: Blood vessels, circulatory system, legs

Specialties and related fields: Cardiology, exercise physiology, hematology, vascular medicine

Definition: The pipeline through which every cell of the body receives oxygen, vitamins, hormones, and the metabolic fuels necessary to sustain life.

Key terms:

arteries: the vessels that carry blood from the heart to all parts of the body

atherosclerosis: the buildup of lipid-containing (fatty) materials beneath or within the inner wall of an artery, which can lead to narrowing or occlusion of the artery

capillaries: minute blood vessels that connect the smallest arteries (arterioles) to the smallest veins (venules); they allow passage of oxygen and nutrients from the arteries into the tissue and passage of waste products from the tissues into the veins

collaterals: small vessels that enlarge to compensate for the obstruction or narrowing of another vessel

heart attack: sudden and permanent damage to a part of the heart muscle as a result of impaired blood flow through the coronary arteries

metabolism: the chemical changes that occur when the body transforms oxygen and nutrients into energy or heat

stroke: permanent damage to part of the brain as a result of impaired blood flow

veins: blood vessels that carry blood from the cells back to the heart

venous thrombosis: the presence of blood clots in the veins, usually in the legs or arms

Structure and Functions

The vascular system is faced with the enormous task of supplying every cell of the human body with a constant supply of oxygen and nutrients needed to sustain life. This elaborate system circulates more than 2,000 gallons of blood per day through more than 12,000 miles of arteries, veins, and capillaries. Moreover, the job of the vascular system is not done when the nutrients arrive at the cell. After the cell uses the nutrients, waste products that are left over from metabolism must be carried away and disposed of before they damage the cell. For this reason, several kinds of vessels exist within the human body that differ in structure and function. They can be broken into three categories: arteries, veins, and capillaries.

The term "arteries" came from ancient times, when arteries were thought to be filled with air. (This misconception evolved because after death much of the blood usually pumped through the arteries had been pumped out, leading scientists of the time to conclude that air, rather than blood, was circulated within them.) Arteries are thick-walled blood vessels that carry oxygen-rich blood from the left side of the heart to all parts of the body. The blood circulating within them is usually moving at high velocities and exerts pressure against the artery walls, creating an expansion of the artery during the contraction of the heart. This expansion, called a pulse, can be palpated in areas where the arteries are large and close to the surface of the skin: in the neck (the carotid artery) or in the wrist (the radial artery). The pressure being exerted against the artery varies greatly. A doctor taking a blood pressure reading is measuring this variation in pressure. A blood pressure of 120/80, for example, would mean that the force from the heart is exerting 120 millimeters of mercury pressure against the artery wall while the heart is contracting (the systolic pressure) and 80 millimeters of mercury when the heart is at rest (the diastolic pressure). Clearly, the artery has to be a very strong structure.

Veins, on the other hand, are thin-walled, almost transparent vessels that return blood to the heart after it has visited the cells. There are far more veins in the body than there are arteries. The blood moving in the veins is under very little pressure and usually is moving quite slowly in comparison to the flow in the arteries. The flow in the veins is slow because most of the force from the contraction of the heart was dissipated when the blood passed through the cell. For this reason, the flow in the veins must be helped along by contraction of the muscles around these blood vessels. For example, with each step, the muscles in the calves of the legs propel the blood in the calf veins upward with great force. For this reason, the calf of the leg is sometimes referred to as the "venous heart." If this pump is not active, blood flow in the veins can stagnate and life-threatening clots can form in the veins.

Another problem for the venous circulation is that its blood is often moving against gravity. If the veins were built like arteries (simple hollow tubes), the blood would flow upward toward the heart with the contraction of the muscles but would fall back down as soon as the contraction stopped. Fortunately, the veins are equipped with one-way valves not found in arteries. These valves open when blood is moving toward the heart and close when blood starts to fall backward. Veins are also different from arteries in that they can expand to several times their normal size. This allows the veins to be used as a storage area for blood. When the body's need for blood is low, such as during a resting state, the veins enlarge and fill with the blood that is not being actively circulated. When the need for blood increases, as during strenuous activity, the stored blood is forced back into active circulation. Because veins have such thin walls and stretch so easily, one might think that they are not as strong as arteries. In reality, veins are strong enough to be used as surgical substitutes for failed arteries and hold up quite well under arterial pressure.

Capillaries are extremely small vessels with very thin walls. These vessels connect the smallest arteries (arterioles) with the smallest veins (venules). Although their size can vary, the average diameter of a capillary is about 8 microns (0.008 millimeter), which is about the size of a single red blood cell. The nutrients carried in the blood pass through tiny pores in the vessel wall directly into the cell, which uses the nutrients to produce energy and heat. During this process, waste products are created that are poisonous to the cell; they must be removed quickly or the cell will die. The waste products then pass from the cell into the capillaries and then into tiny veins that will carry the waste products away.

A trip through the system of arteries, capillaries, and veins—to deliver nutrients to one cell in a calf muscle, for example—would begin in the left ventricle of the heart, where blood is pumped through the aorta (the largest artery) with great force. The aorta has branches that serve the structures of the head and neck (which includes the most important organ—the brain), the upper extremities, the abdomen, and the lower extremities. On this imaginary trip, one passes through the aortic arch and travels down the main artery in the abdomen, called the abdominal aorta. This artery eventually branches into two arteries (at about the level of the navel) that send blood to each leg. This artery continues to branch into smaller and smaller arteries until one reaches the capillaries serving the particular cell of the calf muscle in the leg. Here the nutrients are delivered to the cell. The waste products are dumped back into the capillaries. From the capillaries, one travels into tiny veins called venules. These tiny veins become continually larger until one is finally moving up through a large vein just behind the knee called the popliteal. Soon one is back in the abdomen in the large vein called the vena cava, which enters the heart at the right atrium. The blood then travels through the right ventricle and eventually into another large vessel called the pulmonary artery (the only artery that carries blood that is not oxygenated). This artery leads into the lungs, where the waste products of metabolism are released and exchanged for oxygen. With a new load of oxygen, one travels through the pulmonary veins (the only veins that carry oxygenated blood), into the left atrium of the heart, and into the left ventricle, where the journey began. In a normal person, this entire voyage takes only eighteen to twenty-four seconds.

DISORDERS AND DISEASES

When the vascular system is functioning correctly, all the cells of the body are receiving the right amount of blood at all times. Many problems can arise, however, in the complex functioning of the human organism, and the vasculature must have ways of meeting these challenges. Such problems include the obstruction of vital vessels by plaque formation (a buildup of fatty deposits called atherosclerosis), thrombus (blood clot) formation, and vasospasm (a closing down of a blood vessel in response to cold or trauma). Moreover, some organs in the body cannot survive for more than a few minutes without oxygen before damage occurs. For example, the brain can survive for only a few minutes without oxygen, while the cells in the arms and legs can be deprived of oxygen for a matter of hours without irreversible damage. For this reason, whenever there is a problem the vascular system must be able to set priorities about which systems receive blood flow and which systems do not. When there is a life-threatening problem, the vessels in the arms and legs contract, forcing blood out of the extremities; this allows more flow to reach the brain, where it is most urgently needed. When an artery is narrowed by plaque, the vascular system will compensate by enlarging smaller vessels in the area to help maintain flow. If the artery is totally obstructed, this system of collateral vessels takes over.

While these and other mechanisms work quite well, sudden obstruction or other disease processes involving an artery or vein can result in major problems. The major problems that can result from arterial disease include stroke, myocardial infarction (heart attack), and peripheral artery disease. Problems involving the veins may include deep vein thrombosis, pulmonary embolism, and varicose veins.

A stroke is a condition in which part of the brain is deprived of oxygen long enough to cause permanent damage. The medical term for such an event is a cerebrovascular accident, or CVA. The symptoms may include one-sided weakness or numbness, headache, difficulty in speaking, or transient blindness in one eye. If these symptoms completely resolve within twenty-four hours, the event is referred to as a transient ischemic attack, or TIA. The difference between a TIA and a CVA is that the damage done by the TIA is not permanent. TIAs, however, are often precursors of impending full-blown strokes. Therefore, patients who experience them should see a doctor immediately so that steps can be taken to prevent another, perhaps more severe, episode. The treatment for patients who experience a TIA may include surgery to remove plaque buildup from the carotid artery, bypass surgery (in which another vessel is used to bypass a narrowed area), the use of blood-thinning drugs, or the use of antiplatelet drugs (such as aspirin). Rehabilitation, the use of blood-thinning or antiplatelet drugs, and lifestyle modification are often prescribed for those who have already suffered major strokes.

Myocardial infarction is one of the leading killers in Western societies. A heart attack occurs when blood flow is inadequate to the heart muscle and part of the heart muscle dies. The symptoms include pain in the chest (especially pain that is brought on by exertion), shortness of breath, sweating, nausea, and fatigue. Similar, although usually less severe, symptoms may be present with a condition called angina, in which blood flow to the heart muscle is impaired but there is no permanent damage. Acute treatment for heart attacks can include rest (to reduce additional damage to the heart muscle), treatment with blood-thinning drugs, treatment with drugs that dissolve blood clots, balloon catheters (to help open narrowed arteries), or coronary bypass surgery.

Peripheral artery disease—the narrowing or blockage of arteries in the arms or legs—is also quite common. Symptoms may include pain in the limb, loss of feeling, coolness, and discoloration; in severe cases,

IN THE NEWS: TREATING VASCULAR DISEASE WITH THERAPEUTIC ANGIOGENESIS

Many diseases of the vascular system are associated with decreased perfusion, or the passage of blood through organ vessels; restoration of blood flow is the most effective means to limit damage to ischemic tissue. Therapeutic angiogenesis as related to cardiovascular disease refers to the improvement of myocardial and extremity blood flow and function within ischemic regions where traditional methods of restoring blood vessel structure are not feasible. Angiogenesis refers to the chemical promotion of new vessel growth.

Fibroblast growth factors (FGFs) and vascular endothelial growth factors (VEGFs) have been the most widely studied protein families capable of inducing new vessel growth. Two modes of introducing FGF to the body have been explored: direct injection or implantation of the FGF protein and the induction of individual cells to produce increased amounts of FGF by the incorporation of appropriate deoxyribonucleic acid (DNA) fragments, called gene therapy. The FGF-2 Initiating Revascularization Support Trial (FIRST), described in the *Journal of the American College of Cardiology* in 2000, compared a single intracoronary dose of FGF-2 with placebo in 337 patients. After ninety days, patients receiving FGF did not differ significantly from the placebo group in total exercise time possible, a commonly used indirect measure of restored blood flow. Frequency of angina was also similar in the two groups, indicating that this recombinant (engineered) protein treatment was ineffective. Gene transfer therapies, in which a patient's own cells internally produce new FGF protein, are viewed as holding more promise in eventually translating into a clinically accepted treatment for ischemia. Human studies of FGF gene therapy are ongoing.

—Michael R. King, Ph.D.

tissue loss may result. This disease process is usually progressive. A patient may first notice pain in the calf of the leg that comes on only with walking and goes away as soon as the exercise stops. This condition, called intermittent claudication, indicates that there is minimal narrowing of the arteries in the leg. As more of the artery narrows, the pain occurs even without exercise. Finally, blood flow to the limb is not sufficient to maintain the cells, and tissue begins to die. Treatment of peripheral artery disease may include medication and exercise (during the early stages) and progress to the surgical bypass of narrowed arteries (in later stages). Sometimes arteries in the extremities become clogged by a thrombus instead of plaque. If this is the case, drugs that dissolve blood clots or surgical operations to remove the clot may be used. If treatment for severe peripheral disease is unsuccessful, amputation may be necessary.

The risk factors for developing arterial disease—of the coronary, carotid, or peripheral arteries—include high blood pressure, smoking, diabetes, elevated cholesterol levels, stress, a family history of arterial disease, obesity, and advancing age.

Veins do not develop plaque as do arteries; instead, blood can stagnate and form clots that can obstruct them. When this happens, a condition called venous thrombosis, blood stagnates in the veins behind the clot and a larger clot forms. It is not unusual for clots to fill all the major veins in the leg once this process begins. These clots cause swelling and pain in the leg but do not usually threaten the leg as obstruction of the arteries does. Instead, the danger lies in the possibility of a clot breaking loose and traveling to the lungs. This clot, called a pulmonary embolism, can be fatal. The risk factors for developing venous thrombosis include anything that can slow blood flow in the veins, such as prolonged sitting or standing, a long airplane trip or car trip, a surgical operation, or pregnancy. Injury to the vein can also trigger clots, as can an imbalance of clotting factors in the blood. The best way to prevent venous thrombosis is to keep active.

Another venous problem that strikes as many as one of every four women and one of every five men is a condition most commonly known as varicose veins. The veins become stretched out and elongated to the point where they bulge out when the patient is sitting or standing. Although this is mostly a cosmetic problem, severe cases can lead to blood pooling in the leg and tissue damage.

PERSPECTIVE AND PROSPECTS

The vasculature of the human body has not always been understood, even in recent times. The ancient Egyptians knew about the importance of the heart and the pulse, but this knowledge was not passed on to more modern civilizations. Hippocrates (c. 460-c. 370 B.C.E.) had serious misconceptions about the functions of the circulatory system: He thought that the pulse was caused by movements of the blood vessels. Other great thinkers such as Aristotle and Galen made similar errors in their study of the vascular system, errors that influenced medicine for many years.

In 1628, a doctor in London named William Harvey published a paper introducing his radical theories about how the blood circulates. He changed the way medical people thought about this system by describing it as a closed circuit, with blood being forced through it via contractions of the heart. He postulated that blood passed from the arteries into the veins at the cellular level. It was not until the 1660's, when early microscopes were developed, that this theory could be confirmed.

In 1733, a clergyman named Stephen Hales became the first person to measure blood pressure within the arterial system. He inserted a large, hollow glass tube into the neck artery of a horse. To his amazement, the blood rose 9 feet up the tube. This method of measuring blood pressure was not practical, however, and it was not until the late nineteenth century that the sphygmomanometer was developed to measure blood pressure, utilizing blood pressure cuffs and air pressure.

Another pioneer in the understanding of the vascular system was German physician and biologist Rudolf Virchow, who theorized about how blood clots formed in veins. He concluded that clots formed when the blood flow was slowed down, the vein wall was injured, or an imbalance of clotting factors in the blood existed. These observations were astonishingly correct considering that, at this time, many people still thought blood clots in the veins were composed of pus. Understanding of these principles makes possible modern treatments and prevention techniques.

In the late nineteenth century, modern vascular surgery began with development of techniques to repair blood vessels. By the early twentieth century, methods for connecting the ends of vessels with a watertight suture became commonplace. In 1948, a surgeon in Paris took a saphenous vein and used it to bypass a blockage in an artery in the leg. In the 1950's, the technology necessary to support sustained heart surgeries was introduced, and heart surgery has since become routine. Blood vessels can now be surgically repaired, bypassed, or cleaned out. Laser surgery and clot-dissolving drugs are becoming routine.

—*Steven R. Talbot, R.V.T.*

See also Amputation; Aneurysmectomy; Aneurysms; Angiography; Angioplasty; Arteriosclerosis; Behçet's disease; Biofeedback; Bleeding; Blood and blood disorders; Blood pressure; Blood vessels; Bypass surgery; Carotid arteries; Catheterization; Cholesterol; Circulation; Claudication; Deep vein thrombosis; Diabetes mellitus; Dialysis; Embolism; Endarterectomy; Exercise physiology; Glands; Healing; Hematology; Hematology, pediatric; Hemorrhoid banding and removal; Hemorrhoids; Histology; Hypercholesterolemia; Hyperlipidemia; Ischemia; Klippel-Trenaunay syndrome; Lipids; Lymphatic system; Mitral valve prolapse; Phlebitis; Phlebotomy; Podiatry; Shunts; Stents; Strokes; Sturge-Weber syndrome; Systems and organs; Thrombolytic therapy and TPA; Thrombosis and thrombus; Transfusion; Transient ischemic attacks (TIAs); Varicose vein removal; Varicose veins; Vascular medicine; Vasculitis; Venous insufficiency.

FOR FURTHER INFORMATION:

Hershey, Falls B., Robert W. Barnes, and David S. Sumner, eds. *Noninvasive Diagnosis of Vascular Disease*. Pasadena, Calif.: Appleton Davies, 1984. This book, written for medical personnel, may be difficult reading for the layperson. Nevertheless, it is valuable for its detailed description of the anatomy, physiology, and pathology involved in vascular disease, as well as for its discussion of diagnostic methods.

Loscalzo, Joseph, and Andrew I. Schafer, eds. *Thrombosis and Hemorrhage*. 3d ed. Philadelphia: Lippincott Williams & Wilkins, 2003. Covers an array of relevant topics, including the basic elements of hemostasis, the normal function and response of platelets, thrombotic disorders, and the management of patients with hemorrhagic and thrombotic conditions.

Milady's Standard Textbook of Cosmetology. Clifton Park, N.Y.: Thomson/Delmar Learning, 2008. Although this is a cosmetology textbook, it contains a short and concise chapter on arteries, veins, and capillaries that is very clearly written. Written for a lay audience, this work is an excellent source for gaining a better understanding of the basics of circulation.

Mohrman, David E., and Lois Jane Heller. *Cardiovascular Physiology*. 6th ed. New York: Lange Medical Books/McGraw-Hill, 2006. Provides a thorough overview of the basic concepts of cardiovascular physiology and reviews recent scientific research regarding the vascular system.

Standring, Susan, et al., eds. *Gray's Anatomy*. 40th ed. New York: Churchill Livingstone/Elsevier, 2008.

One of the most complete anatomy reference books available. Contains hundreds of illustrations.

Strandness, D. Eugene, Jr. *Duplex Scanning in Vascular Disorders*. 4th ed. London: Lippincott Williams & Wilkins, 2009. This book is written for medical vascular specialists and is somewhat technical in nature; however, it is well written. The beginning of each chapter defines the importance of that particular subject and the clinical presentation, treatment, and typical course of the vascular disease involved.

VASCULITIS
DISEASE/DISORDER

ANATOMY OR SYSTEM AFFECTED: Abdomen, blood vessels, chest, circulatory system, ears, eyes, gastrointestinal system, hands, immune system, intestines, kidneys, legs, lungs, nerves, nose, respiratory system, skin

SPECIALTIES AND RELATED FIELDS: Cardiology, dermatology, gastroenterology, nephrology, neurology, ophthalmology, otolaryngology, pulmonary medicine, rheumatology

DEFINITION: A number of conditions characterized by inflammation of blood vessels, both arteries and veins, that leads to decreased circulation in the affected tissue or organ, which can damage the tissue or organ. Inflammation may be continuous or spotty and can result in damage to the walls of the blood vessel, leading to destruction of the blood vessel or the formation of an aneurysm.

CAUSES AND SYMPTOMS

There is no definite cause of vasculitis. Some types may be autoimmune in nature, in which the body attacks its own tissues. Some types of vasculitis may be caused by an allergic reaction to a medication, exposure to a toxic chemical, or a virus, such as the hepatitis B and hepatitis C viruses. Vasculitis may occur with connective tissue disease such as rheumatoid arthritis, Sjögren's syndrome, and lupus or with a blood cell cancer such as leukemia or lymphoma.

These conditions are often classified by the size of the blood vessels involved in the condition or by the type of cells involved in the inflammation of the blood vessels. Large vessel vasculitis includes Takayasu arteritis, Behçet's syndrome, polymyalgia rheumatica, and giant cell arteritis. Medium vessel vasculitis includes Buerger's disease, polyarteritis nodosa, Kawasaki disease, cutaneous vasculitis, and primary central nervous system vasculitis. Small vessel vasculitis includes Wegener's granulomatosis, Churg-Strauss arteritis, microscopic polyarteritis/angiitis, hyperallergic vasculitis, Henoch-Schonlein purpura, essential cryoglobinemic vasculitis, hypersensitivity vasculitis, and vasculitis secondary to connective tissue disorders. The types of cells that may be observed in the various vasculitis types are neutrophils, lymphocytes, leukocytes, eosinophils, or granulomatous cells. The two classification systems tend to overlap, and the cell type can change in a type of vasculitis as the condition progresses.

The first symptoms that are reported are usually systemic. They include fatigue, fever, night sweats, weakness, weight loss, anorexia, muscle and joint pain, and numbness. More specific symptoms depend on the type of vasculitis. Some of the types demonstrate only skin lesions, which can be purple spots (purpura), areas of necrosis, or skin ulcers. They include hypersensitivity vasculitis, Buerger's disease, and cutaneous vasculitis. Each type of vasculitis then has its own symptoms based on the part of the body that is affected. Symptoms can include a skin rash, joint or extremity pain, neuropathy, ulcerations of the skin, headache, visual problems, abdominal pain, vomiting, diarrhea, anemia, coughing up blood, muscle pain, conjunctivitis, weakness, heart failure, palpitations, sinus problems, bleeding into the lungs, and abnormal kidney function. Some types of vasculitis are self-limiting, but most are chronic conditions. The damage that vasculitis can cause can be life-threatening.

Vasculitis is diagnosed by blood tests, including a complete blood count (CBC), general chemistry, liver function tests, and kidney function tests. These tests demonstrate what body organs are affected by the vasculitis. Some tests that are commonly abnormal with vasculitis are erythrocyte sedimentation rate (ESR), C-reactive protein (CRP), antinuclear antibody (ANA), and antineutrophil cytoplasmic antibody (ANCA). These tests indicate the presence of inflammation in the body, which is a sign of vasculitis. The most specific test for vasculitis is a biopsy of an affected area of the body, such as the skin or a kidney. The biopsy actually demonstrates the presence of vasculitis. Sometimes, angiograms (X rays of the blood vessels) are performed to look for vasculitis. If kidney problems are suspected, then urine is tested for the presence of microscopic blood and protein.

TREATMENT AND THERAPY

The treatment for vasculitis is based on the type of disease. The most common treatment is the administration of corticosteroid drugs, such as prednisone or solumedrol. They can be given orally or intravenously. Corticosteroids are used to control the inflammation in the blood vessels. Often, other immune system suppressant drugs are administered with the corticosteroids. They include cyclophosphamide (Cytoxan), azathioprine (Imuran), and mycophenolate mofetil (CellCept). These medications can also be administered orally or intravenously. Both of these groups of medications have a number of side effects. Corticosteroids can cause weight gain, diabetes, osteoporosis, insomnia, hypertension, increased risk of infection, mood changes, stomach upset, and cataracts. The immune system suppressant drugs are toxic substances that are also used to treat some types of cancer and to prevent the rejection of transplanted organs. They, too, have many side effects. They can cause hair loss, fatigue, bladder cancer, hemorrhagic cystitis, increased risk of infections, nausea, vomiting, diarrhea, and liver damage.

Usually, vasculitis responds well to one or both of these medications, particularly if it is diagnosed early. If vasculitis does not respond well to this treatment, plasmapheresis can be performed or the medication interferon alpha can be given. Plasmapheresis is a procedure in which plasma is removed from blood previously taken from the body. Removal is done by centrifuging the blood, which is separated into plasma with other immune cells and the red blood cells. The red blood cells are then returned to the patient. Eliminating many of the white blood cells can interfere with the immune response. Interferon alpha is a biologic drug that can affect the immune response. This drug is still being studied for its role in treating vasculitis.

PROSPECTIVE AND PROSPECTS

Although symptoms of conditions that sound like vasculitis have appeared in ancient medical writings, vasculitis was not identified until 1866 by Adolf Kussmaul. Kussmaul noted that the affected patient had nodules under his skin, but on autopsy, he was able to see that there were nodules on the patient's arteries. He called this condition periarteritis nodosa. Kussmaul attributed the arterial nodules to inflammation of the blood vessels, and he considered it to be a novel condition that had not been described previously.

After Kussmaul's description of periarteritis nodosa, other cases of apparent vasculitis were compared to it. However, many of these conditions were actually different types of vasculitis. There are 17 to 20 different types of vasculitis. Giant cell arteritis was described in 1890. Giant cell arteritis is inflammation of the large temporal arteries of the head. It causes localized pain and tenderness, and it can lead to blindness if untreated. It is diagnosed by biopsy of a temporal artery. Polymyalgia rheumatica was first described in 1957, and it occurs in roughly 50 percent of those who develop giant cell arteritis. Polymyalgia rheumatica affects the large arteries of the shoulders and hips and causes muscle pain in the arms and legs.

Takayasu's arteritis, first described in 1908, is inflammation of the aorta and its major branches, the optical arteries. This vasculitis affects young women and can lead to heart failure. Buerger's disease was also described in 1908. It is characterized by severe lack of blood flow to the hands and feet, causing severe pain, blue fingers and toes, and tissue death. Buerger's disease is caused by cigarette smoking. Kawasaki disease was described in 1939. It demonstrates inflammation of the medium-sized arteries of the mucous membranes, lymph nodes, and coronary arteries. This condition occurs only in young children and causes swollen glands in the neck, conjunctivitis, inflammation around the mouth and on the palms of the hands and the bottom of the feet, a skin rash, and aneurysms of the coronary arteries.

Three of the more serious forms of vasculitis are Wegener's granulomatosis, Churg-Strauss syndrome, and microscopic polyarteritis. These conditions can be rapidly fatal unless treated aggressively. All three are associated with the presence of antineutrophil cytoplasmic antibodies in the blood. Wegener's granulomatosis was first described in 1936, and it affects the small blood vessels of the skin, lungs, eyes, sinuses, and kidneys. Churg-Strauss syndrome was described in 1951. It begins with the development of asthma and then progresses to affect the nerves, skin, heart, lungs, gastrointestinal tract, and kidneys. Microscopic polyarteritis was first described in 1948. It affects the smallest blood vessels of the lungs and kidneys. All three conditions can lead to bleeding by the small blood vessels in the lungs and kidney failure.

—*Christine M. Carroll, R.N., B.S.N., M.B.A.*

See also Aneurysmectomy; Aneurysms; Behçet's disease; Bleeding; Blood and blood disorders; Blood vessels; Circulation; Claudication; Inflammation; Varicose vein removal; Varicose veins; Vascular medicine; Vascular system.

FOR FURTHER INFORMATION:

Qontro Medical Guides. *Vasculitis Medical Guide.* Minneapolis: Author, 2008.

Schwar, Sheri Lyn. *Vasculitis: Sick and Tired of Being Sick and Tired.* Lincoln, Nebr.: iUniverse, 2006.

Swart, Myrna. *There Must Be a Reason: My Daughter's Battle With Wegener's Granulomatosis.* Lincoln, Nebr.: iUniverse, 2008.

VASECTOMY

PROCEDURE

ANATOMY OR SYSTEM AFFECTED: Genitals, reproductive system

SPECIALTIES AND RELATED FIELDS: Family medicine, general surgery, urology

DEFINITION: A surgical means of birth control for males that involves the interruption of the tubes that transport sperm to the semen.

KEY TERMS:

ejaculation: the expulsion from a man's erect penis at the time of orgasm of a fluid made up of semen and sperm

elective surgical sterilization: a voluntary operation that is intended to produce permanent birth control

local anesthesia: the injection of medication into the body that renders the immediate area free of pain

scrotum: the genital skin sac that holds the testicles and related structures

semen: fluid produced by a man's prostate gland, which makes up 95 percent of the fluid that is ejaculated *sperm:* a man's reproductive cells, made in the testicles; they carry the man's genetic traits to a woman's egg

*vas (*pl. *vasae): the small, muscular tube that carries sperm from the testicle to the prostate gland

INDICATIONS AND PROCEDURES

The term "vasectomy" describes a minor surgical procedure performed on a man who desires a permanent form of birth control. Vasectomy—which literally means "cutting the tubes"—results in sterilization because it obstructs the passageway through which sperm travel to reach the female ovum. A man's testicles produce both male hormones (that stimulate male characteristics and sex drive) and sperm. A collection of small tubes called the epididymis along each testicle mature and deliver sperm to a single tube called the vas (or vas deferens), which is about the width of a spaghetti noodle. Each vas runs through the scrotum, up the groin on each side, and through the wall of the abdomen, ending in a storage area called the seminal vesicle, which is next to the prostate gland near the base of the penis. From there, the sperm mix with semen from the pros-

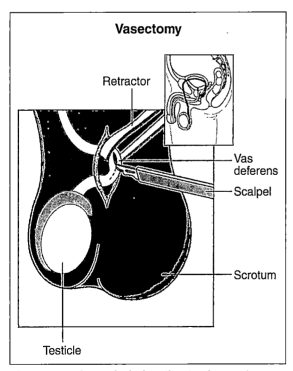

Vasectomy

Retractor

Vas deferens

Scalpel

Scrotum

Testicle

The most popular method of sterilization for men is vasectomy, which involves the severing of the vas deferens, the tube that transports sperm from the testes; the inset shows the location of the vas deferens in the male reproductive system.

tate gland and are expelled from the penis during ejaculation.

Vasectomy occludes (closes off) the vas to block the passage of sperm without affecting the important hormonal functions of the testicle. The surgery is done in the first, straight part of the vas, above the testicle and through the skin of the scrotum, making the procedure relatively easy and safe to perform.

Physicians performing vasectomy come from the specialties of urology, family medicine, general practice, or general surgery. Since the procedure is relatively simple, in comparison with other surgeries, physicians' expertise usually depends more on specific training and interest in performing vasectomies and following up on the procedure than on their particular specialty training.

Vasectomies are usually done on an outpatient basis, either in a physician's office or in a hospital-based or freestanding ambulatory surgery facility. Local anesthesia of the skin and the vasae is produced by an injection into the scrotum, which can be briefly uncomfortable until the medication has taken its full effect (usually after several seconds). Because of anxiety on the part of many men about having any discomfort in this area, many patients and physicians also choose to use sedation in the form of either tranquilizer pills or an injection for both mental and physical relaxation during vasectomy.

A number of techniques can be used safely and effectively by a physician performing a vasectomy, but the procedure can be thought of in terms of accomplishing three basic goals: The first is anesthesia, or the placement of numbing or freezing medication into the scrotum; the second is to gain access to the vas; and the third is its occlusion to prevent the passage of sperm.

Vasectomy can be made almost completely painless when local anesthesia in the form of medication such as lidocaine is used; this drug is similar to the anesthesia commonly used for dental procedures. By blocking the local nerves that send pain messages to the brain, normally painful procedures can be performed with little or no discomfort. A man having a vasectomy will feel the needle used to inject the medication into the skin and then a brief stinging sensation until it takes effect. The rest of the injection into the tubes themselves may or may not cause further discomfort, what some men describe as a pulling sensation.

The standard access procedure that the physician uses can vary with training and experience. It involves making either one incision into the scrotum in the middle of the front side or two incisions, one on either side. The incisions are made after the physician positions the vas directly under the skin, and then the other layers of tissue are separated to expose the vas itself. After each vas is occluded, the incision, which is between 1 and 1.5 centimeters long, must be closed with stitches, usually the type that dissolve and do not have to be removed.

A refinement of the access procedure, called the "no-scalpel" vasectomy, was introduced into the United States in the late 1980's. It originated in China in 1974, and a study comparing it with a standard technique found a more than 80 percent reduction in postoperative complications. It is being adopted only gradually by United States physicians, however, because performing it requires two simple but specially designed surgical instruments and because some physician retraining is required. Many physicians with experience in the new procedure believe that it should become the new standard for the vasectomy access procedure.

The occlusion of the vas is important because it determines the success of the vasectomy in preventing pregnancy. The physician can choose to occlude the vas ends by simple tying, folding back and tying, applying small metal clips, or cauterizing (burning with heat or special electrical current). In addition, one of the vas ends can be covered with a layer of the tissue that surrounds it to form a further barrier to sperm. Although all occlusion methods have been effective, cautery of the opening of the vasae may be the most reliable because it depends less on the technical precision of the physician doing the vasectomy than do the other methods, which can fail if applied too loosely or too tightly.

Finally, some physicians perform an open-ended technique, in which the end of the vas coming from the testicle is left open while only the outgoing end is occluded. This is thought to reduce the amount of backed-up sperm that can cause later complications and to make it easier to perform a vasectomy reversal. Some physicians believe, however, that the rate of vasectomy failure is higher with this technique.

Men from all over the world choose to have vasectomy performed, including about one-half million Americans every year. Vasectomy has been commonly available in the United States since the 1960's and is the fourth most commonly used birth control method overall, with one in eight women stating that they rely on this contraceptive method.

Sometimes men who have undergone vasectomies have, for various reasons, chosen to undergo a proce-

dure to reverse them. In such a procedure, the patient, under general anesthesia, has a one- to two-inch incision made in the scrotum over the site of the previous vasectomy. The ends of the vas deferens are located and cut free of the surrounding scar tissue. A drop of fluid from the testicular end of the vas is placed on a glass slide and examined under an electronic microscope to determine precisely what kind of microsurgery is most appropriate.

Uses and Complications

Most physicians make recommendations to the patient about what should be done, or not done, following a vasectomy, including activity restriction, pain control strategies, and follow-up. A period of rest for about forty-eight hours after a vasectomy helps to prevent pain and complications such as postoperative bleeding into the scrotum, which causes swelling. All sexual activity should be avoided for up to a week. Many men find more relief from an ice pack applied to the scrotum for the first few days following the surgery than from any medication, although acetaminophen (such as Tylenol) or mild prescription narcotics are often helpful as well. Aspirin and ibuprofen, although effective for pain, are generally best avoided in the first few days following a vasectomy because they have a blood-thinning effect that may increase the tendency to bleed. Because aspirin has a longer-lasting blood-thinning effect on platelets (the small blood cells that initiate normal blood clotting and stop minor bleeding), it should also not be taken for about ten days prior to the vasectomy.

Follow-up with a physician should be available in case complications occur in the period immediately following the vasectomy. The physician must also check the semen to ensure that no sperm are present. If sperm remain, it may indicate that one or both vasae remain open or have grown back together, meaning that the procedure has failed and the man remains fertile. If there are no sperm in the semen three to six months after the vasectomy, then it is extremely unlikely that a failure can still occur. Most doctors do not recommend any further follow-up unless a problem arises.

Informed consent means that the patient who will undergo a treatment has been given the opportunity to understand the risks and benefits of that treatment. In the case of vasectomy, the risks are pain, complications, the chance that it will fail, and the possibility that there will be a change of heart and that the man will want to father more children. The benefit is having very reliable, safe, and permanent birth control without ongoing costs or effort required.

The complications of vasectomy are best thought of in terms of those occurring early and late. Early complications include infection and hematoma. Infection is fairly uncommon but can include symptoms of pain, swelling, fever, redness, and abnormal drainage from the vasectomy wound. Treatment consists primarily of antibiotic medication. A hematoma is a collection of blood in a localized area such as the scrotum. Blood vessels in the scrotum that are cut or torn during vasectomy and not tied, clipped, or cauterized can ooze a small or large amount of blood. In the worst case, surgery to remove the blood may be considered to relieve pain and pressure. Fortunately, small hematomas resolve without surgery in a few weeks' time, and the more serious ones are rare, probably occurring in far less than 1 percent of vasectomies.

Later complications include problems with the area between the vasectomy incision and the testicles. Because the sperm are blocked from leaving the vas, and therefore the testicle, they can accumulate and cause three possible problems. First, sperm may back up at the site of the vasectomy and form a knot of sperm and inflamed scar tissue known as a sperm granuloma. It can be a painless lump, tender to pressure, or in rare cases it may be painful enough to require surgery to remove it. If swelling occurs because of accumulated sperm along the collecting area between the straight vas and the testicle (called the epididymis), the area can become tender or painful; this is known as congestive epididymitis. If this process extends backward to the testicle, it is known as orchitis. Fortunately, it is also rare for surgical removal of the entire epididymis to be required for relief of pain; sperm production slows in response to the pressure, and the body reabsorbs old sperm, eventually eliminating the pressure. Therefore, it is usually recommended that congestive epididymitis be treated with anti-inflammatory pain relievers such as ibuprofen, as well as with soaking in a warm bath.

Since there are many misconceptions about the risks and complications of vasectomy, it is useful to point out some problems that are not associated with the procedure. The complications of vasectomy are relatively minor and very rarely require hospitalization. Deaths and major surgical complications are largely unheard of. Impotence, loss of sexual drive, and changes in male characteristics such as beard growth, body hair, and voice do not occur. An apparent link between vasectomy and the hardening of the arteries that causes heart attacks has been disproven since the only such study was publicized in the late 1970's. Although a slight statistical association between vasectomy and cancer of the prostate gland was noted in two studies published in 1993, experts do not believe that vasectomy causes or contributes to prostate cancer because there is no reasonable mechanism for it to do so. Many men with milder forms of prostate cancer never die from it, and the statistics can be misleading because men who have seen a doctor for a vasectomy are also more likely to see a doctor for a prostate examination. Therefore, vasectomy may lead not to a greater risk of prostate cancer but to better detection of this disease.

PERSPECTIVE AND PROSPECTS

Vasectomy has been performed to cause sterility since 1925, but its common use for that purpose started in the 1960's. The concepts of birth control and the desirability of limiting family size became increasingly valued in industrialized countries. Some states in the United States removed legal barriers to sterilization around this time, and the oral contraceptive or birth control pill became available to large numbers of women. These developments and the increased openness to discussion of sexual topics helped to form the basis for what was labeled the "sexual revolution." In this environment, vasectomy became quite popular. It exceeded female sterilization by the early 1970's, driven in part by reports of the side effects of birth control pills. Sterilization for women (also called tubal ligation, literally "tying the tubes") is more invasive than vasectomy because the surgeon must enter the woman's abdomen to occlude the tubes that enable eggs to pass into her uterus. Therefore, vasectomy is somewhat safer when seen in the perspective of family planning. The women's movement of the 1960's placed a new emphasis on the control that women have over their bodies, especially in relation to health and medical decisions. Because the man can assume some of the reproductive responsibility and undergo a safer procedure, vasectomy also has a philosophical advantage for many couples.

Technological innovation by the mid-1970's had produced the first laparoscopic instruments, which enabled a gynecologic surgeon to enter a women's abdomen through two pencil-sized openings and identify and occlude her Fallopian tubes. This procedure, safer than the old one, with visibly smaller scars, and performed by obstetrician-gynecologists (the physicians whom women see most often), quickly became more popular than vasectomy and has remained so ever since. In spite of its high degree of safety, laparoscopic tubal ligation still occasionally results in deaths from general anesthesia and abdominal complications necessitating major surgery. Yet, even though tubal ligation costs three to five times more than vasectomy, it is still done more than twice as often. There are probably several reasons for this discrepancy, one of the most important being that when a woman has to make the sterilization decision alone, only tubal ligation can be chosen. When a woman is single or in a relationship with a lower level of commitment, or when there is a lack of consensus or support for the decision between the two partners, it is often easier for the woman to choose a tubal ligation. When a decision is made by a couple together, however, the risks and benefits give a comparative advantage to the male sterilization procedure.

When a couple makes a well-informed and mutual decision to choose vasectomy, the feelings in the months following the procedure most commonly include an increased sense of relaxation about sex because of lack of fear of unwanted pregnancy and an absence of anxiety and/or side effects related to contraceptive methods. On the other hand, if one of the partners was not ready and feels pressured into acceptance, the vasectomy decision can create irreconcilable conflict in the relationship.

Most doctors and clinics that counsel men about vasectomy emphasize the fact that vasectomy should be regarded as permanent. Every year, thousands of men seek the reversal of their vasectomies. Although the vasae can be surgically "spliced" back together in a safe and minor operation called vasovasostomy, sometimes years after a vasectomy, there are many reasons not to expect a simple reversal of the procedure. Reversal is expensive and often not covered by medical insurance, and the chances of restored fertility (as measured by later pregnancy) are only about 50 percent. The odds of reversal can be improved if the surgeon (usually a urologist) has substantial experience in the procedure, a microsurgical technique is used, and the vasectomy was relatively recent, and perhaps if the open-ended technique was used as well.

Some highly experienced urologists claim a 95 percent success rate in reversals, so patients should be cautioned to seek out a urologist who has extensive experience in performing the procedure. Reversal certainly offers hope to someone who has undergone a divorce or personal tragedy and wants to start a new family, but an ambivalent couple should not be reassured that after va-

sectomy they can change their minds and easily reverse the procedure.

The decision process by a man or a couple to pursue a vasectomy for family planning reasons often begins years before the procedure is actually done. First, they must feel that they have completed their family and be aware of vasectomy as a birth control option. Dissatisfaction with other birth control methods because of inconvenience and real or feared side effects often presses the decision. Discussion about vasectomy with one or more patients who have had one is a very common prerequisite to the decision for many men. Finally, a scare that an unwanted pregnancy can occur—such as a late period or a broken condom discovered too late—or even an actual unplanned pregnancy itself may be the last straw for many couples. The high rates of satisfaction with vasectomy may be attributable to the strong sense of comfort that follows this long and thorough decision process.

—John J. Seidl, M.D.;
updated by R. Baird Shuman, Ph.D.

See also Contraception; Electrocauterization; Men's health; Reproductive system; Sterilization; Testicular surgery; Vas deferens.

FOR FURTHER INFORMATION:
Connell, Elizabeth B. *The Contraception Sourcebook.* Chicago: Contemporary Books, 2002. A straightforward guide that provides comprehensive coverage of each contraceptive method, including a clear and understandable analysis of its advantages and disadvantages as well as a lively discussion of its origins.

Denniston, George C. *Vasectomy.* Victoria, B.C.: Trafford, 2002. Provides a range of information for men who are considering a vasectomy.

Haldar, N., et al. "How Reliable Is a Vasectomy? Long-Term Follow-up of Vasectomised Men." *The Lancet* 356, no. 9223 (July 1, 2000): 43-44. This article discusses the failure rate of vasectomy, which decreases dramatically in the first year following the procedure. The pregnancy rate after vasectomy is about one in two thousand.

Miller, Karl E. "No-Scalpel Technique vs. Standard Incision." *American Family Physician* 61, no. 5 (March 1, 2000): 1464. The major drawbacks to this otherwise safe and effective method of contraception are the adverse effects related to the incision and the delay between the procedure and sterility.

Parker, James N., and Philip M. Parker, eds. *The Official Patient's Sourcebook on Vasectomy.* San Diego,

Calif.: Icon Health, 2002. Draws from public, academic, government, and peer-reviewed research to provide a wide-ranging handbook for patients considering a vasectomy.

Paulson, David. "Diary of a Vasectomy." *American Health* 12 (July, 1993): 70-75. Written in a light and humorous style by a radio talk show host, this article addresses both the emotional and the factual aspects of vasectomy accurately and concisely.

VENEREAL DISEASES. *See* SEXUALLY TRANSMITTED DISEASES (STDs).

VENOUS INSUFFICIENCY

DISEASE/DISORDER

ANATOMY OR SYSTEM AFFECTED: Blood vessels, circulatory system, legs

SPECIALTIES AND RELATED FIELDS: Cardiology, vascular medicine

DEFINITION: An abnormality characterized by decreased blood return from the legs to the trunk that is caused by inefficient valves in the veins.

CAUSES AND SYMPTOMS

Venous insufficiency can be either reversible (acute) or irreversible (chronic). It is caused by conditions that increase the amount of circulating blood combined with a decrease in venous flow and is most commonly manifested by thrombophlebitis, varicose veins, and leg ulcers. Thrombophlebitis and varicose veins may be reversible in acute insufficiency.

Thrombophlebitis is an inflammation of the vein, commonly occurring in the legs. It may impede blood flow, resulting in pain, tenderness, redness, warmth along the vein, and edema (swelling). Thrombi (clots) may also form, enlarge, break off, and produce an

---

INFORMATION ON VENOUS INSUFFICIENCY

CAUSES: Conditions that increase amount of circulating blood and decrease venous flow (e.g., thrombophlebitis, varicose veins, leg ulcers)

SYMPTOMS: Vary; may include achiness, swelling, blue or bulging veins

DURATION: Acute or chronic

TREATMENTS: Leg elevation, warm and moist heat, anticoagulants, elastic stockings or bandages, surgery, debridement

---

embolus (dislodged clot), obstructing circulation and causing death. Varicose veins are large, protruding, and painful veins unable to return blood adequately to the trunk as a result of inefficient valves. They may be caused by pregnancy, congenital valve or vessel defects, obesity, pressure from prolonged standing, and poor posture. Leg ulcers are open, draining, painful wounds resulting from an inadequate supply of oxygen and other nutrients. They may also develop on skin surrounding varicose veins because of the stasis (slowing or halting) of the blood flow.

TREATMENT AND THERAPY

The treatment for thrombophlebitis includes rest; leg elevation; warm, moist heat to decrease pain and discomfort; and anticoagulant (blood-thinning) therapy to assist with circulation and to impede clot formation. Elastic stockings or bandages assist the return of blood to the heart. Drugs may be used to dissolve clots and to dilate vessels, improving circulation.

The conservative treatment of varicose veins includes the use of elastic stockings or bandages and rest. Aggressive treatment may include injecting the vein with sclerosing agents to occlude it and stop blood flow, thereby collapsing it. Surgical treatment may include ligating (tying off) the vein and then stripping and removing it.

Leg ulcer treatment includes debridement (the chemical or surgical removal of dirt or dead cellular tissue), cleansing and dressing the wound with ointments, pressure bandages, and the application of medicated castlike (unna) boots. Skin grafting may be attempted if other measures are not effective.

—*John A. Bavaro, Ed.D., R.N.*

See also Circulation; Deep vein thrombosis; Edema; Embolism; Phlebitis; Thrombosis and thrombus; Ulcer surgery; Ulcers; Varicose vein removal; Varicose veins; Vascular medicine; Vascular system.

FOR FURTHER INFORMATION:

Bergan, John J., and Jeffrey L. Ballard, eds. *Chronic Venous Insufficiency: Diagnosis and Treatment.* New York: Springer, 2000.

Cohen, Barbara J. *Memmler's The Human Body in Health and Disease.* 11th ed. Philadelphia: Wolters Kluwer Health/Lippincott Williams & Wilkins, 2009.

Ernst, Calvin B., and James C. Stanley, eds. *Current Therapy in Vascular Surgery.* 4th ed. St. Louis, Mo.: Mosby, 2001.

Hershey, Falls B., Robert W. Barnes, and David S. Sumner, eds. *Noninvasive Diagnosis of Vascular Disease.* Pasadena, Calif.: Appleton Davies, 1984.

Loscalzo, Joseph, and Andrew I. Schafer, eds. *Thrombosis and Hemorrhage.* 3d ed. Philadelphia: Lippincott Williams & Wilkins, 2003.

Mohrman, David E., and Lois Jane Heller. *Cardiovascular Physiology.* 6th ed. New York: Lange Medical Books/McGraw-Hill, 2006.

VERTIGO

DISEASE/DISORDER

ANATOMY OR SYSTEM AFFECTED: Brain, ears, nervous system

SPECIALTIES AND RELATED FIELDS: Audiology, neurology, otorhinolaryngology

DEFINITION: A sensation of motion or spinning when not moving.

KEY TERMS:

ataxia: coordinated movement difficulties

auditory nerve: the eighth cranial nerve, which conveys information from the ear to the brain

disequilibrium: off-balance sensation

dizziness: non-specific term that includes vertigo, fainting, and disequilibrium

electronystagmography: specialized eye movement measurements

endolymph: inner-ear fluid

labyrinth: mazelike system of canals in the inner ear

Ménière's disease: a disorder affecting endolymph

nystagmus: rhythmic involuntary movements of the eyes

oscillopsia: the sensation of bouncing vision

otoliths: granular bones of the inner ear

otorhinolaryngologist: the ear, nose, and throat (ENT) specialist

proprioception: the ability to locate the body in space

tinnitus: ringing in the ear

vestibular: the inner ear, vision, and nervous systems responsible for balance

CAUSES AND SYMPTOMS

Vertigo is a sensation of spinning or movement. Dizziness and disequilibrium are broader terms that include vertigo in some cases.

Vertigo results from disorders of the inner ear or central nervous system. Inner-ear causes include vestibular injury, labyrinthitis, vestibular neuritis, acute or recurrent vestibulopathy, benign positional vertigo,

Ménière's disease, perilymphatic fistula, and vestibular toxicity from drugs. Labyrinthitis or vestibular nerve dysfunction can result from trauma, cancer (acoustic neuroma), benign tumor, infection, connective tissue disorders, autoimmune disorder, otosclerosis, or middle-ear infection. Central nervous system causes of vertigo include brain stem stroke, cervical vertigo, tumors adjacent to the brain stem, migraines, multiple sclerosis, cranial nerve injury or degeneration, seizure disorders, hereditary familial ataxia, and inflammatory paraneoplastic syndromes. Problems with peripheral nerves and vision can contribute to vertigo.

Three systems work together to provide balance. The first is the inner-ear labyrinth system of tiny canals filled with a fluid called endolymph and tiny bones called otoliths. These canals contain tiny hair cells that sense endolymph movement. Information from the inner ear is conveyed to the brain through the eighth cranial nerve (auditory nerve) as well as branches of the seventh cranial nerve (facial nerve). The second system, vision, provides information to the brain via the optic nerve. The third system is proprioception, the ability to orient the body in space using input from the musculoskeletal system and from peripheral nerves. Specialized areas of the brain process information from these three systems to provide balance and maintain the vestibular ocular reflex and the vestibular spinal reflex. Adaptation to variations in input from these systems allows for activities such as figure skaters being able to tolerate high-speed spins. Balance is also possible with just two of three balance systems, allowing normal individuals to stand with eyes closed and not lose balance.

Disruption of one or more balance systems causes vertigo. Additional symptoms may include tinnitus,

---

INFORMATION ON VERTIGO

CAUSES: Inner ear or central nervous system disorders

SYMPTOMS: Sensation of movement or spinning, sometimes accompanied by tinnitus, nausea, disequilibrium, clumsiness, ataxia

DURATION: Varies depending on cause; may be episodic

TREATMENT: Depends on cause; may include otolith repositioning, inner ear surgery, low-salt diet, medications, vestibular rehabilitation therapy, treatment of underlying diseases

disequilibrium, hearing loss, sensitivity to sound, nausea, blurred vision, oscillopsia, nystagmus, ataxia, clumsiness, or headaches. Symptoms of underlying disease may be present.

Onset and additional symptoms; examination of the ear, nose, and throat; and a general neurological examination will help in diagnosis. Specialized techniques include the Hallpike maneuver (tilting the head over the edge of the examination table) and the fistula test, done by plugging one ear. Testing may include complete eye examination, computed tomogrpahy (CT) scan, magnetic resonance imaging (MRI), electronystagmography, hearing test, and rotational chair testing. Diagnosis of the underlying disorder is necessary for treatment.

Treatment and Therapy

Treatment of vertigo depends on the cause. Ménière's disease and other inner-ear conditions such as vestibular neuronitis may be treated with a salt-restricted diet, diuretics, motion sickness medication, antinausea medication, steroid injections, lifestyle modification including stress reduction, or inner-ear surgery. Otolith repositioning involves specialized physical therapy maneuvers that may be helpful for benign positional vertigo. Perilymphatic fistula may respond to bed rest. Middle-ear infections are treated with antibiotics.

Vertigo requires treatment aimed at correcting the underlying disorder. For example, acoustic neuromas may be treated with surgery and radiation. Symptoms from multiple sclerosis may respond to oral or intravenous steroids.

Diagnosis and treatment of vertigo will require a team of specialists, including a family physician, otorhinolaryngologist, neurologist, audiologist, internist, physical therapist, and occupational therapist.

Vestibular rehabilitation treats vertigo and other balance and dizziness problems through adaptation. Because vision is an important part of the balance system, significant vision impairment might limit rehabilitation effectiveness. Exercises prescribed by a physical or occupational therapist target activities that are problematic and may be done at home, in a rehabilitation center, or both. Exercises include targeted movements such as bending over, walking with one foot in front of the other, or walking with the head turned. Rehabilitation can take several weeks to several months.

Perspective and Prospects

Vertigo and dizziness are common symptoms; 40 percent of Americans may suffer from these conditions in their lifetime. Because of the variety of causes, some otolaryngologists and neurologists focus solely on the diagnosis and treatment of vertigo and dizziness.

Ménière's disease is the best-known cause of vertigo, first presented by Prospère Ménière to the French Academy of Medicine in 1861. Other inner-ear problems cause similar symptoms, but Ménière's disease specifically affects the endolymph fluid, causing vertigo and tinnitus. With modern diagnosis, Ménière's disease is now known to be less common than once thought.

Several famous people may have suffered from Ménière's disease or other forms of vertigo. Julius Caesar was said to have "falling disease" attributed to Ménière's disease or epilepsy. Other famous sufferers include artist Vincent Van Gogh, poet Emily Dickinson, and film star Marilyn Monroe.

Fortunately, vertigo does not usually indicate serious or life-threatening disease; however, it can take time and numerous tests to pinpoint the cause. With patience and persistence, most people can find a treatment or combination of treatments to reduce or eliminate their symptoms.

—E. E. Anderson Penno, M.D., M.S., FRCSC

See also Balance disorders; Brain; Brain disorders; Dizziness and fainting; Ear infections and disorders; Ears; Eye infections and disorders; Eyes; Hypotension; Ménière's disease; Vision; Vision disorders.

For Further Information:

Fauci, Anthony, et al. *Harrison's Principles of Internal Medicine.* 17th ed. New York: McGraw-Hill. 2008. A comprehensive text that includes details on a large number of disorders.

Mayoclinic.com. http://mayoclinic.com. A trusted source for information about a variety of disorders.

National Institutes of Health. http://www.ncbi.nlm .nih.gov/pubmed. An online catalog of peer-reviewed scientific articles.

Poe, Dennis. *The Consumer Handbook on Dizziness and Vertigo.* Sedona, Ariz.: Auricle Ink, 2005. An easy-to-understand book for nonmedical readers.

West, John. *Best and Taylor's Physiological Basis of Medical Practice.* 11th ed. Baltimore: Williams & Wilkins, 1985. A basic science text.

VETERINARY MEDICINE

SPECIALTY

ANATOMY OR SYSTEM AFFECTED: All

SPECIALTIES AND RELATED FIELDS: All

DEFINITION: The health care and medical treatment of animals—both domestic (pets and livestock) and wild (native and exotic species)—which includes preventive health care, sanitary and environmental management, and the treatment of diseases and injuries.

KEY TERMS:

clinical examination: the physical examination of an individual animal, including its medical history and an evaluation of its environment

diagnosis: the determination of what is causing a particular medical problem

epidemiological examination: a systematic explanation of patterns of disease among a group of animals and the use of this information in the treatment of the disease found in one or more of these animals

etiology: the cause of a disease, or the study of such causes

laboratory examination: the use of biochemical, biophysical, or hematological tests in the laboratory to assist in the diagnosis of disease

necropsy: a postmortem (after-death) examination of the animal's body, similar to an autopsy performed on a human corpse

physiological parameters: measurable characteristics determined to represent the normal biochemistry or functioning of a body fluid, organ, or system

subclinical disease: a medical problem with symptoms so slight that it is not diagnosed in a clinical examination

zoonoses: diseases communicable between animals and humans

SCIENCE AND PROFESSION

Animals become sick, get injured, or do not perform as well as they should, just as humans do. Humans, however, have developed a much more sophisticated medical expertise about themselves than they have about the wide variety of other animals. The basics of this medical knowledge apply to other animals, but the physiological differences of each of the many kinds of animal species preclude the application of human medical care. Much of veterinary knowledge has traditionally been concerned with a few common species, such as cats, dogs, cattle, sheep, goats, swine, horses, and some birds. Other species are receiving increasing attention, however, and their medical needs are becoming more widely acknowledged and better understood.

Most of the medical fields concerned with human health apply to veterinary health practice, including anatomy, anesthesiology and pharmacology, biochemistry, cardiovascular medicine, cell biology, dental medicine, dermatology, disease pathology, emergency and critical care, endocrinology, epidemiology, gastroenterology, genetics, geriatric medicine, hematology, immunology, internal medicine, microbiology, nephrology and renal medicine, neurology, obstetrics, oncology, ophthalmology, orthopedics, osteopathic medicine, otorhinolaryngology, physiology, psychiatry, surgery, and urology. There has been much progress in the veterinary applications of these medical fields. In addition, there has been considerable progress in the application of the expertise, techniques, and equipment used in these medical fields to an increasingly wider variety of animal species. This development is attributable to both an improved knowledge of and interest in these other species and an ethical concern for this wider range of species.

Not only have humans become knowledgeable about how to care for less common domestic and wild animals, but it has also become acceptable to do so. As a result, veterinarians have become involved with a much wider range of employment opportunities in government, business, universities, and zoological parks, although most are still in private practice dealing with farm livestock, horses, cats, and dogs. In addition, veterinarians are also working in a wider range of locations, including in the clinic, in the research laboratory, on the farm, in the field, at zoological parks, and in the wild. There are also more employment opportunities for veterinary technicians, paraprofessionals who assist the veterinarian or who carry out certain veterinary duties when the veterinarian is not available.

Veterinary medicine is both a distinct medical field and an extension of human medical fields. It deals with species quite different from humans, the degree of difference ranging from slight (such as primates) to great (such as birds, reptiles, amphibians, and fish). While the medical doctor deals with only one species, the veterinarian is concerned with a multitude of species. Therefore, the medical doctor tends to specialize in a medical field, while the veterinarian tends to specialize in particular kinds of animals. There are some similarities, and many differences, between human medicine and veterinary medicine, with a common ground in zoonoses, those diseases that can be transmitted between humans and other animals. These degrees of similarity and difference among species are a primary concern for the veterinarian and are one of the things that make veterinary medicine such an interesting subject.

In addition to routine clinical work (both in the office and in the field) dealing with farm livestock, domestic pets, and racing horses and dogs, some veterinarians are involved in other kinds of work. Veterinarians may work with exotic pets, exotic livestock (such as ostrich farms or alligator farms), zoological park and aquarium animals, and laboratory animals. They may maintain healthy game herds and flocks (such as deer and turkeys), translocate wild animals from one area to another, work with teams doing scientific research that involves animals, help with efforts to save endangered species (either in the wild or in captivity), work with beached porpoises and whales, and advise government agencies concerned with animal welfare issues.

In addition to treating sick and injured animals, veterinary medicine involves advising on preventive measures, making routine observations of individual animals or groups of animals, evaluating herd management, examining environmental and housing conditions, assisting with births, and performing necropsies. Veterinarians working with laboratory animals, zoological park animals, native game species, or endangered species may also provide advice on reducing stress, assisting with propagation strategies (including various artificial propagation techniques), tranquilization, translocation techniques, the gathering of tissue samples, and other animal welfare matters.

The control of epidemic diseases in farm livestock or native wildlife is also carried out by veterinarians. Also of interest are diseases that may be introduced by imported animals, particularly exotic species. For example, parrots imported for the pet trade are capable of transmitting diseases that could affect poultry, as could migrating native bird species. Imported exotic hoofstock can introduce diseases that could affect farm livestock, as could the importation of farm livestock from already infested areas.

For these reasons, species similar to those on farms and ranches (usually birds and hoofstock) are subjected to medical quarantines and other medical restrictions. The transfer of animals or animal products from one country to another by private citizens is also strictly controlled. Diseases that can be passed to humans by animals, particularly those sold as pets, are another sit-

uation that is closely monitored. Another problem involving both medical doctors and veterinarians is those diseases that can be passed from native wild animals to humans, either directly or through other host species, such as insects.

Veterinarians working in the field on medical problems involving native wildlife, imported exotic species, or endangered species are often on their own, working at remote sites and often carrying their clinics on their backs. Improvisation, creativity, and adventure are often a part of their practice.

Thus, the application of veterinary medicine involves the same kinds of medical fields as those used in human medicine, but the methods, techniques, equipment, medicines, and treatments are different. The amount of difference depends on the species and the area of operation, which in turn ranges from the urban clinic, to the rural farm, to the wilds of remote wilderness areas.

DIAGNOSTIC AND TREATMENT TECHNIQUES

Most medical fields are much better developed for use with humans than with animals because humans know so much more about themselves than they do about the other animal species. Humans constitute only one species—a species that has been studied in depth for quite some time. Unlike human medicine, veterinary medicine is concerned with many animal species, each of which has its own physiological parameters. In addition, different categories of animals—mammals, birds, reptiles, amphibians, and fishes—have significantly different body systems. These different categories and species have to be treated differently when determining whether an animal is normal and healthy and when prescribing treatment for a sick animal.

The best understood groups of animals are the ones that have been of concern to the veterinary profession for the longest period of time, particularly farm livestock and pets. More recently, other groups have received attention, including those used in sporting events, those in zoological parks, laboratory animals, native wildlife, and endangered species. As ethical concerns extend out beyond the human race, more concern has been shown for the health of all animal species. There is much to learn, however, about many species that are not dealt with on a regular basis by veterinarians.

The diagnosis and treatment of an illness or injury depend on the kind of animal being examined. Since the animal cannot tell the owner or the veterinarian what is wrong, it is up to the veterinarian to discover this information. The diagnosis is therefore particularly important. First, the veterinarian must analyze the abnormality. On a clinical level, this means a general physical examination, a special examination of the suspect system or organ, a special examination of the problem area, and a medical history; on a subclinical level, it means laboratory tests and a comparison with peer performance standards. Second, one must analyze the pattern of occurrence of the abnormality in the herd (if necessary), which includes an epidemiological examination; an evaluation of general management, environmental factors, and time of season; nutritional status; and genetics. The veterinarian then categorizes and defines the abnormality, prescribes a treatment, follows up on the treatment, and advises the owner on prevention.

The first step in providing care is to know when an animal is sick. An injury is easier to detect, but it may still be difficult to determine the extent of the injury. Lack of performance may, or may not, be a medical problem. Obviously, an animal is not able to relate any information pertaining to its medical problems. It is easier to determine when an illness is present in animals with which humans are very familiar, such as pets, horses, or livestock. It becomes more difficult with other mammals and birds, and especially with fish, reptiles, and amphibians.

The species of the animal must be known, along with the physiological parameters for that species. The medical history of the individual (and, if applicable, the other individuals with which it is associated, such as a herd) is also necessary. A clinical examination is then used to determine the current medical situation, supplemented by a laboratory examination and an epidemiological examination. From this information, a diagnosis is made and a treatment is prescribed.

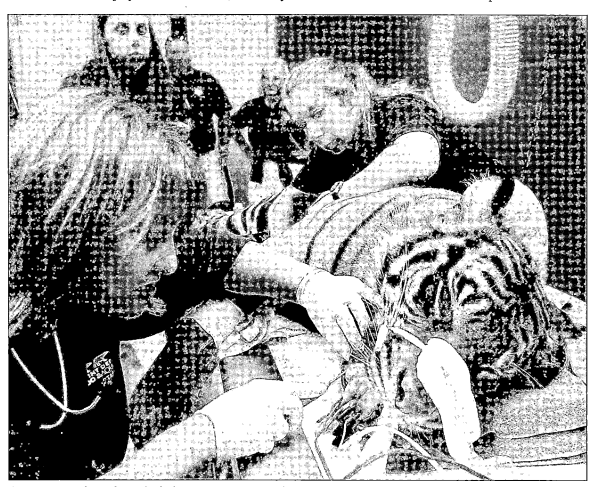

A veterinarian cleans the teeth of a Sumatran tiger. Zoo medicine is a challenging specialty because of the diverse nature of the species that must be treated. (AP/Wide World Photos)

These examinations include consideration of past diseases and treatments, nutrition, behavior, general appearance, skin condition, voice, eating habits, defecation and urination, posture and gait, the inspection of the specific body regions, a physical examination (for example, temperature and pulse), the consideration of environmental factors (such as housing, source of water supply, sanitation, and chemical contaminations), and the consideration of laboratory tests on specimen samples from the animal and the environment.

A diagnosis based on these examinations should provide information on the disease or injury, the etiology of the disease, and the clinical manifestation of the disease, that is, the severity or extensiveness of the disease. From the diagnosis, a treatment can be prescribed. This treatment may involve additional care, surgery, the use of medication, a change in diet, or a change in the animal's environment.

Follow-up on the treatments may also be necessary. For animals, medicines can have side effects, and multiple medicines can have synergistic effects. Another problem is that animals tend to care for themselves by licking, pulling at bandages, and other behaviors that tend to undo what the veterinarian has done. Also, animals are not able to say whether they are feeling better, although this can often be determined by observing the animal's return to normal behavior. Continued monitoring and reexamination by the veterinarian may be necessary.

Preventive health care is as important for animals as it is for humans. This kind of care may include vaccination shots, pills, proper nutrition, dental care, reduction of stress, exercise, sanitation and proper housing, the quarantine of exotic species, or simply observation of behavior.

Low performance may be a medical problem but is difficult to detect because the problem tends to be a subclinical disease. Economically efficient performance of livestock, or peak racing performance in horses and dogs, have become important matters requiring the attention of the veterinarian. The efficient performance of livestock is economically important to the farmer. An assessment of a herd's productivity is usually done by comparing its performance with a standard that is based on known performances of peer herds. Productivity can have several meanings: the amount of milk or meat produced per animal or per hectare, reproductive efficiency, calf survival rate, longevity, and acceptability or quality of the milk or meat at market. Low performance might be caused by a num-

ber of factors: inadequate nutrition, poor genetic inheritance, improper housing, stress, lack of herd management expertise, subclinical diseases, physiological abnormalities, or anatomical problems.

Although some veterinarians specialize in a particular medical field, for the most part, a veterinarian has to be familiar with all medical fields in order to treat an animal. While these fields of medicine are basically the same whether one is treating a human or an animal, it must be kept in mind that each species has different body structures and different physiological parameters. Also, different equipment and techniques are necessary in applying these medical fields to animals. For example, the principles of anesthesiology are well understood, but applying anesthesia to a human is not the same as applying it to a dog, a horse, or an elephant: The gases used, the equipment needed, and the procedures used must be tailored to the particular kind of animal being treated. Similar examples could be given for the application of each medical field.

Most veterinary work is carried out in the clinic, particularly small-animal practice (usually cats, dogs, and other common pets). Large-animal practice (usually farm livestock and horses) is often done at specially designed on-site areas at a farm or ranch. Veterinary schools also have both small-animal and large-animal clinics. While small animals are easily handled, large animals need pens, squeeze cages, tilting tables (tilting from a vertical position, in which the animal is strapped onto it, to a horizontal position), and other equipment to restrain them during the examination. Large-animal veterinarians working on a farm or ranch also use veterinary vehicles that are stocked with whatever the veterinarian normally needs. In rural areas, the veterinarian is too far away from the clinic to go back continually to the clinic for supplies while making rounds from farm to farm. Therefore, their vehicles are specially adapted (by the veterinarian or by commercial companies) as mobile clinics.

PERSPECTIVE AND PROSPECTS

Animal domestication developed around 8000 B.C.E. With humankind's increasing dependency on domestic animals, it became necessary to care for their medical needs. The Mesopotamian Code of Hammurabi (a legal code from about 2200 B.C.E.) mentions payments to animal doctors if they successfully cared for an animal, and punishment if they were not successful. Papyruses from ancient Egypt contain the oldest known veterinary prescriptions (c. 1900 B.C.E.). The first veterinarian known by name was from India (c. 1800 B.C.E.). It was also in India that the first known animal hospitals were established (c. 250 B.C.E.). The Aztecs of ancient America also had animal doctors for the large royal animal collections. Ancient civilizations treated diseases with herbs and rituals, some surgical procedures were performed, and some injuries were treated. Medical instruments were crude, and care was based on magic and folklore. This, however, was not unusual during a time when medicine, science, and religion were integrated into one limited body of knowledge. The fact that an effort was made to care for animals indicates their importance to these early societies.

While medical knowledge increased in ancient China and Greece, veterinary medicine did not. In the Roman and medieval periods, practitioners simply compiled and transcribed what had already been done. Nevertheless, the advances made in medical knowledge were to affect veterinary medicine—for example, the determination that diseases were derived from natural causes rather than divine causes, and improved knowledge of how the body functioned.

The Renaissance brought about a renewed interest in many areas of study, including in veterinary medicine. In particular, there was concern about farm livestock and horses because of their increasing economic importance to society. In addition, much of the medical research conducted during this time was done with animals. Advances in veterinary medicine coincided with those in medicine in general but were eventually made for their own sake. The first short-lived veterinary schools appeared in Spain (c. 1490), and the first modern ones appeared in Europe during the eighteenth century. It was not until the nineteenth century, however, that methodological observation and examination became the foundation for diagnoses, and veterinary medicine passed from the common practitioner to the academic or professional practitioner.

One significant effect of the growth of veterinary medicine and its acceptance among the general public has been the concept of animal rights, which has increased the provision of medical care to pets, exotic animals exhibited at zoological parks, and native wildlife. At the same time, veterinary knowledge has been extended to amphibians, reptiles, and fish, as well as to a larger array of birds and mammals.

—Vernon N. Kisling, Jr., Ph.D.

See also Animal rights vs. research; Education, medical; Ethics; Zoonoses.

For Further Information:

Blood, D. C., O. M. Radostits, and J. A. Henderson. *Veterinary Medicine.* 9th ed. New York: Elsevier, 2000. A textbook on the diseases of cattle, sheep, pigs, goats, and horses. Intended primarily for use by veterinary students.

Ford, Richard B., and Elisa M. Mazzaferro. *Kirk and Bistner's Handbook of Veterinary Procedures and Emergency Treatment.* 8th ed. St. Louis, Mo.: Saunders/Elsevier, 2006. A concise and authoritative reference on the procedures used for the emergency treatment of specific conditions, for interpreting signs of disease, and for interpreting laboratory tests.

Fowler, Murray E., and R. Eric Miller, eds. *Zoo and Wild Animal Medicine.* 6th ed. Philadelphia: Saunders/Elsevier, 2008. A text concerning the veterinary care of nondomestic animals. Covers preventive medicine, sanitation, stress, restraint, and the medical care of mammals, birds, reptiles, and amphibians. More specialized books dealing with these animal groups (in the wild, in zoos, or as pets) are also available.

Kahn, Cynthia M., ed. *The Merck Veterinary Manual.* 50th anniversary ed. Whitehouse Station, N.J.: Merck, 2008. A concise and authoritative reference covering the pathology, clinical findings, and treatment of medical problems related to the various biological body systems. Also covers behavior, clinical values, husbandry, nutrition, toxicology, pharmacology, and zoonoses.

Wallach, Joel D., and William J. Boever. *Diseases of Exotic Animals: Medical and Surgical Management.* Philadelphia: W. B. Saunders, 1983. An authoritative text arranged by broad taxonomic groups within the mammals, birds, reptiles, amphibians, and fishes. Covers biological data, housing, nutrition, restraint, behavior, and medicine for each of these groups.

Viral hemorrhagic fevers
Diseases/disorders
Anatomy or system affected: All
Specialties and related fields: Epidemiology, virology
Definition: Acute zoonotic diseases caused by viruses.
Key terms:
epidemiology: the study of the occurrence, frequency, causes, and distribution of diseases within a population

hemorrhagic: referring to a disease or disorder characterized by abnormal bleeding, often from internal organs, although bleeding may also occur under the skin, in the mucous linings of the nose and throat, and in tear ducts

reservoir species: animals that can carry a virus or bacterium that causes a disease in other species without suffering serious or fatal illness themselves

zoonoses: disorders carried by animal hosts that can be transmitted to humans

CAUSES AND SYMPTOMS

Viral hemorrhagic fevers are caused by a variety of viruses, including members of the Arenaviridae, Bunyaviridae, Flaviviridae, and Filoviridae families, with the last mentioned being the one associated with diseases such as Ebola hemorrhagic fever and Marburg hemorrhagic fever. Many of the hemorrhagic diseases are zoonoses that exist in reservoir species, such as bats, and are transmitted to humans through various modes; others are vector-borne. Crimean-Congo hemorrhagic fever, for example, is carried by ticks; humans become infected when they are bitten. In contrast, Ebola hemorrhagic fever, caused by a filovirus, is suspected of making the leap from animals to humans through the handling and eating of infected wild game, while Lujo fever, which is caused by an arenavirus, apparently infects humans when they inhale dust from rodent droppings. However, some viral hemorrhagic fevers may have the ability to aerosolize and thus may be transmitted person-to-person from an infected patient to caregivers or family members when an infected person sneezes or coughs. Contact with body fluids, such as blood or vomit, from an infected person can also cause the disease to spread.

The initial clinical signs and symptoms for viral hemorrhagic fevers are similar to those of many common illnesses, such as influenza or dysentery, with the patient complaining of a fever, headache, generalized aches and pains, or nausea. In the case of Ebola hemorrhagic fever, clinical signs may include a skin rash or red eyes. It is usually not until several days after the onset of the illness that the hemorrhagic signs, such as bloody diarrhea indicating internal bleeding, appear. Because the symptoms for many hemorrhagic fevers are similar to those of common tropical diseases, initial diagnosis and quarantine efforts may be delayed.

The virulence of the hemorrhagic fevers varies, depending both on the specific viral strain involved and how quickly medical treatment is obtained. Despite the name hemorrhagic fever, it is rarely the blood loss associated with the diseases that causes death but instead the failure of organs such as the kidneys. Some Ebola hemorrhagic fevers have resulted in death rates of close to 90 percent of infected patients, while others have been as low as 20 percent. Similarly, incubation periods vary for the different diseases, from only a few days for some diseases to as long as three weeks for others. The best-known hemorrhagic fever, Ebola, has an incubation period of two to twenty-one days.

TREATMENT AND THERAPY

Treatment for viral hemorrhagic fever varies from disease to disease. In many cases, the only care that can be given is that of relieving the suffering of the patient by treating the symptoms—giving liquids intravenously to replace fluids lost through vomiting or diarrhea, trying to keep electrolytes balanced, and giving drugs that may reduce the patient's fever or body aches. In some cases, patients have been successfully treated with blood transfusions from persons who have survived a similar illness.

Because the exact transmission routes for many hemorrhagic fevers remain unclear, once patients are diagnosed, a strict quarantine must be instituted, with health care workers and family members alike wearing protective clothing to prevent becoming contaminated with any infectious material. When a patient dies, the body must also be handled carefully. In the case of Ebola, the World Health Organization (WHO) recommends cremation as quickly as possible following death.

PERSPECTIVE AND PROSPECTS

As the population has expanded globally and humans encroach upon formerly isolated wildlife habitat, more viral hemorrhagic fevers have been discovered, some-

---

INFORMATION ON VIRAL HEMORRHAGIC FEVERS

CAUSES: Viral infection

SYMPTOMS: Fever, sore throat, generalized body aches, headache, vomiting, diarrhea, rash, red eyes

DURATION: Varies depending on specific disease, from few days to several weeks

TREATMENTS: Primarily supportive care to minimize suffering and alleviate symptoms

times through the case of just one or two persons becoming infected by a previously unknown pathogen and sometimes through devastating outbreaks resulting in many deaths. Despite many years of research, many of these diseases still remain scientific mysteries.

The best-known example, Ebola hemorrhagic fever virus, is now known to exist in multiple locations in Africa. Some strains are comparatively mild; some are extremely virulent, spreading quickly and causing high numbers of deaths within a population. Researchers now know that, as is true with many viruses, patients who have infected by Ebola and survive retain antibodies to that strain of virus for decades. They do not yet know if that means those people are effectively immune to Ebola.

Theoretically, it should be possible to develop vaccines against the viral hemorrhagic diseases, but several factors mitigate such work. First is the reality that although many can be quite devastating in terms of death rates, outbreaks that have occurred to date have been in remote areas or affected very low numbers of persons. It is easy to argue for funding vaccine research work when a disease is widespread, as in the historical example of polio; it becomes much more difficult for researchers when the disease in question is localized in a nonindustrialized country such as the Sudan or Uganda. In recent years, the threat of viruses such as Ebola being utilized for bioterrorism, however, has led to more effort being put into finding effective vaccines and treatments, but for most of the viral hemorrhagic diseases any vaccines or treatments developed to date remain classified as experimental.

—Nancy Farm Mannikko, Ph.D.

See also Bleeding; Centers for Disease Control and Prevention (CDC); Dengue fever; Ebola virus; Emerging infectious diseases; Epidemics and pandemics; Epidemiology; Hemorrhage; Marburg virus; Tropical medicine; Viral infections; Zoonoses.

FOR FURTHER INFORMATION:

Hewlitt, Barry S., and Bonnie L. Hewitt. *Ebola, Culture, and Politics: The Anthropology of an Emerging Disease.* Belmont, Calif.: Thomson Higher Education, 2008. A fascinating book that looks at the social and cultural context in which Ebola emerged as a public health problem that also provides a solid medical explanation of the disease.

Shors, Teri. *Understanding Viruses.* Sudbury, Mass.: Jones and Bartlett, 2008. An introductory textbook intended for undergraduate college students with no prior background in virology, which makes it accessible to the general reader.

Strauss, James H., and Ellen G. Strauss. *Viruses and Human Disease.* San Diego, Calif.: Academic Press, 2007. A textbook intended for college students, but still accessible to the general reader.

VIRAL INFECTIONS

DISEASE/DISORDER

ANATOMY OR SYSTEM AFFECTED: All

SPECIALTIES AND RELATED FIELDS: Epidemiology, family medicine, internal medicine, virology

DEFINITION: A wide range of diseases, from mild (such as the common cold) to fatal (such as rabies, smallpox, and AIDS), caused by viruses, life-forms that function as intracellular parasites.

KEY TERMS:

capsid: the protein coat of a virus, composed of subunits known as capsomeres

envelope: an additional covering found on animal viruses; it is composed of lipids and proteins and surrounds the genome and the protein coat of the virus

genome: the genetic material of a virus; in a virion, the genome consists of deoxyribonucleic acid (DNA) or ribonucleic acid (RNA) and is protected by the capsid

lysogenic (temperate) virus: a virus that integrates its genome into the genome of the host cell; such viruses exist in a latent state and do not produce progeny viruses

lytic virus: a virus that guides the production of progeny viruses and that ultimately causes the death and lysis (disintegration) of the host cell

virion: the form of the virus as it exists outside the host cell

HOW VIRUSES WORK

Viruses are entities that infect the cells of all organisms. Some scientists classify viruses as living organisms based on their ability to reproduce inside an appropriate host cell. Yet, viruses lack cellular structure and have no metabolic capability of their own. They are completely dependent on host cells to reproduce. In addition, some viruses can be crystallized and thus have properties of complex molecules rather than of living organisms.

Viruses can be visualized only with an electron microscope. They are small in size, ranging from approximately 10 to 300 nanometers in either length or diame-

Information on Viral Infections

Causes: Exposure to viruses, usually through contact with infected humans, animals, or vectors
Symptoms: Wide ranging; may include rash, fever, muscle aches, headaches, pain, sore throat
Duration: Acute to chronic
Treatments: Antiviral agents, supportive therapy

ter. Because viruses cannot easily be seen within the host cells that they infect, studies of viral structure often utilize the extracellular form of the virus, called the viral particle or virion.

Viruses are quite variable with respect to size, shape, and biological properties, but they do have some common features. All viruses contain a genome, which is genetic material in the form of either deoxyribonucleic acid (DNA) or ribonucleic acid (RNA). A protein coat known as a capsid that is composed of protein subunits called capsomeres protects the genome of a virus. The capsid is arranged either into a symmetrical structure with spherical (round) or up to twenty-sided (icosahedral) symmetry. Alternatively, the capsid can assume a helical shape.

Some viruses contain additional protein structures that aid in their attachment and penetration of host cells. Other viruses, especially the ones that infect animal cells, are surrounded by a complex membrane structure known as the envelope. While the lipids in the envelope are derived from host cells, the proteins and glycoproteins contained in the envelope are usually viral-specific structures that are encoded by the genetic material of the virus. In animal viruses, the genetic material and protein coat, together called the nucleocapsid, constitute the core of the virus. In addition to these features, some viruses carry enzymes that are necessary for the virus to infect a host cell or to replicate.

Most viruses can infect only one type of host; that is, they display species specificity. The virus that causes rabies is a notable exception since it can infect a variety of mammalian species. All types of organisms—bacteria, protozoa, fungi, plants, and animals—are known to be hosts to viruses. Viruses that infect bacteria are called bacteriophages, or phages. The elucidation of many of the aspects of viral structure and the stages of viral infection was derived from the study of the mechanism by which phages infect their specific bacterial hosts.

Slow virus diseases are a class of viruses that reproduce very slowly, often over months or years. They are difficult to study. A common result of slow virus infections is a condition called spongiform encephalopathy, which is a degeneration of brain cells that ultimately causes death. Recent research has shown that slow viruses cause such diseases as kuru and Creutzfeldt-Jakob disease (CJD) in humans and scrapie in sheep.

Several steps have been identified in the process by which viruses infect host cells. Because they lack motility, viruses must come into contact with host cells by chance. They are transmitted from host to host in the same ways as other microorganisms: through air, water, or food or by physical contact. A common mode of transmission is by aerosols produced when an infected individual coughs, sneezes, or breathes. Virions in the aerosols gain access to the host by means of the respiratory system. Common cold and influenza viruses are transmitted in this manner, as are the viruses that cause common childhood diseases such as chickenpox, measles, and mumps. As a result, these viruses are very contagious; they are easily spread from person to person.

Some viruses, such as the poliomyelitis (polio) virus, can be transmitted in contaminated food or water. The virus gains entry to the host through the mouth and digestive system. Other viruses will also gain entry after contact, which may be direct (person to person) or indirect (via an inanimate object). Viruses will also enter a host if they are directly introduced into the bloodstream, which can occur via a cut or wound or through use of a contaminated needle. Hepatitis B virus and the human immunodeficiency virus (HIV), which causes acquired immunodeficiency syndrome (AIDS), can infect individuals in this manner. Transmission of these viruses occurs at a high rate among intravenous drug users who share needles. In addition to the above methods of transmission, mosquitoes may transmit viruses such as the encephalitis virus and the yellow fever virus.

All viruses must first attach themselves to their respective host cells. This phase of viral infection is sometimes referred to as adsorption. The attachment process is very specific and is controlled (mediated) by receptors present on the host cell, most of which are glycoproteins. It is the specific nature of this attachment process that accounts for the fact that a virus will infect host cells of only one species. Some viruses are also specific for the type of host cell to which they will adsorb. For example, poliovirus adsorbs only to cells of the central nervous system and gastrointestinal tract.

Following adsorption, the virus penetrates the host cell. In the case of bacteriophages, only the viral genome reaches the interior of the host cell; the protein coat of the virus remains outside. In contrast, the entire animal virus penetrates its host cell. Once inside, the viral genome is separated from the protein coat and envelope. During this stage of viral infection, the virus cannot be visualized by electron microscopy.

The viral genome is responsible for the next stages of viral infection. Many viruses begin a process that will eventually result in the replication of the viral genome and the production of progeny viruses. These viruses are referred to as lytic viruses because the death and lysis of the host cell accompany infection. The infecting lytic virus uses many of the host cell's biochemical processes to replicate its DNA or RNA. It also causes the host to make proteins that will constitute the capsids of the newly made viruses. New viral particles assemble spontaneously. In many cases, hundreds of these progeny will be released as the host cell disintegrates. These newly produced viruses are then available to infect other cells. This type of virus causes diseases such as chickenpox and polio. In some cases, progeny viruses are continuously shed from host cells. The host cell remains viable for long periods of time and releases large numbers of viruses.

Some viruses do not produce progeny after they penetrate host cells. Instead of being used to produce new viruses, the genetic material of these viruses becomes part of the host cell genome in a process called integration. These viruses are referred to as lysogenic or temperate viruses. In order for these viruses to integrate into the host cell genome, they must either consist of double-stranded DNA or be capable of forming double-stranded DNA within the host cell. RNA viruses that are capable of lysogeny contain an enzyme known as reverse transcriptase that enables the virus to produce a DNA copy of the viral RNA. These viruses are known as retroviruses. Several medically important viruses, such as some tumor viruses and HIV, belong to this category.

Although integrated into the viral genome, lysogenic viruses do not multiply to produce new viral particles. They remain in an apparently latent state. There is evidence, however, that these viruses can make some types of protein and, in some cases, can alter the properties of their host cells. For example, when a virus called SV40 integrates into the genome of certain host

cells, it will cause these cells to divide rapidly and grow in a manner that resembles tumor cells. Not all lysogenic viruses remain latent. Ultraviolet light is known to cause latent herpesvirus to switch to a lytic mode of infection, an effect known as induction. Other factors, such as stress, may also be responsible for viral induction.

DIAGNOSIS AND TREATMENT

The extent of a viral disease can usually be explained by the biological properties of the particular virus involved. Some viral infections may be mild, such as the common cold, or entirely unnoticed. Other viral infections can be more serious, debilitating, or even fatal, such as polio, influenza, and AIDS. In some cases, viral infection is acute; an individual is sick for a short period of time and then fully recovers. Other viral infections are chronic; the virus persists for long periods of time. The disease that it causes periodically erupts and then subsides.

Diagnosis of viral diseases often relies on an analysis of the symptoms associated with each type of viral infection. Some viral illnesses cause typical rashes such as those seen in chickenpox, measles, and rubella. Influenza virus infection results in typical flulike symptoms, including throat pain, fever, and muscle aches. It is much more difficult to diagnose viral infections when the virus is latent or not actively causing damage to the host. Sometimes it is important to detect individuals who are infected with a latent virus or who are not symptomatic. Such individuals may be carriers of the virus and thus have the potential to transmit the disease to others. It is possible to identify such individuals by testing for the presence of viral proteins or by examining their immune response to the virus.

The major host defense against viral infections in higher organisms is the immune system. Cells of the immune system recognize many disease-causing viruses, either as virions circulating within the host or by the presence of virus-specific proteins on infected host cells. In either case, the virus is eliminated, although damage to host cells is sometimes a natural consequence of this type of protection. This active immune response against the virus will often result in lifelong protection from subsequent infections by the same virus. It is extremely rare for a person who has recovered from measles or mumps to have another occurrence of that particular disease.

Some viruses are not completely eliminated when recovery occurs. Varicella zoster virus is the cause of

---

chickenpox, a common childhood disease. In the United States, more than 90 percent of the population has been infected with this virus by the time they reach adulthood. Chickenpox usually runs its course in about two weeks, and complete clinical recovery is observed. Yet, the virus is not necessarily eliminated. It has been tracked to the nervous system, where it can remain dormant for decades. The virus can be reactivated, usually in older adults or in those individuals whose immune systems are compromised. It will travel via the nerves and cause shingles (herpes zoster). Shingles is a condition characterized by a burning rash, itching, tingling, and pain that may be quite severe.

Vaccines. Vaccines protect against viral infections by utilizing the host's own immune system. For use in vaccines, the virus is either inactivated, and thus is no longer capable of causing an infection, or infectious but of a much milder strain. Viruses are commonly inactivated for vaccine preparation by chemical treatments that essentially kill the virus. The virus is then no longer able to infect and multiply within host cells. These types of vaccines must be administered at repeated time intervals (months or years, depending on the vaccine) to ensure a sufficient level of immunity.

Live viruses are used in some vaccines, but the harmful or pathogenic form of the virus is never employed. Instead, a weaker version of the virus is selected. These weaker variants, called attenuated strains, can sometimes be found when the virus is grown under laboratory conditions. The advantage of live viral vaccines is that the virus can multiply within the host and cause a significantly higher stimulation of the host's immune system than is usually seen with inactivated viral vaccines. Attenuated strains of the poliovirus are used to produce the oral polio vaccine that is commonly administered to infants in the United States. In rare cases, serious problems do occur with live vaccines. A few individuals among the millions who have been vaccinated, or their family contacts, have been known to develop polio as a result of exposure to the live polio vaccine.

Another method of vaccine preparation involves the use of parts of the viral envelope, particularly the viral-coded proteins. These proteins can be mass-produced using modern genetic engineering technology and then incorporated into various vaccine preparations. This method has the advantage of reducing the risks involved with live vaccines.

The important result of vaccination is that the immune system is stimulated to recognize the virus and thus eliminate its harmful form when the virus is next encountered. Vaccination programs have been highly effective in decreasing the incidence of viral diseases in countries where they are administered. The most striking success of a major vaccination program was the virtual global elimination of naturally occurring smallpox by 1976.

For some viral infections, the immune system does not offer adequate protection from the harmful effects

Types of Viral Infection

Family		Conditions
Adenoviruses		Respiratory and eye infections
Arenaviruses		Lassa fever
Coronaviruses		Common cold
Herpesviruses		Cold sores, genital herpes, chickenpox, herpes zoster (shingles), glandular fever, congenital abnormalities (cytomegalovirus)
Orthomyxoviruses		Influenza
Papovaviruses		Warts
Paramyxoviruses		Mumps, measles, rubella
Picornaviruses		Poliomyelitis, viral hepatitis types A and B, respiratory infections, myocarditis
Poxviruses		Cowpox, smallpox (eradicated), molluscum contagiosum
Retroviruses		AIDS, degenerative brain diseases, possibly various kinds of cancer
Rhabdoviruses		Rabies
Togaviruses		Yellow fever, dengue, encephalitis

of the virus. In still other cases, effective vaccines that offer long-term protection against viral infection have not been developed. With some viral infections, an encounter with the virus does not guarantee immunity from future infections: The virus is able to alter its envelope proteins and thus appears different to the immune system when it is encountered again. This is the case with influenza viruses.

Chemical agents. Chemical antiviral agents have also been developed. These chemical agents have been useful because they limit or inhibit important steps in the viral reproductive cycle. For example, acyclovir inhibits the replication of viral DNA in herpesviruses. Among the problems encountered with the use of these chemical agents, however, are their restricted action (they work only for certain viruses) and their toxic effects on the host.

A naturally produced agent with antiviral activity is interferon. Interferon is actually a group of proteins produced by the host during a viral infection. These proteins are active only in the host species in which they are produced. They have the ability to interfere with viral multiplication and are therefore potentially useful agents in the treatment of viral infection and certain human cancers.

Cancer and viruses. The link between viruses and cancer, induced in experimental animals, was established in the early part of the twentieth century. The role of viruses as causative agents of human cancers has been less conclusive. Many viruses are associated with human cancers. They are often integrated into the genomes of cancer cells. Yet, the presence of a virus and its association with a certain type of cancer do not constitute proof that the virus is actually responsible for the cancerous condition. There is evidence that a type of liver cancer is caused by a virus. Hepatocellular carcinoma is thought to be caused by hepatitis B virus. A specific form of leukemia has been linked to human T-cell leukemia viruses. The Epstein-Barr virus is associated with a rare type of cancer, Burkitt's lymphoma. Viruses may be involved in many other types of human cancer, along with other genetic and environmental factors.

The growing evidence for the involvement of viruses in human cancers, either directly or indirectly, provides further impetus for developing an understanding of the biology of these viruses, as well as methods to protect individuals from infection. Molecular biologists continue to elucidate the strategies by which cancer viruses gain entry into host cells and alter the properties and

functions of these cells. Understanding such events will provide important clues that could be utilized to interrupt the processes that cause normal cells to become cancer cells.

Prevention. Very few antiviral agents have proven effective in combating viral illnesses. One of the best approaches in dealing with viral infection is prevention. This can be accomplished by identifying the mode of transmission of the virus and developing measures to block the transmission whenever possible. The most powerful method of preventing viral diseases, however, is through the use of vaccines to immunize individuals against viral infection. Vaccine programs have been tremendously successful in eliminating smallpox worldwide and greatly reducing the number of new cases of polio and chickenpox throughout the Western Hemisphere and Europe. Continued efforts are needed to produce safe and effective vaccines. These vaccines must also be stable and easily administered so that they can be used in parts of the world where populations need protection from serious viral diseases.

Preventive measures cannot be used in all cases. For example, it is extremely difficult to block the transmission of viruses that are carried in the air. There are also many viral diseases for which safe vaccines may not be available. Furthermore, some viruses are able to evade the immune defenses of the host, thus greatly reducing the usefulness of a vaccine. The influenza virus has a strategy for escaping detection by the host's immune system. This virus is able to alter its envelope proteins so that the newer forms are no longer recognized by the immune system of an individual who has recovered from a previous bout with the flu. Thus, an individual who has had one strain of flu is susceptible to another occurrence of the illness caused by a different strain. Although flu vaccines have been developed, their usefulness is limited by the changing nature of the virus.

PERSPECTIVE AND PROSPECTS

From their discovery as the causative agent of tobacco mosaic disease in the late 1890's by the Dutch microbiologist Martinus Beijernick, viruses have been implicated in numerous plant and animal diseases. Human diseases caused by viruses range from very mild to fatal and are often difficult to treat. Epidemics caused by viruses have plagued humankind for centuries. Outbreaks of smallpox, polio, yellow fever, and other viral diseases were once quite commonplace. Viral illnesses such as influenza still appear yearly in epidemic proportions. A severe worldwide outbreak of influenza was responsible for the deaths of 20 million people between 1918 and 1919.

The virus that causes AIDS has the potential to cause millions of deaths worldwide. It is spread relatively easily, and the time between exposure and apparent disease can be a decade or longer. Many experts are working to create a vaccine for AIDS, but they have not yet been successful. The AIDS virus is sending a warning that humans must be careful with viruses.

—Barbara Brennessel, Ph.D.; updated by
L. Fleming Fallon, Jr., M.D., Ph.D., M.P.H.

See also Acquired immunodeficiency syndrome (AIDS); Adenoviruses; Avian influenza; Cancer; Canker sores; Chickenpox; Childhood infectious diseases; Chlamydia; Chronic fatigue syndrome; Cold sores; Common cold; Coronaviruses; Cytomegalovirus (CMV); Diarrhea and dysentery; Disease; Ebola virus; Emerging infectious diseases; Encephalitis; Enteroviruses; Epidemics and pandemics; Epidemiology; Epstein-Barr virus; Fever; Fifth disease; Hand-foot-and-mouth disease; Hanta virus; Hepatitis; Herpes; H1N1 influenza; Human immunodeficiency virus (HIV); Human papillomavirus (HPV); Infection; Influenza; Insect-borne diseases; Keratitis; Marburg virus; Measles; Microbiology; Monkeypox; Mononucleosis; Mumps; Nausea and vomiting; Noroviruses; Parasitic diseases; Pelvic inflammatory disease (PID); Pityriasis rosea; Poliomyelitis; Pulmonary diseases; Rabies; Retroviruses; Rheumatic fever; Rhinoviruses; Roseola; Rotavirus; Rubella; Severe acute respiratory syndrome (SARS); Sexually transmitted diseases (STDs); Shingles; Smallpox; Tonsillitis; Viral hemorrhagic fevers; Warts; West Nile virus; Yellow fever; Zoonoses.

FOR FURTHER INFORMATION:

Biddle, Wayne. *A Field Guide to Germs.* 2d ed. New York: Anchor Books, 2002. This comprehensive book is easily accessible to the nonspecialist and includes a discussion of nearly every virus, bacterium, and fungus known to cause human and nonhuman animal disease. The history of the microbe and the treatment of diseases are included.

Fettner, Ann Giudici. *The Science of Viruses: What They Are, Why They Make Us Sick, How They Will Change the Future.* New York: Quill/William Morrow, 1993. The author of this popular work is a writer who specializes in issues of science and health. In dealing with the topic of viruses and society, she traces the history of viral epidemics through the ages and describes advances in modern virology.

Garrett, Laurie. *The Coming Plague: Newly Emerging Diseases in a World out of Balance.* New York: Penguin, 1995. This book contains an excellent discussion of several viral diseases and the efforts of the World Health Organization to control or eradicate them.

Henig, Robin Marantz. *A Dancing Matrix: Voyages Along the Viral Frontier.* New York: Vintage Books, 1994. The author provides a description of viruses and their relationship to public health and discusses the global impact of viruses from economic, political, and environmental perspectives.

Knipe, David M., and Peter M. Howley, eds. *Fields' Virology.* 5th ed. Philadelphia: Wolters Kluwer Health/Lippincott Williams & Wilkins, 2007. Covers recent discoveries about the replication, molecular biology, pathogenesis, and medical aspects of viruses.

Montagnier, Luc, and Stephen Sartarelli. *Virus: The Co-Discoverer of HIV Tracks Its Rampage and Charts the Future.* New York: W. W. Norton, 2000. This work traces the early life of Luc Montagnier, the co-discoverer of human immunodeficiency virus (HIV), and the events leading up to his famous discovery. Includes a description of the epidemiology and biology of HIV.

Radetsky, Peter. *The Invisible Invaders: Viruses and the Scientists Who Pursue Them.* Rev. ed. Boston: Little, Brown, 1994. The author provides a selected history of virology that highlights important viral diseases such as influenza and hepatitis. The major discoveries in virology are discussed, as are the scientists involved.

Regush, Nicholas. *The Virus Within: A Coming Epidemic.* New York: Plume, 2001. News journalist Regush introduces readers to a virus called human herpesvirus-6 and the debate over whether it might play a role in acquired immunodeficiency syndrome (AIDS), multiple sclerosis, chronic fatigue syndrome, schizophrenia, and several other seemingly unrelated diseases.

Ryan, Frank. *Virus X: Tracking the New Killer Plagues out of the Present and into the Future.* New York: Little, Brown, 1998. The author, a member of both the Royal College of Physicians and the New York Academy of Medicine, painstakingly chronicles numerous outbreaks, including those of hanta virus in the American Southwest in 1993; Ebola virus in Sudan and Zaire in 1976 and in Reston, Virginia, in 1989; and HIV.

Sompayrac, Lauren. *How Pathogenic Viruses Work.*

Boston: Jones and Bartlett, 2002. Engaging exploration of the basics of virology. The author uses twelve of the most common viral infections to demonstrate how viruses "devise" various solutions to stay alive.

Strauss, James, and Ellen Strauss. *Viruses and Human Disease*. 2d ed. Boston: Academic Press/Elsevier, 2008. An undergraduate text that examines virology from a human disease perspective.

Wagner, Edward K., and Martinez J. Hewlett. *Basic Virology*. 3d ed. Malden, Mass.: Blackwell Science, 2008. A very readable undergraduate text covering issues of virology and viral disease, properties of viruses and virus-cell interaction, working with viruses, and replication patterns of specific viruses.

VISION

BIOLOGY

ALSO KNOWN AS: Eyesight, sight

ANATOMY OR SYSTEM AFFECTED: Eyes, nervous system

SPECIALTIES AND RELATED FIELDS: Neurology, ophthalmology, plastic surgery

DEFINITION: One of five special senses. Light enters the eye and is then focused through specialized structures onto the retina, which responds with chemical reactions translating light into nerve impulses that travel to the brain to be interpreted as images.

KEY TERMS:

anterior chamber: the space between the cornea and lens; filled with aqueous

aqueous: watery fluid in the anterior chamber

blindness: legally in the United States, vision less than 20/200 or peripheral vision less than 20 degrees

cones: specialized photoreceptors that sense color and detailed vision in bright light

cornea: the clear central structure on the front of the eye analogous to a vehicle windshield

diplopia: double vision

iris: the colored part of the eye; acts like a shutter to let in more or less light

low vision: impairment of vision requiring visual aids

optic nerve: the largest nerve in the body; takes information from retina to brain

photoreceptors: specialized cells that translate light into electrical information, which is transferred via nerves to the brain

refractive error: a condition requiring corrective lenses

retina: the multilayered structure lining the back of the eye; functions like camera film to sense light and transfer images to the brain

rhodopsin: a chemical within photoreceptors that translates light into electrical impulses

rods: specialized photoreceptors that provide peripheral vision and vision in dim light

strabismus: muscle imbalance between eyes

vitreous: a clear gel that fills the back of the eye between the lens and the retina

STRUCTURE AND FUNCTIONS

Vision is one of five special senses. Vision provides information about the environment and is important in balance. Loss of vision limits activities but is not life-threatening. "Low vision" is a term to describe partial vision loss that can be treated with visual aids such as magnifiers. The word "blind" is often used incorrectly. Criteria for legal blindness varies from country to country and is less than 20/200 in the United States. No light perception means that there is no vision at all.

The most common method to measure vision is the standard eye chart. A vision of 20/20 is considered normal vision. This means that at a standard distance of 20 feet, a person can read a specific line on a standardized eye chart. Vision of 20/40 means that the individual has to be at a distance of 20 feet to see what normally can be seen at 40 feet. When the second number is less than 20—for example, 20/15—then the vision is better than 20/20.

Other vision functions can also be measured. Color vision measures ability to distinguish colors. Red-green color blindness is the most common color deficit. Contrast sensitivity measures ability to distinguish shades of gray. It is possible to read 20/20 but to have reduced visual functions such as reduced contrast sensitivity that would make it difficult to do activities in low light. Stereo vision is made possible by the two eyes working together. Stereo vision is important for tasks such as threading a needle. If vision is impaired in one eye, then stereo vision is reduced. If vision is similar in the two eyes but they are not aligned properly, then double vision (diplopia) results. Peripheral vision is the ability to see to the sides and is measured by visual field testing. Finally, the lens in the eye can focus but becomes weak with age. Focus ability allows the vision to transition between near and far. By forty years or older, the focus ability is usually weak enough that bifocal or reading glasses are needed.

The process of vision begins when light enters the eye. Light travels first through the clear central cornea,

Anatomy of the Eye

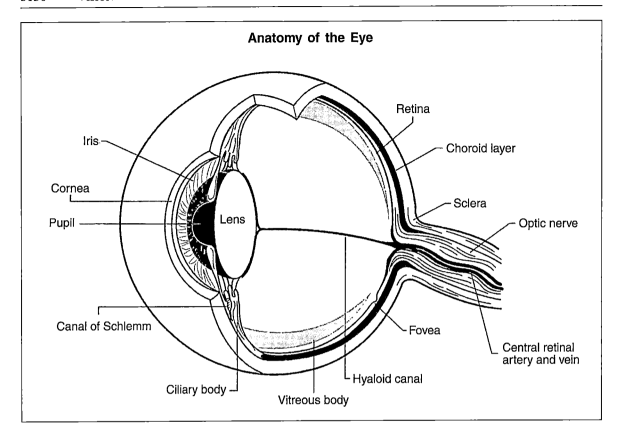

which is analogous to a car windshield. The cornea is approximately 550 microns thick at its thinnest central point. Corneal structure includes collagen connective tissue molecules that are aligned to allow for the cornea to be clear. Light rays entering the eye are parallel and must be focused to allow for vision to be possible. The corneal curvature begins the process of bending the light rays to bring them into focus on the retina at the back of the eye. The cornea provides the majority of focusing power for the eye.

After the cornea, light traverses the anterior chamber, which is filled with a watery substance called aqueous. The anterior chamber is the space between the iris (the colored part of the eye) and the cornea. Light will then travel through the pupil, the space in the center of the iris. The iris is similar to the shutter in a camera and will expand and constrict to let more or less light into the eye. The pupil usually looks dark because the light enters this space but does not exit. The exception is when light bounces off the retina and exits through the pupil, such as happens with red eye effect from a camera flash.

Behind the iris is the lens. The lens focuses light onto the retina and allows transition of vision between far and near. The change in focus, called accommodation, decreases with age. After passing through the lens of the eye, the light enters the posterior chamber, which is filled with a clear gel called vitreous. The posterior chamber is the space between the lens and the retina.

The retina lines the back of the eye and contains approximately 120 million specialized cells called photoreceptors. Photoreceptors around the peripheral retina are called rods and are important for peripheral vision and night vision. The central part of the retina is called the macula, and at the center of the macula is the fovea, which is the most sensitive to color and provides sharp central acuity. The fovea contains approximately 35,000 photoreceptors called cones and no rods. There are about twenty rods for each cone.

The layers of the retina include pigment epithelium, outer segments of the photoreceptor cells, outer nuclear layer, outer plexiform layer, inner nuclear layer, inner plexiform layer, ganglion cell layer, and axon layer. Underneath the retina is the choroid vascular that provides blood flow to the retina. Retinal veins and arteries also nourish the retina. There are no blood vessels in the fovea.

When light strikes the retina, a molecule within the

photoreceptors called rhodopsin undergoes a chemical structural change from a *cis* to a *trans* configuration. This hyperpolarizes the cell, causing an increase in negative charge. The cells within the retina have a hierarchy of on-center and off-center receptive fields that interact to distinguish gradations of light intensity and color. These electrical messages are passed from the photoreceptor cells to bipolar cells to ganglion cells. The ganglion cells then communicate with the visual areas of the brain via the optic nerve.

After light is translated into neural information by retinal cells, information from each eye travels through the optic nerve to the optic chiasm. At the chiasm, the two nerves meet and the central half of each set of nerve fibers crosses and joins with fibers from the fellow eye. The neural pathways continue in parallel to the right and left brain, along the optic tract to the lateral geniculate nucleus and to the primary visual cortex. The visual cortex provides interpretation of the visual images from each eye and fuses them into a single image. A stroke to these areas of the brain will cause an identical defect to the opposite side of the vision in each eye. For example, a right stroke will cause a left field defect that will affect both eyes.

Each eye, also called the globe, is about 24 millimeters long and can distinguish light from 300 nanometers (near ultraviolet) to 2,000 nanometers (near infrared). The globes are positioned within the bony space within the skull called the orbit. Orbital bones are particularly strong around the orbital rim but very thin and weaker toward the back of the orbital roof and orbital floor. This feature protects the eye from trauma, as the orbital bones will fracture before the eye is ruptured. This is called a blow-out fracture.

The orbit contains fatty tissue, connective tissue, the lacrimal gland (important for tearing), and the extraocular muscles. Six extraocular muscles are attached to each eye to provide the ability of the eyes to move synchronously. The inferior oblique, inferior rectus, medial rectus, superior rectus, iris, and lid are supplied by the third nerve. Injury to the third nerve can lead to diplopia, ptosis (droopy lid), and pupil abnormalities. The lateral rectus is supplied by the sixth cranial nerve, and the superior oblique is supplied by the fourth cranial nerve. The oblique muscles provide rotational movement. The extraocular muscles coordinate the eyes to provide a single image. Imbalance of muscles can cause diplopia.

The orbit is covered by the eyelids. To maintain clear vision, the cornea must be covered with a film of tears.

If the cornea becomes too dry or swollen, then it will lose clarity. Disorders of the lacrimal gland and lid disorders can lead to dry eyes, which will impair vision. The lids, lacrimal gland, extraocular muscles, structures within the eye, optic nerve, and brain must all be working properly to provide normal vision.

DISORDERS AND DISEASES

Numerous diseases and disorders can affect vision. The most common disorders are nearsightedness (myopia), farsightedness (hyperopia), and astigmatism, which can be corrected by glasses and contact lenses.

A nearsighted eye is too long or the cornea is too steep, which results in the light from a distance coming to a focal point in front of the retina. The farsighted eye is too short or the cornea is too flat, and light from a distance will come to a focal point past the retina. Astigmatism usually means the cornea is not spherical but is shaped more like a football, with two different radii of curvature. In the astigmatic eye, light from a distance will have two focal points, which results in a tilted image. Refractive errors can be treated with glasses, contact lenses, or laser vision correction.

Uncorrected refractive error or other childhood conditions can lead to amblyopia, also known as a lazy eye. If these problems are not corrected before age seven, then the eye will not develop the proper neural connections and vision is permanently reduced. Treatment with surgery, glasses, or patching can help many patients with amblyopia.

Strabismus is also called a wandering eye or squint. Strabismus commonly develops in childhood and causes an eye turn. Adult causes of strabismus include stroke, thyroid orbitopathy, or trauma. Strabismus can lead to amblyopia in a child or diplopia. Prism glasses, patching, or surgery may be recommended.

The focus ability of the lens, accommodation, decreases with age, resulting in the need for reading glasses or a bifocal eyeglass for reading sometime after the age of forty. Other common eye diseases include cataract, glaucoma, and macular degeneration. Cataract is clouding of the lens and is treated by cataract removal (removal of the lens of the eye) and replacement with a clear lens implant. Glaucoma can be hereditary and involves loss of peripheral vision due to damage to the optic nerve as a result of high eye pressure. Glaucoma can also occur with a normal pressure and, if not treated, will result in tunnel vision. Macular degeneration may be hereditary and can lead to loss of central vision. Vitamins, injections, and laser treatment may sometimes be helpful in the treatment of macular degeneration.

Numerous other eye disorders and diseases can lead to a partial or complete loss of vision. Healthy lifestyle choices such as not smoking, eating a healthy diet, and exercising may help to prevent many eye diseases. Eye examination by a qualified optometrist or ophthalmologist in childhood and routinely throughout life can aid in the early detection of eye disease. Eye disease can often be prevented or treated if detected early.

PERSPECTIVE AND PROSPECTS

Millions of people are affected by eye disease and injury. Americans spend billions of dollars each year, for example, on cataract surgery alone. The Academy of Ophthalmology reports that more than one-half of all eye injuries occur before a person turns twenty-five years old, and up to 160,000 school-age children suffer eye injuries each year in the United States. Many eye injuries can be prevented with proper protective eyewear for sports and other activities, such as using power tools.

Vision has fascinated scientists and writers since classical Greek writers theorized that vision was made possible by light rays emanating from the eyes. Other theories included a process by which images send copies of themselves to the eye. It was the work of Johannes Kepler, Galileo Galilei, Christoph Scheiner, and Willibrord Snellius (Snell) in the seventeenth century that began the true understanding of the vision process.

Some research suggests that many people are more afraid of going blind than of dying, and those with eye disorders such as an eye turn have lower socioeconomic success. However, there are many examples of success in spite of vision loss, including musician Stevie Wonder, artist Claude Monet, and activist Helen Keller. Fortunately, vision loss can often be avoided by proper eye protection and regular eye examinations.

—*E. E. Anderson Penno, M.D., M.S., FRCSC*

See also Albinos; Astigmatism; Behçet's disease; Blindness; Blurred vision; Cataract surgery; Cataracts; Chlamydia; Color blindness; Conjunctivitis; Corneal transplantation; Diabetes mellitus; Eye infections and disorders; Eye surgery; Eyes; Glaucoma; Gonorrhea; Keratitis; Laser use in surgery; Macular degeneration; Microscopy, slitlamp; Myopia; Ophthalmology; Optometry; Optometry, pediatric; Refractive eye surgery; Sense organs; Strabismus; Toxoplasmosis; Transplantation; Vision disorders.

FOR FURTHER INFORMATION:

American Academy of Ophthalmology (AAC). http://www.geteyesmart.org. Web site aimed at the nonmedical reader that is part of the AAC's clinical education resources.

Ferkat, Sharon, and Jennifer S. Weizer. *All About Your Eyes: A Practical Guide in Plain English from the Physicians at the Duke University Eye Center.* Durham, N.C.: Duke University Press, 2006. A text designed for general readers.

West, John B., ed. *Best and Taylor's Physiologic Basis of Medical Practice.* 11th ed. Baltimore: Williams & Wilkins, 1985. Chapter 64, "Vision," offers a detailed description of the physiology of vision.

VISION CORRECTION. *See* REFRACTIVE EYE SURGERY.

VISION DISORDERS
DISEASE/DISORDER
ANATOMY OR SYSTEM AFFECTED: Eyes
SPECIALTIES AND RELATED FIELDS: Geriatrics and gerontology, ophthalmology, optometry
DEFINITION: Poor vision caused by diseases or abnormalities of the eyes.
KEY TERMS:
aqueous fluid: a clear, watery liquid that fills the region inside the front of the eyeball between the lens and cornea
cataract: a loss of transparency in the lens of the eye, commonly associated with aging
cornea: the transparent, curved front surface of the eyeball, which provides protection and focuses light
glaucoma: an increase in the eye's internal pressure that can damage the optic nerve and eventually lead to blindness
laser: a very intense beam of light; used in eye surgery for glaucoma, a detached retina, or hemorrhaging blood vessels
macular degeneration: a deterioration of vision, primarily among the elderly, caused by small hemorrhages in the most sensitive central region of the retina
retina: a thin membrane, lining the inside back surface of the eyeball, where light is transformed into electrical signals that are transmitted to the brain

CAUSES AND SYMPTOMS
The most common defects in human vision are nearsightedness (myopia), farsightedness (hyperopia), and

astigmatism. All three of these conditions are called refractive errors because the cornea-lens focusing system of the eye bends light rays either too much or too little, so that the image formed on the retina is blurred. Fortunately, refractive errors can be corrected by means of eyeglasses or contact lenses. In the United States, almost 60 percent of the population, or about 150 million people, use some form of vision correction, and more than 27 million of them wear contacts.

Myopia and hyperopia are caused by a mismatch between the focusing power of the cornea-lens combination and the length of the eyeball. For a nearsighted person, the incoming light comes to a focus in front of the retina; a diverging lens is needed to move the image farther back. For a farsighted person, the situation is reversed; a converging lens is prescribed to provide extra focusing power.

The problem of astigmatism is attributable to a difference in the focal length of the eye for two perpendicular directions, which can occur if the eyeball is slightly deformed (like a grape being squeezed between two fingers). The curvature of the corneal surface would be different in two perpendicular planes. An optometrist can correct for astigmatism by prescribing glasses with different focal lengths in the two planes. The prescription must specify the angle at which the deformation of the eyeball is maximized.

A vision problem that is common among older adults is the formation of cataracts, in which the lens of the eye becomes cloudy. Cataracts are a normal part of the aging process, like wrinkled skin or gray hair. In rare cases, however, children have them at birth or after an eye injury. Cataracts form on the inside of the lens capsule, not on the surface of the eye. Once started, their growth is irreversible. The only treatment is surgi-

cal removal of the defective eye lens, followed by implantation of an artificial (plastic) replacement. With developments in ophthalmology, such microsurgery has a success rate of better than 95 percent. What causes eye cataracts in the elderly is not yet well understood. One suggested explanation is the Maillard reaction, in which glucose and protein molecules combine when heated to form a brown product. This chemical reaction is responsible for the browning of bread or cookies during baking. The same process is thought to occur even at body temperature, but very slowly over a period of years. It has been suggested that the onset of cataract formation can be delayed by a good diet, regular exercise, and a generally healthy lifestyle.

Glaucoma is a vision problem that afflicts about 2 percent of the adult population, normally after the age of forty. Excessive fluid pressure develops inside the eye, causing damage to the optic nerve. Peripheral vision gradually decreases—a decrease that the patient may not even notice until it is detected by an optometrist during an eye examination. The usual treatments are medicated eyedrops to reduce pressure and laser surgery to improve fluid drainage. Glaucoma has nothing to do with red or watery eyes because these symptoms occur on the exterior of the eyeball.

The retina is a paper-thin membrane at the back of the eye, nourished by a network of tiny blood vessels. A frequent problem encountered by diabetics is the enlargement and possible hemorrhaging of these blood vessels. For older adults, macular degeneration is a condition associated with arteriosclerosis, sometimes leading to retinal bleeding. The most sensitive, central region of the retina deteriorates, causing an irreversible loss in reading ability that cannot be corrected with glasses.

Another retinal problem is its detachment from the back wall of the eye. This is an emergency situation requiring immediate medical attention. A detached retina can be caused by an accumulation of fluid behind the retina resulting from leakage through a small tear in the membrane. It can also come from a blow to the eye, as with a sports injury. Laser surgery has become an effective treatment for the various types of retinal damage.

TREATMENT AND THERAPY
During an eye examination, the optometrist tries to detect any deviations from normal vision. If the patient is nearsighted or farsighted or has astigmatism, appropri-

ate corrective lenses can be prescribed. If cataracts, glaucoma, or a retinal problem exists, the patient will be referred to an ophthalmologist, who has received specialized medical training in eye surgery.

The history of eyeglasses has been traced back to the thirteenth century, when Roger Bacon, a Catholic scholar, wrote about using convex glass to make writing appear larger. Some medieval paintings show elderly noblemen wearing eyeglasses. No significant innovations were made until Benjamin Franklin invented bifocals in 1780, to aid people whose eyes did not focus properly at either near or far distances. Until the late 1940's, prescription eyeglasses were always made out of glass. Then plastic lenses were introduced; they had the advantages of lighter weight and greater resistance to breakage. The main problem with plastic is that it scratches more easily, but coatings have been developed to overcome this drawback. More than 80 percent of the eyeglasses worn in the United States are now made of plastic.

An alternative to eyeglasses came in the 1950's with the development of contact lenses. They were made out of a hard plastic and covered the front of the cornea, floating on a thin layer of tears. They provided good vision but were uncomfortable to insert. Also, hard contacts cannot transmit oxygen and carbon dioxide to nourish the surface of the cornea, causing dryness and irritation for the wearer. Such lenses are now virtually obsolete. Daily-wear soft contact lenses became available in the 1970's. They were much more comfortable than the hard plastic material and were gas-permeable. The soft lenses had an affinity for infection-causing bacteria, however, requiring a tedious, nightly sterilizing procedure with heat or chemicals. The technology of contact lenses continues to evolve. More recent developments are soft contacts for extended wear (up to two weeks without removal), bifocal gas-permeable contacts, and inexpensive, disposable contacts (to be discarded after two or three weeks). Contact lens wearers are cautioned to have regular eye checkups to make sure that the cornea is not being damaged.

Starting in the 1970's, eye specialists began to investigate the possibility of reshaping the eyeball to do away with eyeglasses completely. The first attempt utilized a hard lens pressing directly against the cornea to flatten it, in much the same way that orthodontic braces are used to straighten teeth. The change induced in the shape of the eye generally was only temporary, so lenses still were needed afterward.

A Soviet physician, Svyatoslav Fyodorov, devel-

oped radial keratotomy (RK), a surgical procedure to flatten the cornea permanently. A series of shallow incisions is made in the outer part of the cornea in a radial pattern, like the spokes of a wheel. The center of the cornea is not touched. As the incisions heal, the cornea bulges slightly near the edges, thus reducing its curvature in the middle. In this way, a permanent cure for nearsightedness can be accomplished. In the United States between 1980 and 1993, about 200,000 patients had RK surgery. Nevertheless, the procedure remained controversial. The main problem was that the number of incisions and their depth could overcorrect or undercorrect the original refractive error. Also, some ophthalmologists were concerned about possible long-term aftereffects of scars on the cornea. RK soon decreased in popularity.

Another technique to alter the shape of the cornea is called keratomileusis. The outer half of the patient's cornea is removed and frozen, and then reshaped with a computer-controlled lathe to a predetermined curvature. After thawing, the cornea is sewn back into place, where it acts as a permanent contact lens. Keratomileusis can correct both myopia and hyperopia.

The laser, invented by physicists in the 1960's, is a very intense beam of light that can be adapted particularly well for surgery on the retina of the eye. The light beam passes successively through the transparent cornea, aqueous fluid, and lens without being absorbed. Its energy is then concentrated into a tiny spot on the retina, causing localized vaporization, or "welding," to occur. Laser-assisted in situ keratomileusis (LASIK) became quite popular at the end of the twentieth century. In LASIK surgery, the cornea is reshaped to help patients overcome myopia, hyperopia, or astigmatism. The procedure is done with a cool beam laser that removes thin layers of tissue from selected sites on the cornea to change its curvature. Success rates are high: 90 to 95 percent of the patients get 20/40 vision, and 65 to 75 percent of the patients get 20/20 vision or better. Lasers can also be used to excise leaking blood vessels and to repair or reattach a damaged retina.

Another surgical technique is to use a corneal transplant from an organ donor. The new cornea is shaped to the proper curvature with a lathe and is sewn on top of the patient's own cornea.

The standard treatment for cataracts is surgical removal of the defective lens, followed by implantation of an artificial, plastic lens. Cataract surgery is very common in the United States, comprising more than 40 percent of all eye operations. Ophthalmologists routinely perform cataract surgery using only local anesthetic, so that the patient can go home without an overnight hospital stay.

Glaucoma, a condition of excess pressure in the eye, affects more than two million Americans and has caused approximately 70,000 cases of blindness. The first line of treatment is the use of daily medication in the form of eyedrops to reduce the fluid pressure. Eventually, surgery may be necessary. The procedure used enlarges an opening at the edge of the iris to allow for better drainage of the aqueous fluid between the lens and cornea. The incision can be made with either a miniature scalpel or a laser. Glaucoma damage to the optic nerve cannot be repaired, but prompt treatment can prevent further deterioration of vision.

PERSPECTIVE AND PROSPECTS

The human eye is the most important sense organ for individuals to gather information about their environment. An amazingly high 40 percent of all nerve fibers going to the brain come from the retina of the eye. Any defect or deterioration from normal vision is a serious limitation. During the Middle Ages, few people learned to read and write, so the need for seeing at close range was not important. In modern society, however, people with poor eyesight are greatly handicapped. For example, students, computer operators, airplane pilots, and athletes cannot function without good vision.

Society is gradually becoming more sympathetic to people with handicaps, including blindness. Braille printing, guide dogs, and books recorded on audiotape are helpful developments for the blind. The U.S. Congress in 1992 passed the Americans with Disabilities Act, which mandates improved access for the visually impaired in facilities that serve the general public. Nevertheless, retaining good vision and preventing further deterioration will continue to be a vital part of overall health care.

—*Hans G. Graetzer, Ph.D.*

See also Albinos; Astigmatism; Behçet's disease; Blindness; Blurred vision; Cataract surgery; Cataracts; Chlamydia; Color blindness; Conjunctivitis; Corneal transplantation; Diabetes mellitus; Eye infections and disorders; Eye surgery; Eyes; Glaucoma; Gonorrhea; Keratitis; Laser use in surgery; Macular degeneration; Microscopy, slitlamp; Myopia; Ophthalmology; Optometry; Optometry, pediatric; Refractive eye surgery; Sense organs; Strabismus; Toxoplasmosis; Transplantation; Vision.

FOR FURTHER INFORMATION:

Anshel, Jeffrey. *Healthy Eyes, Better Vision: Everyday Eye Care for the Whole Family.* Los Angeles: Body Press, 1990. A good overview of eye problems typical during childhood, midlife, and old age. The advantages and disadvantages of various types of contact lenses are evaluated. Other topics include eye hazards from work or sports and eye emergencies.

Berns, Michael W. "Laser Surgery." *Scientific American* 264 (June, 1991): 84-90. An excellent article explaining how lasers are used as medical tools. Photographs of blood vessels in the retina of the eye before and after surgery are shown, along with other applications of this technology.

Buettner, Helmut, ed. *Mayo Clinic on Vision and Eye Health: Practical Answers on Glaucoma, Cataracts, Macular Degeneration, and Other Conditions.* Rochester, Minn.: Mayo Foundation for Medical Education and Research, 2002. A helpful handbook on all the medical, social, and emotional facets of vision impairment.

Cassel, Gary H., Michael D. Billig, and Harry G. Randall. *The Eye Book: A Complete Guide to Eye Disorders and Health.* Baltimore: Johns Hopkins University Press, 2001. With particular attention on degeneration of the eye, the combined expertise of three eye care professionals produces a primer on the physiology of the eye and its dysfunctions.

National Foundation for Eye Research. http://www.nfer.org. Provides consumers and professionals with access to developing technology for treating impaired vision.

Parker, James N., and Philip M. Parker, eds. *The 2002 Official Patient's Sourcebook on Myopia.* San Diego, Calif.: Icon Health, 2002. Draws from public, academic, government, and peer-reviewed research to provide a wide-ranging handbook for patients with myopia.

Prevent Blindness America. http://www.preventblindness.org. Founded in 1908, this group is dedicated to fighting blindness and saving sight. Its efforts are focused on promoting a continuum of vision care, public and professional education, certified vision screening training, and community and patient service programs and research.

Ross, Linda M. *Ophthalmic Disorders Sourcebook.* Detroit, Mich.: Omnigraphics, 1997. A popular work that describes such eye diseases as glaucoma, cataracts, macular degeneration, strabismus, and refractive disorders.

Sardegna, Jill, et al. *The Encyclopedia of Blindness and Vision Impairment.* 2d ed. New York: Facts On File, 2002. All aspects of vision impairment are covered in five hundred entries, including health and social issues, surgery and medications, adaptive aids, education, and helpful organizations. Twelve appendixes provide myriad resources for research, support, and services.

Sutton, Amy L., ed. *Eye Care Sourcebook: Basic Consumer Health Information About Eye Care and Eye Disorders.* 3d ed. Detroit, Mich.: Omnigraphics, 2008. A complete guide to eye care that includes such topics as eye anatomy, preventive vision care, refractive disorders and eye diseases, current research and clinical trials, and a list of organizations.

VITAMINS AND MINERALS

BIOLOGY

ANATOMY OR SYSTEM AFFECTED: All

SPECIALTIES AND RELATED FIELDS: Endocrinology, family medicine, internal medicine, nutrition

DEFINITION: Chemicals that supply the body with the means of metabolizing (extracting and using the energy from) the macronutrients (fats, carbohydrates, and proteins) it ingests; essential ingredients of the diet.

KEY TERMS:

fat-soluble vitamins: vitamins that, because of their structure and solubility, migrate to fatty tissues in the body, where they are stored

macronutrients: materials ingested in large amounts to supply the energy and materials for physical bodies

megadose: ten or more times the recommended daily allowance of a nutrient

micronutrients: substances of which only milligrams are needed in the daily diet, such as vitamins and minerals

mineral: an inorganic salt of particular metals or elements needed for good health

recommended daily (or dietary) allowance (RDA): the intake levels of the essential nutrients that are considered adequate to meet the known nutritional needs of most healthy persons

trace elements: elements needed in the diet at levels of less than 100 milligrams per day

vitamin: an organic compound constituent of food that is consumed in relatively small amounts (less than 0.1 gram per kilogram of body weight per day) and that is essential to the maintenance of life

water-soluble vitamins: vitamins that, because of their structure, show strong solubility in water; they normally pass through the body in a relatively short time

STRUCTURE AND FUNCTIONS

Vitamins are organic compounds (that is, compounds made up of carbon, oxygen, nitrogen, sulfur, or hydrogen) that are constituents of food and that are crucial to the maintenance of life and good health. They make possible the production of energy and the formation of coherent body tissues from the macronutrients normally consumed in a regular diet. They are, among other things, coenzymes that serve as oxidizing, reducing, and transfer chemicals at the active sites of enzymes. Vitamins are part of the one hundred or so organic compounds that are of the proper size and stability to be absorbed from the digestive tract into the bloodstream without digestion or breakdown. Nevertheless, they are not produced in the body in amounts large enough to keep a person healthy—because they have always been available in food, there was probably no need for the human metabolism to produce them. Vitamins are synthesized by plants, and therefore plants constitute the principal natural source of these compounds.

Vitamins are divided into two main groups: the water-soluble and the fat-soluble vitamins. Structural differences account for the two types of solubility. Fat-soluble vitamins (such as vitamins A, D, E, and K) consist mainly of hydrocarbon groupings (nonpolar hydrocarbon chains and rings compatible with nonpolar oil and fat) and are structurally similar to fats, whereas water-soluble vitamins have polar hydroxyl (-OH) and carboxyl (-COOH) groups that are attracted to and form hydrogen bonds with water. One of the most important differences between vitamins is the result of their solubility: Fat-soluble vitamins are stored in the body tissues and organs for relatively long periods of time, while water-soluble vitamins are eliminated from the body in a relatively fast manner, sometimes in a matter of hours.

Vitamin A (retinol) maintains the health of eyes, skin, and mucous membranes and is particularly important for good vision in dim light. There are various physiological equivalents to vitamin A, that is, compounds with closely related structures that can be used as the vitamin itself. Beta carotene is a provitamin (a substance that can be easily converted to a vitamin) of vitamin A found in carrots. The vitamin can also be found in liver and liver oils. Lack of vitamin A can cause night or total blindness.

The B vitamins are often considered as a group, called the B complex, because they work together as coenzymes in biochemical reactions leading to growth and energy production. They are water soluble and easily eliminated from food in the cooking process. Members of this group include pyridoxine (B_6), involved in at least sixty enzyme reactions (mostly in the metabolism and synthesis of proteins); thiamine (B_1), a coenzyme in carbohydrate metabolism and involved in energy production, digestion, and nerve activity; riboflavin (B_2), used in obtaining energy from foods; pantothenic acid (B_3), needed for proper growth; niacin (B_4), needed for the production of healthy tissues; cobalamin (B_{12}), involved in the production and growth of red blood cells; and folic acid (B_9), also involved in the production of red blood cells and in metabolism. They are present in various foods, especially meat and dairy products. Deficiency symptoms include anemia, skin disorders, and nervous system disorders.

Vitamin C, or ascorbic acid, is involved in the destruction of invading bacteria, in the synthesis and activity of interferon (which prevents entry of viruses into cells), in decreasing the effect of toxic substances (such as drugs and pollutants), and in the formation of connective tissue. Humans are one of the few species of animals for which ascorbic acid is actually a vitamin, since other species produce it in their metabolic processes. Deficiency symptoms include the degeneration of tissue and scurvy. Vitamin C is found mostly in citrus fruits.

Vitamin D (calciferol) promotes the absorption of calcium and phosphorus through the intestinal wall and into the bloodstream. Its deficiency induces the disease rickets and, in adults, the malformation of bones. Unlike other vitamins, it forms in the body through the action of the sun's ultraviolet light. As with the vitamin B complex, vitamin D has a set of closely related molecular structures, called D_1, D_2, D_3, and so on. All these structures have the same physiological function. Because of limited sun exposure, copious clothing, and indoor living and working conditions, humans need to add vitamin D to their diet, as in fortified milk, cod liver oil, or vitamin supplements.

Vitamin E (alpha tocopherol) is an antioxidant of polyunsaturated fatty acids (fatty acids with numerous double bonds). These fatty acids readily form peroxides, which are particularly damaging because they can lead to runaway oxidation in cells. Vitamin E protects the integrity of cell membranes, which contain considerable amounts of fat. It also helps maintain the integ-

rity of the circulatory and central nervous systems; is involved in the functioning of the kidneys, lungs, liver, and genitalia; and detoxifies poisonous materials absorbed by the body. Since aging, in some theories, is considered to be the cumulative effect of free radicals (reactive atoms) running wild in the body, the antioxidant properties of vitamin E may make it a good candidate for inhibiting aging, or at least preventing premature aging. Its deficiency symptoms in humans are unknown. Vitamin E is present in various foods, especially in grain oils.

Biotin (also called vitamin H) participates in metabolism by acting as a carboxyl carrier for a number of enzymes. Its sources are liver, cereals, and egg yolks. Symptoms of deficiency include alopecia (the loss or absence of hair) and skin rashes.

Vitamin K completes the list of vitamins. It participates in the clotting of blood, and its deficiency can cause hemorrhage and liver damage. This vitamin is commonly found in plants and vegetables.

The term "minerals," when used in a nutritional context, includes all the nutritional chemical elements of foods obtained from macronutrients, except for carbon, hydrogen, nitrogen, oxygen, and sulfur. This term also refers to metal elements combined with others in compounds such as soluble inorganic salts. It is in this combined form that they serve indispensable functions in the body.

Minerals pass slowly through the body and are excreted in the feces, urine, and sweat. Therefore, they must be replaced and an appropriate balance continuously maintained. Because living beings cannot generate minerals in their own bodies, they must obtain them from foods or food supplements. Plants pick up minerals directly from the soil, and animals get them from the plants that they ingest. As opposed to vitamins, which are synthesized by plants, minerals cannot be generated if they are not in the soil. Among their many functions, minerals are components of enzymes, are structural components of body parts such as bones, are involved in maintaining the electrolyte balance in body fluids, and transport materials, as hemoglobin does in blood.

There are seventeen known minerals, although many others may exist. Since most of them are present in the body in relatively small amounts, their functions have been determined through the symptoms of various dietary deficiencies. Minerals can be grouped into two classes. The major elements—calcium, phosphorus, and magnesium—are required in amounts of 1 gram or more per day. The trace elements, such as chlorine, chromium, cobalt, copper, fluorine, iodine, iron, manganese, molybdenum, nickel, selenium, sulfur, vanadium, and zinc, are needed in milligram or microgram quantities each day.

Calcium, probably the best-known mineral, is present in the body in a greater amount than any other mineral: up to 1.5 or 2.0 percent of total body weight, with 99 percent of it in bones and teeth. In the nervous system, it is used to slow down the heartbeat, and it is metabolized in the body by a hormone synthesized from calciferol (vitamin D). Excess calcium can give rise to kidney stones. Its deficiency is common in postmenopausal women, who produce less estrogen. This decrease encourages bone dissolution, and when bones are dissolved, calcium is lost. Calcium is found in milk and dairy products, fish, and green vegetables. Phosphorus, the second most common mineral, is a structural component of bones and soft tissue. It is found in nearly all foods.

Sodium and potassium cations (positively charged atoms) are components of many minerals. They work in the conservation of electrolytic balance in cell fluids. Potassium governs the activity of many cellular enzymes, while sodium keeps the water content of cellular fluids in a healthy balance. For the body to work properly, it needs the appropriate ratio of sodium to potassium. Potassium ions concentrate inside the cell, while sodium ions concentrate outside the cell. Natural unprocessed foods have high sodium-to-potassium ratios. Because sodium and potassium compounds are very soluble in water, however, they dissolve during processing and cooking and are discarded. Sodium is replenished by adding salt to food, but this is not the case with potassium, which is not added to food. Care must be taken in this matter, either by eating more fresh foods or by using a specialized table salt that contains a mixture of sodium chloride and potassium chloride. The retention of sodium leads to water retention and edema (swollen legs and ankles) and to high blood pressure in some individuals. Sodium is mostly found in table salt, and potassium is found in meat, dairy products, and fruit.

Magnesium and chloride ions are the most common minerals in cell fluids, as they regulate fluid balances and electrical charges. Magnesium controls the formation of proteins inside the cell and the transmission of electrical signals from cell to cell. Chloride is present in the stomach as hydrochloric acid, or stomach acid. Magnesium is found in whole-grain cereals, dried

fruits, and leafy green vegetables, and chloride is found in table salt.

Trace elements work in various ways, with most of them incorporated into the structure of enzymes, hormones, and related molecules or acting in conjunction with vitamins. Among the trace elements, one of the more important ones is iron, which is a critical part of the hemoglobin molecule of red blood cells and is involved in oxygen transport. Fluoride, another trace element, helps harden the enamel of teeth to make them resistant to decay; zinc plays an important role in growth, the healing of wounds, and the development of male sex glands; and manganese is needed for healthy bones and a well-functioning nervous system. Iodine is involved in the proper operation of the thyroid gland, chromium is important in the metabolism of glucose, and cobalt aids in cell function. Copper and selenium are other trace elements needed by the body. Most trace elements are found in fish, meat, fruits, and vegetables.

RELATED DISEASES

Vitamin deficiencies are not common in the United States and other Western countries. A well-balanced diet provides ample vitamins of all kinds. Megadoses of vitamins can create harmful effects, however, as a toxic dose exists for many vitamins. For example, vitamin A, when taken in excess, can cause headache, nausea, vomiting, fatigue, swelling, hemorrhage, pain in the arms and legs, and birth defects. An acute deficiency of the vitamin, however, can impair vision and eventually cause blindness. Consequently, there must be a balance in vitamin intake. This balance can be achieved by following the recommended daily (or dietary) allowances (RDAs).

In the United States, the Food and Nutrition Board of the National Academy of Sciences and the National Research Council determined the daily needs for some vitamins and minerals. The Food and Drug Administration (FDA) made these findings the basis for its list of RDAs. These allowances are presented in units of grams or milligrams, and these amounts are determined using international units of biological activity. (Some vitamins come in several forms, all of which are physiologically equivalent.) RDAs do not cover every single vitamin and mineral needed for good health, nor do they cover the more extreme nutritional requirements that result from illness or unusual genetic makeup. They just serve as general guidelines for healthy individuals. For some substances lacking specific RDAs, such as chromium and a handful of other elements, the

FDA lists the daily ranges of these micronutrients that it considers to be safe and effective. RDAs depend on gender, age, weight, and other conditions and are normally presented in food labels as percentages of the daily dietary requirement.

In 2005, the U.S. Department of Agriculture (USDA) updated the Food Guide Pyramid. The new pyramid emphasizes the need for physical activity (thirty minutes of moderate or vigorous exercise per day) and the importance of variety in diet. Consumers can get personalized recommendations, based on their age and gender, at MyPyramid.gov. Unlike the older food pyramids, the 2005 version suggests food quantities in cups and ounces, rather than as servings, which was ambiguous and confusing to consumers. For example, for a 2,000 calorie per day diet, the recommendations are six ounces of whole grains, two and a half cups of vegetables, two cups of fruit, three cups of dairy, and five and a half ounces from the meat and bean subgroup.

The main criticisms of the 2005 food recommendations are that they do not mention any specific foods from which to abstain, that people who do not have Web access cannot obtain personalized recommendations, and that the beef and dairy industry lobbies play a role in the USDA's decisions about these matters. Consumers should keep in mind that the primary role of the USDA is to promote agriculture in the United States. Politics are embedded in decisions made about diets, and recommending that people eat less is not good for business. Some nutritionists and scientists believe that diet matters should be under the auspices of a more neutral party, such as the National Institutes of Health (NIH).

The activity of a vitamin or mineral depends only on its molecular structure, not on its source. Therefore, the synthetic vitamins found in food supplements provide the same nutrients as naturally occurring ones. It is crucial to remember, however, that other substances or nutrients are present in the food that is being consumed to obtain the necessary vitamin and mineral requirements. Authentic food often contains additional substances that enhance the absorption and utilization of its nutrients. For example, the calcium that is naturally present in food is more likely to carry with it any vitamin D or phosphorus that the body might need for its optimum use than is the calcium found in an antacid tablet or a food supplement. A balanced diet provides a diversity of nutrients that no pills can match.

The major medical use of the vitamins is in curing the deficiency diseases—that is, those caused by their absence from the diet. Nine vitamins have been judged by an FDA panel to be safe and effective as over-the-counter drugs. Supplementation is commonly thought of as a means of maintaining nutritional equilibrium in the body.

Many different analytical methods—such as ultraviolet-visible and infrared spectroscopy; paper, thin-layer, and gas-liquid chromatography; and mass spectroscopy—as well as biological assays have been used for the detection and identification of vitamins. They have greatly helped to explain the complex structures of these compounds. These methods are also used in the determination of the vitamin content of a particular food item, providing the consumer with valuable nutritional information.

PERSPECTIVE AND PROSPECTS

Vitamin deficiency diseases such as scurvy, beriberi, and pellagra have plagued the world at least since the existence of written records. The concept of a vitamin or "accessory growth factor" was developed in the early part of the twentieth century. In 1912, Casimir Funk, a Polish biochemist, isolated a dietary growth factor from the outer covering of rice grains and found that, when added to the food of those who had beriberi, it cured the disease. The factor was an organic compound called an amine (that is, a compound containing nitrogen combined with carbon and hydrogen). Funk coined the term "vitamine" (meaning "life-giving amine") for the compound, which is now called thiamin or vitamin B_1. In the next five decades, there was an exciting era of the isolation, identification, and synthesis of vitamins. It was soon found that these compounds were not all amines, and the term was changed to "vitamins." As more information on the structure of vitamins was obtained, names changed from general ones (such as vitamin C) to more specific ones (such as ascorbic acid). These discoveries led to the availability of inexpensive synthetic vitamins and to a dramatic reduction in overt vitamin deficiency disease.

Small amounts of vitamins are essential for good health, but the benefits of taking megadoses of certain vitamins to prevent or cure certain ailments are often debated. Even so, there is evidence that the use of high levels of vitamins can prevent or alleviate a number of diseases. Improvements in the analytical methods used in the detection and identification of vitamins have led to better and more sensitive detection limits for these compounds. The result has been increased knowledge of vitamins and minerals and their function.

In 2002, the American Medical Association endorsed the notion that adults should take a multivitamin daily. This reversed the organization's long-standing antivitamin stance that vitamins were a waste of time and money for all people except pregnant women and for some people with chronic illnesses. The current recommendation, published in the *Journal of the American Medical Association*, acknowledges that vitamins may prevent some kinds of chronic diseases, such as heart disease, cancer, and osteoporosis.

—*Maria Pacheco, Ph.D.;*
Lisa Levin Sobczak, R.N.C.;
updated by LeAnna DeAngelo, Ph.D.

See also Anorexia nervosa; Antioxidants; Beriberi; Bulimia; Cholesterol; Dietary reference intakes (DRIs); Digestion; Eating disorders; Ergogenic aids; Food biochemistry; Food Guide Pyramid; Food poisoning; Hyperlipidemia; Kwashiorkor; Lactose intolerance; Lead poisoning; Macronutrients; Malnutrition; Nutrition; Obesity; Osteoporosis; Phenylketonuria (PKU); Poisoning; Rickets; Scurvy; Self-medication; Supplements; Wilson's disease.

For Further Information:

Balch, James F., and Phyllis A. Balch. *Prescription for Nutritional Healing: A Practical A to Z Reference to Drug-Free Remedies Using Vitamins, Minerals, Herbs, and Food Supplements.* 4th rev. ed. Garden City Park, N.Y.: Avery, 2008. A guide to nutritional, herbal, and complementary therapies. Includes the latest research and theories on treatment of aging, HIV, and a host of other subjects.

Duyff, Roberta Larson. *American Dietetic Association Complete Food and Nutrition Guide.* 3d ed. Hoboken, N.J.: John Wiley & Sons, 2007. The official recommendations of this organization.

Lieberman, Shari, and Nancy Bruning. *Real Vitamin and Mineral Book.* 4th ed. New York: Avery, 2007. Discusses what vitamin and mineral supplements are and why they are needed to protect against disease and aid in mental and physical well-being. Chapters provide factual information on common vitamins, minerals, and other supplements and give recommendations for use with daily nutrition.

Murray, Michael. *The Pill Book Guide to Natural Medicines: Vitamins, Minerals, Nutritional Supplements, Herbs, and Other Natural Products.* New York: Bantam, 2002. An excellent guide that answers questions about the effectiveness and safety of more than two hundred popular natural remedies.

Examines what the product is for and how it works; rates products for safety and effectiveness; discusses possible side effects and drug and food interactions; and covers special concerns for seniors, children, and pregnant women, among other topics.

U.S. Department of Agriculture. http://www.mypyramid.gov. Offers information about nutrition, including personalized guidelines.

Weil, Andrew. *Eight Weeks to Optimum Health: A Proven Program for Taking Full Advantage of Your Body's Natural Healing Power.* Rev. ed. New York: Ballantine Books, 2007. A step-by-step program for enhancing and protecting present and lifelong health, written by a medical researcher. Includes the latest information about personal health and healing.

VITILIGO
DISEASE/DISORDER
ANATOMY OR SYSTEM AFFECTED: Immune system, skin
SPECIALTIES AND RELATED FIELDS: Dermatology, endocrinology
DEFINITION: A disorder that occurs when cells that make pigment (color) in the skin are destroyed, leading to white patches on the body. It may also affect the eyes and the mucous membranes of the mouth and nose, and it may cause hair to gray.
KEY TERMS:
autoimmune disorders: conditions in which the body attacks its own cells and tissues
immune system: a body system in which blood cells, proteins, and organs fight infection and other cellular issues such as cancer through antibody development
melanin: the substance in the skin responsible for color (pigment); tanning from sun exposure is caused by melanin

CAUSES AND SYMPTOMS
There is no known cause for vitiligo, but it may be an autoimmune disease or a disorder in which one or more genes contribute to its development. The white patches that develop on the skin are caused when melanocytes in the skin, cells that produce melanin, are destroyed. The color of the skin is determined by the amount of melanin that the body produces. Contributing factors to the development of vitiligo may include emotional distress, sunburn, or preexisting autoimmune diseases such as hyperthyroidism, but they are not considered causative.

INFORMATION ON VITILIGO

CAUSES: Unknown cause; may be autoimmune disease

SYMPTOMS: Irregular white patches on the skin, most commonly in areas exposed to sun

DURATION: Progressive and lifelong

TREATMENTS: Creams, medicine plus ultraviolet light, skin grafts, tattooing

Vitiligo usually develops before the age of forty and affects all races and sexes equally, with up to 2 percent of the population affected. The disorder may run in families; those with a family history of vitiligo or premature graying of the hair are at an increased risk.

The primary symptom of vitiligo is the loss of pigment in the skin leading to the development of widespread, irregularly shaped white patches on the body. The white patches are more evident in dark-skinned individuals and are much less noticeable in fair-skinned individuals. The patches may develop rapidly. Cycles of depigmentation followed by stable periods may occur throughout the lifetime of the affected individual. The areas commonly affected are the areas exposed to the sun, body folds such as the armpit and groin area, body openings, the area around moles, and areas of previous injury to the skin. Premature graying of the hair, including eyelashes, eyebrows, and beards, may also be symptomatic of vitiligo. The course of the disease is difficult to predict, and the spread of the white patches may spontaneously stop, but in most cases, the entire surface of the body is ultimately affected.

TREATMENT AND THERAPY

If an individual notices areas of skin that are losing color, early graying of hair, or loss of eye color, then a doctor should be consulted. A dermatologist, a doctor who specializes in disease of the skin, is usually the physician of choice to treat vitiligo, but other specialists may be involved. There is no cure for vitiligo. The goal of treatment is to restore color to the skin and stop future depigmentation, if possible.

The diagnosis of vitiligo begins with a thorough patient examination and history, including any family history of vitiligo or autoimmune disease, unusual sun exposure, sunburn or other skin condition in the period of time just prior to onset of the white patches, and recent stress or physical illness. Blood may be drawn to determine if there are thyroid or other blood-related dysfunctions. A referral to an ophthalmologist (a doctor who specializes in the eye) for a comprehensive eye examination for inflammation may be indicated.

Treatment depends on the site and extent of the discolored areas. Therapeutic cosmetics may be used to camouflage white patches and are readily available in most department stores. The use of sunscreen is important to prevent normal skin from becoming increasingly darker than the vitiligo patches, especially in fair-skinned individuals. Sunless tanning preparations may also be used to tint areas of skin.

Topical corticosteroids may be useful in the early stages of the disease. Vitamin D derivatives may be used in conjunction with corticosteroids or with ultraviolet light. Other topical ointments may be used in small areas of vitiligo, although studies are small and side effects including an increased risk of lymphoma and skin cancer are possible. Topical psoralen with ultraviolet A (PUVA therapy), or photochemotherapy, may be effective, although severe sunburn, blistering, and other complications may occur. If more than 20 percent of the body is involved, oral PUVA may be used. Regardless of medical treatment, frequent visits to the doctor's office and careful monitoring are needed.

Narrowband ultraviolet B (UVB) therapy is a newer approach to treating vitiligo. No medicine is needed prior to application of the ultraviolet light. More research is needed, although small clinical trials have shown promise. Depigmentation therapy using monobenzyl ether of hydroquinone twice a day lightens all areas of the skin to match the areas of vitiligo in individuals with depigmentation that affects more than half the body. Autologous skin grafts and tattooing are options that may restore pigmentation or provide color to affected areas.

PERSPECTIVE AND PROSPECTS

Support for the individual experiencing vitiligo is important, as the altered appearance caused by visible white patches may cause emotional distress. The extent of treatment may be determined by the psychological impact of the disease on the individual. Younger people and dark-skinned individuals may find the discoloration more disruptive in their daily lives and seek more aggressive therapies. Support groups are also available in many areas or online through organizations related to vitiligo therapy.

Research is being done to grow melanocytes in the laboratory from the patient's own skin that can be transplanted into the areas of depigmentation. Studies are also being conducted with other medicines, and piperine found in black pepper has been found to be effective at repigmentation of skin in mice. While there are no significant clinical trials, alternative medicines have been tried in individuals with slow-spreading vitiligo. Patients should talk to their doctors before trying any over-the-counter treatments.

—*Patricia Stanfill Edens, Ph.D., R.N., FACHE*
See also Age spots; Albinos; Birthmarks; Dermatology; Dermatology, pediatric; Dermatopathology; Eye infections and disorders; Eyes; Grafts and grafting; Hair; Pigmentation; Plastic surgery; Skin; Skin disorders; Skin lesion removal; Sunburn; Tattoos and body piercing.

FOR FURTHER INFORMATION:

American Academy of Dermatology. "Vitiglio." http://www.aad.org/public/publications/pamphlets/common_vitiligo.html.

Halder, Rebat M., and Jonathan Chappell. "Vitiligo Update." *Seminars in Cutaneous Medicine and Surgery* 28, no. 2 (June, 2009): 86-92.

Isenstein, Arin, Dean Morrell, and Craig Burkhart. "Vitiligo: Treatment Approach in Children." *Pediatric Annals* 38, no. 6 (June, 2009): 339-344.

National Library of Medicine and National Institutes of Health. "Vitiligo." http://www.nlm.nih.gov/medlineplus/print/vitiligo.html.

National Vitiligo Foundation. http://nvfi.org.

Taïeb, Alan, and Mauro Picardo. "Clinical Practice: Vitiligo." *New England Journal of Medicine* 360, no. 2 (January 8, 2009): 160-169.

VOICE AND VOCAL CORD DISORDERS

DISEASE/DISORDER

ANATOMY OR SYSTEM AFFECTED: Respiratory system, throat

SPECIALTIES AND RELATED FIELDS: Otorhinolaryngology, speech pathology

DEFINITION: Physical disorders of the vocal system in the larynx, pharynx, or oral cavity.

CAUSES AND SYMPTOMS

The human vocal apparatus consists of the larynx (voice box), the vocal tract (the pharynx and the nasal and oral cavities), and the nose and mouth (sound radiators). The main sound source is the larynx, containing the vocal cords; the thyroid, forming the projection on the front of the neck known as the Adam's apple; and the arytenoids, which control the size of the glottis (the opening between the vocal cords). The arytenoids are usually well separated to permit breathing; however, they pull together and vibrate during vocalization. Disorders of the vocal system may occur at the larynx or the palate (the roof of the mouth). Such disorders are sometimes caused by nonorganic emotional disturbances.

Laryngitis, or inflammation of the larynx, may be acute or chronic. The acute form may be caused by bacterial infection, chemical agents (such as chlorine), overuse of the vocal cords, or trauma. During acute laryngitis, the membrane lining the larynx swells and secretes a thick mucous substance that obstructs the vocal cords. Vocal strain following prolonged talking or singing may cause chronic hoarseness or roughening of the voice. Abuse of the voice consists of yelling or screaming, being forced to talk loudly in noisy surroundings, or having a faulty vocal technique.

Chronic laryngitis, produced by excessive smoking, alcoholism, or constant abuse of the vocal cords, dries the mucous membrane and often results in nodular growths on the vocal cords. These growths obstruct the normal functioning of the cords or cause erratic vibration. Hoarseness is symptomatic of a vocal cord problem. Sinusitis or any pulmonary disease that results in a chronic cough is particularly damaging to the voice. Chronic bronchitis may permanently injure the vocal apparatus because coughing is particularly traumatic to the vocal folds, which close tightly just prior to the cough and then open abruptly to permit the explosive air blast.

When the palate is not fused, a congenital deformity termed cleft palate, sound in the mouth cavity leaks into the nasal cavity. The resulting speech sounds have a nasal quality. (For normal speech, nasal sounds are produced when the soft palate at the back of the throat opens to allow sound into the nasal cavity.) The speaker with cleft palate may not be able to develop sufficient pressure in the mouth cavity to enunciate stops and fricatives.

Laryngeal granuloma, or contact ulcer, is a vocal cord lesion resulting from the insertion of a tube into the trachea (as with general anesthesia) or from an inappropriate configuration of the vocal cords during speech. This condition is suspected when a patient complains of pain or hoarseness after prolonged talking. Symptoms are slight hoarseness and a peculiar feeling in the throat.

A papilloma, or vocal nodule, is a small, benign,

INFORMATION ON VOICE AND VOCAL CORD DISORDERS

CAUSES: Congenital deformity (e.g., cleft palate); nodules; infection; injury; chemical agents; overuse of vocal cords; abuse of vocal cords (e.g., smoking); emotional disturbances

SYMPTOMS: Hoarseness, discomfort, coughing, difficulty speaking

DURATION: Acute to chronic

TREATMENTS: Surgery, vocal exercises, radiation therapy

wartlike growth (polyp) attached to the vocal cords. It most often occurs in singers, announcers, and people who frequently use their voices strenuously. A patient with a vocal nodule may complain of chronic hoarseness or some ill-defined difficulty in speaking.

Laryngeal carcinoma is a malignant tumor caused by chronic irritation or by alcohol and tobacco abuse. Both types of laryngeal carcinoma—intrinsic, which attacks the vocal cords, and extrinsic, which grows in the area above the vocal cords—produce immediate symptoms of hoarseness, discomfort, and coughing. In the intrinsic form, if the symptoms are diagnosed correctly in the early stages of tumor growth, the patient has a good chance of recovery after the tumor is removed.

TREATMENT AND THERAPY

There are two treatments for chronic laryngitis. Surgery, followed by vocal exercises to correct the cause, will restore the contours of a larynx that has developed polyps or become thickened. In some cases, however, the larynx appears entirely normal but the voice tires or roughens with prolonged use. The problem is repeated vocal cord strain from excessive subglottal pressure or the inappropriate application of breath during phonation. Relief must come from a voice teacher or speech therapist.

A cleft palate is surgically corrected by closing the hole in the palate. When the original palate is inadequate for simple closure, plastic surgery may restore it to its intended purpose, or a prosthesis may be fitted to effect an artificial closure.

Laryngeal granuloma is readily corrected by surgically removing the lesion. When the ulcer occurs as a result of prolonged talking, speech therapy or vocal training will prevent a recurrence. After careful diagnosis, a vocal nodule (polyp) is also removed by means

of surgical forceps. The patient is ordinarily restored to normal talking or singing within two to six weeks. Since nodules usually result from vocal abuse, the cause must also be identified and corrected.

Carcinoma of the larynx can be successfully removed surgically, or treated by radiotherapy, when detected early. The extent of surgical intervention is directly dependent on the site and extent of the tumor. If the tumor is restricted to the surface of the vocal folds, a laryngofissure may be performed, but more extensive penetration requires a laryngectomy. When the tumor is known to be of low malignancy, a hemilaryngectomy and immediate skin graft preserve the natural airway and leave a functional, although inefficient, voice.

—*George R. Plitnik, Ph.D.*

See also Aphasia and dysphasia; Bronchitis; Cleft lip and palate; Cleft lip and palate repair; Hearing loss; Laryngectomy; Laryngitis; Mouth and throat cancer; Nasopharyngeal disorders; Otorhinolaryngology; Pharyngitis; Pharynx; Sinusitis; Sore throat; Speech disorders; Stuttering; Tumor removal; Tumors.

FOR FURTHER INFORMATION:

Colton, Raymond H., Janina K. Casper, and Rebecca Leonard. *Understanding Voice Problems: A Physiological Perspective for Diagnosis and Treatment.* 3d ed. Philadelphia: Lippincott Williams & Wilkins, 2006. This text, which is illustrated with color photographs, addresses the physiopathology behind voice disorders.

Mathieson, Lesley. *Greene and Mathieson's The Voice and Its Disorders.* 6th ed. Philadelphia: Whurr, 2006. A detailed compendium of the normal vocal apparatus, vocal disorders and their correction, and vocal therapies.

Ramig, Lorraine Olson, and Katherine Verdolini. "Treatment Efficacy: Voice Disorders." *Journal of Speech, Language, and Hearing Research* 41, no. 1 (February, 1998): S101-S116. Ramig and Verdolini review the literature on the efficacy of treatment for voice disorders primarily using studies published in peer-reviewed journals.

Rammage, Linda, Murray Morrison, and Hamish Nichol. *Management of the Voice and Its Disorders.* 2d ed. San Diego, Calif.: Singular, 2001. A multidisciplinary book that covers anatomy and physiology, assessment, and treatment for all voice conditions across the human life span.

Rubin, John S., Robert T. Sataloff, and Gwen S. Korovin, eds. *Diagnosis and Treatment of Voice Disorders*. 3d ed. San Diego, Calif.: Plural, 2006. A clinical text that covers basic science, clinical assessment, and management. Topics include laryngeal function during phonation, measurement of vocal fold function, congenital anomalies of the larynx, vocal fold paralysis, and surgical management of benign voice disorders.

Strong, W. J., and G. R. Plitnik. *Music, Speech, Audio*. Provo, Utah: Soundprint, 1992. Comprehensive treatment for the layperson, covering many aspects of human speech, including chapters on vocal sound production, vocal tract effects, speech characteristics, prosodic features, speech defects, degraded speech, machine processing, and singing.

Tucker, Harvey M. *The Larynx*. 2d ed. New York: Thieme Medical, 1993. Includes detailed presentations of the anatomy and physiology of the larynx, as well as of laryngeal pathology and congenital disorders.

VOMITING. See NAUSEA AND VOMITING.

VON WILLEBRAND'S DISEASE
DISEASE/DISORDER
ALSO KNOWN AS: Pseudohemophilia, angiohemophilia, vascular hemophilia
ANATOMY OR SYSTEM AFFECTED: Blood, blood vessels, joints, reproductive system, skin
SPECIALTIES AND RELATED FIELDS: Dentistry, dermatology, family medicine, gastroenterology, gynecology, hematology, vascular medicine
DEFINITION: A genetic disorder characterized by the lack of a clotting factor and manifested by excessive bleeding.

CAUSES AND SYMPTOMS
Von Willebrand's disease (vWD) is a genetic disorder affecting the normal clotting function of platelets in the blood. There are three types of vWD that run in families, all due to inheriting a gene mutation. The pattern of inheritance may be autosomal dominant or autosomal recessive, although with either, both males and females are affected equally; some persons could be carriers of the defective gene without exhibiting any symptoms. There is another form of vWD called acquired Von Willebrand's syndrome. This disease is not caused by inheriting a gene mutation, and thus does not

> ### INFORMATION ON VON WILLEBRAND'S DISEASE
> **CAUSES:** Genetic disorder
> **SYMPTOMS:** Depend on type; may include easy bruising, bleeding gums, frequent nosebleeds, subcutaneous hemorrhages, prolonged bleeding after injury or surgery, menorrhagia in women, spontaneous bleeding, hematomas
> **DURATION:** Chronic
> **TREATMENTS:** DDAVP (desmopressin acetate) nasally or intravenously, intravenous factor VIII and vWF, oral contraceptives, antifibrinolytic drugs, care prior to dental or surgical procedures

run in families. This disease is characterized by the qualitative or quantitative deficiency of von Willebrand factor (vWF). This glycoprotein, present in platelets and the endothelium of blood vessels, facilitates the adhesion of platelets to one another to form a stable clot when there has been injury to a blood vessel. Therefore, patients with vWD exhibit the signs and symptoms of blood clotting abnormality.

Three types of vWD are recognized: type I vWD, with decreased levels of the protein vWF; type II vWD, with normal levels but decreased activity of vWF; and type III vWD, the most severe form of the disease, with a nearly complete deficiency of vWF.

Patients with mild or moderate vWD (type I or type II) can become symptomatic at any age and usually exhibit one or more of the following symptoms: easy bruisability, bleeding gums, frequent nosebleeds, bleeding points under the skin (subcutaneous hemorrhages), prolonged bleeding after injury or surgery of any kind, and, in women, menorrhagia, or excessive bleeding during menstrual periods. Patients with severe type III vWD become symptomatic at an early age and exhibit symptoms similar to hemophilia, with bleeding into and pain in the joints (hemathrosis), spontaneous bleeding into the gastrointestinal tract and from the mucous membranes that is potentially life-threatening, and painful bleeding into the muscles (hematomas). Some patients with type III disease also have multiple episodes of acute gastrointestinal bleeding and are often misdiagnosed. Some patients also have decreased factor VIII, which is deficient in hemophilia. The symptoms of vWD appear to decrease with advancing age, and they are milder in pregnancy, when factor VIII levels are high. Typically, bleeding time is prolonged in all patients with vWD.

The disease is diagnosed in the laboratory using specialized blood tests, such as the von Willebrand factor antigen (which measures the amount of vWF in blood), Ristocetin cofactor (which measures the function of vWF in blood), vWF multimers, and factor VIII levels. A careful family history of the disease should help distinguish it from the rarer hemophilia. A correlation of family history, laboratory findings, and clinical findings may be needed in order to diagnose the condition in mild cases of vWD, in which diagnosis is difficult.

A few cases of acquired vWD have been identified, with antibodies against vWF being present. Such persons may be otherwise healthy or may also exhibit other immune-mediated diseases.

TREATMENT AND THERAPY

The aim of therapy for vWD is to stop the bleeding and to prevent further episodes. Both goals can be met by increasing vWF and/or factor VIII levels in the blood. This result can be achieved by many methods, the most common being the administration of the drug DDAVP (desmopressin acetate) by a nasal or intravenous route. This drug does not seem to have a beneficial effect in type III disease, and these patients may need intravenous infusions of concentrates of factor VIII and vWF. For women with heavy menstrual bleeding, estrogen therapy in the form of oral contraceptive (birth control) pills is a good alternative, as it has been observed that estrogen increases the levels of vWF in the blood. Local antifibrinolytic drugs, which delay the dissolution of the clot, are useful in milder presentations of the disease (such as nosebleeds) or following dental procedures.

Preventive care should be taken by all persons suspected of having vWD. Adequate care and treatment taken prior to any dental procedure or surgical intervention should prevent the excessive loss of blood. Children with the disease are advised against engaging in rough and vigorous sports activities with a high potential for injury. Patients should also be cautioned against the excessive intake of aspirin and other nonsteroidal anti-inflammatory drugs (NSAIDs), as they worsen the symptoms of vWD.

PERSPECTIVE AND PROSPECTS

In 1925, Finnish physician Erik von Willebrand identified a bleeding disorder in the natives of Åland Island and named it after himself. Later, it was found that the disease was caused by a defect in one of the clotting factors, and the factor was also named after the brilliant physician. Today, vWD is recognized as the most common inherited bleeding disorder; it is thought to affect 1 to 3 percent of the population, with an equal distribution between the two sexes. It is important to distinguish this condition from the better-known hemophilia. The diagnosis of vWD in women is significant, as it is a popular misconception that bleeding disorders occur only in men.

The present drug therapy available to combat the disease is quite effective in reducing the bleeding that occurs. Modern-day medicine has reduced the problems of blood infections associated with administration of cryoprecipitates. Further research is being conducted to develop an effective recombinant vWF.

—*Rashmi Ramasubbaiah, M.D., and Venkat Raghavan Tirumala, M.D., M.H.A.*

See also Bleeding; Blood and blood disorders; Circulation; Genetic diseases; Hematology; Hematology, pediatric; Hemophilia; Nosebleeds; Transfusion; Vascular medicine; Vascular system.

FOR FURTHER INFORMATION:
Bellenir, Karen, ed. *Genetic Disorders Sourcebook: Basic Consumer Information About Hereditary Diseases and Disorders*. 3d ed. Detroit, Mich.: Omnigraphics, 2004.
Greer, John, et al., eds. *Wintrobe's Clinical Hematology*. 12th ed. Philadelphia: Wolters Kluwer/Lippincott Williams & Wilkins Health, 2009.
Kasper, Dennis L., et al., eds. *Harrison's Principles of Internal Medicine*. 16th ed. New York: McGraw-Hill, 2005.
Ruggeri, Zaverio M., ed. *Von Willebrand Factor and the Mechanisms of Platelet Function*. New York: Springer, 1998.
Westphal, Robert G., and Dennis M. Smith, Jr., eds. *Treatment of Hemophilia and Von Willebrand's Disease: New Developments*. Arlington, Va.: American Association of Blood Banks, 1990.

WARTS

DISEASE/DISORDER

ANATOMY OR SYSTEM AFFECTED: Feet, genitals, hands, reproductive system, skin

SPECIALTIES AND RELATED FIELDS: Dermatology, gynecology, urology, virology

DEFINITION: A family of generally benign epidermal tumors of the skin and adjacent mucous membranes; genital warts are more serious, sometimes precursors of cervical cancer.

KEY TERMS:

condylomata acuminata: the most common form of genital warts

epidermis: the superficial outer layer of skin, which consists of an outer dead layer and inner living layers of cells

epidermodysplasia verruciformis: the development of numerous small, flat warts that result from a noncontagious, genetic predisposition; they often develop into forms of skin cancer

keratosis: a skin growth that results from the overproduction of keratin, a protein that is the primary component of skin, hair, and nails

myrmeciae: deep plantar warts often found in teenagers; they may occur singly or in small groups

papillomaviruses: small, cuboidal viruses that replicate in the nuclei of epithelial cells

plantar warts: warts that develop on the sole of the foot, usually at points of pressure; they consist of a soft core surrounded by a callouslike ring

verruca: a benign, warty skin lesion caused by a member of the papillomaviruses

CAUSES AND SYMPTOMS

More than fifty different types of wart have been characterized on the basis of the type of lesion or its location. Though all warts are associated with infections by members of the papillomavirus genus, certain forms of warts are associated with specific viral strains or types. Regardless, all warts have certain characteristics in common. Their appearance is usually rough, with an irregular surface. A typical wart is an overgrowth or thickening of surface keratin, a condition sometimes referred to as hyperkeratosis. Generally, warts are painless unless they are found in an area subject to irritation or pressure, as in the genital area or on the soles of the feet.

While the association of warts with an infectious agent has been known since the 1890's, the role played by papillomaviruses was not confirmed until the early 1950's. These are small, cuboidal viruses in which the genetic material is deoxyribonucleic acid (DNA). These viruses are widespread in nature, though they are highly species-specific. Thus human papillomaviruses (HPV), as the name implies, are restricted to human infections.

More than seventy subtypes of HPV have been recognized; development of various forms of warts is associated with specific subtypes. For example, plantar warts are mainly associated with infections by HPV types 1 and 4, while anogenital warts are commonly associated with types 6, 11, 16, and 18. Despite the association of various types of HPV with distinct forms of lesions, certain features of infection are held in common. Thus, all types of HPV exhibit tropism for surface epithelial cells of the skin, specifically for the keratinocytes. Replication of the virus is found mainly within these cells. HPV virus particles may be found on the surface of the wart, resulting in their spread to other mucosal surfaces, including those of another person. The wart itself results from hyperkeratosis and thickening of the upper layers of skin following infection, in addition to hypertrophy (overgrowth) of the underlying basal layer of cells.

The most common types of wart are cutaneous warts. In general, these are encountered during childhood. They fall into three major groups: plantar and deep plantar warts, common warts, and plane or flat warts. Each of these forms of warts is most often associated with specific types of papillomaviruses.

Plantar warts, particularly types of deep plantar warts (myrmeciae), are sometimes referred to as verrucas. They exhibit a rough, raised appearance, with a horny surrounding collar. Often they are found on the sole of the foot, resulting in pain or discomfort when walking. Large numbers of virus particles can be found in the wart tissue, which makes these forms of warts particularly contagious.

Common warts (verruca vulgaris) are generally found on the hands, usually singly or in small groups. Because warts contain viruses, scratching of them may

---

INFORMATION ON WARTS

CAUSES: Papillomavirus infection

SYMPTOMS: Rough patch of skin with irregular surface, pain or discomfort when irritated or rubbed

DURATION: Often chronic

TREATMENTS: Salicylic acid, topical ointments, cryotherapy with liquid nitrogen, surgery

result in spread to other areas of the body. The wart may become quite large, nearly a half-inch in diameter, with a gray, irregular surface.

A type of common wart is the butcher's wart, so called because it was often seen among members of that profession, though it is also found among those in other professions that utilize cutting utensils (such as fishermen). These warts are typically large and cauliflower-shaped and are associated particularly with HPV 7. They are the only form of wart generally associated with this strain of virus.

Plane warts (or verrucae planae) are small, flat papules (pimplelike structures) that may have a slight scalelike appearance. They usually develop on the back of the hands or on the face, generally among children. Variations of these warts are often associated with different strains of papillomaviruses. For example, plane warts associated with HPV 3 are usually small and flat, while those associated with HPV 10 are often larger, with some horny appearance. Plane warts are usually found in groups. They may last for several years, but they eventually undergo spontaneous regression.

Condylomata acuminata, or anogenital warts, are the most common form of warts found in this region, occurring in the soft skin or mucous tissue around the vulva, penis, or anal regions. They usually begin as small, verrucous papules, developing and merging into large, cauliflower-like masses. These warts may also spread into the urethra, anus, and vagina, and even into the cervix. Subclinical or latent infections of the genital tract may occur in women who have anogenital warts. During pregnancy, warts may appear in the genital tract, raising the danger of infection of the baby as it passes through the birth canal. Development of anogenital warts is nearly always the result of infection through sexual intercourse. Their occurrence in children is so rare that the presence of anogenital warts is reason for suspicion of child abuse. As is true for other types of warts, anogenital lesions are associated with particular strains of HPV.

With rare exceptions, warts do not develop into malignancies. Epidermodysplasia verruciformis is a noncontagious, potentially malignant form of wartlike lesion associated with a recessive genetic trait. It is characterized by the development of large numbers of small, flat papules during childhood. Approximately one-third of people with this trait will develop skin cancers at the sites of the warts by the second decade of life. Development of skin cancer is exacerbated by sunlight. Many of these patients have depressed immune

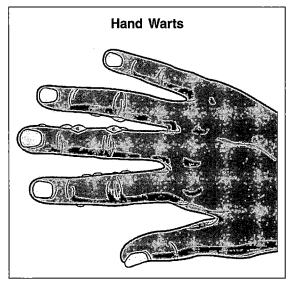

Warts come in more than fifty varieties; a common site is on the fingers of the hand.

systems, further supporting claims of the congenital nature of this form of cancer.

Papillomavirus infections are known to result in malignant transformations of infected cells under certain circumstances. Thus, certain strains of HPV, particularly types 16, 18, and 31, appear to be associated with the development of cervical cancer. Since these viruses are most commonly transmitted through sexual intercourse, this would imply that cervical cancer can be a form of sexually transmitted disease. (It must be emphasized that cancer of the cervix does appear, although less often, in women who are not sexually active.) The association between sexual activity and cervical cancer has been known since the mid-nineteenth century, when it was noted that the disease is more common among married women than among virgins or nuns. The possible role played by HPV in the development of the disease, however, first became apparent in the 1970's. Since then, the consistent finding of HPV DNA in nearly all forms of cervical cancer tissue, coupled with the finding that the expression of certain genes within HPV DNA may cause the transformation of laboratory cells, has strongly supported the suspicion that these viruses are the cause of this form of cancer.

TREATMENT AND THERAPY

In few other areas of medicine is the use of folk tradition as widespread as it is in the treatment of warts. In great part, this fact is attributable to the significant rate of spontaneous regression; as many as 50 percent of warts regress on their own. This feature has sometimes made it difficult to assess the value of alternative treatments. In addition, multiple rounds of treatment are often required in the elimination of warts, treatments that are sometimes uncomfortable or even painful.

Methods for treating warts date nearly as far back in history as the first medical observations. The Roman medical author Celsus (c. 25 B.C.E.-c. 50 C.E.) recommended the use of ash from wine-lees to burn off warts and a mixture of alum and sandarac resin along with a poultice of lentil meal. The Greek physician Galen (129-c. 199 C.E.) reported seeing a treatment that consisted of biting off and sucking plantar warts for their removal; no record indicates the success of the procedure.

Since warts frequently regress on their own, it is not surprising that large numbers of folk cures developed over time. Mary Bunney has cited a number of reported cures over the centuries. For example, in the sixteenth century Sir Francis Bacon reportedly cured his own warts by rubbing them with pork fat, which was then hung out to dry—as the sun melted the fat, so too did the warts disappear. Other folk methods of treatment included rubbing the warts with a green alder stick or with a potato (subsequently buried) and attending wart shrines, as in Japan. Some modern treatments have applied changes in diet, as in the use of various amino acid supplements.

In some instances, folk treatments may contain a factual basis; the willow bark sometimes rubbed on warts contains salicylic acid, a component similar to that found in aspirin. The modern use of a preparation of 16 percent salicylic acid in collodion, sometimes in combination with lactic acid, has had some success. The preparation is used daily by the patient, either by soaking the area or through maintenance of exposure by covering the preparation with a gel or plaster. The salicylic acid preparation apparently does not kill the virus directly. Rather, by destroying the connection between the upper and underlying layers of cells, the portion of the skin containing the virus is removed. In addition, the procedure promotes vascularization of the dermal tissue, aiding the immune response in removing the virus. With a success rate as high as 80 percent, the use of salicylic acid remains the most common daily treatment of warts.

Modern treatment of warts has the goal of maintaining wart-free remissions for as long as possible. Given the nature of the viral infection of the skin area, warts often reappear. In individuals who are immunocom-

promised—that is, lacking an effective immune system—the problem of elimination is even more difficult.

The most common treatment, particularly for those on the hands or feet, is the physical removal of the warts. Cryotherapy using liquid nitrogen is the method used most commonly by physicians. Essentially, the wart is burned off using the supercold "liquid." The liquid nitrogen is applied for five-second to fifteen-second periods, usually about twice a month. The process can be painful and, if not carried out properly, may cause localized scarring. If blistering occurs, as on the soles of the feet, the patient may undergo additional inconvenience. The process may also cause depigmentation in dark-skinned individuals.

On occasion, the wart may be surgically excised. Other than rapid removal, little advantage is observed with this method. The process involves the application of a local anesthetic, followed by surgical removal at the base of the wart. The process has a high rate of recidivism (30 percent), may be painful, and often leaves a scar.

Additional preparations used on occasion in the treatment of warts include formalin and glutaraldehyde. Formalin consists of a 40 percent solution of formaldehyde. More commonly known as a tissue fixative, formalin appears to act by dehydrating the outer layers of tissue. Since many persons may find the treatment irritating and some develop contact dermatitis, a localized allergic reaction, patients should be monitored in their use of formalin. On the other hand, evidence exists that the allergic reaction may be a key element in the elimination of the warts following formalin treatment. Since formalin may be destructive to underlying layers of skin, its use is often confined to treatment of plantar warts, as the keratin layer of skin is thicker on the bottom of the foot. Glutaraldehyde treatment appears to be as effective as the use of formalin. This chemical may combine with keratin, however, causing the area of the skin to turn brown.

A variety of other topical treatments is also available. Cantharidin, an extract of Spanish fly, is often used in the treatment of plantar warts. As with other topical treatments, localized blistering may occur, but scarring is usually minimal. Podophyllin resin is used to treat plantar warts and, by some physicians, in the treatment of anogenital warts. The chemical is an antimitotic agent obtained from the roots of podophyllum. The drug can be extremely irritating and can be absorbed within the body; therefore, it is not used to treat infants or pregnant women. Dinitrochlorobenzene

(DNCB) may be effective in the treatment of warts resistant to removal by other methods. The chemical seems to act through the induction of contact dermatitis. The ensuing immune reaction acts to clear the area of virus-infected cells.

Warts developing in the anogenital region are particularly difficult to treat. They are often small and difficult to find, and the latent, or dormant, virus is difficult to eradicate. Some topical agents are used, including podophyllin and trichloroacetic acid, but neither agent seems to have a cure rate above 50 percent and the warts often recur. Liquid nitrogen cryotherapy is used on occasion, with a cure rate of approximately 70 percent.

Other modern methods for treatment include the use of laser therapy. This procedure utilizes a carbon dioxide laser that vaporizes the tissue. The process can be painful, with a significant period of time required for recovery (from weeks to months). The procedure is more effective in the treatment of plantar warts. Among the drawbacks is the creation of a virus aerosol as the tissue is vaporized.

Immunotherapy as treatment for warts remains disappointing. Some reagents such as DNCB and formalin may act in part through indirect induction of an immune response, but direct stimulation of the immune system has not been particularly successful. Interferon alpha-2a appears to inhibit viruses grown in the laboratory, and use of the chemical in treatment often will cause shrinkage of the lesion. Yet neither the topical use of the chemical in the form of a gel nor the intralesional administration of interferon shows long-term effectiveness.

At best, treatment of warts has a success rate that is anywhere from 50 to 80 percent, depending on the type of wart. The treatment of anogenital warts in particular is often unsatisfactory, with a high rate of recidivism, while treatment of warts on the hands and plantar warts has a greater chance of success. Treatment procedures are often painful; warts often recur. On the other hand, most warts will, with time, disappear on their own. Generally speaking, warts pose no long-term threat to health, with the exception of those caused by oncogenic strains of papillomaviruses. Nevertheless, they can be painful and unsightly. The result is a dilemma with regard to whether, and how, to treat warts.

PERSPECTIVE AND PROSPECTS

Knowledge of warts dates back to the ancient Greeks and Romans; many of the modern terms relating to the nature of warts were first used by medical writers of that period. For example, the Latin word *verruca* re-

ferred to a small hill and was subsequently applied to mean the warts on the skin. The term "wart" itself was derived from the Anglo-Saxon word *wearte*, which referred to a callouslike growth.

As cited by Mary Bunney, the Roman medical writer Celsus recognized three distinct forms of warts: acrochordon, the multiple form of warts often affecting children; thymion, equivalent to the plantar warts and used by that writer to also apply to genital warts; and myrmecia, a deeper form of plantar wart. Celsus also pointed out the spontaneous regression, and reappearance, typical of many forms of warts. He also was aware that some forms of genital warts may be sexually transmitted.

The infectious nature of warts was first noted by Joseph Payne in 1891. Payne, an English physician, reported that he developed warts on his thumb, after it came into contact with an extract from the warts that he had been treating on a patient. In 1894, C. Licht and G. Variot independently demonstrated the transmission of warts by injecting extracts under the skin of volunteers, confirming the infectious nature of material from the wart.

It was during this period, from 1890 to 1910, that the viral nature of many forms of illness was becoming apparent. Though the exact nature of viruses was not understood, and indeed would not be for some decades, it was clear that cell-free filtrates of material from some diseases were still able to transmit the "contagium." Thus, in 1907, the Italian physician G. Ciuffo infected himself with cell-free filtrates of wart extract; the development of warts confirmed their viral nature. In 1950, a team working under Joseph Melnick first visualized the wart virus by using an electron microscope. Though a wide array of warts had been described, once the nature of the virus had been demonstrated it became clear that all warts resulted from infection by similar types of viruses. The wart virus was later grouped with other papillomaviruses.

Papillomaviruses were first described in 1933, when Richard Shope demonstrated that cutaneous papillomatosis in the cottontail rabbit was caused by a papillomavirus. Subsequently, similar viruses were found to cause warts in a variety of animals, and eventually in humans. Difficulty in growing the virus in the laboratory hampered its study for many years. Indeed, it was not until the 1970's, when the virus genome could be cloned in bacteria, that the nature of the viral proteins could be studied in detail.

A possible association between papillomavirus infection and human malignancy dates to as early as 1922, when certain types of infection were found in association with the rare epidermodysplasia verruciformis. It was not until the 1970's, however, that the possibility of papillomaviruses being associated with more common forms of cancer was fully explored. In the 1980's, it became apparent that certain subsets of human papillomaviruses, particularly some associated with genital lesions, may be the etiological agents for some forms of cancer. In particular, cervical carcinoma may result from papillomavirus infection, as viral genetic material is often found in association with these malignant cells. The viral proteins associated directly with malignant transformation continue to be the subject of intense study.

In 2006, the Food and Drug Administration (FDA) approved Gardasil, the first vaccine that prevents HPV infection, for use in girls and women ages nine to twenty-six. Gardasil protects against HPV strains 6, 11, 16, and 18, which together account for a majority of cases of genital warts and cervical cancer. In 2009, Gardasil was approved for the prevention of genital warts and anal cancers in boys and men ages nine to twenty-six. A second HPV vaccine, Ceravix, was approved in 2009. The effectiveness of Gardasil in women over the age of twenty-six remains under study.

—*Richard Adler, Ph.D.*

See also Cancer; Cervical, ovarian, and uterine cancers; Cryosurgery; Dermatology; Dermatopathology; Genital disorders, female; Genital disorders, male; Human papillomavirus (HPV); Malignancy and metastasis; Moles; Sexually transmitted diseases (STDs); Skin; Skin cancer; Skin disorders; Skin lesion removal; Tumor removal; Tumors; Viral infections.

FOR FURTHER INFORMATION:
Brodell, Robert T., and Sandra Marchese Johnson, eds. *Warts: Diagnosis and Management.* Washington, D.C.: Taylor & Francis, 2003. A clinical text that helps make sense out of the large number of competing therapies for warts and discusses recent research in order to present a guide to the diagnosis and management of warts.

Bunney, Mary H., Claire Benton, and Heather Cubie. *Viral Warts: Biology and Treatment.* 2d ed. New York: Oxford University Press, 1992. A thorough overview on the nature and treatment of warts. The text is written in a concise manner and is profusely illustrated.

Fields, Bernard N., and David M. Knipe, eds. *Fields' Fundamental Virology.* 5th ed. Philadelphia: Lippin-cott Williams & Wilkins, 2006. Provides thorough coverage of all major groups of viruses. The section on papillomaviruses is extensive and detailed, and it includes a discussion of the role of these viruses in certain types of cancers.

McCance, Dennis J., ed. *Human Papilloma Viruses.* New York: Elsevier Science, 2002. Examines the pathogenesis and molecular biology of human papillomaviruses.

Tierney, Lawrence M., Stephen J. McPhee, and Maxine A. Papadakis, eds. *Current Medical Diagnosis and Treatment 2007.* New York: McGraw-Hill Medical, 2006. The text contains summaries of the diagnosis and treatment for most major forms of infectious illness. The section on papules (warts) is brief, but it contains an adequate overview of the nature of warts and a good summary of modern methods of treatment.

Turkington, Carol, and Jeffrey S. Dover. *The Encyclopedia of Skin and Skin Disorders.* 3d ed. New York: Facts On File, 2007. More than one thousand entries on skin-related topics, including diseases, treatments, resources and organizations, skin cancer, acne treatment, warts, FDA approvals of new treatments, and remedies for wrinkled skin.

Weedon, David. *Skin Pathology.* 3d ed. New York: Churchill Livingstone/Elsevier, 2010. Text with extensive photographs, covering tissue reaction patterns; the epidermis, dermis, and subcutis; the skin in systemic and miscellaneous diseases; infections and infestations; and tumors, among other topics.

WEANING
PROCEDURE
ANATOMY OR SYSTEM AFFECTED: Gastrointestinal system, stomach

SPECIALTIES AND RELATED FIELDS: Family medicine, nutrition, pediatrics

DEFINITION: The training of an infant to accept food other than breast milk.

KEY TERMS:

engorgement: an uncomfortable, often painful condition in which the breasts are overly full with milk

overfeeding: the provision of more milk or formula for an infant than is necessary; may result in regurgitation

INDICATIONS AND PROCEDURES
For a woman who is well-informed about breastfeeding, the appropriate time to wean her infant will be-

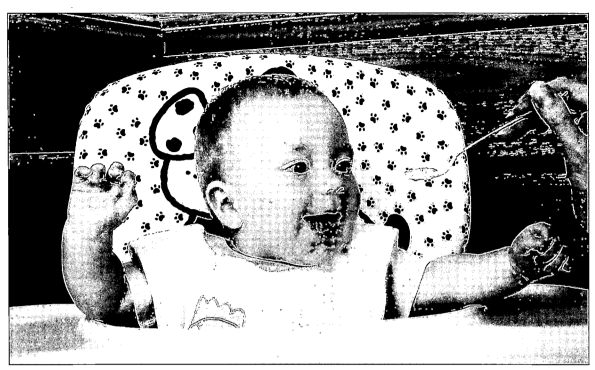

An infant who can sit upright and swallow properly is ready for solid foods, although many more months may pass before complete weaning takes place. (PhotoDisc)

come clear if she is sensitive to the child's cues. Other factors affecting a mother's decision to wean her child include family or cultural pressures, pressure from the partner, and personal beliefs about when weaning should occur. Often, weaning takes place between periods of great developmental activity for the child: between eight to nine months, twelve to fourteen months, eighteen months, two years, or three years of age. Most babies are weaned before nine months of age.

Mothers who want to wean their children from breast milk to a bottle before nine months of age need to prepare the child for the process by introducing a bottle when the infant is about six to eight weeks old. They can do so without compromising the nutrition of breast milk by pumping and offering breast milk occasionally through a bottle. Infants who are not used to the bottle after that age are more reluctant to accept it later. If the mother decides to wean the baby before one year of age, a commercial formula should be used for supplementation. Cow's milk is not appropriate for infants under one year of age. Honey should never be used to sweeten the formula because of the danger of infant botulism.

When a mother decides to wean her child from breast milk, she should supplement one bottle (or cup) of formula for the least important breast-feeding session of the day. This should be done over a period of two days to a week. If weaning is conducted abruptly, the mother's breasts may become painfully engorged with milk. Breast-feeding sessions associated with meals can be easily forgone, as the child has less desire for milk during those times. Gradually, the mother can substitute more breast-feeding sessions with bottle-feeding. Many mothers continue to breast-feed their infants in the morning and/or in the evenings for many months before weaning is completed. This has many advantages, in that both the baby and the mother will have time to adjust to their new feeding schedule. Weaning mothers should continue to drink plenty of fluids, as restricting fluid intake will not prevent engorgement. Typically, this late form of engorgement passes in one or two days after the weaning process begins.

When bottle-feeding babies, mothers should assume the same position with their infants as they did when breast-feeding. Most women cradle their infants in the crook of their arm for comfort and intimacy. The bottle's nipple should have a hole big enough to allow milk to flow in drops when turned upside down. Too big a hole, however, can lead to overfeeding and regurgitation by the baby. Cleanliness is important when bottle-feeding; appropriate methods of formula preparation and the sterilization of bottles must be followed.

Related to weaning is getting an infant to discontinue the use of a pacifier. Just as in weaning a baby from breast milk, this process has to be gradual and gentle. The best time to wean a baby from a pacifier is when he or she becomes more mobile, in order to prevent the pacifier from becoming a habit. The parent can remove the pacifier after the baby is asleep. Gradually, pacifier use can be restricted to nap time and bedtime. Parents should encourage the baby to stop using the pacifier by offering praise and being patient.

Once a baby starts to use a cup, it is important to make sure that the cup is heavy enough to be stable on a flat surface such as a table or high chair tray. The cup needs to be small enough for the baby to hold properly. Special training cups with spill-proof tops are widely available. Using a floor mat often saves the parent time in cleaning up after a spill.

USES AND COMPLICATIONS

If both the mother and the child are comfortable with the timing of the weaning, it can be accomplished with minimal difficulty. Nevertheless, weaning is a time of emotional separation for mother and child, and they may be unwilling to give up the closeness that nursing offers. Hence, it is important to plan comforting, consoling, and play activities to replace breast-feeding. Weaning is best conducted in a gradual manner.

One worry that mothers often express when switching from breast to bottle is uncertainty as to how much milk an infant needs. Parents should avoid overfeeding or feeding infants every time they cry. They should also avoid setting artificial goals such as "the baby must consume 8 ounces," feeding the infant until the goal is reached even though the baby may no longer be hungry. Overfeeding results in obesity.

PERSPECTIVE AND PROSPECTS

In recent years, the American Pediatrics Association has emphasized the importance of breast-feeding through a baby's first year. Physiologically, breast milk helps the infant fight infections by supplying antibodies and by coating the intestines with bacteria-fighting liquids. Developmentally, it has been found that breast-feeding mothers are more likely to engage in frequent interactive behavior with their infants, report that their infants have "easy temperaments," and engage in more flexible caregiving. It has been found that infants who are breast-fed retain an advantage in cognitive ability as measured by intelligence quotient (IQ) tests well into their third year of life.

For a majority of women who end breast-feeding prior to one year, inadequate milk supply and employment are the major reasons cited. Whether the result of choice or necessity, weaning is a natural process and a milestone for both mother and child.

—*Gowri Parameswaran*

See also Bonding; Breast-feeding; Developmental stages; Food poisoning; Malnutrition; Nutrition; Obesity, childhood; Pediatrics; Teething; Thumb sucking.

FOR FURTHER INFORMATION:

Bengson, Diane. *How Weaning Happens*. Schaumburg, Ill.: La Leche League International, 1999. This volume, with accounts from the personal experiences of hundreds of La Leche League mothers, informs mothers of the emotional and physical changes they will encounter when weaning their children.

Bumgarner, Norma Jane. *Mothering Your Nursing Toddler*. Rev. ed. Schaumburg, Ill.: La Leche League International, 2000. This updated volume offers new research into when and how a baby should be weaned and urges mothers who want to nurse beyond the typical few weeks or months to feel comfortable doing so.

Hillis, Anne, and Penelope Stone. *Breast, Bottle, Bowl: The Best Fed Baby Book*. Rev. ed. Pymble, N.S.W.: HarperCollins, 2008. Examines breast-feeding from a nutritional perspective and includes information on weaning and bottle feeding, introducing solids, and the latest recommendations on infant feeding from the World Health Organization.

Markel, Howard, and Frank A. Oski. *The Practical Pediatrician: The A to Z Guide to Your Child's Health, Behavior, and Safety*. New York: W. H. Freeman, 1996. A thorough resource for parents.

Meek, Joan Younger, and Sherill Tippins, eds. *American Academy of Pediatrics New Mother's Guide to Breastfeeding*. New York: Bantam Books, 2006. Excellent overview of breast-feeding, including the process of weaning.

Rolfes, Sharon Rady, Linda Kelly DeBruyne, and Eleanor Noss Whitney. *Life Span Nutrition: Conception Through Life*. 2d ed. St. Paul, Minn.: West, 1998. Chapter 5 of this textbook contains a comprehensive section on breast-feeding. Covers societal support, special medical conditions, physiology, the nutritional characteristics of breast milk, the nutrient requirements for nursing mothers, and the weaning process.

Spock, Benjamin, and Robert Needlman. *Dr. Spock's Baby and Child Care.* 8th ed. New York: Pocket Books, 2004. For more than a half a century, this book has been a virtual bible for parents seeking trustworthy information on child care. Informative, easy to use, and responsive to the changes in society.

WEIGHT LOSS AND GAIN
BIOLOGY
ANATOMY OR SYSTEM AFFECTED: Gastrointestinal system, muscles, musculoskeletal system, psychic-emotional system, stomach

SPECIALTIES AND RELATED FIELDS: Endocrinology, gastroenterology, nutrition, psychology

DEFINITION: Weight loss occurs when more energy is expended than ingested, while weight gain occurs when more energy is ingested than expended; both conditions may exist as a consequence of changes in diet or physical activity or of physical or psychological disease.

KEY TERMS:

basal metabolism: the energy used to fuel the involuntary activities necessary to sustain life (respiration, circulation, and hormonal activity)

energy balance: the state in which kilocalories from ingested food are equal to kilocalories expended

energy-yielding nutrient: nutrients that supply the body with energy (fat provides 9 kilocalories per gram, while carbohydrates and protein provide 4 kilocalories per gram)

kilocalorie: the amount of heat necessary to raise the temperature of a kilogram of water 1 degree Celsius; the unit of measure for the energy content of foods, also called a Calorie

nutrient density: the amount of nutrients provided per kilocalorie of food

wasting: severe weight loss characterized by the loss of muscle tissue and body fat deposits

PROCESS AND EFFECTS

Whether a person gains or loses weight is dependent on the balance of energy expended versus energy ingested. Thus, weight is determined by how many kilocalories are in the foods eaten and how many kilocalories of energy are expended. Normal day-to-day fluctuations in weight are typically minor changes attributed to shifts in body fluid and are not related to energy balance (input versus output). Input kilocalories refer to those from fat, protein, carbohydrates, and alcohol. Although alcohol is not considered an energy-yielding nutrient, it provides 7 kilocalories per gram. Output kilocalories are used to maintain the body's basal metabolism; to chew, digest, and process food; to fuel muscular activity for physical exercise; and to help the body adapt to environmental changes. When energy intake exceeds output, a person gains weight. When energy output exceeds intake, a person loses weight.

Body weight is determined by the amounts of body fat, water, lean tissue (muscle), and bones. Ideally, what people want to lose when dieting is body fat, not lean tissue. It takes approximately 3,500 excess kilocalories to store a pound of body fat, whereas approximately 2,000 to 2,500 kilocalories are required to gain one pound of lean tissue. Any excess food kilocalories—whether from fat, carbohydrates, protein, or alcohol—can be converted into body fat. There is no limit to body fat stores.

During periods of caloric deficit (meaning that input is less than output), a person will lose weight. A deficit of 500 kilocalories per day translates into a loss of about one pound per week. Not all the body weight lost is fat. During a deficit or fasting, the body draws on stores to provide energy. During the first four to six hours without eating, either while sleeping during the night or while awake and active during the day, the body draws its energy primarily from liver carbohydrate stores called glycogen. If no food is consumed after these periods, the body begins to break down muscle (also called lean body tissue) as fuel. Although people lose weight under these circumstances, it is the result of muscle loss and fluid shifts, not fat loss. Body fat supplies fuel during fasting but cannot prevent muscle wasting unless a regular supply of carbohydrates is present. The fat used during fasting is not efficiently metabolized and can cause medical problems if the fast continues for more than a few days. Fat loss can be accomplished by eating balanced regular meals that contain fewer kilocalories than those typically eaten.

Caution should be used before an individual undergoes either a weight loss or a weight gain plan. Starvation diets or very low kilocalorie diets and meal skipping are not wise. These diets promote water and muscle loss, not a steady body fat loss. A reduction in kilocalories of about 500 per day will promote safe, effective fat loss without medical hazards. The central nervous system cannot use stored body fat as fuel, making prolonged fasting a dangerous practice. By consuming a balanced diet that contains all five food groups in moderate portions, exercising, and modifying poor dietary behaviors (such as snacking while watching television), an individual can achieve lasting weight loss. Nutrient-dense foods—those that are low in kilocalories and fat yet still contain ample amounts of vitamins and minerals—should be chosen. Understanding the kilocaloric content of foods is not always necessary if a person uses exchange lists (diabetic exchanges), which are portion-controlled groupings of foods with similar energy contents that can be used to form an adequate diet. Exercise is important because it not only tones the body but also allows for more energy expenditure. Research has shown that regular exercise speeds up the basal metabolic rate, which also helps control weight.

Usually individuals seeking weight gain want to gain muscle, not body fat. Weight gain of this type can be accomplished by physical conditioning and a high kilocalorie diet. The amount of muscle gained is under hormonal control. In healthy individuals, an excess of 700 to 1,000 kilocalories per day is sufficient to add 1 to 2 pounds per week. This excess must be accompanied by exercise training, however, or only body fat deposits will increase.

Healthy individuals desiring weight gain need to exercise and to ingest more kilocalories in order to increase muscle size. Consuming more kilocalories can be problematic, especially for athletes. These individuals must take time to eat perhaps five to six times per day. These individuals should eat more kilocalorically dense foods—the exact foods avoided during weight loss. Emphasis should still be placed on nutrient-wise choices, not simply empty kilocalories. If someone is underweight, increasing fat in the diet is not considered a major heart disease risk because the fat will prevent muscle wastage.

COMPLICATIONS AND DISORDERS

Not all weight gain or loss is voluntary. Weight changes can be warning signs or consequences of disease. Several diseases are frequently accompanied by severe weight loss and wasting, such as acquired immunodeficiency syndrome (AIDS), cancer, colitis, chronic obstructive pulmonary diseases (such as emphysema), cystic fibrosis, and kidney diseases. Wasting is characterized by decreased muscle mass and depleted fat stores. This is a result of inadequacies in both kilocal-

ories and nutrient intake. Lack of appetite, termed anorexia, could be a consequence of disease, drug therapy, or both, complicating a person's desire to eat. Severe weight loss is compounded by other nutrient losses caused by diarrhea, loss of blood, or drug interactions. Individuals with AIDS can experience extreme weight loss, perhaps losing up to 34 percent of ideal body weight.

Thus, with illness a vicious cycle occurs: A lack of adequate food energy promotes the risk of infection; infections require more food energy for healing, further depleting energy reserves; and patients lose more weight, placing them at greater risk for subsequent infections. Extreme weight loss makes AIDS patients prone to other infections, which subsequently compromise weight status because more kilocalories are needed to combat these infections. Similarly, patients with cancer, colitis, and chronic obstructive pulmonary disease who experience weight loss become nutritionally compromised, placing them at risk for infections and delayed wound healing. Extra kilocalories are required to support the labored breathing accompanying chronic obstructive pulmonary disease. People with emphysema, a type of this disease, are often too weak to ingest enough food to prevent weight loss. Diseases of the gastrointestinal tract magnify poor nutritional status because energy-yielding nutrients cannot be absorbed.

Weight loss is also a symptom of cystic fibrosis. Cystic fibrosis is a genetic disorder that affects the pancreas and lungs. Individuals with this disease become malnourished because the normal release of pancreatic digestive enzyme secretions is impaired and because of high nutritional needs to combat lung infections. In an effort to clear congested lungs, individuals with severe cystic fibrosis cough so forcefully that frequently they vomit any food substances that they were able to consume.

Treatment for illness-related weight loss is complex. Individuals do not always want to eat, for both physical and psychological reasons. More frequent meals, higher fat intakes, and even special nutritional supplements are required. In severe cases, intravenous solutions, tube feedings, and hyperalimentation (feeding higher-than-normal amounts of nutrients through tube feeding or veins) may be implemented.

Sudden, dramatic weight loss could be a sign of dehydration. Athletes exercising during hot weather must pay attention to weight loss after practice and replenish fluids immediately. Rapid weight loss in teenagers, especially girls, may be attributable to eating disorders such as anorexia nervosa (self-induced starvation) and bulimia (periods of binge eating followed by intentional vomiting, or purging). Being underweight increases the risk of infections and often causes infertility in women.

Patterns of weight gain or loss are important indicators of childhood growth. Rapid changes may signal illnesses or psychological problems that have manifested themselves as overeating or undereating. Tracking weight gain during pregnancy is also important. Gaining weight too rapidly may be a sign of fluid imbalance forewarning pregnancy complications. Weight gain may precipitate insulin-dependent (type 2) diabetes mellitus. Although people with this type of diabetes are overweight, they are hungry because the energy that they ingest cannot enter the body's cells; consequently they continue to overeat, fostering further weight gain. The location of excess weight on the body is also important. Individuals who gain excess weight in the waist area are considered to be at risk for hypertension, type 2 diabetes, and other disorders.

PERSPECTIVE AND PROSPECTS

It is now well known that weight loss, the predominant goal of people with nonmedical weight-related concerns, cannot usually be achieved and sustained by dieting. It is estimated that one-fifth to one-third of the otherwise healthy adult population in the United States is "on a diet" at any given time. Going on a diet is not the way to get control of weight. Diets can produce weight loss; they rarely produce weight control over the long term. Repeated cycles of weight loss through deprivation of favorite high-calorie foods and weight gain when the motivation to tolerate this deprivation wanes, so-called yo-yo dieting, are hazardous. The cycles usually reduce individual metabolic rates, reduce lean tissue, discourage the individual, and make subsequent weight loss extremely difficult.

Weight management is a long-term endeavor resulting from myriad short-term decisions. Success comes with setting and achieving realistic goals. Family or group support, positive and tolerant attitudes, regular meals representative of all food groups, and behavioral modification will sustain healthy weight. Twenty to thirty minutes of exercising the large muscle groups, every other day, can prove a modest, effective way to burn fat and increase one's metabolic rate. It also produces more lean muscle tissue, a goal for both dieters and gainers.

Whether weight gain or loss is the goal, healthful eating habits require one to make wise choices and understand that weight control is a lifestyle, not a quick fix. Individuals experiencing a weight gain or loss who are not voluntarily altering exercise or food intake should have a thorough physical examination to determine the root cause.

—*Wendy L. Stuhldreher, Ph.D., R.D.;*
Paul Moglia, Ph.D.;
updated by LeAnna DeAngelo, Ph.D.

See also Acquired immunodeficiency syndrome (AIDS); Alcoholism; Anorexia nervosa; Appetite loss; Bariatric surgery; Bulimia; Cancer; Cholesterol; Colitis; Cystic fibrosis; Diabetes mellitus; Dietary reference intakes (DRIs); Eating disorders; Emphysema; Food Guide Pyramid; Growth; Hyperadiposis; Hyperlipidemia; Malnutrition; Metabolic disorders; Metabolic syndrome; Metabolism; Nutrition; Obesity; Obesity, childhood; Pregnancy and gestation; Vitamins and minerals; Weight loss medications.

FOR FURTHER INFORMATION:

Barasi, Mary E. *Human Nutrition: A Health Perspective.* 2d ed. New York: Oxford University Press, 2003. A text that emphasizes basic nutrition information and the application of this information to health maintenance and disease prevention.

"Best Diets." *Consumer Reports* 70, no. 6 (June, 2005): 18-22. This independent, nonprofit group provides ratings and recommendations for some of the top advertised diets, including Weight Watchers, Slim-Fast, the Zone, the Dean Ornish diet, and Atkins.

Brownell, Kelly D. *The LEARN Program for Weight Management.* 10th ed. Dallas, Tex.: American Health, 2004. A popular workbook, presenting a how-to, stepwise program for weight management utilizing sound principles and user-friendly format. Recommended for those who want to start a realistic program on their own or with others. Contains many behavioral suggestions and much nontechnical nutritional information.

Rolfes, Sharon Rady, Kathryn Pinna, and Eleanor Noss Whitney. *Understanding Normal and Clinical Nutrition.* 8th ed. Belmont, Calif.: Thomson/Wadsworth, 2009. Offers an introductory normal nutrition section with a chapter on weight control and a section on nutrition during disease which contains information on how illness impairs nutritional status and how proper nutritional support can aid in recovery or improve quality of life.

Stransky, Fred W., and R. Todd Haight. *The Good News About Nutrition, Exercise, and Weight Control.* Troy, Mich.: Momentum Books, 2001. This volume offers helpful hints on weight loss, nutrition, and health.

Summerfield, Liane. *Nutrition, Exercise, and Behavior: An Integrated Approach to Weight Management.* Pacific Grove, Calif.: Wadsworth/Thomson Learning, 2000. This text presents the basic principles of weight management and examines the role that nutrition and physical fitness play in weight control.

Wardlaw, Gordon M., and Anne M. Smith. *Contemporary Nutrition.* 7th ed. New York: McGraw-Hill, 2008. This easy-to-read introductory nutrition text has chapters on energy balance and weight control.

WEIGHT LOSS MEDICATIONS

TREATMENT

ANATOMY OR SYSTEM AFFECTED: Brain, endocrine system

SPECIALTIES AND RELATED FIELDS: Endocrinology, family medicine, internal medicine, nutrition

DEFINITION: The use of drugs to assist in weight loss.

INDICATIONS AND PROCEDURES

By the mid-1990's, several drugs had come onto the market showing promise in helping people achieve weight loss. The most widely sought and prescribed of these were Fen-Phen (combining serotonergic fenfluramine and amphetamine-like phentermine) and Redux (dexfenfluramine, with similar properties and actions to fenfluramine). Fen-Phen inhibited the brain's utilization of the neurochemical serotonin, which acts on the brain's appetite control center in the hypothalamus, and suppressed appetite directly, much as traditional over-the-counter diet pills do. Other drugs, less widely used, included phentermine, mazindol, and fluoxetine.

The hope and early evidence were that these medications would produce improved cardiac function, cholesterol and triglyceride profiles, blood sugar concentrations, and blood pressure; assist in the treatment of bulimia; and reduce weight in the obese and prevent weight gain in those at high risk for it, such as individuals who recently have quit smoking. The drugs were intended to assist those with morbid obesity, obese persons with serious medical conditions, and obese persons who had failed to manage their weight using more conservative nutritional and behavioral methods. At no point did researchers intend the medications as quick fixes for those unwilling to exercise or unwilling to change their eating habits. Nevertheless, many physicians prescribed them to patients who were not significantly obese or who were merely overweight.

USES AND COMPLICATIONS

Multiple studies across many different populations have tended to show the same results: Measurable weight loss in those taking the drugs was between 5 and 15 percent, with weight regained one year after patients had stopped taking the drug. The medications had few initial side effects—dry mouth, constipation, and drowsiness being the most common—and were unlikely to become physically addicting.

Health providers across all disciplines were particularly concerned, however, that some patients were coming to rely on these medications as alternatives to the sustained, hard work of developing lifestyle habits of healthy, proportional eating and exercise. In addition, concerns grew over the drugs' potential to cause neurotoxicity and primary pulmonary hypertension. Fen-Phen, in particular, was responsible for numerous reports of valvular heart disease and pulmonary hypertension.

PERSPECTIVE AND PROSPECTS

In 1997, the Food and Drug Administration (FDA) withdrew approval of Fen-Phen and Redux for treating obesity, and their marketing and distribution were discontinued. Class-action lawsuits were filed—former Fen-Phen users alone have filed approximately fifty thousand lawsuits against the makers of the drug—and large settlements were reached for those who had used Fen-Phen and other such drugs.

The government then set its sights on dietary products containing ephedra. Manufacturers claimed that ephedra, a botanical source of ephedrine, is a "fat-burning" supplement that could boost energy and enhance athletic performance, but reports began to surface about seizures, strokes, heart attacks, and even deaths in otherwise healthy users. In 2003, the FDA banned the use of ephedra.

—*Paul Moglia, Ph.D.;*
updated by LeAnna DeAngelo, Ph.D.

See also Addiction; Anorexia nervosa; Appetite loss; Bariatric surgery; Bulimia; Caffeine; Eating disorders; Malnutrition; Nutrition; Obesity; Obesity, childhood; Weight loss and gain.

FOR FURTHER INFORMATION:

Berke, Ethan M., and Nancy E. Morden. "Medical Management of Obesity." *American Family Physician* 62, no. 2 (July 15, 2000): 419-427.

Finn, R. "Pharmacotherapy May Help Some Obese Teens." *Internal Medicine News* 38, no. 19 (June, 2005): 45.

Marcovitz, Hal. *Diet Drugs.* Farmington Hills, Mich.: Lucent Books, 2007.

Mitchell, Deborah R., and David Dodson. *The Diet Pill Guide: A Consumer's Book to Prescription and Over-the-Counter Weight-Loss Pills and Supplements.* New York: St. Martin's Griffin, 2002.

Peikin, Steven R. *The Complete Book of Diet Drugs: Everything You Need to Know About Today's Prescription and Over-the-Counter Weight Loss Products.* New York: Kensington Books, 2002.

Whelan, S., and T. A. Wadden. "Combining Behavioral and Pharmacological Treatments for Obesity." *Obesity Research* 10, no. 6 (June, 2002): 560-574.

WELL-BABY EXAMINATIONS

PROCEDURE

ANATOMY OR SYSTEM AFFECTED: All

SPECIALTIES AND RELATED FIELDS: Neonatology, nursing, pediatrics, perinatology

DEFINITION: The art and scientific procedure of the pediatric physical examination.

KEY TERMS:

alopecia: hair loss

dehydration: excessive loss of the body's water content; in infants, manifests as increased pulse, sunken fontanelle, decreased blood pressure, dry mucous membranes, and decreased skin turgor

periodic breathing: rapid breathing followed by several seconds of no breathing; more than ten-second pauses are abnormal

trichotillomania: excessive hair pulling

INDICATIONS AND PROCEDURES

A pediatrician or nurse practitioner usually performs the routine physical examination of an infant. Because the child may be frightened, some steps in the examination may be performed while the baby is being held in the parent's lap. If the baby or child is ill, the health care provider will look for signs of dehydration and possible lethargic mental status. Dehydration is always checked in cases where fever is present. A child's normal oral temperature is similar to an adult's (98.6 degrees Fahrenheit). A rectal temperature will typically be 1 degree higher. It is not uncommon for a young child to have a temperature of 105 degrees with even a minor infection.

Respiration and pulse are measured. Young children and infants breathe with their diaphragm; therefore, the movements of the abdomen can be counted. Periodic breathing is common in infants. Respiratory rates for newborns are 30 to 50 respirations per minute. Toddlers average rates of 20 to 40 respirations per minute. The pulse of a newborn baby is detected best over the brachial artery. The rate is usually in the range of 120 to 160 beats per minute; this figure declines as the child grows older.

Blood pressure, length, weight, and head circumference are measured and checked against charts showing norms. Infants are weighed without clothing and are measured on a firm table. The head is measured at the maximum point of the occipital protuberance posteriorly and at the mid forehead anteriorly. The shape of the child's head, such as flatness or swelling, is observed. Hair is checked for quantity, color, texture, and infestations. The presence of a fungus can be indicated by alopecia (hair loss), but this cause must be distinguished from trichotillomania. Hypothyroidism can be indicated by dry, coarse hair.

An eye examination can give information about systemic problems and about the eyes themselves. The eyes are observed working together; reaction to light, pupil size, cornea haziness, excess tearing, vision, visual fields, and the distance between the eyes are checked. Observations for nystagmus (involuntary movement of the eyes) and for the abnormal upward outward eye slant and epicanthal folds associated with Down syndrome are also made. Newborns have about 20/400 vision, which improves to 20/40 by six months of age.

During an ear examination, the tympanic membrane is checked for perforations, color, lucency, and bulging (indicating pus and/or fluid) in the middle ear. A rough hearing acuity may be determined by eliciting from the child a startle reflex to sound.

The nose is checked interiorly, and the nasal mucus is checked for watery discharge (indicating allergy) and mucopurulent discharge (indicating infection). The nasal septum and passages are also checked, and any foreign bodies are removed.

The oral cavity examination consists of checking the lips for asymmetry, fissures, clefts, lesions, and color. The tongue is examined for color, size, coating, and dryness. The tonsils are observed for signs of infection and color, while the palate is observed for arch and possible lesions. The throat is examined for signs of inflammation and other problems. The neck is checked for tilt and range of motion. The thyroid gland is palpitated and evaluated for symmetry, consistency, and surface characteristics. Any other swellings are noted and their causes determined.

The neurologic examination is extensive and begins with an assessment of a child's milestones. An infant's primitive reflexes—Moro, asymmetric tonic neck, Babinski, palmar grasp, rooting, and parachute reflexes—are checked. Cranial nerves that can be assessed at the child's stage of development may be assessed. General sensation and response to touch and muscle tone and movement are checked for unusual responses. The musculoskeletal system and extremities are checked for gross deformities and congenital anomalies. Gait and stance are observed, as well as muscle tone and range of motion. Posture in older children may be observed for spinal curvatures.

The lungs are checked to evaluate air movement, to identify breath sounds and chest sounds, and to inspect the shape of the chest. The physician will note any physical deformities and listen to rhythms that could indicate abnormal blood circulation. Indications of circulatory system problems in infants are cyanosis, clubbing of fingers or toes, tachycardia (rapid heart rate), peripheral edema, and tachypnea (rapid breathing). Examination of the abdominal contour and auscultation and palpation of the abdomen are done. In newborns, the genitals are checked for ambiguity, and the rectal area is checked for fissures or anal prolapse. Skin is checked for color, pigmentation, rashes, or burns.

Vaccinations—either oral or by injection—and boosters are a part of some well-baby visits. Occasionally, blood or urine samples are taken for analysis.

USES AND COMPLICATIONS

The challenge of keeping the child calm enough for the clinician to perform a valid exam is important in the diagnostic process. Although an older child can usually be examined easily in standard adult order, this does not work well for pediatric patients. The younger the patient, the more important it is that crucially affected areas be examined first, before the child becomes upset or cries. Clinicians and parents should work together to minimize a child's fears during the examination.

—*Patricia A. Ainsa, M.P.H., Ph.D.*

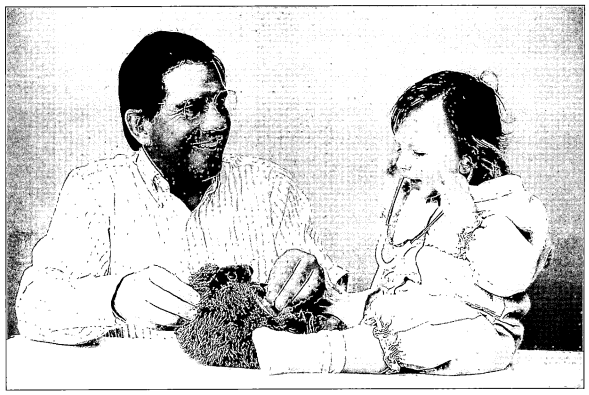

Well-baby examinations assess a young child's health and development. (PhotoDisc)

See also Bones and the skeleton; Cardiology, pediatric; Childhood infectious diseases; Cognitive development; Colic; Cradle cap; Dermatology, pediatric; Developmental disorders; Developmental stages; Diagnosis; Diaper rash; Endocrine system; Endocrinology, pediatric; Failure to thrive; Gastroenterology, pediatric; Gastrointestinal system; Growth; Immune system; Immunization and vaccination; Motor skill development; Neonatology; Nervous system; Neurology, pediatric; Obesity, childhood; Physical examination; Pulmonary medicine, pediatric; Reflexes, primitive; Reproductive system; Respiration; Screening; Signs and symptoms; Umbilical cord; Urinary system; Urology, pediatric; Weight loss and gain.

FOR FURTHER INFORMATION:

Albright, Elizabeth K. *Pediatric History and Physical Examination*. Updated and revised ed. Laguna Hills, Calif.: Current Clinical Strategies, 2003. This handbook teaches the fine art of history and physical examination of children. It is organized by disease and symptom, featuring a complete review of history, physical examination, and differential diagnosis for each disease.

Barness, Lewis A. *Manual of Pediatric Physical Diagnosis*. 6th ed. St. Louis, Mo.: Mosby Medical, 1991. Topics discussed include diagnosing pediatric disease through physical examination. Includes an index and illustrations.

Hay, William W., Jr., et al., eds. *Current Diagnosis and Treatment in Pediatrics*. 19th ed. New York: Lange Medical Books/McGraw-Hill, 2009. Easy-to-read and comprehensive general pediatrics book aimed at a wide audience, ranging from the medical student to the practicing pediatrician. Chapters are organized by pediatric subspecialty.

Sanghavi, Darshak. *A Map of the Child: A Pediatrician's Tour of the Body*. New York: Henry Holt, 2003. A comprehensive tour of a child's eight vital organs, beginning with the lungs and proceeding through the heart, blood, bones, brain, skin, gonads, and gut. Interspersed with personal stories of children with disorders and afflictions and how medical science was or was not able to intervene.

Schwartz, M. William, ed. *Schwartz's Clinical Handbook of Pediatrics*. 4th ed. Philadelphia: Wolters Kluwer/Lippincott Williams & Wilkins, 2009. A guide to assessing and managing seventy-four common problems in children. Each chapter has information on symptoms, differential diagnosis, laboratory assessment, and treatments, plus suggested readings and tables of normal lab values.

Zitelli, Basil J., and Holly W. Davis, eds. *Atlas of Pediatric Physical Diagnosis*. 5th ed. St. Louis, Mo.: Mosby/Elsevier, 2007. This is an excellent book, and although it is not quite as comprehensive as a major textbook of medicine, it is very concise and readable.

WEST NILE VIRUS
DISEASE/DISORDER
ALSO KNOWN AS: West Nile encephalitis, West Nile meningitis

ANATOMY OR SYSTEM AFFECTED: Brain, nervous system, psychic-emotional system

SPECIALTIES AND RELATED FIELDS: Environmental health, epidemiology, neurology, pathology, public health, virology

DEFINITION: A mosquito-borne virus affecting humans, birds, and possibly other warm-blooded animals.

KEY TERMS:
arbovirus: any virus transmitted by an arthropod such as a mosquito or fly; the term is an abbreviation of "arthropod-borne virus"

emerging disease: a disease whose incidence in target organisms such as humans has suddenly increased

encephalitis: any disease that manifests symptoms of swelling of the meninges, or linings of the brain

meninges: the three protective layers or linings of the brain, called the pia mater, dura mater, and subarachnoid

CAUSES AND SYMPTOMS
For most of the twentieth century following its discovery in Uganda, West Nile virus, an organism that can cause severe inflammation of the spinal cord and brain, was known only in Africa, southeast Europe, and southwest Asia. As the century came to a close, however, the potentially fatal disease emerged in the Western Hemisphere, in the New York City metropolitan area. Since then, it has spread across the continental United States, seven Canadian provinces, Mexico, the Caribbean, and parts of Central America. One of the hallmarks of the disease is dead birds, such as crows, who are also susceptible to the virus.

The first North American cases of the mosquito-borne West Nile virus were found in patients from New York in 1999, and its resurgence in following summers indicates that this disease has become established. The virus is a member of the Japanese encephalitis complex most closely related to St. Louis encephalitis, which also occurs in North America. This group of encephalitis viruses includes the Japanese, Murray Valley, and Stratford complex of viruses. The West Nile virus is also called West Nile encephalitis or West Nile meningitis.

The West Nile virus is called an arbovirus, which is an abbreviation for "arthropod-borne virus." Mosquitoes are the only known agents of transmission of the virus. Other blood-feeding animals, such as ticks and flies, may carry the virus, but so far none of them has been shown to transmit the viral disease to humans. The disease cannot be transmitted from one person to another or between animals and humans other than through a vector mosquito.

A potential transmission cycle begins when a mosquito becomes infected with the disease by feeding on an infected animal, usually a bird or mammal. The virus enters the mosquito's bloodstream and is eventually carried to its salivary glands. The virus incubates within the salivary glands for an unknown period of time. During the mosquito's next blood meal, some of the saliva containing the virus may be injected. Once inside the individual, the virus multiplies and is carried via the bloodstream to all the tissues of the body. In about 1 in 150 individuals, some of the virus makes its way past the blood-brain barrier and into the brain. In humans, the pathology of the West Nile virus disease manifests as a type of encephalitis, a swelling of the meninges, or tissue linings, of the brain.

The first symptoms of infection usually appear within three to fifteen days following exposure, and they may include fever, headache, general body aches, swollen lymph glands, and sometimes a skin rash. In more serious cases, symptoms such as high fever, stiffness, disorientation, stupor, coma, tremors, convulsions, and muscle weakness and paralysis may progressively occur.

TREATMENT AND THERAPY

Severely infected individuals are hospitalized and treated with a battery of life-support therapies, including intravenous fluids, ventilation to aid breathing, and inoculations to prevent the occurrence of pneumonia and other secondary infections. In many cases, the symptoms may last several weeks. In severe cases, brain damage and other neurological disorders may be permanent. Fatalities result from swelling of the brain and associated neurological pathologies. At present, there is no treatment for the disease.

PERSPECTIVE AND PROSPECTS

West Nile virus is a classic emerging disease. It was first isolated in 1937 in the West Nile Valley of Uganda in humans and animals, notably horses and birds. The virus quickly spread throughout much of interior Africa, following the course of the Nile River southward into Uganda and neighboring countries, then westward into the Republic of the Congo, then still farther south into Botswana and Zimbabwe. Spreading northward along the Nile River, the virus reached Egypt in 1950, then spread across the Middle East, Eurasia, and Oceania. By 1997, the virus was documented in Italy, France, and Romania. The first cases of West Nile virus in North America were reported in the early summer of 1999 in New York. Twelve states reported cases in 2001, and all states but Alaska and Hawaii had reported the disease by 2005. The numbers of both infections and fatalities in the United States appear to have stabilized at about 3,000 cases and 200 deaths per year. The number of reported cases in Canada peaked in 2003 at about 1,400; by 2005, only 200 persons were diagnosed.

The transmission and fatality rates in humans are actually very low, for several reasons. First, the incidence of infected mosquitoes in an area is typically small, generally on the order of about 1 percent or less, even in regions that have had a long history of West Nile virus. Second, acquiring the virus from the bite of an infected mosquito is not certain, as particles of the virus may or may not be transmitted into the human bloodstream during the blood meal. Finally, small amounts of virus

---

INFORMATION ON WEST NILE VIRUS

CAUSES: Viral infection transmitted by mosquitoes

SYMPTOMS: Fever, headache, body aches, swollen lymph glands, sometimes rash; in severe cases, high fever, stiffness, tremors, convulsions, muscle weakness and paralysis, disorientation, stupor, brain swelling, coma, sometimes death

DURATION: Several weeks

TREATMENTS: In severe cases, hospitalization and life-support therapies (intravenous fluids, ventilation, inoculations against secondary infections)

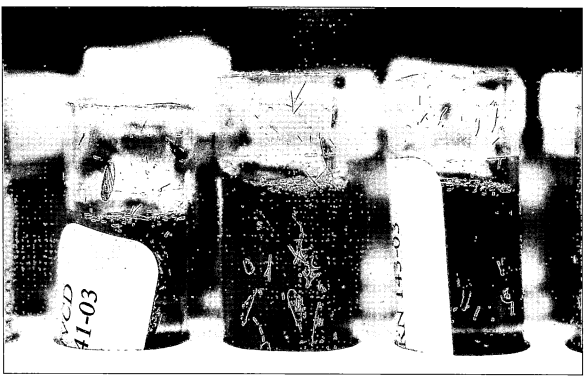

Vials are filled with mosquitoes to be tested for the presence of West Nile virus in California in August, 2003. (AP/Wide World Photos)

may not produce the "full-blown" disease in humans. The Centers for Disease Control and Prevention (CDC) suggest that about 1 in 150 people bitten by an infected mosquito becomes severely ill with the disease. Healthy people may simply fight off the viral infection without manifesting any symptoms at all. Others experience a variety of generally mild, flulike symptoms, which may include malaise, aching bones, and headaches.

CDC estimates of fatality rates are uncertain but suggest that one in one thousand infected people actually dies from the disease, but some estimates place the fatality rate at 3 to 15 percent. As with many viral diseases, the effect of West Nile virus increases with age; the young and healthy seem to develop very few symptoms and almost no residual traces of the disease, but people fifty and older or individuals with compromised immune systems are most at risk. Individuals who survive exposure apparently develop a long-term immunity to the virus.

At present, the only way to prevent becoming infected with West Nile virus is to avoid being outdoors in areas where mosquitoes are plentiful or, alternately, to confine outdoor activities to midday hours, when mosquitoes are least active. When outdoors, one should use a recommended mosquito repellant and wear long pants and a long-sleeved shirt.

Among mammals, horses seem most susceptible to the West Nile virus, but the virus has also been documented in dogs, cats, rabbits, skunks, bats, chipmunks, mice, and squirrels. At least seventy species of birds have been found with the disease, of which sparrows, ducks, pigeons, starlings, and crows are the best-known examples. Of these animals, crows seem most at risk, or at least seem to show the highest incidence of infection and mortality, but this may reflect their size and coloration, both factors making them easily seen. Despite public concern over the incidence of West Nile virus in birds and other mammals, tests have shown that the virus cannot be transmitted simply by handling dead birds. There are no records of animal-to-animal or animal-to-human transmission of West Nile virus. However, it is always advisable to wear gloves and avoid the animal's body fluids when handling animals found dead or known to be infected with West Nile virus.

—Dwight G. Smith, Ph.D.;
updated by David M. Lawrence

See also Brain; Brain disorders; Emerging infectious diseases; Encephalitis; Epidemics and pandemics; Insect-borne diseases; Meningitis; Nervous system; Neurology; Neurology, pediatric; Viral infections; Zoonoses.

FOR FURTHER INFORMATION:

Despommier, Dickson D. *West Nile Story*. New York: Apple Tree, 2001. A general but very readable account for the nonscientist and scientist about the appearance and subsequent spread of West Nile virus.

Emerging Infectious Diseases Journal 7, no. 4 (August, 2001). A special edition on West Nile virus.

Giesecke, Johan. *Modern Infectious Disease Epidemiology*. 2d ed. New York: Oxford University Press, 2002. An introduction to the biology and epidemiology of infectious diseases.

Lashley, Felissa R. "West Nile Virus." In *Emerging Infectious Diseases: Trends and Issues*, edited by Lashley and Jerry D. Durham. New York: Springer, 2002. Provides updated information on West Nile virus.

Sfakianos, Jeffrey N. *West Nile Virus*. Rev. ed. Philadelphia: Chelsea House, 2005. Discusses the initial panic surrounding the spread of West Nile virus in the United States, the structure and transmission of the virus, diagnosis and treatment of infections, and prevention strategies.

White, Dennis J., and Dale L. Morse, eds. *West Nile Virus: Detection, Surveillance, and Control*. New York: New York Academy of Sciences, 2003. Another excellent account of the impact and importance of West Nile virus, with emphasis on detection and control protocols.

WHEEZING
DISEASE/DISORDER

ALSO KNOWN AS: Sibilant rhonchi
ANATOMY OR SYSTEM AFFECTED: Chest, lungs, respiratory system
SPECIALTIES AND RELATED FIELDS: Emergency medicine, family medicine, pulmonary medicine
DEFINITION: Noise produced in the respiratory tract when air passes through narrowed or partially blocked breathing tubes.

CAUSES AND SYMPTOMS

Wheezing is a whistling or grating noise created when a person's breathing passages are narrowed or blocked. It

---

INFORMATION ON WHEEZING
CAUSES: Asthma, emphysema, bronchitis, pneumonia, allergies, smoking, inhalation of fumes or foreign matter
SYMPTOMS: Noisy breathing; often chest tightness or shortness of breath
DURATION: Often chronic with acute episodes
TREATMENTS: Depends on cause; antibiotics, antihistamines, bronchodilators, corticosteroids, drinking warm liquids, inhaling moist and heated air

can be accompanied by tightness in the chest or shortness of breath, as well as anxiety due to difficulty breathing.

Wheezing is a symptom of several disorders. The most common causes of chronic wheezing are asthma and emphysema. Temporary wheezing due to obstruction by mucus can be caused by bronchitis, pneumonia, viral infections, and allergies as well as smoking and inhalation of fumes or foreign matter. The exact timing of the wheeze can give clues to its cause. Bronchitis causes a noise at the very end of a complete exhalation. Wheezing at the start of exhalation usually indicates asthma or emphysema. Wheezing only when inhaling is a sign of asthma.

Conditions such as gastroesophageal reflux disease, vocal cord dysfunction, and genetic disorders that affect the lungs, such as cystic fibrosis, can also cause wheezing. Patients with heart failure often develop cardiac asthma caused by a pulmonary edema, in which fluid builds up in the lungs because of inefficient pumping of the heart. Less commonly, wheezing may be a symptom of tumors, joint disorders, or heart aneurysms. Radiation therapy for cancer or other diseases can also cause the airways to constrict.

TREATMENT AND THERAPY

Treatment for wheezing involves treating the underlying disorder. Doctors may do blood work or administer X rays, and antibiotics and antihistimines may be prescribed for allergies or infections.

Medicines are often given to manage the discomfort and anxiety this symptom causes. For chronic wheezing, respiratory inhalers are usually prescribed. Bronchodilators give temporary relief by relaxing the airways. Bronchodilators can cause dependence, however, and patients should be monitored continually by a doctor. More severe symptoms may require regular use of corticosteroid inhalers, which reduce inflammation in the airways and make them less likely to constrict.

For mild wheezing, drinking warm liquids and inhaling moist, heated air, such as from a vaporizer or a hot shower, is helpful. Severe wheezing may require hospitalization and use of a strong bronchodilator, an oxygen tent, or a respiratory tube.

PERSPECTIVE AND PROSPECTS

The Western use of bronchodilators for treatment of bronchitis and asthma began in the nineteenth century, although Indian medicine had used plant derivatives for similar effect for thousands of years. Corticosteroids became standard treatment during the 1970's.

Although wheezing is a well-managed symptom, determining the precise cause is often extremely difficult. This is especially true for doctors with limited resources in developing countries, where pneumonia is the most common respiratory cause of child mortality.

—Caroline M. Small

See also Allergies; Aneurysms; Antihistimines; Asbestos exposure; Aspergillosis; Asthma; Bronchi; Bronchiolitis; Bronchitis; Chronic obstructive pulmonary disease (COPD); Corticosteroids; Croup; Cystic fibrosis; Emergency medicine; Emergency medicine, pediatric; Emphysema; Environmental diseases; Heart failure; Hyperbaric oxygen therapy; Hyperventilation; Inflammation; Interstitial pulmonary fibrosis (IPF); Lung cancer; Lungs; Multiple chemical sensitivity syndrome; Oxygen therapy; Pneumonia; Pulmonary diseases; Pulmonary medicine; Pulmonary medicine, pediatric; Radiation therapy; Respiration; Signs and symptoms; Smoking; Steroids.

FOR FURTHER INFORMATION:

Barnes, Peter J., and Simon Godfrey. *Asthma and Wheezing in Children*. New York: Taylor & Francis, 1999.

Bruck, Laura, and Brenna H. Mayer, eds. *Respiratory Care Made Incredibly Easy!* Philadelphia: Lippincott Williams & Wilkins, 2005.

Silverman, Michael, ed. *Childhood Asthma and Other Wheezing Disorders*. New York: Oxford University Press, 2002.

WHIPLASH
DISEASE/DISORDER

ANATOMY OR SYSTEM AFFECTED: Head, ligaments, neck, spine

SPECIALTIES AND RELATED FIELDS: Orthopedics, physical therapy

DEFINITION: An injury to the muscles and ligaments in the neck that is usually the result of riding inside a motor vehicle that is hit from behind.

CAUSES AND SYMPTOMS

When a moving car collides with an obstacle, the driver and passengers suddenly feel themselves thrown forward. If an occupant's head hits the dashboard or windshield, then serious injury can result. Seat belts, a padded dashboard, and air bags can reduce the severity of the impact. Conversely, when a car is hit by another vehicle from behind, the occupants will feel an extra forward push against the trunk of their body while the head snaps backward. This so-called whiplash effect is like the crack of a whip made by the driver of a team of horses, in which the whip handle is rapidly moved forward while the end of the rope snaps backward. In a rear-end automobile collision, if a person's head flies backward beyond its normal range of motion, then the muscles and ligaments of the neck can be damaged. The person may not feel pain right away, but it can show up after a delay of some days. In severe cases, vertebrae of the spine can be knocked out of alignment or fractured. Most commonly, injury occurs at the junction of the fourth and fifth vertebrae. The upper four vertebrae are flexible and act as the lash, while the lower ones act as the handle of the whip.

TREATMENT AND THERAPY

Various treatments for whiplash are available, depending on the severity of the injury. Physically demanding

---

INFORMATION ON WHIPLASH

CAUSES: Usually an automobile collision

SYMPTOMS: Neck pain (sometimes delayed), muscle spasms; in severe cases, fracture or misalignment of vertebrae

DURATION: Acute

TREATMENTS: Initial avoidance of activity, aspirin or other anti-inflammatory drugs, neck collar to limit motion, physical therapy (heat treatment, massage, stretching exercises)

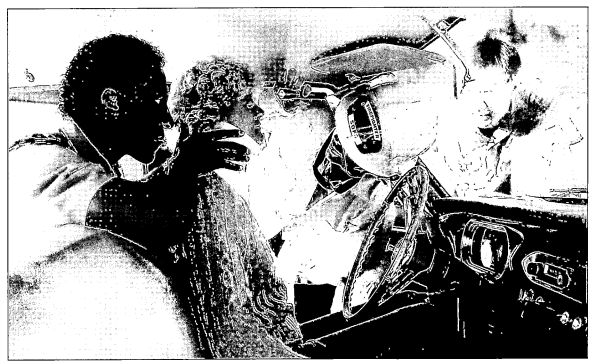

Following a rear-end collision, a brace may be used to stabilize the neck. (PhotoDisc)

activities such as sports or heavy lifting should be avoided. For pain control, aspirin or other anti-inflammatory drugs can be taken. If muscle spasms occur, then a physician may prescribe physical therapy, which includes heat treatment, massage, and stretching exercises. Wearing a neck collar can be useful to limit the motion of the head so that the muscles and ligaments can heal.

Perspective and Prospects
Most automobiles have a headrest attached to the top of each seatback. Its purpose is to prevent an occupant's head from snapping backward in a rear-end collision. Whiplash injuries happen frequently in cases such as a multiple-car pileup on an interstate highway. Slower speeds and a greater distance between cars are especially important during foggy driving conditions or on an icy road.

Whiplash injury is not limited to car accidents. In football, a quarterback sometimes is tackled from behind, causing the same effect as a car collision from the rear. On the ski slope, a skier may lose control and crash into someone who has stopped to rest. During the snow season, some mountain towns have a tubing hill where people can slide down on inflated inner tubes, with frequent collisions resulting. Any activity that causes excessive flexion of the neck muscles and ligaments can result in whiplash injury.

—*Hans G. Graetzer, Ph.D.*

See also Accidents; Head and neck disorders; Headaches; Ligaments; Muscle sprains, spasms, and disorders; Muscles; Physical rehabilitation; Spine, vertebrae, and disks; Sports medicine.

For Further Information:
American Medical Association. *American Medical Association Family Medical Guide.* 4th rev. ed. Hoboken, N.J.: John Wiley & Sons, 2004.

Foreman, Stephen M., and Arthur C. Croft. *Whiplash Injuries: The Cervical Acceleration/Deceleration Syndrome.* 3d ed. Philadelphia: Lippincott Williams & Wilkins, 2002.

Kasper, Dennis L., et al., eds. *Harrison's Principles of Internal Medicine.* 16th ed. New York: McGraw-Hill, 2005.

Komaroff, Anthony, ed. *Harvard Medical School Family Health Guide.* New York: Free Press, 2005.

Rook, Jack L. *Whiplash Injuries.* Philadelphia: Butterworth-Heinemann, 2003.

WHOOPING COUGH

DISEASE/DISORDER

ALSO KNOWN AS: Pertussis

ANATOMY OR SYSTEM AFFECTED: Chest, heart, neck, respiratory system, throat

SPECIALTIES AND RELATED FIELDS: Bacteriology, critical care, family medicine, otorhinolaryngology, pediatrics

DEFINITION: A highly contagious respiratory disease characterized by uncontrollable coughing that ends in a loud whoop as the patient attempts to inhale.

KEY TERMS:

catarrhal stage: the early stage of pertussis, characterized by sneezing and dry cough

DPT vaccine: a trivalent vaccine that provides immunization against diphtheria, pertussis, and tetanus

dyspnea: difficulty in breathing

epiglottis: tissue that lies over the larynx to prevent food from entering the windpipe

paroxysmal stage: the second stage of pertussis, characterized by deep, rapid coughing accompanied by sharp intakes of breath with sound of "whooping"

CAUSES AND SYMPTOMS

The etiological agent of whooping cough is *Bordetella pertussis*, a small, gram-negative, rod-shaped bacterium. A similar organism, *Bordetella parapertussis*, causes a less severe form of the disease. Symptoms and tissue damage are the result of a toxin secreted by the organism.

The diagnosis of pertussis is primarily clinical, based on the characteristic whoop that accompanies the paroxysmal stage. The most definitive diagnosis involves the actual isolation of the organism. Most pathogenic strains of *Bordetella* are fastidious in their requirements. Nasal swabs from the patient are obtained, with the organism grown on a special Bordet-Gengou medium.

The clinical manifestation of whooping cough is arbitrarily divided into the catarrhal, paroxysmal, and convalescent stages. The average incubation period following exposure is about seven days. During this period, the patient develops a dry cough, often accompanied by sneezing. A mild fever may be present. Early symptoms resemble those of bronchitis or influenza.

The severity of the cough gradually increases over the next ten to fourteen days; it may be triggered by exercise or even eating. As the patient enters the paroxysmal stage, the cough becomes deeper and more pronounced. It is often characterized as a series of short

bursts, followed by a whooping sound as the patient attempts to inhale; the sound itself is caused by possible spasm of the epiglottis.

Large quantities of mucus may be expelled during the coughing spells, which in severe cases may occur forty to fifty times a day. The patient may exhibit dyspnea and become cyanotic from lack of air. In infants, choking is common during this stage and can prove fatal. The severity of the cough has also been known to result in hemorrhaging from the throat.

The paroxysmal stage of the disease lasts from four to six weeks. Gradually, the cough disappears as the patient enters the convalescent stage. The entire period of illness may last six to eight weeks, with the cough persisting for months afterward.

The disease is highly contagious, with the agent passing from person to person by means of respiratory droplets. The patient is most infectious during both the catarrhal stage and the early portion of the paroxysmal stage, a period lasting two to three weeks.

TREATMENT AND THERAPY

Routine treatment of whooping cough consists of bed rest and the provision of adequate food and water. Infants are most at risk and are generally hospitalized. The administration of oxygen may be helpful in the relief of dyspnea and cyanosis. If there is prolonged vomiting, intravenous therapy may be necessary. Administration of corticosteroids has also been shown to ameliorate the severity of the cough.

Because paroxysmal symptoms are associated with production of a toxin secondary to the initial infection, antibiotics are of little help. An antibiotic such as erythromycin, however, may be administered to reduce secondary infections or to limit transmission to other persons. If erythromycin is administered early during the development of the disease, during the incubation

---

INFORMATION ON WHOOPING COUGH

CAUSES: Bacterial infection

SYMPTOMS: Dry, hacking cough that becomes deep and uncontrollable, followed by whooping sound upon inhalation; fever; excess mucus production

DURATION: Six to eight weeks

TREATMENTS: Antibiotics (erythromycin), supportive therapy

3166 • WHOOPING COUGH

period, or even during the first week of the catarrhal stage, it may prevent the disease or limit its severity. Persons coming into contact with the patient should also receive a course of antibiotic treatment.

Immunoglobulin is available, but its effectiveness is in dispute. Active immunization with pertussis vaccine is recommended to protect against the initial infection. Usually, this is a portion of the DPT vaccine administered in a series of injections beginning at about two months of age.

PERSPECTIVE AND PROSPECTS

The earliest known description of whooping cough was that by G. Baillou in 1578. It was Robert Watt, an English physician, who in 1813 provided the first complete clinical description of the disease. Watt also described the results of autopsies that he had performed on children who had died of the disease during his thirty years of observations; two of these children were his own. Watt also noted the highly contagious nature of whooping cough.

In 1906, Jules Bordet and his brother-in-law, Octave Gengou, isolated the infectious agent from the sputum of Bordet's son, who had contracted the disease. Known initially as *Haemophilus pertussis*, the organism was eventually renamed *Bordetella pertussis* after its discoverer. Bordet also determined that the virulent nature of the disease resulted from the production of a toxin. The special substance needed to grow the organism in the laboratory became known as Bordet-Gengou medium.

Initial attempts to develop a pertussis vaccine by Bordet and Gengou using inactivated toxin were largely unsuccessful. In the 1940's, however, an inactivated whole cell suspension was introduced and proved effective in immunizing children against the disease. In the United States, the pertussis vaccine was combined with inactivated diphtheria and tetanus preparations into a trivalent vaccine, DPT, that proved effective in immunizing children against all three diseases simultaneously.

Because of side effects in some children receiving the pertussis preparation, such as fever, vomiting, and mild seizures, questions developed as to the safety of the vaccine. In 1997, a new vaccine, DTaP, was introduced after researchers learned it was much less likely to cause the adverse reactions found with the DPT vaccine. The *a* in DTaP stands for "acellular," which means

there are no whole bacteria in the vaccine. While the DPT vaccine uses whole, inactivate pertussis bacteria, the DTaP uses only the parts of the bacteria that help children develop immunity to it. Since human beings represent the only reservoir of whooping cough, the disease may eventually face eradication.

—*Richard Adler, Ph.D.*

See also Antibiotics; Bacterial infections; Childhood infectious diseases; Coughing; Immunization and vaccination; Lungs; Pulmonary diseases; Pulmonary medicine; Pulmonary medicine, pediatric; Respiration; Wheezing.

FOR FURTHER INFORMATION:

Behrman, Richard E., Robert M. Kliegman, and Hal B. Jenson, eds. *Nelson Textbook of Pediatrics*. 18th ed. Philadelphia: Saunders/Elsevier, 2007. Text covering all medical and surgical disorders in children, with authoritative information on genetics, endocrinology, etiology, epidemiology, pathology, pathophysiology, clinical manifestations, diagnosis, prevention, treatment, and prognosis.

Cohen, Jonathan, and William Powderly, eds. *Infectious Diseases*. 2d ed. St. Louis, Mo.: Mosby, 2004. This book discusses syndromes by body system, special problems, HIV and AIDS, anti-infective therapy, and clinical microbiology. Includes helpful illustrations, bibliographical references, and an index.

Kimball, Chad T. *Childhood Diseases and Disorders Sourcebook: Basic Consumer Health Information About Medical Problems Often Encountered in Preadolescent Children*. Detroit, Mich.: Omnigraphics, 2003. Offers basic facts about serious diseases, illnesses and infections, and other chronic conditions in children and discusses frequently used diagnostic tests, surgeries, and medications.

Ryan, Kenneth J., and C. George Ray, eds. *Sherris Medical Microbiology: An Introduction to Infectious Diseases*. 4th ed. New York: McGraw-Hill, 2004. An introductory text focusing on infectious diseases. Aimed at the medical professional.

Woolf, Alan D., et al., eds. *The Children's Hospital Guide to Your Child's Health and Development*. Cambridge, Mass.: Perseus, 2002. An authoritative and comprehensive guide to children's health, providing a guide to every common illness or condition that affects children and a carefully designed emergency section.

WILSON'S DISEASE

DISEASE/DISORDER

ALSO KNOWN AS: Hepatolenticular degeneration

ANATOMY OR SYSTEM AFFECTED: Brain, liver, nervous system, psychic-emotional system

SPECIALTIES AND RELATED FIELDS: Biochemistry, gastroenterology, internal medicine, neurology

DEFINITION: An inherited disease of abnormal copper metabolism, leading to copper accumulation and toxicity in the liver and brain.

CAUSES AND SYMPTOMS

Wilson's disease is an autosomal recessive disorder of copper metabolism, resulting in excess copper accumulation and toxicity in the body. The gene in Wilson's disease is located on chromosome 13 and codes for a copper-transporting protein. The normal mechanism of elimination of excess copper in humans is excretion of extra copper in the bile for loss in the stool. The genetic mutation in this disease causes defective, reduced excretion of copper into the bile by the liver. The resultant excessive copper accumulation in the liver and brain causes liver damage and neurologic as well as psychiatric abnormalities.

Wilson's disease typically manifests itself between the ages of ten and forty, although it may also appear in earlier childhood as well as later in life. Typical signs and symptoms are related to damage to the liver and brain. Liver involvement in Wilson's disease may vary from hepatitis or chronic cirrhosis to acute liver failure. Neurologic symptoms and signs often involve areas of brain that control movement. Patients may have slurred speech, tremor and rigidity in the extremities, and dystonia, a syndrome of sustained muscle contractions

causing abnormal postures or movements. Other symptoms include seizures, mental changes, and transient periods of coma. Psychiatric abnormalities may also be prominent and may be the initial presentation. Behavioral changes include impaired school performance, labile moods, depression, and psychosis.

Useful screening tests for Wilson's disease include serum ceruloplasmin, twenty-four-hour urine copper, and slitlamp examination for Kayser-Fleischer rings. Blood ceruloplasmin is usually low in Wilson's disease, although approximately 10 to 25 percent of patients will have a normal value. Urinary copper values are typically elevated in symptomatic patients. Kayser-Fleisher rings, which are caused by copper deposits in the cornea of the eye, can be detected reliably only by slitlamp microscopy examination. They are almost always seen in patients with neurologic or psychiatric symptoms but may not be present in patients with symptoms related to liver damage. The gold standard for diagnosis in Wilson's disease is liver biopsy, which reveals an elevated amount of copper in the liver.

TREATMENT AND THERAPY

Given the diverse initial presentations of Wilson's disease, early diagnosis is often difficult. It is important, however, because effective treatments exist. Treatment is aimed toward the prevention of copper accumulation, the reduction of copper absorption through promotion of its excretion in the urine or bile, or a combination of these mechanisms. Pharmacologic treatments include penicillamine and trientine, two drugs that act by removing copper (chelating agents); zinc, which blocks copper absorption; and tetrathiomolybdate, which is experimental. Liver transplantation can be helpful in the patient with end-stage liver disease.

—Winona Tse, M.D.

See also Genetic diseases; Liver disorders; Liver transplantation; Metabolic disorders; Metabolism; Nervous system; Neurology; Neurology, pediatric; Vitamins and minerals.

INFORMATION ON WILSON'S DISEASE

CAUSES: Genetic defect in copper metabolism

SYMPTOMS: Liver damage (hepatitis, cirrhosis, liver failure); neurologic problems (slurred speech, tremor, rigidity in extremities, dystonia, seizures, mental changes, transient periods of coma); psychiatric abnormalities (behavioral changes, moodiness, depression, psychosis)

DURATION: Chronic

TREATMENTS: Chelating agents (penicillamine, trientine), zinc, tetrathiomolybdate, liver transplantation

---

FOR FURTHER INFORMATION:

Brewer, George J. *Wilson's Disease: A Clinician's Guide to Recognition, Diagnosis, and Management.* Boston: Kluwer Academic, 2001.

Hoogenraad, Tjaard U. *Wilson's Disease.* Philadelphia: W. B. Saunders, 1996.

Parker, James N., and Philip M. Parker, eds. *The 2002 Official Patient's Sourcebook on Wilson's Disease.* San Diego, Calif.: Icon Health, 2002.

Rowland, Lewis P., ed. *Merritt's Textbook of Neurology*. 12th ed. Philadelphia: Lippincott Williams & Wilkins, 2010.

Schilsky, M. L. "Diagnosis and Treatment of Wilson's Disease." *Pediatric Transplantation* 6 (2002): 15-19.

WISDOM TEETH

ANATOMY

ALSO KNOWN AS: Third molars

ANATOMY OR SYSTEM AFFECTED: Gums, mouth, teeth

SPECIALTIES AND RELATED FIELDS: Dentistry

DEFINITION: The common term for the permanent third molars, which usually appear between the ages of seventeen and twenty-four.

STRUCTURE AND FUNCTIONS

The third molars are called wisdom teeth because they appear much later than the other permanent teeth, at an age when people are supposedly wiser than they were as children. The average number of wisdom teeth is four, but it is possible to have more or less. They come in behind the second molars on the upper left, upper right, lower left, and lower right. Wisdom teeth are no longer considered necessary. People now eat soft diets and have better dental care, which prevents decay and molar loss. Thus, the second molars are sufficient.

Wisdom teeth become impacted if the tooth cannot erupt because of gum or bone hardness and/or lack of space. Impacted wisdom teeth fall into four categories: Mesioangular refers to a tooth that is angled forward toward the front of the mouth; vertical refers to a tooth that does not fully erupt through the gum line; horizontal refers to a tooth that angles forward, growing into the roots of the second molar; and distoangular refers to a tooth that is angled backward.

DISORDERS AND DISEASES

Wisdom teeth may become infected when saliva, bacteria, or food particles collect around them, causing pain, decay, swelling, and, in severe cases, trismus (inability to open the mouth fully). The infection can spread to the cheek and neck. In rare cases, the infection has been linked to heart disease. Infected wisdom teeth are usually extracted.

Wisdom teeth may also be removed even if no infection is present, such as when a younger patient is having lengthy orthodontic treatment to straighten teeth, as unremoved wisdom teeth may erupt and damage the straightened teeth. Also, older patients who need dentures should have any latent wisdom teeth removed. Should wisdom teeth erupt beneath a denture, it could cause severe irritation. The patient could suffer considerable pain and must replace the dentures, as the shape of the jaw will have changed.

There is a possibility of nerve damage during tooth extraction. Two nerves are close to the lower wisdom teeth. One of them, the inferior alveolar nerve, supplies sensation to the lower teeth on the right and the left side of the mouth, and a sense of touch to the right and left half of the chin and lower lip. The second nerve, the lengual, supplies a sense of touch and taste to the tongue and the gums. Injury can occur as a result of a faulty extraction or by a dental drill. Such injuries are rare, but damage can be prolonged or permanent.

Treatment after extraction usually consists of packing gauze pads in the hole for half an hour to control bleeding. Swelling is controlled by the use of cold packs. After twenty-four hours, rinsing with warm saltwater every two hours will help healing. For minor discomfort, aspirin or ibuprofen can be taken.

PERSPECTIVE AND PROSPECTS

Researchers from the United States and Australia have made stem cell studies on the dental pulp found in extracted wisdom teeth. These stem cells have the potential to save injured teeth and grow jawbone. As research progresses, it may be possible to use these stem cells to restore cells damaged by conditions such as Parkinson's disease.

—*Billie M. Taylor, M.S.E., M.L.S.*

See also Dental diseases; Dentistry; Dentistry, pediatric; Dentures; Orthodontics; Teeth; Tooth extraction; Toothache.

FOR FURTHER INFORMATION:

Fields, Helen, and Margaret Mannix. "Not so Wise Wisdom Teeth." *U.S. News and World Report* 139, no. 12 (October 13, 2005): 53.

Goldie, Maria Perno. "Stem Cell Research: A New Era." *Access* 19, no. 9 (November, 2005): 28-30.

"Hold On to Your Wisdom Teeth." *Consumer Reports on Health* 5, no. 8 (August, 1993): 84-85.

"Just Ask Us." *Current Health* 27, no. 2 (October, 2000): 94.

Steinmeh, Eric. "Yanking Those Wisdom Isn't Always Necessary." *Health* 19, no. 8 (October, 2005): 91.

WISKOTT-ALDRICH SYNDROME

DISEASE/DISORDER

ALSO KNOWN AS: Aldrich syndrome, eczema-thrombocytopenia-immunodeficiency syndrome

ANATOMY OR SYSTEM AFFECTED: Blood, ears, immune system, lungs, skin

SPECIALTIES AND RELATED FIELDS: Dermatology, genetics, immunology, oncology, pediatrics

DEFINITION: An X-linked genetic disorder characterized by thrombocytopenia, infections, and eczema in childhood.

CAUSES AND SYMPTOMS

Wiskott-Aldrich syndrome is a rare primary inherited immunodeficiency disorder, involving both T and Bdf lymphocytes. Also, the disease is characterized by the deficiency of platelets, which are integral cells required for blood clotting. In the classical form, it is manifested soon after birth and through the first year of life, with the symptoms of recurrent sinopulmonary infections (from a decreased immune system); bleeding into the skin, bowels, gums, or joints (from defective platelets); and eczematous scaly skin rash. Autoimmune manifestations in the form of anemia and or malignancies such as lymphoma or leukemia later in adolescence or young adulthood are also reported.

The disease is seen in its classical form as a result of ineffective production of Wiskott-Aldrich syndrome protein (WASP), which determines the severity of the disease. The greater is the deficiency of the WASP, the more severe is the disease. Defective production of WASP is caused by a mutation or error in the WASP gene, located on the short arm of the X chromosome. This mutation is inherited in an X-linked recessive fashion, and therefore, primarily boys are affected by the disease. In extremely rare cases involving girls, similar genetic mutations have not been noted.

Wiskott-Aldrich syndrome is suspected in any male child who has bleeding, typically bloody diarrhea in infancy. Older children may even have a low platelet count and abnormally small platelets when a routine blood smear is done during an infection. Otitis media, sinusitis, and pneumonia are quite common infections for these children, and viral infections are also seen as a result of the abnormal immune response.

The clinical presentation depends on the severity of the WASP deficiency and may differ from patient to patient. It may range from just thrombocytopenia (low platelet count) to all three classic symptoms of eczema, recurrent infections (because of immunodeficiency), and bleeding (because of low platelets). The disease X-linked thrombocytopenia is now considered a different form of Wiskott-Aldrich syndrome. The first presentation of the disease is usually within the first year of life, soon after birth, and most often is as a result of immunodeficiency or thrombocytopenia. The most characteristic feature of Wiskott-Aldrich syndrome is reduced platelets. Also, a defect in the function of platelets is noticed in some forms of the disease, manifested as bleeding gums, prolonged epistaxis (nosebleeds), or bleeding into joints or bowels.

Eczema is a common symptom of Wiskott-Aldrich syndrome. It may be localized or generalized, with itchy rashes all over the body. Scratching of such rashes might lead to bleeding and infections. Recurrent infections are common in the syndrome because of the deficiency of T and B lymphocytes (white blood cells). As both T and B cells are affected, the infections may be attributable to bacteria, fungi, or viruses. Other manifestations of the disease are autoimmune anemia, leukemia, and lymphoma, which are seen more often in older boys and adults.

A diagnosis of Wiskott-Aldrich syndrome must be considered in any boy with unusual bleeding, recurrent infections, and eczema. The characteristic platelet features of low count and abnormally small size are also evident in the cord blood of a newborn. The blood test for platelet count and size is, therefore, the most useful one. In older children, other tests such as serum immunological studies for antibodies and negative skin tests for T cell function are done. Confirmation of the diagnosis is by measuring the levels of WASP in the blood or by detecting WASP gene mutation through genetic studies.

In families with a boy diagnosed with Wiskott-Aldrich syndrome, prenatal testing of the mother be-

---

INFORMATION ON WISKOTT-ALDRICH SYNDROME

CAUSES: Genetic protein deficiency affecting lymphocytes and platelets

SYMPTOMS: Thrombocytopenia; eczema; recurrent sinus and pulmonary infections; bleeding into skin, bowels, gums, or joints

DURATION: Chronic

TREATMENTS: Blood and platelet transfusions, antibiotics, intravenous immunoglobulins, removal of spleen, bone marrow transplantation, cord blood stem cell transplantation

3170 • WOMEN'S HEALTH

fore subsequent pregnancies should be performed by amniocentesis or chorionic villus sampling, as there is a 50 percent chance of a mother transferring the abnormal gene to her baby.

TREATMENT AND THERAPY

The treatment of Wiskott-Aldrich syndrome is prolonged and involves multiple approaches. Family support is of vital importance in the treatment of chronic illnesses. Bleeding often results in anemia that requires blood transfusions for correction. To counter recurrent infections, these boys require appropriate antibiotics, which must be determined after careful culture and sensitivity tests. As a result of the abnormality of the immune system, vaccinations might not prove very effective. In fact, live virus vaccines are contraindicated in these patients and must be avoided. Instead, patients are given intravenous immunoglobulins (IVIGs), or preformed antibodies, to decrease the chances of bacterial infections. The treatment of eczema involves avoiding frequent bathing and applying bath oils and moisturizing creams after a bath; topical steroids are often helpful. Systemic antibiotics are of help in some cases of eczema. Platelet deficiency is corrected by transfusing platelets into the bloodstream. Surgical removal of the spleen is of some beneficial effect in checking the thrombocytopenia. Avoiding allergens is an important way to prevent the exacerbation of eczema. Bone marrow transplantation and cord blood stem cell transplantation are the only methods of curing the disease permanently.

PERSPECTIVE AND PROSPECTS

In 1937, Alfred Wiskott first discovered this disease in three brothers with low platelet counts. In 1954, Robert Anderson Aldrich identified it as an X-linked recessive disease. When the disease was first identified, the prognosis was dismal, with a life expectancy of just two to three years. The discovery of and advances in antibiotics, immunoglobulins, bone marrow transplantations, and cord blood stem cell transplantation have improved the prognosis greatly. Today, it is not unusual to see patients with Wiskott-Aldrich syndrome lead productive lives as adults without developing the complications of the disease.

—*Rashmi Ramasubbaiah, M.D.*

See also Autoimmune disorders; Bleeding; Blood and blood disorders; Bone marrow transplantation; Eczema; Genetic diseases; Hematology; Hematology, pediatric; Immune system; Immunodeficiency disorders;

Immunology; Immunopathology; Stem cells; Thrombocytopenia.

FOR FURTHER INFORMATION:

Frazier, Margeret Schell, and Jeanette Wist Drzymkowski. *Essentials of Human Diseases and Conditions.* 4th ed. St. Louis, Mo.: Saunders/Elsevier, 2009.

Greer, John, et al., eds. *Wintrobe's Clinical Hematology.* 12th ed. Philadelphia: Wolters Kluwer/Lippincott Williams & Wilkins Health, 2009.

Kasper, Dennis L., et al., eds. *Harrison's Principles of Internal Medicine.* 16th ed. New York: McGraw-Hill, 2005.

Porter, Robert S., et al., eds. *The Merck Manual Home Health Handbook.* Whitehouse Station, N.J.: Merck Research Laboratories, 2009.

WOMEN'S HEALTH

OVERVIEW

ANATOMY OR SYSTEM AFFECTED: All

SPECIALTIES AND RELATED FIELDS: All

DEFINITION: Issues related to the well-being of women, including but not limited to reproductive health.

KEY TERMS:

biopsy: removal of tissue for the purpose of examination under a microscope

bronchoscopy: the insertion of a tube for the evaluation of the bronchi in the lungs

osteoporosis: thinning of bone that occurs primarily in postmenopausal women

placebo: an inactive substance provided to research subjects to compare the effectiveness of a medication to the inactive substance

postmenopausal: time in the adult female's life that occurs after the menstrual cycle has been absent for more than one year as a result of hormone changes or after surgical removal of the uterus

MAJOR HEALTH CONCERNS

Women continue to live longer than men. In the United States, the life expectancy of a woman is 79.5 years. Living to an advanced age increases the risk of developing diseases such as stroke, osteoporosis, and rheumatoid arthritis. Many of the health issues that women face are preventable with lifestyle changes.

Heart disease. In the United States, heart disease causes approximately 22 percent of deaths in women. It is the leading cause of death and disability in women over the age of fifty. More than half of women who experience sudden cardiac death did not have symptoms of heart disease. Women generally develop heart disease ten years later in life than do men. Women who survive heart disease have worse long-term outcomes than do men. Approximately 35 percent of women who have had a heart attack will have a second heart attack within six years. Of women with heart disease, 46 percent will become disabled from heart failure and 11 percent will suffer a stroke.

Obesity, high low-density lipoprotein (LDL) cholesterol, high blood pressure (hypertension), inactivity, smoking, and diabetes are known risk factors for the development of heart disease. The percentage of overweight women in the United States continues to increase. In women, being overweight (greater than 20 percent over ideal body weight) is related to an increased risk of heart attack, heart failure, sudden cardiac death, chest pain, and abnormal heart rhythms.

Identification of heart disease has been based primarily on studies with men. The screening for high cholesterol in healthy females under the age of forty-five is considered controversial. In 2004, recommendations were made for lifestyle changes and the use of medications in women with elevated LDL cholesterol levels in the presence of cardiac risk factors. Studies have since shown that women do not receive adequate treatment for high cholesterol despite these recommendations. Blood pressure control in women has shown a risk reduction comparable to men in the development of heart disease. These findings have led to recommendations for all women to have their blood pressure monitored periodically. In studies, physical activity has shown a small decrease in the risk for heart disease in women. Studies have shown that women who stop smoking will decrease their heart disease risk by 50 to 80 percent within five years compared to those who continue to smoke.

The classic symptoms of crushing chest pain and shortness of breath are based on male experiences of heart attack. Women often experience what is called atypical chest pain. Women often complain of tightness in the chest that goes into their neck, back, shoulders, or throat, or they may not experience any discomfort in the chest. The lack of classical symptoms often causes misdiagnosis or delayed diagnosis, which increases the risk of mortality.

The treatment of heart disease should begin with prevention. Modifiable risk factors, such as being overweight, smoking, and inactivity, account for 90 percent of heart attacks. Low-dose aspirin and vitamin E are of-ten recommended for the prevention of heart attacks; however, research has not shown these to be beneficial for women. Underlying disorders that contribute to heart disease, such as high blood pressure and heart valve disease, must be treated.

Lung cancer. In women, lung cancer is the second leading cause of death and the most common cause of cancer death. The majority of lung cancers are caused by cigarette smoking. Women tend to develop lung cancer at a younger age and with fewer cigarettes smoked than men. Nonsmoking women are more likely to develop lung cancer than are nonsmoking men. Aggressive types of lung cancer that are more difficult to treat are more common in women. The five-year survival rate for lung cancer is less than 15 percent.

Lung cancer may have few symptoms until the disease is advanced. Cough is a common complaint in smokers but often ignored. Coughing up blood is reason for a medical evaluation. Other complaints may include shortness of breath or hoarseness. Late symptoms include weight loss and fatigue.

Routine screening for lung cancer has not been recommended. Chest X rays are often obtained on a regular basis for smokers. Research has not found screening to be an effective method for diagnosis or improvement of outcomes. Computed tomography (CT) scans are used to further evaluate abnormal chest X rays. The diagnosis of lung cancer is made by biopsy or bronchoscopy.

Treatment for lung cancer should be preventive, with abstinence from smoking or smoking cessation. Lung cancer treatment includes surgery, chemotherapy, and/or radiation. Surgery includes the removal of the tumor and lung tissue. An entire lung or sections of lung may be removed. Chemotherapy in lung cancer may extend the survival time by four to twenty-four months, depending on the type of cancer. Radiation is used to decrease discomfort by shrinking the size of the tumor.

Breast cancer. Breast cancer is the most common form of cancer in women. It is the second leading cause of cancer death in women between the ages of thirty-five and fifty-four. The rate of five-year survival has increased to 96 percent, compared to 72 percent in the 1940's. The survival rate has been attributed to earlier diagnosis, as well as expanded options for treatment.

The exact cause of breast cancer is unknown, but some types are sensitive to the female hormone, estrogen. The risk for breast cancer increases with a prolonged number of menstrual cycle years, not having children, or delaying childbirth until after age thirty.

Other risk factors include obesity, oral contraceptives, and hormone therapy.

The suspicion of breast cancer occurs with certain lumps in the breast or an abnormal mammogram. Mammograms are considered less accurate in the detection of breast cancer in women under the age of thirty-five. Prior to age thirty-five, the density of breast tissue makes the mammogram of less value. The diagnosis of breast cancer requires a biopsy either in radiology with a special needle or during a surgical procedure. Early detection is important, with regular mammograms recommended after the age of forty.

Treatment of breast cancer may include surgery, chemotherapy, hormone therapy, and/or radiation. A lumpectomy is the surgical removal of a small tumor with the maximum preservation of breast tissue. A mastectomy is the removal of the tumor, breast tissue, and lymph nodes under the arm. The additional surgical removal of underlying chest muscles is less common than in the past. Chemotherapy is the administration of toxic medications to kill the rapidly growing cancer cells; however, chemotherapy drugs also kill rapidly growing normal cells, which causes the common side effects of hair loss, mouth soreness, and nausea and vomiting. In postmenopausal women who have estrogen-sensitive breast cancer, hormone therapy is used. Radiation is administered to prevent or treat local recurrences of breast cancer. It is also used before surgery in some women with breast cancer.

Stroke. Stroke occurs more frequently in men but causes death more often in women. Stroke occurs in young adults but is most common after the age of sixty-five. A stroke is caused by a sudden disruption of the blood supply in the brain. Strokes may be caused by hemorrhage or a blood clot. A blood clot may occur in the brain or may travel from a remote part of the body (such as the heart) to the brain. Stroke is a leading cause of long-term disability.

Risk factors for stroke that may be controlled are high blood pressure, heart disease, diabetes, cigarette smoking, obesity, and inactivity. The number of cigarettes smoked is related to the level of risk for stroke. Risk factors specific to females include migraine headaches, mitral valve prolapse, lupus, and the use of oral contraceptives.

As with heart disease, the majority of women may experience atypical symptoms of stroke. Men generally experience loss of balance and numbness or loss of function in one side of the body. Women may experience change in their level of alertness, headache, or chest pain. Diagnosis is made by CT scan of the brain or by evaluation of the blood flow in the brain (cerebral angiography). Treatment may include medications and/or surgery, depending on the cause of the stroke.

Like many other diseases, prevention of stroke should be a priority. Individuals should be encouraged to lose weight, stop smoking, and become physically active. Aspirin or other drugs to prevent blood clots have not proven to be effective methods to prevent stroke in healthy individuals.

Osteoporosis. Normal bones are broken down and rebuilt throughout an individual's life. In women, the loss of estrogen during menopause causes increased bone loss. Eight million women in the United States have osteoporosis. Half of the fractures attributable to loss of bone were in women without osteoporosis. Approximately 50 percent of those with osteoporosis-induced hip fractures will not regain their previous capabilities. Risk factors for osteoporosis include inactivity, smoking, excess alcohol usage, early menopause, inadequate dietary calcium, and body weight less than 127 pounds.

Diagnosis is made using a bone mineral density (BMD) scan. BMD scans evaluate certain bones and compare them to "normal" bone based on the age and sex of the individual. This comparison is reported as a standardized score. The scan is recommended for all women over the age of sixty-five, regardless of risk factors.

Preventive treatment includes lifelong physical activities that involve weight-bearing, which improve the strength of bones. The average adult woman in the United States gets only one-third to one-half of the daily recommended requirements of 1,000 to 1,500 milligrams of calcium. Supplemental calcium should be taken with meals. Vitamin D supplementation is recommended for women over the age of sixty. Results from studies have suggested that strict compliance with calcium and vitamin D recommendations is necessary in order to reduce hip fractures. Prescription medications for the treatment of osteoporosis have been shown to reduce the risk of fractures significantly as early as six months after beginning therapy. Hormones, other than estrogen, have been found to reduce the risk of osteoporosis in women with fewer negative effects.

Cervical cancer. Cervical cancer is the most preventable cancer in women. The rates of cervical cancer have decreased in the United States, but it is still the fourth most common type of cancer in females. Cervical cancer usually occurs between the ages of forty and fifty, but rarely before age twenty, with more than four thousand deaths each year. Risk factors for cervical cancer include early age of first vaginal intercourse, multiple sexual partners, multiple pregnancies, previous sexually transmitted infection of human papillomavirus (HPV), and cigarette smoking.

Early detection of cervical cancer is associated with 75 percent to 90 percent cure rates. Diagnosis of cervical cancer is initially made by Pap testing, with a biopsy for confirmation. In 2002, new Pap screening guidelines were released by the American College of Obstetricians and Gynecologists (ACOG) and by the American Cancer Society (ACS). Prior to these guidelines, sexually active females were given annual Pap tests. The newer guidelines recommend that the initial screening occur between the ages of eighteen and twenty-one, or within three years of the first vaginal intercourse. After three or more normal Pap tests, healthy, low-risk women may receive less frequent screenings based on provider recommendation. There may be no symptoms of cervical cancer. Early symptoms may include abnormal bleeding or discharge. Late symptoms may include pelvic pain and weight loss.

Prevention of cervical cancer requires abstinence from intercourse or the consistent use of condoms to prevent the transmission of HPV. In 2006, a vaccine was approved by the Food and Drug Administration (FDA) for the prevention of certain strains of HPV in females aged nine to twenty-six. It is a series of three vaccines given over a six-month period that will likely be recommended at age eleven or twelve when other booster shots are due. The vaccine will prevent approximately 70 percent of HPV infections associated with cervical cancer.

Treatment depends on the extent of the cancer. Early cervical cancer may require treatments in a health care provider's office, which may include freezing or removal of cervical tissue. More aggressive cancer may require surgery (hysterectomy) and/or radiation. Radiation may be implanted into the vagina during surgery or may consist of radiation exposure during outpatient treatment over several weeks.

RESEARCH

In response to the lack of medical research conducted on women, the National Institutes of Health (NIH) established the Office of Research on Women's Health in 1990. The following year, the Women's Health Initiative was launched with the purpose of understanding the main causes of illness, disability, and death in

postmenopausal women between the ages of fifty and seventy-nine. The fifteen-year study included 161,808 women from all races and socioeconomic classes.

Prior to the Women's Health Initiative, long-term hormone therapy was routinely prescribed for postmenopausal women. An estimated six million postmenopausal women in the United States were taking it. These women often had not had menopausal symptoms, such as hot flashes, for years. It was thought that hormone therapy was heart-protective. The Postmenopausal Estrogen/Progestin Interventions (PEPI) Trial was a three-year study that examined the effects of hormone therapy on cardiovascular risk factors. At the end of the study, recommendations were made for hormone therapy as treatment for the prevention of cardiovascular disease in postmenopausal women. A second study, the Heart and Estrogen/Progestin Replacement Study (HERS), was conducted with women with known heart disease. Initial recommendations were that women already on hormone therapy could continue but that women who had heart disease should not begin it in order to prevent further heart problems. After another 2.7 years of follow-up with these women, the study recommended that continued hormone therapy could not be recommended as a result of increased cardiac events.

Several studies were conducted under the Women's Health Initiative. The first study was the Hormone Therapy Trial, which evaluated the effect of hormone therapy on the prevention of heart disease and osteoporosis. Hormone therapy was also evaluated for its potential to increase the risk of breast cancer. The study participants were women who had not had a hysterectomy compared with those who had had a hysterectomy prior to the study. The women who had not had a hysterectomy were given combination hormone therapy of estrogen and progestin. The women who had had a hysterectomy were given estrogen replacement only. In 2002, the study was stopped for the women taking the combination therapy because the risks of the therapy outweighed the possible benefits. The study found that these women had a greater risk of heart attack, blood clots, stroke, and breast cancer. Nevertheless, they did experience less colorectal cancer and fewer osteoporosis-related hip fractures than did the other group. In 2004, the estrogen-only group stopped their medication. The study recommended that hormone therapy should not be used to prevent heart disease in women.

The second study, the Dietary Modification Trial, was a study of 48,835 women aged fifty to seventy-nine who were followed for eight to twelve years. The purpose was to evaluate the effect of diet on heart disease, breast cancer, and colorectal cancer. One group continued their usual eating habits, kept a food diary, and completed health information every six months. These women were given general nutrition guidelines. The second group decreased the fat content of their diet by 20 percent and increased the daily servings of fruits, vegetables, and grains to meet or exceed established recommendations. They attended group meetings led by specialists that focused on nutrition. These participants recorded their food intake throughout the study. A low-fat diet did not provide protection against colorectal cancer or heart disease. The effect of a low-fat diet on the reduction of breast cancer risk was not considered statistically significant, meaning that the results may have occurred by chance rather than from the diet change. A mild decrease in the risk of breast cancer was found only in women who had previously eaten a high-fat diet.

Another study of the Women's Health Initiative, the Calcium/Vitamin D Supplementation Trial, evaluated the effect of calcium and vitamin D supplements on osteoporosis-related fractures and colorectal cancer in 36,282 postmenopausal women. In the study, participants took either 1,000 milligrams of calcium carbonate and 400 international units (IU) of vitamin D or a placebo. If they were already taking calcium supplements prior to the study, then they were allowed to continue them. At the end of the seven-year study, calcium with vitamin D was found to slow the progression of bone density loss and perhaps help prevent hip fractures. The supplements were not found to have a protective effect against colorectal cancer.

The Observational Study was an eight- to twelve-year study that followed 93,676 women. The purpose of the study was to examine the relationships among medical history, risk factors, and health behavior with certain diseases and outcomes. This study found that postmenopausal breast cancer survivors had an increased risk of broken bones compared to postmenopausal women who had never had breast cancer. The study also found that 11.1 percent of women in the study had experienced physical and/or emotional abuse in the year prior to the study. Prior to this study, there had been little information about the incidence of abuse in women over the age of fifty. The study also reported that women with emotional support systems were more likely to participate in mammograms and breast cancer screening than were women who lacked emotional

support. Finally, the study reported a link between depression and the risk for heart disease in postmenopausal women.

The final study in the Women's Health Initiative was conducted with the Centers for Disease Control and Prevention (CDC). It was a five-year study designed to develop community health interventions that would assist women over the age of forty develop healthy behaviors.

PERSPECTIVE AND PROSPECTS

In *Everything You Always Wanted to Know About Sex* (1969), American physician David Reuben wrote that menopause was the loss of womanhood and functionality as females. Historically, medical research has generally been conducted with males. If females were included in the studies, then the results were grouped with those of the males. This clustering of results prevented the identification of sex differences. In 1990, the NIH established the Office of Research on Women's Health in response to the lack of information about women and health. The Women's Health Initiative, a fifteen-year research study, began in 1991.

In 1993, Congress passed legislation requiring that women be included in all research studies funded by the NIH. Prior to this legislation, women were excluded if they were in their potential childbearing years in order to prevent the risk of drug-related birth defects. The following year, Congress also mandated the establishment of the FDA Office of Women's Health. The purpose of this office was to require the inclusion of women in studies. Studies have since demonstrated that women experience increased side effects and often more serious consequences from medications as compared to men. The exact mechanisms of these events are unknown.

In 2001, the Institute of Medicine (IOM) published its acknowledgment of the impact of an individual's sex on disease and treatment. (According to the IOM, the terms "sex" and "gender" are not interchangeable; sex is the biologic classification of male or female based on chromosomal makeup, XX or XY, while gender is the social representation of being male or female.) The IOM reported that available evidence suggests differences at the cellular level in males and females. These differences have been linked to particular disease entities as well as to outcome differences based on sex.

In June, 2006, the first vaccine was approved to prevent four strains of HPV that are associated with 70 percent of cervical cancers. In October, 2006, studies reported further risks associated with postmenopausal hormone therapy. Studies found an increased risk of ovarian cancer in women who used estrogen for ten or more years. The Women's Health Initiative Extension Study has been funded through 2010. The study will continue to follow participants regarding their individual health status through surveys and questionnaires.

—*Amy Webb Bull, D.S.N., A.P.N.*

See also Abortion; Amenorrhea; Amniocentesis; Anorexia nervosa; Assisted reproductive technologies; Bonding; Botox; Breast biopsy; Breast cancer; Breast disorders; Breast-feeding; Breast surgery; Breasts, female; Bulimia; Cancer; Cervical, ovarian, and uterine cancers; Cervical procedures; Cesarean section; Childbirth; Childbirth complications; Chlamydia; Chorionic villus sampling; Chronic fatigue syndrome; Circumcision, female, and genital mutilation; Clinical trials; Colon cancer; Contraception; Cystitis; Domestic violence; Dysmenorrhea; Eating disorders; Ectopic pregnancy; Endometrial biopsy; Endometriosis; Episiotomy; Face lift and blepharoplasty; Fibrocystic breast condition; Gamete intrafallopian transfer (GIFT); Gender reassignment surgery; Genital disorders, female; Gestational diabetes; Gynecology; Heart attack; Heart disease; Hermaphroditism and pseudohermaphroditism; Hip fracture repair; Hip replacement; Hormone therapy; Hormones; Hot flashes; Human papillomavirus (HPV); Hysterectomy; In vitro fertilization; Incontinence; Infertility, female; Kyphosis; Lung cancer; Mammography; Mastectomy and lumpectomy; Mastitis; Menopause; Menorrhagia; Men's health; Menstruation; Miscarriage; Mitral valve prolapse; Multiple births; Nutrition; Obesity; Obesity, childhood; Obstetrics; Osteoporosis; Ovarian cysts; Ovaries; Pap test; Pelvic inflammatory disease (PID); Plastic surgery; Polycystic ovary syndrome; Postpartum depression; Preeclampsia and eclampsia; Pregnancy and gestation; Premature birth; Premenstrual syndrome (PMS); Puberty and adolescence; Rape and sexual assault; Screening; Sexuality; Sexually transmitted diseases (STDs); Sterilization; Stretch marks; Strokes; Systemic lupus erythematosus (SLE); Toxemia; Toxic shock syndrome; Toxoplasmosis; Tubal ligation; Urinary disorders; Uterus; Vitamins and minerals; Weight loss and gain; Weight loss medications; Wrinkles.

FOR FURTHER INFORMATION:

American Heart Association. "Heart Disease and Stroke Statistics: 2010 Update." http://www.americanheart .org/statistics. Provides the most recent statistical evidence from data on the incidence of heart disease and stroke by gender and race.

Dibble, Suzanne L., and Patricia A. Robertson. *Lesbian Health 101: A Clinician's Guide.* San Francisco: UCSF Nursing Press, 2010. The first comprehensive textbook on lesbian health for clinicians and students. Helpful to general readers as well. Also provides insight into women's health in general.

Eastwood, Jo-Ann, and Lynn V. Doering. "Gender Differences in Coronary Artery Disease." *Journal of Cardiovascular Nursing* 20, no. 5 (September/October, 2005): 340-351. Written for nurses caring for individuals with heart disease.

Gupta, Nelly Edmonson. "What You Should Know About the HPV Vaccine." *Clinical Advisor* 9, no. 7 (July, 2006): 46-48. An interview with two physicians about the new HPV vaccine that prevents the major cause of cervical cancer. Written in conversational style that is easy to follow.

Hobson, Katherine. "Hello, His and Her Health Care." *U.S. News and World Report* 140, no. 8 (March 6, 2006): 74-76. A short article about the recognition of gender differences in health issues.

Institute of Medicine. *Exploring the Biological Contributions to Human Health: Does Sex Matter?* http://www.nap.edu/catalog/10028.html. This work is written in an easy-to-understand style with explanations for scientific information.

Leppert, Phyllis C., and Jeffrey F. Peipert, eds. *Primary Care for Women.* 2d ed. Philadelphia: Lippincott Williams & Wilkins, 2004. A textbook written for primary care providers of women.

National Institutes of Health. "Women's Health." http://health.nih.gov/category/womenshealth. This site provides links to other Web sites with information and resources on a variety of issues related to women's health.

Sinclair, Barbara Peterson. "Women and the Health Care System." In *Women's Health: A Primary Care Clinical Guide,* edited by Ellis Quinn Youngkin and Marcia Szmania Davis. 3d ed. Upper Saddle River, N.J.: Pearson/Prentice Hall, 2004. Historical information about women and the American health system.

Women's Health: A Guide to Health Promotion and Disorder Management. Philadelphia: Lippincott Williams & Wilkins, 2005. A textbook written for primary care providers of women.

WORLD HEALTH ORGANIZATION
ORGANIZATION
DEFINITION: A specialized agency of the United Nations that fights illness and disease all over the globe.
KEY TERMS:
ecology: a branch of science concerned with the relationships among organisms and their environments
ecosystem: an ecological community considered together with the nonliving factors of its environment
epidemic: an unarrested spread of something, as of a disease
epidemiology: a science that deals with the incidence, distribution, and control of disease in a population
etiology: the investigation of the causes of any disease
meningitis: inflammation of a membrane that envelops the brain or spine, often caused by bacteria
pandemic: pertaining to a high proportion of a population
vaccine: any substance for preventive inoculation to build immunity

FUNCTIONS AND RESPONSIBILITIES
The World Health Organization (WHO) is a specialized agency of the United Nations. With its headquarters in Geneva, Switzerland, the organization has grown from 26 member countries in 1948 to more than 190 in 2003, improving health conditions on every continent of the earth. It functions under the aegis of the United Nations' Economic and Social Council. The governing body of WHO is the World Health Assembly, which is composed of delegations from all member states. The assembly decides the policies, programs, and budget of the organization. It selects the countries that will place one member each on its twenty-four-member executive board, which oversees the programs and budget for the coming year. These plans are presented for approval by the director general, who, with a staff of two thousand, is responsible for conducting investigations and surveys.

The World Health Organization is divided into six regional subdivisions working in Europe, the Americas, Africa, the middle eastern Mediterranean, southeastern Asia, and the western Pacific. These regional organizations have headquarters in Copenhagen, Denmark; Washington, D.C.; Brazzaville, Congo; Alexandria, Egypt; New Delhi, India; and Manila, the Philippines, respectively.

The regular budget is contributed directly to WHO by its member states. The United Nations also devotes many resources to the Fund for Technical Assistance to Underdeveloped Countries, of which a substantial part is for health work. Other financial sources are individual donations for promoting good health practices and eradicating malaria. Despite these incomes, there is a continual drain on funds because many underdeveloped countries cannot afford to pay for the drugs, vaccines, or technical medical assistance that they receive.

One of WHO's enduring achievements has been to communicate to the world an understanding and acceptance of the idea of a common, basic list of drugs. The model Essential Drug List has been a powerful tool in providing scientific justification for the improvement of health standards and practices through publicity, workshops, and training in the developing world. The first list of essential drugs was published in 1977 and included 205 drugs; the list published in 1999 contained 306 preparations. Drugs are included based on recommendations of expert committees from both developing and developed countries. The committees consist of clinical pharmacologists, health officials, and university professors. The drugs are chosen for efficacy, safety, quality, and stability. By emphasizing generic agents, the list has stimulated international competition among drug suppliers and brought down prices—an important consideration since some countries spend 40 percent of their slim health budgets on drugs.

WHO concerns itself with the needs of those billions of people in the world who are still without regular access to the most basic drugs at the primary health care level. It seeks to establish equitable access to essential drugs for people. The organization has helped more than 90 percent of its member nations to develop a partly or fully developed essential drugs policy. The Essential Drug List is a valuable resource for countries trying to develop their own national lists. Changes have been made in the list for several reasons, including oversight or omission, accumulation of more conclusive evidence of the therapeutic advantages of various drugs, and changes in the perceived role of the list itself.

WHO attacks communicable diseases in every country through prevention, control, and treatment. The cornerstone of prevention and control is education. Public information is of crucial importance in controlling epidemics. Also vital to many populations is information on nutrition, breast-feeding, personal hygiene, cleanliness, and the use of safe water. Stress is placed on the public's ability to play an important role in prevention and early detection. With full and accurate information, symptoms may be correctly interpreted and conditions correctly diagnosed, thus preventing the spread of disease.

Various WHO commissions continue working on projects to improve health standards. Efforts continue for increasing the number of trained medical personnel in many countries. Systems for selecting, procuring, storing, and distributing drugs and supplies more efficiently are continually being refined. WHO is cognizant of a global range of concerns, from promoting a healthy environment to revising guidelines for ethical conduct in research on an international level.

EFFORTS AROUND THE WORLD

The World Health Organization monitors the spread or decline of disease all over the world. An example of how beneficial such knowledge can be when applied internationally is the organization's work on inoculation in Egypt and Brazil. Public information services led to the success. In 1973, a study supported by WHO to test the effectiveness of a newly perfected meningitis vaccine was conducted in Egypt, with 250,000 school-

children participating. After the first year, it was clear that the vaccine was extremely effective.

Then a major meningitis epidemic broke out in Brazil. King Faisal of Saudi Arabia, aware of the successful results in Alexandria, Egypt, donated 4 million U.S. dollars to send the vaccine to Brazil in order to reduce international concern. Immunization against meningitis was later carried out in Sudan, with the population of Khartoum and surrounding areas receiving vaccinations in 1987 when the disease began to break out across the country.

In Saudi Arabia, vaccination against meningitis is particularly important in preventing disease at the time of the annual pilgrimage to the holy city of Mecca. The health authorities ask that all pilgrims be vaccinated against meningitis before they arrive in Saudi Arabia, and, if they have not done so, then they are offered vaccination on arrival. People living in the pilgrimage area—in the cities of Jeddah, Mecca, and Medina—who come into contact with the pilgrims are also vaccinated against meningitis regularly; thus, no cases are expected among them.

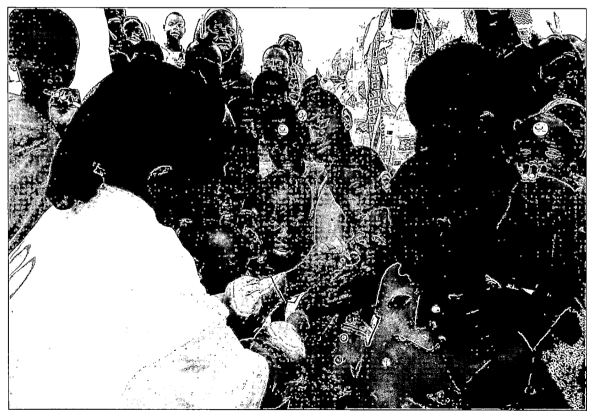

A World Health Organization (WHO) official gives a dose of polio vaccine to Somali children in Somalia in 2000. (AP/Wide World Photos)

The exchange of information has also led to spectacular success in Egypt in the control of diarrheal diseases. Authorities have used a proven method: After recognizing the seriousness of the problem, they have developed a simple preventive message and have used public personalities to deliver it. Egypt has also made effective use of all information channels, employing various methods to give the same message. Egypt's national program to control diarrheal diseases is recognized as one of the best in the world. It has demonstrated the value of using the media for advocating health. The country is no longer concentrating only on curing these diseases but instead is giving equal emphasis to prevention. These practices are also used to educate mothers about nutrition, breast-feeding, personal hygiene, cleanliness, and the use of safe water for drinking, cooking, and bathing.

Vaccinating newborns against the hepatitis B virus, a contagious infection of the liver, is another successful campaign by WHO. Immunizing poor children is an ongoing, worldwide program. Medical experts are also looking ahead at trying to take care of the orphaned children of the victims of acquired immunodeficiency syndrome (AIDS).

Prenatal care and safe childbirth practices are also global concerns of WHO, which contends that there is no need to die in giving birth. Every time a woman in Africa becomes pregnant, her risk of dying as a result is more than one hundred times greater than for a woman in the industrialized world. Conferences are held regularly in order to try to stop this waste of life. Involved in the exchanges and preparations are public health officials, midwives, doctors, and the representatives of nongovernmental agencies.

It is estimated that south of the Sahara, 150,000 women die every year as the result of becoming pregnant. Epidemiological studies have brought together twenty-two French-speaking governments in Africa to act to reduce maternal mortality. Apart from such specific causes as excessive blood clots, difficult confinements, infections, and other complications, factors in maternal mortality include anemia, malnutrition, malaria, or simply overwork—many African women toil twelve to fourteen hours a day.

WHO contends that the heavy price that African women pay for maternity is not inevitable. There are inexpensive methods that can put a stop to such tragedy. Some of the most important are family planning, prenatal and postnatal care, supervision of the confinement, and recourse to well-equipped and well-staffed primary health care centers. To achieve these goals, WHO coordinates the mobilization of resources with the help of both national commitment and international cooperation.

Heavy publicity and effort attend the multifaceted WHO campaign to cope with the dramatic rise in the global AIDS toll. Statistics show that human immunodeficiency virus (HIV) infection has spread rapidly among women and children in sub-Saharan Africa and in Asia. In 2001, an estimated 19 million women worldwide lived with AIDS; 15 million of that number resided in sub-Saharan Africa. Millions of HIV-infected babies are being born to these women. AIDS is the leading cause of death of women aged twenty to forty in some central African cities. AIDS has also eroded many of the gains developing countries made in decreasing infant mortality rates during the 1980's and 1990's. Globally, by the end of 2001, there were approximately 14 million children orphaned after one or both parents died of AIDS.

Experts working in the field of AIDS have noted that one of the greatest obstacles to prevention is the general lack of basic health care in the developing world, as well as among the poor in urban cities. A lack of resources and medicine compounds the seriousness of AIDS in countries such as Zaire and Tanzania. At times, there is not the money to buy medicine, even if the supply of medicine existed. Experts also note that women's status and their typical lack of control in their own sexuality have dire consequences for the AIDS epidemic in developing countries.

Without a cure for AIDS in sight, common treatments are the drugs zidovudine (formerly known as azidothymidine, or AZT) and standard sulfa drugs for *Pneumocystis carinii*, a type of pneumonia seen in immunocompromised patients. Unfortunately, access to these medications is severely limited for people with AIDS in Africa and Asia. Even elsewhere in the world, zidovudine is an expensive option. WHO continues to promote better distribution and use of sulfa drugs in the developing world. It is also financing drug development studies for promising agents in these countries. In 2003, WHO announced its ambitious "3 by 5" program—getting three million people on critically important antiretroviral (ARV) therapy by the end of 2005. Only 300,000 people globally had access to ARV, but experts estimated that five to six million people infected with HIV in the developing world needed it. The initiative fell short of its goal, but the number of people receiving ARV tripled.

The fight against communicable diseases continues to be fought and won on various fronts. Oral rehydration tablets to cope with diarrhea among children, for example, have proven effective, reducing infant mortality in many countries by 50 percent. Early in the 1950's, Professor Samir Najjar of Lebanon produced a formula for oral rehydration that differed only slightly from the present oral rehydration formula. Then in 1962, a hospital training course in oral rehydration was organized in Alexandria, Egypt, another pioneering effort. Eventually, oral rehydration salts became the standard worldwide treatment of diarrhea in the 1970's.

PERSPECTIVE AND PROSPECTS

The World Health Organization's efforts to fight diseases of all kinds and to improve health are so impressive that international successes in all fields seem almost inevitable. Yet the world's health problems also have a larger cause, one that is more difficult to solve. It is now increasingly evident that many diseases stem from the degradation to the environment caused by humans. The harmful effects of industrial development on the global ecosystem are now better known. Some of these ecological wounds are depletion of the ozone layer, acid rain, changes in climate, deforestation, and chemical pollution.

In Europe, thirty-two member nations of WHO have agreed to a single health policy, including environmental issues. It contains measurable objectives to which each nation has agreed to be publicly accountable on an annual basis. The program is called Health for All, and it is based on four sweeping policy goals. The goals have thirty-eight targets supported by more than one hundred measurable indicators, all of which are aimed at achieving a symbolic health standard and improving the environment of Europe.

Communicable diseases are a continual problem. Susceptible populations have to be monitored for their appearance, and the latest medical information and practices need to be made accessible. Like environmental problems, the spread of diseases must be prevented, controlled, treated, and, wherever possible, eradicated completely.

The polio vaccine has been so effective that the illness has been eradicated in the United States, but in tropical areas the disease remains. The Sabin oral vaccine confers long-lasting immunity and is easy to administer. It is now routinely used to immunize children and adults against polio throughout the world. WHO has exploited this advantage and undertaken a program

to eradicate polio globally. To date, this program has been highly successful, eliminating polio in all but 7 countries worldwide, down from more than 125 countries when the Global Polio Eradication Initiative was launched in 1988. The seven countries with remaining indigenous poliovirus are Nigeria, India, Pakistan, Egypt, Afghanistan, Niger, and Somalia.

The World Health Organization plans to use the same type of intensive immunization program for polio in other areas of the world, including areas where the incidence is high: Africa, China, and India. Millions more children have also been immunized against diphtheria, pertussis (whooping cough), measles, and tetanus. Using advanced biotechnology, scientists are working on keeping vaccines cool in transit to recipients in the tropics.

Still other endeavors by WHO are "no tobacco" days, vaccination programs against hepatitis B virus, laws to facilitate the distribution of drugs and medical supplies, the reduction of prices charged by manufacturers, the provision of more X-ray machines, the elimination of iron deficiency among the destitute, and advanced research on amino acids. For example, researchers predict that within thirty years the number of tobacco-related deaths will rise to 10 million per year. This will make tobacco the single biggest cause of death worldwide. About 500 million people will die because of tobacco-related disease, based on current long-term trends. Smoking can reduce the lives of persons aged thirty-five to sixty-nine by fifteen to twenty years, the NCI Cancer Weekly reported in 1990, and each year, 3 million die from the habit. Furthermore, children's health is at risk from adult smoking. If women stopped smoking, it is estimated that fetal and infant deaths would drop by 10 percent.

In the area of nutrition, WHO is helping to publicize the fact that requirements for each amino acid may be higher than professionally recommended. Amino acids are the molecular units that combine to make proteins. Adult humans need eight amino acids in the diet. Other amino acids required for protein synthesis are manufactured in the body and do not need to be consumed in food. If new, higher levels are accepted, as WHO recommends, better protein nutrition could be achieved and food aid programs could be improved.

—Walter Appleton

See also Acquired immunodeficiency syndrome (AIDS); Centers for Disease Control and Prevention (CDC); Childbirth; Childbirth complications; Childhood infectious diseases; Diarrhea and dysentery;

Environmental diseases; Environmental health; Epidemiology; Ethics; Hepatitis; Immunization and vaccination; Malnutrition; Meningitis; National Institutes of Health (NIH); Nutrition; Poliomyelitis; Preventive medicine; Tropical medicine; Tuberculosis.

FOR FURTHER INFORMATION:

Beigbeder, Yves. *The World Health Organization.* Boston: M. Nijhoff, 1998. This work, written by a former World Health Organization official, presents a broad outline of the activities and evolution of WHO. Research was based on the official documentation of WHO, both open and restricted.

Burci, Gian Luca, and Claude-Henri Vignes. *World Health Organization.* Frederick, Md.: Aspen, 2004. Discusses the founding, structure, relations, and functions of WHO.

Grahame, Deborah A. *World Health Organization.* Milwaukee: Gareth Stevens, 2003. A book for young adults that traces the history and importance of WHO.

Lee, Kelley. *Historical Dictionary of the World Health Organization.* Lanham, Md.: Rowman & Littlefield, 1998. An excellent reference that brings together a broad range of data on WHO and covers key offices, programs, events, and individuals. Also provides a brief history, a chronology of key events, a comprehensive bibliography of primary and secondary sources, and extensive appendixes of basic documents and organizational structures.

WORMS

DISEASE/DISORDER

ANATOMY OR SYSTEM AFFECTED: Abdomen, gastrointestinal system, intestines, respiratory system

SPECIALTIES AND RELATED FIELDS: Gastroenterology, internal medicine, pediatrics, public health

DEFINITION: Invertebrates, usually roundworms or flatworms, that act as human parasites.

In common usage, the term "worm" includes many other wormlike organisms, a few with medical importance: Some fly larvae (or maggots) can cause human infections, some caterpillars are covered with irritating hairs, and leeches have had a place in medical history (of misuse to "bleed" victims and, more recently, of help with swelling or the reattachment of limbs). To control many parasitic worms, a society must be affluent enough to provide water treatment, plumbing, and sewage treatment; fuel to cook fish and meat thoroughly; and regular medical care for the general population.

Flatworms. Flatworms are primitive organisms in the phylum Platyhelminthes. The class Turbellaria are mostly free-living, planaria-like worms, although some are in intermediate stages of becoming parasitic. Tapeworms in the class Cestoda and flukes in the class Trematoda are the most serious parasitic worms, particularly in tropical and subtropical regions. Flukes that are medically important to humans are in the order Digenea. Schistosomes are flukes that live in the blood system; other adult flukes live in bile ducts, in the lungs, or along the digestive tract. A few are known to infect the body cavity, urogenital system, or eyes of victims. Control requires understanding not only the effect that the adults have on a human host but also the complex life cycle that flukes have developed to ensure a continuous chain of offspring in successive hosts.

Blood flukes affect more than 200 million people and are second only to malaria as a world health problem. The human blood fluke, *Schistosoma mansoni*, has both male and female individuals and is long and hairlike. This blood fluke feeds on blood and clings to the walls of small veins in the large intestine. The strategy of all parasitic worms is to produce vast numbers of eggs. Some of these breach the intestinal wall and pass out with human wastes into the environment. Modern plumbing and sewage treatment can stop the fluke life cycle at this point. In poorer tropical countries, however, the fluke eggs are soon washed into ponds, ditches, or rice paddies, where they immediately hatch. The larvae, coated with cilia, swim about in search of a snail. Boring into the flesh of the snail, the larva sheds its cilia and develops into a sporocyst. This sporocyst absorbs nutrients and asexually subdivides; eventually, as many as 200,000 tadpolelike cercarias will develop from the one larva. Erupting through the surface of the snail, the cercarias swarm near the water surface. People working in rice paddies or wading or swimming in streams are infected when the cercaria bores through the skin to reach a blood vessel and complete its life cycle.

The Chinese liver fluke, *Clonorchis sinensis*, represents a life history involving two intermediate hosts. In this more representative fluke, the adults are hermaphroditic—possessing both male and female organs. Large numbers of eggs are released from the host's liver into the bile duct, where they pass through the digestive tract and are shed in the feces. When the eggs are washed into the bottoms of ponds, streams, and pad-

ARTHROPOD-BORNE WORM (HELMINTHIC) DISEASES

Contracted Through Ingesting Arthropod Host

Disease	Parasite	Arthropod Host
Broad tapeworm	Dibothriocephalus latus	Crustaceans eaten by fish that in turn are eaten by humans
Dog tapeworm	Dipylidium caninum	Dog flea Pulex irritans and lice
Dracunculosus or guinea worm	Dracunculus medinensis	Copepod crustaceans: Cyclops species
Oriental lung fluke	Paragonimus westermani	Snails via crabs and crayfish
Rodent tapeworm	Hymenolepis diminuta	Fleas including Xenopsylla cheopis; also roaches, moth and beetle larvae
Spiny-headed worm	Macracanthorhynchus hirudinaceus	Beetle larvae

Contracted from Blood-Sucking Flies

Disease	Parasite	Principal Vectors
Acanthocheilonemasis	Acanthocheilonema perstans	Biting midges: Culicoides austeni and C. grahami
Bancroft's filariasis	Wuchereria bancrofti	Mosquitoes: Culex pipiens quinquefasciatus and other Culex, Aedes, Anopheles, and Mansonia species
Brug's filariasis	Brugia malayi,	Mosquitoes: Mansonia, Anopheles, Aedes, and Armigeres species
Dog heartworm	Dirofilaria immitis	Mosquitoes: Culex pipiens, Aedes aegypti, and others
Loiasis or African eyeworm	Loa loa	Mango flies: Chrysops dimidiatus and C. silaceus
Onchocerciasis	Onchocerca volvulus	Black flies: Simulium damnosum, S. neavei, S. ochraceum, and others
Ozzard's filariasis	Mansonella ozzardi	Biting midge Culicoides furens

dies, many are eaten by snails. This releases the larva, which burrows into the snail's tissues and becomes a sporocyst. The sporocyst subdivides into redia, an active feeding stage that eventually develops many cercariae. The cercariae erupt from the snail and swim through the water to infect native fish. The cercariae encyst in the meat of the fish and wait until the fish is eaten by a human or other mammal. If the fish is not thoroughly cooked, the cyst coating will be digested in the intestine and the young fluke will emerge. From there, it will eventually move to the smaller bile passages of the liver. Using its suckers to anchor, the fluke feeds on

blood, causing both anemia and liver blockage. Chronic infection over twenty to thirty years results in a significant incidence of biliary cancer.

Tapeworms are unique parasitic flatworms, with adults specialized for living in the digestive tract of vertebrates. By relying on the host's digestive system, tapeworms have lost all evidence of an alimentary canal in both larval and adult stages. A tapeworm possesses a head with hooks and suckers by which it hangs on the gut lining. Bags called proglottids are constantly budded off; younger ones nearer the neck show developing testes and ovaries, while the most distant proglottids are large sacs of maturing eggs. One common large tapeworm of humans is the beef tapeworm. When eggs are shed with human feces, some eggs may find their way to vegetation and be eaten by cattle. The tapeworm egg coating is digested, and the larval tapeworm migrates across the intestinal wall and flows with the blood to the muscle. There it grows into a tapeworm bladder, which can be seen as measly beef by meat inspectors. When such meat is not thoroughly cooked, digestion releases the enclosed tapeworm, which begins to grow in the intestine of the new host. Mature beef tapeworms can grow to 10 meters in length and release thousands of egg-laden proglottids.

Roundworms. Most roundworms, of the phylum Nematoda, are free-living. They are widely distributed across the land, streams, and oceans. The large *Ascaris lumbricoides* is a roundworm parasite that invades the human intestine. A mature female worm can produce 200,000 eggs a day, which are expelled with the host's feces. These minute eggs are easily washed through the soil and ingested by a new host. Hatching in the small intestine, the baby worms burrow into the body and are soon in the bloodstream or lymph. Fine capillaries of the lungs eventually filter them out; the worms bore across into the bronchial tubes, where they are coughed up and then swallowed, returning the roundworms to the intestine to mature. Damage occurs when the worms migrate through the body or when infestations are very large and cause blockage, especially in small children. Among the more serious diseases caused by roundworms are elephantiasis and trichinosis.

—*John Richard Schrock, Ph.D.*

See also Elephantiasis; Insect-borne diseases; Parasitic diseases; Pinworms; Roundworms; Schistosomiasis; Tapeworms; Trichinosis; Tropical medicine; Zoonoses.

FOR FURTHER INFORMATION:

Desowitz, Robert S. *New Guinea Tapeworms and Jewish Grandmothers: Tales of Parasites and People.* New York: W. W. Norton, 1987. This collection of essays by a distinguished professor of tropical medicine focuses on parasitic diseases. These profiles of schistosomes, tapeworms, and filarial worms are readable true stories.

Goddard, Jerome. *Physician's Guide to Arthropods of Medical Importance.* 4th ed. Boca Raton, Fla.: CRC Press, 2003. Nontechnical description of a wide variety of arthropods and conditions related to their stings or bites. Topics include allergy to venoms and the signs and symptoms of arthropod-borne diseases.

Roberts, Larry S., and John Janovy, Jr., eds. *Gerald D. Schmidt and Larry S. Roberts' Foundations of Parasitology.* 7th ed. Boston: McGraw-Hill Higher Education, 2005. A graduate-level textbook covering all aspects of parasitology. The book is well illustrated, but sensitive readers may be disturbed by many of the case study photographs.

Salyers, Abigail A., and Dixie D. Whitt. *Bacterial Pathogenesis: A Molecular Approach.* 2d ed. Washington, D.C.: ASM Press, 2002. Examines the molecular mechanism involved in bacterial-host interactions that can produce infectious disease. Introductory chapters discuss host-parasite relationships.

Zeibig, Elizabeth A. *Clinical Parasitology: A Practical Approach.* Philadelphia: W. B. Saunders, 1997. Presents all the guidelines needed to perform, read, and interpret parasitology tests. Each chapter contains thorough descriptions of parasitic forms, drawings with structures labeled, typical characteristics, and look-alike parasites.

WOUNDS
DISEASE/DISORDER
ANATOMY OR SYSTEM AFFECTED: All
SPECIALTIES AND RELATED FIELDS: Critical care, emergency medicine, family medicine, internal medicine
DEFINITION: Disruptions or breaks in the continuity of any body tissue.

Wounds might arise because of violence, accident, or intentional procedure, such as surgery. They may be classified according to the instrument responsible, such as a knife, bullet, or shrapnel, or according to the way in which they occurred, such as a burn or a crushing wound.

Surgeons describe wounds according to their general appearance. A wound may be described as incised, when a sharp cutting instrument is involved; lacerated, when damage is due to a jagged instrument; contused, when the edges are cut; avulsed, when part of the tissue is torn apart; punctured, when the outer opening is rather small; penetrating; and nonpenetrating, when the external tissue remains intact. Fractures are also classified in several terms, such as spiral, impacted, and comminuted. The depth of the tissue injury classifies burns as first, second, or third degree.

Generally, wounds may be classified as open or

closed. Closed wounds involve no external hemorrhage, and their degree of seriousness is related to the force of the blow and its direction, the age of the victim, and other physiological and anatomical factors. Normally, internal hemorrhage stops abruptly, with the blood and fluid absorbed within a few days. More bleeding occurs when larger internal vessels are damaged, with subsequent collection of the blood in the tissues forming a hematoma that may take several weeks to be absorbed. The impact on a body part may result in damage to a part that is not directly involved at the time of impact. Thus, a fall on an outstretched hand may injure not only the flesh and bones of the hand itself but also the scaphoid part of the wrist, or even the elbow or shoulder. During a car accident, a stationary body part may be heavily affected by the transmission of impact from a relatively mobile part; when occurring in the neck, this type of injury is commonly known as whiplash. First aid procedures for fractures, sprains, and strains include ice packs, crutches, elevation, and splinting.

Infections resulting from wounds. Open wounds take place when the skin and/or mucous membranes are broken, thus allowing the invasion of hazardous foreign material, such as bacteria or dirt, into the tissues. This invasion may lead to infection, which is particularly serious when the disruption of the skin is considerable. Generally, injuries from sharp instruments (such as a needle, knife, or bullet) cause little tissue damage, except to the part that they penetrate. The great danger lies in the injury of a vital organ and from the foreign objects that are on the surface of the instrument. Injuries from irregular objects (such as bomb fragments or a jagged knife) create much more damage, which leads to longer recuperation periods. Skin is elastic and well supplied with blood, which means that superficial cuts heal easily. The subcutaneous fatty tissues and muscles are not as rich in blood supply, and their damage is more serious and long-lasting, especially because it is easier for infection to occur. Fragmentation of bone in

an open wound is particularly troublesome, since the fragments cannot survive without blood and will act as foreign substances, thus creating a serious infection. Injuries to joints, nerves, or major capillaries (such as arteries) will complicate the state of the open wound.

The contamination of the wound may start immediately after the causative incident. Nonbacterial contamination is more serious when organic substances are involved. In bacterial contamination, the most serious results are seen with virulent bacteria that are nourished by dead tissue and organic foreign material, sometimes leading to gas gangrene. Such infection generally spreads unchecked and can be stopped only by surgical removal or amputation, in order to avoid death. Other infections are caused by streptococcal and staphylococcal bacteria and are characterized by the local production of pus. Finally, tetanus is another type of wound infection. It starts with serious muscle spasms a few days after the injury and, left untreated, often leads to death.

The healing process. When an open wound occurs, the tissues are cut and the edges of the wound separate, pulled apart by the elasticity of the skin. Blood flowing from the wound fills the resulting cavity, fibrin is produced, and the blood clots, creating a scab. During the first twenty-four hours after the injury, the scab shrinks, drawing the edges of the skin together. Special cells called histiocytes and macrophages digest the debris in the wound, such as blood seepage, dead cells, and other foreign bodies. Connective tissue cells called fibroblasts grow inward from the margins of the wound to close the cavity. The fibroblasts produce a protein called collagen that provides strength to the new skin.

The red-colored capillaries slowly disappear and are replaced by white collagen. Thus, upon removal of the scab a layer of reddish granulation tissue appears, which covers the subcutaneous tissue. A thin, gray membrane extends outward from the skin edges and covers the whole surface. Contraction brings the epithelial sheets from the two sides together, and eventually the skin around the wound is reproduced. Wounds that cross normal skin creases become depressed below the level of the surrounding skin. The resulting scars, which are very low in capillaries, do not become tanned with sunlight exposure, and they produce neither hair nor sweat, which is indicative of skin that is less than fully functional. They are much whiter than the surrounding skin.

Treatment. Medical treatment of wounds requires first the control of bleeding by bandaging. Dead tissue is removed surgically through amputation. Sutured wounds heal faster because stitches bring the skin edges together. Foreign material in a wound may be absorbed by the tissues, which is exactly what happens when catgut is used to close the wounded tissue. Disinfection is particularly helpful in the healing process. In the case of small cuts, methods of disinfection include the external use of oxidizing agents (such as hydrogen peroxide) and of nonpolar ointments (such as petroleum jelly) to combat the invading polar bacteria. Body factors are also crucial in the overall healing; these include age, the concurrent presence of diseases, and nutrition that includes adequate quantities of protein and antioxidants, such as vitamin C. Hospitals take elaborate precautions to prevent infections through sterilization, good air filtration, the use of ultraviolet light to kill bacteria in the operating room, and the administration of antibiotics. The skin in the area of any surgery is treated with antiseptics and is carefully protected with sterilized cloth.

—*Soraya Ghayourmanesh, Ph.D.*

See also Amputation; Bites and stings; Bleeding; Bruises; Burns and scalds; Concussion; First aid; Fracture and dislocation; Fracture repair; Frostbite; Gangrene; Grafts and grafting; Healing; Infection; Laceration repair; Lesions; Necrotizing fasciitis; Plastic surgery; Shock; Skin; Tetanus; Toxic shock syndrome; Transfusion.

FOR FURTHER INFORMATION:

American Academy of Orthopaedic Surgeons. *Emergency Care and Transportation of the Sick and Injured.* Edited by Benjamin Gulli, Les Chatelain, and Chris Stratford. 9th ed. Sudbury, Mass.: Jones and Bartlett, 2005. Includes new and expanded coverage of patient assessment, anatomy and physiology, stroke and seizure, trauma injuries, and special chapters on pediatrics and geriatrics.

Handal, Kathleen A. *The American Red Cross First Aid and Safety Handbook.* Boston: Little, Brown, 1992. A comprehensive, fully illustrated guide outlining basic first aid and emergency care steps to be taken until medical assistance can be obtained. Updated materials can also be obtained directly from local Red Cross Association chapters listed in telephone books.

Krohmer, Jon R., ed. *American College of Emergency Physicians First Aid Manual.* 2d ed. New York: DK, 2004. An excellent reference guide illustrated with photographs and written in a clear, step-by-step for-

mat. Covers many first aid methods, from resuscitation of conscious and unconscious choking victims, to how to deal with bleeding, shock, spinal injuries, poisoning, seizures, fractures, and bandages.

Subbarao, Italo, et al., eds. *American Medical Association Handbook of First Aid and Emergency Care.* Rev. ed. New York: Random House Reference, 2009. Covering urgent emergency situations as well as the common injuries and ailments that occur in every family, this AMA guide takes the reader step by step through basic first aid techniques.

Thygerson, Alton L. *First Aid and Emergency Care Workbook.* Boston: Jones and Bartlett, 1987. Concise information packed into a workbook format, produced in cooperation with the National Safety Council. Charts, drawings, photographs, and tables outline common emergency care, covering a wide range of topics for the general public.

Youngson, R. M. *First Aid.* New York: HarperCollins, 2003. Gives clear, step-by-step instructions for the handling of accidents or illness of all types and degrees of severity.

WRINKLES

DISEASE/DISORDER

ANATOMY OR SYSTEM AFFECTED: Skin

SPECIALTIES AND RELATED FIELDS: Dermatology, plastic surgery

DEFINITION: Lines in the skin caused by structural changes over time.

CAUSES AND SYMPTOMS

All human body fibers are formed by specialized cells in the tissues and can be classified as inelastic or elastic. Inelastic fibers are rigid and provide support to the surrounding tissue, while elastic fibers are more mal-

---

INFORMATION ON WRINKLES

CAUSES: Aging process, prolonged exposure to wind and ultraviolet light, smoking

SYMPTOMS: Lines in skin (particularly on face or hands), decreased skin elasticity

DURATION: Chronic

TREATMENTS: Collagen injections; topical application of vitamin C, collagen amino acids, or copper peptides; topical application of growth factors and hormones; chemical peels; plastic surgery

leable. With the passage of time, inelastic fibers tend to become even tougher because of structural changes that occur in collagen, the major protein found in skin, bones, and ligaments. The dermis, the inner layer of the skin, contains large amounts of collagen, which is responsible for the skin's mechanical characteristics, such as strength and texture. The skin cells that make and reproduce damaged collagen are called fibroblasts.

As a person ages, collagen tends to form crosslinks between different parts of the molecule or between similar molecules that are near each other, thus creating a rigidity that leads to skin sagging and wrinkling. Moreover, the recoiling ability of elastic fibers appears to be reduced, a condition that is often enhanced by calcification. Skin wrinkling is much more pronounced with prolonged exposure to wind and ultraviolet light. The effect appears to be cumulative along with collagen degeneration and epidermis thinning, as seen with people of outdoor professions. Other studies suggest that heavy cigarette smoking contributes to the risk of wrinkling.

Treatment and Therapy

Application of collagen-containing creams does not seem to create a desired change because the applied collagen molecules are too large to penetrate the dermis. Such applications only temporarily cover wrinkles. Injecting collagen under the wrinkles in a way that pushes the groove up, causing it to become smooth, has some positive cosmetic effect but also serious drawbacks. The main problem comes from the animal source of the collagen, which may lead to serious allergic reactions by the immune system and may, in rare cases, trigger a long-lasting autoimmune disease. Moreover, the smoothing effect of the injections appears to be brief because of the inability of the animal collagen to integrate itself into the skin's collagen mesh. Better results are observed when biotechnology-synthesized collagen is used or when the patient's own fibroblasts are removed, grown in a laboratory, and reinjected into the body. The careful administration of vitamin C, collagen amino acids, or very small quantities of copper peptides appears to stimulate the skin to produce more collagen. In addition, the topical application of growth factors and hormones that enhance the collagen-forming process of cells seems to give favorable results.

In the News: Dermal Fillers Restylane and Juvéderm

Antiaging and cosmetic dermatology have been gaining in popularity for years as people try to look younger and improve their appearance. Dermal fillers are one of the most recent options in this field.

In December, 2003, the Food and Drug Administration (FDA) approved the first of six non-animal-derived hyaluronic acid dermal fillers for the treatment of wrinkles. These products, of which Restylane and Juvéderm have become the most popular, are injected into the mid- to deep dermis of the skin to fill in wrinkles and make the skin appear more smooth. Hyaluronic acid is one of the components of collagen, the substance that gives skin its strength and texture. Products containing it have almost completely replaced animal-derived collagen fillers for a variety of reasons: Hyaluronic acid fillers do not require skin allergy testing before use, the effects last for several months longer than collagen, and they are more pliable products that lead to a more natural look. After four to six months, they are absorbed into the body.

In addition to treatment of deep wrinkles, dermal fillers have also been used in lip enhancement. They have a very real advantage over products such as Botox, in that they do not paralyze the facial muscles. A more natural facial expression and facial movement can therefore be expected with dermal fillers.

Some controversy exists over which product leads to better results. Juvéderm is available in three formulations and Restylane in one. The products behave similarly but vary slightly in concentration and cross-linking of the polysaccharide. This leads to variations in consistency. Many dermatologists and plastic surgeons believe that the stiffer formulations such as Restylane and Juvéderm Ultra Plus are best suited for areas that need added bulk and substance, such as the nasolabial folds. Juvéderm and Juvéderm Ultra are softer products and are often used in areas such as the lips to give a more natural feel.

—*Karen Nagel, R.Ph., Ph.D.*

By the early twenty-first century, two treatments were gaining widespread attention as new "fixes" for wrinkles: Botox and Artefill. Botox is a laboratory-refined strain of botulinum toxin, the cause for botulism and a highly poisonous substance, that is given in very small doses. It is injected into the facial muscles that cause wrinkling and works by paralyzing them. The effect lasts for approximately three months, and side effects can include numbness and swelling. The Food and Drug Administration (FDA) approved it for cosmetic use in 2002. Artefill works by combining collagen with tiny plastic beads of polymethyl methacylate (PMMA), which is injected into wrinkled areas. PMMA spheres, about the thickness of a human hair, settle in wrinkles as the collagen gradually absorbs into the body. The spheres then stimulate the body's own collagen to encapsulate them. The effects are expected to be more permanent than those of Botox; researchers are hoping that the injection will last for several years. Patients have reported some problems with lumps on the face following the procedure, and critics note that no studies of the treatment's long-term effects have taken place.

Chemical peels have been used to correct facial wrinkling in face lift or eyelid surgeries. A mixture of chemicals is applied to the skin, leading to extreme swelling and consequent peeling of the old skin, thus providing a fresh skin in two weeks. Carbon dioxide lasers were first developed in 1964, but experiments that combined them with computer technology did not begin until the 1990's. This resurfacing technique, which affects an area of skin no more than one hair in thickness for no more than one-thousandth of a second, works in a way similar to chemical peel. It is considered best for patients of fair to medium complexion who have good healing qualities and who have not used Accutane in the previous year.

—*Soraya Ghayourmanesh, Ph.D.*

See also Aging; Botox; Collagen; Dermatology; Face lift and blepharoplasty; Plastic surgery; Skin; Skin disorders.

FOR FURTHER INFORMATION:

Freinkel, Ruth K., and David T. Woodley, eds. *Biology of the Skin.* New York: Parthenon, 2001.

Lewis, Wendy. *The Beauty Battle: The Insider's Guide to Wrinkle Rescue and Cosmetic Perfection from Head to Toe.* Berkeley, Calif.: Laurel Glen Books, 2003.

Turkington, Carol, and Jeffrey S. Dover. *The Encyclopedia of Skin and Skin Disorders.* 3d ed. New York: Facts On File, 2007.

X RAYS. *See* IMAGING AND RADIOLOGY.

XENOTRANSPLANTATION
PROCEDURE
ANATOMY OR SYSTEM AFFECTED: All

SPECIALTIES AND RELATED FIELDS: Biotechnology, ethics, general surgery, immunology

DEFINITION: The transfer of cells, tissues, or organs from nonhuman animal donors to human recipients for therapeutic purposes.

KEY TERMS:

gene: a piece of deoxyribonucleic acid (DNA), or sometimes ribonucleic acid (RNA), that directs a specific activity within a cell, such as the production of a protein

genetic engineering: the transfer of genes, often from one species to another

rejection: the destruction of transplanted organs by the immune system

INDICATIONS AND PROCEDURES

The transplantation of organs from human donors to human recipients has been established practice in medicine since the first successful kidney transplant was performed in 1954. Its applications have been limited, however, for two major reasons. First, the demand for human-donated organs always exceeds the supply. Second, the human body naturally rejects transplants. When the immune system recognizes compounds on the surfaces of cells from any source that is "not self," a chain reaction begins. Antibodies attack foreign proteins and mark them for destruction by white blood cells. Enzymes attack the walls of blood vessels in a transplanted organ, destroying it within hours. To prevent rejection, transplant recipients must take immunosuppressive drugs for months or years. Blocking their immune response, however, makes transplant patients susceptible to infections, some of which can be deadly.

Xenotransplantation—the transfer of cells, tissues, or organs from nonhuman animal donors to human recipients for therapeutic purposes—might solve both of these problems. A large supply of organs can, in theory, be farmed in animals such as pigs. Also, theoretically, organs can be tailor-made to prevent rejection. Genetic engineering techniques should be able to replace animal proteins and sugars on the surfaces of cells with human ones, thus creating an organ that the recipient's immune system is tricked into accepting as "self."

This genetic engineering is accomplished by trans-ferring genes from humans to animals specially bred and farmed to serve as organ donors. To achieve this, a fertilized egg is removed from the uterus of a female donor animal. Next, human protein-coding genes are inserted into the nucleus of the fertilized egg. Finally, the egg is returned to the animal's uterus and allowed to develop normally. If the human genetic material is preserved and activated, then the cells of the animal that develops from the egg will manufacture human proteins on the surfaces of its cells.

USES AND COMPLICATIONS

One concern about xenotransplantation is that new diseases might be introduced into humans from other animals. All animals carry endogenous viruses that are part of their genetic makeup. Endogenous viruses are harmless in their natural hosts, but they can prove deadly when they cross from one species to another. For example, the Hong Kong flu virus lay harmlessly in waterbirds for many years. It then struck chickens and caused massive deaths on poultry farms, and now it infects and sometimes kills people. How the virus migrated to humans remains unknown. Also, diseases can be minor in some animals but major in humans. The herpesvirus B is one example. It gives monkeys mild cold sores but causes fatal encephalitis in people. The concern is that a virus imported into the human population through xenotransplantation might subsequently spread through other means, such as blood, air, water, or food.

Issues of morality, ethics, and religion also arise. Although the genetic makeup of other primates most closely matches that of humans, many people believe that using apes and monkeys as organ donors would be morally unacceptable. One answer to such objections is to use animals that are routinely raised and slaughtered for food. Pigs are easy to breed and care for, and they produce large litters. Their size and weight are similar to humans. Few people object to killing pigs. Much xenotransplantation research involves the development of pigs as potential organ donors. If pig cells can be induced to display human proteins on their surfaces, then the human body will, in theory, accept organs donated from them.

Animals used as transplant donors could not come from ordinary farms because the possibility of transferring infections would be too great. The animals would need to be raised in germ-free medical facilities. Animal rights advocates condemn organ farms as cruel. Despite such objections, public opinion supports further research on xenotransplantation. In a 1998 survey sponsored by the National Kidney Foundation, nearly two-thirds of respondents judged xenotransplantation an acceptable alternative to human donor transplants.

PERSPECTIVE AND PROSPECTS

Xenotransplantation is not a new idea. In 1906, with no knowledge of the immune system, French surgeon Mathieu Jaboulay transplanted a kidney from a pig and a liver from a goat to human patients, both of whom died. In 1964, Thomas Starzl at the University of Pittsburgh transplanted baboon kidneys into two humans. Both patients died from infections accompanied by kidney failure. That same year, a chimpanzee-to-human transplant fared a little better. The patient lived for nine months before the kidney failed.

In 1984, a child the press called "Baby Fae" was born prematurely with a severely malformed heart. She could not live long without a transplant. No human heart small enough was available, so surgeons at Loma Linda University in California gave Baby Fae the heart of a baboon. The operation went well, but Fae died of organ rejection and infection after the surgery.

In 1992, two liver transplants from baboons were attempted. The livers functioned well, but the patients died from infections. That same year, two women received livers from pigs. The transplants were not meant to be permanent but were intended as "bridges" until human donors could be found. In both women, the livers functioned well, but one woman died before a human organ could be located.

In 1995, British scientists succeeded in transplanting pig hearts into monkeys. Half the monkeys survived for forty days, but long-term survival was not achieved, and attempts to transplant whole organs declined after that. Instead, researchers turned to cell transplants. Since 1995, brain cells from pigs have been used with some success in the experimental treatment of people with Parkinson's disease. In 2002, researchers in Virginia announced that they had successfully bred pigs lacking a specific sugar molecule on their cell surfaces known to trigger the rejection response in humans. Xenotransplantation advocates hope that this and similar developments will spur further progress in the field.

—*Faith Hickman Brynie, Ph.D.*

See also Animal rights vs. research; Cloning; Ethics; Genetic engineering; Grafts and grafting; Heart transplantation; Immune system; Immunology; Kidney transplantation; Liver transplantation; Systems and organs; Transplantation; Zoonoses.

FOR FURTHER INFORMATION:

Brynie, Faith Hickman. *101 Questions About Your Immune System You Felt Defenseless to Answer . . . Until Now.* Brookfield, Conn.: Twenty-first Century Books, 2000.

Cooper, David K. C., and Robert P. Lanza. *Xeno: The Promise of Transplanting Animal Organs into Humans.* New York: Oxford University Press, 2003.

Munson, Ronald. *Raising the Dead: Organ Transplants, Ethics, and Society.* New York: Oxford University Press, 2004.

YEAST INFECTIONS. *See* CANDIDIASIS.

YELLOW FEVER
DISEASE/DISORDER
ANATOMY OR SYSTEM AFFECTED: Blood, circulatory system, liver

SPECIALTIES AND RELATED FIELDS: Environmental health, epidemiology, public health, virology

DEFINITION: An acute tropical and subtropical disease spread by infected mosquitoes from human to human or from infected monkeys to humans.

KEY TERMS:

endemic: referring to a disease that has a reservoir in a particular area and that can be expected to occur at some time and level of intensity

epidemic: an incidence of a disease well in excess of the constant rate expected in an area where it is endemic

flaviviruses: a family of ribonucleic acid (RNA) viruses that are transmitted by an arthropod vector; examples include yellow fever, dengue, and St. Louis and Japanese tick-borne encephalitis

hemorrhage: excessive or heavy and uncontrollable bleeding from blood vessels

jaundice: a yellowish skin discoloration symptomatic of yellow fever and other diseases that affect the production and processing of bile

zoonosis: a disease that can be transmitted by animals such as vertebrates to humans; sylvan yellow fever is transmitted from vertebrate reservoirs such as monkeys to humans via mosquitoes

CAUSES AND SYMPTOMS

Yellow fever is a viral disease of humans spread by infected mosquitoes. The infectious agent is a flavivirus. Yellow fever is primarily a disease of tropical and pantropical areas of South America and sub-Saharan Africa. The absence of yellow fever from Asia is curious but may be explained by the lack of suitable reservoirs. Two types of yellow fever are recognized, sylvan yellow fever and urban yellow fever.

Both types are highly communicable, but neither is directly transmitted via personal contact between humans. A human contracts the disease through the bite of an infected mosquito that, in turn, has taken a blood meal from an infected monkey or other human. The viral incubation period within the mosquito is nine to twelve days. The virus then appears in the saliva and can be transmitted during the mosquito's next blood meal. Thereafter, the mosquito carries the virus throughout its life.

Sylvan yellow fever is also known as jungle yellow fever. Forest monkeys are its primary reservoir, but marmosets and marsupials may also harbor the disease. Sylvan yellow fever is spread from monkey to monkey by the bite of infected *Sabethes* or *Haemagogus* mosquitoes, which breed in water-filled tree holes.

People who visit or work in rain-forest environs, such as miners, engineers, wildlife biologists, and foresters, are at risk of contracting the disease. Sylvan yellow fever is rare or nonexistent outside tropical rain forests, but cases are reported every year in areas where it is endemic.

Urban yellow fever is spread by the *Aedes aegypti* mosquito, which is the main reservoir of the disease, along with humans. *Aedes* commonly lives and breeds in trash dumps and waste places around human habitations. Urban yellow fever often results in thousands of cases and high fatality rates.

In humans, the first symptoms of yellow fever typically appear from three to six days following the bite of an infected mosquito. Symptoms vary widely; the mildest cases may pass unnoticed, but in more severe cases the patient shows a number of flulike symptoms, such as muscle aches, backaches, headache, high fever, chills, nausea, and vomiting. Liver damage may occur as early as the fourth or fifth day of the illness, leading to progressive and extensive jaundice. In the most severe cases, periods of nausea, vomiting, renal failure, and extensive bleeding (hemorrhage) may prove fatal. The fatality rate may range from as low as 5 percent in indigenous populations to 50 percent or more during epidemics. Higher fatality rates are typically seen in nonindigenous people.

Clinical diagnosis of yellow fever is aided by isolation of the virus in mice, by microscopic examination

---

INFORMATION ON YELLOW FEVER

CAUSES: Viral infection transmitted by mosquitoes

SYMPTOMS: Vary widely; may include muscle aches, backaches, headache, high fever, chills, nausea, vomiting, liver damage leading to jaundice, kidney failure

DURATION: Several weeks, sometimes fatal

TREATMENTS: Alleviation of symptoms through oxygen support, medications for fever and pain, vitamin K supplements, replacement fluids, dialysis for kidney failure

of liver tissue for necrotic lesions that characterize this disease, by detection of the yellow fever viral antigen in blood or liver tissue fluid of the infected patient, or by detection of the viral genome in liver tissue. Diagnosis can also be determined serologically through the detection of specific antibodies.

TREATMENT AND THERAPY

There is no specific antiviral drug for yellow fever, so treatment goals include providing symptom relief, such as oxygen support, medications to reduce fever and pain, and the administration of vitamin K and replacement fluids. Dialysis may be required for patients suffering from kidney failure. Complete recovery may take several weeks, after which the individual has a lifelong immunity to yellow fever.

PERSPECTIVE AND PROSPECTS

Yellow fever has long been a dreaded tropical and subtropical disease of humans. Throughout the centuries of exploration, yellow fever epidemics occurred with alarming regularity, and high fatality rates were seen among nonindigenous visitors and settlers in regions where the disease is endemic. The presence of yellow fever on a ship was indicated by flying the fever flag or yellow jack.

Despite modern medical advances, yellow fever remains a problem in many areas. Small numbers of cases of sylvan yellow fever occur every year in certain areas of Amazonia and northern South American countries, including Peru and Bolivia. In central Africa, the yellow fever belt extends from Ethiopia westward through Senegal, Sudan, and Ghana. Both occasional cases and epidemics occur irregularly. Between 1986 and 1988, for example, thirty thousand cases of yellow fever were reported in Nigeria, and ten thousand people died.

Walter Reed was the first to describe the epidemiology of yellow fever and to recognize the importance of the mosquito vector in its spread. His research elucidated control and eradication measures that provide containment during epidemics. It was largely through his insights that yellow fever was eliminated from urban areas and was one of the main reasons that the Panama Canal could be completed by the United States after the failure of the French effort led by Ferdinand de Lesseps, the architect of the Suez Canal.

The traditional and still most effective method of preventing urban yellow fever is the eradication of the *Aedes aegypti* mosquito vector. Control measures involve a combination of insecticide spraying and the cleanup or removal of potential breeding sites. The prevention of yellow fever can also be achieved through the vaccination of all people within the endemic regions. A single vaccination with an attenuated strain of virus grown in chick embryos has been shown to be effective for thirty or more years, but revaccination is recommended every ten years.

The elimination of sylvan yellow fever is probably impossible because of the difficulty of eradicating jungle populations of *Sabethes* and *Haemagogus* mosquitoes. Prevention must therefore be achieved through defensive measures for people who work in or visit jungle areas, including immunization and the use of protective clothing, netting, and mosquito repellents.

—*Dwight G. Smith, Ph.D.*

See also Bites and stings; Epidemiology; Insectborne diseases; Jaundice; Tropical medicine; Viral infections; Zoonoses.

FOR FURTHER INFORMATION:

Delaporte, François. *The History of Yellow Fever: An Essay on the Birth of Tropical Medicine*. Translated by Arthur Goldhammer. Cambridge, Mass.: MIT Press, 1991. Delaporte stresses the impact of yellow fever and its treatment via alternate strategies in Cuba and North America.

Heymann, David L., ed. *Control of Communicable Diseases Manual*. 19th ed. Washington, D.C.: American Public Health Association, 2008. This pocket-sized handbook on communicable diseases presents a nice summary of the causes, impact, and control of yellow fever.

Kettle, D. S., ed. *Medical and Veterinary Entomology*. 2d ed. Wallingford, England: CAB International, 1995. Provides succinct summaries of yellow fever and other human diseases.

Murphy, Jim. *An American Plague: The True and Terrifying Story of the Yellow Fever Epidemic of 1793*. New York: Clarion Books, 2003. Aimed at the high school reader, this slim book describes the medical and emotional devastation wrought by yellow fever in postrevolutionary America.

Wills, Christopher. *Yellow Fever, Black Goddess: The Coevolution of People and Plagues*. Reading, Mass.: Addison-Wesley, 1996. Wills offers a highly readable description of the impact of yellow fever and other diseases on human civilization.

Yoga

Treatment

Anatomy or system affected: Muscles, nervous system, psychic-emotional system

Specialties and related fields: Alternative medicine, preventive medicine

Definition: An ancient Indian system of physical exercises, breath control, and meditation aimed at attaining bodily and mental control and well-being.

Introduction

The word "yoga" comes from the Sanskrit word *Yuj*, meaning to "yoke," "join," or "unite." The word implies joining or integrating all aspects of the body with mind to achieve a healthy and balanced life. The true purpose of the ancient practices of yoga is to bring a proper balance between the physical and mental aspects of a person and to awaken the subtle energies of the body. Yoga cultivates muscular strength, endurance, and flexibility and enhances the practitioner's mental acuity. Meditative breathing calms a person's nerves and sharpens a person's focus. With regular yoga practice, individuals are known to gain physical health, mental relaxation, and inner tranquillity.

Yoga has been practiced in India, in one form or another, for more than four thousand years. More than two thousand years ago, the Indian scholar Patanjali codified the various yoga practices into a written collection called the *Yoga Sutras*. According to Patanjali, there are three critical components of yoga: physical postures (*asanas*), breath control (*pranayama*), and meditation. The main purpose of *asanas* and *pranayam* is to cleanse the body, unlock energy paths, and raise the level of consciousness. Yoga styles have come to include a strong component of meditation to enhance the union of mind, body, and soul. Patanjali showed how, through the practice of yoga, one can gain mastery over mind and emotion. Advanced yoga practitioners are known to have incredible control over several autonomic functions such as respiration, heart rate, and blood flow. Many of the bodily functions previously thought to be involuntary can be controlled in a relaxed state achieved through the regular practice of yoga.

Yoga *asanas* offer a simple yet profound technique for promoting muscle flexibility and deep relaxation. Practicing a variety of *asanas*, in combination with *pranayam*, is believed to clear the nervous system, causing energy to flow without obstruction and ensuring its even distribution through the body during *pranayam*. Advanced practitioners of yoga claim to experience a feeling of a pure state of joy while practicing the various yoga *asanas*. Yoga *asanas* are designed to switch constantly from one posture to another. Holding the most intense *asanas* builds strength and endurance, while flexing postures are known to provide muscles with a greater range of motion in the hip and shoulder joints.

There are many forms and schools of yoga. The form most commonly practiced in Western countries is hatha yoga. It places special emphasis on physical postures, which are integrated with breath control and meditation. Hatha yoga thus emphasizes a balance of mind, body, and spirit.

Health Benefits

Research, mostly done in India, suggests a wide variety of positive health effects from the daily practice of

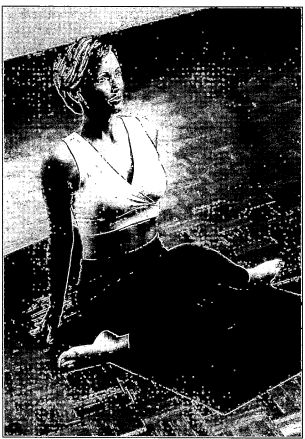

The movements and positions of yoga have been recognized within medicine for their promotion of flexibility and strength. (© Bruce Shippee/Dreamstime.com)

yoga, including, but not limited to, pain reduction in arthritis and carpal tunnel syndrome, reduction of coronary artery disease, and relief from asthma and other respiratory ailments. Situated in Bangalore, India, the Swami Vivekananda Yoga Anusandhana Samsthana (SVYASA) University, treats people with such ailments as asthma, arthritis, heart disease, high blood pressure, psychiatric ailments, and eating disorders. The center uses an integrated approach of yoga therapies that includes *asanas*, chanting, *kriya* (yoga cleansing techniques), meditation, *pranayam*, and lectures on yoga philosophy. The system has been shown to benefit people with asthma, mental retardation, rheumatoid arthritis, and type 1 diabetes mellitus. It is believed to improve visual perception, manual dexterity, and spatial memory.

With support from other organizations, SVYASA has been engaged in a vast variety of research, including the use of yoga to treat obsessive-compulsive disorder; the effects of yoga on people with multiple sclerosis; and the use of yoga for assessing alertness, ability to focus, flexibility, balance, quality of life, and fatigue in healthy elderly people. *Pranayam* has been shown to lower blood pressure in people with hypertension, to alleviate discomfort from gastritis, and to reduce stress and anxiety.

One difficulty with the work in India, however, has been a lack of rigor in research design and protocol. For example, the yoga practices are traditionally combined with chanting, discourse, and other activities, and it is difficult to determine the effects of such extra variables when comparing the results of one study with another.

PERSPECTIVE AND PROSPECTS

With growing interest in alternative therapies, several individuals and institutions have recently initiated extensive studies on the effects of yoga. For example, researchers at Ball State University found that fifteen weeks of yoga training brought a 10 percent improvement in lung capacity. Yoga has been found to help fight cardiovascular disease when used in conjunction with other lifestyle changes, such as a low-fat diet. The National Institutes of Health (NIH) is supporting research on yoga, including its use for treating insomnia and chronic lower back pain.

In a study at the University of Iowa, some patients with chronic fatigue syndrome were shown to benefit from yoga. Yoga prevailed among numerous conventional and alternative therapies as an effective fatigue fighter. At the end of the two-year study, yoga was the only therapy linked to a statistically significant positive outcome by linear regression analysis.

Marian Garfinkel, a yoga teacher turned researcher, has demonstrated that practicing certain yoga postures can relieve the symptoms of carpal tunnel syndrome, the common ailment resulting from repetitive hand activities such as typing. Patients practicing prescribed yoga postures showed significant improvement in grip strength and suffered less pain. There was also improvement on a nerve test used to measure the severity of carpal tunnel syndrome. Studies are in progress to observe the effect of yoga on osteoarthritis of the knee and on repetitive strain injuries.

Because each patient is unique, with different abilities and weaknesses, a yoga approach should be tailored to specific problems as well as specific potentials. It is also important to look at the studies in which yoga did not prove effective and to determine which variables led to these failures.

—*Tulsi B. Saral, Ph.D.*

See also Alternative medicine; Carpal tunnel syndrome; Chronic fatigue syndrome; Hypertension; Meditation; Stress; Stress reduction.

FOR FURTHER INFORMATION:

Birkel, Dee Ann. *Hatha Yoga: Developing the Body, Mind, and Inner Self.* 3d ed. Dubuque, Iowa: Eddie Bowers, 2000.

Garfinkel, M. S., et al. "Yoga-Based Intervention for Carpal Tunnel Syndrome." *Journal of the American Medical Association* 280 (1998): 1601-1603.

Iyengar, B. K. S. *Light on Yoga.* Rev. ed. New York: HarperCollins, 2001.

Mishra, Rammurti S. *Fundamentals of Yoga: A Handbook of Theory, Practice, and Application.* Reprint. New York: Julian Press, 1987.

ZOONOSES

DISEASE/DISORDER

ANATOMY OR SYSTEM AFFECTED: All

SPECIALTIES AND RELATED FIELDS: Bacteriology, epidemiology, public health, virology

DEFINITION: Diseases that can be transferred to humans from their primary animal hosts, including farm animals, laboratory research animals, tropical insects and animals, and common house pets, and including poliomyelitis, malaria, rabies, and toxoplasmosis.

KEY TERMS:

inoculate: to introduce immunologically active material in order to treat or prevent a disease

malaise: a feeling of lack of health or debility, often indicating or accompanying the onset of illness

mycobacterium: any of a genus of nonmotile aerobic bacteria that are difficult to stain and include numerous saprophytes and the organisms causing tuberculosis and leprosy

organism: a complex structure of interdependent and subordinate elements whose relations and properties are largely determined by their function as a whole

pathogen: a specific causative agent (as a bacterium or virus) of disease

rabies: an acute virus disease of the nervous system of warm-blooded animals, usually transmitted through the bite of a rabid animal

toxoplasma: any of a genus of parasitic microorganisms that are typically serious pathogens of vertebrates

toxoplasmosis: the infection of humans, other mammals, or birds with disease caused by toxoplasmas that invade the tissues and may seriously damage the central nervous system, especially that of an infant

tuberculosis: a highly variable, communicable disease of humans and some other vertebrates caused by the tubercle bacillus; characterized by toxic symptoms of allergic manifestations that in humans primarily affect the lungs

vaccinate: to administer a vaccine, usually by injection

vaccine: a preparation of killed microorganisms or living, virulent organisms that is administered to produce or increase immunity to a particular disease

CAUSES AND SYMPTOMS

There are many types of contact between humans and animals. Some produce pleasure, such as stroking a kitten's fur; some have strictly utilitarian considerations, such as farming or meat processing; and some are to help animals themselves, such as the veterinary sciences. Unfortunately, some also result in the transmission of infectious diseases to humans, which are called zoonoses. The most common symptoms of zoonoses are headache, fevers, general malaise, diarrhea or bloody stool, and sometimes skin rashes, eruptions, or inflammation (in the event of a bite or sting).

Approximately 150 types of zoonoses can be transmitted either directly or indirectly to human beings. Direct exposure results from coming in contact with an infected animal or its excrement, blood, or saliva. Indirect exposure results from being bitten by an insect carrying an infected animal's blood. In either case, a disease may or may not develop.

Although many diseases transmissible to humans from animals now can be cured, it is important to avoid the methods of transmittal, especially the handling of infected animals. Humans must wash their hands after handling animals, especially after cleaning cages or litter boxes. Small children should be discouraged from kissing and cuddling pets. In rural or mountainous areas, humans should be discouraged from handling wild animals. In some communities, especially rural areas, keeping wild animals such as wolves or raccoons as pets is popular. Unfortunately, wild animals can carry many serious diseases that can be passed to humans, notably rabies.

Incubation periods for zoonoses can range from a few days to several years. If it is suspected that a human has contracted a disease from an animal, it is important to seek medical attention. Most zoonoses can be diagnosed and treated. In most cases, treatment will clear up the disease with no lasting aftereffects. If the infected person waits too long for treatment, however, therapy may take longer, and problems may persist. In rare cases, surgery is necessary, and in even rarer cases, death can occur.

INFORMATION ON ZOONOSES

CAUSES: Diseases transferred to humans from animal hosts

SYMPTOMS: Headache; fever; general malaise; diarrhea or bloody stool; rashes, eruptions, or inflammation (from bite or sting)

DURATION: Acute to chronic

TREATMENTS: Depend on cause; may include supportive therapy, antibiotics, antiviral drugs, antifungal agents

Zoonoses vary greatly in their sources and symptoms. Among the most important of these diseases are anthrax, brucellosis, cat-scratch fever, encephalitis, Lyme disease, malaria, cattle tuberculosis, plague, rabies, ringworm, Rocky Mountain spotted fever, roundworm, salmonella poisoning, sporotrichosis, and toxoplasmosis.

Anthrax is an infectious disease of warm-blooded animals such as cattle or sheep, caused by the bacterium *Bacillus anthracis*. The disease can be transmitted to humans by the handling of infected products, such as the animals' hair. The disease is characterized by lesions in the lungs and by external ulcerating nodules.

Brucellosis is characterized by repeated fevers accompanied by weakness and joint pain. It is contracted from the amniotic and fetal membranes of pregnant and newborn animals. More typical in farm animals, it can also be present in dogs that are bred. While it is not fatal, it does cause severe flulike symptoms. It can be difficult to treat and cure completely.

Not as serious as toxoplasmosis, which can also be transmitted through a bite or scratch from a cat, cat-scratch fever is a bacterial infection that can result when a human is bitten, nipped, or scratched by a feline. Symptoms include a blistery inflammation at the site of the infection, fever, malaise, and sometimes swelling of the lymph nodes. Such symptoms appear two to thirty days after the skin is broken and generally last about a month. The infection will generally clear up on its own, but, after washing the affected area with soap and water, a consultation with a physician is recommended. Approximately twenty thousand people are infected annually with cat-scratch fever, mostly children. It is important for parents to instruct children not to play roughly with cats.

The bite of mosquitoes infected with encephalitis can cause this disease in humans. The illness is an infection of the lining of the brain; symptoms include a high fever, general malaise, and usually a very strong headache. Another disease transmitted by the bite of mosquitoes is malaria, which is caused by sporozoan parasites. Symptoms include intermittent chills and fever. Malaria may persist for years, and once the disease has been contracted, those affected are discouraged from donating blood, to avoid passing it on to others.

Lyme disease is an insect-related disease that is usually caused by the bite of a deerfly or tick. The disease was named for an area of Connecticut where it was first discovered. A doctor treating patients with flulike symptoms and skin inflammations realized that patients complaining of the symptoms had all been walking in woody areas and had been in contact with brush, weeds, and flowers where the tiny ticks and deerflies could have been harbored. The insects preyed on deer and other animals in the area, then probably jumped off or were brushed off the host animal into the grass. (Bitten animals may become infected with the disease as well.) Cases of Lyme disease have been found in almost every state, with the highest percentage being reported in the Midwest and on the East Coast. Although humans can develop the disease from a tick or deerfly bite, there is no evidence yet that a bite or scratch from an infected animal can transmit the disease.

The bacterium *Borrelia burgdorferi* is responsible for Lyme disease. Its symptoms include inflammation, skin lesions and redness, joint inflammation, fever, fatigue, general malaise, and headaches or a stiff neck. These symptoms may last for weeks after the bite. Nerve-related disorders and heart ailments may follow the preliminary symptoms. Early treatment is a fourteen-day regimen of antibiotics, which can then be followed by treatment with antimicrobial agents until symptoms cease. Later stages of Lyme disease, such as arthritis and heart disorders, can be treated with penicillin-type antibiotics. Nevertheless, joint and muscle pain may persist for several weeks.

Rocky Mountain spotted fever is another disease caused by tick bites. The disease is found in all areas of the United States, not only in the Rocky Mountains. Symptoms include headache, fever, and skin rash. Early diagnosis and antibiotic treatment are very important in order to prevent more serious complications.

An infection that often strikes herded animals such as cows, deer, or elk is a subspecies of tuberculosis caused by *Mycobacterium bovis*. Individuals who come in contact with such animals, such as veterinarians, farmers, and slaughterhouse workers, are most susceptible to this disease because they breathe in the tiny droplets of bacteria. In addition to lung infections, other diseases are reported to be associated with the *M. bovis* bacterium. Treatment for infected individuals is with antibiotics.

Plague is an infectious disease transmitted by the bite of a rodent flea infected with the bacillus *Yersinia pestis*. Two forms of plague affected millions of humans in Asia and Europe during the Middle Ages and continue to occur today, although not in epidemic form. Bubonic plague results in the formation of buboes, or swellings of the lymph glands. The Black Death was caused by the same bacterium and was probably pneumonic plague; this form is transmissible between people and is characterized by black patches appearing on the skin of its victims. Both types cause fevers and heavy coughing. Before the discovery of antibiotics, most victims died from this very contagious disease.

Rabies is an acute viral disease of the nervous system of warm-blooded animals, usually transmitted through the bite of the infected animal. Rabies can be found in a small number of animal species across the world. There are two main types: urban rabies, carried mainly by domesticated animals such as dogs; and sylvatic rabies, carried by wild animals such as bats. Symptoms of the disease include fever, nausea, vomiting, shortness of breath, abdominal pain, and a cough. If left untreated, the muscles become paralyzed and breathing and heartbeats stop, causing death. There are three methods of treating the disease: vaccination of people at risk of exposure before any exposure has occurred; animal control and immunization, especially preexposure immunization; and postinfection treatment, usually a series of expensive, painful shots.

Generally, the incubation period for rabies in humans is three weeks to three months. There have been cases, however, in which the victim was bitten by a rabid animal a year before the onset of the disease. Two documented cases showed that the victims were bitten by infected dogs while traveling in Asia six or seven years prior to the onset of the illness. Worldwide, approximately eighteen thousand people per year are treated for possible rabies infection. While domesticated animals, such as dogs and cats, can be treated against the development of rabies, it is difficult to inoculate wild animals, mostly because vaccines are not licensed for use on them. One method to attempt to control rabies in wild animals is the use of edible bait laced with vaccine.

Ringworm is a skin disease caused by a fungus, not a worm. The fungus usually occurs on exposed skin, especially the scalp, and looks inflamed and scaly. Diagnosis in animals is made by exposing the hair or fur to an ultraviolet lamp (the infected area will appear greenish in color). In humans, antifungal soaps or drugs will cure the disease.

Salmonella bacteria in food cause gastroenteritis, inflammation of the mucous membrane of the stomach and intestine. Symptoms of the disease are severe, bloody diarrhea and sometimes dehydration. The illness is very contagious and often spread rapidly in day-care or home settings. Although salmonella bacteria are usually found in uncooked meat, they can also be present in pet turtles raised on farms. Thus parents buying pet turtles for their children may unknowingly bring the disease into their homes. Many of these strains of salmonella are quite resistant to commonly used antibiotics, thus making treatment difficult and allowing the disease to spread. When this information came to the attention of the United States government, the shipping of live turtles from their farms was banned and various laws were enacted to restrict the interstate and international trade of the reptiles. Shipment of turtle eggs is still allowed, however, and as many as 20 percent of these eggs may carry the bacteria.

Most spider bites result in redness and itchiness or soreness at the site. They usually heal by themselves in a few days. The bites of some venomous spiders, however, such as the brown recluse, or violin, spider (Loxosceles reclusa), can cause serious complications in humans. Symptoms of the bite of a brown recluse spider include an eruption that turns black in the center, surrounded with a characteristic bull's-eye pattern of red, white, and blue circles. The sore is accompanied by flulike symptoms, weight loss, and extreme fatigue. If treatment is not sought, the flesh at the site becomes gangrenous, and surgery is necessary.

Almost all newborn puppies carry roundworms, and because children love to cuddle puppies, the children often pick up the worms without knowing it. Symptoms in humans are a cough, fever, headache, and poor appetite. Treatment for both humans and puppies is with anthelminthic (worm-destroying) drugs. It is important that all puppies be seen by a veterinarian when very young.

Sporotrichosis is a fungal infection transmitted by cats. The fungus is found as mold on decaying vegetation, soil, and timber, usually found along southern U.S. waterways and in places with similar climates. Left untreated, the fungus can spread throughout the human body. The organism enters the body through a cut or abrasion in the skin or through inhalation of the fungus. Therefore, it is a good idea to wash one's hands after handling cats.

Protozoan toxoplasmas are found in undercooked meat, on unwashed raw fruits, and in the feces of cats, and cause a condition called toxoplasmosis. The toxoplasmas may enter the human body through the skin or by respiration. Extreme care should be taken, especially by pregnant women, when disposing of used cat litter. In pregnant women, the disease invades fetal tissues, causing damage to the baby's central nervous system. The antibiotic spiramycin is effective in combating the disease's effects. Toxoplasmosis also poses a threat to AIDS patients as a major cause of encephalitis (inflammation of the brain or brain's lining). Experiments have been conducted with the drug clindamycin in treating toxoplasmic encephalitis in AIDS or HIV-positive patients; however, such side effects as diarrhea and rashes have resulted.

Treatment and Therapy

Zoonoses are transmitted either directly from an animal (by handling it or coming in contact with its feces or saliva) or indirectly (by being bitten or stung by an insect that is carrying tainted blood from an infected animal). Symptoms of infection in humans usually consist of headache, fevers, general malaise, nausea, diarrhea, and skin eruptions or inflammation. If any of these symptoms is present after receiving an animal bite or scratch, or even after handling an animal, a visit to medical personnel is necessary.

Prevention plays the largest part in avoiding transmission of these diseases. People should wash their hands after touching or being in contact with animals, even if they do not appear to be sick or infected. Parents should instruct children to be careful when playing with pets. Humans should not care for wild animals as house pets. Hunters and hikers should take care when traveling through wooded areas so as not to pick up ticks or other insects; wearing clothing that covers the body, with socks rolled over pant legs and gloves fitting over long sleeves, can help in these instances. Finally, pregnant women should avoid contact with animal feces (someone else, for example, should change the cat's litterbox) in order to avoid contracting toxoplasmosis.

Perspective and Prospects

Zoonoses have been in existence ever since humans and other animals have been together. There is probably no way to completely eliminate such diseases from the human world. Since zoonoses can be transmitted in any environment in which animals and humans live, work, or play together, such eradication would be impossible. It is, therefore, extremely important for people to take precautions when handling animals or animal by-products (such as meat).

Although there are approximately 150 known zoonoses, new diseases that are transmissible between humans and animals are being identified. Most zoonoses

are relatively rare and can be treated once a proper diagnosis is made by medical personnel. With common sense and precautionary measures, the contraction of such diseases can be controlled.

—*Carol A. Holloway*

See also Anthrax; Babesiosis; Bacterial infections; Bites and stings; Chagas' disease; Chronic wasting disease (CWD); Creutzfeldt-Jakob disease (CJD); Ebola virus; Ehrlichiosis; Emerging infectious diseases; Encephalitis; Food poisoning; Fungal infections; Influenza; Insect-borne diseases; Leishmaniasis; Lice, mites, and ticks; Lyme disease; Malaria; Monkeypox; Parasitic diseases; Pinworms; Plague; Poliomyelitis; Prion diseases; Protozoan diseases; Rabies; Rocky Mountain spotted fever; Roundworms; Salmonella infection; Schistosomiasis; Severe acute respiratory syndrome (SARS); Tapeworms; Toxoplasmosis; Tuberculosis; Typhus; Viral infections; West Nile virus; Worms; Xenotransplantation; Yellow fever.

For Further Information:

Biddle, Wayne. *A Field Guide to Germs.* 2d ed. New York: Anchor Books, 2002. This comprehensive book is easily accessible to the nonspecialist and includes a discussion of nearly every virus, bacterium, and fungus known to cause human and nonhuman animal disease.

Folkenberg, Judy. "Pet Ownership: Risky Business?" *FDA Consumer* 24 (April, 1990): 28-30. This three-page article focuses on a list of the most common zoonoses transmitted from domesticated animals, such as house pets. The targeted audience consists of adults who are contemplating becoming pet owners.

Hugh-Jones, Martin E., William T. Hubbert, and Harry V. Hagstad. *Zoonoses: Recognition, Control, and Prevention.* Malden, Mass.: Blackwell, 2008. Preceding synopses of parasitic, fungal, and viral agents are sections on the principles and history of zoonosis recognition, new disease agents, and advances in control and prevention.

"Human Rabies: Strain Identification Reveals Lengthy Incubation." *The Lancet* 337, no. 8745 (April 6, 1991): 822. In this clinical article, virus-typing techniques are presented to show the many strains of rabies. Case histories of victims who did not demonstrate any symptoms for several years after infection are cited.

Krauss, Hartmut, et al. *Zoonoses: Infectious Diseases Transmissible from Animals to Humans.* 3d ed. Washington, D.C.: ASM Press, 2003. Explores the myriad infections introduced by human-animal contact.

Palmer, S. R., Lord Soulsby, and D. I. H. Simpson, eds. *Zoonoses: Biology, Clinical Practice, and Public Health Control*. New York: Oxford University Press, 2003. This volume covers the history, scientific basis for control, microbiology of the causative agent, pathogenesis, clinical features, symptoms and signs, diagnosis, treatment, and prognosis for each disease.

"Salmonella and Pet Turtles." *Child Health Newsletter* 8 (April, 1991): 21. This article highlights the dangers lurking in pet turtles and their eggs, with a warning to adults seeking to buy such pets for their children. A list of symptoms is presented, along with contagion issues.

Schlossberg, David, ed. *Infections of Leisure*. 4th ed. Washington, D.C.: ASM Press, 2009. This volume brings together a collection of essays, each addressing a different setting for the transmission of disease. Chapter titles include "At the Shore," "Freshwater: From Lakes to Hot Tubs," "The Camper's Uninvited Guests," and "Perils of the Garden."

Swabe, Joanna. *Animals, Disease, and Human Society: Human-Animal Relations and the Rise of Veterinary Medicine*. New York: Routledge, 1999. This book takes a historical perspective on zoonoses, discussing such things as the intensification of livestock production and the domestication of animals and how these trends have effected disease transmission.

Woodruff, Bradley A., Thomas R. Eng, and Jeffrey L. Jones. "Human Exposure to Rabies from Pet Wild Raccoons in South Carolina and West Virginia, 1987 Through 1988." *American Journal of Public Health* 81, no. 10 (October, 1991): 1328. This clinical article focuses on the risk of transmission of rabies to humans as a result of attempts to domesticate wild animals.

"Zoonoses: Unseen Dangers." *Current Health* 17 (March 2, 1991): 11-13. This three-page article is written for the general reader and highlights the basic manners in which zoonoses can be transmitted— through family pets, hunting, hiking, and wildlife. Prevention tips are given in an inset box.

GLOSSARY

Abandonment: The failure of a health care provider to continue emergency medical treatment.

Abdomen: The part of the body between the thorax (chest) and the pelvis.

Abortion: Termination of a pregnancy before the stage of viability (about twenty weeks); may occur from natural causes (spontaneous abortion) or may be induced by medical intervention.

Abscess: A pocket of infection or inflammation.

Absorption: A process transporting digested food from the small intestine into blood vessels, blood, and body cells.

Abutment: A tooth protected by a crown that serves to anchor one end of a bridge.

Acetylcholine: A chemical released by motor neuron terminals that causes muscle contraction.

Acid: A water-soluble compound with a pH between 0.0 and 6.9 that contains hydrogen and can donate hydrogen ions (protons) to other substances.

Acid-base balance: The ratio of carbonic acid to base bicarbonate, with a pH between 7.35 and 7.45.

Acid-base chemistry: The interaction between acids and bases in the cells of the body, the proper functioning of which is crucial in digestive metabolism, respiration, and the buffering capacity of body fluids.

Acid reflux disease: A chronic digestive disorder in which the lower esophageal sphincter (LES), designed to keep digestive juices in the stomach, relaxes and permits gastric acid to rise into the esophagus, causing a burning sensation.

Acidosis: A state of excess acidity in the body's fluids; metabolic acidosis involves the kidneys, while respiratory acidosis involves the lungs.

Acne: A group of skin disorders; acne vulgaris usually affects teenagers, while acne rosacea usually afflicts older people.

Acoustic neuroma: A benign tumor of the auditory nerve.

Acquired immunodeficiency syndrome (AIDS): A progressive loss of immune function and susceptibility to secondary infections that arises from chronic infection with the human immunodeficiency virus (HIV).

ACTH. *See* Adrenocorticotropin (ACTH).

Action potential: An electrochemical event in which nerve cells send signals along their cellular extensions in the nervous system.

Active euthanasia: The administration of a drug or some other means that directly causes death.

Active immunity: Immunity resulting from antibody production following exposure to an antigen.

Activities of daily living: General personal care activities such as eating, dressing, and bathing.

Acupressure: An ancient Chinese mode of therapy performed by applying pressure to specific points on the body.

Acupuncture: Insertion of long, fine needles at particular points on the body located along one of fourteen major meridian lines, thought to be the major channels of life force. Developed by the Chinese.

Acute: Referring to a disease process of sudden onset and short duration.

Acute confusion: A transient condition caused by social and/or biological stressors, which may include inattention, disorganized thinking, other mental impairments, and emotional problems.

Acute rejection: The rejection of a transplanted organ by cells of the immune system; acute rejection is common days to weeks after cadaveric organ transplants and can usually be treated successfully with antilymphocytic drugs.

Acute respiratory distress syndrome (ARDS): Respiratory failure caused by filling of the lungs with fluid from the capillaries, leading to a shortage of oxygen in the body that can eventually lead to death if not treated.

Adaptation: A decreased sensitivity to a stimulus, even though the stimulus may still be present, resulting in slowing of nerve impulses until the impulses stabilize or stop entirely.

Addiction: A psychological and sometimes physiological process whereby an organism comes to depend on a substance; characterized by a persistent need to use the substance, increases in the dosage used in order to counteract tolerance, and withdrawal symptoms when the substance is withheld or the dosage is reduced.

Addison's disease: A chronic condition in which the adrenal glands do not produce adequate amounts of corticosteroid hormones.

Adenohypophysis: Another name for the anterior lobe of the pituitary gland.

Adenoids: A group of lymph nodes located above the tonsils, at the back of the nasal passage; usually disappear after childhood but are sometimes surgically removed (adenoidectomy) if they become swollen and cause blockage or infection.

Adenosine triphosphate (ATP): A high-energy compound found in the cell that provides energy for all bodily functions.

Adenoviruses: Medium-sized viruses that can cause respiratory infections and diarrhea by infecting the tissue linings of the respiratory and urinary tracts, the intestines, and the eyes.

Adhesion: The "gluing" together by scar tissue of internal organs and tissues, often caused by endometriosis or infections; a common cause of pelvic pain.

Adipose tissue: Fat; a soft tissue of the body composed of cells (adipocytes) that contain triglyceride, a compound consisting of glycerol and fatty acids.

Adjustment (chiropractic): A thrust delivered into the spine or its articulations in order to reestablish normal joint and nerve function.

Adjuvant therapy: Therapy used in addition to surgery in order to control the growth of remaining cancer cells.

Adrenal glands: Small organs near the kidneys that are responsible for the production of certain sex hormones, including testosterone and small amounts of estrogen, and of hormones involved in metabolism and stress responses.

Adrenalectomy: Surgical removal of one or both of the adrenal glands.

Adrenocorticotropin (ACTH): A hormone made in the pituitary gland in the brain that stimulates the adrenal cortex to make steroid hormones.

Adrenoleukodystrophy: A variable X-linked genetic disorder with symptoms ranging from adrenal insufficiency to progressive neurological deterioration.

Advanced life support (ALS): Procedures to sustain life such as intravenous therapy, pharmacology, cardiac monitoring, and electrical defibrillation.

Adverse reaction: An undesirable event caused by the taking of a drug; onset could be immediate or develop over time.

Aerobic exercise: Exercise that requires oxygen for energy production and that can be sustained for prolonged periods of time; involves large muscle groups, increases the heart rate and/or breathing rate, and is rhythmic and continuous.

Aerobic respiration: The chemical reactions that use oxygen to produce energy.

Aerospace medicine: The medical specialty concerned for the health of the operating crews and passengers of air and space vehicles.

Affective disorders: Mental conditions characterized by a primary disturbance of mood as distinct from thinking or behavior.

Ageism: Discrimination against individuals based on their age; the overlooking of individuals' abilities to make positive contributions to society because of their age.

Agglutination: A clumping of blood cells caused by antibodies joining with antigens on the cell surfaces.

Aging: The process of growing older, which begins at conception and eventually leads to death; the gradual effects of aging include changes in every organ and body system.

Agnosia: Inability to identify objects or persons using one or more of the senses, even though the basic sensory modalities are not defective.

Agonist: A drug that acts in a similar fashion to a hormone or neurotransmitter normally found in the body.

AIDS. *See* Acquired immunodeficiency syndrome (AIDS).

Akathisia: An unpleasant sensation of "inner" restlessness that compels the patient to move or walk.

Albinos: Individuals who have an inherited defect in the production of melanin characterized by a lack of pigmentation.

Alcohol: An organic compound containing a hydroxyl group attached to a carbon atom; ethyl alcohol is the compound found in alcoholic beverages.

Alcoholism: The compulsive drinking of and dependency on alcoholic beverages; viewed as psychological in origin, it can be arrested but not cured.

Aldosterone: A hormone produced by the adrenal gland that helps regulate the salt (sodium) and water balance in the body by increasing both sodium and water retention.

Alkalosis: A condition of abnormally low carbon dioxide levels that results from hyperventilation (rapid breathing).

Alkylating agents: Drugs that introduce alkyl groups to biologically important cell constituents, whose function is then impaired.

Alleles: Alternate forms of a gene; an individual has two alleles of each gene (one from each parent), which may be the same or different.

Allergen: A substance (such as pollen, dust, or animal dander) that causes an allergic reaction.

Allergic rhinitis: Acute or seasonal nasal stuffiness and sneezing that follows the exposure to allergens like pollen or animal dander; hay fever is one form of allergic rhinitis.

Allergies: Exaggerated immune reactions to materials that are intrinsically harmless; the body's release of pharmacologically active chemicals during allergic reactions may result in discomfort, tissue damage, or, in severe responses, death.

Allied health: A designation used to describe the services and personnel that support the providers of direct patient care within the larger health care system.

Allogeneic: Of the same species.

Allograft: A graft of tissue from one individual to another individual, usually between close relatives.

Alloimmunization: Immunization by means of antibodies from another person.

Allopathic medicine: The traditional course of study leading to a doctorate in medicine; most practicing physicians are allopathic physicians.

Alopecia: Hair loss, especially if noticeable or significant.

ALS. *See* Advanced life support; Amyotrophic lateral sclerosis.

Alternative medicine: Any of a variety of nontraditional therapies and treatments (such as acupuncture, herbal medicine, and homeopathy) that are not practiced by the established medical community. These alternative treatments range in the degree to which their efficacy and legitimacy have been accepted, from highly experimental and non-science-based to well established.

Altitude sickness: A condition resulting from altitude-related hypoxia (low oxygen levels).

Alveolar cell: Also known as an acinar cell; the fundamental secretory unit of the mammary glandular tissue.

Alveoli: Tiny air sacs deep within the lungs.

Alzheimer's disease: A progressive disease characterized by a loss of brain cells; it causes increasing memory impairment and cognitive deficits.

AMA. *See* American Medical Association (AMA).

Ambulatory care: Health care provided outside the hospital, usually in a clinic, office, or home.

Amebiasis: Infection of the colon or associated organs by the parasite *Entamoeba histolytica.*

Amenorrhea: A lack of menstruation in girls by the age of eighteen or its suppression, often as a result of overly strenuous exercise, rapid weight loss or gain, or emotional trauma.

American Board of Emergency Medicine: The agency certifying medical doctors as emergency medicine specialists; sets criteria for training and knowledge to become board certified in emergency medicine.

American College of Emergency Physicians: Supports quality emergency care and promotes the interests of emergency physicians.

American Medical Association (AMA): The largest voluntary association of physicians in the United States, with most of its members engaging directly in the practice of medicine.

Amino acid: The fundamental building block of proteins; there are twenty amino acids.

Amnesia: An impairment of memory, which may be total or limited, sudden or gradual.

Amniocentesis: A procedure in which a small amount of fluid is removed from the amniotic sac of a pregnant woman to detect abnormalities that may be present in the fetus.

Amniotic fluid: Fluid within the amniotic cavity produced by the amniotic sac during the early embryonic period (two to eight weeks) and later by the fetus' lungs and kidneys; it protects the fetus from injury and helps to maintain a stable temperature.

Amniotic sac: A thin, tough, membranous sac that contains amniotic fluid and the embryo or fetus of mammals, birds, and reptiles.

Amputation: Surgical removal of all or part of a limb or digit (finger or toe), often as a last resort to prevent fatal infection from gangrene.

Amygdala: Front portion of the temporal lobe of the brain.

Amylase: The enzyme responsible for breaking down carbohydrates in the small intestine; amylase enters the intestinal tract from the salivary glands and the pancreas.

Amyloidosis: A condition characterized by the deposit of waxy substances in animal organs.

Amyotrophic lateral sclerosis (ALS): Also called Lou Gehrig's disease; the most common form of motor neuron disease, in which the nerves that control muscle movement degenerate in the brain and spinal cord.

Anabolic steroids: A class of steroids that stimulate body reactions to build up more complex molecules and structures from simpler molecules; most are synthetic derivatives of testosterone.

Anaerobic: Occurring in the absence of oxygen.

Anal incontinence: The inability to control defecation.

Anal intraepithelial neoplasia: Precursor lesions to the development of anal cancer.

Analgesic: A medication (such as aspirin) that reduces or eliminates pain.

Analyte: Any chemical substance undergoing measurement; includes charged electrolytes found in the blood, such as sodium or potassium.

Anaphylaxis: Severe allergic reaction involving the circulatory and respiratory systems; often fatal without immediate treatment.

Anastomosis: The surgical connection of one tubular organ to another.

Anatomy: The structure of the human body—its parts, systems, and organs.

Androgens: Hormones that regulate sexual differentiation and the development and maintenance of male sex characteristics.

Andrology: The study of the physiological functions relating to male reproductive capacity.

Anemia: A condition characterized by a deficiency of red blood cells or hemoglobin; anemia is sometimes caused by a decrease in hemoglobin production, an increase in cell destruction, or blood loss.

Anesthesia: A state characterized by the loss of sensation, caused by or resulting from drugs that induce pharmacological depression of normal nerve function.

Anesthesiology: The branch of medicine specializing in the application of anesthetics.

Anesthetic: A pharmacologic agent used to block nerve conduction and reduce sensations.

Anesthetist: A health care specialist who administers anesthetics.

Aneuploidy: An abnormal number of chromosomes.

Aneurysm: A localized enlargement of a vessel, usually an artery, caused by the stretching of a weak place in the vessel wall.

Aneurysmectomy: Surgical removal of an aneurysm.

Angina: Pain in the chest caused by insufficient blood flow to the heart muscle.

Angiography: A radiological technique for visualizing the interior of the arteries; involves the placement of a catheter in an artery and the injection of dye.

Angioplasty: Compression of arterial plaque by insertion of a catheter into the artery and inflation of a balloon at the end of the catheter.

Anomia: An inability to remember the names of persons or objects even though the patient sees and recognizes the persons or objects.

Anorectal: Associated with the anal portion of the large intestine.

Anorexia nervosa: An eating disorder characterized by a compulsive aversion to food, caused by a fear of obesity and a distorted body image, that may result in severe malnutrition.

Anoscopy: Examination of the anal canal via a small tubal instrument inserted a few inches into the anus.

Anosmia: A complete loss in the ability to detect odors.

Anoxia: Oxygen deprivation.

Antagonist: A drug that acts to block the effects of a hormone or neurotransmitter normally found in the body.

Anterior: Toward the front of the body.

Anterior chamber: Space between the cornea and lens; filled with aqueous humor.

Anthropology: The study of human culture.

Antibiotic: Any substance that destroys or inhibits the growth of microorganisms, such as bacteria.

Antibody: A protein produced in the body by the immune system that recognizes and binds selectively to foreign material (antigens) to facilitate their elimination; antibodies combat bacterial, viral, chemical, and other invasive agents in the body.

Anticholinergic: Referring to drugs that oppose the action of acetylcholine in nerve-impulse transmission.

Anticoagulant: A drug that reduces the clotting of the blood.

Anticonvulsant: An agent that prevents or relieves seizures.

Antidepressants: A group of drugs used for the treatment of clinical depression.

Antidote: Anything that counteracts the effect of a substance.

Antiemetic: A drug that prevents or relieves the symptoms of nausea and/or vomiting.

Antifungal agent: A drug that kills or inhibits the growth of fungi.

Antigen: A molecule that induces the production of antibodies; antigens are generally proteins.

Antihistamines: Over-the-counter and prescription drugs that reduce the effects of histamines, thus treating allergy symptoms.

Antihypertensive drugs: Medicines designed to reduce and control elevated blood pressure.

Anti-inflammatory drugs: Drugs that counter the effects of inflammation, either locally or throughout the body; the three classes of these drugs are steroidal, immunosuppressant, and nonsteroidal.

Antimetabolites: Chemotherapeutic agents that act by inhibiting enzymes in the DNA synthetic pathway or by incorporating in DNA itself.

Antioxidants: Chemicals that destroy free radicals or neutralize them before they can do damage to a cell's mechanism; they are produced as a by-product of a normal process of metabolism.

Antiserum: The fluid portion of blood that contains specific antibodies.

Anxiety: A condition characterized by nervousness or agitation.

Anxiety disorders: Problems in which physical and emotional uneasiness, apprehension, and fear are the dominant symptoms.

Aorta: A large artery from the left ventricle of the heart that supplies oxygenated blood to the body.

Aphasia: The total absence of such language skills as speaking, reading, writing, and comprehension.

Apheresis: The removal of whole blood from a donor, followed by its separation into components, the retention of the desired component, and the return of the recombined remaining elements.

Aphrodisiacs: Substances thought to induce sexual desire or lust or to enhance sexual performance.

Apnea: Lack of airflow for more than ten seconds.

Apothecary: A pharmacist or druggist.

Appendectomy: The surgical removal of the vermiform appendix.

Appendicitis: Inflammation of the vermiform appendix, which may require its removal.

Aqueous humor: A clear, watery liquid that fills the region inside the front of the eyeball between the lens and cornea; also called the vitreous humor.

Arch bar: A pliable piece of metal that is fitted along the teeth to prevent jaw movement.

ARDS. *See* Acute respiratory distress syndrome (ARDS).

Areola: The pigmented tissue immediately surrounding the nipple.

Aromatherapy: The use of scents to facilitate physical, mental, and emotional well-being.

Arrhythmia: A heart rhythm that is abnormal, either in speed or in force.

Arteries: Vessels that take blood away from the heart and toward the tissues.

Arteriosclerosis: Hardening and thickening of the walls of the arteries caused by a buildup of fatty deposits or plaques; also called atherosclerosis.

Arteriovenous malformation: A condition in which the capillary beds that connect the arteries and the veins are abnormal or defective, resulting in malnourishment of tissues, especially in the brain and spinal cord.

Arthritis: Joint inflammation.

Arthroconidia: Asexual fungal spores that are made by the segmentation of preexisting fungal hyphae.

Arthroplasty: Replacement or repair of a joint using metal or plastic parts.

Arthropods: Small animals including mites, ticks, insects, and related organisms that may be vectors to animal or human hosts.

Arthroscopy: The use of an endoscope to examine the interior of a joint.

Articulation: A joint between two bones of the skeleton; also called an arthrosis.

Artificial nutrition and hydration: The medical intervention of giving a patient nutrients and/or fluids through a tube placed in the stomach, the intestine, or a vein.

Asbestos: A term for a group of naturally occurring silicate minerals with long, thin fibers; exposure can cause respiratory disease.

Aseptic techniques: Sterilization and other procedures that allow surgeons to operate in a germ-free environment.

Asperger's syndrome: A pervasive developmental disorder involving clinically significant impairment in social interactions and repetitive or stereotyped patterns of behavior, but no particular problem with cognitive functioning.

Asphyxiation: An impaired exchange of oxygen and carbon dioxide in the lungs; if prolonged, this condition leads to death.

Aspiration: The breathing of material into the lungs (such as vomit or food particles); also, the removal of a substance using suction or a needle and syringe.

Assessment: The systematic process of collecting, validating, and communicating patient data; these data will include information gathered from the patient's history and the results of physical examination and laboratory tests.

Assisted reproductive technologies: A range of medical procedures that are used to assist couples in conception and prenatal care, with special focus on infertility and its cure.

Asthma: A disorder of the lungs, experienced as wheezing and mucus blockage of the bronchi.

Astigmatism: A visual disorder in which either the cornea of the eye or the lens is not symmetrical.

Asymptomatic: Lacking or without any symptoms.

Ataxia: An inability to coordinate the muscles in voluntary movement.

Atherosclerosis: A process in which plaque builds up on the walls of blood vessels.

Athlete's foot: A contagious fungal infection of the skin on the feet.

Atom: The smallest chemically and biologically active unit of matter; composed of electrons enclosing an atomic nucleus containing protons and neutrons.

ATP. *See* Adenosine triphosphate (ATP).

Atrial fibrillation: Abnormal heart rhythm or muscle contractions in the atria as a result of disorganized electrical impulses.

Atrioventricular (A-V) node: A small region of specialized heart muscle cells that receives the electrical impulse from the atria and begins its transmission to the ventricles.

Atrium (*pl.* atria): One of the two upper chambers of the heart; the right atrium receives blood returning through the veins, while the left atrium receives oxygenated blood from the lungs.

Atrophy: The wasting of tissue, an organ, or an entire body as the result of a decrease in the size and/or number of the cells within that tissue, organ, or body.

Attenuation: The weakening or elimination of the pathogenic properties of a microorganism; ideally, the organism is rendered harmless.

Audiology: The study of hearing disorders and hearing loss.

Audiometer: A calibrated electronic device for the purpose of measuring human hearing to determine the magnitude of loss and the probable rehabilitative course.

Auditory nerve: The nerve that conducts impulses originating in hair cells of the cochlea to the brain for processing as the sensation of sound.

Auditory system: The human hearing mechanism, including the pinna, the external ear canal, the middle-ear structures, the cochlea, and the ascending neural pathway that terminates in the auditory cortex of the brain.

Aura: Sensory symptoms that may precede a seizure, a migraine or cluster headache, or a psychotic episode.

Aural rehabilitation: A program for hearing-impaired individuals that may include auditory prosthesis, auditory training, and speech reading training.

Auscultation: Active listening, usually with the aid of a stethoscope, to sounds generated by the body.

Autism: An emotional disturbance found in children in which communication, social interactions, and language skills are severely impaired.

Autoantibody: An antibody produced against tissue antigens within a host; self-antigens.

Autograft: A graft of tissue transferred from one part of an individual's body to another.

Autoimmune disorders: Disorders in which the immune system starts to attack the body's cells as foreign matter.

Autologous: Self-derived.

Automated external defibrillator (AED): A portable and automated device that can deliver lifesaving shocks to the heart.

Autonomic nervous system: The division of the nervous system that regulates involuntary actions, such as vital functions; comprises the sympathetic and parasympathetic systems.

Autopsy: Examination of a dead body to determine cause of death.

Autosomal dominant gene: A gene (other than the X or Y chromosome) that needs to be on only one chromosome in order to be expressed.

Autosomal recessive gene: A gene (other than the X or Y chromosome) that must be on both chromosomes in order to be expressed.

Autosomes: All chromosomes, except the X and Y chromosomes (sex chromosomes), that determine body traits.

Autotransplantation: The transplantation of tissue or organs in which the recipient serves as his or her own donor (such as a skin graft); may also refer to transplantation between genetically identical individuals (identical twins).

A-V node. *See* Atrioventricular (A-V) node.

Axon: The cellular extension of the neuron that conducts electrical information, transmitting it to the dendrite of the next neuron through the synaptic gap between them.

AZT. *See* Zidovudine.

B lymphocyte: A blood and lymphatic cell that plays a role in the secretion of antibodies.

Babesiosis: A parasitic disease that is transmitted to humans by the bite of an infected tick.

Bacillus Calmette-Guérin (BCG): A weakened version of *Mycobacterium bovis*, which is used in vaccines to protect against tuberculosis; also, the vaccine itself.

Bacteremia: A condition in which bacteria enter the bloodstream and thus can be disseminated throughout the body.

Bacteria: Single-celled microorganisms that exist throughout the environment.

Bacterial endocarditis: Bacterial infection of the heart, which may scar or destroy a valve.

Bacteriology: The study of bacteria.

Balloon catheterization: The use of a balloonlike device on the tip of a catheter to widen blood vessels, as in angioplasty.

Bariatric surgery: Any surgical procedure changing the structure of the digestive system in order to achieve weight reduction.

Bariatrics: The medical management of obesity and related conditions.

Barium study: A medical procedure in which the patient drinks a liquid barium sulfate mixture prior to undergoing an X-ray examination of the chest and abdomen; used to identify problems in the upper gastrointestinal tract.

Barrel chest: A rounded chest in which the anterior and posterior diameter is increased.

Barrier method: The use of a contraceptive that physically prevents sperm from meeting the ovum, including the male condom, female condom, diaphragm, cervical cap, and vaginal sponge.

Basal cell carcinoma: The most common type of skin cancer; it grows slowly and seldom spreads beneath the skin.

Basal cells: Cells at the base of the epidermis that migrate upward and become the principal source of epidermal tissue.

Basal ganglia: A group of interconnected deep brain nuclei that includes striatum, pallidum, subthalamic nucleus, and substantia nigra.

Base: A water-soluble compound with a pH between 7.1 and 14.0 that contains a hydroxyl group and can accept hydrogen ions (protons) from acids; it can combine with acids to form salts and water and turns litmus blue.

Basic life support (BLS): A variety of life-support procedures, including rescue breathing and chest compressions, often given to a heart attack victim by the first person responding to the patient; public training in such procedures is available from the Red Cross and the American Heart Association.

Batten's disease: A progressive neurological disruption and deterioration of intellectual and physical development caused by mutated genes.

BCG. *See* Bacillus Calmette-Guérin (BCG).

Becquerel: The international unit of radioactivity, defined as a radioactive sample that is decaying at the rate of one nucleus disintegration per second.

Bed-wetting: Enuresis; a condition characterized by an inability of the bladder to contain urine during sleep, often a developmental condition in children.

Bedsores: Sores caused by sustained pressure, with restricted blood flow to the skin.

Behçet's disease: A multisystem disease characterized by recurrent oral and genital ulcers.

Bell's palsy: A sudden paralysis of one side of the face, including muscles of the eyelid.

Beneficence: A principle of medical ethics which requires that actions be taken for the patient's good.

Benign: Referring to a tumor made of a mass of cells that do not leave the site where they develop.

Benign senescent forgetfulness: A common source of frustration in old age, associated with memory impairment; unlike dementia, it does not interfere with the individual's social and professional activities.

Benzodiazepine: Any of a group of drugs with strong sedative and hypnotic action.

Bereavement: The general, overall process of mourning and grieving; considered to have progressive stages that include anticipation, grieving, mourning, postmourning, depression, loneliness, and reentry into society.

Beriberi: A serious vitamin deficiency caused by an inadequate intake of thiamine (B_1).

Bicarbonate: An incompletely neutralized carbonic acid lacking one hydrogen atom.

Biguanide: A medication to lower blood glucose by increasing sensitivity to insulin and possibly lowering the liver's glucose production.

Bile: Fluid produced by the liver and stored in the gallbladder to be secreted into the intestine; contains salts, bile pigments (bilirubin), cholesterol, and other waste products.

Biliary colic: A distinct pain syndrome characterized by severe intermittent waves of right-sided, upper abdominal pain, often brought on by the ingestion of fatty foods; pain occurs when a gallstone obstructs the outflow of bile and usually resolves when the gallstone moves away from the outflow area.

Bilirubin: A yellow-brown component of bile created when the liver breaks down old red blood cells.

Bioengineering: The combination of biological principles and engineering concepts and/or methodology to improve knowledge in both areas.

Biofeedback: Receiving information about involuntary bodily responses in an effort to modify these responses to some extent, thus learning how to reduce stress and induce or maintain other positive behavior.

Bioflavonoids: Active flavonoids that work synergistically with vitamin C; they are not vitamins but are sometimes referred as vitamin P.

Bioinformatics: A computational discipline that provides the tools needed to study whole genomes and proteomes.

Biological sciences: Natural sciences that deal with the structure and behavior of living organisms; includes disciplines such as zoology, genetics, cell biology, biochemistry and molecular biology, and anatomy and physiology.

Biological weapons: Biological agents or toxins produced by biological agents that are used as weapons.

Biomechanics: The application of mechanical principles to the living body, specifically of forces used by muscles and gravity on the skeletal structure and how biomaterials such as collagen or elastin behave under those conditions.

Biomedicine: The branch of medical science concerned with the capacity of human beings to survive and function in abnormally stressful environments, as well as with the protective modification of such environments.

Bionics: The medical application of biological and engineering knowledge to the design of artificial systems that act in the place of natural systems.

Biophysics: The application of the theories and laws of physics to the study of biological processes.

Biopsy: The removal of tissue from a suspected site of disease, such as cancer, in order to identify abnormal cells under microscopic examination.

Biopsychosocial model: A model that examines the effects of illness on all spheres in which the patient functions—the biological sphere, the psychological sphere, and the social sphere.

Biostatistics: The application of statistical analyses to the study of biological data.

Biotechnology: The medical application of biological and engineering knowledge at the molecular and genetic levels of natural systems in order to diagnose, treat, cure, or learn more about diseases.

Biphasic reaction: Delayed allergic reaction to an allergen, between one and four hours after the initial reaction.

Bipolar disorder: A syndrome characterized by alternating periods of mania and depression; formerly called manic-depressive disorder.

Birth defect: A genetic abnormality in the tissue development of a certain body part of the fetus; in some cases the defect is minor, but in others it may be medically dangerous to the fetus and/or the mother.

Blackout: Memory loss, usually as a result of taking substances known to disrupt memory, in which the affected person may function as if aware of what is happening, despite having no memory of activities.

Bladder: The organ that stores urine until it is discharged from the body.

Blastocyst: A small, hollow ball of cells that typifies one of the early embryonic stages in humans.

Blepharoplasty: The removal of excess tissue around the eyelids.

Blindness: Loss of sight; legal blindness in the United States means vision less than 20/200 or peripheral vision less than 20 degrees.

Blood: The fluid that circulates in the veins and arteries, carrying oxygen and nutrients through the body, transporting waste materials to excretory channels, and participating in the body's defense against infection.

Blood bank: A temporary storehouse of blood, kept at reduced temperatures, for transfusions into persons needing an additional supply; such transfers are vital in surgery and in unexpected emergency procedures.

Blood group system: A classification of individuals into groups on the basis of their possession or nonpossession of specific blood substances.

Blood pressure: A measure of how much the fluid in the blood vessels pushes against the walls of the vessels.

Blood testing: The withdrawal of blood from an individual and its analysis for one of many purposes, including blood typing and a search for acquired or genetic disease indicators.

Blood type: A blood classification group based on the presence or absence of certain antigens on red blood cells.

Blood typing: The identification of the blood-group substances of individuals so as to classify them in specific blood groups; individuals may have blood types A, B, AB, or O and be Rh negative or Rh positive.

BLS. *See* Basic life support (BLS).

Body dysmorphic disorder: A psychiatric somatoform disorder resulting in exaggerated preoccupation with an imagined or minor defect in physical appearance that causes significant impairment of social functioning.

Body mass index (BMI): Weight in kilograms divided by height in meters, squared (kg/m^2).

Bolus: Food that has been mixed with saliva and formed into a ball; the bolus passes from the mouth to the stomach through a process called swallowing, or deglutition.

Bone grafting: The transplantation of a section of bone from one part of the body to another, or from one individual to another.

Bone marrow: The soft substance that fills the cavities within bones and that is the site of blood cell production.

Bone marrow transplantation: The removal of bone marrow from an immunologically matched individual for infusion into a patient whose bone marrow has been destroyed.

Bone scan: A diagnostic technique using a radioactive tracer that is strongly absorbed by a tumor, whose location then can be detected by radiation counters.

Bones: Hard tissues that form the skeleton, providing support while allowing flexibility.

Botox: A neurotoxin produced by bacteria that causes botulism in very high doses and is also used as a therapeutic agent for a variety of conditions.

Botulism: Food poisoning caused by bacteria that produce a toxin that is absorbed by the digestive tract and spread to the central nervous system.

Bowman's capsule: The group of cells in the kidneys that forms the cup of a nephron; fluids that seep from glomerular capillaries into the hollow wall of the capsule will be transformed into urine during their passage through the renal tubule leading from the capsule.

Bowman's glands: One of three sources in the nasal cavity of the mucus that moistens the membranes of the olfactory center, thereby allowing odoriferous molecules to adhere to the olfactory hairs; located between olfactory supporting cells.

Bradycardia: Slowness of the heartbeat.

Brain: The most complex organ in the body, which is used for thinking, learning, remembering, seeing, hearing, and many other conscious and subconscious functions.

Brain death: Irreversible brain damage so extensive that the organ enjoys no potential for recovery and can no longer maintain the body's internal functions.

Brain stem: The medulla oblongata, pons, and mesencephalon portions of the brain, which perform motor, sensory, and reflex functions (such as respiration) and which contain the corticospinal and reticulospinal tracts.

Breast: The mammary gland, along with the nipple in front of it and the surrounding fatty tissue.

Breast biopsy: The surgical removal of a lump or tissue from the breast to determine whether it is malignant.

Breast cancer: Malignancy occurring in breast tissue and possibly involving the associated lymph nodes.

Breech position: A commonly encountered abnormal fetal presentation in which the buttocks is delivered first, rather than the head; may require a cesarean section.

Bronchi: The right and left branches from the trachea that supply air into the lungs.

Bronchioles: Small conducting tubes in the lungs that carry air to the alveoli.

Bronchitis: An inflammation of the bronchial tree of the lungs.

Bronchoscopy: The visual examination of the respiratory system using a flexible tube composed of optic fibers.

Buffer: A solution that contains components that enable a solution to resist large changes in pH when small quantities of acids and bases are added.

Bulbourethral gland: The bulbous portion of the male urethra adjacent to the prostate gland.

Bulimia: A compulsive eating disorder characterized by food binges and purges (either through self-induced vomiting or the use of laxatives).

Bulla: A blister that develops on the surface of the lung; also called a bleb.

Bunion: A swelling of the big toe caused by an inflamed bursa, often a complication of ill-fitting footwear.

Burkitt's lymphoma: A highly aggressive lymphoma often presenting in extranodal sites or as an acute leukemia.

Bursa: A connective tissue sac filled with fluid that reduces friction at joints.

Bursitis: An inflammation of a bursa, one of the membranes that surround joints.

Bypass graft: A surgical procedure that reroutes blood around an obstruction, usually caused by atherosclerosis; the "new" artery can be either plastic or constructed from an expendable, healthy section of vein in another part of the patient's body.

Bypass surgery: Heart surgery to bypass a clogged artery by use of an unclogged vein, usually taken from the leg.

CABG. *See* Coronary artery bypass graft (CABG).

Caffeine: An addictive chemical substance found in foods such as coffee, tea, chocolate, and some soft drinks.

Calcification: The deposit of lime salts in organic tissue, leading to the buildup of calcium in the arterial wall.

Calcitonin: A hormone made and released by the thyroid gland that lowers the level of calcium in the blood by stimulating the formation of bone.

Calculi (*sing.* calculus): Any of a variety of stones formed by calcium deposits, cholesterol, and other materials that may accumulate in the kidneys, in the gallbladder, or elsewhere in the urinary or digestive tract.

Callus: An area of skin that has become thick and hard in response to repeated friction and pressure; also a bony deposit formed between and around the broken ends of a fractured bone during healing.

Calorie: The basic unit of energy; the amount of heat needed to raise the temperature of 1 kilogram of water by 1 degree Celsius.

Campylobacter infection: An acute disease, often spontaneously resolving, caused by bacterial infection; sometimes called food poisoning.

Canaliculus: A small canal linking the upper and lower puncta (tear duct openings) to the lacrimal sac.

Cancer: Inappropriate and uncontrollable cell growth within specialized tissues, which threatens normal cell and organ function.

Candidiasis: An overgrowth of the fungus *Candida albicans*, which may affect the vagina, mouth, or skin; commonly called a yeast infection.

Canker sores: Small, round ulcers of the mucous membranes that line the mouth.

Cannula: A tube used to drain body fluids or to administer medications.

Capacitation: A change in sperm when in the female reproductive tract that causes them to swim more vigorously.

Capillaries: Minute blood vessels that connect the smallest arteries (arterioles) to the smallest veins (venules); they allow passage of oxygen and nutrients from the arteries into the tissues and passage of waste products from the tissues into the veins.

Capsid: The protein shell of a virus.

Carbohydrates: A group of organic compounds that includes the sugars and the starches; one of three classes of nutrients and a basic source of energy.

Carbon dioxide: The gas produced by the body from the use of oxygen; carbon dioxide and the hydrogen ions that it can create may become toxic if not excreted by the body.

Carcinogen: A chemical or radiation that causes changes in genes, leading to the cancerous state in a cell.

Carcinoma: A malignant neoplasm arising from the epithelial cells that make up the surface layers of skin or other membranes.

Cardiac: Related to the heart.

Cardiac arrest: The cessation of heart contractions or insufficient contractions to pump blood to the brain and other vital organs.

Cardiac catheterization: The guidance of a catheter into the heart or great blood vessels to measure function, assess problems, and identify treatment options.

Cardiac muscle: A type of muscle, found only in the heart, that makes up the major portion of the heart; involved in the movement of blood through the body.

Cardiac rehabilitation: The activities that ensure the physical, mental, and social conditions necessary for returning cardiac patients to good health.

Cardiology: The branch of medicine specializing in the diagnosis and treatment of heart disease.

Cardiomyopathy: A serious acute or chronic disease in which the heart becomes inflamed; it may result from multiple causes, including viral infection, and may involve obstructive damage.

Cardiopulmonary resuscitation (CPR): A method of restoring normal breathing to a patient in cardiac arrest using chest compressions and artificial ventilation.

Cardiovascular: Relating to or involving the heart and blood vessels.

Cardiovascular disease: Any of a group of diseases that affect the heart, including coronary artery disease, hypertension, congestive heart failure, congenital heart defects, and valvular heart disease.

Carotenoids: A group of fat-soluble pigments found in plants that have a strong antioxidant capability.

Carpal tunnel syndrome: Tingling and pain in the thumb, index, and middle fingers caused by pressure on a nerve that passes through an area in the hand called the carpal tunnel.

Carpus: The wrist.

Carrier: A person infected by an organism who can transmit that organism to other people but who is asymptomatic.

Cartilage: A strong, flexible connective tissue that lines the end of bones at a joint, providing a cushioning effect, and for other body structures supports the nose, ears, or bronchial tubes.

Case management: An interdisciplinary approach to medical care characterized by the inclusion of physical, psychological, social, emotional, familial, financial, and historical data in patient treatment.

Casuistry: A form of moral reasoning whereby specific cases about which there is moral uncertainty are compared to other cases about which there is moral certainty.

Catalysis: An increase in the speed of a chemical reaction.

Cataract: A dark region in the lens of the eye that causes gradual loss of vision.

Cataract surgery: The removal of an eye lens with cataracts and the implantation of a plastic replacement using microsurgery.

Catheter: A flexible tube that is inserted into a small opening or incision in the body.

Catheterization: The insertion of a tube into a cavity of the body to withdraw fluids from or introduce fluids into that cavity.

Cathode-ray tube (CRT): A display device used for the presentation of nuclear medicine data; it displays images in real time.

Cauterization: A means of sealing blood vessels with heat, used to prevent bleeding.

Cavities: Disintegrations in tooth enamel; also called tooth decay or dental caries.

CDC. *See* Centers for Disease Control and Prevention (CDC).

Cecum: The dividing passageway between the small intestine and the large intestine (or colon).

Cell: The basic functional unit of the body, which contains a set of genes and all the other materials necessary for carrying out the processes of life.

Cellular biology: The study of the processes that take place within a cell.

Cellular respiration: The chemical reactions that produce energy in the cell; these reactions can be aerobic or anaerobic.

Cellular transformation: The process in which a cell becomes cancerous, which begins with abnormal changes in gene expression and cell differentiation.

Cellulitis: Infection of the skin and underlying tissue.

Cementum: The outer covering of the root of a tooth.

Centers for Disease Control and Prevention (CDC): The government agency charged with monitoring the spread of infectious diseases in the United States.

Central nervous system: The brain and spinal cord.

Centrifugation: The spinning of blood or another fluid to separate out certain components for laboratory analysis.

Cerebellum: The part of the brain in the lower rear of the head located just above the brain stem; controls balance, coordination, and motion.

Cerebral palsy: A group of nonprogressive disorders of the upper neurologic system resulting in abnormal muscle tone and lack of muscular control.

Cerebrospinal fluid (CSF): The extracellular fluid of the central nervous system; it flows through the ventricles of the brain and the central canal of the spinal cord, circulating nutrients and providing a cushion for the brain.

Cerebrum: The largest and uppermost section of the brain, which integrates memory, speech, writing, and emotional responses.

Certification: The formal notice of certain privileges and abilities after completion of certain training and testing.

Cerumen: Earwax; secreted by glands at the outer third of the ear canal.

Cervical vertebrae: The first seven bones of the spinal column, located in the neck.

Cervix: The entrance to the uterus from the vagina; it secretes mucus, which appears as vaginal discharge.

Cesarean section: Delivery of a baby through the lower abdomen by means of surgery.

Chagas' disease: An acute disease that is most common in children and caused by the protozoan *Trypanosoma cruzi*.

Charge: The quantity of electricity responsible for attraction and repulsion among atoms and molecules.

Chemical energy: The energy locked up in the chemical bonds that hold the atoms of a molecule together; food molecules, such as glucose, contain considerable energy in their bonds.

Chemical weapons: Synthetic chemical agents used as weapons, or devices used to disseminate them.

Chemoreception: Sensitivity to chemical stimuli.

Chemoreceptors: Specific structures that respond to chemical stimuli, producing such sensations as taste and odor.

Chemotherapeutic index: For antibiotics, the ratio of the maximum dose that can be administered without causing serious damage to a person to the minimum dose that will cause serious damage to the infecting microorganism; a measure of selective toxicity.

Chemotherapy: The use of chemicals to kill or inhibit the growth of cancer cells.

Chest: The region of the body from the diaphragm to the neck, both within the rib cage (heart and lungs) and in front of it (breasts and muscles).

Chest compression: Pressure applied to the bottom half of the breastbone to pump blood from a heart in cardiac arrest.

Chiari malformations: A group of disorders where the cerebellum, the part of the brain in the lower rear of the head that controls motion, extends below the opening of the spinal canal (the foramen magnum).

Chickenpox: A very contagious but mild disease caused by the herpes zoster virus whose symptoms include fever, abdominal pain, and skin eruptions.

Chiropractic: Manipulation of the musculoskeletal and nervous structures (often the spine) to allow the body to use its natural recuperative systems to restore or maintain health.

Chlamydia: A sexually transmitted disease characterized by discharge, pain, and swelling of the genitals; if a pregnant woman is infected, the disease can infect her infant's eyes during childbirth.

Choking: A condition in which the breathing passage (windpipe) is obstructed.

Cholecystectomy: The surgical procedure that results in the removal of the gallbladder in its entirety. The two main techniques are the traditional open method and the laparoscopically aided method.

Cholecystitis: Inflammation or bacterial infection of the gallbladder, usually caused by the presence of gallstones.

Cholelithiasis: The formation of gallstones in the gallbladder or the ducts that connect the gallbladder to the liver or small intestine.

Cholera: An infection of the small intestine caused by *Vibrio cholerae*, a comma-shaped bacterium.

Cholesterol: A waxy essential substance present in all cells and transported in the blood.

Chondrocyte: A cell found disseminated at different locations throughout cartilage.

Chordee: The downward curvature of the penis, most apparent on erection, caused by the shortness of the skin on the downward side of the penile shaft.

Chorionic villi: The fingerlike projections of the placenta that function in oxygen, nutrient, and waste transportation between a fetus and its mother.

Chorionic villus sampling: Removal of a small portion of chorionic villi for genetic analysis.

Chromosomal abnormality: Any change to the number, shape, or appearance of the forty-six chromosomes in each human cell; the presence of many such abnormalities will prevent the normal development of an individual and lead to miscarriage.

Chromosomes: The parts of a cell's nucleus that contain genetic information, made of DNA covered with protein; each human cell has twenty-three pairs of chromosomes.

Chronic: Referring to a lingering or long-term disease process.

Chronic fatigue syndrome: A multifaceted disease state characterized by debilitating fatigue.

Chronic obstructive pulmonary disease (COPD): A progressive, irreversible disease of the lungs that causes expiratory airflow obstruction; the most common form is a combination of chronic bronchitis and emphysema.

Chronic rejection: The rejection of a transplanted organ months or years after transplantation.

Chronic wasting disease (CWD): A neurological disease of deer and elk caused by an infectious protein particle called a prion.

Chronobiology: The study of the timing of biological processes (such as growth, development, aging, and accompanying cycles) within an individual.

Chyle: The product that results from the emulsification of fat by pancreatic juice during the digestive process.

Chyme: The semiliquid state of food as it is found in the stomach and first part of the small intestine.

Cilia: Hairlike structures on cells that sweep mucus, containing bacteria and foreign particles, out of the airways.

Ciliary body: A ring of tissue that surrounds the eye; the uveal portion of this tissue contains the ciliary muscle that adjusts the degree of curvature of the lens.

Circadian rhythm: A cyclical variation in a biological process or behavior that has a duration of slightly greater than twenty-four hours.

Circulation: The flow of blood throughout the body; the circulatory system consists of the heart, lungs, arteries, and veins.

Circulator: The worker in the operating room whose responsibility is to keep records and to open sterile supplies for the team members wearing gowns and gloves.

Circumcision: Surgical removal of an area surrounding a body part, most often used to denote removal of the male foreskin (prepuce).

Cirrhosis: A condition of the liver in which injured or dead cells are replaced with scar tissue.

Claudication: Muscle cramps that occur when arterial blood flow does not meet the muscles' demand for oxygen.

Cleavage: The process by which the fertilized egg undergoes a series of rapid cell divisions, which results in the formation of a blastocyst.

Cleft lip: Incomplete fusion of the two sides of the lips during embryonic development; often associated with cleft palate.

Cleft palate: Incomplete fusion of the two sides of the palate in the mouth during embryonic development.

Clinic: A site for outpatient care.

Clinical examination: The physical examination of a patient, including medical history and an evaluation of environment.

Clinical laboratory: A general term for those areas of a medical facility where analyses of body fluids are performed.

Clinical trial: A research study to compare standard treatment against potentially better treatment.

Cloning: The making of identical copies; the techniques that genetic engineers use to recombine DNA from different sources and to reproduce those fragments in bacteria or other organisms.

Clot: A clumping of platelets, blood, fibrin, and clotting factors that normally accumulates in damaged tissue as part of the body's healing process; also called a thrombus.

Clotting factors: Chemicals circulating in the blood that are necessary for the process of blood clotting.

Cluster headaches: Headaches characterized by intense pain behind one eye.

CME. *See* Continuing medical education (CME).

Coagulation: The process of blood clotting.

Coccidioidomycosis: A fungal infection acquired by inhaling the spores of particular soil-based fungi; it initially attacks the lungs and often resolves without causing symptoms, but the infection can cause pneumonia and disseminate throughout the body.

Cochlea: A structure in the inner ear that receives sound vibrations from the ossicles and transmits them to the auditory nerve.

Cognitive: Relating to the mental process by which knowledge is acquired.

Cognitive functioning: A general term describing mental processes such as awareness, knowing, reasoning, problem-solving, judging, and imagining.

Cold sores: Thin-walled vesicles around the mouth that are infectious.

Colitis: Inflammation of the large intestine (colon), which usually is associated with bloody diarrhea and fever.

Collagen: A protein found in bone and other connective tissues; collagen fibers are well suited for support and protection because they are sturdy, are flexible, and resist stretch.

Collaterals: Small vessels that enlarge to compensate for the obstruction or narrowing of another vessel.

Collecting duct: Tubular canal that transports milk from the milk duct to the nipple.

Collimator: A device used for restricting and directing gamma rays by passing them through a grid made of metal, which absorbs the rays.

Colon: The large intestine, divided from the small intestine by the cecum (a controlled passageway) and ending at the sigmoid, which leads food waste into the rectum.

Colon therapy: The irrigation of the colon with water in order to detoxify it.

Colonoscopy: An endoscopic procedure used for visualization of the large intestine.

Color blindness: A genetic condition of the eye in which the patient is unable to distinguish between some colors.

Colostomy: The surgical creation of an artificial opening for the colon.

Colostrum: Thin, yellow milky secretions of the mammary gland just a few days before and after childbirth; it contains more proteins and less fat and carbohydrates than does milk.

Coma: A loss of consciousness from which a person cannot be aroused; a symptom signifying a variety of possible causes.

Commissurotomy: The severing of the corpus callosum, the fiber tract joining the two cerebral hemispheres.

Common cold: An acute respiratory tract infection including stuffy or running nose, sore throat, sneezing, fever, wheezing, and nasal pressure headache.

Communicative skills: Those skills required to express thoughts, desires, and feelings effectively through verbal and nonverbal communication.

Complement: A series of about twenty serum proteins that, when sequentially activated by immune complexes, may trigger cell damage.

Complication: A secondary medical problem that develops from an existing problem.

Compound: To mix or combine; to make by combining parts or elements.

Compulsion: A persistent, irresistible urge to perform a stereotyped behavior or irrational act, often accompanied by repetitive thoughts (obsessions) about the behavior.

Computed tomography (CT) scanning: A method of displaying the outline of a tumor or other structure, utilizing a computer to combine information from multiple X-ray beams.

Conception: A process encompassing all the events from fertilization of an egg to its first cell divisions.

Concordance: The inheritance of the same trait by both twins.

Concussion: Temporary neural dysfunction, causing confusion, dizziness, nausea, headache, lethargy, and short-term amnesia; often results when the head is struck by a hard blow or shaken violently.

Conductive loss: A hearing loss caused by an outer-ear or middle-ear problem that results in reduced transmission of sound.

Cones: Specialized photoreceptors that sense color and detailed vision in bright light.

Confidential: Referring to a situation distinguished by the willing disclosure of intimate, potentially damaging information because of assurances that the information will be protected from general distribution or unauthorized disclosure.

Congenital: Referring to a condition present at birth.

Congenital adrenal hyperplasia: A family of genetic conditions that affect hormone production by the adrenal glands.

Congenital disorders: Abnormalities present at birth that occurred during fetal development as a result of genetic errors, exposure to toxins and microorganisms, illness, or unknown causes.

Congenital heart disease: Conditions resulting from malformations of the heart that occur during embryonic and fetal development.

Congestive heart failure: Abnormal heart function characterized by circulatory congestion caused by cardiac disorders, especially myocardial infarction of the ventricles.

Conjunctivitis: An inflammation of the white part of the eye, the conjunctiva.

Connective tissue: The tissue in the body that binds and supports body parts, such as tendons and ligaments.

Conscious: Having an awareness of one's existence, behavior, and surroundings.

Constipation: The slow passage of feces through the bowels or the presence of hard feces.

Contact dermatitis: A common skin allergy characterized by inflamed skin; it occurs when skin comes in contact with substances such as poison ivy or allergenic cosmetics.

Contact lens: A small, shell-like glass or plastic lens that rests directly on the external surface of the eye; used to correct refractive error as an alternative to spectacles, to protect the eye, or to serve as a prosthetic device promoting a more normal appearance of a disfigured eye.

Continuing medical education (CME): Medical coursework given by hospitals, medical societies, and conferences.

Continuous care: Services provided for extended periods of time, such as shifts of eight, ten, twelve, or twenty-four hours.

Contraception: Avoidance of conception by either natural means (such as abstinence) or artificial means (use of condoms, spermicides, diaphragms, intrauterine devices, or chemical hormone regulators such as birth control pills).

Contraction: A squeezing action of the muscles, such as the squeezing of the uterus that results in birth.

Contraindication: A condition that makes a particular treatment not advisable; contraindications may be absolute (should never be used) or relative (should be used only with caution when the benefits outweigh the potential problems).

Control group: A group of patients receiving either a standard treatment or a placebo, allowing comparison with the experimental treatment.

Contusion: A bruise; injury to tissue without breaking the skin.

Convulsion: An instance of amplitude-random and high-frequency electrical activity in the brain.

Cooper's ligament: Projections of breast parenchyma covered by fibrous connective tissue that extend from the skin to the deep layer of superficial fascia.

COPD. *See* Chronic obstructive pulmonary disease (COPD).

Cornea: The curved, transparent front surface of the eyeball, which provides protection and partial light focusing.

Cornelia de Lange syndrome: A disorder with distinctive physical abnormalities and mental retardation usually apparent at birth.

Coronary arteries: The arteries that supply blood to the heart muscle.

Coronary artery bypass graft (CABG): A surgical procedure in which a blocked coronary artery is bypassed using a vein or artery; this intervention provides a blood supply to areas beyond the distal attachment of the graft.

Coronary artery disease: Formation of fatty deposits or plaque on the blood vessel walls; results in a narrowing of the coronary arteries and a concomitant reduction of oxygen supply to the heart muscle.

Coronaviruses: Viruses frequently infecting the upper respiratory system and capable of producing either the common cold or severe acute respiratory syndrome (SARS).

Coroner: An officer, often a layperson, who holds inquests in regard to violent, sudden, or unexplained deaths.

Corpora cavernosa: Two parallel erectile cylinders on the upper side of the penis that are filled with blood during an erection.

Corpus luteum: A yellow cell mass produced from a graafian follicle after the release of an egg.

Corpus spongiosum: A third cylinder in the penis below the corpora cavernosa; the urethra passes through it, and the glans penis forms the front end of the cylinder.

Corpuscle: A minute particle; a protoplasmic cell floating free in the blood.

Correlation: A number between -1 and +1 that describes the strength and direction of the relationship between two variables.

Corrosives: Having a burning (caustic) and locally destructive effect.

Cortex: The outer layer of the adrenal gland; the area that produces steroid hormones.

Corticosteroid: A fatlike molecule (or steroid), produced by the adrenal gland or made synthetically, that can be used to treat inflammation.

Cortisol: A glucocorticoid that raises blood sugar levels, elevated in response to physical or psychological stress.

Cosmetic surgery: The application of plastic surgical techniques to alter the patient's appearance.

CPR. *See* Cardiopulmonary resuscitation (CPR).

Craniotomy: Any surgical incision into the cranium.

Creatine phosphate: An energy-containing molecule present in significant quantities in muscle tissue; energy is stored in a high-energy bond similar to that of ATP.

Creatinine: A nitrogen-containing by-product of metabolism; levels of creatinine may be indicative of kidney function.

Cretinism: Severe hypothyroidism, in which infants are born with insufficiently developed thyroid tissue.

Critical care: A multiprofessional health care specialty that cares for patients with severe, life-threatening illness and injury.

Crohn's disease: A chronic inflammation of the bowel, often as a result of an autoimmune disease.

Croup: A respiratory disease that causes a severe, barking cough.

Crown: That portion of the tooth, normally covered with enamel, which is exposed in the oral cavity above the gingiva (gum).

CRT. *See* Cathode-ray tube (CRT).

Cryogenic agent: One of various mediums used to achieve the low temperatures needed to produce therapeutic effects.

Cryoprobe: An instrument used by physicians to apply cryogenic agents to diseased tissue; cryoprobes have differently shaped tips that affect the size and depth of the freezing.

Cryosurgery: The destruction of tissue by the application of extreme cold.

Cryotherapy: Use of cold temperatures to treat disease.

Crypt: A pit or cavity in the surface of a body organ (such as a tonsil).

CSF. *See* Cerebrospinal fluid (CSF).

CT scanning. *See* Computed tomography (CT) scanning.

Culdocentesis: Retrieval of a small amount of fluid, by means of needle aspiration, from the rectovaginal pouch for diagnostic purposes.

Culture: A medium for growing bacteria in laboratory conditions.

Current: The flow of electrical charges through space or a material.

Cusp: The conical projection of the chewing surface of the tooth.

Cuspid: The longest anterior tooth; also called the canine tooth or the eyetooth.

Cutaneous: Pertaining to the skin.

Cuticle: Cutaneous or skin tissue that surrounds the nail plate on its proximal sides and provides a protective barrier to the nail bed; it is attached to the proximal nail fold and to the nail plate.

CWD. *See* Chronic wasting disease (CWD).

Cyanosis: A bluish skin color resulting from poor oxygenation of the blood.

Cybernetics: A field of study, closely associated with bionics, which is concerned with communication and control in living systems and their application to artificial systems.

Cyst: A swelling or nodule containing fluid or soft material, resulting from a blocked duct or abnormal growth in fluid-producing tissue.

Cystectomy: Surgical removal of the urinary bladder or the gallbladder; also, surgical removal of a cyst.

Cystic fibrosis: A genetic disease that affects the exocrine glands and most physical systems of the body, resulting in death usually between the ages of sixteen and thirty.

Cystitis: Inflammation of the bladder, primarily caused by bacterial infection and resulting in pain, urgency in urination, and sometimes hematuria (blood in the urine).

Cystoscopy: Use of an endoscope to examine the urinary bladder.

Cytokine: Small, regulatory protein of the immune system that mediate cell interactions.

Cytopathology: The study of disease states as they manifest themselves within cells.

Cytoskeleton: A network of filaments (including microtubules, microfilaments, and intermediate filaments) that supports the cytoplasm and extensions of the cell surface.

D & C. *See* Dilation and curettage (D & C).

Date rape: A forced sexual act during a date.

Debridement: The removal of all foreign material and contaminated and devitalized tissues from or adjacent to a traumatic or infected lesion until surrounding tissue is exposed.

Decompression surgery: Removal of tissue or bone pressing against the spinal cord or a nerve in order to make more space and relieve pressure.

Decongestants: Drugs that are taken in order to break up congested mucus, fluids commonly found in the sinuses during allergic reactions and colds, in order to reduce swelling in the sinuses.

Decubitus ulcer: Ulceration of the skin and subcutaneous tissues resulting from protein deficiency and prolonged, unrelieved pressure on bony prominences.

Deep tendon reflex: A brisk contraction of a muscle responding to a sudden stretch produced by a sharp tap of a rubber hammer on a tendon insertion of a muscle.

Deep vein thrombosis: The formation of a blood clot (thrombus) in a deep vein that prevents blood circulation.

Defibrillation: The application of electrical energy through the chest in order to correct abnormal heart function and restore a normal heart rhythm.

Delayed primary closure: A procedure in which the wound is left open four to six days and then sewn closed; used for infected or contaminated wounds.

Dementia: Impairment/loss of intellect and personality due to loss or damage of neurons in the brain.

Demyelination: A loss of the fatty, white substance that coats nerves.

Dendrite: The extension of the neuron that receives electrical information from neurotransmitters.

Dengue fever: A flulike viral illness, contracted by humans through the bite of an infected *Aedes* mosquito.

Dental arch: The arched bony part of the upper and lower jaws in which the teeth are found.

Dentin: The substance that constitutes the major portion of the tooth internally.

Dentistry: The study, diagnosis, treatment, and maintenance of the teeth, gums, and other parts of the oral anatomy; also known as odontology.

Deoxyribonucleic acid (DNA): A long, spiral-shaped molecule in chromosomes; the sequence of DNA subunits contains the genetic information of the cell and organism.

Department of Health and Human Services: A federal organization, headed by a member of the U.S. president's cabinet, concerned with the health of the nation's citizens.

Dependence: A condition related to maladaptive substance use and characterized by tolerance, withdrawal, and contrived use despite psychosocial or physical impairment because of use of the substance or efforts to acquire it.

Depression: A condition characterized by persistent feelings of despair, weight change, sleep problems, thoughts of death, thinking difficulties, diminished interest or pleasure in activities, and agitation or listlessness.

Dermatitis: A general term for nonspecific skin irritations that may be caused by bacteria, viruses, or fungi.

Dermatology: The study of the skin: its chemistry, physiology, histopathology, cutaneous lesions, and the relationships of these lesions to systemic disease.

Dermatopathology: The study of diseased skin tissue.

Dermatoses: Disorders of the skin.

Dermis: The second layer of skin, immediately below the epidermis; it contains blood and lymphatic vessels, nerves, glands, and (usually) hair follicles.

Detoxification: The process by which toxic substances are removed from the body, often as a function of the body's natural responses over time; in alternative medicine, such methods as juice therapy or colon therapy may be used to aid this process.

Development: The process of progressive change that takes place as one matures from birth to death; development can be gradual (as on a continuum) or ordered (as in distinctly different stages).

Developmental disorders: A group of conditions that indicate significant delays in or a lack of social skill development, with deficiencies in adaptive behaviors, poor language skills, and a limited capacity to communicate effectively.

Diabetes mellitus: A hormonal disorder in which the pancreas is unable to produce sufficient insulin to process and maintain a proper level of sugar in the blood; if left untreated, may lead to circulatory problems, heart disease, blindness, dementia, kidney failure, and death.

Diabetic nephropathy: Kidney disease associated with long-standing diabetes.

Diagnosis: The act of identifying a specific disease using signs and symptoms as evidence.

Diagnostic: Relating to the determination of the nature of a disease.

Dialysis: The filtration of crystalloid from colloid substances; most commonly used to refer to the medical procedure performed periodically on individuals whose kidneys have failed to remove waste products and other toxic substances that build up in the blood.

Diaphragm: The muscular partition that separates the abdominal and thoracic cavities; also, a contraceptive device that covers the cervix.

Diarrhea: Loose, watery, and copious bowel movements.

Diastole: The period of relaxation of the heart between beats.

Diastolic blood pressure: The pressure of the blood within the artery while the heart is at rest.

Diathermy: The heating of body tissues because of the resistance to the passage of high-frequency electromagnetic radiation, electric current, or ultrasonic waves; also known as electrocoagulation.

DIC. *See* Disseminated intravascular coagulation (DIC).

Dietary reference intake (DRI): The amount of nutrients needed daily by a healthy person to maintain health; age and gender affect the listed DRIs.

Differentiation: The process of gradual change of tissues in the embryo or fetus.

Diffusion: The process in which substances move from an area of high concentration to an area of low concentration; if given enough time, the concentration of the substance will be the same everywhere.

DiGeorge syndrome: A pediatric syndrome caused by a missing piece of chromosome 22 and characterized by congenital heart defects, the absence or hypoplasia of the thymus and parathyroid glands, cleft palate, and dysmorphic facial features.

Digestion: The chemical breakdown of food materials in the stomach and small intestine and the absorption into the bloodstream of essential nutrients through the intestinal walls.

Digit: A finger or toe.

Dilation: The opening of the cervix to allow passage of the fetus through the birth canal.

Dilation and curettage (D & C): Dilation of the cervix to allow scraping of tissue from the endometrium (lining of the uterus); used to diagnose and treat disease and as an abortion method.

Diminished capacity: Partial insanity; a legal determination that a defendant does not have the ability to achieve the state of mind required to commit a crime.

Diopter: A unit of power of a lens equal to the reciprocal of the focal length of the lens in meters.

Diphtheria: A highly contagious bacterial infection that usually affects the respiratory system.

Diploid: Containing a double set of chromosomes.

Diplopia: Double vision.

Dipstick: A chemically treated paper strip used for the chemical analysis of urine or saliva.

Disarticulation: The amputation of a limb through a joint, without cutting the bone.

Disease: An abnormal condition of the body, with characteristic symptoms associated with it.

Disequilibrium: The sensation of being off-balance.

Disintegrative disorder: Deterioration in functioning following a period of normal development.

Disk: A soft, cushionlike structure that lies between bony vertebrae from the base of the skull to the sacrum of the pelvis; it has a soft liquid in the center and is surrounded by a thickened ligament.

Disk prolapse: The protrusion (herniation) of intervertebral disk material, which may press on spinal nerves.

Dislipidemia: Abnormal blood lipid levels, especially

characterized by high serum triglycerides and very low-density lipoproteins (VLDLs) and depressed serum high-density lipoprotein (HDL) cholesterol.

Dislocation: The forceful separation of bones in a joint.

Disorder: An abnormal physical or mental condition.

Disseminated intravascular coagulation (DIC): A hemorrhagic disorder that occurs as a complication of several different disease states and results from abnormally initiated and accelerated blood clotting.

Distal: Away from the point of origin.

Diuresis: Increased formation and excretion of urine.

Diuretic: A drug that stimulates the kidneys to eliminate more salt and water from the body.

Diverticulitis: The painful inflammation of diverticula.

Diverticulosis: A disease involving multiple out-pouchings, or diverticuli, of the wall of the colon.

Diverticulum: A pouchlike, weakened region of the colon wall, which can cause pain and bleeding.

Dizygotes: Fraternal twins; born from two ova separately fertilized by two sperm.

Dizziness: A nonspecific term that includes vertigo, fainting, and disequilibrium.

DNA. *See* Deoxyribonucleic acid (DNA).

DNA testing: A technique for identifying a person based on matching unique gene-bearing proteins from an organic sample taken from that person (such as hair, blood, or tissue) with another organic sample.

Domestic violence: Assaultive behavior intended to punish, dominate, or control another in an intimate family relationship; physicians are often best able to identify situations of domestic violence and assist victims to implement preventive interventions.

Dominant allele: The version of a gene that produces a recognizable trait in offspring when present in only one of the two chromosomes of a pair.

Dominant genetic disease: A disease caused by a mutation in a gene that need be inherited from only one parent in order to exert its effect.

Dopaminergic: Related to the brain's neurotransmitter dopamine, which plays a role in such processes as mood, movement, and psychological functioning.

Doppler shift: The increase in frequency of sound waves as the source of the waves approaches the observer or instrument; Doppler techniques are often used to assess blood flow in body channels such as veins.

Down syndrome: An inherited disease caused by a defect in chromosome 21 that produces moderate to severe mental retardation.

DRI. *See* Dietary reference intake (DRI).

Drug: Any chemical substance that can be ingested into the body to modify bodily functions and responses.

Drug interactions: The chemical effects of taking drugs in combination, where the effects will reduce, magnify, or alter the desired effects of one or more of the drugs.

Duodenum: The initial part of the small intestine, where most of the digestion of food occurs.

Duplex scan: An ultrasound representation of echo images of tissues and blood vessels combined with a Doppler representation of blood-flow patterns.

Dura mater: Tissue layer between the brain and skull.

Durable power of attorney: Designation of a person who will have legal authority to make health care decisions if the patient becomes incapable of making decisions for himself or herself.

Dwarfism: Underdevelopment of the body, most often caused by a variety of genetic or endocrinological dysfunctions and resulting in either proportionate or disproportionate development, sometimes accompanied by other physical abnormalities and/or mental deficiencies.

Dys-: A prefix denoting wrong, painful, or difficult.

Dysfunction: The disordered or impaired function of a body system, organ, or tissue.

Dyskinesia: A neurologic disorder causing difficulty in the performance of voluntary movements.

Dyslexia: Severe reading disability in children with average to above-average intelligence.

Dysmenorrhea: Painful menstruation; primary dysmenorrhea is generally harmless and occurs in young women, while secondary dysmenorrhea may be caused by endometriosis, pelvic inflammatory disease, or tumors.

Dysmorphic: Abnormal in shape or appearance.

Dyspareunia: Painful sexual intercourse.

Dyspepsia: A general term applied to several forms of indigestion.

Dysphasia: A disturbance of such language skills as speaking, reading, writing, and comprehension.

Dysplasia: Any form of abnormal tissue development.

Dyspnea: Abnormal or uncomfortable breathing.

Dystrophy: A progressive condition that occurs when required nutrients do not reach tissues or organs, causing an inability of these structures to carry out their proper functions.

Dysuria: Painful or difficult urination, often the result of urinary tract infection or obstruction.

E. coli. See *Escherichia coli.*

Eardrum: The membrane separating the outer ear canal from the middle ear that changes sound waves into movements of ossicles; also called the tympanic membrane.

Ears: The organs responsible for both hearing and balance.

Eating disorder: An emotional disorder centering on body image that leads to a misuse of food, such as overeating, overeating and purging (bulimia), or undereating (anorexia nervosa).

Ecchymosis: Bleeding into the skin, subcutaneous tissue, or mucous membranes, resulting in bruising.

ECG waves: The repeated deflections of an electrocardiogram; one complete wave consists of a P wave, followed by a QRS complex, and then a T wave and represents one complete cardiac cycle, or heartbeat.

Echocardiogram: A graph of cardiac motion and heart valve closure produced by sending sound waves to the heart and recording their deflections.

Echocardiography: The use of sound waves to record activities within the heart and great arteries and to examine heart structures.

Eclampsia: Hypertension induced by pregnancy, in its convulsive form.

Ecology: A branch of science concerned with the relationships between organisms and their environments.

Ecosystem: An ecological community considered together with the nonliving factors of its environment.

-ectomy: A suffix denoting surgical removal; for example, an appendectomy is the removal of the appendix.

Ectopic pregnancy: The development of a fertilized egg in a Fallopian tube instead of the uterus; can be fatal to the mother unless it is corrected surgically.

Eczema: A skin disorder characterized by reddening, swelling, blistering, crusting, and scabbing; also called dermatitis.

Edema: The abnormal accumulation of fluid in tissues or cavities of the body, resulting in swelling.

EEG. *See* Electroencephalography (EEG).

Effector: A general term referring to skeletal, smooth, and cardiac muscles or glands that respond to impulses produced by the nervous system.

Efficacy: The extent to which a drug or procedure works as expected under ideal conditions, such as in the laboratory; efficacy must be proven before a drug or procedure may be applied in a clinical environment.

Ehrlichiosis: Infection by one of a group of intracellular bacteria transmitted to humans through tick bites.

Ejaculation: The release of sperm from the male's body during sexual activity.

Elastin: A protein that forms the main substance of yellow elastic fibers within connective tissue such as ligaments.

Elbow: The joint between the upper arm and the forearm.

Electric anesthesia: The use of pulses of electricity to deaden nerve cells or cause unconsciousness.

Electrical shock: The physical effect of an electrical current entering the body and the resulting damage.

Electrocardiography (ECG or EKG): The recording of heartbeat activity using electrodes attached to the chest.

Electrocauterization: The use of a high-frequency electrical current or electrically heated metal to sear tissue.

Electroconvulsive therapy: The use of electric shocks to induce seizure in depressed patients as a form of treatment.

Electrodermal response biofeedback: The monitoring and displaying of information about the conductivity of the skin; used for anxiety reduction, asthma treatment, and the treatment of sleep disorders.

Electroencephalography (EEG): The recording of brain-wave activity using electrodes attached to the scalp.

Electrolytes: Chemicals that, when dissolved in water, dissociate to form positive and negative ions so that the resulting solution is an electrical conductor.

Electromyograph: An instrument that is capable of monitoring and displaying information about electrochemical activity in a group of muscle fibers.

Electromyography (EMG): An electrodiagnostic technique for recording the extracellular activity (action and evoked potentials) of skeletal muscles at rest, during voluntary contractions, and during electrical stimulation.

Electron: A tiny particle with an electronic charge; a component of an atom.

Electron volt: A unit of energy defined as the energy acquired by an electron traveling through a potential difference of 1 volt.

Elephantiasis: A grossly disfiguring disease caused by a roundworm parasite; it is the advanced stage of the disease Bancroft's filariasis, contracted through roundworms.

Embolism: The blockage of an artery by matter (such as a blood clot) that has broken off from another area.

Embolus: Any particle in the arterial or venous system that travels with the flow of blood and eventually lodges in the lungs, brain, or other organ or blood vessel.

Embryo: In humans, the cells growing from conception until the eighth week of pregnancy.

Embryology: The study of the development of the (human) organism from conception to birth.

Emergency medical services: The complete chain of human and physical resources that provides patient care in cases of sudden illness or injury.

Emergency medicine: The branch of medicine that addresses conditions (such as cardiac arrest, severe wounds, poisoning, or seizures) requiring immediate medical treatment.

Emergency room (ER): A health care facility where rapid evaluation and treatment of sudden illnesses, accidents, and traumas occurs.

Emerging diseases: Those diseases that newly appear in a populace, or have been in existence for some time but are rapidly increasing in incidence, geographic range, or surface as new drug-resistant strains of viruses, bacteria, or parasitic species.

Emetic: Something that causes vomiting (emesis).

EMG. *See* Electromyography (EMG).

Emphysema: A disease characterized by an increase in the size of air spaces at the terminal ends of bronchioles in the lungs, which reduces the ability of the lungs to exchange oxygen and carbon dioxide.

Enamel: The tissue that covers the crown of the tooth; the hardest tissue in the body.

Encephalitis: Inflammation of the brain resulting in a variety of usually serious symptoms and sometimes death.

Encephalopathy: Any abnormality in the structure or function of the brain.

End-stage renal disease: The final phase of long-standing kidney disease, characterized by a nearly complete loss of kidney function.

Endarterectomy: A surgical technique for excising atherosclerotic plaque or the diseased endothelial lining of an artery.

Endemic disease: A disease that is usually present in a specific population such that the frequency of disease occurrence does not fluctuate greatly.

Endocarditis: Inflammation of the lining of the heart and its valves.

Endocrine: Referring to a process in which cells from an organ or gland secrete substances into the blood, which in turn act on cells elsewhere in the body.

Endocrine glands: Ductless glands that secrete hormones directly into the bloodstream.

Endocrine pancreas: Specialized secretory tissue dispersed within the pancreas called islets of Langerhans, which are responsible for the secretion of glucagon and insulin.

Endocrine system: The system of glands located throughout the body that produces hormones and secretes them directly into the blood for delivery by the circulatory system.

Endocrinology: The study of the endocrine system, the glands that produce hormones and the functioning of those hormones.

Endodontic disease: Diseases of the dental pulp found within teeth and diseases of the surrounding tissues, the gums.

Endodontics: The dental specialty that treats diseases of infected pulp tissue.

Endogenous: Something occurring or naturally found within the body.

Endolymph: Inner ear fluid.

Endometrial biopsy: A procedure designed to obtain a sample of the uterine lining (endometrium) for diagnostic analysis.

Endometriosis: A female reproductive disease in which cells from the uterine lining (the endometrium) grow outside the uterus, causing severe pain and sometimes infertility or the need for hysterectomy.

Endoplasmic reticulum: A system of cytoplasmic membrane-bound sacs that, with attached ribosomes, synthesize proteins destined to enter membranes or to be stored or secreted.

Endoscope: A lighted, flexible, hollow instrument used for examination and the placement of surgical instruments.

Endoscopic retrograde cholangiopancreatography (ERCP): An endoscopic procedure in which dye is injected into the common bile duct and pancreatic ducts for visualization with X rays.

Endoscopy: The process of passing a flexible fiber-optic instrument into an area of the body (such as the gastrointestinal tract) to allow visualization.

Endospore: A modified bacterial cell that is extraordinarily resistant to heat, desiccation, and other environmental extremes.

Endothelium: The inner surface of the cornea, which is separated from the rest of the eye by a layer of transparent fluid.

Endotracheal tube: A flexible tube inserted through the mouth or nose into the trachea (windpipe) to carry anesthetic gas and oxygen directly to the lungs.

Enema: Any one of a variety of procedures for cleaning out the lower colon or injecting food or diagnostic substances.

Energy: A measure of a system's capacity to do work.

Enteroviruses: A class of viruses capable of infecting multiple organ systems, such as the central nervous system, the skin, the eyes, and the heart.

Enuresis. *See* Bed-wetting.

Environment: The biological, physical, cultural, and mental factors that influence health; anything external to an individual.

Environmental diseases: Conditions and diseases resulting from largely human-mediated hazards in both the natural and artificial environments.

Environmental health: The control of all factors in the physical environment that exercise, or may exercise, a deleterious effect on human physical development, health, and survival.

Environmental medicine: The branch of medical science that addresses the impact of chemical and physical stressors and biological hazards on the individual or group in a community.

Environmental toxicology: The study of the impact of chemical pollutants on biological organisms; human health is the primary consideration, but the specialty also examines the effects of toxins on nonhuman organisms.

Enzyme: A protein secreted by a cell that acts as a catalyst to induce chemical changes in other substances, remaining apparently unchanged itself in the process.

Enzyme therapy: The administration of enzymes to aid digestive problems.

Epidemic: A widespread, rapid occurrence of an infectious disease in a community or region at a particular time.

Epidemiology: The study of the occurrence, frequency, causes, and distribution of diseases within a population.

Epidermis: The outer layer of the skin, consisting of a dead superficial layer and an underlying cellular section.

Epididymis: An organ attached to the testis in which newly formed sperm reach maturity (that is, become capable of fertilizing an egg).

Epidural anesthesia: Anesthesia produced by injecting a local anesthetic between the vertebrae and beneath the ligamentum flavum into the extradural space; also known as extradural anesthesia.

Epilepsy: Uncontrollable excessive activity in either all or part of the central nervous system.

Epinephrine: A hormone that acts as a vasoconstrictor and cardiac stimulant.

Episiotomy: Surgical incision into the area between the anus and the vagina to enlarge the vaginal opening during childbirth.

Epi-Pen: A device that administers a prescribed dose of injectable epinephrine.

Epithelia: Tissues that originate in broad, flat surfaces, usually lining the surfaces of the body and organs.

ER. *See* Emergency room (ER).

ERCP. *See* Endoscopic retrograde cholangiopancreatography (ERCP).

Erectile dysfunction: A disorder whereby a male cannot achieve or maintain an erection suitable for sexual intercourse.

Erection: A complex phenomenon involving nerves, blood vessels, and the mind that leads to the entrapment of blood in the penis, making it rigid.

Ergonomics: The science of the relationship between the human form and its biomechanical environment.

Erythema multiforme: A skin disorder that produces multiple skin lesions and results from an allergic reaction or infection.

Erythema nodosum: Inflammation of the fatty layer of the skin resulting in red, painful bumps, usually located on the front of the legs.

Erythematous: Related to or marked by reddening.

Erythrocyte: The nonnucleated, disk-shaped blood cell that contains hemoglobin; also called a red blood cell.

Escherichia coli: A common bacterium that inhabits the human intestinal tract; used by genetic engineers to carry and propagate cloned DNA fragments and to produce proteins from the cloned genes.

Esophagectomy: Surgical removal of all or part of the esophagus.

Esophagus: The muscular tube through which food passes from the throat to the stomach.

Essential nutrient: A substance that must be included in the diet because it cannot be synthesized by the body.

Ester: The relatively non-water-soluble compound formed when an alcohol reacts with a carboxylic acid.

Estrogen: The female sex hormone produced by the ovaries and the adrenal gland that is responsible for the development of female secondary sex characteristics; the three types naturally produced by the body are estradiol, estrone, and estriol.

Ether: A volatile liquid that causes unconsciousness when inhaled.

Ethics: A philosophical discipline that attempts to analyze systematically the way in which moral decisions are made; in medicine, ethics involves defining appropriate patient care, humane biological research, an equitable distribution of scarce medical resources, and a just health care delivery system.

Etiology: The investigation of the causes of any disease.

Eustachian tube: The tube connecting the middle ear to the back of the throat; air exchange through this tube equalizes air pressure in the middle ear with the outside air pressure.

Euthanasia: The medical inducement of death to relieve suffering; though performed routinely on non-human animals, euthanasia on humans is against the law in most, but not all, societies.

Evidence-based medicine: A method of basing clinical medical practice decisions on systematic reviews of published medical studies.

Evolution: A theory that explains the development of all organisms from simple ancestor organisms.

Excision: The surgical removal of an organ or tissue.

Excisional biopsy: Biopsy by incision to excise and completely remove an entire lesion, including adjacent portions of normal tissue.

Exercise: Physical movement that boosts metabolism and strengthens the body.

Exercise physiology: The science that studies the effects on the body of various intensities and types of physical activity, including cellular metabolism, cardiovascular responses, respiratory responses, neural and hormonal adaptations, and muscular adaptations to exercise.

Exocrine glands: Glands that excrete their products into tubes or ducts.

Exogenous: Originating outside the body.

Expiration: The act of breathing out, which partly collapses the lungs.

Extended care: Long-term, ongoing medical care for individuals with serious, chronic, or terminal conditions; may be performed in a medical or hospice facility or at the individual's home.

Extended care facility: A facility that can be found in several settings, outside the home, where specialized medical care can be rendered under a physician's orders.

Extension: Movement that increases the angle between the bones, causing them to move further apart; straightening or extension of the ankle occurs when the toes point away from the shin.

Exteroreceptors: Sensory receptors generally located on the skin or body surfaces that supply the brain with information about the external environment in which the body is located.

Extracellular fluid: The internal environment of the human body that surrounds the cells; the fluid contains ions, gases, and the nutrients needed by cells for proper functioning and is constantly circulated throughout the body by the blood and into tissues by diffusion.

Extracellular respiration: The process of oxygen transport from the lungs to the cells and carbon dioxide transport from cells back to the lungs.

Extracorporeal: Pertaining to something occurring outside the body, such as therapy.

Extubation: Removal of a breathing tube.

Eyes: The body structures that receive and transform information about objects into neural impulses that can be translated by the brain into visual images.

Face lift: The separation of the skin of the face from the underlying fascia and its tightening until the desired degree of wrinkle elimination is achieved; also called rhytidectomy.

Facial nerve: The seventh cranial nerve pair, which relays signals from the face and the front region of the tongue up to the pons of the brain stem; conducts impulses related to taste, salivation, and facial expression.

Fallopian tube: One of the two tubes through which egg cells travel from the ovaries, in which they originate, to the uterus.

Family medicine: The branch of medical practice concerned with treating individuals comprehensively on a long-term basis, often along with, or in the context of, all members of that person's immediate family.

Farsightedness: The inability of the eye to focus on close objects; also called hyperopia.

Fas ligand: A membrane protein that is a member of the tumor necrosis factor family of signaling proteins; binds to a Fas receptor and induces programmed cell death.

Fascia: Connective tissues such as tendons and ligaments.

Fasciculation: A brief, spontaneous contraction of muscle fibers associated with disorders of the lower motor neurons.

Fasciectomy: Surgical removal of any part of the fascia.

Fatigue: A general symptom of tiredness, malaise, depression, and sometimes anxiety associated with many diseases and disorders; in some cases, no specific cause can be found.

Fats: A group of organic compounds, also called lipids, that store energy; one of three classes of nutrients.

Fatty acid: An organic compound that is composed of a long hydrocarbon chain with a carboxyl group at one end.

Favorable: Indicating that a better outcome is more likely to occur.

FDG-PET. *See* Fluorodeoxyglucose-positron emission tomography (FDG-PET).

Fecalith: A hardened piece of fecal matter that often begins the events leading to appendectomy by blocking the appendix.

Fee-for-service: The traditional way of paying for medical care by billing patients when services are rendered (in contrast to a health maintenance organization).

Feedback: A system in which two parts of the body communicate and control each other, often through hormones; through such a system, hormones trigger other hormones' production (stimulatory feedback) or inhibition (inhibitory feedback).

Femur: The thigh bone.

Fenestration: The surgical opening of a passage in a closed or narrowing ear canal in order to allow sound to pass.

Fermentation: A chemical reaction that splits complex organic compounds into relatively simple substances.

Fertilization: The process in which the sperm head penetrates the ovum, resulting in the formation of an embryo.

Fetal alcohol syndrome: Growth retardation and mental or physical abnormalities in a child resulting from alcohol consumption by the mother during pregnancy.

Fetal surgery: Surgical intervention in utero, before birth, if the fetus has a life-threatening condition or congenital abnormality that can be alleviated.

Fetal tissue transplantation: The controversial use of tissue from aborted human fetuses to replace damaged tissue in patients with diseases in which the patient's own tissue has been destroyed (such as Parkinson's disease or diabetes mellitus).

Fetus: The unborn child from the eighth week after fertilization until birth.

Fever: A symptom associated with a variety of diseases and disorders, characterized by body temperature above normal.

Fiber: Food material derived from plant substances that retain the full structure of their cell walls despite the chemical effects of the digestive process.

Fiber optics: The transmission of light through thin, flexible tubes.

Fibrillation: Rapid and chaotic contractions of the heart muscle.

Fibrin: A fibrous insoluble protein formed from fibrinogen by the action of thrombin, especially in the clotting of blood.

Fibrinogen: A protein produced in the liver that is present in blood plasma and is converted to fibrin during the clotting of blood.

Fibrinolysis: The breakdown of fibrin, a major component of blood clots, that occurs after the broken vessel wall has healed; fibrinolytic agents are used to dissolve unwanted clots.

Fibroblast: A cell in connective tissue that gives rise to other cells that form binding and supportive tissue of the body.

Fibrocystic breast condition: A noncancerous breast condition affecting approximately 60 percent of all women, the majority of whom are premenopausal; now considered to be a normal physiologic variant.

Fibromyalgia: A connective, soft tissue disease involving chronic, spontaneous, and widespread musculoskeletal pain, as well as recurrent fatigue and sleep disturbance.

Fibrosis: Development of scar tissue consisting of excess fibrous connective tissue.

Fibula: The smaller of the two bones in the lower leg, on the lateral side.

Fight-or-flight response: A stressful biochemical reaction in animals, usually involving the adrenal hormone epinephrine, that prepares the animal for confrontation with predators or competitors.

Filiform papillae: The small, rounded projections that form the tough, yet velvetlike, texture of the tongue surface; lacking any chemoreceptors, these papillae do not function in the process of taste.

Filovirus: A member of the family Filoviridae, characterized by a filamentous form of the virus, and causing severe hemorrhagic fever in humans.

Filtrate: Water and small solute molecules filtered from the blood by the glomerulus of the nephron.

Fistula: Any of a variety of abnormal openings from an internal organ to the body's surface.

Flagellum: A long, whiplike structure at the base of the sperm that propels it forward.

Flavivirus: A member of the family Flaviridae of single-strand RNA viruses that spread via mosquitoes and ticks.

Flexion: A bending movement that decreases the angle of the joint and brings two bones closer together; for example, flexion of the ankle pulls the foot closer to the shin.

Flora: The microorganisms that are commonly found on or in the human body; also called microflora.

Fluid: An intracellular or extracellular solution of water and other substances, the concentrations of which must be regulated to achieve proper physiological functioning.

Fluorescein: A brightly colored dye used for diagnostic purposes.

Fluorodeoxyglucose-positron emission tomography (FDG-PET): A molecular imaging method in which radioactive sugar (FDG) is injected, accumulates in tissues with hypermetabolism, and is detected by its positron emission.

Fluoroscopy: Examination of the deep structures of the body by means of a fluoroscope, which renders visible X-ray shadows by projecting them on a screen.

fMRI. *See* Functional magnetic resonance imaging (fMRI).

Foliate papillae: The folded papillae found on the soft edges of the tongue and just ahead of the V shape formed by the vallate papillae; although found in the regions that detect bitter or sour tastes, foliate papillae are not specific receptors for bitter or sour tastes.

Follicle: A small, saclike cavity for secretion or excretion, such as a hair follicle; also, spherical structures in the ovary that contain the maturing ova (eggs).

Food allergy: An abnormal response by the immune system to some foods, causing mild to severe symptoms that may become life-threatening.

Food biochemistry: The breakdown of food by cells, a process in which nutrients are converted to energy and other components needed by the body.

Food group: Category of organic material from plants or animals that share similar characteristics.

Food poisoning: Food-borne illness caused by bacteria, viruses, or parasites consumed in food and resulting in acute gastrointestinal disturbance that may include diarrhea, nausea, vomiting, and abdominal discomfort.

Foramen magnum: An opening at the bottom of the skull where the nerves from the brain pass through and connect with the spinal cord.

Forearm: The region from the elbow joint to the wrist; also called the antebrachium.

Foremilk: The milk released early in a nursing session, which is low in fat and rich in nutrients.

Forensic: Having to do with a court of justice; forensic medicine and its various subspecialties apply medical science to the purposes of the law.

Forensic autopsy: A systematic investigation to determine the cause of death, providing the pathologist with information to state an informed opinion about the manner and mechanism of death in cases that are of public interest.

Forensic pathology: The branch of medicine that applies medical knowledge to legal situations, particularly crimes; forensic specialists, for example, gather data to determine the causes and circumstances surrounding a death that is believed to be a homicide.

Forensic toxicology: The branch of toxicology that interacts regularly with the legal community and law enforcement.

Fourier transform: A mathematical method that allows MRI to utilize one radio frequency pulse and thereby examine all wavelengths, as opposed to examining each wavelength individually with a continuous wave.

Fracture: A break in a bone, which may be partial or complete.

Free radical theory: The idea that aging may be brought about by the production within the body of very reactive chemicals (free radicals) that damage chromosomes and other cell parts.

Frequency: The number of complete events per period of time; for example, sound is measured in cycles per second, and one cycle per second is equal to 1 hertz.

Frontal lobe: The area of the brain in the front of the skull, responsible for executive functions; each cerebral hemisphere has one frontal lobe.

Frontotemporal dementia (FTD): A group of neuro-degenerative disorders that affect the frontal and temporal lobes of the brain.

Frostbite: Localized freezing of tissue, usually of extremities exposed to low temperatures.

Frozen section: An extremely thin tissue section cut by a specially designed instrument called a microtome from tissue that has been rapidly frozen, for the purpose of microscopic evaluation and rendering a diagnosis.

Full-term: Referring to a gestation period of nine months.

Functional disease: A derangement in the way that normal anatomy operates; also, a disorder without any known organic basis (sometimes suggesting that the basis may be psychological).

Functional magnetic resonance imaging (fMRI): A radiologic technique that shows regional oxygen uptake, indicating brain activity.

Fungal infections: Infections caused by fungi, ranging from minor skin disease to serious, disseminated disease of the lungs and other organs.

Fungiform papillae: The papillae scattered about the tongue surface, in no specific array, that are responsive to tastant molecules; they do not exhibit specificity for a particular type of taste.

Fungus (pl. fungi): A plantlike organism that does not produce its own food through photosynthesis, instead living as a heterotroph that absorbs complex carbon compounds from other living or dead organisms.

Gallstones: Particles of cholesterol and other substances that form in the gallbladder when the solubility of bile components is altered.

Gamete intrafallopian transfer (GIFT): A treatment for infertility in which sperm and eggs are introduced surgically into a Fallopian tube, where fertilization (and subsequent implantation in the uterus) are expected to occur naturally.

Gametes: The reproductive cells in either sex (the sperm and the ova).

Gamma camera: A type of radiation-detection instrument that detects gamma rays external to the body and makes an image of the radionuclide distribution in body organs; also known as a scintillation camera.

Gamma ray: A type of electromagnetic radiation that has the same physical properties as X rays but is emitted by unstable nuclei in their decay process; gamma rays are capable of penetrating soft tissue,

thereby allowing their detection outside the body to produce images of organs.

Ganglion: A benign swelling or nodule surrounding a tendon, usually in the wrists, fingers, or feet.

Gangrene: Necrosis (tissue death) caused by obstruction of the blood supply; it may be localized to a small area or involve an entire extremity.

Gas exchange: The movement of oxygen and carbon dioxide across the membrane of the lungs and into the blood and tissues; other gases, such as nitrogen, may also cross the membrane.

Gastrectomy: Surgical removal of all or part of the stomach.

Gastric: Pertaining to the stomach.

Gastritis: Any inflammation of the stomach.

Gastroenteritis: An acute infectious process affecting the gastrointestinal system, usually leading to abdominal discomfort and diarrhea.

Gastroenterology: The medical specialty devoted to care of the digestive tract and related organs.

Gastrointestinal: Referring to the stomach and to the small and large intestines.

Gastrointestinal system: The gastrointestinal tract together with the salivary glands, pancreas, liver, and gallbladder.

Gastrointestinal tract: The digestive tract; a tubelike series of organs that includes the mouth, pharynx, esophagus, stomach, small intestine, large intestine, and anus.

Gastrostomy: Surgical incision into the stomach.

Gaucher's disease: A congenital disorder caused by a defect in lipid metabolism and characterized by cell hyperplasia in the liver, spleen, and bone marrow.

Gender: Strictly speaking, the behavioral and social aspects of being one sex versus the other; loosely used to refer to the biological and physical aspects of being male or female as well.

Gender identity: The mental view of oneself as male or female.

Gender identity disorder: A psychiatric classification describing persons experiencing a strong and persistent incongruity between their anatomy and the gender with which they identify.

Gender reassignment surgery: Also known as sex reassignment surgery; surgery aimed to alter a person's physical sexual characteristics to resemble that of the other gender.

Gender role: Behaviors and self-presentations that are associated with being male or female and that one uses to identify or recognize others as male or female; also implies societal and/or cultural expectations.

Gene: The basic unit of inheritance; at the molecular level, a gene consists of a segment of DNA that codes for a particular protein.

Gene regulation: The control of whether a gene is active (that is, encoding messenger RNA and protein) or inactive (that is, not encoding RNA or protein), a process often affected by hormones.

General anesthesia: Anesthesia that induces unconsciousness.

General practice: A primary care field in which health care is provided by physicians who usually have completed less than three years of residency training.

Generic drugs: Copycat versions of brand-name originals that are no longer protected by patents.

Genetic: Imparted at conception and incorporated into every cell of an organism.

Genetic counseling: Physician-provided advice to a couple who plan to have a child who might inherit a condition or disorder.

Genetic disease: A disease state that exists because of a decrease in or the absence of normal protein activity as the result of an alteration in the information carried in DNA.

Genetic engineering: A group of scientific techniques that allow scientists to alter genes; also called recombinant DNA research.

Genetic screening: A program designed to determine whether individuals are carriers of or are affected by a particular genetic disease.

Genetics: The study of the hereditary transmission of characteristics.

Genome: The total complement of genes inherited by an organism.

Genomics: The study of whole genomes.

Genotype: The genetic makeup of an individual; it is usually expressed as a list of alleles.

Genus: A category, below a family and above a species, used to classify living organisms and fossils.

Geriatrics: The branch of medicine that treats the conditions and diseases associated with aging and old age.

German measles. *See* Rubella.

Gerontology: The branch of medicine focused on the process of aging and the conditions and diseases that affect the elderly.

Gestation: The period from conception to birth in which the fetus reaches full development in order to survive outside the mother's body.

Gestational diabetes: A medical condition in which diabetes mellitus first occurs during pregnancy.

GIFT. *See* Gamete intrafallopian transfer (GIFT).

Gigantism: A rare endocrine disorder characterized by an overgrowth of all bones and body tissues.

Gingiva: The gum tissue surrounding the neck of the tooth.

Gingivitis: A superficial inflammation of the gums associated with the destructive buildup of dental plaque; if left untreated, it can result in periodontitis.

Gland: An organ or area of the body that produces, stores, and secretes fluids, exerting a profound effect on growth, energy production, chemical balance, reproduction, and health.

Glans penis: The head of the penis; also called the glans.

Glasses: A pair of ophthalmic lenses held together with a frame or mounting; also called spectacles.

Glaucoma: An eye disease characterized by increased intraocular pressure, which can lead to degeneration of the optic nerve and ultimately blindness if left untreated.

Glial cells: Nonexcitable cells of the nervous system; they include astrocytes, microglial cells, oligodendrocytes, and Schwann cells.

Glomerular filtration: The first step in urine formation; passive filtration in which fluids and solids dissolved in the fluid (solutes) are forced through a membrane, resulting in filtration of the blood.

Glomerulonephritis: Inflammation of the glomeruli, the clusters of blood vessels and nerves found throughout the kidney.

Glomerulus (*pl.* glomeruli): One of the very small units in the kidney, in which blood is filtered through a membrane.

Glossopharyngeal nerve: The ninth cranial nerve, which relays signals pertaining to or controlling salivation; it sends neurological information to and from the posterior region of the tongue to the medulla oblongata of the brain stem.

Glucagon: A pancreatic hormone that signals an elevated concentration of glucose circulating in the blood.

Glucocorticoids: Steroid hormones that regulate the metabolism of glucose and other organic molecules.

Gluconeogenesis: The synthesis within the body of glucose from noncarbohydrate precursors.

Glucosuria: A condition in which the concentration of blood glucose exceeds the ability of the kidney to reabsorb it; as a result, glucose spills into the urine, taking with it body water and electrolytes.

Gluten: A protein found in wheat, barley, and rye grains.

Gluten intolerance: A chronic, immune-mediated condition of progressive, itchy skin lesions triggered by ingestion of gluten.

Glycerol: A three-carbon alcohol that has one hydroxyl compound on each carbon atom.

Glycogen: The form that glucose takes when it is stored in the muscles and liver.

Glycogen storage diseases: Inherited metabolic disorders that lead to the accumulation of an abnormal amount or type of glycogen in the liver, muscles, and heart.

Glycolysis: The chemical process of splitting a molecule of glucose in order to obtain energy for other cellular processes; at times of intense activity, glycolysis produces most of the energy used by muscles.

Glycoprotein: A protein to which is attached one or more sugar molecules.

Goiter: Enlargement of the thyroid gland in the neck.

Golgi complex: A system of membrane sacs in which proteins are chemically modified, sorted, and routed to various cellular destinations.

Gonad: The male or female organ (testis or ovary, respectively) in which the essential gametes are formed for reproduction.

Gonadotrophin: A hormone secreted by the pituitary gland; the primary gonadotrophins are luteinizing hormone (LH) and follicle-stimulating hormone (FSH).

Goniometry: The measurement of angles, particularly those for the range of motion of a joint.

Gonorrhea: An infection of the urogenital tract that is a common sexually transmitted disease.

Gout: Painful arthritis of the peripheral joints, often in the big toe, caused by uric acid buildup.

Graafian follicle: Any of the ovarian follicles that produce eggs.

Graft-versus-host disease: A genetic incompatibility between tissues in which immune system cells from the grafted tissue attack host tissue.

Grafting: A surgical graft of skin from one part of the body to another or from one individual to another.

Gram staining: The use of a stain to classify bacteria as either gram-positive (they retain the primary stain of crystal violet when subjected to treatment with a decolorizer) or gram-negative (no coloration).

Grand mal: A type of epileptic seizure characterized by severe convulsions, body stiffening, and loss of consciousness during which victims fall down.

Granulocyte: A white blood cell characterized by large numbers of cytoplasmic granules, including neutrophils, eosinophils, and basophils.

Granuloma: A nodular, inflammatory lesion that is usually small, firm, and persistent and contains proliferated macrophages.

Graves' disease: A common type of hyperthyroidism in which the thyroid gland produces an oversupply of hormone.

Gross pathology: The study of that which is visible to the naked eye (macroscopic) during inspection.

Growth: The development of the human body from conception to adulthood.

Guillain-Barré syndrome: An acute degeneration of peripheral motor and sensory nerves, known to physicians as acute inflammatory demyelinating polyneuropathy, a common cause of acute generalized paralysis.

Gum disease: Inflammation of the soft tissue that surrounds the teeth; in advanced disease, there is also loss of bone that holds the teeth in place.

Gustation: The ability to taste, which is independent of smell (olfaction) or textural and temperature enhancements; ageusia, or apogeusia, is the loss of taste sensation.

Gynecology: The branch of medicine that focuses on the conditions and disorders affecting the female reproductive system.

Hair: Threadlike outgrowths of nonliving, mostly proteinaceous material that covers much of the body of humans and other mammals.

Hair transplantation: The surgical relocation of healthy hair follicles to a part of the scalp where shrunken follicles are producing short, thin hair or no hair.

Half-life: The time required for half of the nuclei in a radioactive sample to decay.

Halitosis: Bad breath, usually the result of drinking alcohol, smoking, and eating pungent foods but sometimes the result of bacteria.

Hallucinations: The perception of sensations without relevant external stimuli.

Hallucis: The big toe; the flexor hallucis longus is a muscle that flexes the big toe.

Hammertoe: An abnormality of the tendon in a toe that causes the main joint to curve upward and can be painful as a result of shoe pressure.

Haploid: Containing only a single set of chromosomes; mature gametes are haploid.

Hard palate: The bony portion of the roof of the mouth, contiguous with the soft palate.

Harelip. *See* Cleft lip.

Hashimoto's thyroiditis: An inflammation of the thyroid gland caused when abnormal blood antibodies and white blood cells infiltrate and attack thyroidal cells.

HDLs. *See* High-density lipoproteins.

Headaches: Pain localized in the head or neck, often caused by tension but also the result of a range of disorders.

Healing: The process of mending damaged tissue by which an organism restores itself to health.

Health: A condition in which all functions of the body, mind, and spirit are normally active.

Health care system: The collection of services in a given country that provide hospital, emergency, preventative, and other outpatient care to citizens.

Health insurance: The promise by a company to pay specified costs related to the health care of an individual or group of individuals who pay premium fees.

Health maintenance: The practice of anticipating, finding, preventing, and/or dealing with potential or established medical problems at the earliest possible stage to minimize adverse effects on the patient.

Health maintenance organization (HMO): A group of general practitioners, specialists, and allied health professionals who provide medical services to subscribers who pay a regular maintenance fee.

Hearing loss: Loss of sensitivity to sound pressure changes as a result of congenital factors, disease, traumatic injury, noise exposure, or aging.

Heart: The muscle that pumps blood through the body by means of rhythmic contractions.

Heart attack: Sudden and permanent damage to a part of the heart muscle as a result of impaired blood flow through the coronary arteries; the common term for myocardial infarction.

Heart block: A delay or blockage of the electrical signal traveling through the heart muscle, which upsets the synchronization between contractions of the upper and lower chambers.

Heart failure: A condition in which the heart cannot pump enough blood to meet the body's needs.

Heart rate: The number of times the heart contracts, or beats, per minute.

Heart transplantation: The removal of a diseased heart and its replacement with a healthy donor heart.

Heart valve replacement: A surgical procedure involving the removal of a defective heart valve and its replacement with another tissue valve or with a mechanical valve.

Heartburn: The presence of a burning sensation in the chest and throat caused by the reflux of stomach acids.

Heat: The transfer of energy across a boundary because of a temperature difference.

Heat exhaustion: Mild shock caused by a decrease in the amount of fluid in the blood.

Heatstroke: A medical emergency in which high body temperatures result in organ damage.

Heel spur: A bony outgrowth on the heel of the foot.

Heimlich maneuver: An emergency technique used to prevent suffocation when the airway becomes blocked.

Helminths: A general term for roundworms (nematodes) and flatworms (platyhelminths), many of which are parasites of humans and animals.

Hematology: The study of the blood, including its normal constituents and such blood disorders as anemia, leukemia, and hemophilia.

Hematoma: A localized collection of clotted blood in an organ or tissue as a result of internal bleeding.

Hematopoiesis: The production of red and white cells and platelets, which occurs mainly in bone marrow; also called hematosis.

Hematuria: The abnormal presence of blood in the urine.

Hemiplegia: Paralysis or weakness on one side of the body.

Hemochromatosis: A multisystem disease characterized by increased iron absorption and storage.

Hemodialysis: The removal of toxins from blood through the process of dialysis.

Hemodynamics: The study of blood circulation.

Hemoglobin: The oxygen-carrying iron-containing pigment present in red blood cells that is responsible for oxygen exchange in cells and tissues.

Hemolysis: Breakdown of red blood cells and the release of hemoglobin.

Hemolytic anemia: Anemia resulting from hemolysis, the excessive destruction of red blood cells.

Hemophilia: A hereditary blood defect (occurring almost exclusively in males) characterized by delayed clotting of the blood and consequent difficulty in controlling bleeding even after minor injuries.

Hemorrhage: The loss of a large amount of blood in a short period of time.

Hemorrhagic fever: A disease in humans or other animals characterized by a high fever and a bleeding disorder, affecting multiple organ systems and, if severe, leading to death.

Hemorrhoids: Dilated blood vessels in the anus or rectum that are itchy and painful.

Hemostasis: The stopping of blood flow through the blood vessels, usually as a result of blood clotting.

Hepatic: Of or referring to the liver.

Hepatitis: Inflammation of the liver.

Hepatitis A virus: The virus associated with certain forms of hepatitis; generally contracted through fecal contamination of food and water.

Hepatitis B virus: The agent associated with severe forms of viral hepatitis; contracted through contaminated blood or hypodermic needles or through contaminated body fluids.

Hepatitis C virus: Formerly referred to as the etiological agent for non-A, non-B viral hepatitis; most often passed in contaminated blood.

Hepato-: A prefix denoting an association with the liver; for example, a hepatocyte is a liver cell.

Hepatocyte: The functional cell of the liver.

Herbal medicine: A nontraditional form of medicine that uses different types of herbs for therapy and health maintenance.

Hernia: A pouch of intestines and/or vital organs of the abdomen that protrudes through the abdominal wall.

Herpes: A family of viruses that cause several diseases, including infectious mononucleosis, cold sores, genital herpes, and chickenpox.

Heterosexual: Being principally attracted to and aroused by opposite-gender persons.

Heterozygous: Having two different alleles for a particular gene.

Heuristics: Methods used to aid and guide in the discovery of a disease process when incomplete knowledge exists.

Hiatal hernia: A condition in which a portion of the stomach protrudes into the chest cavity through an opening in the diaphragm.

High-density lipoproteins (HDLs): A form of cholesterol in the blood that appears to be associated with a lower risk of arterial and heart disease.

Hindmilk: The milk released late in a nursing session, which is higher in fat content.

Hippocratic oath: A document written in the fifth century B.C.E. to offer guidelines for the emerging medical profession.

Hirsutism: Excessive hair growth.

Histamine: A compound released during allergic reactions that causes many of the symptoms of allergies.

Histamine II blockers: Various drugs that combat the chemical action of ulcers by reducing the secretion of gastric juices, or "stomach acids."

Histiocytosis: A group of relatively rare blood disorders characterized by the abnormal accumulation of white blood cells called histiocytes, leading to a wide range of adverse bodily responses.

Histocompatibility: Tissue compatibility, as determined by histocompatibility protein antigens present on the cell membranes of all tissue cells.

Histology: The branch of medicine that focuses on the study of cells and tissues as they relate to their function.

Histopathology: The histologic or microscopic description of abnormal pathologic tissue changes; these changes can be seen under the microscope.

HIV. *See* Human immunodeficiency virus (HIV).

HLAs. *See* Human leukocyte antigens (HLAs).

HMO. *See* Health maintenance organization (HMO).

Hodgkin's disease: A neoplastic disorder originating in the tissues of the lymphatic system, recognized by distinctive histologic changes and defined by the presence of Reed-Sternberg cells.

Holistic: The philosophy that individuals function as complete units or integrated systems and are not understood merely through their parts.

Holistic medicine: An approach to the practice of medicine based on the philosophy that treatment must occur taking into consideration the entire organism, both physiological and psychological.

Home care: The provision of outside services to a patient living in a home setting.

Homeopathy: A nontraditional approach to treatment based on a theory of Samuel Hahnemann, called the "law of similars," positing that substances which provoke disease may be used in small doses to treat the disease.

Homeostasis: The maintenance of a constant internal environment; the systems of the body work together to maintain constant temperature, pH, oxygen availability, water content, ion concentrations, and so on.

Homosexual: Being principally attracted to and aroused by persons of one's own gender; two synonymous terms are "gay," which can refer to all homosexuals or to homosexual males exclusively, and "lesbian," which refers only to homosexual females.

Homozygous: Having two identical alleles of a particular gene.

H1N1 influenza: An acute respiratory infection caused by the H1N1 subtype of the influenza A virus.

Hormone: A substance that creates a specific effect in an organ distant from its site of production.

Hormone receptor: A molecule contained in or on a cell that allows it to respond to a hormone; if receptors are not present, the hormone will have no effect.

Hormone therapy: The use of hormones as treatment, especially the use of estrogens, with or without progesterone, to treat menopausal symptoms.

Hospice: A program designed to ease the suffering and grief for terminally ill patients and their families; care can be rendered in the home or in a special hospice setting with special emphasis on the relief of pain.

Hospital: An institution focused on the management, prevention, and treatment of illness, utilizing a staff of medical and allied health professionals to provide medical, surgical, and psychiatric treatments, along with emergency care and evaluation.

Host: The body of the person or animal infected with a pathogen, especially a parasite.

Host-defense mechanisms: Immunological methods that the body uses to protect against external infectious agents and to maintain internal homeostasis, such as skin, sweat, urine, tears, phagocytes, and "helpful" bacteria.

Host-versus-graft disease: A tissue rejection in which the immune system cells of the graft recipient attack the grafted tissue from a donor individual.

Hot flashes: Temporary sensations of warmth experienced by perimenopausal and postmenopausal women in which the upper body feels hot, the skin turns red, and sweating occurs.

HPV. *See* Human papillomavirus (HPV).

Human immunodeficiency virus (HIV): The virus that causes acquired immunodeficiency syndrome (AIDS); it may be transmitted through blood or semen.

Human leukocyte antigens (HLAs): Structures located on the surface of each cell that are unique to an individual; also called transplantation antigens.

Human papillomavirus (HPV): A common virus affecting skin and mucosal surfaces; some types are implicated in cervical and anal cancer.

Humerus: The bone that forms the structural beam of the upper arm.

Huntington's disease: A genetic disease characterized by uncoordinated movements as a result of neuron degeneration.

Hydro-: A prefix denoting water or fluid.

Hydrocarbon: An organic compound composed of only hydrogen and carbon atoms that does not dissolve in water (water-insoluble).

Hydrocele: A fluid-filled area around the testis often caused by infection or inflammation.

Hydrocelectomy: Surgical removal of a hydrocele.

Hydrocephalus: An excessive collection of cerebrospinal fluid in the brain.

Hydrocortisone: Pharmaceutical term for cortisol.

Hydrophilic: "Water-loving" or water-attracting; a term given to molecules or regions of molecules that interact favorably with water.

Hydrophobic: "Water-hating" or "water-repelling"; a term given to molecules or regions of molecules that do not interact favorably with water.

Hydrotherapy: A form of treatment that uses water, externally, to aid in recovery or ease pain.

Hygiene: The science of health and the prevention of disease.

Hyper-: A prefix denoting "high" or more than normal.

Hyperalimentation: Intravenous fluid providing nutrition.

Hyperandrogenism: Higher-than-normal levels of androgens in the blood.

Hyperglycemia: High blood glucose.

Hyperinsulinemia: Abnormally high serum insulin concentration.

Hyperlipidemia: The presence of abnormally large amounts of lipids in the blood.

Hypernatremia: A high salt concentration in the blood that can result in seizure and coma.

Hyperopia: The inability of the eye to focus on close objects; also called farsightedness.

Hyperparathyroidism: The excessive, uncontrolled secretion of parathyroid hormone.

Hyperplasia: A proliferation of cells in response to either normal or abnormal physiological processes.

Hypersensitivity: An overreaction by the immune system to the presence of certain antigens; this overreaction often results in some damage to the person as well as the antigen.

Hypertension: High blood pressure; a systolic pressure of at least 140 or a diastolic pressure of at least 90.

Hyperthermia: The elevation of the body core temperature of an organism above a normal range.

Hypertrophy: The growth of a tissue or organ as a result of an increase in the size of existing cells.

Hyperventilation: Breathing at a faster rate than what is needed for metabolism, resulting in the exhalation of carbon dioxide faster than it is produced.

Hyphae: The long, filamentous, often branching cells of many fungi.

Hypnosis: The induction of an altered state of consciousness.

Hypo-: A prefix denoting "low" or less than normal.

Hypocalcemia: Low blood levels of calcium.

Hypochondriasis: A condition in which patients believe strongly that they are suffering from one or more serious illnesses, even when this belief is unsupported by medical evidence.

Hypodermis: The layer of fat under the dermis that contains carotene.

Hypoglycemia: A condition in which the concentration of glucose in the blood is too low to meet the needs of key organs, especially the brain.

Hypoparathyroidism: The reduced secretion of parathyroid hormone.

Hypospadias: An abnormal urethral opening in the penis, either on the underside or on the perineum.

Hypotension: Decrease in blood pressure to the point that insufficient blood flow causes symptoms.

Hypothalamus: The region of the brain called the diencephalon, forming the floor of the third ventricle, including neighboring, associated nuclei.

Hypothermia: A subnormal body temperature; clinically, it is a sustained cooling of the body to lower-than-normal temperatures.

Hypothyroidism: A condition in which the thyroid gland produces an insufficient supply of hormone.

Hypoxia: A deficiency in the amount of oxygen reaching the body tissues.

Hysterectomy: The surgical removal of the uterus. In a total hysterectomy, the uterus, ovaries, and Fallopian tubes are removed.

Iatrogenic: Referring to a complication or negative reaction resulting from physician intervention or contracted as a result of actions taken in a clinical setting.

Idiopathic: Referring to a medical condition with no known cause.

IgE. *See* Immunoglobulin E (IgE).

Ileostomy: The surgical creation of a fistula through which the lower part of the small intestine (ileum) passes to create an artificial bowel.

Ileum: The lower third of the small intestine, which joins with the colon.

Illicit drugs: Drugs that are illegal to possess, have addiction potential, and lack approved medical uses.

Imaging: Any one of a wide variety of technologies for creating visual depictions of the internal structures of the body, including (among others) X radiation, MRI, CT scanning, PET scanning, ultrasonography, and radionuclide scanning.

Immune response: The reaction of an intricate system of cells, which identify, attack, immobilize, and remove foreign tissue from the body through chemical signals.

Immune system: A body system (including the thymus, bone marrow, and lymph tissues) and processes that protect the body from foreign substances by identifying and destroying them.

Immunity: Resistance to infection by a particular disease-causing microorganism, often acquired by vaccination.

Immunization: The process of creating an immunity to a disease through the introduction of vaccines or other agents designed to produce the immunity.

Immunoassay: The use of antibody-antigen recognition as the basis of a medically useful method of detecting and measuring a substance in body fluids.

Immunocompromised: Referring to a condition in which the immune system is impaired in some way, such as being not fully developed, deficient, or suppressed.

Immunodeficiency disorders: Genetic or acquired disorders in which the normal functioning of the immune system is disturbed.

Immunoglobulin: The globulin fraction of serum protein.

Immunoglobulin E (IgE): A type of antibody associated with the release of granules from basophils and mast cells; ordinarily, a relatively rare antibody, but in patients with atopic dermatitis, levels can be significantly higher than in the general population.

Immunology: The branch of medicine that studies the immune system: its function and processes and agents that affect its function either positively or negatively, including allergies.

Immunopathology: The study of conditions or diseases that impair the immune system.

Immunosuppression: A decrease in the effectiveness of the immune system; drugs are sometimes used to depress the immune system in order to lower the probability of rejection in organ transplantation.

Immunotherapy: Therapy using antibodies or other immune system components or using antigens designed to stimulate an immune response.

Implant: A section of endometrial tissue found outside the uterus; also, an artificial part or device inserted surgically in a part of the body (such as a breast).

Implantation: The process in which the embryo attaches to the uterine lining; also, the surgical process of adding an artificial body part, such as a pacemaker.

Impotence: The inability to achieve or maintain an erection.

In utero: A Latin term meaning "in the womb."

In vitro fertilization: Fertilization of an ovum outside the female body, in an artificial culture in a test tube or dish.

In vivo fertilization: Fertilization of an ovum naturally, within the female body.

Incidence: The number of new illnesses or events occurring over a specified period of time among a specific population.

Incision: A cut made with a scalpel.

Incisional biopsy: The biopsy of a selected sample of lesion.

Incisor: One of the front teeth, used primarily to cut or shear food with a scissoring motion.

Incontinence: The inability to control the expulsion of urine or feces.

Incubation period: The time between first exposure to an organism and onset of symptoms.

Incubator: In the nursery, a Plexiglas unit that encloses the premature or sick infant to allow strict temperature regulation.

Incus: A small bone within the middle ear; also called the anvil because of its shape.

Indigestion: A digestive disorder characterized by a burning sensation in the chest and throat, sometimes by abdominal pain, bloating, nausea, vomiting, and diarrhea; also called dyspepsia.

Infant: A young child from birth to twelve months of age.

Infarction: Damage resulting from insufficient blood supply to a tissue or organ.

Infection: The invasion of healthy tissue by a pathogenic microorganism, resulting in the production of toxins and subsequent injury of tissue.

Infectious disease: A disease that is capable of being transmitted; often caused by a microorganism.

Infectivity: The ability of an organism to enter and reproduce within a host.

Inferior: Situated below another part; for example, the ankle bones are inferior to the bones of the lower leg.

Infiltration: Movement of fluid into the tissue.

Inflammation: Irritation caused by such things as infection, injury, allergy, or toxins; symptoms include redness, swelling, warmth, pain, and drainage.

Influenza: Any one of a group of serious respiratory diseases caused by viruses; different strains of the "flu" have been responsible for worldwide epidemics.

Informed consent: The process of educating a patient fully about the purpose, benefits, and risks of a clinical trial or procedure and of obtaining authorization to perform it.

Inguinal hernia: The most common form of hernia, in which the hernial sac protrudes into the lower groin area.

Inhalant: Medication that is inhaled into the lungs.

Inheritance: The passage of traits from parents to offspring in discrete units called genes.

Injection: Administration into the skin, muscle, or blood vessels via needle.

Inner ear: An organ that includes the cochlea (for detection of sound) and the labyrinth (for detection of movement).

Inoculate: To introduce immunologically active material in order to treat or prevent a disease.

Inotropic agent: A drug that improves the ability of the heart muscle to contract.

Inpatient care: Evaluation and treatment services requiring an overnight stay in a medical facility.

Insane: In legal terms, a state wherein a person is said to be incapable of appreciating the wrongfulness of certain acts or of conforming to the requirements of the law.

Insemination: The placement of semen in the female reproductive tract, which may occur naturally as a result of sexual intercourse or artificially as a result of a medical procedure.

Insomnia: Disturbed sleep; insomnia can be caused by many factors, such as dysfunctional sleep cycle, breathing problems, leg jerking, underlying medical and psychiatric disorders, and the side effects of medication.

Inspiration: The act of breathing in, which expands the lungs.

Instinctual drives: Libido (the seeking of gratification of sexual impulses) and aggression (the seeking of gratification of destructive impulses).

Insulin: A hormone secreted by the pancreas that is essential in regulating blood glucose, as well as in assimilating carbohydrates for growth and energy.

Integrase: A virally encoded enzyme that catalyzes the integration of viral double-stranded DNA into the host genome.

Intensive care: Continuous medical treatment involving vigilant monitoring of the vital signs of patients with grave physical conditions.

Interferons: A family of proteins; some induce an antiviral state within a cell, while others serve to regulate aspects of the immune response.

Intermittent care: Services provided one or more times a week with each visit limited in time.

Intermittent claudication: Pain that comes and goes in the leg as a result of poor circulation in the arteries of the lower extremities.

Internal medicine: The branch of medicine that focuses on the diagnosis and treatment of diseases, particularly of the internal organs, in adults; practitioners of internal medicine, called internists, often act as primary care physicians.

Internship: A synonym for the first year of residency training for a variety of master's- and doctoral-level practitioners in diverse fields.

Interstitial: Referring to the spaces within the tissues or other structures of the body, but not the large body cavities.

Interstitial pulmonary fibrosis (IPF): A disease characterized by scarring and thickening of lung tissue, which causes breathing difficulty.

Intervertebral disks: Flattened disks of fibrocartilage that separate the vertebrae and allow cushioned flexibility of the spinal column.

Intervertebral foramina: Openings between two adjacent vertebrae to permit the exit of nerve structures from the spinal cord.

Intestinal lumen: The inner cavity of the intestine, which represents the food (chyme) compartment.

Intestines: The section of the gut between the anus and the stomach, consisting of the rectum, colon, and small bowel (subdivided into the ileus, jejunum, and duodenum).

Intoxication: Poisoning of the body by toxins, such as drugs; also, alcohol intoxication (drunkenness).

Intracellular fluid: The fluid within cells.

Intraocular pressure: The degree of firmness of the eyeball, as controlled by the proper secretion and drainage of the aqueous humor.

Intravascular fluid: The fluid carried within the blood vessels; it is in a constant state of motion because of the pumping action of the heart.

Intravenous (IV) therapy: The introduction of medication into a vein with a special needle.

Intraventricular hemorrhage: Bleeding into or around the normal fluid spaces within the brain.

Intubation: The introduction of a tube into a body cavity, as into the larynx.

Invasive: Referring to any process (such as disease) that spreads throughout an area of the body or any procedure (such as diagnostic or therapeutic surgery) that requires entry into the body through the skin.

Involuntary muscle contractions: Muscle contractions that occur unconsciously, such as those of the intestines.

Ionization: A process in which a neutral atom loses one or more of its orbital electrons because of light, heat, or electrical collisions.

Ions: Small chemical substances that have a positive or negative charge; the most important ions with a positive charge are sodium, potassium, hydrogen, and calcium, while the most important negative ion is chloride.

Ipecac: A plant extract that will induce vomiting when orally administered; the syrup can be used to induce vomiting after ingestion of a poisonous substance.

IPF. *See* Interstitial pulmonary fibrosis (IPF).

Iris: The circular pigmented membrane behind the cornea, perforated by the pupil; the most anterior portion of the vascular tunic of the eye.

Iron-deficiency anemia: Anemia characterized by low serum iron concentration.

Ischemia: A local anemia or area of diminished or insufficient blood supply caused by mechanical obstruction of the blood supply (commonly, the narrowing of an artery).

Islets of Langerhans: Clusters of cells scattered throughout the pancreas; they produce three hormones involved in sugar metabolism: insulin, glucagon, and somatostatin.

Isokinetic: Referring to the resistance training that provides muscular overload at a constant preset speed.

Isotonic: A solution that causes no change in cell volume.

Isotypes: The different classes of antibodies.

Itching: An irritating skin sensation that provokes a desire to scratch the affected area; also called pruritus.

-itis: A suffix denoting inflammation; for example, laryngitis is an inflammation of the larynx.

IV therapy. *See* Intravenous (IV) therapy.

Jaundice: A yellowish coloration of the skin and mucous membranes caused by high levels of bilirubin in the blood; the result of liver malfunction.

Jejunum: A region of the small intestine located below the duodenum.

Jet lag: The malaise, headache, fatigue, gastrointestinal disorders, and other symptoms that may result from traveling across several time zones within a few hours.

Joint: The conjunction of two or more bones.

Joint replacement. *See* Arthroplasty.

Karyotype: An analysis of the chromosomes from the cells of an individual; it can be used to predict the chromosomal set of a fetus or the presence of a large chromosomal abnormality.

Keratin: An extremely tough protein that is the chief constituent of the epidermis, hair, nails, and tooth enamel.

Keratinocytes: Matrix basal epithelial cells that differentiate, fill with keratin, and form the dead horny substance making up the nail plate.

Keratitis: A state of inflammation of the cornea that may cause partial or total opacity, leading to loss of vision.

Keratoses: Wartlike growths caused by the excessive production of the skin protein keratin, usually occurring in elderly people.

Keratotomy: Surgical incision into the cornea of the eye to correct myopia (nearsightedness) or astigmatism.

Ketones: The by-products of fat metabolism; their presence may be indicative of diabetes mellitus.

Kidney transplantation: A surgical procedure that replaces the recipient's diseased, nonfunctioning kidney with a donated one.

Kidneys: The organs that control the amount and composition of body water by separating the blood into waste products (which leave the body as urine) and nutrients (which are returned to the blood).

Kilocalorie: The unit measurement of food energy, defined as the amount of heat needed to raise the temperature of 1 kilogram of water 1 degree Celsius; also known as a Calorie.

Kinase: An enzyme that catalyzes the transfer of phosphate from adenosine triphosphate (ATP) to another molecule.

Kinesiology: The study of the body's movement and the function of structures involved in that movement.

Klippel-Trenaunay syndrome: A rare congenital syndrome characterized by hemangiomas of the vascular system that can affect bone or soft tissue throughout the body.

Kluver-Bucy syndrome: A series of symptoms following temporal-lobe removal, such as psychic blindness, abnormal oral tendencies, and changes in sexuality.

Knee: The joint between the thigh and the lower leg.

Knockout mouse: A mouse in which a specific gene has been inactivated or "knocked out."

Koch's postulates: Criteria for judging whether given bacteria cause a given disease, including that the bacteria must be present in every case, that they must be isolated from the host and grown in pure culture, that the disease must be reproduced when the culture is inoculated into a healthy susceptible host, and that the bacteria must be recoverable from the experimentally infected host.

Kupffer cells: Specialized cells in the liver that perform the function of removing bacterial debris from the blood that has circulated throughout the body.

Kwashiorkor: A protein-deficiency disease that may affect young children in developing countries.

L-dopa (L-dihydroxyphenylalanine or levodopa): An amino acid that is the parent compound for dopamine; used to treat parkinsonism.

Labia: The folds of tissue along the external portion of a woman's vagina and urethra.

Labor: The physiological process by which the fetus and placenta are expelled from the uterus; labor involves strong uterine contractions.

Laboratory tests: The collection and analysis of body fluids such as blood and urine in order to establish a diagnosis or to monitor a treatment regimen.

Labyrinth: A structure consisting of three fluid-filled, semicircular canals at right angles to one another in the inner ear; they monitor the position and movement of the head.

Laceration: A torn, jagged wound, or an unintentional cut (as opposed to an incision).

Lacrimal: Pertaining to the secretion and conduction of tears.

Lacteals: Lymphatic capillaries in the villi of the small intestine that absorb fat, producing a milky substance called chyle.

Lactiferous duct: A single excretory duct from each lobe of mammary glandular tissue that converges yet opens separately at the tip of the nipple; the mammary gland has fifteen to twenty lactiferous ducts.

Lamellar keratoplasty: The partial removal or transplantation of a portion of the cornea; usually possible in younger patients or those with less advanced disorders.

Lamina (*pl.* laminae): An arch of the vertebral bones.

Laminaria: A type of seaweed that absorbs water and swells; it can be used to dilate the cervix.

Laminectomy: Surgical removal of part or all of a lamina to relieve pressure on the spinal cord; sometimes called fusion surgery.

Laparoscopy: A surgical procedure in which an instrument is inserted into the abdominal cavity through tiny incisions in the abdomen; usually performed without hospitalization.

Laparotomy: A surgical procedure, often exploratory in nature, carried out through the abdominal wall; it may be used to correct endometriosis.

Laryngectomy: Surgical removal of all or part of the larynx.

Laryngitis: Inflammation of the larynx, characterized by hoarseness in the voice and sometimes the inability to speak.

Larynx: The voice organ, lying between the pharynx and the trachea; commonly called the voice box.

Laser: An acronym for "light amplification by stimulated emission of radiation"; a laser produces a high-intensity light beam at a single wavelength.

Latent: Lying hidden or undeveloped within a person; unrevealed.

Lateral: On the outer side; for example, toward the little toe when in reference to the leg.

LDLs. *See* Low-density lipoproteins.

Lead poisoning: Poisoning as the result of ingestion or inhalation of abnormally high levels of lead, which disrupts kidney function and damages the nervous system.

Learning disabilities: A variety of disorders involving the failure to learn an academic skill despite normal levels of intelligence.

Leg: The lower extremity, excluding the foot; the upper leg runs from the hip to the knee, and the lower leg runs from the knee to the ankle.

Legionnaires' disease: Acute bacterial pneumonia that resembles influenza and that may prove fatal to older persons or those individuals with previous lung damage.

Leishmaniasis: One of several diseases associated with the single-celled protozoan genus *Leishmania*,

transmitted by the bite of a sandfly, that cause ulcers in the skin or internal organs.

Lens: A transparent, flexible structure, convex on both surfaces and lying directly behind the iris of the eye; it focuses light rays onto the retina.

Leprosy: A bacterial infection that affects the skin and nerves, causing symptoms ranging from numbness to disfigurement.

Lesion: A visible local tissue abnormality such as a wound, sore, rash, or boil, that can be benign, cancerous, gross, occult, or primary.

Leukemia: A condition characterized by the presence of an increased number of leukocytes in the blood, with the specific disorder classified according to the predominant proliferating cells, the clinical course, and the duration of the disease.

Leukocyte: A white or colorless blood corpuscle.

Leukodystrophy: A group of genetic disorders characterized by progressive deterioration of the white matter (myelin sheath) of the brain.

Leukopenia: An abnormal decrease in white blood cells.

Liability: Responsibility for wrongdoing.

Ligament: A tough, rubber band-like structure that connects one bone to another and prevents the abnormal motion of these bones in relationship to each other.

Light therapy: A nontraditional form of therapy that employs light to alleviate symptoms such as depression.

Lingual: Related to the tongue; in dentistry, the inner sides or faces of the teeth.

Lipases: Enzymes secreted by the pancreas into the small intestine that break down fatty materials (triglycerides) in the first intestinal stage of digestion.

Lipids: Any of a group of fatty substances including triglycerides, phospholipids, and sterols (such as cholesterol).

Lipopolysaccharide (LPS): A major component of the cell walls of gram-negative bacteria; the toxicity of LPS is associated with illnesses caused by gram-negative organisms.

Lipoproteins: Lipid aggregates that transport fat and cholesteryl esters in the circulation; associated apolipoproteins determine how rapidly they are taken up by the liver or other tissues.

Liposuction: A cosmetic method for removing body fat by a surgical vacuuming procedure.

Lithium: A drug used in the treatment of bipolar disorder.

Lithotripsy: Pulverization of stones (calculi) located in the kidneys, bladder, or urethra by means of high-frequency sound waves.

Liver: A vital organ that controls blood sugar levels; metabolizes carbohydrates, lipids, and proteins; stores blood, iron, and some vitamins; degrades steroid hormones; and inactivates and/or excretes certain drugs and toxins.

Liver transplantation: Surgery performed to replace a diseased, nonfunctional liver with one that is healthy and capable of carrying out normal liver functions.

Living will: A legally binding document instructing a physician whether or not to prolong life by externally administered life-support systems if the patient is unable to express his or her decision concerning physician-recommended forms of medical treatment.

Lobectomy: The removal of a lobe of the brain, or a major part of a lobe.

Lobotomy: The separation of either an entire lobe or a major part of a lobe from the rest of the brain.

Lobule: Small gland that, when sent appropriate hormonal cues, produces breast milk.

Local anesthesia: The injection of medication into the body that renders the immediate area free of pain, allowing surgery in that area to be performed.

Lockjaw. *See* Tetanus.

Long-term care: Health care or personal care performed for someone who is chronically unable to provide his or her own care; the cornerstone of assisted living.

Loss-of-control syndrome: A pattern of behavior characterized by violent and emotional outbursts, occasionally associated with temporal-lobe seizures.

Lou Gehrig's disease. *See* Amyotrophic lateral sclerosis (ALS).

Low-density lipoproteins (LDLs): A form of cholesterol in the blood that appears to be associated with a higher risk of arterial and heart disease.

Lower extremities: The legs (thighs, lower legs, and feet), which are attached to the pelvis at the hip joint and which consist of muscles, bones, blood vessels, lymph vessels, nerves, skin, and toenails.

LPS. *See* Lipopolysaccharide (LPS).

Lumbar puncture: A procedure to extract cerebrospinal fluid from the lumbar region of the spine (between the ribs and the pelvis), usually to diagnose disease (such as meningitis) or to administer therapeutic drugs (in leukemia treatment, for example).

Lumbar vertebrae: The five bones of the spinal column in the lower back, which experience the greatest stress in the spine.

Lumen: The space within an artery, vein, or other tube.

Lumpectomy: Surgical removal of a lump, often in the female breast.

Lungs: Vital organs that allow gas exchange between an organism and its environment.

Lunula: A whitish, crescent-shaped area at the end of the proximal nail fold that marks the end of the nail matrix and is the site of mitosis and nail growth.

Lupus: Systemic lupus erythematosus; a chronic inflammatory disease characterized by an arthritic condition and a rash.

Lyme disease: Lyme disease involves a mild-to-serious infection caused by the bacteria *Borrelia burgdorferi*, which is spread by the bite of infected ticks.

Lymph: The straw-colored fluid of the lymphatic system containing infection-fighting lymphocytes; as much as 1 to 2 liters is collected from tissue each day and returned to the bloodstream.

Lymph node: A small, oval structure that filters tissue fluids; lymph nodes are found in areas such as the armpits, groin, mouth, and neck, and serve as sites of immune response.

Lymphadenectomy: The removal of lymph nodes, one or more in a group.

Lymphadenopathy: Enlarged lymph nodes, which may be caused by any disorder related to the lymphatic vessels or lymph nodes.

Lymphatic system: A major part of the body's immune system, consisting of lymphatic vessels and lymph nodes, that transports lymph through tissues and organs and drains it back into the bloodstream.

Lymphocyte: A small white blood cell constituting about 25 percent of all blood cells; two basic types are B cells (antibody production) and T cells (cellular immunity).

Lymphoma: A group of cancers that affect lymphatic tissue.

Lysosome: An organelle inside cells that contains a variety of enzymes for breaking down cellular constituents.

Lysosyme: An enzyme found in body secretions that destroys bacteria by breaking down their walls.

Macrophage: A white blood cell that engulfs foreign substances and stimulates other immune cells.

Macular degeneration: The progressive breakdown of the macula, the part of the eye that allows for detailed sight in the center of the field of vision, with a dense concentration of rods and cones.

Magnetic field therapy: A practical and inexpensive modality that uses magnets to relieve chronic and acute pain incurred through overuse or trauma.

Magnetic resonance imaging (MRI): A type of scan that uses radio waves and a powerful magnet to produce detailed computer images.

Malabsorption: The abnormal utilization of nutrients from food.

Malaise: A feeling of lack of health or debility, often indicating or accompanying the onset of illness.

Malaria: A serious parasitic infection spread by mosquitoes and characterized by fever, chills, sweating, vomiting, and damage to the kidneys, brain, and liver.

Malignancy: Any condition that becomes progressively worse, especially the growth of a cancerous tumor.

Malignant melanoma: A fast-growing, highly dangerous form of skin cancer.

Malleus: A small bone within the middle ear; also called the hammer because of its shape.

Malnutrition: A physical state characterized by an imbalance of dietary proteins, carbohydrates, fats, vitamins, and minerals, given an individual's physical activity and health needs.

Malocclusion: A condition in which the teeth of the upper and lower jaws do not fit together properly.

Malpractice: The failure to care for patients in accordance with professional standards, for which injured patients are allowed to sue for compensation.

Malpractice insurance: Insurance policies held by physicians in order to protect them financially in the event of a patient-initiated lawsuit alleging incidents of improper medical decisions or incompetence.

Mammary gland: Group of milk-producing cells consisting of lobules and ducts.

Mammography: The use of X rays to image the female breast, primarily in the detection and diagnosis of malignant breast tumors before they can be felt.

Mandible: The lower jaw, which is hinged to the skull.

Manic-depressive disorder. *See* Bipolar disorder.

MAOIs. *See* Monoamine oxidase inhibitors (MAOIs).

Maple syrup urine disease (MSUD): A recessive autosomal genetic disease resulting in the absence, partial activity, or inactivity of a multisubunit enzyme responsible for metabolizing the branched chain amino acids leucine, isoleucine, and valine.

Marasmus: The condition that results from consuming a diet that is deficient in both energy and protein.

Marijuana: A plant containing a psychoactive substance with the potential for both recreational abuse and medical use.

Mass spectrometry: A very sensitive technique that accurately measures protein or peptide mass.

Mast cells: Cells in connective tissue capable of releasing chemicals that cause allergic reactions.

Mastectomy: Surgical removal of the female breast.

Mastication: The act of chewing food.

Mastitis: Infection of the breast, which results in inflammation, tenderness, swelling, and pain.

Mastoidectomy: The surgical removal of the temporal or mastoid bone, which is located behind the ear.

Materia Medica: The homeopathic pharmacopoeia, a list of remedies with their associated symptoms and uses.

Matrix: Organic or inorganic material occurring in connective tissues but located outside the cells.

Maxilla: The upper jaw, which is fixed to the skull.

Maxillofacial surgery: Surgery of the face and neck, a form of cosmetic and reconstructive surgery.

Maximal oxygen uptake: The maximum rate of oxygen consumption during exercise.

MCAT. *See* Medical College Admission Test (MCAT).

Measles: A childhood infectious disease, also known as rubeola, characterized by a rash and fever; it can be controlled through immunization.

Mechanoreceptors: Sensory receptors that, when mechanically deformed (such as being pressed on), send nerve impulses causing sensations of pressure and touch.

Medial: Closer to an imaginary midline dividing the body into equal right and left halves than another part.

Medicaid: A health care program in the United States made available to those with low-level income or who are disabled and unable to pay health insurance premiums.

Medical College Admission Test (MCAT): A test of problem-solving skills taken by all candidates to medical school in the United States; used to predict which students will be successful.

Medicare: A U.S. federal program that covers many of the hospital costs and doctor bills for elderly and disabled persons and those with end-stage renal (kidney) disease.

Medicine: The science and art of diagnosing, treating, curing, and preventing disease; relieving pain; and improving and preserving health. Also, any drug or other substance used in treating disease, healing, or relieving pain.

Meditation: A mental exercise to enhance personal understanding of the self and the universe.

Medulla: The central portion of the adrenal gland, the area that produces epinephrine (adrenaline).

Megadose: Ten or more times the recommended daily allowance of a nutrient, such as a vitamin.

Megaloblastic anemia: Anemia caused by the failure of red blood cells to mature; also known as pernicious anemia, Addisonian anemia, or maturation failure.

Meiosis: A special kind of cell division whereby four cells are produced; each cell has only half of the original number of chromosomes; meiosis produces the sex cells (eggs and sperm).

Meissner's corpuscles: Receptors at which the sense of a light touch or low-frequency vibrations are detected; also called corpuscles of touch.

Melanin: A polymer made up of several compounds (including the amino acid tyrosine) that causes pigmentation in the skin, hair, and eyes.

Melanoma: Cancer of the melanocytes, the cells that produce melanin.

Melatonin: A hormone produced by the pineal gland within the epithalamus of the forebrain; it is usually released into the blood during the night phase of the light-dark cycle.

Membrane: A thin layer of lipid and protein molecules that controls transport of molecules and ions between the cell and its exterior and between membrane-bound compartments within the cell.

Menarche: The first menstrual cycle.

Ménière's disease: A progressive dysfunction of the inner ear that causes recurrent episodes of hearing loss, tinnitus, severe dizziness, and ear pressure.

Meningitis: The inflammation of the protective tissues surrounding the brain and the spinal cord.

Menopause: The permanent cessation of the menstrual cycle, signifying the conclusion of a woman's reproductive life.

Menorrhagia: Excessive or prolonged bleeding during menstruation.

Menstruation: The cyclic bleeding that normally occurs, usually in the absence of pregnancy, during the reproductive period of the human female; typically occurs at twenty-eight day intervals.

Mental retardation: A condition characterized by a below-average intelligence quotient (IQ) and deficits in adaptive functioning before the age of eighteen years; the degree of retardation ranges from mild to severe.

Meridians: Designated channels in the body that react to acupuncture or acupressure stimulation.

Merkel's disks: Sensory receptors in the skin located in deeper layers of the epidermis; also called tactile disks.

Mesothelioma: A malignancy originating from the mesothelial surfaces (the lining cells) of the pleural and peritoneal cavities, the pericardium, or the tunica vaginalis.

Messenger ribonucleic acid (mRNA): A single-stranded RNA that arises from and is complementary to double-stranded deoxyribonucleic acid (DNA); it passes from the nucleus to the cytoplasm, where its information is translated into proteins.

Metabolic equivalent (MET): A unit used to estimate the metabolic cost of physical activity; 1 MET is equal to 3.5 milliliters of oxygen consumed per kilogram of body weight per minute.

Metabolic rate: A measurement of the Calories (kilocalories) that are converted into heat energy in order to maintain body temperature and/or for physical exertion.

Metabolic syndrome: A constellation of metabolic changes that affect most major organ systems and may impinge on practically all systems of the body, beginning with excess weight or obesity.

Metabolism: The chemical and physical processes involved in the interconversion of foods and the maintenance of life.

Metabolites: The molecular breakdown products of a substance.

Metastasis: The transfer of disease-producing cells to other parts of the body.

Metastasize: To spread by means of the bloodstream to other parts of the body.

Methicillin-resistant *Staphylococcus aureus* (MRSA) infection: An infection caused by virulent and destructive bacteria that is resistant to common antibiotics and difficult to treat.

Methotrexate: A powerful drug, originally developed to treat cancer, that is used to treat patients with severe cases of psoriasis.

Microarrays: Miniature plastic or glass chips upon which tiny amounts of biological material are permanently spotted in a grid-like array.

Microbiology: The study of organisms too small to be seen by the unaided human eye, especially the identification, transmission, and control of microorganisms that cause disease.

Microcephaly: Abnormal smallness of the head.

Microorganism: An organism that is too small to be seen without a magnifying lens; also known as a microbe.

Microscopy: The use of a microscope to make extremely small objects appear larger.

Microsurgery: Surgery done with the aid of a microscope.

Micturition: The act of urinating.

Middle ear: The air-filled cavity in which vibrations are transmitted from the eardrum to the inner ear via the ossicles.

Migraine headaches: Severe, incapacitating headaches that may be preceded by nausea and vomiting or by visual, sensory, and motor disturbances.

Milk duct: Tubular canal that transports breast milk from the lobule to the collecting duct.

Milk line: A line that originates as a primitive milk streak on each front side of the fetus; it extends from axilla to vulva, where rudimentary breast tissues or nipples could be located.

Mineralocorticoids: Steroid hormones that regulate the body levels of sodium and potassium.

Minerals: Inorganic compounds that are essential for human life; seventeen are required in the diet.

Miscarriage: The expulsion of the embryo or fetus before it is viable outside the uterus; also called spontaneous abortion.

Mitochondrion: A membrane-bound cytoplasmic organelle that constitutes the primary location of oxidative reactions providing energy for cellular activities.

Mitosis: The type of cell division that occurs in nonsex cells, which conserves chromosome number by equal allocation to each of the newly formed cells.

Mitral valve: The valve between the heart's left auricle and ventricle.

Mitral valve prolapse: The inability of the mitral valve in the heart to close properly; also called mitral insufficiency.

Modality: The ability to distinguish one sensation from another; the ability to discriminate light or heavy touch, pain, pressure, vibratory, or hot and cold sensations from one another.

Molars: The back teeth, which are used to grind food into smaller portions prior to swallowing.

Molecular biology: The study of the interactions that occur among the molecules making up living organisms.

Molecule: A collection of atoms bonded together; normally neutral because it has an equal number of protons and electrons.

Momentum: The product of mass and velocity for a particle; inverse with wavelength (the distance between peaks of a wave).

Monkeypox: A rare disease, originating in the rain forests of Central and West Africa, that affects animals and humans and is caused by a virus.

Monoamine oxidase inhibitors (MAOIs): A class of drugs that relieve the symptoms of depression by inhibiting the enzyme that deactivates the brain chemical monoamine oxidase.

Monoclonal antibodies: Antibodies (proteins that protect the body against disease-causing foreign bodies such as bacteria and viruses) produced in large quantities from cloned cells.

Mononucleosis: An infectious respiratory illness caused by the Epstein-Barr virus.

Monozygotes: Identical twins; born of a single ovum that divides after a single sperm fertilizes it.

Morbid obesity: Excessive accumulation of fat (more than 100 pounds overweight or 100 percent overweight).

Morbidity: In medical statistics, the occurrence of clinical disease, in contrast to mortality (death) and occurrence (which includes subclinical infections).

Mordant: A chemical that acts to fix a stain within a physical structure; the role played by iodine in Gram staining.

Morgellons disease: A skin disorder characterized by a pattern of dermatologic symptoms described as insect-like sensations, with skin lesions varying from very minor to disfiguring, and associated with disabling fatigue, joint pain, and various neuropsychiatric symptoms.

Morgue: A place, usually cooled, where dead bodies are temporarily kept, pending proper identification, autopsy, or burial.

Mortality: Relating to death.

Motility: Spontaneous motion, such as of the gastrointestinal tract or of sperm.

Motion sickness: A feeling of nausea brought on by motion.

Motor: Referring to parts of the nervous system having to do with movement production.

Motor neuron: A nerve that functions either directly or indirectly to control movement in a target organ.

Motor neuron diseases: Progressive, debilitating, and eventually fatal diseases affecting nerve cells in muscles.

Motor weakness: Muscle weakness resulting from the failure of motor nerves.

MRI. *See* Magnetic resonance imaging (MRI).

mRNA. *See* Messenger ribonucleic acid (mRNA).

MRSA infection. *See* Methicillin-resistant *Staphylococcus aureus* (MRSA) infection.

MSUD. *See* Maple syrup urine disease (MSUD).

Mucopolysaccharidosis (MPS): A genetic disorder characterized by accumulations of mucopolysaccharides in tissues.

Mucosa: The tissue lining the interior of the gastrointestinal tract, through which nutrients pass into the bloodstream.

Mucous membrane: The soft, pink layer of cells that produce mucus to keep body structures lubricated; found in the eyelids and in the respiratory and urinary tracts.

Mucus: A fluid excreted by many body membranes as a lubricant.

Müllerian ducts: The pair of tubes in the early embryo that will develop into the internal female organs (uterus, oviducts, and upper vagina).

Multiple sclerosis (MS): An incurable, debilitating disease of the nervous system.

Multipotent: Referring to stem cells derived from adults that may develop into one of several types of tissue.

Mumps: An infectious, viral childhood disease characterized by swelling of the salivary glands in front of and below the ears.

Murmur: The sound made by blood flowing backward through a heart valve.

Muscle: A bundle of contractile cells that is responsible for the movement of organs and body parts.

Muscle contraction: The shortening of a muscle that results in movement of a particular body part.

Muscle fibers: Elongated muscle cells that make up skeletal, cardiac, and smooth muscles.

Muscle relaxant: Any of a number of medications that can be used either to paralyze the muscles of the patient temporarily before a medical procedure or to alleviate neuromuscular pain and spasms.

Muscular dystrophy: A group of progressive genetic diseases that attack the muscles.

Musculature: The arrangement of skeletal muscles in the body.

Musculoskeletal: Pertaining to or comprising the skeleton and the muscles.

Mutagen: A chemical or an ionizing radiation that causes a change in the nucleotide sequence of the DNA of a gene, possibly affecting the gene's normal expression.

Mutation: Damage to a gene that changes how it works.

Myasthenia gravis: A disorder in which the nicotinic acetylcholine receptors located in junctions between nerve cells and muscles are attacked by the immune system, causing exhaustion of the muscles.

Mycetoma: A progressive and chronic fungal or bacterial infection that causes overgrowth of the infected tissue and the formation of sinuses filled with the infecting organism.

Myco-: A prefix denoting fungus.

Mycobacterium: Any of a genus of nonmotile aerobic bacteria that are difficult to stain and include numerous saprophytes and the organisms causing tuberculosis and leprosy.

Mycosis: Any disease of humans, plants, or animals caused by a fungus.

Myocardial infarction. *See* Heart attack.

Myocardium: The muscle tissue that forms the walls of the heart, varying in thickness in the upper and lower regions.

Myoclonus: Involuntary twitching or spasm of muscle.

Myomectomy: Surgical removal of a noncancerous muscle tumor (myoma).

Myopia: The inability of the eye to focus on distant objects; also called nearsightedness.

Myringotomy: Incision of the tympanic membrane, used to drain fluid and reduce middle-ear pressure.

NAD. *See* Nicotinamide adenine dinucleotide (NAD).

Narcolepsy: An apparently inherited disorder of the nervous system characterized by brief, numerous, and overwhelming attacks of sleepiness throughout the day.

Narcotics: A group of potent painkilling drugs characterized by their ability to cause the user to develop tolerance and therefore dependency (physical addiction); such drugs include morphine, codeine, heroin, and other opium-like compounds.

Nasogastric tube: A tube fed through the nose to the stomach.

Nasopharyngeal: Referring to the nose and pharynx (the upper part of the throat that leads from the mouth to the esophagus).

Nausea: An unpleasant sensation followed by stomach and intestinal discomfort, which may lead to vomiting.

Nearsightedness: The inability of the eye to focus on distant objects; also called myopia.

Necropsy: A postmortem (after-death) examination of an animal's body, similar to an autopsy performed on a human corpse.

Necrosis: Tissue damage occurring as a result of cell death.

Needle biopsy: The obtaining of tissue fragments by the puncture of a tumor, through a large-caliber needle, syringe, and plunger; the tissue within the lumen of the needle is obtained through the rotation and withdrawal of the needle.

Negative feedback: A homeostatic control system designed to respond to a stress by returning body conditions to normal physiologic levels.

Negligence: Failure to perform an important or necessary medical technique, or the performance of such a technique in a careless or unskilled manner so as to cause further injury.

Neonatal intensive care unit: A hospital nursery with advanced equipment and specially trained staff to maintain the vital functions of sick newborns and to monitor their progress closely.

Neonatal period: The first month of life; derived from the Greek *neo* (meaning "new") and the Latin *natum* (meaning "birth").

Neonate: A newborn infant.

Neonatology: The study of diseases, conditions, and treatments of newborns (infants between the time of birth and approximately one month of age).

Neoplasm: An uncontrolled growth of cells, which can develop into a tumor; may be malignant (cancerous) or benign.

Nephrectomy: Kidney removal.

Nephritis: Any disease or pathology of the kidney that results in inflammation.

Nephrology: The study of kidney diseases.

Nephron: A tiny blood-processing unit located in the kidneys (composed of the renal corpuscle, the loop of Henle, and renal tubules) that carries out the processes that form urine; each kidney contains approximately one million nephrons.

Nephrotic syndrome: An abnormal condition of the kidneys characterized by a variety of conditions, including edema and proteinuria; often accompanies glomerular dysfunction and diabetes.

Nephroureterectomy: A procedure similar to a radical nephrectomy, with the additional removal of the ureter and a cuff of the bladder; performed to treat transitional cell carcinomas of the ureters and the pelvis of the kidneys.

Nerve: A bundle of sensory and motor neurons held together by layers of connective tissue.

Nerve compression: Excessive pressure causing a nerve to be pinched.

Nervous system: The bodily system that receives and interprets stimuli and transmits impulses to and from the brain and other organs.

Neural tube: The embryonic structure that gives rise to the central nervous system.

Neuralgia: Pain associated with a nerve, often caused by inflammation or injury.

Neuritis: An inflammatory or degenerative lesion of a nerve, marked by pain and the loss of normal reflexes.

Neurofibrillary tangles: A hallmark lesion of Alzheimer's disease and several other disorders consisting of intracellular aggregates of the structural protein tau.

Neuroglial cell: A supportive cell for neurons within the central nervous system of animals.

Neuroleptic: An agent that modifies psychotic behavior.

Neurologic: Dealing with the nervous system and its disorders.

Neurology: The study of the central nervous system, which is composed of the brain and spinal cord.

Neuromuscular electrical stimulation (NMES): The application of electrical and current to elicit a muscle contraction.

Neuromusculoskeletal: Pertaining to the interrelationship between the body's nerves, muscles, and skeleton.

Neuron: The principal nervous system cell that conducts electrical information from its dendritic extensions, through its cell body, to its axonal extensions, and on to other cells and is capable of releasing neurotransmitters.

Neuropathy: Any disorder of the nerves.

Neuroscience: The scientific specialization that seeks to understand mental processes, occurrences, and disturbances in terms of underlying mechanisms in the brain and the nervous system.

Neurosis: A psychic disturbance and defect from childhood that develops into a particular pattern of emotional illness and dysfunctional behavior.

Neurosurgery: Surgery to correct disorders of the nervous system, including the brain.

Neurotoxicity: An excessive or unwanted effect of too much anesthetic drug on the nerves.

Neurotransmitter: A chemical substance released by one nerve cell to stimulate or inhibit the function of an adjacent nerve cell; a chemical message released by a neuron.

Neutrophil: A circulating white blood cell that serves as one of the principal phagocytes for the immune system.

Nicotinamide adenine dinucleotide (NAD): A molecule used to hold pairs of electrons when they have been removed from a molecule by some biological process; the empty molecule is denoted by NAD+, while it is denoted as NADH when it is carrying electrons.

Nicotine: A colorless, poisonous alkaloid derived from tobacco plants.

Niemann-Pick disease: This lipid disease group, resulting from inactive sphingomyelinase and cholesterol-modifying enzymes, causes lipid buildup in the brain and other organs, mental and physical debilitation, and a short life span.

Night sweats: Hot flashes that occur at night, typically during sleep.

Nitrous oxide: A chemical compound that at room temperature forms a colorless gas (also known as laughing gas) used to produce anesthesia and analgesia during surgery.

NMES. *See* Neuromuscular electrical stimulation (NMES).

Nocturia: Involuntary nighttime urination.

Nondisjunction: A malfunction of mitosis, resulting in cells with an abnormal chromosome number.

Noninvasive: Referring to a procedure that does not require entering the body.

Nonmaleficence: A principle of medical ethics which requires that the actions taken not harm the patient.

Nonsteroidal anti-inflammatory drugs (NSAIDs): Drugs such as ibuprofen that are used to reduce swelling and pain.

Normal: A term of reference that can mean average (as in statistically normal), functional (as in adaptive), or socially appropriate (as in within cultural bounds of acceptability).

Noroviruses: A family of viruses that cause acute gastroenteritis.

Novocaine: A local anesthetic, commonly used in dentistry, whose chemical structure is similar to cocaine.

NSAIDs. *See* Nonsteroidal anti-inflammatory drugs (NSAIDs).

Nuclear medicine: The branch of medicine that employs radioactive substances to diagnose or treat disease.

Nucleic acids: Very large molecules, located on DNA molecules, that control the synthesis of proteins and carry basic information determining heredity.

Nucleolus: A nuclear structure formed through the activity of chromosome segments in the production of ribosomal RNA and the assembly of ribosomal subunits.

Nucleoprotein: A virally encoded protein that is directly associated with the viral nucleic acid.

Nucleotide: A chemical subunit of DNA; different sequences of linked nucleotides spell out instructions for the assembly of proteins.

Nucleus: A large spherical mass occupying up to one-third of the volume of a typical plant or animal cell; also, the dense, positively charged, central core of an atom, containing its massive protons and neutrons.

Null hypothesis: A statement about populations that can be tested statistically which presupposes that there are no differences in the terms of some numerical measure.

Nulliparity: Having never given birth to a viable infant.

Numbness: A reduction or loss of feeling in an area of skin.

Nursing: The profession of providing health care that assists a patient to recover from an illness, injury, or surgical or other procedure, performed in a variety of settings. Also, the act of breast-feeding.

Nursing home: A type of extended care facility that can be classified as either skilled or intermediate, depending on the type of care; physicians oversee medical care that is rendered around the clock by a nursing staff.

Nutrients: Substances needed by the body for maintenance, growth, and repair; the six classes of nutrients are carbohydrates, fats, proteins, vitamins, minerals, and water.

Nutrition: The study of those substances found in foods that are needed by the body for maintenance, growth, and repair, as well as those substances that increase the risk of disease.

Nystagmus: Rhythmic involuntary movements of the eyes.

Obesity: A medical condition defined as being in excess of 20 percent above ideal weight.

Obsession: A recurrent and persistent thought or impulse associated with continuous and involuntary preoccupation that cannot be expunged by logic or reasoning.

Obsessive-compulsive disorder: An anxiety disorder characterized by intrusive and unwanted thoughts and/or the need to perform ritualized behaviors.

Obstetrics: The branch of medicine specializing in the problems and needs of pregnant women and their fetuses from conception through delivery and postnatal care.

Obstruction: Partial or complete blockage of the gastrointestinal tract.

Obstructive sleep apnea: Periods of interrupted breathing during sleep due to airway obstruction in the nose or throat.

Occlusion: The fit of the upper and lower teeth when they are brought together; also, the blockage of any vessel in the body, which may be caused by a thrombus or other embolus.

Occult blood: Fecal blood, as detected by microscopic or chemical testing.

Occupational health: Those health disciplines collectively concerned with the conditions, diseases, and injuries that occur within or as a result of the work setting.

Occupational medicine: A medical specialty focused on providing all levels of preventive medical services to working men and women in order to preserve, maintain, or restore health and well-being.

Occupational toxicology: A subspecialty of environmental toxicology that focuses on the effects of chemicals on the health of a workplace population.

Odontology: The study of teeth.

Oedipus complex: The experience of having sexual feelings toward the parent of the opposite sex that can occur in young children.

Olfaction: The sense of smell; a process in which nerve impulses caused by chemicals interacting with chemoreceptors in the nose arrive in the olfactory center of the brain and are classified as certain kinds of odor.

Olfactory adaptation: The relatively quick response to and subsequent fatigue of the sense of smell that allows the presence of odoriferous chemicals to be recognized quickly and then become less and less noticed until they are soon ignored.

Olfactory bulb: An extension of the brain located below the frontal lobes of the cerebrum and above the ethmoid bone (extending back from nose); one of a pair of gray masses into which the olfactory nerves

terminate, thus serving as the first synaptic sites in olfactory neural pathways.

Olfactory knobs: Unmyelinated, tiny, rounded nerve endings of the sensory cells found at the mucus-coated olfactory membrane; each knob has five to eight extensions, called olfactory hairs, that branch out into the nasal cavity and monitor the environment.

Oncogene: A gene or DNA segment that can cause cancer.

Oncology: The branch of medicine specializing in the study of tumors, especially malignant tumors, and their treatment.

Onychomycosis: Common nail disorder in which fungal organisms invade the nail bed, causing progressive changes in the color, texture, and structure of the nail.

Oocyte: A female germ cell that differentiates to become a mature ova.

Oophorectomy: Removal of the ovaries, which is often necessary in cases of severe endometriosis.

Oophoritis: Inflammation of the ovary.

Operating room: A room in which surgical procedures are performed.

Operator: A person who induces a hypnotic state; synonymous with "hypnotist" and "suggestor."

Ophthalmology: The branch of medicine concerned with the study of the eye and its structures, disorders, conditions, and treatments.

Opioids: Pain medications derived from opiates, such as morphine, oxycodone, codeine, and fentanyl, intended to control severe pain.

Opportunistic infections: Potentially life-threatening diseases occurring in persons with a weakened immune system, caused by microorganisms that typically do not cause severe illnesses in an otherwise healthy person.

Optic disc: The portion of the optic nerve at its point of entrance into the rear of the eye.

Optic nerve: The nerve that takes information from retina to brain; largest nerve in the body.

Optical fiber: A very thin thread made of high-purity glass, plastic, or quartz; used to transmit light from a laser into the body.

Optometry: The practice of diagnosing visual problems and diagnosing correctional devices such as eyeglasses and contact lenses.

Oral hygiene: Care of the teeth and mouth.

Oral surgery: The dental specialty that surgically removes diseased teeth and oral tissues and treats bone fractures of the jaws.

Orchiectomy: Surgical removal of the testicle for benign or malignant conditions.

Orchiopexy: Fixation of the testicle to the internal lining of the scrotum to eliminate the possibility of testicular torsion.

Orchitis: Inflammation of the testis.

Organelles: Specialized parts of cells.

Organic: Pertaining to, arising from, or affecting a body organ.

Organic brain syndromes: Clusters of behavioral and psychological symptoms involving impaired brain function, where etiology is unknown; includes delirium, delusions, amnesia, intoxication, and dementias.

Organic disease: A disease caused or accompanied by an alteration in the structure of the tissues or organs.

Organic mental disorders: Mental and emotional disturbances from transient or permanent brain dysfunction, with known organic etiology; includes drug or alcohol ingestion, infection, trauma, and cardiovascular disease.

Organism: A complex structure of interdependent and subordinate elements whose relations and properties are largely determined by their function as a whole.

Organs. *See* Systems and organs.

Oroprioception: Ability to locate the body in space.

Orthodontics: The branch of dentistry that diagnoses and treats malformed teeth.

Orthognathic surgery: Jaw reconstruction.

Orthopedics: The branch of medicine that specializes in the surgical repair or correction of injured or malformed bones and joints and the structures (such as muscles) associated with them.

Orthotic device: A podiatric appliance or prosthesis that is used to correct a foot deformity.

Orthotopic: Referring to the placement of a transplanted organ in the position occupied by the original organ.

Oscillopsia: Sensation of bouncing vision.

Oscilloscope: An instrument that displays a visual representation of electrical variations on the fluorescent screen of a cathode-ray tube.

Osmosis: The diffusion of molecules through a semipermeable membrane until there is an equal concentration on either side of the membrane.

Ossicles: Three small bones in the middle ear that transmit vibrations from the eardrum to the fluid of the inner ear.

Ossification: The formation of bone tissue.

Osteoarthritis: A degenerative process in which components of the joints undergo thinning, resulting in loss of motion, pain, and often inflammation in the later stages.

Osteoblast: A bone cell that can produce and form bone matrix; osteoblasts are responsible for new bone formation.

Osteoclast: A large bone cell that can destroy bone matrix by dissolving the mineral crystals.

Osteocyte: The primary living cell of mature bone tissue.

Osteomyelitis: Infection of bone.

Osteopathic medicine: A form of medicine, founded by Andrew Taylor Still in 1874, that emphasizes the health of the musculoskeletal system as well as a holistic approach to the functioning of the body.

Osteoporosis: A loss of bone mass accompanied by increasing fragility and brittleness.

Ostomy: A popular term for any operation that results in a stoma.

Otitis: Any inflammation of the outer or middle ear.

Oto-: A combining form indicating "ear."

Otoliths: Granular bones of the inner ear.

Otologist: A medical doctor who specializes in diseases and disorders of the ear.

-otomy: A suffix meaning an opening or incision in an organ or structure; for example, a ureterotomy is an opening in the ureter.

Otorhinolaryngology: The branch of medicine concerned with the diseases, conditions, and treatment of the ear, nose, and throat.

Otosclerosis: A condition in which the stapes becomes progressively more rigid and hearing loss results.

Otoscope: An instrument for viewing the ear canal and the eardrum.

Outer ear: The visible, fleshy part of the ear and the ear canal; it transmits sound waves to the eardrum.

Outpatient care: Evaluation and treatment services not requiring an overnight stay in a medical facility.

Ovarian cysts: Benign growths in the ovaries, which may cause pain.

Ovariectomy: The removal of the ovaries.

Ovaries: The pair of structures in the female that produce ova (eggs) and hormones.

Over-the-counter drugs: Pharmaceutical products, vitamins, herbal remedies, and other medicines that can be purchased without a doctor's prescription.

Oviducts: The pair of tubes leading from the top of the uterus upward toward the ovaries; also called the Fallopian tubes.

Ovulation: The release of an ovum from its follicle in the ovary.

Ovum (*pl.* ova): The female gamete; a large round cell that carries the female's chromosomes and is released from the ovaries during ovulation.

Oxidation-reduction: The transfer of electron(s) from one now-positive substance (oxidation) to one now-negative (reduction).

Oxygen therapy: Application of pure or high-oxygen gas to assist in recovery from oxygen deprivation (as in respiratory diseases).

Oxygenation: The process of getting oxygen into the bloodstream.

Oxytocin: The maternal pituitary hormone that regulates milk production and uterine contraction.

Pacemaker: A device surgically implanted in a patient suffering from heart disease in order to maintain a healthy heartbeat; also, a region of the heart called the sinoatrial (S-A) node, which maintains the regular heartbeat.

Pacinian corpuscles: Receptors at which the sensations of heavy touch or deep pressure originate; also called lamellated corpuscles.

Paget's disease: A disorder characterized by a progressive thickening and weakening of the bones.

Pain: Physical distress that is often associated with disorder and injury.

Pain management: The alleviation of pain, either completely or to a point of tolerance, by means of a variety of therapies, both chemical (as with drugs) and physical (as with exercise therapy).

Palliative treatments: Therapies that reduce symptoms without completely eradicating a disorder.

Palpation: Application of the hands, or touching, to determine the size, texture, consistency, and location of body structures.

Palpitation: The sensation of being aware of one's own heartbeat, usually because the heart is beating rapidly or more forcefully than normal.

Palsy: Partial or complete paralysis of a nerve followed by muscle weakness and wasting.

Pancreas: A secretory organ, located behind the stomach and connected to the duodenum, that produces enzymes to digest food and insulin to metabolize sugar.

Pancreatitis: Inflammation of the pancreas.

Pandemic: An epidemic prevalent throughout a country, a continent, or the world.

Panic attack: A sudden feeling of intense apprehension, fear, doom, and/or terror that can cause shortness of breath, palpitations, chest pain, chills, nausea, and light-headedness.

Pap smear: A simple diagnostic test for the presence of cervical cancer involving the removal of cervical tissue cells and the subsequent biopsy of these cells.

Papillomaviruses: Small, cuboidal viruses that replicate in the nuclei of epithelial cells.

Paralysis: The loss of muscle function or sensation as a result of trauma or disease.

Paramedic: A person who is not generally a physician but is trained to provide emergency treatment in critical situations, such as resuscitation after a heart attack or seizure, arrest of bleeding, dressing wounds, and setting broken bones.

Paramedical: Related to the science or practice of medicine.

Paranoia: Pervasive distrust and suspiciousness of others and a tendency to interpret others' motives as malevolent.

Paraplegia: Partial or complete paralysis of both legs caused by damage to the spinal cord.

Parasite: An organism whose principal food source is another living organism; in medicine, the term refers to both unicellular and multicellular animals.

Parasympathetic nervous system: The part of the autonomic nervous system that stimulates digestion, slows the heart, and dilates blood vessels, acting in opposition to sympathetic nerves.

Parathyroid gland: One of four small endocrine glands, situated underneath the thyroid gland, whose main product is parathyroid hormone; this hormone is responsible for the regulation of serum calcium levels.

Parathyroidectomy: Removal of part or all of one or both of the parathyroid glands.

Parenteral: Administered by injection or infusion.

Parkinson's disease: A disease in which the dopamine-secreting cells of the midbrain degenerate, resulting in uncontrolled movement and rigidity.

Paroxysm: An uncontrolled spasm or convulsion that may be violent.

Parturition: The process or action of giving birth.

Passive euthanasia: Ending life by refusing or withdrawing life-sustaining medical treatment.

Passive immunity: Immunity resulting from the introduction of preformed antibodies.

Pathogen: An agent that is capable of causing a disease, including viruses, bacteria, protozoa, rickettsia, or parasitic worms.

Pathogenicity: The ability of an organism to cause disease.

Pathologic: Pertaining to the study of disease and the development of abnormal conditions.

Pathology: The study of the nature and consequences of disease.

Pathophysiology: An alteration in function as seen in disease.

Patient advocacy: The representation of the patient's interest in medical diagnosis and treatment decisions, in which the health care provider acts as an information source and counselor for the patient.

Patient assessment: The systematic gathering of information in order to determine the nature of a patient's illness.

Pediatric: Pertaining to neonates, infants, and children up to the age of twelve.

Pediatrics: The branch of medicine specializing in the conditions, diseases, and development of infants and children.

Pedodontics: The dental specialty that treats children.

Pelvic inflammatory disease (PID): An infection of the female reproductive organs that may be caused by a sexually transmitted disease.

Penis: The male genital organ containing the urethra, through which both urine and semen pass; sufficient erection of the penis is required for intercourse.

Pepsin: A substance in the stomach that breaks down most proteins.

Peptic ulcer: Open sores that develop in the lining of the stomach as a result of excessive secretion of gastric juices.

Peptidoglycans: Repeating units of sugar derivatives that make up a rigid layer of bacterial cell walls; found in both gram-positive and gram-negative cells.

Percussion: Gentle tapping by the medical examiner's finger, which has been positioned on the patient; a hollow sound is heard over air-filled structures, while a dull thud is heard over solid areas or liquid-filled structures.

Percutaneous transluminal coronary angioplasty (PTCA): A procedure undertaken to increase the internal diameter of a coronary artery by inflating a small balloonlike device at the site or sites where the artery has narrowed because of plaque buildup.

Perforation: An abnormal opening, such as a hole in the wall of the colon.

Perfusion: The flow of blood through the lungs or other vessels in the body.

Perfusionist: A health care specialist who operates extracorporeal circulation equipment when it is necessary to support or replace a patient's circulatory or respiratory function.

Peri-: A prefix denoting "around," either in a literal sense (as in "pericarditis") or in a figurative sense (as in "perinatal").

Pericarditis: A disease of the membrane that surrounds the heart, caused by an inflammation that can lead to constriction of the heart muscle.

Pericardium: A fluid-filled conical sac of fibrous tissue that surrounds the heart and the roots of the great blood vessels.

Perinatology: The branch of medicine that treats the mother and child during the late stages of pregnancy and the first month or so following birth.

Perineum: The short bridge of flesh between the anus and vagina in women and the anus and base of the penis in men.

Period: The length of one complete cycle of a rhythm; ultradian rhythms are about twenty-four hours (twenty to twenty-eight hours), and infradian rhythms are longer than twenty-eight hours.

Periodontics: The dental specialty that treats the diseases of the supporting tissues of the teeth.

Periodontitis: The inflammation and infection of the gums, which may cause loss of the supporting bone and eventually tooth loss.

Periodontium: Those tissues supporting the tooth in the jaws, including the gingiva, the jawbone, and the periodontal ligament that attaches the root of the tooth into the jaw.

Periosteum: The thick, fibrous membrane that covers the entire surface of a bone except for the cartilage within joints.

Peripheral: Referring to a part of the body away from the center.

Peripheral nervous system: A system consisting of the nerves not located in the central nervous system (brain and spinal cord); these nerves carry impulses from the central nervous system to the target muscles and relay sensory impulses from the rest of the body to the central nervous system.

Peripheral vision: Side vision, or the visual perception to all sides of the central object being viewed.

Peristalsis: The wavelike muscular contractions that move food and waste products through the intestines; problems with peristalsis are called motility disorders.

Peritoneal cavity: The abdominal cavity, which contains the visceral organs.

Peritoneal dialysis: The removal of toxins from blood by dialysis in the peritoneal cavity.

Peritoneum: The membrane lining the walls of the abdominal cavity and enclosing the viscera.

Peritonitis: Infection of the abdominal (peritoneal) cavity in which the visceral organs are found.

Peroxisome: A membrane-bound organelle that contains reaction systems linking biochemical pathways taking place elsewhere in the cell; also called a microbody.

Personality disorders: Pervasive, inflexible patterns of perceiving, thinking, and behaving that cause long-term distress or impairment, beginning in adolescence and persisting into adulthood.

Pertussis: A serious bacterial infection of the respiratory tract that usually strikes very young children; commonly known as whooping cough.

Pervasive developmental disorders: Disorders characterized by severe, impaired social interaction or communication skills, or stereotyped behavior, interests, and activities.

PET scanning. *See* Positron emission tomography (PET) scanning.

Petechiae (*sing*. petechia): Minute, pinhead-sized spots caused by hemorrhage or bleeding into the skin.

Petit mal: A mild type of epileptic seizure characterized by a very short lapse of consciousness, usually without convulsions or falling.

Peyer's patches: Lymphatic nodules in the ileum of the intestine; Peyer's patches are one kind of mucosal associated lymphoid tissue (MALT), which, unlike lymph nodes, is not enclosed by tissue capsules.

pH: A value that represents the relative acidity or alkalinity of a solution; values below pH 7.0 are acidic, while values above pH 7.0 are basic.

Phagocyte: Any cell capable of surrounding, ingesting, and digesting microbes or cell debris; in a certain sense, phagocytes function as scavengers.

Phagocytosis: The ingestion and destruction of a pathogen or abnormal tissue by specialized white blood cells known as phagocytes.

Pharmaceutical: Of or relating to pharmacy; a medicinal drug.

Pharmaceutical care: The responsible provision of drug therapy to improve a patient's quality of life.

Pharmacist: A person with a license to dispense or sell drugs prescribed by a medical practitioner, such as a dentist, physician, or veterinarian.

Pharmacodynamics: Changes in tissue sensitivity or physiologic systems in response to pharmacological substances.

Pharmacognosy: The preparation of medicinal agents from natural sources.

Pharmacokinetics: The action of pharmacological substances within a biological system; pharmacologic substance absorption, distribution, metabolism, and elimination by an organism.

Pharmacology: The science that deals with the chemistry, effects, and therapeutic use of drugs.

Pharmacy: The art or profession of preparing and dispensing drugs and medicine.

Pharyngitis: Inflammation of the pharynx.

Pharynx: The throat; the part of the respiratory-digestive passage that extends from the nasal cavity to the larynx (voice box).

Phenylketonuria (PKU): A genetic disease characterized by the absence of the enzyme that breaks down the amino acid phenylalanine; the resulting buildup can lead to brain damage.

Phimosis: The narrowing of the opening of the skin covering the head of the penis sufficient to prevent retraction of the skin back over the glans.

Phlebitis: The inflammation of a vein, often in the legs; may be accompanied by blood clots.

Phlebotomy: The act or practice of opening a vein for letting blood.

Phobia: Any abnormal or exaggerated fear of a particular object or situation.

Photism: In synesthesia, a vivid light or color sensation induced by a different sensory stimulus.

Photocoagulation: The condensation of protein material by the controlled use of an intense beam of light (such as a xenon arc light or argon laser).

Photon: A particle of light whose energy depends on its wavelength (that is, its color); many billions of individual photons make up a light beam.

Photophobia: Dread or avoidance of light.

Photoreception: Sensitivity to light.

Photoreceptor: A light-responsive nerve cell or receptor that is located in the retina of the eye.

Phrenic: Of or relating to the diaphragm.

Phylogenetics: The building of evolutionary trees, such as to describe accurately the base-by-base changes in a particular protein from different species.

Physiatry: The branch of medicine dealing with the

prevention, diagnosis, and treatment of disease or injury and the rehabilitation from resultant impairments and disabilities; it uses physical agents such as light, heat, cold, water, electricity, therapeutic exercise, mechanical apparatus, and pharmaceutical agents.

Physical deconditioning: A condition that results when a person who has previously been exercising (has become conditioned) stops exercising for a significant period of time.

Physical examination: A step in the diagnostic process in which the physician makes general observations about the patient and examines structures of the patient's body through touching (palpation), tapping (percussion), and listening, usually with the aid of a stethoscope (auscultation).

Physical modalities: The physical means of addressing a disease, which include heat, cold, electricity, exercises, braces, assistive devices, and biofeedback.

Physical rehabilitation: The discipline devoted to the restoration of normal bodily function, primarily of the muscles and skeleton.

Physical sciences: The branch of natural science that analyzes the nature and properties of energy and nonliving matter; includes disciplines such as physics, chemistry, astronomy, and geology.

Physician assistant: A health care provider who works under the supervision of a licensed physician and who is trained to perform physical examinations, diagnose illnesses, interpret laboratory tests, set fractures, and assist in surgeries.

Physiological: Characteristic of or appropriate to an organism's healthy or normal functioning.

Physiology: The study of how the body functions, both at the cellular level and at the anatomical level.

Phytochemicals: Nonnutritive chemicals produced by plants that provide health benefits to humans who eat foods derived from them.

PID. *See* Pelvic inflammatory disease (PID).

Pigmentation: The color of the skin, hair, and eyes, caused by the degree and distribution of melanin in the skin.

Piles: A common term for hemorrhoids.

Pilosebaceous: Referring to hair follicles and the sebaceous glands.

Pimple: The common term for a papule (a solid elevation in the skin) or a pustule (a papule containing pus).

Pituitary gland: A very small gland at the base of the brain that is referred to as the master gland; with the hypothalamus, it regulates most of the endocrine systems.

PKU. *See* Phenylketonuria (PKU).

Placebo: An inactive substance resembling the experimental drug that might be given to a control group, especially when no standard treatment exists.

Placenta: The oval, spongy tissue containing blood vessels that provides the fetus with nutrients and oxygen from the mother via the umbilicus.

Plague: A serious, and sometimes fatal, bacterial infection transmitted by fleas.

Plaintiff: A person or corporation that brings legal action against another person or corporation.

Plantar: Having to do with the sole of the foot.

Plantar warts: Warts that develop on the soles of the feet, usually at points of pressure; such a wart consists of a soft core surrounded by a calluslike ring.

Plaque: The fatty material composed of cholesterol, degenerating cells, and proteinaceous substances that can build up in the wall of any artery; also, an accumulation of decomposing matter on the teeth that promotes tooth decay.

Plasma: The fluid portion of blood, in which white and red blood cells are suspended and that contains water, proteins, minerals, nutrients, hormones, and wastes.

Plasma proteins: Any proteins found in the plasma of blood, which include those proteins necessary for blood clotting and some necessary for the transport of other molecules; most are produced by the liver.

Plasmin: An enzyme present in the blood that can dissolve clots; plasmin is normally found in its inactive form, plasminogen, until needed.

Plastic surgery: Surgery performed to repair defects of the skin and underlying tissues caused by injury or malformations.

Plasticity: A phenomenon of many animal nervous systems, particularly those in higher vertebrates, in which central nervous system neurons grow in patterns based on input information.

Platelets: Specialized blood-clotting particles that travel in the blood and become sticky when they come in contact with a damaged blood vessel.

Pleura: A serous membrane that covers and protects the lungs.

Pleurisy: The inflammation and swelling of the pleurae, the membranes that enclose the lungs and line the chest cavity.

Pluripotent: Referring to stem cells that have the capacity to develop into most of the specialized tissues of the body, but not an entire individual.

PMS. *See* Premenstrual syndrome (PMS).

Pneumocystis pneumonia: A form of pneumonia caused by the single-celled parasite *Pneumocystis carinii*; dangerous mainly to persons with impaired immune systems, particularly patients with AIDS.

Pneumonia: An inflammation of the lungs or bronchial passageways caused by viral or bacterial infection.

Pneumothorax: The collapse of a lung or portion of a lung due to the introduction of air or another gas or of fluid into the pleural space surrounding the lungs.

Podiatry: The branch of medicine that treats diseases and conditions of the foot.

Poisoning: Exposure to any substance in a quantity sufficient to cause health problems.

Poisonous plants: Plants that cause gastrointestinal or dermatological reactions in humans.

Poliomyelitis: A viral illness that may cause meningitis and permanent paralysis; it can be prevented through immunization.

Polycystic kidney disease: A genetic disorder characterized by multiple, bilateral, grapelike clusters of fluid-filled cysts that slowly replace much of the mass of the kidney, reducing kidney function and leading to renal failure.

Polycystic ovary syndrome: A complex disorder related to dysfunctional ovulation, endocrine abnormalities, and multiple cysts on the ovary that result in fertility difficulties; related to obesity and diabetes and poses increased risk for cardiovascular disease.

Polycythemia: An abnormal increase in red blood cells.

Polydactyly: A congenital anomaly characterized by excess fingers or toes.

Polymerase chain reaction: A technique that multiplies small amounts of genetic material (DNA) into amounts that can be detected by specific genetic probes.

Polymethylmethacrylate: A material used in the fixation of bones.

Polypharmacy: The prescription of many drugs at one time, often resulting in excessive use of medications and adverse drug interactions.

Polyps: Abnormal growths arising from mucous membranes anywhere in the body.

Polyspermy: Entry of more than one sperm into an egg, resulting in too many sets of chromosomes.

Population: All the people, research animals, or other items of interest in a particular study.

Porphyria: One of several rare, genetic disorders caused by the accumulation of substances called porphyrins.

Portacaval: Referring to a type of shunt used to carry blood from the portal vein to the inferior vena cava, allowing blood to bypass the liver.

Portal system: A system of veins, unique to the liver, that carry nutrient-rich blood from the digestive organs to the liver.

Positive feedback: Physiological process in which a product feeds back to stimulate the process, resulting in additional production or the continuation of that process.

Positron emission tomography (PET) scanning: A technique for creating three-dimensional images of tissues in the body by tracking radioisotopes injected into the body, allowing for diagnosis of tumors or metabolic diseases and conditions, especially of the brain.

Positrons: A type of radiation, similar to electrons but with positive charge, emitted by radioactive atoms.

Posterior: Toward the back or rear of the body or any structure.

Postnasal drip: The discharge of nasal mucus into the back of the throat.

Postoperative: Referring to a the period of time following a surgical procedure.

Postpartum depression: Depression following childbirth brought on by hormonal changes and sometimes by underlying social or emotional problems.

Potency: The effectiveness of a drug.

Prader-Willi syndrome: A disorder caused by a deletion in chromosome 15, characterized by developmental and cognitive delays, overeating resulting in obesity, and behavioral difficulties.

Preeclampsia: Hypertension induced by pregnancy, in its nonconvulsive form.

Pregnancy: The development of an embryo or fetus within the uterus, which begins with conception.

Premature: Referring to a birth that is less than full term.

Premenstrual syndrome (PMS): A common condition involving tension, irritability, headaches, depression, and bloating in the week prior to menstruation.

Premolars: The teeth between the cuspids and the molars, used in crushing and grinding food; also called bicuspids.

Prep: A short form of the word "prepare"; to prep means to wash and shave the surgical area and to clean the skin surface immediately before a surgical procedure.

Prescription drugs: Medicines that can be obtained only with the prescription of a doctor.

Presenilins: Proteins linked to several forms of inherited Alzheimer's disease, which are believed to play a role in the production of Aβ.

Pressure: The measure of how much a gas or a liquid pushes on the walls of its container.

Prevalence: The number of individuals at a particular time who have a disease or a given characteristic.

Preventive medicine: An approach to health care that emphasizes behaviors and therapies (such as exercise and proper diet) designed to minimize contraction of disease before it happens.

Prima facie: The concept that one ethical principle is morally binding unless the action it requires violates another equal or greater principle.

Primary care: General medical services provided in family practice, internal medicine, pediatrics, geriatrics, obstetrics, and emergency care (in contrast to specialties, such as urology or cardiac surgery).

Primary infection: A person's first infection with a particular agent such as a virus.

Privacy: The state of being free from unwanted or unauthorized observation, company, or other intrusion.

Probability: A number varying between 0 (for an impossible event) to 1 (for an absolutely certain event).

Procedure: Any medical treatment that involves physical manipulation or invasion of the body.

Proctology: The study and treatment of diseases of the rectum.

Prodromal: Sensation before an event occurs.

Professional licensing: State-granted privileges to health care and other professionals allowing them to deliver services or to participate in certain activities; a privilege that is revocable and subject to censure; a privilege usually granted only after thorough examination of the skill and practice of a person seeking licensure.

Progesterone or progestin: A hormone produced in the ovaries, adrenal gland, and placenta (of pregnant women) that prepares for and sustains pregnancy.

Prognosis: The predicted outcome of a disease.

Prolactin: A hormone secreted from the anterior pituitary gland that signals the breast to start and sustain milk production.

Prone: The position of the body when lying face downward, on the abdomen.

Prophylactic treatment: A treatment focusing on preventing disease, illness, or their symptoms from occurring.

Prostaglandins: Chemical messengers that are not carried in the blood and that function only locally; they cause pain, contractions, and a variety of other effects.

Prostate gland: An accessory reproductive gland whose main function is to secrete into semen vital additive components that increase the fertilizing potential of sperm.

Prosthesis: A fabricated, artificial substitute for a missing part of the body, such as a limb.

Prosthetist: An individual skilled in constructing and fitting prostheses.

Prosthodontics: The dental specialty that restores missing teeth with fixed or removable dentures.

Prostoglandular carcinoma: The general pathological nomenclature for cancers located in the prostate gland.

Protein: Large molecules made up of amino acids connected by peptide bonds; the sequence of amino acids in a protein determines its three-dimensional structure.

Protein kinase: An enzyme type that often is encoded by oncogenes; this enzyme attaches phosphate molecules to certain amino acids on specifically targeted proteins.

Proteinuria: The presence of protein (typically albumin) in the urine.

Proteome: The complete set of proteins in a particular cell type.

Proteomics: The study of proteomes.

Protozoan (*pl.* protozoa): A single-celled organism that is more closely related to animals than are bacteria and is often a vector of disease; only a few drugs are available that will kill protozoa without harming their animal hosts.

Provider: The medical practitioner within a clinic or hospital; providers may be physicians, nurses, dentists, or other licensed health care professionals.

Proving: The testing of a substance or remedy on healthy volunteers (provers), who take repeated doses and record in detail any symptoms produced by it.

Proximal: Toward the origin.

Psoriasis: A chronic skin disease characterized by red, scaly patches overlaid with thick, silvery gray scales.

Psyche: The human mind, which according to Sigmund Freud is divided into id, ego, and superego; the id contains instincts and repressed feelings, the ego directs everyday behavior, and the superego guides the ego.

Psychedelic drugs: Substances that cause alterations in perception and thinking, such as changes in awareness, sense of self, or hallucinations.

Psychiatry: The branch of medicine, practiced by physicians, that treats emotional and behavioral problems through both medication and non-drug therapies such as counseling.

Psychoanalysis: A form of treatment for mental illness that employs interviews designed to elicit information from the patient, which the analyst then interprets in the light of theories developed by Sigmund Freud.

Psychoanalyst: A person, usually a psychiatrist, who has received several years of postgraduate training and supervised practice in using psychoanalysis to diagnose and treat clients; psychoanalysts are often, but not always, medical doctors.

Psychogenic: Psychological (rather than physical) in origin; set off by psychologically stressful events.

Psychosis: A condition occurring where a person is severely out of touch with reality and unable to function in an adaptive manner.

Psychosomatic: Referring to physical symptoms caused or aggravated by psychological factors.

Psychosurgery: The surgical removal or destruction of part of the brain of depressed patients as a form of treatment.

Psychotherapy: Treatment using the mind, body, and behavior to remedy problems related to disordered behavior or thinking, emotional problems, or disease.

Psychotic: Referred to a disabling mental state characterized by poor reality testing (inaccurate perceptions, confusion, disorientation) and disorganized speech, behavior, and emotional experience.

Psychotropic drugs: Substances primarily affecting behavior, perception, and other psychological functions.

PTCA. *See* Percutaneous transluminal coronary angioplasty (PTCA).

Ptosis: Downward drooping or sagging of tissue, caused by the influence of gravity or the loss of muscular or other support.

Puberty: The physiological sequence of events by which a child is transformed into an adult; the growth of secondary sexual characteristics occurs, reproductive functions begin, and the differences between males and females are accentuated.

Public health: Preventive measures intended to improve the health of all persons in a community.

Pulmonary: Related to the lungs and breathing.

Pulmonary edema: Accumulation of fluid in the lungs, which may lead to death.

Pulmonary hypertension: A rare disorder of the pulmonary circulation occurring mostly in young and middle-aged women.

Pulmonary medicine: The field of medicine concerned with all the diseases that may afflict the lungs or in which the lungs may be involved.

Pulmonary nodules: Small, round growths on the lung that contain either trapped microorganisms or cancer cells.

Pulp: The internal, living tissue of the tooth, consisting of nerves, blood vessels, and dental cells.

Pulse: The rhythmical dilation of an artery, produced by the increased volume of blood forced into the vessel by the contraction of the heart; the frequency of the pulse corresponds to the heart rate.

Pulsed laser: A laser technique used to deliver a light beam of high power for a very short time in order to localize the heating effect without damaging surrounding tissue.

Pupil: The opening at the center of the iris through which light passes.

Pyelonephritis: Inflammation of the kidney as the result of a bacterial infection in the bladder.

Pyloric stenosis: A narrowing of the passageway between the stomach and the duodenum.

Pyorrhea: The second stage of gingivitis.

Pyridostigmine bromide: A chemical that prevents damage from possible nerve gas exposure.

Pyrogens: Protein substances that appear at the outset of the process that leads to a fever reaction.

Qi gong: A Chinese meditative exercise that improves cardiovascular circulation, restores deep breathing, and relieves stress.

Quadriplegia: Partial or complete paralysis of the arms, legs, and trunk caused by damage to the spinal cord in the neck.

Quantum theory: The theory that energy, momentum, and other physical quantities appear in indivisible units of finite quantity.

Quickening: The stage during a pregnancy when the mother begins to feel the movements of the fetus, usually in the second trimester.

Rabies: A viral infection, usually transmitted through the bite of a rabid animal, that attacks the nervous system; it can be cured through immediate immunization but is nearly always fatal once symptoms occur.

Radial: Toward the edge of the forearm and hand containing the radius and thumb.

Radiation dose: The amount of radiation absorbed, depending on the intensity of the source and the time of exposure; measured in units of rads or grays.

Radiation sickness: Acute, sometimes fatal illness that occurs with exposure to a sudden, large dose of radiation.

Radiation therapy: The use of radiation to kill cancer cells or shrink cancerous growth; when high and full doses of radiation (measured in units called rads) are used, the patient is said to be given a "megavoltage."

Radical surgery: Any surgery that removes all of the organ or tissue affected by a disease, as well as tissue surrounding the area, in an attempt to eradicate the disease.

Radiculopathy: Pain distributed along a specific pathway resulting from irritation of a nerve root.

Radioimmunoassay: The quantitative measurement of a hormone using an unlabeled hormone to inhibit the binding of a radiolabeled hormone to an antibody.

Radioimmunotherapy: A cancer therapy using radionuclides; the radionuclides attach themselves to antibodies that tend to target cancer cells in the body, thus eradicating the cancer cells through selective irradiation.

Radioisotope. *See* Radionuclide.

Radiology: The branch of medicine that focuses on imaging technologies such as X rays, magnetic resonance imaging (MRI), scanning techniques, and ultrasonography.

Radionucleotide scanning: A technique that develops an image of an internal bodily structure by detecting radiation emitted from a substance injected into the body to see how the bodily structure reacts to it.

Radionuclide: An unstable atomic nucleus that, in the process of decay, emits radiation.

Radiopharmaceutical: A sterile, radioactively tagged compound that is administered to a patient for diagnostic or therapeutic purposes.

Radius: The shorter of the two forearm bones, on the thumb side.

Random sample: A sample in which every member of the population has the same probability of being included.

Rash: A skin disorder, usually temporary, characterized by red, inflamed areas or spots; generally a symptom of an underlying condition, such as a skin disease, autoimmune disorder, infectious disease, or bleeding disorder.

RDA. *See* Recommended daily (or dietary) allowance (RDA).

Receptor: A molecular structure at the cell surface or inside the cell that is capable of combining with hormones or neurotransmitters and causing a change in cell metabolism.

Recessive allele: A version of a gene that must be present on both chromosomes of a pair in order to produce a recognizable trait in offspring.

Recessive genetic disease: A disease caused by a mutation in a gene that must be inherited from both parents in order for an individual to show the symptoms of the disease; such a disease may show up only occasionally in a family history, especially if the mutation is rare.

Recombinant DNA technology: Manipulation of genetic material or DNA whereby pieces of DNA are separated and interchanged in order to obtain a desired result.

Recombination: The reciprocal exchange of segments between the two chromosomes of a pair, producing new combinations of alleles.

Recommended daily (or dietary) allowance (RDA): Former term for dietary reference intake (DRI).

Reconstructive surgery: Surgery designed to rebuild or replace a body part malformed at birth, damaged as a result of injury, or surgically removed for therapeutic reasons.

Recovery room: The room where a patient returns to full consciousness after a surgical procedure; in an outpatient facility, patients can change clothes in the recovery room, which may serve double duty as the preoperative waiting room.

Rectal prolapse: The protrusion of the rectum through the anus.

Rectum: The intestinal storage area for feces between the colon and anus.

Recurrence: The appearance of an infection or disease after initial treatment has been completed.

Red blood cells: Blood cells that contain hemoglobin; their role is to transport oxygen.

Reduction: The restoration of a fractured bone to its normal position; also a decrease in the total volume or mass of breast tissue, usually to correct undesirable ptosis.

Reed-Sternberg cell: A large, atypical macrophage with multiple nuclei; found in patients with Hodgkin's disease.

Referred pain: Pain that is felt somewhere other than at the site of injury or disease, as a result of neural pathways.

Reflux: The abnormal backward flow of a fluid (such as bile or urine).

Refraction: The bending of light rays by the cornea and lens to form an image on the retina.

Regeneration: The renewal, regrowth, or restoration of destroyed or missing tissue; the production of new tissue.

Regional anesthesia: Insensibility caused by the interruption of nerve conduction in a region of the body.

Regression: Reverting to a pattern of behavior seen at an earlier age of development.

Regurgitation: The leakage of blood backward through a valve; also vomiting.

Rehabilitation: The restoration of normal form and function after injury or illness; the restoration of the ill or injured patient to optimal functional level in the home and community in relation to physical, psychosocial, vocational, and recreational activity.

Reiter's syndrome: An autoimmune disorder with associated symptoms of arthritis, urethritis, conjunctivitis, and ulcerations of the skin and mouth.

Rejection: A cellular and chemical attack by the immune system on transplanted tissues or organs, which are recognized as foreign to the body.

Reliability: The concept that repeated tests will produce the same result.

Renal: Referring to the kidneys.

Renal cell carcinoma: Cancer of the small tubules of the kidney; generally known as kidney cancer.

Renal failure: The inability of the kidneys to process waste products in the blood and excrete them through the urine.

Renal pelvis: The central pocket or sac of each kidney, which collects urine from all nephrons and channels it into the ureter.

Renal tubule: The tubular portion of a nephron that allows renal fluid to flow from the Bowman's capsule to the renal pelvis; these tubules, shaped like hairpins, are crucially important in the production of urine.

Repertory: In homeopathy, a published index of symptoms, with each heading listing the drugs known to cause the symptom.

Replication: The process by which the DNA of a cell is duplicated so that the information stored there can be passed on to new cells after cell division.

Reproductive system: The organs of the female (the vagina, uterus, Fallopian tubes, ovaries, and mammary glands) and the male (the penis, testes, vas deferens, and prostate gland) that are involved in the production or feeding of offspring.

Reservoir: An animal population that is infected with a disease that can be transmitted either to other animals or to humans; also called an alternate host.

Residency: A course of clinical medical education undertaken after receiving an M.D. or D.O. degree and leading to certification in a generalist or specialist branch of medicine.

Resorption: The process in which bones dissolve and return their components to the body fluids.

Respect for autonomy: A principle of medical ethics which requires that the autonomous decisions of patients be honored.

Respiration: A process that includes both air conduction (the act of breathing) and gas exchange (oxygen and carbon dioxide transfer between the air and blood).

Respirator: A machine that inflates and deflates the lungs, imitating normal breathing; connected to patient through a tube placed into the windpipe.

Respiratory diseases: Any of a wide variety of diseases that affect the lungs and/or the process of respiration, including emphysema, lung cancer, and pneumonia.

Respiratory distress syndrome: A life-threatening illness primarily of premature infants; immature lungs lack a vital substance that keeps the tiny air sacs (alveoli) from collapsing upon exhalation.

Rest pain: Pain noted in the most distal portion of the extremity at rest, relieved by analgesics.

Restless legs syndrome: A sensorimotor disorder characterized by uncomfortable and even painful sensations in the limbs, especially the legs, when at rest or trying to sleep.

Restoration: An item or material that is used to restore the structure and function of a compromised tooth.

Restriction endonuclease: An enzyme that responds to a specific, short sequence of nucleotides within a DNA molecule by binding to that sequence and breaking the DNA strands near the sequence.

Resuscitation: The return of a person to consciousness or the restoration of a person's vital signs after an injury, seizure, or heart attack by means of artificial respiration, cardiopulmonary resuscitation (CPR), electrical shock treatment, chemicals, or other means.

Retina: A thin membrane at the back of the eyeball where light is converted into nerve impulses that travel to the brain.

Retrocochlear hearing loss: Any disruption of neural information processing beyond the cochlea.

Retroviruses: RNA viruses that replicate by synthesizing a double-stranded DNA molecule that integrates into the host genome; they are known to infect virtually all animals and sometimes cause serious disease, including cancer.

Revascularization: Procedures to reestablish the circulation to a diseased portion of the body.

Reverse transcriptase: An enzyme that synthesizes double-stranded DNA from single-stranded RNA.

Reye's syndrome: A somewhat rare, noncontagious disease of the liver and central nervous system that strikes individuals under the age of eighteen.

Rh factor: Any one of several "factors," or elements present in the blood, according to one system of blood-type classification; the presence of the D factor can cause erythroblastosis fetalis, a type of hemolytic disease of the newborn.

Rh0(D) immune globulin (human): A type of gamma globulin protein injected into Rh-negative mothers who may have an Rh-positive fetus in order to protect the fetus from an immune reaction.

Rheumatic fever: A complication of untreated streptococcal infections characterized by swollen joints, rashes, fever, and sometimes heart disorders; evidence of heart valve damage may emerge later in life.

Rheumatoid arthritis: A disease affecting the muscles, cartilage, and joints characterized by stiffness, pain, and swelling.

Rheumatology: The study and treatment of rheumatoid arthritis and related diseases.

Rhinitis: Inflammation of the mucous membrane that lines the nose, resulting from an allergic reaction or a common cold virus.

Rhinoplasty: Surgical alteration of the structure of the nose, performed for both therapeutic and cosmetic reasons.

Rhinovirus: A microorganism causing respiratory illness; one of the most prevalent causes of the common cold.

Rhodopsin: A chemical within photoreceptors that translates light into electrical impulses.

Ribonucleic acid (RNA): The material contained in the core of many viruses that is responsible for directing the replication of the virus inside the host cell.

Ribosome: A cytoplasmic particle assembled from ribosomal RNA and ribosomal proteins that uses messenger RNA molecules as directions for synthesizing proteins.

Ribs: The bones that support the chest and define its outline.

Rickets: A deficiency in vitamin D, calcium, and phosphorus that results in soft bones.

Risk assessment: The process that establishes whether a health risk exists for a population exposed to a toxic substance.

Risk factors: The situations, circumstances, or conditions that increase the probability of the occurrence of disease or accident.

RNA. *See* Ribonucleic acid (RNA).

Rods: Specialized photoreceptors that provide peripheral vision and vision in dim light.

Root: That portion of the tooth which is below the crown and is embedded in a bony socket of the jaw.

Root canal treatment: Surgery to save a tooth whose pulp has become diseased or has died.

Root hair plexus: A network of sensory receptors located at hair roots that generates an impulse when hairs are moved.

Rosacea: The chronic inflammation of facial skin; also known as acne rosacea or adult acne.

Roseola: A common and contagious childhood disease characterized by high fever and a skin rash.

Rotator cuff surgery: The surgical correction of a muscle tear within the shoulder.

Roundworm: Intestinal parasites in humans that thrive in the gastrointestinal tract.

Rubella: A mild, contagious viral illness that is dangerous only when contracted by women during the early months of pregnancy, when it is likely to cause birth defects; also called German measles.

Rubeola. *See* Measles.

Rubinstein-Taybi syndrome: A syndrome typically characterized by small skeletal stature, mental retardation, and large thumbs and toes.

Ruffini endings: Sensory receptors that respond to heavy and continuous touch and pressure; also called type II cutaneous mechanoreceptors or the end organs of Ruffini.

Rule of nines: A system for designating areas of the body, represented by various body parts; used in determining the extent of a burn.

S-A node. *See* Sinoatrial (S-A) node.

Salicylates: A group of drugs that includes aspirin and related compounds used to relieve pain, reduce inflammation, and lower fever.

Salivary glands: The glands that produce saliva, a watery substance in the mouth that helps break down food.

Salmonella: Bacteria that cause a general infection of the gastrointestinal tract and lymphatic system when ingested.

Sample: The members of a population that are actually studied or whose characteristics are measured.

Sanatorium: An institution designed for the treatment of chronic illnesses, such as tuberculosis.

Sanitation: The application of measures designed to protect public health.

Saphenous vein: Vein from the upper leg that is often used to bypass a blocked coronary artery.

Saponification: A reaction in which a strong basic solution splits a molecule into a carboxylic acid unit and an alcohol unit.

Sarcoidosis: An inflammatory disease, characterized by noncaseating granulomas, of unknown cause, affecting multiple systems, especially the lungs, lymph nodes, skin, and eyes.

Sarcoma: A malignant tumor originating in connective tissue, including bone and muscle.

Sarin: A nerve gas that can cause convulsions and death.

SARS. *See* Severe acute respiratory syndrome (SARS).

Scabies: Skin infestation by mites, causing a rash and severe itching.

Scarlet fever: An acute, contagious childhood disease caused by bacterial infection.

Schistosomiasis: A chronic illness caused by parasitic worms that live in the blood vessels around the liver and bladder.

Schizophrenia: A mental disturbance characterized by psychotic features during the active phase and deteriorated functioning in occupational, social, or self-care abilities.

Schwann cell: A supportive cell for neurons in the peripheral nervous system of vertebrate animals that wraps around and insulates axons using the protein myelin.

Sciatica: Painful inflammation of one of the sciatic nerves.

SCID. *See* Severe combined immunodeficiency syndrome (SCID).

Scientific method: A method of scientific investigation involving observation, the formation of a hypothesis (a possible explanation), experimentation, and the reevaluation of data.

Scintillation: The production of flashes emitted by luminescent substances when excited by high-energy radiation.

Sclera: The opaque portion of the outer layer of the eye; commonly referred to as the "white of the eye."

Scleroderma: A rare autoimmune connective tissue disorder affecting various organs.

Scoliosis: Abnormal curvature of the spine, which is often progressive.

Screening: A strategy used by physicians and public health professionals to diagnose disease or the potential for disease at an early stage, when it may be treatable or preventable; may be a mandatory procedure for a specific population or a voluntary activity requested by individuals.

Scrotum: The genital skin sac that holds the testicles and related structures.

Scrub: To wash one's hands and forearms in preparation for donning gown and gloves, which protect the patient from the surgeon and staff and protect the surgeon and staff from the patient.

Scurvy: A disease caused by a prolonged inadequate intake of vitamin C.

Seasonal affective disorder: A depression that undergoes a seasonal fluctuation as a result of various factors, both unknown and known.

Sebaceous glands: Glands in the skin that usually open into the hair follicles.

Sebum: A semifluid, fatty substance secreted by the sebaceous glands into the hair follicles.

Secondary infection: A bacterial, viral, or other infection that results from or follows another disease.

Sedation: The use of medication to calm patients who are agitated or anxious, to relieve pain, or to relax patients experiencing discomfort from a device being used to support care (for example, a breathing tube inserted down the throat).

Seizure: A sudden, violent, and involuntary contraction of a group of muscles; may be paroxysmal and episodic, also called a convulsion.

Selective serotonin reuptake inhibitors (SSRIs): A class of antidepressant drugs that work by inhibiting the neurotransmitter serotonin, thus making more of it available to brain cells.

Semen: Fluid produced by a man's prostate gland that makes up 95 percent of the fluid that is ejaculated.

Seminoma: The most common cancer of the testes.

Semipermeable membrane: A barrier that allows some materials to pass but blocks others.

Semisynthetic: Referring to natural products, such as antibiotics, that have been chemically modified to be more useful for a particular application.

Senile plaques: A hallmark lesion of Alzheimer's disease, composed of $A\beta$ amyloid.

Senility: An outmoded term for dementia often applied to the elderly.

Sense organs: Specialized structures anatomically suited to a particular sense—the eyes for vision, the nose for smell (olfaction), the taste buds for taste, the ears for hearing and balance, and the skin for such cutaneous sensations as warmth, cold, light touch, deep pressure, and pain.

Sensitivity: The ability of a screening technique to identify correctly people who have a disease.

Sensorineural hearing loss: The loss of sensory or neural tissue of the auditory system as a result of disease, age, and acquired or congenital factors.

Sensory: Referring to perception by the senses: touch, sight, hearing, smell, and other senses such as hunger.

Sepsis: An infection in the circulating blood.

Septic pyelophlebitis: Inflammation of the veins that carry blood away from the kidneys.

Septic shock: A dangerous condition in which there is tissue damage and a dramatic drop in blood pressure as a result of septicemia.

Septicemia: Serious, systemic infection of the blood with pathogens that have spread from an infection in a part of the body, characteristically causing fever, chills, prostration, pain, headache, nausea, and/or diarrhea.

Septum: A membrane that serves as a wall of separation; in the heart, the interatrial septum divides the two atria, and the interventricular septum divides the two ventricles.

Serology: The branch of medicine specializing in the clear portion of the blood called the serum, often focused on analysis of the serum as a means of diagnosing disease.

Seronegative: The test result seen when blood does not contain the specific antibody or antigen being sought and the particular antigen-antibody reaction is not present.

Seropositive: The test result seen when blood contains the specific antibody or antigen being sought and the particular antigen-antibody reaction is present.

Serotonin: An abundant chemical nerve signal in the brain that is involved in modulating aggression.

Serotype: A subgroup member within a larger species; similar, but not identical, to other members of the species.

Serum: The fluid part of blood, without red blood cells and clotting factors.

Set point: A mechanism, thought to be formed by a series of feedback systems, for maintaining such characteristics as temperature and body weight.

Severe acute respiratory syndrome (SARS): A recently recognized type of pneumonia caused by a novel coronavirus that may progress to respiratory failure and death.

Severe combined immunodeficiency syndrome (SCID): A syndrome in which the immune system is unable to produce T and B lymphocytes, resulting in catastrophic failure of the immune system.

Sex change surgery: A set of procedures designed to convert the secondary sexual characteristics of an anatomic male to those of a female or an anatomic female to those of a male.

Sex glands: The ovaries in the female and the testes in the male, which secrete hormones involved in reproduction.

Sex steroids: Steroid hormones such as androgens and estrogens that influence the activity of sexual organs and activity.

Sexual differentiation: The process by which an embryo becomes male or female under the influence of genetic and hormonal factors.

Sexually transmitted disease (STD): Any disease that can be acquired through sexual contact or passed from a pregnant woman to her fetus, including syphilis, gonorrhea, chlamydia, herpes, and AIDS.

Shigellosis: An intestinal infection caused by *Shigella* bacteria.

Shingles: A disease of the central nervous system characterized by painful red blisters that join together and rapidly rupture and become crusted.

Shock: A life-threatening condition in which the heart is unable to pump enough blood to the vital organs; symptoms include rapid and shallow breathing, clammy skin, low blood pressure, and dizziness.

Shock wave: A miniature explosion caused by intense local heating with a laser beam; used to fragment stones in the kidney or gallbladder.

Shunt: An opening established by surgery to maintain easy access to an internal area of the body for various purposes, such as application of medication or drainage of excess body fluids.

Sickle cell disease: An inherited blood disorder in which abnormally high amounts of hemoglobin cause red blood cells to become sickle-shaped and block capillaries.

Side effect: A secondary and usually adverse effect (as of a drug); also known as an adverse effect or reaction.

SIDS. *See* Sudden infant death syndrome (SIDS).

Sigmoidoscopy: Endoscopy performed on the lower section of the colon.

Sign: Objective evidence of disease; a finding noted by the physician during the course of the physical examination.

Signal-averaged electrocardiogram: A sophisticated ECG that detects subtle and potentially lethal cardiac conduction defects.

Silicone: A plastic made primarily of silicon polymer.

Sinoatrial (S-A) node: A cluster of cells above the right atrium that emit electrical signals that initiate contractions of the heart; also called natural pacemaker cells.

Sinusitis: The inflammation of the lining of the nasal sinuses.

Sjögren's syndrome: An autoimmune disorder resulting in the loss of tears and saliva.

Skeletal muscle: A type of muscle that attaches to bone and causes movement of body parts; the only type that is under conscious, voluntary control.

Skeleton: The bony framework of the body.

Skilled home care: Medically necessary care that requires a service by a professional such as a nurse or physical therapist.

Skin: The largest organ of the body, which is vital to the survival of an organism for its protection against dehydration and abrasion, regulation of body temperature, and sensory reception.

Skin biopsy: A removal of a piece of skin for the purpose of further microscopic examination.

Sleep apnea: A sleep disorder characterized by intermittent cessation of airflow through the upper airway.

Sleep disorder: Any abnormal pattern of sleep that threatens normal function, including conditions that cause too much as well as too little sleep, and that may be both organic and nonorganic in origin.

Sleeping sickness: An infectious protozoan disease transmitted through the bite of a tsetse fly.

Slipped disk: A supportive ligament surrounding a vertebra in the neck or back that has broken through the spinal column and into the spinal canal; also called a herniated disk or a ruptured disk.

Small intestine: The region of gut between the stomach and the colon that comprises the duodenum, jejunum, and ileum; also called the small bowel.

Smallpox: A contagious, often-fatal viral infection that has been eradicated through vaccination but that remains a bioterrorist threat.

Smegma: A pasty accumulation of shed skin cells and secretions of the sweat glands, which collects in the moist areas of the foreskin-covered base of the glans (in men) and around the clitoris and labia minora (in women).

Smell: A special sense in which chemicals interact with receptor sites in specialized structures of the nasal cavity and the resulting nerve impulses are classified as certain kinds of odor.

Smooth muscle: Muscle that, when viewed under a microscope, does not have striations, which are stripes seen in skeletal muscle cells; smooth muscle contracts involuntarily and is related to the functioning of the stomach, intestines, and urinary bladder; involved in the movement of food through the digestive tract.

Sodium pentothal: A fast-acting anesthetic that is injected into the vein; first developed for military hospitals during World War II.

Soft palate: A structure of mucous membrane, muscle fibers, and mucous glands suspended from the posterior border of the hard palate in the mouth.

Soma: The body of a cell, where the cell's genetic material and other vital structures are located.

Somatoform disorder: A mental disorder whose symptoms focus on the physical body.

Sonography: The use of sound waves deflected from internal body organs to find growing masses (including fetuses) and abnormal lesions; also called ultrasound.

Sore throat: Discomfort and/or pain experienced in the throat, which sometimes indicates the presence of a more serious disorder.

Spastic: Characterized by uncontrollable spasms.

Spasticity: A rigidity or resistance to passive limb movement, usually occuring in limbs that are weak, that respond in an impaired way to voluntary control, and whose weakness is thought to be due to observed lesions in the upper motor neurons.

Specialist: Any physician who practices in a specialty other than the generalist areas of family practice, general internal medicine, general pediatrics, or obstetrics and gynecology.

Specific gravity: The density of a solution relative to that of water; abnormal values can be indicative of elevated sugar or protein levels in urine.

Specificity: The ability of a screening technique to identify correctly people who do not have a disease.

Spectrum of activity: The range of microbial species that can be inhibited by an antibiotic; broad-spectrum antibiotics can control more than one kind of infection, but narrow-spectrum antibiotics avoid unintentional damage to the normal microbiota.

Speech disorder: A dysfunction in the brain-coordinated use of speech organs, such as problems with language, vocal quality, articulation, fluency, and dementia.

Sperm: The male gamete; the mature sperm has an oval head that contains the male's chromosomes and a long tail that allows it to swim in fluid.

Spermicide: A chemical that kills sperm after they are ejaculated.

Sphincter: A ringlike muscle that acts as a one-way valve to control the flow of fluids and waste.

Sphincterectomy: Surgical removal of a sphincter.

Sphygmomanometer: A device that uses a column of mercury to measure blood pressure.

Spina bifida: A genetic abnormality in which the spine has failed to fuse, sometimes exposing the spinal cord and nerves.

Spinal anesthesia: The injection of an anesthetic at the base of the spine to produce loss of feeling in the lower part of the body and legs; also known as a subarachnoid block.

Spinal canal: A tube or tunnel that runs down the spine and contains the spinal cord, which carries the nerves from the brain to the body.

Spinal cord: A cord in the trunk containing nerve cells that transmit impulses to and from the brain.

Spinal nerves: Pairs of nerves connected to the spinal cord and numbered according to the level at which they emerge from the cord; each spinal nerve attaches to the spinal cord by an anterior and a posterior root.

Spinal stenosis: A condition in which the diameter of the spinal canal is decreased and thus compromises the spinal cord and spinal nerve roots.

Spinal tap. *See* Lumbar puncture.

Spine: The combined spinal cord and the vertebral (spinal) column.

Spinous processes: Bony projections from vertebrae (horizontally in the neck, tilting downward in the thoracic area, and horizontally in the lumbar area) that are connected to one another by the interspinous and supraspinous ligaments and that control extremes of trunk motion.

Spleen: A lymphatic organ, found between the stomach and the diaphragm, that destroys old blood cells and filters foreign material from the blood.

Splenectomy: Surgical removal of the spleen.

Spondylitis: Inflammation and stiffening of the joints between the vertebrae of the spine.

Spondylosis: A condition characterized by restriction of movement of the vertebral bones; occurs naturally as a child grows.

Spontaneously resolve: To get better without any treatment.

Sports medicine: A medical subspecialty concerned with the care and prevention of athletic injuries, primarily those related to the musculoskeletal system.

Sprain: An injury in which ligaments are stretched or torn.

Squamous cell carcinoma: A form of skin cancer starting as a small, painless lump and often resembling a wart; common in fair-skinned individuals, especially in later life.

Staging: A numerical classification system used by physicians to describe how far a cancerous growth has advanced.

Staining: The artificial coloring of tissue sections and cells to facilitate their microscopic study.

Stapedectomy: The surgical removal of all or part of the stapes or innermost ossicle of the ear.

Stapes: A small bone within the middle ear; also called the stirrup because of its shape.

Staphylococcal infections: A variety of infections caused by staphylococcus bacteria, including boils, abscesses, pneumonia, bone infections, and toxic shock syndrome.

STD. *See* Sexually transmitted disease (STD).

Stem cell: A master cell from which other blood cells develop; these cells are located primarily in the bone marrow.

Stenosis: An abnormal narrowing or constriction of a canal or passageway in the body caused by the buildup of cholesterol, fats, or other substances (plaque); the swelling or overgrowth of cells, tissue, or an organ; or a deformity.

Stents: Wire mesh tubes permanently implanted to prop open arteries or veins.

Stereotaxic computed tomography: A method of imaging using a series of X rays that are compiled by a computer to give a three-dimensional image of internal structures.

Sterile field: An area in which only sterile supplies may be placed and which only those wearing sterile gowns and gloves may touch; includes the surgical wound, the surgical drapes, and the extra tables.

Sterilization: Any procedure that makes it impossible for a person to reproduce, whether chemical or surgical.

Sternum: The breastbone, which is found in the midline of the chest cavity and lying over the heart.

Steroids: A class of fat-soluble chemicals that are structurally related to one another and share the same chemical skeleton; includes hormones, drugs, and other molecules.

Sterol: A steroid that has long side chains of carbone compounds attached to it and contains at least one hydroxyl group; cholesterol is one type of sterol.

Stethoscope: An instrument for listening to sounds in the body, such as the heartbeat.

Stevens-Johnson syndrome: A severe immune response-mediated hypersensitivity reaction to either particular drugs or infections; causes rashes, sloughing of the skin, and the disruption of mucous membranes.

Stillbirth: A condition in which a fetus has died within the uterus and is born after the twenty-eighth week of pregnancy.

Stimulus: Anything capable of producing a response.

Stoma: A surgically created passage between the intestines and the outer skin.

Stone: A deposit of cholesterol and calcium that may form in the gallbladder, kidneys, ureters, bladder, or urethra; also called a calculus (*pl.* calculi).

Stool: The waste matter of digestion excreted from the body through the anus or a stoma.

Strabismus: Muscle imbalance between the eyes.

Strain: An injury in which muscles or tendons are stretched or torn.

Stratum corneum: The outermost layer of the epidermis; its cells are normally dead, hard, and constantly removed by normal bathing.

Strep throat: A contagious bacterial infection by streptococcal bacteria that causes inflammation of the pharynx.

Streptococcal infections: A variety of infections caused by streptococcus bacteria, including tonsillitis, strep throat, pneumonia, endocarditis, urinary tract infections, and otitis media.

Stress: Physical, environmental, or psychological strain experienced by an individual that requires adjustment.

Stress reduction: A set of procedures with the goal of decreasing bodily and mental tension by increasing rest and coping skills.

Stricture: The narrowing of a passageway.

Stridor: The harsh, high-pitched sound produced by turbulent airflow through a partially obstructed airway.

Stroke: Permanent damage to part of the brain as a result of impaired blood flow.

Stroke volume: The blood volume leaving either the right or the left side of the heart with each beat; each side usually ejects the same volume per beat.

Sturge-Weber syndrome: A disorder associated with partial facial disfigurement that involves vascular accumulations that affect the central nervous system.

Stuttering: The repetition of sounds or syllables or the inability to formulate words in a spoken sentence.

Subclinical: Referring to a medical problem in which the patient has no symptoms of disease or symptoms so slight that the disease is not diagnosed.

Subcutaneous: Under the skin.

Subdural hematoma: Collection of blood (clotted and partially clotted) in the subdural space between brain tissue and the dura mater.

Subluxation: An incomplete or partial dislocation of a joint, which creates abnormal neurological and physiological symptoms in neuromusculoskeletal structures and/or other body systems via interference with nerve impulse transmission.

Substance abuse: Ongoing, chronic ingestion of a substance (usually drugs such as alcohol, nicotine, or narcotics), which threatens health and may cause death if not arrested.

Substantia nigra: A clump of cells located near the base of the cerebral hemispheres that secrete the neurotransmitter dopamine; plays a role in movement, reward, and addiction.

Substrates: Reactants that enzymes convert into products; every enzyme is specific for one specific substrate.

Succussion: Violent shaking at each stage of dilution in the preparation of a homeopathic remedy.

Sudden infant death syndrome (SIDS): The abrupt death of any infant or young child in which postmortem examination fails to demonstrate an adequate cause.

Suggestion: A communication that evokes a nonvoluntary response reflecting the ideational content of the communication.

Superinfection: An infection caused by destruction of the normal microbiota by antibiotic therapy, which allows for proliferation of a pathogen other than the one targeted by the antibiotic.

Superior: Above another part or closer to the head; the ankle bones are superior to the bones of the feet.

Supine: Lying face-upward.

Suppressor T cell: A type of T lymphocyte that is believed to modulate the immune response.

Suprachiasmatic nuclei: Two clusters of nerve cell bodies located in the hypothalamus of the forebrain; these structures display circadian rhythms and seem to be the source of rhythmicity for many of the body's other cycles.

Surgery: The treatment of diseases or disorders by physical intervention, which usually involves cutting into the skin and other tissues.

Surgical pathology: The branch of pathology that deals with the interpretation of biopsies.

Surgical team: The people working together in the operating room during a surgical procedure, including the surgeon, first assistant, surgical technologist, anesthesiologist and/or anesthetist, and circulator.

Surgical technologist: A surgical team member whose primary functions are to prepare surgical instruments and hand them to the surgeon as needed and to prevent infection by maintaining a sterile field in the operating room.

Suspiciousness: A range of symptoms from increasing distrust of others to paranoid delusions of conspiracies.

Suture: A thread used to unite parts of the body.

Sympathectomy: The surgical process of removing or destroying nerves that may be afflicted by frostbite or other injury.

Sympathetic nervous system: The division of the autonomic nervous system concerned primarily with preparing the individual to expend energy.

Symptom: Subjective evidence of disease, provided by the patient.

Symptomatic disease: A disease or disorder that displays overt symptoms.

Symptomatic treatment: A treatment focusing on aborting disease, illness, or their symptoms once they have occurred.

Synapse: An area of close contact between nerve cells that is the functional junction where one cell communicates with another.

Syndactyly: A congenital anomaly characterized by the fusion of the fingers or toes.

Syndrome: A group or pattern of recognizable symptoms or conditions that occur together and indicate a specific disease, psychological disorder, or other abnormal condition.

Synergistic effects: The combined effects of drugs interacting with one another, such that the effects of the drugs together have a compounded effect, greater than that of any one alone.

Synesthete: A person who experiences synesthesia by virtue of having a second sensation evoked by a single stimulus.

Synovial: Referring to the lubricating fluid in the joints or the membrane surrounding the joints.

Synovium: The cellular lining of a joint, having a blood supply and a nerve supply; the synovium secretes fluid for lubrication and protects against injury and injurious agents.

Syphilis: A serious sexually transmitted disease that can be fatal if left untreated.

Systemic: Affecting the entire body.

Systems and organs: Groups of tissues and organs dedicated to particular functions, all of which must work together to perform efficiently.

Systole: The period of contraction of the heart when blood moves out of the heart chambers and into the arteries.

Systolic blood pressure: The pressure of the blood within the artery while the heart is contracting.

T lymphocyte: A type of immune cell that kills host cells infected by bacteria or viruses or produces a chemical compound that mediates the host cells' destruction.

Tachycardia: Rapid beating of the heart.

Tachypnea: Rapid breathing greater than twenty breaths per minute.

Tapeworm: An intestinal parasite in humans transmitted through eating improperly cooked or raw pork, beef, or fish or by being bitten by a larva-carrying flea.

Target heart rate range: A heart rate range that is to be maintained during exercise training.

Tarsus: The ankle.

Tartar: Hardened, mineralized layers of dental plaque.

Taste: A special sense in which chemicals interact with receptor sites in specialized structures of the tongue, and the resulting nerve impulses are classified as certain kinds of taste.

Taste bud: A special sensing structure for taste found on taste-responsive papillae; taste buds are made of three cell types—gustatory or taste cells, supporting cells, and basal cells.

Taste cell: The cellular compartment of a taste bud that contains chemoreceptors; taste hairs, one type of chemoreceptor, are found at the taste pore (or entry point) of a taste cell.

Teeth: Structures that aid animals in processing food prior to swallowing, bringing food into the mouth and grinding; may also be used for defense, the killing of prey, and displays of either hostility or pleasure.

Temporal lobes: Lateral portions of the brain cerebrum; responsible for language, memory, and emotion.

Temporomandibular joint (TMJ): The hinged joint that attaches the head of the mandible to the skull.

Tendinitis: Inflammation of a tendon or a tough band of tissue that connects muscle to the bone.

Tendon: A structure of tough connective tissue that attaches a muscle to a bone.

Tensile strength: The greatest stress that can be placed on a tissue without tearing it apart; it is relative to the strength of a tissue.

Teratogens: Substances that induce congenital malformations when embryonic tissues and organs are exposed to them.

Teratology: The study of congenital malformations.

Testes (*sing.* testis): The male reproductive organs, a pair of gonads that are suspended in the scrotum and produce sperm; also known as the testicles.

Testicular torsion: Twisting of the testicle in the scrotum, with compromise of the blood supply to the testicle, as a result of spermatic cord rotation.

Testosterone: The male sex hormone that gives rise to male fertility and secondary sexual characteristics, such as body hair and musculature.

Tetanus: An often fatal nervous system disease characterized by painful, sustained, and violent muscle spasms; it can be prevented through vaccination.

Thalassemia: An inherited form of anemia in which red blood cells contain less hemoglobin than normal.

Thalidomide: A sedative and sleep-inducing drug that was found to produce phocomelia (a birth defect in which hands or feet are attached to the body by short, flipperlike stumps) in developing fetuses.

Thanatology: The study and investigation of life-threatening actions, terminal illness, suicide, homicide, death, dying, grief, and bereavement.

Therapeutics: The use of chemicals in the diagnosis, prevention, or treatment of disease.

Thermogenesis: The combustion of fuels to provide energy in excess of that required to perform biological work in order to maintain body temperature.

Thermoregulatory set point: The ultimate neural control that maintains the human internal body temperature at 37 degrees Celsius and can either raise or lower it as a defense mechanism against disease.

Thigh: The upper segment of the leg, from the hip joint to the knee.

Thoracic: Pertaining to the chest.

Thoracic duct: The largest lymphatic vessel, which collects lymphatic fluid and returns it to the bloodstream at the left subclavian vein in the region of the neck.

Thorax: The part of the trunk above the diaphragm, containing the ribs; also called the chest.

Thrombin: An enzyme that facilitates the clotting of blood by catalyzing a conversion of fibrinogen to fibrin.

Thrombocytes: Small, irregularly shaped cells in the blood that participate in blood clotting; also called platelets.

Thrombocytopenia: A bleeding disorder in which the blood contains an abnormally low count of functional platelets (thrombocytes).

Thromboembolism: The blockage of a blood vessel by a fragment that has broken off from a thrombus in another blood vessel.

Thrombolytic drugs: A group of drugs that dissolve blood clots by increasing the level of plasmin in the blood.

Thrombosis: The act of complete clotting of an artery or vein, through which no blood can then flow.

Thrombus: A blood clot that has formed inside an intact blood vessel; a thrombus can be life-threatening if it occludes a vessel that supplies the heart or brain.

Thymus: The lymphatic gland in which T lymphocytes mature; located in humans just below the thyroid.

Thyroid gland: A gland found in the neck that secretes the hormones responsible for the synthesis and breakdown of proteins and the metabolism of carbohydrates.

Thyroidectomy: Surgical removal of the thyroid gland.

Thyroxine: The chief hormone of the thyroid gland, an iodine-containing derivative of the amino acid tyrosine.

TIA. *See* Transient ischemic attack (TIA).

Tibia: The larger of the two bones in the lower leg, on the medial side.

Tincture: A homeopathic remedy in liquid form, normally with alcohol and water as a solvent; the most concentrated form is called the mother tincture, from which all dilutions are made.

Tinnitus: An auditory sensation originating in the head, without external stimulation; also called ringing in the ears.

Tissue: A specialized region of cells that forms organs within the body; the four principal types are epithelial, connective, nervous, and muscular; tissues have specific functions.

Tissue culture: A diagnostic method in which cells from plant or animal tissues bathed in sustaining liquid solution form a monolayer on a container that can be inoculated and observed for deterioration or destruction by replicating viruses.

Tissue plasminogen activator (TPA or tPA): A substance produced by the body to prevent abnormal blood clots by stimulating the formation of plasmin from plasminogen; can also be administered to dissolve blood clots.

Tissue typing: The process of identifying a person's transplantation antigens.

TMJ. *See* Temporomandibular joint (TMJ).

Tolerance: With repeated substance abuse, the need for increasing amounts of a substance to achieve the same effect.

Tomography: All types of body-section imaging techniques; that is, a visual representation restricted to a specified section or "cut" of tissue within an organ.

Tonometer: An instrument used to measure the eye's intraocular pressure, thus checking for the presence of glaucoma.

Tonsillectomy: Surgical removal of one or both tonsils.

Tonsillitis: Infection and inflammation of the tonsils; if severe or chronic, it may require removal of the tonsils.

Tonsils: Masses of lymphatic tissue lying on either side of the entrance to the throat near the back of the tongue.

Tooth decay: The common term for dental caries.

Tooth extraction: The surgical removal of a tooth because it is damaged by decay, disease, or trauma; threatening the health of other teeth; or near the site of significant disease.

Tooth pulp: The tissue at the center of teeth, surrounded by dentin.

Toothache: Pain in the teeth or gums ranging from a dull, throbbing sensation to intense, sharp pains.

Tophus (*pl.* tophi): A lump in the cartilage or joints of chronic gout suffers, caused by crystals of uric acid.

Topical: Referring to treatments or procedures applied directly to the skin or mucous membranes that affect primarily the area in which they are applied.

Tort: A wrongful act for which civil courts, rather than criminal courts, are empowered to render justice.

Totipotence: The capacity for cells of a given tissue type to regenerate and replace killed or damaged cells within a given body region.

Touch: A special sense in which nerve endings and specialized structures in the skin and other tissues send the brain data about the organism's environment, both internal and external.

Toxemia: The presence of toxins in the blood produced by bacteria, which may be ingested or caused by an infection in the body; also called blood poisoning or septicemia.

Toxic shock syndrome: A potentially fatal infection causing failure of multiple organs of the body, most notably associated with tampon use.

Toxicokinetics: The study of the time course of chemical absorption, distribution, metabolism, and elimination of toxic chemicals in the body; when the chemicals considered are therapeutic drugs, the correct term is "pharmacokinetics."

Toxicology: The science devoted to the study of poisons.

Toxin: A poisonous substance that is a product of the chemical processes of a living organism.

Toxoid: A toxin that has been chemically treated to eliminate its toxic properties but that retains the same antigens as the original.

Toxoplasmosis: An infection caused by parasitic microorganisms that invade tissues and that may cause damage to the central nervous system, especially in fetuses.

TPA or tPA. *See* Tissue plasminogen activator.

Trace elements: Elements needed in the diet at levels of less than 100 milligrams per day.

Trace evidence: Minute, often microscopic, signs or indications of an event or a presence.

Tracer: A radioactive substance introduced into the body, the progress of which may be followed by means of an external radioactive detector; it must not affect the process that it is used to measure.

Trachea: The tube that leads from the throat to the lungs; commonly called the windpipe.

Tracheostomy: Surgical creation of an opening in the trachea.

Trachoma: A contagious eye infection, leading to blindness, that affects millions of people in developing countries.

Tract: A collection of nerve fibers (axons) in the brain or spinal cord that all have the same place of origin and the same place of termination.

Transcription: The process by which the information stored in DNA is copied into the structure of RNA for transport to the cytoplasm.

Transducer (probe): A device designed to transfer ultrasound waves into the body noninvasively, receive the returning echoes, and transform those echoes into electrical voltages.

Transference: The unconscious tendency of a person to re-create preexisting nonfunctional relationship patterns with others; psychoanalytic treatment depends on the development of transference between client and analyst.

Transfusion: Injection directly into the bloodstream of a large amount of blood or blood components, usually to correct loss of blood as a result of injury or during surgery.

Transgender: A general term for persons who deviate from masculine and feminine gender norms.

Transient ischemic attack (TIA): A brief loss of blood to the brain, accompanied by temporary impairment of vision and numbness.

Transitional cell carcinoma: Cancer arising from the lining of the urine collection system of the kidneys, ureters, and bladder.

Translation: The process by which the copied information in RNA is utilized in the production of a protein.

Transmission: The mode of acquiring a disease.

Transplantation: The movement of one part of the body (such as an organ) or one area of tissue to another, either within the same individual or from one individual to another.

Transsexuals: Individuals who genuinely believe that they exist in the body of the wrong sex, despite the fact that they are anatomically normal.

Transverse processes: Projections from the sides of vertebrae, to which are attached muscles and ligaments, that assist in motor function by enhancing leverage and limiting extremes of motion.

Transvestism: Also called cross-dressing; wearing clothing deemed appropriate for a person of the gender to which one is not socially and culturally identified.

Trauma: Physical injury to bodily tissue.

Trauma center: An emergency room (ER) that meets certain criteria for the delivery of care to those suffering severe injuries.

Treatment: Any specific procedure used for the cure or improvement of a disease or pathological condition.

Trephination: The opening of a hole in the skull.

Trephine: A specialized surgical instrument that is used to cut a perfectly vertical incision in bone or corneal tissue.

Triage: A process in which patient needs are evaluated and prioritized by a health care team and preliminary treatment plans are made.

Trichomoniasis: A sexually transmitted disease in which motile *Trichomonas vaginalis* protozoans become established in the genitourinary tract of men and women.

Tricyclics: Medications used to relieve the symptoms of depression.

Trimester: An arbitrary division of a human pregnancy into three-month divisions based on development changes in the fetus over time.

Triple test: A blood test that screens for genetic defects.

Trisomy: The presence of an extra chromosome.

Tropical medicine: The area of medicine concerned particularly with diseases, often arthropod-borne (such as malaria, yellow fever, or schistosomiasis), that thrive in tropical latitudes.

Trunk: The central part of the body, to which the extremities are attached.

Tubal ligation: A procedure for rendering a woman sterile by cutting, constricting, or otherwise blocking the Fallopian tubes so that sperm cannot reach the ovum.

Tuberculosis: A chronic, highly infectious lung disease.

Tubular reabsorption: The process of returning important solutes that were filtered out of the blood back into the blood; these important solutes include glucose, amino acids, vitamins, and most ions.

Tubular secretion: The process of tubular reabsorption in reverse; important solutes moved from the filtrate to the urine include hydrogen and potassium ions, organic acids, ammonia, and creatine.

Tumor: An abnormal mass of tissue that may be malignant (growing larger) or benign (not spreading).

Turgor: Fullness and firmness; the quality of normal skin in a healthy young person.

Twins: The presence of two fetuses in the womb.

Tympanic membrane: The eardrum, which separates the external ear canal from the middle ear and ossicles and which transmits sound vibration to the ossicles.

Tympanoplasty: A surgical procedure to repair the tympanic membrane.

Typhoid fever and typhus: Acute infectious diseases caused by bacteria or rickettsiae.

Ulcer: A lesion that destroys tissue.

Ulcerative colitis: An inflammatory disease that causes ulcers in the large intestine.

Ulna: The larger of the two forearm bones, forming the principal part of the elbow joint with the humerus.

Ulnar: Toward the edge of the forearm and hand containing the ulna and little finger.

Ultrasonic: Referring to any frequency of sound that is higher than the audible range—that is, higher than 20,000 cycles per second (20 kilohertz).

Ultrasonography: An imaging technique that employs sound waves to form an image, still or moving, of internal organs.

Ultraviolet radiation: Radiation that is potentially damaging to the skin; it is not visible to humans.

Umbilicus: The cord that contains the blood vessels connecting the fetus to the placenta.

Unconsciousness: A state in which an individual is unaware of either surroundings or self and lacks response to stimuli; includes sleep, fainting, and coma.

Universal coverage: Inclusion of all persons in health insurance, without exception.

Upper arm: The region from the shoulder joint to the elbow joint; also called the brachium.

Upper extremities: The arms (upper arms, forearms, and hands), which are attached to the shoulder blade at the shoulder joint and which consist of muscles, bones, blood vessels, lymph vessels, nerves, skin, and fingernails.

Urea: A waste product of protein metabolism, that represents the form in which nitrogen is eliminated from the body.

Uremia: The presence of excessive amounts of urea and other nitrogenous waste products in the blood.

Ureter: Either of the two tubes that carry urine from the kidneys to the bladder.

Ureterolithotomy: The surgical removal of a stone in the ureter.

Urethra: The tube that drains from the bladder to outside the body; in the male, the urethra passes through the penis and carries sperm during ejaculation, while in the female, the urethra opens in front of the vagina but does not have a reproductive function.

Urethritis: Inflammation or infection of the urethra as a result of bacterial infection.

Urethroplasty: Surgical repair of the urethra.

-uria: A suffix meaning the presence of a substance in urine; for example, hematuria refers to blood in the urine.

Urinalysis: Laboratory analysis of urine to determine presence, absence, or quantity of compounds that may point to disease.

Urinary bladder: A stretchable, muscular sac that functions to store urine.

Urinary system: A system, composed of the kidneys, ureters, urinary bladder, and urethra, that removes body waste, maintains the proper amount of body water, and regulates the acid-base balance of the blood.

Urinary tract infections (UTIs): Infections of the bladder, kidneys, urethra, and ureters (which connect the bladder to the kidneys); infection may be limited to one area of these organs or spread throughout the urinary tract.

Urine: Fluid collected in the kidneys that contains metabolic wastes, including urea and salts.

Urolithiasis: The formation of stones in the urinary tract.

Urology: The branch of medicine specializing in the urinary tracts of both sexes, and the genitourinary tract of the male.

Uterus: The organ that supports the embryo during its development.

UTIs. *See* Urinary tract infections (UTIs).

Uvea: The iris and ciliary body of the eye.

Uveitis: Inflammation of the uvea of the eye.

Vaccination: Induction of immunity in organisms by ingestion or injection of an etiological agent.

Vaccine: Any substance used for preventive inoculation to build immunity.

Vaccinia: A virus that causes a poxlike illness in cattle (cowpox); it serves as a smallpox vaccine in humans because of its similarity to the smallpox virus.

Vagina: The tube-shaped cavity of the female into which the male's penis is inserted during intercourse and through which a baby is delivered; the diaphragm, cervical cap, vaginal sponge, or spermicide can be inserted into the vagina as contraceptives.

Vaginitis: Inflammation and infection of the vagina.

Vagotomy: Surgical incision into the vagus nerve.

Vagus nerve: The tenth cranial nerve, which carries taste messages from the limited number of taste buds located in obscure sites such as the palate, epiglottis, uvula, and other structures at the entrance of the esophagus; also sends important information from the thoracic and abdominal viscera to the brain.

Valgus: A musculoskeletal deformity in which a limb is twisted outward from the body.

Validity, selective: A preliminary indication of a screening technique's capability to identify persons with preclinical disease as test-positive and those without preclinical disease as test-negative.

Vallate papillae: The seven to ten papillae mounds arranged in a V shape that can be seen when the tongue is fully extended; these taste sensors lack taste specificity.

Valves: Structures that close periodically to allow the passage of blood, such as those that connect heart chambers to each other and to the great arteries.

Variable: Any quantity that varies, such as height or cholesterol level.

Varicocele: An enlarged vein surrounding the testicle as a result of incompetent venous valves; most commonly found surrounding the left testicle.

Varicosis: The distension of superficial veins, often in the legs; also known as varicose veins.

Varus: A musculoskeletal deformity in which a limb is twisted toward the body.

Vas deferens: The duct that carries the male seminal fluid.

Vascular: Relating to or containing blood vessels.

Vascular medicine: The diagnosis and management of diseases of the arteries, veins, and lymphatic system, exclusive of the heart and lungs.

Vascular system: The pipeline through which every cell of the body receives oxygen, vitamins, hormones, and the metabolic fuels necessary to sustain life.

Vascularized transplant: Transplanted tissue or organs that must have blood vessels reattached in the recipient in order to function (such as a kidney); corneal or bone marrow transplants are examples of nonvascularized transplants.

Vasculature: All the blood vessels, including the arteries (blood vessels carrying oxygenated blood away from the heart), the capillaries (the smallest blood vessels, where fluid and nutrients are exchanged between arteries and veins), and the veins (blood vessels that return deoxygenated blood to the heart).

Vasculitis: A number of conditions characterized by inflammation of blood vessels, both arteries and veins, that leads to decreased circulation in the affected tissue or organ, which can damage the tissue or organ.

Vasectomy: A surgical procedure to render a male sterile by cutting the two vas deferens, the ducts carrying sperm from the testes to the seminal vesicles.

Vasoconstriction: A decrease in the diameter of vessels transporting blood throughout the body, reducing blood flow and oxygen transport.

Vasodilation: An increase in the diameter of arteries, which decreases the amount of work required for the heart to move blood.

Vector: An organism, usually an insect or other arthropod, that transmits a disease from one host to another; the vector may itself be a host in which the pathogen multiplies, or it may merely transmit the pathogen mechanically.

Veins: Blood vessels that carry blood from the cells back to the heart.

Vena cava: A large vein that carries deoxygenated blood into the right atrium of the heart from the lower half of the body.

Venereal disease: Former term for sexually transmitted disease (STD).

Venipuncture: A method of obtaining blood from a vein using a tourniquet, needle, and syringe.

Venous insufficiency: An abnormality characterized by decreased blood return from the legs to the trunk that is caused by inefficient valves in the veins.

Venous thrombosis: The presence of blood clots in the veins, usually in the legs or arms.

Ventricles: The two lower chambers of the heart; the right ventricle pumps blood to the lungs, and the left ventricle pumps oxygenated blood to the body.

Ventriculoperitoneal: Referring to a type of shunt used to carry cerebrospinal fluid from the brain to the abdominal cavity.

Vertebra: A bony structure in the back with a central spinal canal surrounded by an arch; the back part of the arch (the lamina) and the front part of the arch (the pedicle) are joined together by muscles, ligaments, and cartilage for motion, stability, and posture.

Vertigo: A sensation of motion or spinning when not moving.

Vesicle: A fluid-filled blister.

Vestibular: Referring to the parts of the ear concerned with balance.

Veterinary medicine: The health care and medical treatment of animals, both domestic (pets and livestock) and wild (native and exotic species); includes preventive health care, sanitary and environmental management, and the treatment of diseases and injuries.

Villi: Fingerlike projections on the intestinal lining that absorb essential body nutrients after enzymes break down chyme.

Virilization: The development of masculine sex characteristics in a female.

Virion: A single virus particle.

Virulence: Level of aggressiveness of an organism.

Virus: A subcellular particle that enters cells and causes cellular damage; it uses cellular mechanisms to reproduce itself.

Visual acuity: Clarity or clearness in vision.

Vital organs: Organs of the body essential to life, usually considered to be the brain, the heart, the lungs, the liver, and sometimes the kidneys.

Vitamins: Organic compounds, essential for life but required in very minute quantities, that participate in biochemical reactions and help to release energy from the three classes of nutrients.

Vitiligo: A disorder that occurs when cells that make pigment in the skin are destroyed, leading to white patches on the body; may also affect the eyes and the mucous membranes of the mouth and nose and cause hair to gray.

Vitrectomy: Surgical removal of the vitreous humor.

Vitreous humor: The clear, jellylike substance that fills the eyeball; also called the aqueous humor.

Voltage: Energy per unit charge; typical biological voltages range from hundredths to tenths of a volt.

Voluntary euthanasia: A patient's consent to a decision that results in the shortening of his or her life.

Vomiting: The regurgitation of the contents of the stomach.

Von Neumann machine: A cellular automaton or machine that can think and self-replicate; based on the attempts of the physicist John von Neumann to duplicate the human nervous system in computers.

Von Willebrand's disease: A genetic disorder characterized by the lack of a clotting factor and manifested by excessive bleeding.

Wart: A generally benign tumor of the skin and mucous membranes caused by a papillomavirus.

Wasting: Severe weight loss characterized by the loss of both muscle tissue and body-fat deposits.

Wavelength: A property used to measure colors in the spectrum of light from infrared to ultraviolet; usually expressed in units of microns (1 micron is equal to one-millionth of a meter).

Wedge argument: A logically contrived argument supporting a morally acceptable action that subsequently leads to other actions that are considered morally unacceptable.

Whiplash: Injury to the ligaments, joints, and soft tissues of the neck region of the spine due to a sudden, violent jerking motion.

White blood cells: Colorless, large blood cells that work together to combat infections.

WHO. *See* World Health Organization (WHO).

Whole blood: Blood from which none of the elements has been removed.

Wilson's disease: An inherited disease of abnormal copper metabolism, leading to copper accumulation and toxicity in the liver and brain.

Wiskott-Aldrich syndrome: An X-linked genetic disorder characterized by thrombocytopenia, infections, and eczema in childhood.

Withdrawal: A physical and mental condition following decreased intake of an abusable substance, with symptoms ranging from anxiety to convulsions.

Wolffian ducts: The pair of tubes in the early embryo that will develop into the internal male organs (the epididymis, the vas deferens, and the seminal vesicles).

Work: A form of energy transfer; it may take the form of mechanical work (force multiplied by distance), electrical work (moving an electric charge against a voltage gradient), or chemical work (chemical synthesis or maintaining a difference in concentration across a membrane).

World Health Organization (WHO): A specialized agency of the United Nations that fights illness and disease all over the globe.

Worms: Invertebrates, usually flatworms or roundworms, that act as human parasites.

Wounds: Injuries classified as open or closed depending on whether the skin is broken; types of open wounds include abrasions, lacerations, avulsions, punctures, and incisions.

X and Y chromosomes: The chromosomes that determine genetic sex; males carry an XY pair and females carry an XX pair.

X radiology: The use of ionizing radiation of short wavelength to detect abnormalities in primarily dense portions of the body.

X-ray tube: A high-voltage electronic device used to produce X rays; X-ray tubes are used in X-ray machines, fluoroscopes, and CT scanners.

X rays: Penetrating radiation produced by means of a high-voltage machine; useful for both the diagnosis and the treatment of cancerous tissue.

Xanthomatosis: A condition in which fatty deposits appear anywhere in the body, including various areas of the skin, internal organs, eyes, and tendons.

Xenobiotics: Drugs and chemical compounds foreign to the body; the terms "xenobiotic," "toxin," "drug," and "chemical" are used interchangeably when discussing toxicology, since all substances are poisonous at some concentration.

Xenotransplantation: The transplantation of tissue or organs between different species (such as baboon to human).

Yang: The Chinese concept of the positive, male element of the universe.

Yeast infection: Candidiasis, an infection caused by the fungus *Candida albicans*; commonly infects the vaginal area and causes intense itching.

Yellow fever: An acute viral infection of the liver, kidneys, and heart muscle transmitted by *Aedes aegypti* mosquitoes.

Yin: The Chinese concept of the negative, female element of the universe.

Yoga: A mental discipline, originating in India, designed to master consciousness, to offer spiritual insight, and to induce tranquillity.

Zeugmatography: A name applied to MRI characterizing the close relationship of nuclear magnetic forces and electromagnetic waves (from the Greek *zeugma*, meaning "to yoke together").

Zidovudine: A drug, formerly known as azidothymidine (AZT), used to treat HIV infection; it interferes with the functioning of the virus's reverse transcriptase enzyme.

Zona pellucida: A translucent layer surrounding the mammalian egg; it promotes fertilization by causing the acrosome reaction in the sperm and also prevents polyspermy.

Zoonoses: Diseases communicable between animals and humans.

Zygoma: The cheekbone.

Zygote: A fertilized ovum before multicelluar development begins.

Symptoms and Warning Signs

Warning Signs of Common Diseases

Cancer

Forms of cancer differ by age, race, and sex, but the most common cancers in industrialized countries are lung, reproductive organ (prostate gland, breast, uterus), and colon. Early detection is critical. Signs may include the following:

Breast lump or nipple discharge
Change in bowel habits (unexplained by diet or medications)
Change in color, shape, size or texture of a skin mole
Chronic cough
Difficulty urinating
Noninfectious swollen glands (lymph nodes)
Vaginal bleeding between periods or in menopausal women

Diabetes

This disease has two forms. Type 1 begins in childhood or early adulthood, is usually detected quickly in pediatric visits, and requires insulin injections from the start, along with dietary restrictions. Type 2 presents itself in adulthood, usually without obvious symptoms at first. This form can be treated with diet and perhaps by medications; insulin is usually a last resort. It is important to recognize type 2 diabetes by these signs:

Blurry vision
Excessive thirst
Excessive urination

Frequent vaginal yeast infections
Unexplained weight change

Hypertension

High blood pressure is known as the "silent killer," as few symptoms present themselves. **Note:** This diagnosis depends on having several blood pressure readings higher than 140/90 on different occasions after rest. Risk factors include the following:

Diabetes
Family history of hypertension
Increased age (although younger for African Americans)
Kidney disease
Medication side effect
Obesity
Poor diet (high sodium; low potassium, magnesium, calcium)
Sleep apnea

Strokes and Ministrokes

Ministrokes are often overlooked but are warnings of possible vascular problems. Their symptoms are sudden and short-lived (lasting one to two hours):

Disorders of equilibrium (balance), movement, speech, vision
Heaviness or weakness of limbs
Numbness
Continuation of symptoms beyond twenty-four hours implies that a stroke has occurred

Symptoms and Possible Conditions

Abdominal Pain

- **DIFFUSE, NONLOCALIZED**
  Gastroenteritis (stomach or intestinal infection)
- **LOWER LEFT SIDE**
  Appendicitis (rarely)
  Diverticulitis
  Hernia
  Kidney stones
  Pelvic infection

- **LOWER RIGHT SIDE**
  Appendicitis
  Kidney stones
- **UPPER LEFT SIDE**
  Kidney stones
  Ulcer
- **UPPER RIGHT SIDE**
  Gallbladder inflammation or infection
  Kidney stones

Abdominal Pain *(cont.)*
- **UPPER RIGHT SIDE** *(cont.)*
  Liver disorder
  Ulcer

Back Pain (Lower Back)
  Arthritis
  Herniated disk
  Kidney stones
  Muscle injury
  Sciatica

Blood
- **IN PHLEGM (COUGHING UP BLOOD)**
  Blood clot in lung
  Bronchitis
  Lung cancer
  Pneumonia
  Tuberculosis
- **IN STOOL**
  Anal fissure
  Colorectal cancer
  Hemorrhoids
  Ulcer
  Ulcerative colitis or Crohn's disease
- **IN URINE**
  Bladder infection
  Kidney stones

Breast Disorder
- **DISCHARGE**
  Breast cancer
  Contraceptive use
  Hormone therapy
  Medication side effect
- **SWELLING AND/OR PAIN**
  Benign tumors or cysts
  Cancer
  Trauma

Chest Pain
- **DEEP, DULL, POORLY LOCALIZED**
  Angina
  Gallbladder inflammation or infection
- **SHARP, WELL LOCALIZED**
  Hernia
  Muscle injury
  Rib fracture
  Shingles
  Ulcer

Constipation
  Colorectal cancer (sudden onset of constipation)
  Dehydration
  Hemorrhoids
  Impaction
  Medication side effect

Cough
  Allergy
  Bronchitis
  Emphysema
  Pneumonia

Diarrhea
  Antibiotics and other drugs
  Appendicitis
  Colorectal cancer
  Diverticular disease
  Food intolerance
  Infections
  Ulcerative colitis or Crohn's disease

Dizziness
  Anemia
  Anxiety
  Heart-related problem
  Inner-ear problem
  Low blood pressure
  Low blood sugar
  Ministroke

Eye Discomfort
- **BURNING**
  Dryness
- **DISCHARGE**
  Allergic conjunctivitis
  Bacterial or viral conjunctivitis
- **ITCHING**
  Allergy
- **PAIN**
  Foreign object
  Infection
  Inflammation
  Trauma
- **REDNESS**
  Conjunctivitis
  Corneal disorder
  Glaucoma

Fainting
Anxiety
Blood pressure drop
Heart-related problem
Low blood sugar

Fatigue
Anxiety
Depression
Malnutrition
Obesity
Poor physical conditioning
Sleep disturbance

Fever
Bacterial infection
Fungal infection
Viral infection

Gas (Flatulence)
Food intolerance
Peptic ulcer

Headache
Eyestrain
Migraine headache
Sinusitis
Tension headache

Heart Palpitations
Anemia
Anxiety
Arrhythmias (abnormal heartbeat)
Heart valve dysfunction
Hyperthyroidism (overactive thyroid)

Heartburn
Food intolerance
Gallbladder inflammation or infection
Gastric (acid) reflux
Medication side effect
Ulcer

Jaundice
Excess vitamin A
Gallbladder inflammation or infection
Hepatitis
Liver inflammation or infection
Medication

Nasal Discharge
• **CLEAR**
Allergies
• **DISCOLORED**
Sinus infection

Nausea and Vomiting
Appendicitis
Early pregnancy
Food intolerance or poisoning
Gallbladder inflammation or infection
Gastric intestinal infection
Hepatitis
Ulcer

Nosebleed
Aspirin or blood thinner
Sinus infection
Spontaneous small blood vessel rupture
Trauma

Penile Discharge (Pus)
Infection (bladder or prostate)
Sexually transmitted disease (STD)

Rectal Bleeding
Anal fissure
Colitis
Colorectal cancer
Diverticulosis
Hemorrhoids

Seizures
Alcohol or drug withdrawal
Epilepsy
High fever
Low blood sugar
Low potassium

Shortness of Breath
Anemia
Anxiety
Asthma
Blood clot in lungs
Bronchitis
Collapsed lung
Congestive heart failure
Heart attack
Pneumonia

Sinus Pain and Pressure
Allergy
Infection

Swallowing Difficulty
Allergic reaction
Infection (yeast)
Neurological disease
Strep throat
Tonsillitis

Swollen Ankles
Arthritis
Congestive heart failure
Excessive salt intake
Kidney failure
Malnutrition

Swollen Glands
Infection
Leukemia
Lymphoma

Swollen Joints
- CHRONIC
  Arthritis
  Trauma
- SUDDEN
  Gout
  Infection
  Lyme disease
  Trauma

Tremor
Alcoholism
Anxiety
Benign old-age condition
Dementia
Medication
Multiple sclerosis
Parkinson's disease

Urination Disorder
- DIFFICULTY
  Enlarged prostate gland
  Infection and inflammation
  Sexually transmitted disease (STD)

Urination Disorder (cont.)
- FREQUENCY (INCONTINENCE)
  Alcohol
  Bladder cancer
  Caffeine
  Diabetes
  Diuretic drugs
  Infection (bladder or prostate)
  Pregnancy

Vaginal Bleeding
- PREMENOPAUSE
  Cervical cancer
  Cervical polyps or warts
  Ectopic pregnancy
  Impending miscarriage
  Infection
- POSTMENOPAUSE
  Cervical cancer
  Infection
  Uterine cancer

Vaginal Discomfort
- DISCHARGE
  Infection
- ITCHING
  Dryness
  Yeast infection
- PAIN
  Dryness
  Infection or inflammation
  Psychological muscular contractions

Weight Gain
Diabetes
Hypothyroidism (underactive thyroid)
Medication

Weight Loss
Alcoholism
Anorexia
Depression
Hyperthyroidism (overactive thyroid)
Loss of appetite (medication)

—*Mel Siegel, M.A.;*
Connie Rizzo, M.D., Ph.D., consultant

Diseases and Other Medical Conditions

Abscess: A pocket of infection or inflammation.

Acid reflux disease: The regurgitation or bathing of the lower esophagus with acid from the stomach.

Acidosis: A state of excess acidity in the body's fluids; metabolic acidosis involves the kidneys, while respiratory acidosis involves the lungs.

Acne: A group of skin disorders, the most common of which, acne vulgaris, usually affects teenagers; another form, acne rosacea, usually afflicts older people.

Acquired immunodeficiency syndrome (AIDS): A progressive loss of immune function and susceptibility to secondary infections that arises from chronic infection with human immunodeficiency virus (HIV).

Acute infection: Infection characterized by a rapid onset and generally followed by a relatively rapid resolution.

Acute lymphocytic leukemia (ALL): A rapidly developing form of leukemia affecting lymphocytes and characterized by the rapid production of immature lymphoblasts.

Acute myeloid leukemia (AML): Rapidly development form of leukemia characterized by large numbers of immature granulocytes in the circulation. The disease is found most frequently among persons exposed to high doses of radiation.

Acute respiratory distress syndrome (ARDS): Respiratory failure caused by filling of the lungs with fluid from the capillaries, leading to a shortage of oxygen in the body that can eventually lead to death if not treated.

ADD. *See* Attention-deficit disorder (ADD).

Addiction: A psychological and physiological process whereby an organism comes to depend on a substance.

Addison's disease: A chronic condition in which the adrenal glands do not produce adequate amounts of corticosteroid hormones.

Adenoviruses: Medium-sized viruses that can cause respiratory infections and diarrhea by infecting the tissue linings of the respiratory and urinary tracts, the intestines, and the eyes.

Adhesion: The "gluing" together by scar tissue of internal organs and tissues, often caused by endometriosis or infections; a common cause of pelvic pain.

Adrenoleukodystrophy: A variable X-linked genetic disorder with symptoms ranging from adrenal insufficiency to progressive neurological deterioration.

Affective disorders: Mental conditions characterized by a primary disturbance of mood, as distinct from thinking or behavior.

African sleeping sickness: Disease resulting from infection by the parasite *Trypanosoma brucei* and characterized by headache, sleep, and progression into coma.

Age spots: Benign lesions, also known as liver spots or solar lentigo, found on sun-exposed skin. Age spots are seen in more than 90 percent of Caucasians sixty-five years of age and older; they typically represent no immediate danger.

Agnosia: Inability to identify objects or persons using one or more of the senses, even though the basic sensory modalities are not defective.

AIDS. *See* Acquired immunodeficiency syndrome (AIDS).

Albinos: Individuals who have an inherited defect in the production of melanin characterized by a lack of pigmentation.

Alcoholism: The compulsive drinking of and dependency on alcoholic beverages; it can be arrested but not cured.

Alkalosis: A condition of abnormally low carbon dioxide levels that results from hyperventilation (rapid breathing).

ALL. *See* Acute lymphocytic leukemia (ALL).

Allergies: Exaggerated immune reactions to materials that are intrinsically harmless; the body's release of pharmacologically active chemicals during allergic reactions may result in discomfort, tissue damage, or, in severe responses, death.

Alopecia: Loss of hair as a result of skin disease, endocrine disorders, or chemotherapy.

Alopecia areata: The formation of round bald spots on the head or other portions of the body; of unknown cause, but generally self-limiting.

Altitude sickness: A condition resulting from altitude-related hypoxia (low oxygen levels).

Alzheimer's disease: A progressive disease resulting in the loss of higher cognitive function; the most common form of dementia.

Amebiasis: Infection of the colon or associated organs by the parasite *Entamoeba histolytica*.

Amenorrhea: Lack of menstruation in girls by the age of eighteen or its suppression, often as a result of overly strenuous exercise, rapid weight loss or gain, or emotional trauma.

AML. *See* Acute myeloid leukemia (AML).

Amnesia: An impairment of memory, which may be total or limited, sudden or gradual.

Amyloidosis: A condition characterized by the deposit of waxy substances in animal organs.

Amyotrophic lateral sclerosis: A progressive, degenerative neurological disorder that affects the cells in the brain and spinal cord.

Anal cancer: Cancer affecting the lower alimentary tract, including the interior anal canal from the anorectal ring to the anal verge with 5 centimeters of skin extending beyond, including the perianal skin.

Ancylostomiasis: Any infection by the hookworm *Ancylostoma*.

Andersen's disease: A congenital glycogen storage disease characterized by glycogen deposition in the liver and spleen.

Anemia: A condition characterized by a deficiency of red blood cells or hemoglobin; may be caused by a decrease in hemoglobin production, an increase in cell destruction, or blood loss.

Anemic anoxia: An oxygen deficiency in tissues resulting from lack of red blood cells or a deficiency in the oxygen carrier hemoglobin.

Anergy: A condition in which an immune response cannot occur.

Aneurysm: A localized enlargement of a vessel, usually an artery, caused by the stretching of a weak place in the vessel wall.

Angiitis: Inflammation of a blood vessel.

Angina: Chest pain often caused by coronary artery disease.

Angiosclerosis: Hardening of a blood vessel wall; also known as atherosclerosis.

Aniseikonia: A condition in which each eye observes the same object as a different size.

Ankyloglossia: A defect of the muscle in the mouth in which movement of the tongue and speech are impaired.

Ankylosing spondylitis: A chronic progressive disease characterized by fusion of the spine and joints.

Anodontia: A congenital disorder in which one or several teeth do not develop.

Anomia: An inability to remember the names of persons or objects even though the patient sees and recognizes those persons or objects.

Anorexia nervosa: An eating disorder characterized by a compulsive aversion to food, caused by a fear of obesity and a distorted body image; may result in severe malnutrition.

Anosmia: A complete loss in the ability to detect odors.

Anuria: Decrease or blockage of urine production or secretion, generally the result of kidney dysfunction or failure.

Anxiety: Heightened fear or tension that causes psychological and physical distress; the American Psychiatric Association recognizes six types of anxiety disorders, which can be treated with medications or through counseling.

Aortic atresia: A congenital heart defect characterized by the absence of the normal valve opening into the aorta.

Aortic regurgitation: The backflow of blood from the aorta into the left ventricle.

Aortic stenosis: Narrowing of the aortic valve, resulting in decreased cardiac output.

Aortitis: Inflammation of the aorta, often a result of tertiary syphilis.

Aortopulmonary fenestration: An opening or "window" between the pulmonary artery and the aorta, resulting in the combining of oxygenated blood with deoxygenated blood.

Apareunia: Lack of ability to perform sexual intercourse.

Apert's syndrome: Congenital fusion of fingers and toes, generally accompanied by facial abnormalities.

Aphasia: The total absence of such language skills as speaking, reading, writing, and comprehension.

Aplasia: Congenital absence of a tissue or organ.

Apophysitis: Inflammation or swelling of a projection from a bone; generally found on the foot.

Appendicitis: Inflammation of the vermiform appendix, which may require its removal.

Arachnodactyly: The congenital formation of long, spiderlike fingers or toes; often associated with Marfan's syndrome.

ARDS. *See* Acute respiratory distress syndrome (ARDS).

Arrhythmia: A heart rhythm that is abnormal, either in speed or in force.

Arteriosclerosis: Also called atherosclerotic disease or "hardening of the arteries," a generalized disease that causes narrowing of the arteries because of deposits on the arterial walls; may lead to a multitude of serious medical conditions, notably stroke and heart attack.

Arthritis: A group of more than one hundred inflammatory diseases that damage joints and their surrounding structures, resulting in symptomatic pain, disability, and systemwide inflammation.

Arthropod-borne diseases: Diseases transmitted to humans and animals by arthropods (insects and spiders).

Ascites praecox: Accumulation of fluid within the peritoneal cavity.

Aseptic fever: Fever not associated with an infectious agent.

Asherman's syndrome: Amenorrhea resulting from adhesions in the endometrial lining.

Asperger's syndrome: A pervasive developmental disorder involving clinically significant impairment in social interactions and repetitive or stereotyped patterns of behavior, but no particular problem with cognitive functioning.

Aspergillosis: An inflammatory condition following infection by members of the fungal genus *Aspergillus*; infection is usually opportunistic and may affect any organ.

Asphyxia neonatorum: Inability of a newborn to begin to breathe; may result from placental dysfunction or from inappropriate responses to analgesics.

Asphyxiation: An impaired exchange of oxygen and carbon dioxide in the lungs; if prolonged, this condition leads to death.

Aspiration pneumonia: Inflammation of the lungs resulting from inhalation of gastric acid.

Asplenia: Absence of a spleen.

Astereognosis: Inability to identify objects by touch alone.

Asthenia: Weakness.

Asthenopia: Weakness of muscles in the eye, resulting in tiredness and headache.

Asthma: A chronic inflammatory obstructive pulmonary disease that obstructs the airways to the lungs and makes it difficult or, in severe attacks, nearly impossible to breathe.

Asthmatic eosinophilia: An allergic response to fungi characterized by bronchospasms and pneumonia in which fungal casts containing eosinophils build up in the lungs or chest cavity.

Astigmatism: A visual disorder in which either the cornea of the eye or the lens is not symmetrical.

Astroblastoma: A malignant tumor of the brain or spinal cord in which the growth is wrapped around blood vessels.

Astrocytoma: A central nervous system tumor originating with an astroglial cell.

Astrocytosis: A buildup in concentration of glial cells in the brain; often associated with or resulting from tissue damage.

Ataxia: An inability to coordinate the muscles in voluntary movement.

Ataxia-telangiectasia: A congenital disorder generally associated with an immunoglobulin defect and characterized by degeneration of the cerebellum.

Ataxic dysarthria: Abnormal speech associated with neuromuscular disorders.

Ateliosis: Dwarfism associated with lack of development of the adenohypophysis.

Atelorachidia: Defective formation of the spinal cord.

Athetosis: Involuntary movement of the arms or legs, a condition often observed in persons with cerebral palsy.

Athlete's foot: A contagious fungal infection of the skin on the feet; also known as tinea pedia.

Athlete's heart: An enlarged heart sometimes found in athletes; the condition is normal and generally results from endurance training.

Atresia: The absence of a normal opening or the failure of a structure to be tubular.

Atrial fibrillation: Abnormal heart rhythm or muscle contractions in the atria as a result of disorganized electrical impulses.

Atrial septal defect: A congenital malformation of the heart in which an opening is found between the two atria.

Atrial standstill: The inability of either of the atria to contract; usually the result of an electrical malfunction of the nerve impulse.

Atrial tachycardia: Extremely rapid heartbeat resulting from an electrical abnormality in the upper portion of the heart.

Atrioventricular dissociation: Condition in which the chambers of the heart contract in an uncoordinated fashion.

Atrophoderma: Degeneration of the skin characterized by a decrease in thickness; often a result of the aging process.

Atrophy: A wasting away or decrease in size and/or activity of a body part because of disease or other influences such as inactivity.

Attention-deficit disorder (ADD): A condition characterized by an inability to focus attention or to inhibit impulsive, hyperactive behavior; it is associated with poor academic performance and behavioral problems in children.

Auras: Warning sensations of varying kinds received by the patient prior to a seizure, migraine, or psychotic episode.

Autism: A lifelong mental disability characterized by difficulty with social relationships, difficulty with language and communication, preoccupation with repetitive or stereotyped behaviors and interests, and a general resistance to changes in routine.

Autoimmune disorders: Disorders in which the immune system attacks the body's cells as foreign matter.

Babesiosis: A parasitic disease that is transmitted to humans by the bite of an infected tick.

Bacteremia: A condition in which bacteria enter the bloodstream and thus can be disseminated throughout the body.

Balance disorders: Problems with balance that may be described by sufferers as dizziness or vertigo and usually are associated with the inner ear; balance disorders may result in falls and other accidents.

Barrett's syndrome: A condition characterized by ulcerous lesion formation in the lower esophagus; most commonly associated with untreated acid reflux.

Basal cell carcinoma: The most common type of skin cancer, usually the result of sun exposure; it grows slowly and seldom spreads beneath the skin.

Basophilic adenoma: A tumor found in the pituitary gland characterized by cells that stain using basic dyes.

Bassen-Kornzweig syndrome: A congenital disorder of lipid metabolism characterized by abnormally low concentrations of certain serum lipids.

Bathycardia: A congenital condition in which the heart is situated low in the thoracic cavity.

Batten's disease: A childhood disorder resulting from defects in fatty acid metabolism.

Battledore placenta: A condition characterized by attachment of the umbilical cord near the margin of the placenta.

Battle's sign: A swelling or hemorrhagic area behind the ear, possibly indicating a fracture.

Becker's muscular dystrophy: A congenital form of progressive muscular weakness; unlike the more common Duchenne's muscular dystrophy, Becker's MD is not a sex-linked trait and has a better prognosis.

Beckwith-Wiedemann syndrome: A congenital disorder resulting in enlargement of the adrenal cortex, and possible dysplasia of the renal medulla.

Beckwith's syndrome: A congenital disorder resulting in neonatal hypoglycemia and the excessive production of insulin.

Bedsores: Sores caused by sustained pressure with restricted blood flow to the skin.

Bed-wetting: A condition characterized by an inability of the bladder to contain urine during sleep; often a developmental condition in children.

Bednar's aphthae: Ulcerated patches on the palates of infants who place contaminated items in their mouths.

Behçet's disease: A multisystem disease characterized by recurrent oral and genital ulcers.

Bell's palsy: A sudden paralysis of one side of the face, including muscles of the eyelid.

Bence-Jones protein: The secretion of antibody light chains in the urine; associated with certain forms of multiple myeloma.

Benign prostatic hypertrophy: Nonmalignant enlargement of the prostate gland; most commonly found among men over the age of fifty.

Benign senescent forgetfulness: A common source of frustration in old age associated with memory impairment; unlike dementia, it does not interfere with the individual's social and professional activities.

Berger's disease: A kidney disorder resulting from the deposition of IgA antibodies within the glomerulus.

Berger's paresthesia: Weakness or loss of feeling in the limbs in the absence of any obvious organic etiology.

Beriberi: A serious vitamin deficiency caused by an inadequate intake of thiamine (vitamin B_{12}).

Berlock dermatitis: Hyperpigmentation of the skin; usually the result of an allergic response to oils found in perfumes.

Bernard-Soulier syndrome: The inability of platelets to aggregate and form a clot; a congenital condition associated with the lack of production of a surface glycoprotein.

Biliary colic: A distinct pain syndrome characterized by severe intermittent waves of right-sided, upper abdominal pain, often brought on by the ingestion of fatty foods; pain occurs when a gallstone obstructs the outflow of bile and usually resolves when the gallstone moves away from the outflow area.

Bipolar disorder: A syndrome characterized by alternating periods of mania and depression; formerly called manic-depressive disorder.

Birth defect: A genetic abnormality in the tissue development of a certain body part of the fetus; in some cases, the defect is minor, but in others it may be medically dangerous to the fetus and/or the mother.

Birthmarks: Spots or marks on the skin that are present at birth or shortly thereafter.

Blackout: Memory loss, usually as a result of taking substances known to disrupt memory; the affected person may function as if aware of what is happening but later have no memory of those activities.

Bleeding: Damage or disruption to hemostasis (the normal absence of bleeding), resulting in loss of blood or abnormal clotting.

Blindness: The absence of vision, or its extreme impairment to the extent that activity is limited; about 95 percent of all blindness is caused by eye diseases, the rest by injuries.

Blisters: Fluid-filled areas on the skin caused by tears between the upper layers.

Bloom's disease: A congenital recessive trait characterized by growth retardation and sensitivity to sunlight; found primarily among Ashkenazi Jews.

Blue baby syndrome: A congenital heart disease consisting of four distinct defects that result in poorly oxygenated blood being delivered to tissues, thereby causing a bluish discoloration of the skin and mucous membranes upon birth.

Blurred vision: A decrease in clarity of vision (visual acuity).

Body dysmorphic disorder: A psychiatric somatoform disorder resulting in exaggerated preoccupation with an imagined or minor defect in physical appearance that causes significant impairment of social functioning.

Boil: A localized abscess filled with pus that has developed in a hair follicle.

Bone cancer: Cancer that may have originated in bone or have spread there from another site in the body.

Botulism: Food poisoning caused by bacteria that produce a toxin which is absorbed by the digestive tract and spread to the central nervous system.

Bovine spongiform encephalopathy (BSE): Another name for mad cow disease; a prion infection of the brain.

Bradycardia: Slowness of the heartbeat.

Bradyesthesia: Inability to perceive objects at a normal pace.

Bradypnea: Slow rate of breathing.

Brain death: Brain damage so extensive that the organ enjoys no potential for recovery and can no longer maintain the body's internal functions.

Breast cancer: Malignancy occurring in breast tissue and possibly involving the associated lymph nodes.

Bronchiolitis: Inflammation of the bronchioles that affects breathing and the transfer of oxygen to the bloodstream.

Bronchitis: An inflammation of the bronchial tree of the lungs.

Bruton's agammaglobulinemia: A sex-linked congenital disorder characterized by the inability to synthesize serum antibodies.

BSE. *See* Bovine spongiform encephalopathy (BSE).

Bucardia: Abnormal enlargement of the heart.

Budd-Chiari syndrome: Enlargement of the liver associated with venous obstruction.

Bulimia: A compulsive eating disorder characterized by food binges and purges (through either self-induced vomiting or the use of laxatives).

Bullous myringitis: Inflammation of the ear accompanied by formation of fluid-filled sacs.

Bunion: Swelling of the big toe caused by an inflamed bursa; often a complication of ill-fitting footwear.

Buphthalmos: A congenital form of glaucoma.

Burkitt's lymphoma: A highly aggressive lymphoma often presenting in extranodal sites or as an acute leukemia.

Burnett's syndrome: Alkalosis as a result of excessive consumption of calcium-containing products such as milk or food supplements.

Burns: Injury to the skin and other tissues caused by contact with dry heat (fire), chemicals, electricity, lightning, or radiation.

Burping: The mouth release of gas brought up from the stomach.

Bursitis: An inflammation of a bursa, one of the membranes that surround joints.

Byssinosis: A respiratory illness cause by allergic reactions to contaminants in cotton or other plant fibers; primarily an occupational disease.

Byzantine arch palate: A congenital abnormality in which the roof of the mouth does not fuse properly.

Cachexia: Severe emaciation as a result of improper diet or disease.

Cacodemonomania: A psychological disturbance in which the patient believes he is possessed by demons.

Cacosemia: A hallucinogenic disorder in which the patient incorrectly believes that there is a foul odor in the environment.

Calabar swelling: Swollen tissue resulting from the underlying presence of a parasitic worm; both the worm and the swelling may migrate.

Calcification: Abnormal accumulation of calcium in tissue.

Calluses: Areas of thickened skin that form as a result of constant pressure or friction over a bony prominence.

***Campylobacter* infection:** An acute disease, often spontaneously resolving, caused by bacterial infection; sometimes called food poisoning.

Canavan's disease: Congenital progressive degeneration of the central nervous system characterized by a spongy appearance of the white matter; found primarily among Ashkenazi Jews.

Cancer: Inappropriate and uncontrollable cell growth within one of the specialized tissues of the body, threatening normal cell and organ function and in serious cases traveling via the bloodstream to other areas of the body.

Candidiasis: An acute or chronic fungal infection of humans and animals that can be superficial or deep-seated; caused by a species of the fungus *Candida*.

Candiru fever: A viral infection transmitted through the bite of a sandfly.

Canker sores: Small, round ulcers of the mucous membranes that line the mouth.

Cannabism: A hallucinogenic condition associated with the excessive use of marijuana.

Caplan's syndrome: A condition characterized by the formation of intrapulmonary nodules.

Carcinoma: A malignant neoplasm arising from epithelial cells making up the surface layers of the skin or other membranes.

Cardiomyopathy: A serious acute or chronic disease in which the heart becomes inflamed; may result from multiple causes, including viral infection, and may involve obstructive damage.

Cardiovascular disease: Any of a group of diseases that affect the heart, including coronary artery disease, hypertension, congestive heart failure, congenital heart defects, and valvular heart disease.

Carpal tunnel syndrome: Tingling and pain in the thumb, index, and middle fingers caused by pressure on a nerve that passes through an area in the hand called the carpal tunnel.

Cartilage hair hypoplasia: A mitochondrial defect characterized by dwarfism and malignancy; most

common among the Amish, with one in nineteen carrying the recessive gene.

Cat-eye syndrome: A congenital abnormality characterized by pupils that resemble those of a cat, as well as mental retardation and heart defects; most commonly the result of a trisomy 22.

Cataract: A dark region in the lens of the eye that causes gradual loss of vision.

Cavities: Disintegrations in tooth enamel; also called tooth decay or dental caries.

Cerebral palsy: A group of nonprogressive disorders of the upper neurologic system resulting in abnormal muscle tone and lack of muscular control.

Chagas' disease: An acute, febrile disease, most common in children and caused by the protozoan *Trypanosoma cruzi*; the infection may be asymptomatic or characterized by edema and swollen lymph nodes.

Chagres fever: A Central American viral disease transmitted by the bite of a sandfly; characterized by headache, fever, and nausea.

Chalazion: Swelling of the eyelid, usually resulting from an obstruction of the meibomian glands.

Chancre: an ulcerated lesion of the skin, most commonly observed on the penis as a result of primary syphilis.

Chancroid: A sexually transmitted disease associated with infection by *Hemophilus ducreyi*; the lesion bears some physical resemblance to the chancre of syphilis.

Chickenpox: A highly infectious viral disease occurring primarily in children; characterized by weakness, fever, and a generalized body rash.

Childbirth complications: The difficulties that can occur during childbirth, either for the mother or for the baby.

Childhood infectious diseases: A group of diseases including diphtheria, tetanus, measles, polio, rubella (German measles), mumps, and pertussis (whooping cough).

Chiari malformations: A group of disorders where the cerebellum, the part of the brain in the lower rear of the head that controls motion, extends below the opening of the spinal canal (the foramen magnum).

Chlamydia: A sexually transmitted disease caused by members of the bacterial genus *Chlamydia* and characterized by discharge, pain, and swelling of the genitals; if a pregnant woman is infected, the disease can infect her infant's eyes during childbirth.

Choking: A condition in which the breathing passage (windpipe) is obstructed.

Cholecystitis: Inflammation or bacterial infection of the gallbladder, usually caused by the presence of gallstones.

Cholera: An infection of the small intestine caused by *Vibrio cholerae*, a comma-shaped bacterium.

Chronic disease: Disease characterized by a slow progression, lasting months to years.

Chronic fatigue syndrome: A multifaceted disease state characterized by debilitating fatigue.

Chronic obstructive pulmonary disease (COPD): A progressive, irreversible disease of the lungs that causes expiratory airflow obstruction.

Chronic wasting disease (CWD): A neurological disease of deer and elk caused by an infectious protein particle called a prion.

Cirrhosis: A condition of the liver in which injured or dead cells are replaced with scar tissue.

Claudication: Muscle cramps that occur when arterial blood flow does not meet the muscles' demand for oxygen.

Cleft lip: Incomplete fusion of the two sides of the lips during embryonic development; often associated with cleft palate.

Cleft palate: Incomplete fusion of the two sides of the palate in the mouth during embryonic development.

Closed head injury: Contusion or concussion within the central nervous system that occurs within the skull, showing no obvious external damage.

Clot: A clumping of platelets, blood, fibrin, and clotting factors that normally accumulates in damaged tissue as part of the body's healing process; also called a thrombus.

Cluster headache: A headache characterized by intense pain behind one eye.

CMV. *See* Cytomegalovirus (CMV).

Coccidioidomycosis: A fungal infection acquired by inhaling the spores of particular soil-based fungi; it initially attacks the lungs and often resolves without causing symptoms, but the infection can cause pneumonia and disseminate throughout the body.

Cold agglutinin disease: Primarily found in patients with certain forms of pneumonia and various blood disorders; characterized by serum antibodies that cause the agglutination of red blood cells at temperatures below 37 degrees Celsius.

Cold sores: Infectious lesions around the mouth that are characterized by thin-walled vesicles.

Colic: As a general term, a paroxysm of acute abdominal pain caused by spasm, obstruction, or twisting of a hollow abdominal organ; infantile colic is a group of behaviors displayed by young infants including crying, facial grimacing, fist clenching, and drawing up of the legs over the abdomen.

Colitis: A potentially fatal but manageable disease of the colon that inflames and ulcerates the bowel lining; occurs in both acute and chronic forms.

Collagen vascular disease: Inflammation of small blood vessels, possibly resulting in a variety of conditions such as arthritis, pleuritis, and vasculitis.

Color blindness: A genetic eye condition in which the patient is unable to distinguish between some colors; the most common form, Daltonism, is a sex-linked recessive trait in which red and green cannot be distinguished.

Colorectal cancer: Cancer occurring in the large intestine or rectum; the second deadliest type of malignancy.

Coma: A loss of consciousness from which a person cannot be aroused; a symptom signifying a variety of possible causes.

Common cold: A class of viral respiratory infections that form the world's most prevalent illnesses.

Compulsion: A persistent, irresistible urge to perform a stereotyped behavior or irrational act, often accompanied by repetitious thoughts (obsessions) about the behavior.

Concussion: Temporary neural dysfunction, causing confusion, dizziness, nausea, headache, lethargy, and short-term amnesia; often results when the head is struck by a hard blow or shaken violently.

Congenital adrenal hyperplasia: A family of genetic conditions that affect hormone production by the adrenal glands.

Congenital disorders: Abnormalities present at birth; may be due to a genetic defect, exposure to a toxic or infectious agent in utero, or a deficiency/lack of a substance necessary for fetal development.

Congenital heart disease: A number of conditions resulting from malformations of the heart that occur during embryonic and fetal development.

Congenital syphilis: Syphilis that is acquired by the developing fetus as a result of passage of the spirochete across the placenta.

Congestive heart failure: Abnormal heart function characterized by circulatory congestion caused by cardiac disorders, especially myocardial infarction (heart attack) of the ventricles.

Conjoined twins: Twins who are joined to varying extents as a result of incomplete separation of cells early in embryonic development.

Conjunctivitis: An inflammation of the white part of the eye, the conjunctiva.

Conn's syndrome: Excessive production of the hormone aldosterone, resulting in headache, fatigue, and possible mineral depletion.

Constipation: The slow passage of feces through the bowels or the presence of hard feces.

Contact dermatitis: A common skin allergy characterized by inflamed skin; occurs when skin comes in contact with substances such as poison ivy or allergenic cosmetics.

Contracture: Abnormal and generally permanent bending or twisting of a joint; generally the result of muscle damage or atrophy.

Contusion: An injury to tissue without breaking of the skin.

Convulsion: An instance of high-frequency and amplitude-random electrical activity in the brain.

Cooley's anemia: A form of congenital thalassemia in which abnormal hemoglobin is unable to properly transport oxygen.

COPD. *See* Chronic obstructive pulmonary disease (COPD).

Cornelia de Lange syndrome: A multiple congenital anomaly syndrome of unknown origin characterized by a distinctive facial appearance, prenatal and postnatal growth deficiencies, feeding difficulties, psychomotor delay, multiple behavioral problems, and malformations of the upper extremities.

Corns: Small painful areas of thickened skin, which may be flat or slightly elevated with a smooth and hard surface, that form as a result of constant pressure or friction over a bony prominence.

Coronary artery disease: A disease that results in a narrowing of the coronary arteries and a concomitant reduction of oxygen supply to the heart muscle.

Coronaviruses: Viruses frequently infecting the upper respiratory system and capable of producing either the common cold or severe acute respiratory syndrome (SARS).

Costen's syndrome: A condition in which the jaw may be subjected to severe pain as a result of mandibular displacement.

Coughing: A physiological act in which air is forcibly expelled from the lungs.

Cowpox: A mild disease of cattle generally characterized by lesions on the udder; its similarity to smallpox resulted in the use of the causative virus as the first smallpox vaccine.

Cradle cap: A common condition on the scalp of infants in which thick scales develop.

Craniosynostosis: The premature closing of the open areas between the bones in an infant's skull; also known as craniostosis.

Cretinism: Retardation of mental and physical growth arising from prenatal or neonatal hypothyroidism.

Creutzfeldt-Jakob disease: A human central nervous system disorder caused by prions that is characterized by distinctive lesions in the brain, progressive dementia, lack of coordination, and eventual death.

Crohn's disease: A chronic disease process in which the bowel becomes inflamed, leading to scarring and narrowing of the intestines; an autoimmune manifestation of ulcerative colitis.

Croup: An inflammation of the larynx, throat, and upper bronchial tubes causing hoarseness, cough, and difficult breathing; refers to a condition rather than any specific disease and generally results from a viral infection in children.

CWD. *See* Chronic wasting disease (CWD).

Cyanosis: Dark blue discoloration of the skin and nail beds resulting from decreases in the oxygenation of the hemoglobin of arterial red blood cells.

Cyst: A swelling or nodule containing fluid or soft material resulting from a blocked duct or abnormal growth in fluid-producing tissue.

Cystic fibrosis: A genetic disease that affects the exocrine glands and most physical systems of the body, resulting in death usually between the ages of sixteen and thirty.

Cystinosis: Congenital defect in the metabolism of the amino acid complex cystine; characterized by cystine deposition in organs such as the liver and spleen.

Cystitis: An inflammation of the bladder, primarily caused by bacteria and resulting in pain, a sense of urgency to urinate, and sometimes hematuria (blood in the urine).

Cystofibroma: A fibrous tumor associated with a cyst.

Cytomegalovirus (CMV): A viral disease normally producing mild symptoms in healthy individuals but severe infections in the immunocompromised and sometimes malformations or fetal death with congenital infection; results from infection by cytomegalovirus, a type of herpesvirus.

Dead fetus syndrome: A coagulation disorder in women resulting from the death of a fetus in utero.

Debility: Any weakness or loss of physical abilities.

Deep vein thrombosis: The formation of a blood clot (thrombus) in a deep vein that prevents blood circulation.

Dehydration: Excessive loss of body water, which is often accompanied by disturbances in electrolyte balance.

Delusions: False beliefs regarding the self or persons or objects outside the self that persist despite the facts; common in paranoia, schizophrenia, and psychotic depressed states.

Dementias: Disorders characterized by a general deterioration of intellectual and emotional functioning; may involve problems with memory, judgment, and emotional responses and personality changes.

Dengue fever: A flulike viral illness, contracted by humans through the bite of an infected *Aedes* mosquito.

Dental diseases: Diseases that affect the teeth (such as dental caries) or the gums (such as gingivitis, pyorrhea, and cancer).

Depression: A condition characterized by persistent feelings of despair, weight change, sleep problems, thoughts of death, thinking difficulties, diminished interest or pleasure in activities, and agitation or listlessness.

Dermatitis: A general term for nonspecific skin irritations that may be caused by bacteria, viruses, or fungi.

Developmental disorders: A group of conditions that indicate significant delays in or a lack of social skill development with deficiencies in adaptive behaviors, poor language skills, and a limited capacity to communicate effectively.

Diabetes mellitus: A hormonal disorder in which the pancreas is unable to produce or utilize sufficient insulin to process and maintain a proper level of sugar in the blood; if left untreated, may lead to circulatory problems, heart disease, blindness, dementia, kidney failure, and death.

Diaper rash: A skin condition characterized by irritation in the diaper area that can vary from slight redness to severe inflammation with sores or blisters.

Diarrhea: Loose, watery, and copious bowel movements.

DIC. *See* Disseminated intravascular coagulation (DIC).

DiGeorge syndrome: A congenital disease whose symptoms commonly include recurrent infections, heart defects, facial anomalies, and low serum calcium levels; characterized by the lack of a thymus gland.

Diphtheria: A highly contagious bacterial infection that usually affects the respiratory system.

Disk prolapse: The protrusion (herniation) of intervertebral disk material, which may press on spinal nerves.

Dislocation: The forceful separation of bones in a joint.

Disseminated intravascular coagulation (DIC): A hemorrhagic disorder that occurs as a complication of several different disease states and results from abnormally initiated and accelerated blood clotting.

Diverticulitis: A painful condition in which diverticuli (outpouchings of the wall of the colon) become inflamed.

Diverticulosis: A disease involving multiple outpouchings, called diverticuli, in the wall of the colon.

Dizziness: A feeling of light-headedness and unsteadiness, sometimes accompanied by a feeling of spinning or other spatial motion.

Dohle-Heller disease: Inflammation of the aorta resulting from tertiary syphilis.

Domestic violence: Assaultive behavior intended to punish, dominate, or control another in an intimate family relationship; physicians are often best able to identify situations of domestic violence and assist victims to implement preventive interventions.

Donath-Landsteiner syndrome: A blood disorder characterized by destruction of red blood cells upon exposure to cold; sometimes associated with syphilis.

Dorsalgia: Pain in the upper back.

Down syndrome: A congenital abnormality characterized by moderate to severe mental retardation and a distinctive physical appearance; caused by a chromosomal aberration, the result of either an error during embryonic cell division or the inheritance of defective chromosomal material.

Dracunculiasis: A parasitic infection caused by the nematode *Dracunculus*; characteristics include ulcers on the legs or feet.

Dressler's syndrome: An autoimmune disease in which the body reacts against the pericardium; usually occurs as a result of heart attack or cardiac surgery.

Dropsy: The abnormal accumulation of fluid in a body cavity or joint.

Drug resistance: The ability of a pathogen, formerly susceptible to a particular medication, to change in such a way that it is no longer affected by it.

Dubin-Johnson syndrome: A congenital disorder resulting in the abnormal excretion of organic molecules by the liver.

Duchenne-Aran disease: Degeneration of the spinal cord resulting in weakness of the upper limbs; often associated with exposure to toxins.

Duchenne's paralysis: Progressive neurological and motor weakness involving facial and laryngeal muscles.

Dwarfism: Underdevelopment of the body, most often caused by a variety of genetic or endocrine dysfunctions and resulting in either proportionate or disproportionate development, sometimes accompanied by other physical abnormalities and/or mental deficiencies.

Dysentery: An intestinal infection characterized by severe diarrhea.

Dysesthesia: A distortion of any sense, especially that of touch.

Dyskinesia: Abnormal involuntary movements with different causes and clinical presentations.

Dyslexia: Severe reading disability in children with average to above-average intelligence.

Dysmenorrhea: Painful menstruation; primary dysmenorrhea is generally harmless and occurs in young women, while secondary dysmenorrhea may be caused by endometriosis, pelvic inflammatory disease, or tumors.

Dysostosis: A defect in the ossification of cartilage during development.

Dyspareunia: Painful sexual intercourse.

Dyspepsia: A general term applied to several forms of indigestion.

Dysphasia: A disturbance of such language skills as speaking, reading, writing, and comprehension.

Dystrophy: A developmental defect associated with muscles, often resulting from malnutrition.

Dysuria: Difficulty in or pain associated with urination.

E. coli infection: Infection with *Escherichia coli*, a rod-shaped, anaerobic, self-propelling bacterium of the family Enterobacteriaceae; it normally inhabits mammal intestines without ill effect, but some strains can cause life-threatening illness.

Earache: Pain or discomfort in the ear.

Eating disorders: A set of emotional disorders centering on body image that lead to the misuse of food in a variety of ways (overeating, overeating and purging, undereating) that severely threaten the physical and mental well-being of the individual.

Eaton-Lambert's syndrome: Muscle weakness that often accompanies lung cancer.

Ebola virus: A virus responsible for a severe and often fatal hemorrhagic fever.

Ebstein's anomaly: Hereditary defect of the heart in which the tricuspid valve may be displaced into the right ventricle.

Ecchymoma: Swelling associated with a bruise.

Ecchymosis: A bruise.

Eclampsia: Hypertension induced by pregnancy, in its convulsive form.

Ectopic pregnancy: The development of a fertilized egg in a Fallopian tube instead of in the uterus; may be fatal to the mother unless corrected surgically.

Eczema: A skin disorder characterized by reddening, swelling, blistering, crusting, and scabbing; also called dermatitis.

Edema: The accumulation of fluid in body tissues, which may indicate a variety of diseases, including cardiovascular, kidney, liver, and medication problems.

Edwards syndrome: Trisomy 18, characterized by severe mental retardation and abnormalities of bone structures; generally, infants with the syndrome do not survive more than a few months after birth.

Ehrlichiosis: Infection by one of a group of intracellular bacteria transmitted to humans through tick bites.

Electrical shock: The physical effect of an electrical current entering the body and the resulting damage.

Elephantiasis: A grossly disfiguring disease caused by a roundworm parasite; the advanced stage of the disease Bancroft's filariasis.

Embolus: Any particle in the arterial or venous system that travels with the flow of blood, eventually lodging in the lungs, brain, or other organ or blood vessel.

Emerging diseases: Those diseases that newly appear in a populace, or have been in existence for some time but are rapidly increasing in incidence, geographic range, or surface as new drug-resistant strains of viruses, bacteria, or parasitic species.

Emery-Dreifuss syndrome: A congenital disorder characterized by cardiac arrhythmia as well as contraction of the joints.

Emphysema: A lung disease characterized by enlargement of the small bronchioles or alveoli, the destruction of alveoli, decreased elastic recoil of these structures, and the trapping of air in the lungs; results in shortness of breath, reduced oxygen to the body, and a variety of serious and eventually fatal complications.

Encephalitis: Inflammation of the brain caused by viral infection or complications from another disease and resulting in a variety of serious symptoms and sometimes death.

End-stage renal disease: Stage 5 of chronic kidney disease; causes irreversible damage to and near-complete failure of the kidneys.

Endocarditis: Inflammatory lesions of the endocardium, the lining of the heart.

Endocrine disorders: Breakdowns in the normal functioning of the endocrine system, which controls the metabolic processes of the body.

Endodontic disease: A number of diseases of the dental pulp found within teeth and of the surrounding tissues, the gums.

Endometriosis: A female reproductive disease in which cells from the uterine lining (the endometrium) grow outside the uterus, causing severe pain and sometimes infertility or the need for hysterectomy.

Enteroviruses: A class of viruses capable of infecting multiple organ systems, such as the central nervous system, the skin, the eyes, and the heart.

Enuresis: Bed-wetting.

Environmental diseases: A wide variety of conditions and diseases resulting from largely human-mediated hazards in both natural and artificial (for example, home and workplace) environments.

Epidemic: A widespread, rapid occurrence of an infectious disease in a community or region at a particular time.

Epilepsy: A serious neurologic disease characterized by seizures, which may involve convulsions and loss of consciousness.

Erectile dysfunction: A disorder whereby a male cannot achieve an erection suitable for sexual intercourse.

Erythema: Reddening of the skin resulting from the dilation of capillaries; may result from local infections or insect bites.

Erythralgia: Reddening of and pain associated with the skin.

Erythremia: An abnormal increase in the numbers of red blood cells.

Erythroblastosis: A condition in which immature blood cells are found in the circulation.

Ewing's sarcoma: A rare bone cancer involving any part of the skeleton but found commonly in the long bones, pelvis, and ribs of children and young adults.

Factitious disorders: Psychophysiological disorders in which individuals intentionally produce their symptoms in order to play the role of patient.

Failure to thrive: A disorder of early childhood growth that includes disturbances in psychosocial skills and development; usually associated with metabolic disturbances.

Fainting: Loss of consciousness as a result of insufficient amounts of blood reaching the brain.

Fanconi's anemia: A congenital disorder in children resulting in blood and bone abnormalities and an increased risk of developing cancer.

Fanconi's syndrome: A combination of disorders resulting from kidney dysfunction and characterized by acidosis or bone disorders; may be either congenital or acquired as a result of toxin exposure.

Farsightedness: The inability of the eye to focus on close objects; also called hyperopia.

Fasciculation: Uncontrolled twitching of a muscle group within the skin.

Fascioliasis: Infection by the liver fluke *Fasciola hepatica*; characterized by jaundice, fever, and chronic liver damage.

Fatigue: A general symptom of tiredness, malaise, depression, and sometimes anxiety associated with many diseases and disorders; in some cases, no specific cause can be found.

Fatty liver disease: Accumulation of lipids in the liver; often associated with obesity, alcohol overconsumption, or toxin exposure.

Felty's syndrome: Enlargement of the spleen; often a result of rheumatoid arthritis.

Fetal alcohol syndrome: Growth retardation and mental or physical abnormalities in a child resulting from alcohol consumption by the mother during pregnancy.

Fever: A symptom associated with a variety of diseases and disorders and characterized by a body temperature above normal (98.6 degrees Fahrenheit or 37 degrees Celsius); usually considered very serious at 104 degrees Fahrenheit (40 degrees Celsius) and higher.

Fibrocystic breast condition: A noncancerous breast condition affecting approximately 60 percent of all women, the majority of whom are premenopausal; now considered to be a normal physiologic variant.

Fibromyalgia: A chronic, spontaneous, and widespread musculoskeletal pain disorder with multiple, specific, and intense pain sites; also characterized by recurrent fatigue and sleep disturbance.

Fifth disease: An infectious disease of children characterized by an erythematous (reddish) rash and low-grade fever; associated with infection by a parvovirus.

Flat feet: A congenital or acquired flatness of the longitudinal arches of the feet.

Food allergies: An abnormal response by the immune system to some foods, causing mild to severe symptoms that may become life-threatening.

Food poisoning: Food-borne illness caused by bacteria, viruses, or parasites consumed in food and resulting in acute gastrointestinal disturbance that may include diarrhea, nausea, vomiting, and abdominal discomfort.

Fracture: A break in a bone, which may be partial or complete.

Fragile X syndrome: A genetic disorder of variable expression, with mental retardation being the most common feature.

Frontotemporal dementia (FTD): A group of neurodegenerative disorders that affect the frontal and temporal lobes of the brain.

Frostbite: Localized freezing of tissue, usually of extremities exposed to low temperatures.

Fructosemia: An inborn error of metabolism in which eating foods containing fructose or sucrose will result in high blood fructose levels.

Fungal infections: Infections caused by fungi ranging from minor skin diseases to serious, disseminated diseases of the lungs and other organs; patients whose immune systems are impaired are at greater risk of serious fungal infections.

Gallbladder diseases: A family of disorders affecting the gallbladder, usually causing abdominal pain but occasionally symptomless.

Gallstones: Particles of cholesterol and other substances that form in the gallbladder when the solubility of bile components is altered.

Gangrene: Necrosis (tissue death) resulting from blood loss and bacterial invasion followed by putrefaction; may be initiated by a variety of diseases and conditions and if left untreated may result in amputation or death.

Gastritis: Inflammation of the stomach.

Gastroenteritis: An acute infectious process affecting the gastrointestinal system, usually leading to abdominal discomfort and diarrhea.

Gaucher's disease: A congenital disorder characterized by a defect in lipid metabolism and character-ized by cell hyperplasia in the liver, spleen, and bone marrow.

Gender identity disorder: A psychiatric classification describing persons experiencing a strong and persistent incongruity between their anatomy and the gender with which they identify.

Genetic diseases: A variety of disorders transmitted from parent to child through chromosomal material.

Gerstmann-Straussler syndrome: Progressive neurological disease associated with prion infection.

Gestational diabetes: A medical condition in which diabetes, or unregulated blood glucose, first occurs during pregnancy.

Giardiasis: An acute or chronic parasitic infection of the gastrointestinal system caused by the protozoan *Giardia lamblia.*

Gigantism: A rare endocrine disorder characterized by an overgrowth of all bones and body tissues.

Gingivitis: Superficial inflammation of the gums, associated with the destructive buildup of dental plaque; if left untreated, it can result in periodontitis.

Glaucoma: A group of eye diseases characterized by an increase in intraocular pressure; early diagnosis can allow management of the disease, while late diagnosis may result in impaired vision or blindness.

Glomerulonephritis: Inflammation of the glomeruli, the clusters of blood vessels and nerves found throughout the kidney.

Glucosuria: A condition in which the concentration of blood glucose exceeds the ability of the kidney to reabsorb it; as a result, glucose spills into the urine, taking with it body water and electrolytes.

Gluten intolerance: A chronic, immune-mediated condition of progressive, itchy skin lesions triggered by ingestion of gluten.

Glycogen storage diseases: Inherited metabolic disorders that lead to the accumulation of an abnormal amount or type of glycogen in the liver or in muscle and heart tissue.

Goiter: Enlargement of the thyroid gland in the neck.

Gonadal dysgenesis: Any of a variety of conditions in which genital organs do not develop properly.

Gonorrhea: An infection of the urogenital tract that is a common sexually transmitted disease; results from infection by the bacterium *Neisseria gonorrheae.*

Goodpasture's syndrome: Chronic form of glomerulonephritis.

Gout: Painful arthritis of the peripheral joints, often in the big toe.

Graft rejection: Rejection of a graft by the host, generally resulting from tissue incompatibility.

Graft-versus-host disease: A transplantation response in which cells from the graft react against host tissue; most commonly associated with bone marrow transplantation in which the donor and recipient tissues are not compatible.

Grand mal seizure: A type of epileptic seizure characterized by severe convulsions, body stiffening, and loss of consciousness during which victims fall down; also called tonic-clonic seizure.

Granulocytopenia: An unusual decrease in the numbers of white blood cells.

Granulocytosis: An unusual increase in the numbers of white blood cells.

Granuloma: A nodular, inflammatory lesion that is usually small, firm, and persistent and that contains proliferated macrophages.

Graves' disease: A common type of hyperthyroidism in which the thyroid gland produces an oversupply of hormone.

Gravidarum chloasma: Skin discoloration in a woman during pregnancy.

Gray hair: The reduction in hair pigmentation that is a natural by-product of aging.

Gray syndrome: A cyanotic appearance in infants, often the result of an adverse reaction to antibiotics.

Grocer's itch: A skin condition resulting from contact with insects found in food.

Gronblad-Strandberg's syndrome: A congenital disorder resulting in the breakdown of connective tissue; symptoms include breakdown of the retina and premature aging.

Growth failure: A defect in physical development associated with any of a multitude of causes.

Guillain-Barr syndrome: An acute degeneration of peripheral motor and sensory nerves, known to physicians as acute inflammatory demyelinating polyneuropathy; a common cause of acute generalized paralysis.

Gulf War syndrome: A popular term used to describe collectively a variety of symptoms, not a specific disease, suffered by veterans of the 1991 Persian Gulf War.

Gunther's disease: A congenital disorder of porphyrin metabolism, resulting in unusual sensitivity to sunlight.

Hailey-Hailey disease: A congenital skin condition characterized by chronic ulcer formation.

Hairy-cell leukemia: A type of leukemia characterized by hairlike structures on the surface of cells in the bone marrow.

Hairy leukoplakia: The formation of white plaques on the tongue. Most commonly found in patients with immunodeficiency disorders.

Hairy nevus: A mole with hair formation.

Halitosis: Bad breath, usually the result of drinking alcohol, smoking, or eating pungent foods.

Hallervorden-Spatz syndrome: A neurological disease of children characterized by muscle rigidity; associated with iron deposition in the brain.

Hallucination: The perception of sensations without relevant external stimuli.

Hallux rigidus: Condition of limited mobility of the big toe.

Hammertoe: An abnormality of the tendon in a toe that causes the main joint to curve upward and creates pain; often the result of shoe pressure.

Hantavirus: An often-fatal virus carried by rodents that causes influenza-like symptoms and respiratory failure.

Hartnup's disease: A pellagra-like condition resulting from the metabolic inability to absorb amino acids.

Hashimoto's thyroiditis: Inflammation of the thyroid gland that occurs when abnormal blood antibodies and white blood cells infiltrate and attack thyroidal cells.

Haverhill fever: An infection associated with *Streptobacillus moniliformis* and characterized by fever, headache, chills, and a rash; transmitted by a rodent bite.

Headache: Pain localized in the head or neck; often caused by tension but may result from a range of disorders.

Hearing loss: Loss of sensitivity to sound pressure changes as a result of congenital factors, disease, traumatic injury, noise exposure, or aging.

Heart attack: Sudden and permanent damage to a part of the heart muscle as a result of impaired blood flow through the coronary arteries; the common term for myocardial infarction.

Heart block: A delay or blockage of the electrical signal traveling through the heart muscle, which upsets the synchronization between contractions of the upper and lower chambers.

Heart disease: One of the leading causes of death in many industrialized nations; includes atherosclerotic disease, coronary artery disease, cardiac arrhythmias, and stenosis.

Heart failure: A condition in which the heart cannot pump enough blood to meet the needs of the body because its ability to contract is impaired.

Heartburn: The presence of a burning sensation in the chest and throat caused by the reflux of stomach acids.

Heat exhaustion: Mild shock caused by a decrease in the amount of fluid in the blood.

Heat stroke: A medical emergency in which high body temperatures result in organ damage.

Heel spur: A bony outgrowth on the heel of the foot.

Hematomas: Localized, semisolid masses of pooled blood in tissue, caused by spontaneous or post-trauma blood leakage through the vessel walls of arteries, capillaries, or veins and subsequent clotting in surrounding tissue.

Hematuria: The presence of blood or red blood cells in the urine.

Hemeralopia: Condition in which exposure to bright light results in blurred vision.

Hemiparesis: Weakness on one side of the body.

Hemiplegia: Paralysis on one side of the body.

Hemochromatosis: A multisystem disease characterized by increased iron absorption and storage.

Hemoglobin C disease: A congenital disorder characterized by hemoglobin C, a variant of normal hemoglobin; it may be asymptomatic or cause jaundice.

Hemoglobin M disease: A condition in which an abnormal form of iron in the hemoglobin molecule prevents proper oxygen transport.

Hemoglobinemia: The abnormal presence of hemoglobin in circulation, rather than exclusively within red blood cells.

Hemolytic anemia: A chronic disorder characterized by the abnormal breakdown of red blood cells.

Hemolytic disease of the newborn: The destruction of red blood cells in a fetus by antibodies transferred from the mother; also known as erythroblastosis fetalis.

Hemophilia: A hereditary blood defect occurring almost exclusively in males and characterized by delayed clotting of the blood and consequent difficulty in controlling bleeding even after minor injuries.

Hemoptysis: The expiration of blood while coughing; usually the result of a respiratory infection, though sometimes indicative of more severe problems.

Hemorrhage: Loss of blood from an area of the body.

Hemorrhagic shock: Shock associated with the loss of large quantities of blood.

Hemorrhoids: Dilated blood vessels in the anus or rectum that are itchy and painful.

Hemosiderosis: The abnormal deposition of iron in tissues; usually the result of lysis of red blood cells.

Hepatitis: An inflammatory condition of the liver characterized by discomfort, jaundice, and liver enlargement; often bacterial, viral, or immunological in origin, but may also result from the use of alcohol or other toxic drugs.

Hermaphroditism: A condition in which both testicular and ovarian tissues are found in an individual with ambiguous urogenital development; caused by developmental defects.

Hernia: A pouch of intestines and/or vital organs of the abdomen that protrudes through the abdominal wall.

Herpes: A family of viruses that cause several diseases, including infectious mononucleosis, cold sores, genital herpes, and chickenpox.

Hiccups: Involuntary, spasmodic contractions of the diaphragm and simultaneous closure of the glottis.

His-Werner disease: Also called trench fever; an infection associated with louse-borne rickettsia.

Histiocytosis: The overproduction of macrophages.

Hives: The presence of pink swellings called wheals that may occur in groups on any part of the skin.

Hodgkin's disease: A neoplastic disorder originating in the tissues of the lymphatic system, recognized by distinctive histologic changes and defined by the presence of Reed-Sternberg cells.

H1N1 influenza: An acute respiratory infection caused by the H1N1 subtype of the influenza A virus.

Hot flashes: Temporary sensations of warmth experienced by perimenopausal and postmenopausal women in which the upper body feels hot, the skin turns red, and sweating occurs.

Huntington's disease: An autosomal dominant genetic disease in which patients experience uncoordinated movements as a result of the degeneration of neurons.

Hurler's syndrome: A congenital disease characterized by the buildup of mucopolysaccharides within cells as a result of metabolic defects; an example of the class of diseases known as mucopolysaccharidoses.

Hurthle cell carcinoma: A type of thyroid tumor.

Hutchinson's disease: A skin condition characterized by small red spots forming circles; also known as angioma serpiginosum.

Hyaline membrane disease: The inability to dissolve hyaline membrane in the lungs of premature infants; results from a lack of production of tissue surfactant.

Hydatidosis: Infection by the tapeworm *Echinococcus*.

Hydradenitis: Inflammation of the sweat glands.

Hydramnios: The buildup of excess amniotic fluid during pregnancy; generally associated with diabetes or toxemia in the pregnant woman.

Hydrocele: A fluid-filled area around the testis or other sac; often caused by infection or inflammation.

Hydrocephalus: A collection of excessive amounts of cerebrospinal fluid (CSF) within the cranial cavity; may cause increased pressure within the brain and skull, leading to brain tissue damage and, in infants, enlargement of the skull.

Hyperadiposis: Having excess body fat; exceeding 200 percent of standard body weight as defined on a height-weight table.

Hyperbarism: A condition that results from a sudden increase in atmospheric pressure.

Hyper-beta-alaninemia: A congenital disorder characterized by an inability to produce the enzyme beta-alanine alpha-ketoglutarate transferase.

Hyperbetalipoproteinemia: A congenital disorder of lipid metabolism characterized by high levels of serum cholesterol.

Hyperbilirubinemia: The buildup of bilirubin in serum, often resulting in jaundice; usually associated with liver damage or bile duct obstruction.

Hyperlipidemia: The presence of abnormally large amounts of lipids (fats) in the blood.

Hypernatremia: A high salt concentration in the blood that can result in seizure and coma.

Hyperopia: The inability of the eye to focus on close objects; also called farsightedness.

Hyperparathyroidism: The excessive, uncontrolled secretion of parathyroid hormone.

Hyperplasia: A proliferation of cells in response to either normal or abnormal physiological processes.

Hypertension: A condition in which the blood pressure is higher than what is considered normal.

Hyperthermia: The elevation of the body core temperature of an organism above a normal range.

Hypertonia: An abnormal increase in muscle strength; sometimes associated with trisomy 18.

Hypochondriasis: Unwarranted belief about or anxiety regarding having a serious disease that is based on a subjective interpretation of physical symptoms or sensations; the belief or anxiety is maintained despite appropriate medical assurances that there is no serious disease.

Hypoglycemia: A condition in which the concentration of glucose in the blood is too low to meet the needs of key organs, especially the brain.

Hypoparathyroidism: Reduced secretion of parathyroid hormone.

Hypospadias: An abnormal urethral opening in the penis, either on the underside or on the perineum.

Hypothermia: A decrease in the body core temperature of an organism below a normal range.

Hypothyroidism: A condition in which the thyroid gland produces an insufficient supply of hormone.

Hypoxia: An inadequate supply of oxygen to tissues caused by either oxygen delivery not being sufficient for tissue requirements or because utilization of oxygen is ineffective.

I cell disease: A congenital lysosomal storage disease in children resulting in eventual respiratory and cardiac failure.

Iatrogenic disorders: Health problems caused by medical treatments.

IBS. *See* Irritable bowel syndrome (IBS).

Immunodeficiency disorders: Genetic or acquired disorders in which the normal functioning of the immune system is disturbed.

Impetigo: One of several severe skin infections caused by bacteria.

Impotence: The inability to achieve an erection.

Incontinence: The inability to control the expulsion of urine or feces.

Indifference-to-pain syndrome: A congenital malformation of nerve endings in the skin, resulting in a lack of sensitivity to pain.

Indigestion: A digestive disorder characterized by a burning sensation in the chest and throat and sometimes by abdominal pain, bloating, nausea, vomiting, and diarrhea; also called dyspepsia.

Infarction: A localized area of tissue damage or necrosis caused by absence of blood supply and oxygen to the part.

Infection: Invasion of the body by disease-causing organisms such as bacteria, viruses, fungi, and parasites; symptoms may include pain, swelling, fever, and loss of normal function.

Infertility: The inability to achieve a desired pregnancy as a result of dysfunction of female and/or male reproductive organs or biochemistry.

Inflammation: The reaction of blood-filled living tissue to injury.

Influenza: An acute respiratory infection caused by an influenza virus.

Insomnia: Disturbed sleep; may be caused by a dysfunctional sleep cycle, breathing problems, leg jerking, underlying medical and psychiatric disorders, or the side effects of medication.

Insulin resistance syndrome: A reduced sensitivity to the action of insulin, which brings glucose into body tissues to be used as a source of energy.

Interstitial pulmonary fibrosis: A disease characterized by scarring and thickening of lung tissue, which causes breathing difficulty.

Intraventricular hemorrhage: Bleeding into or around the normal cerebrospinal fluid spaces within the brain.

Iron-deficiency anemia: Anemia characterized by low serum iron concentration.

Irritable bowel syndrome (IBS): A common intestinal disorder characterized by abdominal pain and cramps, altered bowel habits (diarrhea or constipation), bloating, and nausea.

Ischemia: A local anemia or area of diminished or insufficient blood supply caused by obstruction of the blood supply, commonly the narrowing of an artery.

Itching: An unpleasant sensation on or in the skin that causes a desire to scratch or rub the affected area.

Jaundice: A yellowish coloration visible on the skin.

Jet lag: Malaise, headache, fatigue, gastrointestinal disorders, and other symptoms that may result from traveling across several time zones within a few hours.

Juvenile rheumatoid arthritis: A usually chronic autoimmune disease of unknown cause, characterized by joint swelling, pain, and sometimes the destruction of joints.

Kala-azar: A disease associated with sandfly transmission of the protozoan *Leishmania*; characterized by malfunction of the liver and spleen.

Kaposi's sarcoma: The presence of cancer cells in tissues, causing lesions on the skin and/or mucous membranes and spreading to other organs in the body; an opportunistic disease often associated with AIDS.

Keratitis: Inflammation of the cornea that may cause partial or total opacity, leading to loss of vision.

Keratoses: Wartlike growths caused by the excessive production of the skin protein keratin, usually occurring in elderly people.

Kleine-Levin syndrome: A complex of symptoms including very long sleep periods and abnormal hyperactivity.

Klinefelter syndrome: A male chromosomal disorder causing infertility and significant female attributes.

Klippel-Feil syndrome: A congenital lack of cervical vertebrae resulting in a short neck and limited head movement.

Klippel-Trenaunay syndrome: A rare congenital syndrome characterized by hemangiomas of the vascular system but that can affect bone or soft tissue throughout the body.

Kluver-Bucy syndrome: Behavioral disorder characterized by lack of emotional activity or responses similar to that often observed in patients with Alzheimer's disease.

Kwashiorkor: A protein deficiency disease that may affect young children in developing countries.

Kyphosis: A marked increase of the normal curvature of the thoracic vertebrae or upper back; sometimes referred to as dowager's hump because of its prevalence in elderly women.

Lactose intolerance: An inability to break down and absorb lactose (milk sugar), resulting in stomach pain, gas, and diarrhea if lactose is consumed.

Laryngitis: Inflammation of the larynx characterized by hoarseness in the voice and sometimes the inability to speak.

Lead poisoning: Poisoning as the result of the ingestion or inhalation of abnormally high levels of lead, which disrupts kidney function and damages the nervous system.

Learning disabilities: A variety of disorders involving the failure to learn an academic skill despite a normal level of intelligence.

Legionnaires' disease: Acute bacterial pneumonia resulting from infection with members of the genus *Legionella* that resembles influenza and may prove fatal to older persons or those individuals with previous lung damage; also known as Pontiac fever.

Leishmaniasis: One of several diseases associated with the single-celled protozoan species *Leishmania*, transmitted by the bite of a sandfly; these diseases cause ulcers in the skin or internal organs.

Lennox-Gastaut syndrome: A condition of unknown cause characterized by seizures and mental retardation.

Lentigo maligna melanoma: A type of melanoma that generally develops from a facial freckle and is observed only in the elderly.

Leprosy: A bacterial infection that affects the skin and nerves, causing symptoms ranging from mild numbness to gross disfiguration.

Leptospirosis: Any of a variety of diseases associated with infection by members of the genus *Leptospira.*

Leriche's syndrome: The chronic lack of oxygen to vascular tissue, which results in gangrene or other tissue disorders; occlusions within the aorta are not uncommon.

Lesch-Nyhan syndrome: A congenital disorder of purine metabolism, resulting in mental retardation and often self-mutilation.

Lesions: Damaged areas of tissue as a result of injury or disease.

Letterer-Siwe syndrome: Variety of malignant histiocyte (macrophage) disorders which begin during infancy; probably of congenital origin, though the specific cause is unknown.

Leukemia: A family of cancers that affect the blood, characterized by an increase in the number of white blood cells.

Leukopenia: An abnormal decrease in white blood cells.

Lisping: The defective pronunciation of the sibilants "s" and "z," usually substituted with a "th" sound.

Listeria **infections:** Infections caused by the bacterium *Listeria monocytogenes.*

Liver cancer: Malignancies of the liver, which may be primary (arising in the organ itself) but are more likely to be secondary (metastasizing from another site).

Lung cancer: The appearance of malignant tumors in the lungs, which is usually associated with cigarette smoking.

Lupus: Systemic lupus erythematosus; a chronic inflammatory disease characterized by arthritis and a rash.

Lyme disease: A mild-to-serious infection caused by the bacteria *Borrelia burgdorferi* that is spread by the bite of infected ticks of the genus *Ixodes.*

Lymphadenopathy: Enlarged lymph nodes.

Lymphogranuloma venereum: A sexually transmitted disease associated with infection by *Chlamydia trachomatis* and characterized by ulcerative genital lesions.

Lymphoid interstitial pneumonia: Lobar pneumonia characterized by the infiltration of lymphocytes and macrophages; often associated with immunosuppression caused by AIDS.

Lymphoma: A group of cancers characterized by the unchecked multiplication of lymphatic tissue cells.

Macular degeneration: The progressive breakdown of the macula, the part of the eye that allows for detailed sight in the center of the field of vision, with a dense concentration of rods and cones.

Mad cow disease: A spongiform encephalopathy that affects cattle but may be transmissible to humans, leading to new variant Creutzfeldt-Jakob disease (nvCJD).

Malabsorption: The impaired absorption of nutrients from food into the bloodstream.

Malaise: A feeling of lack of health or debility, often indicating or accompanying the onset of illness.

Malaria: A serious parasitic infection borne by mosquitoes in tropical and subtropical regions and characterized by recurrent bouts of severe fever, chills, sweating, vomiting, and damage to kidneys, blood, brain, and liver.

Malnutrition: A physical state characterized by an imbalance of dietary proteins, carbohydrates, fats, vitamins, and minerals, given an individual's physical activity and health needs.

Maple syrup urine disease (MSUD): A recessive autosomal genetic disease resulting in the absence, partial activity, or inactivity of a multisubunit enzyme responsible for metabolizing the branched chain amino acids leucine, isoleucine, and valine.

Marasmus: The condition that results from consuming a diet deficient in both caloric intake and protein.

Marfan syndrome: A condition in which the connective tissue does not form correctly and tends to be too flexible, leading to such characteristics as unusually long fingers or arms, loose joints, and disorders of the heart, eyes, and spinal column.

Mastitis: Infection of the breast, which results in inflammation, tenderness, swelling, and pain.

Measles: A highly contagious disease contracted through a virus transmitted in respiratory secretions and characterized by a spreading skin rash.

Megaloblastic anemia: Anemia caused by the failure of red blood cells to mature; also known as pernicious anemia, Addisonian anemia, or maturation failure.

Melanoma: Cancer of the melanocytes, the cells that produce the skin pigment melanin.

Meningism: Irritation or mild inflammation within the central nervous system, resulting in symptoms that resemble those of meningitis.

Meningitis: An inflammation of the meninges of the brain and spinal cord.

Menorrhagia: Excessive or prolonged bleeding during menstruation.

Mental retardation: A condition characterized by a below-average intelligence quotient (IQ) and deficits in adaptive functioning before the age of eighteen years; the degree of retardation ranges from mild to severe.

Meralgia: Pain in the thigh region.

Mercury poisoning: Poisoning resulting from the ingestion or inhalation of mercury; symptoms include tremors, slurred speech, pain, vomiting, and occasionally a metallic taste in the mouth.

Merergasia: Mental instability in which excessive anxiety is exhibited.

Merkel cell carcinoma: Rapidly progressing carcinoma of the skin, usually the result of excessive exposure to sunlight.

Meromelia: Congenital absence of a portion of a limb.

Mesenchymoma: A type of cancer that originates within mesenchymal tissue, that of mesodermal origin.

Mesothelioma: A malignancy originating from the mesothelial surfaces (the lining cells) of the pleural and peritoneal cavities, the pericardium, or the tunica vaginalis.

Metabolic alkalosis: An increase in the pH of tissue fluids, often resulting from excessive use of bicarbonate or excessive vomiting and loss of acid.

Metabolic syndrome: A complex medical disorder characterized by dyslipidemia (high triglycerides and low high-density lipoproteins), insulin resistance, abdominal obesity, and high blood pressure.

Methicillin-resistant *Staphylococcus aureus* (MRSA) infection: An infection caused by a virulent and destructive bacteria that is resistant to common antibiotics and difficult to treat.

Midlife crisis: The emotional, psychological, physical, spiritual, and relationship crises that may arise during the transition from early to later adulthood.

Migraine headache: A severe, incapacitating headache that may be preceded by nausea and vomiting or by visual, sensory, and motor disturbances.

Milk fever: General term for fever that accompanies lactation.

Mineral deficiency: Absence of required minerals in tissue; generally the result of poor dietary habits but can be associated with a congenital or acquired inability to absorb minerals properly.

Miscarriage: The expulsion of the embryo or fetus before it is viable outside the uterus; also called spontaneous abortion.

Mitral valve prolapse: The inability of the mitral valve in the heart to close properly; also called mitral insufficiency.

Möbius syndrome: A congenital disorder characterized by bilateral facial palsy.

Mold and mildew: Growths of fungi that can be parasitic on plants and humans.

Moles: Nonmalignant marks, pigmented spots, or growths on the skin.

Monkeypox: A mild infection caused by members of the poxvirus family; may be transmitted to rodents and, on occasion, to humans.

Mononucleosis: An infectious respiratory illness caused by the Epstein-Barr virus that produces lymph node enlargement.

Monosomy: A condition in which one chromosome from the human diploid total of forty-six is missing.

Morgellons disease: A skin disorder characterized by a pattern of dermatologic symptoms described as insect-like sensations, with skin lesions varying from very minor to disfiguring, and associated with disabling fatigue, joint pain, and various neuropsychiatric symptoms.

Motion sickness: A disorder characterized by nausea, vomiting, and vertigo and caused by a combination of repetitive back-and-forth and up-and-down movements.

Motor neuron diseases: Progressive, debilitating, and eventually fatal diseases affecting nerve cells in muscles.

Motor seizure: Unusual electrical discharge in the brain that results in the involuntary movement of a muscle.

Motor weakness: Muscle weakness resulting from the failure of motor nerves.

MRSA infection. *See* Methicillin-resistant *Staphylococcus aureus* (MRSA) infection.

MSUD. *See* Maple syrup urine disease (MSUD).

Mucoepidermoid carcinoma: Cancer of glandular tissues, such as within the salivary glands.

Mucolipidosis: Any of several metabolic disorders characterized by excessive accumulation of lipids in tissues.

Mucopolysaccharidosis (MPS): A genetic disorder characterized by accumulations of mucopolysaccharides in tissues; six distinct classes have been described, with specific symptoms associated with each type.

Multiple chemical sensitivity syndrome: An increasing intolerance to commonly encountered chemicals at concentrations well tolerated by most people.

Multiple myeloma: Cancer of the bone marrow characterized by the overproduction of a clone of lymphocytes or plasma cells.

Multiple sclerosis (MS): A debilitating disease affecting the central nervous system that is caused by the degeneration of myelin; symptoms can be mild (such as limb numbness) or severe (such as paralysis and loss of vision).

Mumps: An acute, contagious childhood disease caused by a virus and characterized by swollen salivary glands.

Münchausen syndrome by proxy: A disorder in which a parent fabricates, simulates, or induces a medical condition in a child in order to receive attention and acknowledgment as the source of information about the child's health.

Murmur: Fluttering or echo associated with the heartbeat; though generally benign, may be a sign of a more significant disorder.

Muscular dystrophy: A group of progressive genetic diseases that attack the muscles.

Mutation: Any genetic change; depending upon the site of the mutation, expression of a gene product may be altered.

Mutism: The inability to speak.

Myasthenia gravis: A disorder characterized by selective muscle fatigue following repeated use and caused by an abnormal immune reaction to specific receptors on the muscle surface.

Myopia: The inability of the eye to focus on distant objects; also called nearsightedness.

Narcolepsy: An apparently inherited disorder of the nervous system characterized by brief, numerous, and overwhelming attacks of sleepiness throughout the day.

Nausea: An unpleasant sensation followed by stomach and intestinal discomfort, which may lead to vomiting.

Nearsightedness: The inability of the eye to focus on distant objects; also called myopia.

Necrosis: Tissue damage occurring as a result of cell death.

Necrotizing fasciitis: An invasive bacterial infection that occurs in the connective tissue between the skin and muscle, cutting off blood flow; popularly known as infection by flesh-eating bacteria.

Nephritis: Any disease or pathology of the kidney that results in inflammation.

Nephrotic syndrome: A kidney abnormality characterized by a variety of conditions, including edema and proteinuria; often accompanies glomerular dysfunction and diabetes mellitus.

Neuritis: An inflammatory or degenerative lesion of a nerve, marked by pain and the loss of normal reflexes.

Neurofibromatosis: A genetic disease affecting the nervous system, skin, and bones that produces multiple nerve tumors (neurofibromas), deeply pigmented areas of skin (café-au-lait spots), and bone deformities.

Neurosis: A chronic mental disorder characterized by distressing and unacceptable anxiety.

Niemann-Pick disease: A group of several lipid storage diseases that cause an enlarged liver and spleen and the accumulation of fatlike sphingomyelin and cholesterol.

Nightmares: Anxiety-provoking, scary, unpleasant, and frightening dreams that disturb sleep; children having nightmares may cry in their sleep or awake in an emotionally upset, typically anxious state.

Nocturia: Involuntary nighttime urination.

Noroviruses: Viruses that cause acute gastroenteritis.

Nosebleed: Bleeding from the nose, often the result of irritation of or trauma to the nasal mucosa.

Numbness: A reduction or loss of feeling in an area of skin.

Obesity: A condition in which the body carries abnormal or unhealthy amounts of fat tissue, leading the individual to weigh in excess of 20 percent more than his or her ideal weight.

Obsession: A recurrent, unwelcome, and intrusive thought.

Obsessive-compulsive disorder: An anxiety disorder characterized by intrusive and unwanted thoughts and/or the need to perform ritualized behaviors.

Obstruction: Partial or complete closure of the channels through which food or blood normally passes; may be silent or may cause either acute and life-threatening or chronic and debilitating illness.

Oophoritis: Inflammation of the ovary.

Opportunistic infections: Potentially life-threatening diseases occurring in persons with a weakened immune system by microorganisms that typically do not cause severe illnesses in an otherwise healthy person.

Orchitis: Inflammation of the testis.

Osteoarthritis: A degenerative disease of the joints and surrounding tissues.

Osteochondritis juvenilis: The disturbance of the blood supply to the tops of the thigh bones, resulting in their destruction.

Osteogenesis imperfecta: A genetic disorder of variable severity that results in frequent bone breaks.

Osteomyelitis: A secondary bacterial infection of the bone and bone marrow.

Osteoporosis: A loss of bone mass accompanied by increasing fragility and brittleness.

Otitis: Any inflammation of the outer or middle ear.

Otosclerosis: A condition in which the stapes becomes progressively more rigid and hearing loss results.

Ovarian cysts: Benign growths in the ovaries that may cause pain.

Paget's disease: A disorder characterized by a progressive thickening and weakening of the bones.

Pain: Physical distress often associated with a disorder or injury.

Palsy: Partial or complete paralysis of a nerve, followed by muscle weakness and wasting.

Pancreatitis: Inflammation of the pancreas, which may be acute or chronic.

Pandemic: An epidemic prevalent throughout a country, a continent, or the world.

Panic attack: A sudden feeling of intense apprehension, fear, doom, and/or terror that can cause shortness of breath, palpitations, chest pain, chills, nausea, and light-headedness.

Paralysis: Loss of muscle function or sensation as a result of trauma or disease.

Paranoia: A psychological disorder characterized by pervasive distrust and suspiciousness of others and a tendency to interpret others' motives as malevolent.

Paraplegia: Partial or complete paralysis of both legs caused by damage to the spinal cord.

Parasite: An organism whose principal food source is another living organism; in medicine, the term refers to both unicellular and multicellular animals.

Parkinson's disease: A progressive neurological disease characterized by tremor, slow movement, and muscle rigidity.

Patau's syndrome: Trisomy 13, resulting in significant central nervous system and cardiac abnormalities; rarely do infants with this syndrome survive the first year of life.

Pellagra: A deficiency of niacin (vitamin B3), characterized by dermatitis, diarrhea, dementia, and death.

Pelvic inflammatory disease (PID): An infection of the female reproductive organs that may be caused by a sexually transmitted disease.

Peptic ulcers: Open sores that develop on the mucous membranes that line the gastrointestinal tract and are caused by excessive secretion of gastric juices, particularly from the pancreas into the intestine.

Pericarditis: A disease of the membrane that surrounds the heart, caused by an inflammation that can lead to constriction of the heart muscle.

Pericholangitis: Inflammation of the bile ducts in the liver.

Pericholitis: Inflammation of tissue around the colon.

Pericoronitis: Inflammation of the gum around the crown of a tooth; often associated with infection following the development of molars.

Periodontitis: Inflammation and infection of the gums, which may cause loss of the supporting bone and eventually tooth loss.

Peritonitis: Infection of the abdominal (peritoneal) cavity in which the visceral organs are found.

Pernicious anemia: Hemoglobin deficiency associated with the inability to properly absorb vitamin B12 in the diet.

Personality disorders: Pervasive, inflexible patterns of perceiving, thinking, and behaving that cause long-term distress or impairment, beginning in adolescence and persisting into adulthood.

Pertussis: A serious bacterial infection of the respiratory tract that usually strikes very young children; commonly known as whooping cough.

Petit mal seizure: A mild type of epileptic seizure characterized by a very short lapse of consciousness, usually without convulsions or falling.

Pharyngitis: Inflammation of the pharynx (throat).

Phenylketonuria (PKU): A genetic disease characterized by an absence of the enzyme that breaks down the amino acid phenylalanine; the resulting buildup can lead to brain damage.

Phlebitis: The inflammation of a vein, often in the legs; may be accompanied by blood clots.

Phobia: Any abnormal or exaggerated fear of a particular object or situation.

Pinworm: A common parasitic nematode that resembles a white thread approximately 0.5 inch in length.

PKU. *See* Phenylketonuria (PKU).

Plague: A serious, and sometimes fatal, bacterial infection with *Yersinia pestis* transmitted by fleas.

Plaque, arterial: Fatty deposits within arterial walls.

Plaque, dental: Various kinds of bacteria that live in the mouth; stick to each other and then to the tooth surface, both above and below the gums; and cause tooth decay and gum disease.

Pleurisy: The inflammation and swelling of the pleurae, the membranes that enclose the lungs and line the chest cavity.

PML. *See* Progressive multifocal leukoencephalopathy (PML).

PMS. *See* Premenstrual syndrome (PMS).

Pneumocystis pneumonia: A form of pneumonia caused by the single-celled parasite *Pneumocystis carinii*; dangerous mainly to persons with impaired immune systems, particularly patients with AIDS.

Pneumonia: An inflammation of the lungs or bronchial passageways caused by a viral or bacterial infection.

Pneumothorax: The collapse of a lung or portion of a lung caused by the introduction of air or another gas or of fluid into the pleural space surrounding the lungs.

Poisoning: Exposure to any substance in a quantity sufficient to cause health problems.

Poisonous plants: Plants that cause gastrointestinal or dermatological reactions in humans.

Poliomyelitis: A viral illness that may cause meningitis and permanent paralysis; can be prevented through immunization.

Polycystic kidney disease: A genetic disorder characterized by multiple, bilateral, grapelike clusters of fluid-filled cysts that slowly replace much of the mass of the kidney, reducing kidney function and leading to renal failure.

Polycystic ovary syndrome: A complex disorder related to dysfunctional ovulation, endocrine abnormalities, and multiple cysts on the ovary that result in fertility difficulties; related to obesity and diabetes and poses increased risk for cardiovascular disease.

Polydactyly: A congenital dominant trait in which more than five fingers or toes are present on a limb.

Polydipsea: Extreme thirst, often associated with diabetes mellitus.

Polyesthesia: A dysesthesia in which a single object seems to be felt in several different places.

Polyposis: A condition in which numerous polyps are present.

Polyps: Abnormal growths arising from mucous membranes anywhere in the body.

Polyuria: The excretion of excessive urine.

Pompe's disease: A congenital glycogen storage disease that is generally fatal in children but less severe in adults.

Porphyria: One of several rare genetic disorders caused by the accumulation of substances called porphyrins; often characterized by nervous system damage and unusual sensitivity to light.

Postpartum depression: In a woman, the feeling of being emotionally down or miserable following the birth of a child; most cases are mild and transient, but severe depression may occur.

Post-traumatic stress disorder: Intense fear, helplessness, or horror following a traumatic event, with accompanying reexperiencing, avoidance, and arousal.

Prader-Willi syndrome: A disorder caused by a deletion in chromosome 15; characterized by developmental and cognitive delays, overeating resulting in obesity, and behavioral difficulties.

Precocious puberty: The early onset of puberty caused by the premature secretion of sex hormones, resulting in the commencement of sexual maturation prior to age eight in girls and age ten in boys.

Preeclampsia: A serious complication of pregnancy, occurring anytime from the middle stages of pregnancy to just after birth, characterized by hypertension and proteinuria.

Pregnancy luteoma: Hyperplasia of ovarian cells, generally occuring during the third trimester of pregnancy.

Premature birth: Childbirth occurring before the thirty-eighth week of pregnancy.

Premenstrual syndrome (PMS): A common condition involving tension, irritability, headaches, depression, and bloating in the week prior to menstruation.

Prion diseases: Neurological diseases associated with abnormal forms of prions, intracellular proteins of unknown function; examples include Creutzfeldt-Jacob disease and bovine spongiform encephalopathy (mad cow disease).

Progeria: Rare disorders characterized by many aspects of premature aging.

Progressive multifocal leukoencephalopathy (PML): A degenerative central nervous system disease resulting from infection by an SV40-like virus; rare and generally found in persons who are immunoincompetent.

Prostate cancer: Malignancy occurring in the prostate gland, which is the most deadly cancer for men in the United States.

Proteinuria: The elimination of abnormally high amounts of protein in the urine, typically defined as the excretion of more than 150 milligrams of protein in the urine per day.

Pseudohermaphroditism: A condition in which either testicular tissues or ovarian tissues, but not both, are found in an individual with ambiguous urogenital development; caused by developmental defects.

Psoriasis: A chronic skin disease characterized by red, scaly patches overlaid with thick, silvery gray scales.

Psychosis: A severe mental disorder in which the individual loses contact with reality and suffers from such symptoms as delusions and hallucinations.

Psychosomatic disorders: Physical disorders influenced by psychological stressors, or disorders characterized by symptoms that result from unconscious psychological factors instead of underlying medical conditions.

Ptosis: Downward drooping or sagging of tissue, caused by the influence of gravity or the loss of muscular or other support.

Puerperal fever: A potentially fatal uterine infection following childbirth; historically associated with streptococcal contamination as a result of physicians treating patients sequentially without maintaining aseptic conditions.

Pulmonary diseases: Diseases of the lungs, which may be serious or fatal; common pulmonary diseases include those caused by infection (bronchitis, pneumonia, tuberculosis), tobacco smoke (emphysema, lung cancer), and allergies (asthma).

Pulmonary edema: A lung ailment in which the pressure in the blood vessels in the lungs exceeds the pressure in the air sacs, resulting in fluid being pushed from the blood into the lungs.

Punch-drunk: A condition characterized by slow movement and slurred speech that is often associated with injuries to the brain; the origin of the term is its association with boxers injured by repeated punches to the head.

Pus: A creamy tissue exudate composed primarily of white blood cells.

Pyelonephritis: Inflammation of the kidney, usually as the result of a bacterial infection in the bladder.

Pygomelus: A fetal mutation resulting in an extra limb, generally attached to the buttocks.

Pyloric stenosis: A narrowing of the passageway between the stomach and the duodenum.

Pyorrhea: The second stage of gingivitis.

Pyrenemia: The presence of nucleated red blood cells in the circulation; often associated with infections that result in the rapid production and release of cells from the bone marrow.

Pyrosis: Another term for heartburn.

Quadriplegia: Partial or complete paralysis of the arms, legs, and trunk caused by damage to the spinal cord in the neck.

Quincke's disease: Subcutaneous swelling associated with interruption of the blood supply and tissue death.

Rabies: A virus that attacks the nerve cells and is most often transmitted to humans by the bite of an infected animal; once symptoms occur in humans, the disease is nearly always fatal.

Rachitis: Inflammation of the vertebral column.

Radiation sickness: An acute, sometimes fatal illness that occurs with exposure to a sudden, large dose of radiation.

Radiculopathy: Pain distributed along a specific pathway resulting from irritation of a nerve root.

Ramsay Hunt syndrome: Ear pain and vertigo associated with viral infection of nerve ganglia that radiate to the face.

Rash: A skin disorder, usually temporary, characterized by red, inflamed areas or spots; generally a symptom of an underlying condition, such as a skin disease, autoimmune disorder, infectious disease, or bleeding disorder.

Red neck syndrome: An allergic reaction to antibiotics characterized by a rash affecting the upper body.

Reiter's syndrome: An autoimmune disorder with associated symptoms of arthritis, urethritis, conjunctivitis, and ulcerations of the skin and mouth.

Renal failure: The inability of the kidneys to process waste products in the blood and excrete them through the urine.

Respiratory distress syndrome: A life-threatening illness primarily of premature infants; immature lungs lack a vital substance that keeps the tiny air sacs (alveoli) from collapsing upon exhalation.

Restless legs syndrome: A sensorimotor disorder characterized by uncomfortable and even painful sensations in the limbs, especially the legs, when at rest or trying to sleep.

Retroviruses: RNA viruses that replicate by synthesizing a double-stranded DNA molecule that integrates into the host genome; known to infect virtually all animals and sometimes cause serious disease, including cancer.

Rett's syndrome: A congenital disease of the central nervous system characterized by significantly reduced brain size in children as well as motor and respiratory abnormalities.

Reye's syndrome: A somewhat rare, noncontagious disease of the liver and central nervous system that strikes individuals under the age of eighteen; generally associated with previous infection by Epstein-Barr virus or chickenpox.

Rh incompatibility: The destruction of red blood cells in an Rh-positive fetus by antibodies transferred from an Rh-negative mother.

Rhabdomyosarcoma: A malignant tumor that originates from striated (voluntary) muscle tissue.

Rheumatic fever: An inflammatory disease of the heart that may follow a streptococcal throat infection.

Rheumatoid arthritis: A disease affecting the muscles, cartilage, and joints and characterized by stiffness, pain, and swelling.

Rhinitis: A discharge from the nose caused by inflammation of the internal nasal structures.

Rhizomelia: Abnormality in the length of arms or legs.

Rickets: A disorder involving the softening and weakening of a child's bones; primarily caused by lack of vitamin D and/or lack of calcium or phosphate.

Rickettsialpox: An infectious disease caused by *Rickettsia akari* and characterized by a rash, fever, headache, and muscle aches.

Rigor mortis: Muscle rigidity that occurs after death.

Ringworm: A group of fungal diseases caused by several species of dermatophytes and characterized by itching, scaling, and sometimes painful lesions.

Ritter's disease: Staphylococcal infection of the newborn characterized by a spreading rash and the exfoliation of skin.

Rocky Mountain spotted fever: An acute febrile illness caused by *Rickettsia rickettsii.*

Rosacea: The chronic inflammation of facial skin; also known as acne rosacea or adult acne.

Roseola: A common and contagious childhood disease characterized by high fever and a skin rash.

Roundworms: Intestinal parasites in humans that thrive in the gastrointestinal tract.

Rubella: An acute, contagious childhood disease caused by a virus and characterized by a rash; also called German measles.

Russell's syndrome: A congenital disorder characterized by dwarfism accompanied by facial and skeletal abnormalities.

Saber-sheath trachea: An abnormally shaped trachea, generally resulting from chronic pulmonary obstruction.

St. Vitus' dance: Involuntary movement and jerking of the limbs and face, usually as a complication of rheumatic fever; also known as Sydenham's chorea.

Salmonella infection: A broad spectrum of clinical diseases caused by many types of salmonella bacteria.

Salpingitis: Inflammation of the Fallopian tubes, often associated with infections.

Sandhoff's disease: A form of Tay-Sachs disease resulting from the defective metabolism of carbohydrates; generally resulting from defects in the hexosaminidase enzymes.

Sarcoidosis: An inflammatory disease characterized by noncaseating granulomas of unknown cause affecting multiple systems, especially the lungs, lymph nodes, skin, and eyes.

Sarcoma: A malignant tumor originating in connective tissue, including bone and muscle.

Sarcopenia: Reduction in muscle mass with aging that is associated with weakness, decreased physiological functioning, and decreased physical activity; can result in functional impairment, disability, loss of independence, and increased risk of fall-related fractures.

SARS. *See* Severe acute respiratory syndrome (SARS).

Scabies: Skin infestation by mites, causing a rash and severe itching.

Scald: Injury to the skin and other tissues caused by contact with moist heat (steam or hot liquid).

Scaphocephaly: A congenital malformation of the skull characterized by a long, narrow appearance; the result of early closure and blockage of lateral development.

Scarlet fever: An acute, contagious childhood disease caused by a bacterial infection.

Schistosomiasis: A chronic illness caused by parasitic worms that live in the blood vessels around the liver and bladder.

Schizophrenia: A mental disturbance characterized by psychotic features during the active phase and by deteriorated functioning in occupational, social, or self-care abilities.

Sciatica: Painful inflammation of one of the sciatic nerves.

SCID. *See* Severe combined immunodeficiency syndrome (SCID).

Scleroderma: A rare autoimmune connective tissue disorder affecting various organs.

Scoliosis: Abnormal curvature of the spine that is often progressive.

Scurvy: A disease caused by a prolonged inadequate intake of vitamin C.

Seasonal affective disorder: A form of major depressive disorder believed to exhibit two forms: winter depression, beginning in late fall or winter, and spring-onset, which continues through summer and fall.

Seizure: A sudden, violent, and involuntary contraction of a group of muscles that may be paroxysmal and episodic; also called a convulsion.

Septic pyelophlebitis: Inflammation of the veins that carry blood away from the kidneys.

Septic shock: A dangerous condition in which there is tissue damage and a dramatic drop in blood pressure as a result of septicemia.

Septicemia: Serious, systemic infection of the blood with pathogens that have spread from an infection in a part of the body, characteristically causing fever, chills, prostration, pain, headache, nausea, and diarrhea.

Severe acute respiratory syndrome (SARS): A newly recognized type of pneumonia caused by a coronavirus that may progress to respiratory failure and death.

Severe combined immunodeficiency syndrome (SCID): A syndrome in which the immune system is unable to produce T and B cells, resulting in catastrophic failure of the immune system.

Sexual dysfunction: The persistent inability of a man to achieve and maintain an erection adequate for vaginal penetration and the successful completion of intercourse or a disinterest in sex because of inadequate or unpleasurable sensation during intercourse.

Sexually transmitted diseases (STDs): Diseases acquired through sexual contact or passed from a pregnant woman to her fetus; include syphilis, gonorrhea, chlamydia, genital herpes, genital warts, viral hepatitis, and AIDS.

Shigellosis: An intestinal infection caused by *Shigella* bacteria.

Shingles: A disease of the central nervous system characterized by painful red blisters that join together and rapidly rupture and become crusted; caused by reactivation of the varicella zoster virus, the same virus that causes chickenpox.

Shock: A life-threatening condition that may occur in response to any circumstance that causes the heart to be unable to pump enough blood to supply the vital organs.

Sickle cell disease: A genetic red blood cell disorder in which illness is attributable to the dysfunction of hemoglobin.

Side effects: Unwanted, unintended changes to healthy cells, tissue, or organs caused by drugs, medical treatments, or existing medical conditions.

SIDS. *See* Sudden infant death syndrome (SIDS).

Signs: Characteristics of a disease state perceived by someone other than the affected individual.

Sinusitis: Inflammation of the lining of the nasal sinuses.

Sjögren's syndrome: An autoimmune disorder resulting in the loss of tears and saliva.

Skin cancer: Malignancy of the skin caused by the ultraviolet radiation in sunlight; sometimes spreads to the internal organs.

Sleep apnea: A sleep disorder characterized by intermittent cessation of airflow through the upper airway.

Sleep disorder: Any abnormal pattern of sleep that threatens normal function, including conditions that cause too much as well as too little sleep; may be both organic and nonorganic in origin.

Sleepwalking: Repeated episodes of arising from bed during sleep and walking about, without being conscious of the episodes or remembering them.

Slipped disk: A supportive ligament surrounding a vertebra in the neck or back that has broken through the spinal column and into the spinal canal; also called a herniated disk or a ruptured disk.

Smallpox: A contagious, often-fatal viral infection that has been eradicated through vaccination but that remains a bioterrorist threat.

Sneezing: A physiological act in which air is expelled forcibly through the nose via a reflex spasm of chest and pharynx muscles.

Soiling: The passage of fecal material into inappropriate places, usually underclothes.

Sore throat: Discomfort and/or pain experienced in

the throat, which sometimes indicates the presence of a more serious disorder.

Speech disorders: Conditions characterized by dysfunction in the brain-coordinated use of speech organs, such as problems with language, vocal quality, articulation, fluency, and dementia.

Spina bifida: A birth defect that results from a mistake early in the development of the spinal cord.

Spondylosis: A condition characterized by restriction of movement of the vertebral bones; occurs naturally as a child grows.

Sprain: An injury in which ligaments are stretched or torn.

Squamous cell carcinoma: A form of skin cancer starting as a small, painless lump and often resembling a wart; common in fair-skinned individuals, especially in later life.

Staphylococcal infections: A variety of infections caused by *Staphylococcus* bacteria, including boils, abscesses, pneumonia, bone infections, and toxic shock syndrome.

STDs. *See* Sexually transmitted diseases (STDs).

Stenosis: An abnormal narrowing or constriction of a canal or passageway in the body that is caused by the buildup of cholesterol, fats, or other substances; the swelling or overgrowth of cells, tissue, or an organ; or a deformity.

Stevens-Johnson syndrome: A severe immune response-mediated hypersensitivity reaction to either particular drugs or infections that causes rashes, sloughing of the skin, and disruption of mucous membranes.

Stillbirth: A condition in which a fetus has died within the uterus and is born after the twenty-eighth week of pregnancy.

Stones: Hard deposits of material in the body associated with urine and bile.

Strabismus: Improper alignment or crossing of the eyes.

Strain: An injury in which muscles or tendons are stretched or torn.

Strep throat: An acute, contagious, bacterial infection of the throat that often spreads to the ears and sinuses and that can seriously damage the heart and kidneys.

Stress: A psychophysiological response to perceived pressures in the environment, including danger; prolonged stress contributes to hormonal imbalances, immune system collapse, susceptibility to disease, cancer, and death.

Stretch marks: Whitish lines or lesions on the skin caused by excessive stretching or tension on the skin; may occur with rapid weight gain, as with pregnancy.

Stroke: A severe reduction or cessation of blood flow to the brain, resulting in a variety of serious and often permanent impairments, depending on the area of the brain affected.

Stuttering: The repetition of sounds or syllables or the inability to formulate words in a spoken sentence.

Subacute sclerosing panencephalitis: A rare central nervous system condition associated with previous infection by the measles virus.

Subdural hematoma: Collection of blood (clotted and partially clotted) in the subdural space between the brain and skull.

Sudden infant death syndrome (SIDS): The abrupt death of any infant or young child in which postmortem examination fails to demonstrate an adequate cause.

Suicide: The deliberate taking of one's own life; usually the result of a mental disorder, although sometimes deliberated in the face of life-threatening physical illness.

Sunburn: An inflammation of the skin produced by excessive exposure to the sun, sunlamps, or occupational light sources.

Symptoms: Characteristics of a disease state perceived by the affected individual.

Syndactyly: A congenital anomaly characterized by fusion of the fingers or toes.

Syndrome: A group or pattern of recognizable symptoms or conditions that occur together and indicate a specific disease, psychological disorder, or other abnormal condition.

Synesthesia: A phenomenon wherein one sensory stimulus—a word or a musical note, for example—automatically induces a second, unstimulated sensory perception, typically a color.

Syphilis: A sexually transmitted disease caused by the spirochete bacterium *Treponema palladum* that can progress from a genital lesion to a systemic disorder involving multiple organs.

Tachycardia: Rapid beating of the heart.

Tapeworms: Intestinal parasites in humans transmitted through eating improperly cooked or raw pork, beef, or fish or by being bitten by a larva-carrying flea.

Taussig-Bing's syndrome: A congenital heart defect characterized by transposition of the pulmonary artery and aorta.

Tay-Sachs disease: An inherited disorder in which products of fat metabolism (gangliosides) accumulate in and destroy the brain and spinal cord.

Telangiectasia: Dilation of the lymphatic or blood vessels; associated with tumors or other forms of blockage.

Temporomandibular joint (TMJ) syndrome: A disorder that produces pain and stiffness in the joint between the lower jawbone (mandible) and the temporal bone of the skull.

Tendinitis: Inflammation of a tendon or tendon sheath.

Tentorial herniation: Extension of brain tissue into the tentorial notch as a result of tumor growth or swelling.

Teratogenesis: The formation of embryonic defects.

Testicles, undescended: Testicles that neither reside in nor can be manipulated into the scrotum.

Testicular torsion: A twisting or rotation of the testicle (testis) or spermatic cord on its long axis, causing acute pain and swelling.

Tetanus: An often fatal disease of the nervous system characterized by painful, sustained, and violent muscle spasms.

Tetany: Cramping or twitching of muscles, generally as a result of calcium loss.

Thalassemia: Any of a variety of inherited forms of anemia in which red blood cells contain an abnormal form of hemoglobin.

Thromboembolism: The blockage of a blood vessel by a fragment that has broken off from a thrombus in another blood vessel.

Thrombosis: The act of complete clotting of an artery or vein, through which no blood can then flow.

Thrombus: A blood clot that has formed inside an intact blood vessel; may be life-threatening if it occludes a vessel that supplies the heart or brain.

TIA. *See* Transient ischemic attack (TIA).

Tics: Small, brief, recurrent, inappropriate, compulsive jerking movements or twitches, often set off by stressful events.

Tinnitus: An auditory sensation originating in the head, without external stimulation.

TMJ syndrome. *See* Temporomandibular joint (TMJ) syndrome.

Tonsillitis: Inflammation, infection, and enlargement of the palatine tonsils (two small masses of lymphoid tissue located on either side of the back of the throat) and frequently of the pharyngeal tonsils, or adenoids, which are located high in the throat above the soft palate.

Tooth decay: The common term for dental caries.

Toothache: Pain in the teeth or gums ranging from a dull, throbbing sensation to intense, sharp pains.

Torticollis: A form of muscle rigidity in which the neck muscles contract involuntarily, causing spasms and abnormal movements and posture of the neck and head.

Tourette's syndrome: A disorder characterized by recurrent, multiple motor tics and one or more vocal tics that causes stress and impairs social functioning.

Toxemia: A common disorder of pregnancy characterized by hypertension and proteinuria.

Toxic shock syndrome: A potentially fatal bacterial infection causing the failure of multiple organs; most notably associated with tampon use.

Toxoplasmosis: An infection caused by parasitic microorganisms that invade tissues and cause damage to the central nervous system, especially in fetuses.

Trachoma: A bacterial infection of the eyes that causes blindness.

Transient ischemic attack (TIA): A temporary, brief loss of blood to the brain, accompanied by temporary impairment of vision, numbness, or other symptoms; may herald a stroke.

Trauma: Any injury that results from a physical or psychological event.

Travelers' diarrhea: Severe diarrhea resulting from bacterial infection or poisoning; commonly associated with toxin production by *Escherichia coli*.

Treacher Collins syndrome: A hereditary disorder characterized by facial dysostosis.

Trench mouth: A periodontal disorder characterized by ulceration of the gums; usually associated with poor oral hygiene.

Trisomy: A genetic aberration in which there is an extra chromosome, resulting in a human complement of forty-seven; the most common form is trisomy 21, resulting in Down syndrome.

Trisomy C syndrome: A congenital syndrome resulting from a third copy of chromosome 8; characterized by an abnormally shaped head and possible other skeletal abnormalities as well as sometimes mild to severe mental and motor retardation.

Trousseau's sign: Reddening of the skin when a finger is drawn across the area; characteristic of some nervous system disorders.

Trypanosomiasis: Infection by a member of the genus *Trypanosoma*; includes Chagas' disease and sleeping sickness.

Tuberculosis: A chronic, highly infectious lung disease that can destroy tissue.

Tumors: Abnormal growths of bodily tissues caused by genetic changes within normal cells; may be benign (noninvasive) or malignant (invasive).

Turner syndrome: The most common sex chromosome abnormality in females; results from a missing X chromosome, in which case the person is considered XO.

Typhoid fever: An acute infectious disease caused by the bacterium *Salmonella typhi*.

Typhus: An acute infectious disease caused by *Rickettsia prowazekii*.

Ulcerative colitis: An inflammatory disease that causes ulcers in the large intestine.

Ulcers: Lesions that destroy tissue; peptic ulcers are open sores that develop on the mucous membranes that line the gastrointestinal tract and are caused by excessive secretion of gastric juices, particularly from the pancreas into the intestine.

Unconsciousness: A state in which an individual is unaware of either surroundings or self and lacks response to stimuli; includes sleep, fainting, and coma.

Uremia: A condition that occurs when an excess of urea and other waste elements accumulates in the blood as the result of reduced or inadequate kidney function, or both.

Ureteritis: Inflammation of a ureter, possibly as a result of an infection or blockage.

Urethritis: Inflammation or infection of the urethra as a result of bacterial infection.

Urinary tract infections (UTIs): Infections of the bladder, kidneys, urethra, and ureters; may be limited to one area of these organs or spread throughout the urinary tract.

Urolithiasis: The formation of stones in the urinary tract.

UTIs. *See* Urinary tract infections (UTIs).

Uveitis: Inflammation of the uvea of the eye.

Vaccinia: A member of the poxvirus family whose similarity to the smallpox virus resulted in its use in the smallpox vaccine.

Valgus: A musculoskeletal deformity in which a limb is twisted outward from the body.

Van Bogaert-Bertrand syndrome: Progressive degeneration of the nervous system characterized by the spongy appearance of white matter; also known as Canavan's disease.

Varicocele: An enlarged vein surrounding the testicle as a result of incompetent venous valves; most commonly found surrounding the left testicle.

Varicose veins: The distension of superficial veins, usually affecting the legs and causing the appearance of twisted, swollen, blue veins, especially on the backs of the calves.

Vasculitis: A number of conditions characterized by inflammation of blood vessels, both arteries and veins, that leads to decreased circulation in the affected tissue or organ, which can damage the tissue or organ.

Venous insufficiency: An abnormality characterized by decreased blood return from the legs to the trunk; caused by inefficient valves in the veins.

Venous thrombosis: The presence of blood clots in the veins, usually in the legs or arms.

Vertigo: A sensation of motion or spinning when not moving.

Viral hemorrhagic fevers: Acute zoonotic diseases caused by viruses and characterized by internal and external bleeding.

Vitiligo: A disorder that occurs when cells that make pigment in the skin are destroyed, leading to white patches on the body; may also affect the eyes and the mucous membranes of the mouth and nose and cause hair to gray.

Vomiting: Regurgitation of contents of the stomach.

Von Recklinghausen's tumor: A tumor associated with smooth muscle and surrounding tissue.

Von Willebrand's disease: A genetic disorder characterized by the lack of a clotting factor and manifested by excessive bleeding.

Warts: Generally benign tumors of the skin and mucous membranes caused by a papillomavirus.

Whiplash: Injury to the ligaments, joints, and soft tissues of the neck region of the spine as the result of a sudden, violent jerking motion.

Whooping cough: A highly contagious respiratory disease characterized by uncontrollable coughing that ends in a loud whoop as the patient attempts to inhale; also known as pertussis.

Wilson's disease: An inherited disease of abnormal copper metabolism, leading to copper accumulation and toxicity in the liver and brain; causes liver damage and neurologic and psychiatric abnormalities.

Wolf-Herschorn syndrome: A congenital disorder of infants characterized by mental and growth retardation; other symptoms may include cleft lip and cardiac abnormalities.

Wolff-Parkinson-White syndrome: A heart disorder resulting from an extra electrical pathway emanating from the atrioventricular (A-V) node; characterized by tachycardia.

Woolsorter's disease: A form of inhalation anthrax common among handlers of spore-contaminated wool.

Worms: Invertebrates, such as flatworms or roundworms, that can act as human parasites.

Wounds: Disruptions or breaks in the continuity of any body tissue.

Wrinkles: Lines in the skin caused by structural changes over time.

Wryneck: A twisted or stiff neck that may either result from congenital abnormalities or be acquired as a result of muscle spasm.

X-linked diseases: Diseases associated with mutations of genes found on the X chromosome; also referred to as sex-linked diseases.

Xanthomatosis: A condition in which fatty deposits appear anywhere in the body, including various areas of the skin, internal organs, eyes, and tendons.

Xanthosis: Yellowish discoloration of the skin; most commonly associated with eating large quantities of carotene-containing vegetables.

Xeroderma pigmentosum: A congenital disease characterized by extreme sensitivity to sunlight; symptoms include the formation of tumors or keratoses on the skin.

Xerostomia: Dryness of the mouth resulting from lack of production by the salivary glands.

Xerotic keratitis: Inflammation of the cornea.

XYY syndrome: Trisomy caused by an extra Y chromosome; such males are often larger than average in height.

Yeast infection: An infection caused by the fungus *Candida albicans*, also known as candidiasis; commonly occurs in the vaginal area and causes intense itching.

Yellow fever: An acute viral infection of the liver, kidneys, and heart muscle transmitted by *Aedes aegypti* mosquitoes.

Zoonoses: Diseases that can be transferred to humans from their primary animal hosts, including farm animals, laboratory research animals, tropical insects and animals, and common house pets; they include poliomyelitis, malaria, rabies, and toxoplasmosis.

—Richard Adler, Ph.D.; updated by Tracy Irons-Georges

PHARMACEUTICAL LIST

Brand names are capitalized and generics are lowercased. The most common uses are presented here; other uses may apply when appropriate.

Abilify (aripiprazole)
Bipolar disorders
Mania
Psychosis
Schizophrenia

Abreva (docosonal)
Facial herpes
Oral herpes
Skin infections

acarbose (Precose)
Type 2 diabetes

Accupril (quinapril)
Heart failure
Hypertension

Accutane (isotretinoin)
Severe acne

acetaminophen (Tylenol, Children's Tylenol, Tylenol with Codeine)
Fever
Pain

Actonel (risedronate)
Osteoporosis
Paget's disease (bone disease)

Actos (pioglitazone oral)
Type 2 diabetes

Acuvail (ketorolac tromethamine)
Postoperative ocular inflammation

acyclovir (Zovirax)
Chickenpox
Herpes

Adderall (amphetamine)
Attention-deficit hyperactivity disorder (ADHD)

Advil (ibuprofen)
Arthritis
Menstrual cramps
Minor aches and pains

albuterol (Combivent, Proventil, Ventolin)
Bronchial asthma

Aldactone (spironolactone)
Edema
Hypertension

Aleve (naproxin sodium)
Arthritis
Menstrual cramps

Allegra (fexofenadine)
Allergies

Alli (orlistat)
Obesity

alprazolam (Xanax)
Anxiety
Panic disorder

Altace (ramipril)
Arrhythmia
Heart failure
Hypertension

Alupent (metaproterenol sulfate)
Bronchial asthma

amantadine (Symmetrel)
Influenza
Parkinson's disease

Ambien CR (zolpidem tartrate)
Insomnia

amoxicillin (Amoxil, Augmentin)
Pneumonia
Sinusitis

ampicillin (Unasyn)
Abdominal infections
Gynecological infections
Skin infections

Anafranil (clomipramine)
Obsessive-compulsive disorder (OCD)

Antivert (meclizine)
Motion sickness
Vertigo

Aricept (donepezil)
Mild to moderate Alzheimer's dementia

aripiprazole (Abilify)
Bipolar disorders
Mania
Psychosis
Schizophrenia

aspirin salicylate (Bayer, Ecotrin)
Arthritis
Fever
Pain
Rheumatism

Atenolol (tenormin)
Angina
Hypertension

Atripla (efavirenz, emtricitabine, and tenofovir)
Human immunodeficiency virus (HIV) infections

Augmentin (amoxicillin)
Pneumonia
Sinusitis

Axid (nizatidine)
Acid reflux
Ulcers

azithromycin (Zithromax, Zmax)
Pneumonia
Sinusitis

Azmacort (triamcinolone acetonide)
Asthma

Azulfidine (sulfasalazine)
Arthritis
Colitis

bacitracin/polymixin b (Polysporin)
Minor cuts, scrapes, and burns

Bactrim (sulfamethoxazole)
Infections

Bayer (aspirin salicylate)
Fever
Pain

belladonna alkaloids/phenobarbital (Donnatal)
Intestinal inflammation
Irritable bowel syndrome

Benadryl Allergy (diphenhydramine)
Allergies
Colds

Bentyl (dicyclomine)
Irritable bowel syndrome

benzoyl peroxide (Benzac)
Acne

betamethasone (Diprolene, Lotrisone, Luxiq, Taclonex)
Dermatosis
Fungal skin infections
Psoriasis

bismuth subsalicylate (Pepto-Bismol)
Diarrhea

Boniva (ibandronate)
Osteoporosis

Brethine (terbutaline sulfate)
Asthma
Chronic bronchitis
Emphysema

bromocriptine (Parlodel)
Parkinson's disease

buproprion (Wellbutrin)
Depression

Buspar (buspirone)
Depression

calcium polycabophil (Fibercon)
Constipation
Diarrhea

Cambia (diclofenac potassium)
Migraine headaches

carbamazepine (Tegretol)
Neuralgia
Seizures

carbidopa (Sinemet)
Parkinson's disease

Cardizem LA (diltiazem)
Angina
Hypertension

Cardura (doxazosine)
Hypertension
Urinary retention

cefaclor (Ceclor CD)
Bronchitis
Pharyngitis
Skin infections
Tonsillitis

Cefprozil (cefzil)
Infections

Ceftin (cefuroxime)
Infections

Celebrex (celecoxib)
Pain
Painful menstruation
Osteoarthritis
Rheumatoid arthritis

Celexa (citalopram)
Depression

chlorpromazine (Thorazine)
Mania
Nausea
Psychosis

chlorpropamide (Diabinese)
Diabetes

cholestyramine (Questran)
Cholesterol and triglygeride control

cimetidine (Tagamet)
Ulcers

ciprofloxacin (Cipro)
Infections

clarithromycin (Biaxin)
Duodenal ulcers

clotrimazole betamethasone (Lotrisone, Mycelex Troches)
Fungal skin infections

clozapine (Clozaril)
Schizophrenia

codeine (Promethazine with Codeine, Soma Compound with Codeine, Tussi-Organidin, Tylenol with Codeine)
Congestion
Cough
Pain

Combivir (lamivudine and zidovudine)
Human immunodeficiency virus (HIV) infections

Corgard (nadolol)
Angina
Hypertension

Coumadin (warfarin sodium)
Blood thinner

Cozaar (losartan potassium)
Diabetes
Hypertension

Crestor (rosuvastatin)
Cholesterol reduction

cromolyn sodium (Crolom, Intal, Nasalcrom)
Asthma
Conjunctivis
Nasal allergies

Cymbalta (duloxetine)
Chronic pain
Depression
Diabetic pain

Darvocet (acetaminophen and propoxyphene)
Fever
Pain

Demerol (meperidine)
Moderate to severe pain

Depakote (divalproex sodium)
Bipolar disorders
Mania
Migraine headaches
Seizure disorders

Depo-Provera (medroxyprogesterone acetate)
Injectable contraception

dexamethasone (Ciprodex, Decadron, TobraDex)
Ear infections
Eye infections
Steroid-responsive disorders

Diabeta (glyburide)
Diabetes

Diabinese (chloropropamide)
Diabetes

diazepam (Valium)
Anxiety
Convulsive disorders
Muscle spasms

diclofenac potassium (Cambia)
Migraine headaches

Diflucan (flucanazole)
Infections of esophagus, pharnyx

digoxin (Lanoxin)
Heart failure

Dilantin (phenytoin sodium)
Seizures

diltazem (Cardizem LA, Dilacor XR, Tiazac)
Angina
Hypertension

diphenhydramine (Benadryl Allergy, Nytol, Sominex)
Colds or upper respiratory allergies (Benadryl)
Insomnia (Nytol, Sominex)

docosonal (Abreva)
Facial herpes
Oral herpes
Skin infections

Donnatal (belladonna alkaloids/phenobarbital)
Intestinal inflammation
Irritable bowel syndrome

Dovonex (calcipotriene)
Plaque psoriasis

doxycycline (Doryx, Monodox, Vibramycin)
Acne
Infections

Dumyrox (fluvoxamine)
Obsessive-compulsive disorder (OCD)

E.E.S. (erythromycin ethylsuccinate)
Infections

Ecotrin (aspirin salicylate)
Arthritis
Coagulation disorders
Juvenile rheumatoid arthritis
Rheumatoid arthritis

Effexor XR (venlafaxine)
Anxiety
Depression
Panic disorder

Elavil (amitriptyline)
Bulimia
Chronic pain
Depression

Eldepryl (selegiline)
Parkinson's disease

Embeda (morphine and naltrexone)
Chronic pain

Enbrel (etanercept)
Arthritis
Inflammation of the vertebrae
Juvenile rheumatoid arthritis
Psoriasis
Rheumatoid arthritis

Epipen (epinephrine)
Emergency treatment of allergic reactions

Epivir HBV (lamivudine)
Chronic hepatitis B

Epzicom (abacavir sulfate and lamivudine)
Human immunodeficiency virus (HIV) infections

erythromycin (Benzamycin, Ery-Tab, Eryc, PCE)
Acne
Infections

erythromycin ethylsuccinate (E.E.S., Pediazole)
Ear infections in children (Pediazole)
Infections (E.E.S.)

Estrace (estradiol)
Menopausal disorders
Osteoporosis

Estraderm (estradiol)
Menopausal disorders
Osteoporosis

estradiol (Combipatch, Estrace, Estraderm, Femring, Vivelle)
Menopausal disorders
Osteoporosis

estrogens (Premarin, Prempro)
Menopausal disorders
Osteoporosis

ethinyl estradiol (Alesse, Fem HRT, Lo/Ovral, Mircette, Seasonale, Tri-Levlen, Yasmin)
Oral contraception

Evista (raloxifene)
Bone disorders
Osteoporosis

famotidine (Pepcid, Pepcid AC)
Heartburn
Indigestion
Ulcers

Flomax (tamsulosin)
Enlarged prostate

Flumadine (rimantadine)
Influenza A

fluoxetine (Prozac)
Bulimia
Depression
Obsessive-compulsive disorder (OCD)
Panic disorder

fluvoxamine (Dumyrox, Faverin, Fevarin, Luvox)
Obsessive-compulsive disorder (OCD)

Forteo (teriparitide)
Postmenopausal osteoporosis

Fosamax (alendronate)
Bone disorders
Osteoporosis
Paget's disease (bone disease)

furosemide (Lasix)
Edema
Hypertension

gabapentin (Gabarone, Neurontin)
Epilepsy
Fibromyalgia
Neuropathic pain
Restless legs syndrome
Seizures

gemfibrozil (Lopid)
Lipid control

glipizide (Glucotrol XL, Metaglip)
Type 2 diabetes

Glucophage XR (metformin)
Type 2 diabetes

Glucotrol XL. *See* **glipizide**

glyburide (Diabeta, Glucovance, Micronasse)
Type 2 diabetes

H1N1 vaccine
Influenza A

Heparin (heparin sodium)
Anticoagulation therapy

hepatitis B vaccine (Comvax, Engerix B, Pediarix, Recombivax HB, Twinrix)
Hepatitis immunization

Humulin (insulin isophane suspension)
Diabetes

hydrochlorothiazide (Atacand HCT, Diovan HCT, Dyazide, Hyzaar, Lopressor HCT)
Hypertension

hydrocortisone (various)
Dermatosis (Westcort)
Eye infections (Cortisporin Ophthalmic)
Hemorrhoids (Anusol HC Suppositories)

ibuprofen (Advil)
Menstrual cramps
Minor arthritic pain

Imodium (loperamide)
Diarrhea

Inderal (propranolol)
Angina
Congestive heart failure and arrhythmias
Hypertension
Migraine headaches

iron sulfate (Feosol, Fer-in-Sol, Fero-Folic 500, Slow Fe)
Iron deficiency
Iron-deficiency anemia

isosorbide dinitrate (Bidil, Dilatrate-SR, Isordil)
Mild angina
Heart failure

isosorbide mononitrate (Imdur, Ismo, Monoket)
Mild angina

isotretinoin (Accutane)
Severe acne

itraconazole (Sporanox)
Fungal infections

Kadian (morphine sulfate)
Severe pain

K-Dur (potassium chloride)
Hypokalemia

ketoconazole (Nizoral)
Fungal skin infections

Klonopin (clonazepam)
Restless legs syndrome
Seizures

lactase (Lactaid)
Lactose intolerance

Lamasil (terbinafine)
Skin infections

Lasix (furosemide)
Edema
Hypertension

Levaquin (levofloxacin)
Infections

levodopa (Parcopa, Sinemet, Stalevo)
Parkinson's disease

levoflaxin (Levaquin, Quixin)
Bacterial conjunctivitis
Infections

levonorgestrel (Alesse, Levlite, Seasonale, Tri-Levlen)
Oral contraception

Levothroid (levothyroxine sodium)
Hypothyroidism

levothyroxine sodium (Levothroid, Synthroid)
Hypothyroidism

Lexapro (escitalopram)
Anxiety
Depression

Librium (chlordiazepoxide)
Anxiety

lisinopril (Zestril)
Heart failure
Hypertension

lithium carbonate (Lithobid)
Mania

Lithobid. *See* **lithium carbonate**

Livalo (pitavastatin)
High cholesterol

Lopressor (metoprolol tartrate)
Angina
Congestive heart failure and arrhythmias
Hypertension

Lotrisone (betamethasone)
Fungal skin infections
Skin infections

Lunelle (progestin plus estrogen)
Injectable contraception

Lunesta (eszopicione)
Insomnia

Luvox (fluvoxamine)
Obsessive-compulsive disorder (OCD)

Lyrica (pregabalin)
Diabetic pain
Epilepsy
Fibromyalgia
Neuropathic pain
Restless legs syndrome

Lysteda (tranexamic acid)
Heavy menstrual bleeding

Maxair Autohaler (pirbuterol)
Asthma
Bronchial spasm

Metamucil (psyllium husk)
Constipation

miconazole (Monistat 1, Monistat 3, Monistat 7)
Vaginal candidiasis

Minipress (prazosin)
Hypertension

Minocin (minocycline)
Acne
Bacterial infections

minocycline. *See* **Minocin**

Mirapex (pramipexole)
Parkinson's disease
Restless legs syndrome

Monistat. *See* **miconazole**

morphine. *See* **Embeda, Kadian, MS Contin**

Motrin (ibuprofen)
Arthritis
Fever
Juvenile rheumatoid arthritis
Menstrual cramps
Pain
Rheumatoid arthritis

MS Contin (morphine sulfate)
Severe pain

Namenda (memantine)
Moderate to severe Alzheimer's dementia

Naprosyn (naproxen)
Arthritis
Inflammation of the joints
Juvenile rheumatoid arthritis
Menstrual cramps
Pain
Rheumatoid arthritis

Neosporin Plus (neomycin)
Infections

Neurontin (gabapentin)
Epilepsy
Fibromyalgia
Neuropathic pain
Restless legs syndrome
Seizures

Nicorette (nicotine polacrilex)
Aid in smoking cessation

Nicotrol (nicotine transdermal patch)
Aid in smoking cessation

nitroglycerin (Nitro-Bid EXT, Nitrolingual, Nitrostat)
Angina

Nizoral (ketoconazole)
Skin infections

Nonsteroidal anti-inflammatory drugs (NSAIDs)
Arthritis
Inflammation
Joint pain
Rheumatism

Norvasc (amlodipine)
Angina
Hypertension

NSAIDs. *See* **Nonsteroidal anti-inflammatory drugs (NSAIDs)**

nystatin (Mycostatin, Mytrex with Nystatin and Triamcinolone Acetonide)
Candidiasis

ofloxacin (Floxin, Floxin Otic, Ocuflox)
Infections

omeprazole (Prilosec, Prilosec OTC, Zegerid)
Frequent heartburn (Prilosec OTC)
Ulcers (Prilosec, Zegerid)

Onglyza (saxagliptin)
Type 2 diabetes

orlistat (Alli, Xenical)
Obesity

Os-Cal (calcium)
Calcium supplement

oxycodone (Combunox, Oxycontin, OxylR, Percocet, Percodan, Tylox)
Pain

paroxetine (Paxil CR)
Anxiety
Depression
Obsessive-compulsive disorder (OCD)
Panic disorder
Premenstrual anxiety disorder
Social anxiety disorder

Paxil CR. *See* **paroxetine**

penicillin V (Veetids)
Penicillin-sensitive infections

Pepcid (famotidine)
Acid reflux
Ulcers

Percocet (oxycodone and acetaminophen)
Pain

phenytoin (Dilantin)
Seizures

Plan B One-Step (levonorgestrel)
Oral contraception

Pneumovax 23 (pneumococcal vaccine polyvalent)
Pneumococcal immunization

polycarbophil. *See* **calcium polycarbophil**

3306 • PHARMACEUTICAL LIST

polymyxin b (Cortisporin, Cortisporin Ophthalmic, Neosporin Plus, Polysporin)
Dermatosis
Eye inflammation and infection
Infection
Minor pain

Polysporin (bacitracin and polymixin b)
Infections

potassium chloride (K-Tab, Slow-K)
Hyperkalemia

PrandiMet (repaglinide and metformin HCl)
Type 2 diabetes

Pravachol (pravastatin sodium)
Adjunct to diet for heart conditions

prednisolone (Blephamide)
Eye inflammation and infection

Precose (acarbose)
Type 2 diabetes

Prilosec (omeprazole)
Chronic heartburn
Gastroesophageal reflux disease (GERD)
Ulcers

procainamide (Procanibid)
Arrhythmias

Procardia XL (dihydropyridine)
Angina
Hypertension

propranolol (Inderal)
Angina
Arrhythmias
Hypertension
Migraine headaches

Proventil (albuterol)
Bronchial asthma

Provera (medroxyprogesterone acetate)
Amenorrhea
Menopausal disorders

Provigil (modafinil)
Chronic fatigue
Narcolepsy
Sleep apnea

Prozac (fluoxetine)
Bulimia
Depression
Obsessive-compulsive disorder (OCD)
Panic disorder

pseudoephedrine (Allegra-D, Clarinex-D, Dimetapp, Sudafed, Zytrec-D)
Allergies
Cough
Nasal congestion

psyllium (Konsyl, Metamucil, Semmaprompt)
Constipation

Questran (cholestyramine resin)
Cholesterol or triglyceride level reduction

quinapril (Accupril)
Heart failure
Hypertension

Quinidex (quinidine sulfate)
Arrhythmias

raloxifene (Evista)
Bone disorders
Osteoporosis

ranitidine (Zantac)
Gastric reflux
Ulcers

Reglan (metoclopramide)
Gastrointestinal disorders
Nausea

Remicade (infliximab)
Arthritis
Colorectal disorders
Crohn's disease
Inflammation of the joints
Ulcerative colitis

Renova (tretinoin)
Acne
Skin discoloration
Wrinkles

Risperdal (benzisoxazole)
Bipolar disorders
Mania
Psychosis
Schizophrenia

ropinirole hydrochloride (Requip)
Parkinson's disease
Restless legs syndrome

rosiglitazone (Avandia)
Diabetes

Sarafem (fluoxetine)
Premenstrual disorder

Savella (milnacipran)
Fibromyalgia

Seasonale (levonorgestrel)
Oral contraception

senna (Senokot)
Constipation

Septra (sulfamethoxazole)
Infections

Seroquel (dibenzothiazepine)
Bipolar disorders
Mania
Psychosis
Schizophrenia

sertraline (Zoloft)
Depression
Obsessive-compulsive disorder (OCD)
Panic disorder
Post-traumatic stress disorder (PTSD)
Premenstrual disorder
Social anxiety disorder

Sinemet (carbidopa)
Parkinson's disease

Sinequan (doxepin)
Anxiety
Depression

Singulair (montelukast sodium)
Asthma

Slow-K (potassium chloride)
Hypokalemia

Stelazine (trifluoperazine)
Anxiety
Psychosis

Sudafed (pseudoephedrine HCl)
Nasal congestion

sulfamethoxazole (Bactrim, Septra)
Infections

Sumavel DosePro (sumatriptan injection)
Cluster headaches
Migraine headaches

sympathomimetic appetite suppressant (Adipex, Atti-Plex P, Bontril, Didrex, Fastin, Ionamin, Melfiat, Meridia, Phentercot, Tenuate, Tenuate Dospan)
Appetite suppressant

Tagamet (cimetidine)
Ulcers

Tamiflu (oseltamivir)
Influenza in infants

tamoxifen (Nolvadex)
Breast cancer

Tegetrol (carbamazepine)
Neuralgia
Seizure disorders

testosterone (Androgel)
Low testosterone

Tranxene (clorazapate dipotassium)
Anxiety

trifluoperazine (Stelazine)
Anxiety
Psychosis

Tums (calcium carbonate)
Calcium supplement
Hyperacidity

Tylenol (acetaminophen)
Fever
Minor aches and pains

Tylenol with Codeine (acetaminophen plus codeine)
Mild to moderately severe pain

Valium (diazepam)
Anxiety
Seizure disorders
Spasms

valproic acid (Depakene)
Absence seizures

verapamil (Calan)
Angina
Arrhythmias
Hypertension

Viagra (sildenafil citrate)
Erectile dysfunction

Vicodin (acetaminophen and hydrocodone)
Pain

Vytorin (ezetimibe and simvastatin)
Cholesterol control

warfarin sodium (Coumadin)
Blood thinner

Wellbutrin XL (buproprion HCl)
Depression

Xenical (orlistat)
Obesity

Yasmin (drospirenone)
Oral contraception

Zantac (ranitidine)
Ulcers

Zerit (stavudine)
Human immunodeficiency virus (HIV)-1 infection

Zestril (lisinopril)
Arrhythmias
Hypertension

Zithromax (azithromycin)
Infections

Zmax (azithromycin)
Pneumonia
Sinusitis

Zocor (simvastatin)
Cholesterol control

Zoloft (sertraline)
Anxiety
Depression
Obsessive-compulsive disorder (OCD)
Panic disorder
Premenstrual disorder

Zovirax (acyclovir)
Chickenpox
Herpes

Zyloprim (allopurinol)
Gout
Hyperuricemia

Zyprexa (olanzapine)
Bipolar disorders
Mania
Psychosis
Schizophrenia

—Mel Siegel, M.A.,
and Connie Rizzo, M.D., Ph.D. (consultant);
updated by Desiree Dreeuws

TYPES OF HEALTH CARE PROVIDERS

Acupuncturists
Training and Degrees: Program in acupuncture or
Chinese medicine, preferably one approved by
the Accreditation Commission for Acupuncture
and Oriental Medicine (ACAOM)
—Diplomate in Acupuncture (Dipl.Ac.) or
Master of Science (M.S.)
Duties: Pain reduction and health balance in the
body through the use of thin needles inserted at
specific points
Specializations: None

Biotechnologists
Training and Degrees: Undergraduate degree
program; graduate degree recommended
—Bachelor of Science (B.S.), Master of Science
(M.S.)
Duties: The performance of research or application
studies in the field of biology
Specializations: All medical fields

Chiropractors
Training and Degrees: Two years of premedical
studies (minimum), followed by four years of
chiropractic school
—Doctor of Chiropractic (D.C.)
Duties: The mechanical manipulation of the spinal
column for the maintenance of health
Specializations: The use of radiology or
physiotherapy to supplement manipulation

Counselors
Training and Degrees: Varies; may range from
personal experience to specialized training
—Bachelor of Arts (B.A.) or Bachelor of
Science (B.S.), with possible advanced degree
Duties: One-on-one work with a patient to deal
with specific emotional problems
Specializations: All areas of health care

Cytologists
Training and Degrees: Undergraduate degree
program, followed by graduate program and
postgraduate training
—Doctor of Philosophy (Ph.D.) or Doctor of
Medicine (M.D.)
Duties: The microscopic study of cells or tissue
Specializations:
Hematology (the observation and study of blood cells
or tissues associated with blood cell formation)
Histology (the observation and study of tissue)

Dentists
Training and Degrees: Two years of undergraduate
studies (minimum), followed by three to four
years of dental college
—Doctor of Dental Surgery (D.D.S.) or Doctor
of Dental Medicine (D.M.D.)
Duties: The repair, restoration, and cleaning of teeth
Specializations:
Endodontics (the diagnosis and treatment of
diseases of dental pulp and tissue)
Oral pathology or surgery (the diagnosis and
surgical repair of oral disorders)
Orthodontics (the diagnosis and treatment of
tooth irregularities)
Pedodontics (the diagnosis and treatment of the
dental problems of children)
Periodontics (the diagnosis and treatment of
disorders in tissue surrounding teeth)
Prosthodontics (the production of artificial
devices for tooth replacement)

Dietetic Technicians
Training and Degrees: A two-year dietetic program
—Associate degree in a program approved by
the American Dietetic Association
Duties: The assessment, design, and
implementation of nutritional programs
Specializations:
Dietitian (a person trained in nutritional care)
Geriatric dietician (a person trained in the
nutritional care of the elderly)
Pediatric dietician (a person trained in the
nutritional care of children)

Immunologists
Training and Degrees: Undergraduate degree
program; graduate or professional program
—Master of Science (M.S.); Doctor of
Philosophy (Ph.D.)

3310 • Types of Health Care Providers

Duties: The observation and study of the body's immune system
Specializations: None

Interns
Training and Degrees: The completion of a postgraduate program in the field of health care —Master of Science (M.S.) or doctoral degree
Duties: The learning of medical procedures under the supervision of residents or other physicians
Specializations: All areas of health care

Laboratory Technicians
Training and Degrees: A two-year or four-year school —Associate degree, Bachelor of Science (B.S.) or Master of Science (M.S.)
Duties: The collection, preparation, and testing of tissues or fluids for diagnostic purposes; the carrying out of medical procedures under the direction of physicians
Specializations: Many medical fields

Medical Doctors
Training and Degrees: Undergraduate degree program followed by medical school; specializations are generally based on training that begins during the years as a resident —Doctor of Medicine (M.D.)
Duties: The assessment and diagnosis of medical problems; the administration of procedures or drugs for treatment
Specializations:
Anesthesiology (the administration of anesthetics for the relief or prevention of pain)
Cardiology (the diagnosis and treatment of disorders of the heart)
Dermatology (the diagnosis and treatment of skin disorders)
Family practice (the diagnosis and treatment of disorders among all individuals, rather than specialization based on age or sex)
Gastroenterology (the study of disorders of the stomach and intestinal tract)
Geriatrics (the treatment of disorders of the elderly)
Gynecology (the diagnosis and treatment of disorders of the female reproductive system)
Internal medicine (the diagnosis and treatment of disorders affecting internal organs)
Nephrology (the diagnosis and treatment of disorders associated with the kidneys)

Obstetrics (the diagnosis and treatment of disorders dealing with pregnancy and childbirth)
Oncology (the diagnosis and treatment of tumors)
Ophthalmology (the diagnosis and treatment of disorders associated with the eyes)
Pediatrics (the diagnosis and treatment of disorders of children)
Plastic surgery (the surgical repair or restoration of visible areas of the body)
Proctology (the diagnosis and treatment of disorders affecting the anus, colon, or rectum)
Psychiatry (the diagnosis and treatment of mental disorders)
Pulmonology (the diagnosis and treatment of disorders of the lungs or respiratory system)
Rheumatology (the diagnosis and treatment of disorders affecting connective tissue)
Urology (the diagnosis and treatment of disorders affecting the urinary tract)
Vascular medicine (the diagnosis and treatment of disorders associated with the circulatory system)

Microbiologists
Training and Degrees: Undergraduate degree program; graduate degree recommended —Bachelor of Science (B.S.), Master of Science (M.S.)
Duties: The research, maintenance, or identification of microorganisms
Specializations:
Bacteriology (the identification and study of bacteria)
Mycology (the identification and study of molds)
Virology (the identification and study of viruses)

Midwives
Training and Degrees: Program in midwifery; registration and license to practice
Duties: The supervision of pregnancy, labor, delivery, and the postpartum period, in addition to counseling and family planning
Specialization: Certified nurse midwife (a person who is certified as both a nurse and a midwife)

Nurses
Training and Degrees: Undergraduate degree program, followed by study at an approved school of nursing; passage of the National Council Licensure Examination (NCLEX-RN) is required to become a Registered Nurse —Associate Degree in Nursing (A.D.N.),

Bachelor of Science in Nursing (B.S.N.) (four-year program), Master of Science in Nursing (M.S.N.), Registered Nurse (R.N.)

Duties: The administration of medical treatments recommended by physicians; the monitoring and facilitation of medical care

Specializations:

Clinical nurse specialist (R.N. with experience in dealing with overall health care; requires M.S.N.)

Nurse educator (R.N. trained in the teaching of nurses)

Nurse practitioner (R.N. with advanced training and experience in a particular branch of nursing)

Obstetric nurse (R.N. specializing in pregnancy and childbirth)

Pediatric nurse (R.N. trained in the nursing care of children)

Surgical nurse (R.N. trained to assist during surgical procedures)

Optometrists

Training and Degrees: Two years of undergraduate studies (minimum), followed by four years of optometry college; state license
—Doctor of Optometry (D.O.)

Duties: Testing of the eyes for visual acuity; the prescription of corrective lenses

Specialization: Optician (a person who makes or sells corrective lenses)

Osteopaths

Training and Degrees: Undergraduate degree program, followed by medical school and an internship, or graduation from a college of osteopathy
—Doctor of Medicine (M.D.), Doctor of Osteopathy (D.O.)

Duties: The manipulation of body structures as supplemental treatment for disease

Specialization: Doctor of Medicine (M.D.)

Pathologists

Training and Degrees: Undergraduate degree program, followed by medical school
—Doctor of Medicine (M.D.)

Duties: The observation of the effects of disease on the body

Specializations:

Autopsy (the determination of the cause of death)

Clinical pathology (the assessment of disease states as reflected in changes within the body)

Pharmacists

Training and Degrees: A two-year undergraduate program, followed by a two-year to three-year program in an approved school of pharmacy; state license
—Doctor of Pharmacology (Pharm.D.)

Duties: The formulation and dispensation of medications

Specializations: None

Pharmacologists

Training and Degrees: Undergraduate degree program; graduate program
—Master of Science (M.S.); Doctor of Philosophy (Ph.D.)

Duties: The study of the properties and use of drugs or other pharmacologic agents

Specializations: None

Physical Therapists

Training and Degrees: Undergraduate program in physical therapy, or a one-year certified course in conjunction with a degree program in a related field

Duties: The testing and treatment of persons who are physically handicapped, either temporarily or permanently

Specializations: None

Physician Assistants

Training and Degrees: A two-year program for national certification by the American Association of Physician Assistants (AAPA)

Duties: The provision of assistance as requested by supervising physicians

Specializations:

Radiology (providing aid during X-ray and related procedures)

Surgery (assisting surgeons during operations)

Podiatrists

Training and Degrees: Two years of premedical studies (minimum), followed by four years of podiatry school; state license
—Doctor of Podiatric Medicine (D.P.M.)

Duties: The treatment of foot disorders

Specializations: None

Psychological Assistants

Training and Degrees: Undergraduate degree program, graduate degree, and an internship —Master's degree or higher

Duties: The administration of psychological tests or their assessment under the supervision of psychologists

Specializations:
Child psychology (the assessment of children)
Clinical psychology (the assessment of behavioral disorders)
Educational psychology (the preparation and administration of tests)

Psychologists

Training and Degrees: Undergraduate degree program, graduate degree, an internship, and postdoctoral experience
—Doctor of Philosophy (Ph.D.), Doctor of Psychology (Psy.D.), Doctor of Education (Ed.D.)

Duties: The assessment, diagnosis, and administration of psychological tests and treatments for mental disorders and physical conditions that are affected by mental conditions

Specializations:
Child psychology (the diagnosis and treatment of emotional disorders in children)
Clinical psychology (the diagnosis and treatment of personality or behavioral disorders)
Educational psychology (the application of psychology to education or testing procedures)

Radiologists

Training and Degrees: Undergraduate degree program, followed by medical school and generally a residency in radiology
—Doctor of Medicine (M.D.)

Duties: The use of radioactive materials for the diagnosis and treatment of disease

Specializations:
Diagnostic radiology (the use of radioactive materials for imaging)
Nuclear medicine (the performance of diagnostic procedures and imaging involving the internal use of radiochemicals)
Therapeutic radiology (the use of radiochemicals for the treatment of disorders)

Residents

Training and Degrees: Undergraduate degree program, followed by medical school and one year of internship
—Doctor of Medicine (M.D.)

Duties: Clinical duties in hospitals in any of several specialties

Specializations: All medical fields

Respiratory Therapists

Training and Degrees: Undergraduate degree from a school approved by American Medical Association, with training appropriate for passing the registry examination
—Associate degree or Bachelor of Science (B.S.)

Duties: The carrying out of treatments designed to improve or correct functions of the respiratory tract, under the direction of physicians

Specialization: Registered respiratory therapist (the graduate of an advanced program from the National Board of Respiratory Care)

Toxicologists

Training and Degrees: Undergraduate degree program; graduate program
—Master of Science (M.S.), Doctor of Philosophy (Ph.D.)

Duties: The study of poisonous compounds

Specializations: None

MEDICAL JOURNALS

The journals below are arranged alphabetically by official abbreviation; the full journal title follows.

Abbreviation	Full Title
AACN Clin Issues	*AACN Clinical Issues*
Acad Med	*Academic Medicine: Journal of the Association of American Medical Colleges*
Acad Psychiatry	*Academic Psychiatry*
Acta Diabetol	*Acta Diabetologica*
Acta Med Scand	*Acta Medica Scandinavica* (to 1988)
Acta Neurol Scand	*Acta Neurologica Scandinavica*
Acta Neurol Scand Suppl	*Acta Neurologica Scandinavica. Supplement*
Acta Obstet Gynecol Scand	*Acta Obstetrica et Gynecologica Scandinavica*
Acta Ophthalmol	*Acta Ophthalmologica*
Acta Ophthalmol Suppl	*Acta Ophthalmologica. Supplement*
Acta Paediatr	*Acta Paediatrica*
Acta Paediatr Scand	*Acta Paediatrica Scandinavica* (to 1991). Continued by *Acta Paediatrica*
Acta Paediatr Scand Suppl	*Acta Paediatrica Scandinavica. Supplement* (to 1992)
Acta Paediatr Suppl	*Acta Paediatrica. Supplement*
Acta Psychiatr Scand	*Acta Psychiatrica Scandinavica*
Acta Psychiatr Scand Suppl	*Acta Psychiatrica Scandinavica. Supplement*
Addict Behav	*Addictive Behaviors*
Addiction	*Addiction*
Adv Mind Body Med	*Advances in Mind-Body Medicine*
Age Ageing	*Age and Ageing*
Aggress and Violent Behav	*Aggression and Violent Behavior*
AIDS	*AIDS*
AIDS Care	*AIDS Care*
AIDS Res Hum	*AIDS Research and Human Retroviruses*
AJR Am J Roentgenol	*American Journal of Roentgenology*
Alcohol	*Alcohol*

Abbreviation	Full Title
Alcohol Health Res World	*Alcohol Health and Research World*
Alcoholism Treat Q	*Alcoholism Treatment Quarterly*
Alter Ther Health Med	*Alternative Therapies in Health and Medicine*
Am Ann Deaf	*American Annals of the Deaf*
Am Fam Physician	*American Family Physician*
Am Heart J	*American Heart Journal*
Am Ind Hyg Assoc J	*American Industrial Hygiene Association Journal*
Am J Addict	*American Journal on Addictions*
Am J Audiol	*American Journal of Audiology*
Am J Cardiol	*American Journal of Cardiology*
Am J Clin Nutr	*American Journal of Clinical Nutrition*
Am J Clin Pathol	*American Journal of Clinical Pathology*
Am J Dis Child	*American Journal of Diseases of Children* (to 1993). Continued by *Archives of Pediatrics and Adolescent Medicine*
Am J Electroneurodiagnostic Technol	*American Journal of Electroneurodiagnostic Technology*
Am J Epidemiol	*American Journal of Epidemiology*
Am J Fam Ther	*American Journal of Family Therapy*
Am J Gastroenterol	*American Journal of Gastroenterology*
Am J Health Promot	*American Journal of Health Promotion*
Am J Health Stud	*American Journal of Health Studies*
Am J Hematol	*American Journal of Hematology*
Am J Hum Genet	*American Journal of Human Genetics*
Am J Hypertens	*American Journal of Hypertension*
Am J Infect Control	*American Journal of Infection Control*
Am J Med	*American Journal of Medicine*
Am J Nurs	*American Journal of Nursing*
Am J Obstet	*American Journal of Obstetrics and Gynecology*
Am J Occup Ther	*American Journal of Occupational Therapy*
Am J Ophthalmol	*American Journal of Ophthalmology*
Am J Orthopsychiatry	*American Journal of Orthopsychiatry* (to 1990)
Am J Pathol	*American Journal of Pathology*

Abbreviation	Full Title
Am J Phys Med	American Journal of Physical Medicine (to 1987). Continued by American Journal of Physiology—Endocrinology and Metabolism
Am J Phys Med Rehabil	American Journal of Physical Medicine and Rehabilitation
Am J Physiol Cell Physiol	American Journal of Physiology—Cell Physiology
Am J Physiol Endocrinol Metab	American Journal of Physiology—Endocrinology and Metabolism
Am J Physiol Gastrointest Liver Physiol	American Journal of Physiology—Gastrointestinal and Liver Physiology
Am J Physiol Heart Circ Physiol	American Journal of Physiology—Heart and Circulatory Physiology
Am J Physiol Lung Cell Mol Physiol	American Journal of Physiology—Lung Cellular and Molecular Physiology
Am J Physiol Regul Integr Comp Physiol	American Journal of Physiology—Regulatory, Integrative, and Comparative Physiology
Am J Physiol Renal Physiol	American Journal of Physiology—Renal Physiology
Am J Prev Med	American Journal of Preventive Medicine
Am J Psychiatry	American Journal of Psychiatry, The
Am J Psychoanal	American Journal of Psychoanalysis, The
Am J Psychol	American Journal of Psychology
Am J Psychother	American Journal of Psychotherapy
Am J Public Health	American Journal of Public Health
Am J Respir Crit Care Med	American Journal of Respiratory and Critical Care Medicine
Am J Sci	American Journal of Science
Am J Speech Lang Pathol	American Journal of Speech-Language Pathology
Am J Sports Med	American Journal of Sports Medicine
Am J Surg	American Journal of Surgery, The
Am Lab	American Laboratory
Am Med News	American Medical News
Am Rev Respir Dis	American Review of Respiratory Disease (to 1993). Continued by American Journal of Respiratory and Critical Care Medicine
Am Surg	American Surgeon
Ambul Surg	Ambulatory Surgery
Anal Biochem	Analytical Biochemistry
Anat Embryol (Berl)	Anatomy and Embryology (Berlin)
Ann Biomed Eng	Annals of Biomedical Engineering
Ann Clin Psychiatry	Annals of Clinical Psychiatry

Abbreviation	Full Title
Ann Diagn Paediatr Pathol	Annals of Diagnostic Paediatric Pathology
Ann Emerg Med	Annals of Emergency Medicine
Ann Epidemiol	Annals of Epidemiology
Ann Hematol	Annals of Hematology
Ann Hum Genet	Annals of Human Genetics
Ann Intern Med	Annals of Internal Medicine
Ann Nutr Metab	Annals of Nutrition and Metabolism
Ann Occup Hyg	Annals of Occupational Hygiene, The
Ann Otol Rhinol Laryngol	Annals of Otology, Rhinology, and Laryngology
Ann Sci	Annals of Science
Ann Surg	Annals of Surgery
Ann Thorac Surg	Annals of Thoracic Surgery, The
Annu Rev Biochem	Annual Review of Biochemistry
Annu Rev Biomed Eng	Annual Review of Biomedical Engineering
Annu Rev Genet	Annual Review of Genetics
Annu Rev Immunol	Annual Review of Immunology
Annu Rev Med	Annual Review of Medicine
Annu Rev Microbi	Annual Review of Microbiology
Annu Rev Neurosci	Annual Review of Neuroscience
Annu Rev Nutr	Annual Review of Nutrition
Annu Rev Pharmacol Toxicol	Annual Review of Pharmacology and Toxicology
Annu Rev Psychol	Annual Review of Psychology
Annu Rev Public Health	Annual Review of Public Health
ANS Adv Nurs Sci	ANS, Advances in Nursing Science
Antimicrob Agents Chemother	Antimicrobial Agents and Chemotherapy
Aphasiology	Aphasiology
Apoptosis	Apoptosis
Appetite	Appetite
Appl Environ Microbiol	Applied and Environmental Microbiology
Appl Microbiol Biotechnol	Applied Microbiology and Biotechnology
Appl Nurs Res	Applied Nursing Research
Appl Psychophysiol Biofeedback	Applied Psychophysiology and Biofeedback

Abbreviation	Full Title
Appl Radiat Isot	Applied Radiation and Isotopes
Appl Radiol	Applied Radiology
Arch Biochem Biophys	Archives of Biochemistry and Biophysics
Arch Clin Neuropsychol	Archives of Clinical Neuropsychology
Arch Dis Child	Archives of Disease in Childhood
Arch Environ Contam Toxicol	Archives of Environmental Contamination and Toxicology
Arch Environ Health	Archives of Environmental Health
Arch Gen Psychiatry	Archives of General Psychiatry
Arch Gerontol Geriatr	Archives of Gerontology and Geriatrics
Arch Gynecol Obstet	Archives of Gynecology and Obstetrics
Arch Intern Med	Archives of Internal Medicine
Arch Med Res	Archives of Medical Research
Arch Microbiol	Archives of Microbiology
Arch Neurol	Archives of Neurology
Arch Ophthal	Archives of Ophthalmology
Arch Otolaryngol	Archives of Otolaryngology (to 1985). Continued by Archives of Otolaryngology—Head and Neck Surgery
Arch Otolaryngol Head Neck Surg	Archives of Otolaryngology—Head and Neck Surgery
Arch Pathol Lab Med	Archives of Pathology and Laboratory Medicine
Arch Pediatr Adolesc Med	Archives of Pediatrics and Adolescent Medicine
Arch Phys Med Rehabil	Archives of Physical Medicine and Rehabilitation
Arch Surg	Archives of Surgery
Arch Virol	Archives of Virology
Arch Womens Ment Health	Archives of Women's Mental Health
Arterioscler Thromb Vasc Biol	Arteriosclerosis, Thrombosis, and Vascular Biology
Asia Pac J Clin Nutr	Asia Pacific Journal of Clinical Nutrition
Atherosclerosis	Atherosclerosis
Auris Nasus Larynx	Auris Nasus Larynx
Aust J Rural Health	Australian Journal of Rural Health
Aust N Z J Ment Health Nurs	Australian and New Zealand Journal of Mental Health Nursing
Aust N Z J Psychiatry	Australian and New Zealand Journal of Psychiatry
Aust Occup Ther J	Australian Occupational Therapy Journal

Abbreviation	Full Title
Australas Psychiatry	Australasian Psychiatry
Auton Neurosci	Autonomic Neuroscience
Behav Brain Res	Behavioural Brain Research
Behav Brain Sci	Behavioral and Brain Sciences
Biochem Educ	Biochemical Education
Biochem Eng J	Biochemical Engineering Journal
Biochem Genet	Biochemical Genetics
Biochem J	Biochemical Journal
Biochem Med Metab Biol	Biochemical Medicine and Metabolic Biology
Biochem Pharmacol	Biochemical Pharmacology
Biochemistry	Biochemistry
Biol Cell	Biology of the Cell
Biol Psychiatry	Biological Psychiatry
Biol Psychol	Biological Psychology
Biol Reprod	Biology of Reproduction
Biomed Instrum Technol	Biomedical Instrumentation and Technology
Biomed Pharmacother	Biomedicine & Pharmacotherapy
Biotech Histochem	Biotechnic & Histochemistry
Biotechnol Appl Biochem	Biotechnology and Applied Biochemistry
Blood	Blood
Blood Cells Mol Dis	Blood Cells, Molecules, and Diseases
BMJ	BMJ
Bone	Bone
Br J Clin Psychol	British Journal of Clinical Psychology
Br J Educ Psychol	British Journal of Educational Psychology
Br J Med Psychol	British Journal of Medical Psychology
Br J Nutr	British Journal of Nutrition
Br J Occup Ther	British Journal of Occupational Therapy
Br J Psychol	British Journal of Psychology
Br Med J	British Medical Journal (to 1988). Continued by BMJ
Brain	Brain: A Journal of Neurology

Abbreviation	Full Title
Brain Behav Evol	Brain, Behavior, and Evolution
Brain Behav Immun	Brain, Behavior, and Immunity
Brain Inj	Brain Injury
Brain Res	Brain Research
Brain Res Bull	Brain Research Bulletin
Bull Environ Contam Toxicol	Bulletin of Environmental Contamination and Toxicology
Bull Hist Med	Bulletin of the History of Medicine
Bull Inst Pasteur	Bulletin de l'Institut Pasteur
Bull Med Libr Assoc	Bulletin of the Medical Library Association
Bull World Health	Bulletin of the World Health Organization/Bulletin de l'Organisation Mondiale de la Santé
Burns	Burns
CA Cancer J Clin	CA: A Cancer Journal for Clinicians
Camb Q Healthc Ethics	Cambridge Quarterly of Healthcare Ethics
Can J Med Lab Sc	Canadian Journal of Medical Laboratory Science
Can J Med Radiat Technol	Canadian Journal of Medical Radiation Technology
Can J Occup Ther	Canadian Journal of Occupational Therapy
Can J Public Health	Canadian Journal of Public Health/Revue Canadienne de Santé Publique
Can J Respir Ther	CJRT: The Canadian Journal of Respiratory Therapy
Can Med Assoc J	Canadian Medical Association Journal
Can Nurse	Canadian Nurse/L'infirmière Canadienne
Cancer	Cancer
Cancer Causes Control	Cancer Causes & Control
Cancer Cytopathol	Cancer Cytopathology
Cancer Detect Prev	Cancer Detection and Prevention
Cancer Genet Cytogenet	Cancer Genetics and Cytogenetics
Cancer Nurs	Cancer Nursing
Cancer Res	Cancer Research
Carcinogenesis	Carcinogenesis
Cardiovasc Pathol	Cardiovascular Pathology
Cardiovasc Radiat Med	Cardiovascular Radiation Medicine
Cardiovasc Res	Cardiovascular Research

Abbreviation	Full Title
Cardiovasc Surg	Cardiovascular Surgery
Cell	Cell
Cell Biol Int	Cell Biology International
Cell Biol Toxicol	Cell Biology and Toxicology
Cell Immunol	Cellular Immunology
Cell Microbiol	Cellular Microbiology
Cell Physiol Biochem	Cellular Physiology and Biochemistry
Cell Prolif	Cell Proliferation
Cell Tissue Res	Cell and Tissue Research
Cell Transplant	Cell Transplantation
Chem Res Toxicol	Chemical Research in Toxicology
Chest	Chest
Child Psychiatry Hum Dev	Child Psychiatry and Human Development
Circ Res	Circulation Research
Circulation	Circulation
Clin Biochem	Clinical Biochemistry
Clin Chem	Clinical Chemistry
Clin Child Fam Psychol Rev	Clinical Child and Family Psychology Review
Clin Dermatol	Clinics in Dermatology
Clin Diagn Lab Immunol	Clinical and Diagnostic Laboratory Immunology
Clin Diagn Virol	Clinical and Diagnostic Virology
Clin Electroencephalogr	Clinical Electroencephalography
Clin Exp Immunol	Clinical and Experimental Immunology
Clin Eye Vis Care	Clinical Eye and Vision Care
Clin Immunol	Clinical Immunology
Clin Immunol Immunopathol	Clinical Immunology and Immunopathology
Clin Immunol Newslett	Clinical Immunology Newsletter
Clin Kinesiol	Clinical Kinesiology: Journal of the American Kinesiotherapy Association
Clin Lab Sci	Clinical Laboratory Science
Clin Med Res	Clinical Medicine & Research
Clin Microbiol Newslett	Clinical Microbiology Newsletter

Abbreviation	Full Title
Clin Microbiol Rev	Clinical Microbiology Reviews
Clin Neurol Neurosurg	Clinical Neurology and Neurosurgery
Clin Neurophysiol	Clinical Neurophysiology
Clin Nurs Res	Clinical Nursing Research
Clin Nurse Spec	Clinical Nurse Specialist
Clin Psychol Rev	Clinical Psychology Review
Community Ment Health J	Community Mental Health Journal
Comp Biochem Physiol C Pharmacol Toxicol Endocrinol	Comparative Biochemistry and Physiology, Part C: Pharmacology, Toxicology, and Endocrinology
Comp Hematol Int	Comparative Hematology International
Comput Biol Med	Computers in Biology and Medicine
Comput Biomed Res	Computers and Biomedical Research
Comput Human Behav	Computers in Human Behavior
Comput Med Imaging Graph	Computerized Medical Imaging and Graphics
Comput Nurs	Computers in Nursing
Conscious Cogn	Consciousness and Cognition
Contemp Fam Ther	Contemporary Family Therapy
Contraception	Contraception
Crit Rev Oncol Hem	Critical Reviews in Oncology/Hematology
Cult Med Psychiatry	Culture, Medicine, and Psychiatry
Curr Gastroenterol Rep	Current Gastroenterology Reports
Curr Genet	Current Genetics
Curr Microbiol	Current Microbiology
Curr Oncol Rep	Current Oncology Reports
Curr Opin Biotechnol	Current Opinion in Biotechnology
Curr Opin Cell Biol	Current Opinion in Cell Biology
Curr Opin Genet Dev	Current Opinion in Genetics & Development
Curr Opin Immunol	Current Opinion in Immunology
Curr Opin HIV AIDS	Current Opinion in HIV/AIDS
Curr Opin Microbiol	Current Opinion in Microbiology
Curr Opin Neurobiol	Current Opinion in Neurobiology
Curr Opin Oncol	Current Opinion in Oncology

Abbreviation	Full Title
Cytogenet Cell Genet	Cytogenetics and Cell Genetics
Cytokine	Cytokine
Dent Assist	Dental Assistant
Dent Mater	Dental Materials
Dermatol Nurs	Dermatology Nursing
Dev Comp Immunol	Developmental and Comparative Immunology
Dev Neurosci	Developmental Neuroscience
Diabetes Obes Metab	Diabetes, Obesity & Metabolism
Diabetes Res Clin Pract	Diabetes Research and Clinical Practice
Diabetologia	Diabetologia
Diagn Microbiol Infect Dis	Diagnostic Microbiology and Infectious Disease
Dig Dis Sci	Digestive Diseases and Sciences
Dis Colon Rectum	Diseases of the Colon and Rectum
Dis Manag Clin Outcome	Disease Management and Clinical Outcomes
Disabil Rehabil	Disability and Rehabilitation
Drug Alcohol Rev	Drug and Alcohol Review
Drug Metab Dispos	Drug Metabolism and Disposition
Drug Topics	Drug Topics
Drugs	Drugs
Dysphagia	Dysphagia
Ear Hear	Ear and Hearing
Ecotoxicol Environ Saf	Ecotoxicology and Environmental Safety
Educ Gerontol	Educational Gerontology
Electroencephalogr Clin Neurophysiol	Electroencephalography and Clinical Neurophysiology
Emerg Med	Emergency Medicine
Emerg Med Serv	Emergency Medical Services
Environ Microbiol	Environmental Microbiology
Environ Pollut	Environmental Pollution
Environ Toxicol Pharmacol	Environmental Toxicology and Pharmacology
Epidemiol Infect	Epidemiology and Infection

Abbreviation	Full Title
Epilepsy Res	Epilepsy Research
Eur Addict Res	European Addiction Research
Eur Arch Psychiatry Clin Neurosci	European Archives of Psychiatry and Clinical Neuroscience
Eur Child Adolesc Psychiatry	European Child & Adolescent Psychiatry
Eur Heart J	European Heart Journal
Eur J Biochem	European Journal of Biochemistry
Eur J Cancer	European Journal of Cancer
Eur J Cancer Care	European Journal of Cancer Care
Eur J Cardiothorac Surg	European Journal of Cardio-Thoracic Surgery
Eur J Clin Nutr	European Journal of Clinical Nutrition
Eur J Epidemiol	European Journal of Epidemiology
Eur J Heart Fail	European Journal of Heart Failure
Eur J Intern Med	European Journal of Internal Medicine
Eur J Neurosci	European Journal of Neuroscience
Eur J Nutr	European Journal of Nutrition
Eur J Obstet Gynecol Reprod Biol	European Journal of Obstetrics & Gynecology and Reproductive Biology
Eur J Pain	European Journal of Pain
Eur J Pediatr	European Journal of Pediatrics
Eur J Pharm Biopharm	European Journal of Pharmaceutics and Biopharmaceutics
Eur J Pharm Sci	European Journal of Pharmaceutical Sciences
Eur J Pharmacol	European Journal of Pharmacology
Eur J Radiol	European Journal of Radiology
Eur Neuropsychopharmacol	European Neuropsychopharmacology
Eur Psychiatry	European Psychiatry
Evid Based Med	Evidence-Based Medicine
FASEB J	FASEB Journal
Fed Proc	Federation Proceedings (to 1987). Continued by FASEB Journal
FEMS Immunol Med Microbiol	FEMS Immunology and Medical Microbiology
FEMS Microbiol Ecol	FEMS Microbiology Ecology
Fertil Steril	Fertility and Sterility

Abbreviation	Full Title
Food Chem Toxicol	Food and Chemical Toxicology
Food Microbiol	Food Microbiology
Forensic Sci Int	Forensic Science International
Found Sci	Foundations of Science
Free Radic Biol Med	Free Radical Biology and Medicine
Front Neuroendocrinol	Frontiers in Neuroendocrinology
Fundam Appl Toxicol	Fundamental and Applied Toxicology
Fungal Genet Biol	Fungal Genetics and Biology
Gait Posture	Gait and Posture
Gastroenterology	Gastroenterology
Gen Comp Endocrinol	General and Comparative Endocrinology
Gen Hosp Psychiatry	General Hospital Psychiatry
Gen Pharmacol	General Pharmacology
Gene	Gene
Genesis	Genesis: The Journal of Genetics and Development
Genet Res	Genetical Research
Genetica	Genetica
Genetics	Genetics
Geriatr Nurs	Geriatric Nursing
Geriatrics	Geriatrics
Gerontologist	Gerontologist
Gerontology	Gerontology
Gynecol Oncol	Gynecologic Oncology
Health	Health
Health Aff .	Health Affairs
Health Place	Health & Place
Health Care Manage Rev	Health Care Management Review
Health Care Women Int	Health Care for Women International
Health Educ Behav	Health Education and Behavior
Health Prog	Health Progress
Hear Res	Hearing Research

Abbreviation	Full Title
Heart Lung	*Heart and Lung*
Hematol Cell Ther	*Hematology and Cell Therapy*
Hepatol Res	*Hepatology Research*
Heredity	*Heredity*
HIV Med	*HIV Medicine*
Holist Nurs Pract	*Holistic Nursing Practice*
Home Healthc Nurse	*Home Healthcare Nurse*
Horm Behav	*Hormones and Behavior*
Hosp Health Netw	*Hospitals and Health Networks*
Hosp Pract	*Hospital Practice*
Hospitals	*Hospitals*
Hum Gene Ther	*Human Gene Therapy*
Hum Genet	*Human Genetics*
Hum Immunol	*Human Immunology*
Hum Mol Genet	*Human Molecular Genetics*
Hypertension	*Hypertension*
Immunity	*Immunity*
Immunogenetics	*Immunogenetics*
Immunol Cell Biol	*Immunology and Cell Biology*
Immunol Today	*Immunology Today*
Immunology	*Immunology*
Immunomethods	*ImmunoMethods*
Immunopharmacology	*Immunopharmacology*
Immunotechnology	*Immunotechnology*
Infect Immun	*Infection and Immunity*
Injury	*Injury*
Int Arch Occup Environ Health	*International Archives of Occupational and Environmental Health*
Int Immunol	*International Immunology*
Int J Biochem Cell Biol	*International Journal of Biochemistry and Cell Biology, The*
Int J Cardiol	*International Journal of Cardiology*
Int J Dev Neurosci	*International Journal of Developmental Neuroscience*

Abbreviation	Full Title
Int J Eat Disord	*International Journal of Eating Disorders*
Int J Epidemiol	*International Journal of Epidemiology*
Int J Fatigue	*International Journal of Fatigue*
Int J Food Microbiol	*International Journal of Food Microbiology*
Int J Gynaecol Obstet	*International Journal of Gynecology and Obstetrics*
Int J Hematol	*International Journal of Hematology*
Int J Immunopharmacol	*International Journal of Immunopharmacology*
Int J Med Inform	*International Journal of Medical Informatics*
Int J Nurs Pract	*International Journal of Nursing Practice*
Int J Nurs Stud	*International Journal of Nursing Studies*
Int J Palliat Nurs	*International Journal of Palliative Nursing*
Int J Parasitol	*International Journal for Parasitology*
Int J Pediatr Otorhinolaryngol	*International Journal of Pediatric Otorhinolaryngology*
Int J Pharm	*International Journal of Pharmaceutics*
Int J Psychoanal	*International Journal of Psycho-Analysis*
Int J Psychophysiol	*International Journal of Psychophysiology*
Int J Qual Health Care	*International Journal for Quality in Health Care*
Int J Radiat Oncol Biol Phys	*International Journal of Radiation Oncology, Biology, Physics*
Int J Stress Manag	*International Journal of Stress Management*
Int Nurs Rev	*International Nursing Review*
Integr Med	*Integrative Medicine*
Intensive Care Med	*Intensive Care Medicine*
Intensive Crit Care Nurs	*Intensive & Critical Care Nursing*
Intervent Cardiol Newslett	*Interventional Cardiology Newsletter*
Invest Ophthalmol Vis Sci	*Investigative Ophthalmology & Visual Science*
Issues Compr Pediatr Nurs	*Issues in Comprehensive Pediatric Nursing*
Issues Ment Health Nurs	*Issues in Mental Health Nursing*
J Abnorm Child Psychol	*Journal of Abnormal Child Psychology*
J Adolesc Health	*Journal of Adolescent Health*
J Adv Nurs	*Journal of Advanced Nursing*
J Affect Disord	*Journal of Affective Disorders*

Abbreviation	Full Title
J Allergy Clin Immunol	*Journal of Allergy and Clinical Immunology*
J Allied Health	*Journal of Allied Health*
J Am Acad Audiol	*Journal of the American Academy of Audiology*
J Am Acad Child Psychiatry	*Journal of the American Academy of Child Psychiatry*
J Am Assoc Audiol	*Journal of the American Association of Audiology*
J Am Coll Cardiol	*Journal of the American College of Cardiology*
J Am Coll Surg	*Journal of the American College of Surgeons*
J Am Dent Assoc	*Journal of the American Dental Association*
J Am Diet Assoc	*Journal of the American Dietetic Association*
J Am Geriatr Soc	*Journal of the American Geriatrics Society*
J Am Soc Echocardiogr	*Journal of the American Society of Echocardiography*
J Am Soc Nephrol	*Journal of the American Society of Nephrology*
J Anxiety Disord	*Journal of Anxiety Disorders*
J Appl Dev Psychol	*Journal of Applied Developmental Psychology*
J Appl Psychoanal Stud	*Journal of Applied Psychoanalytic Studies*
J Athl Train	*Journal of Athletic Training*
J Autism Dev Disord	*Journal of Autism and Developmental Disorders*
J Autoimmun	*Journal of Autoimmunity*
J Back Musculoskelet Rehabil	*Journal of Back and Musculoskeletal Rehabilitation*
J Bacteriol	*Journal of Bacteriology*
J Behav Med	*Journal of Behavioral Medicine*
J Behav Ther Exp Psychiatry	*Journal of Behavior Therapy and Experimental Psychiatry*
J Biochem	*Journal of Biochemistry*
J Biotechnol	*Journal of Biotechnology*
J Bone Joint Surg	*Journal of Bone and Joint Surgery*
J Burn Care Rehabil	*Journal of Burn Care and Rehabilitation*
J Can Diet Assoc	*Journal of the Canadian Dietetic Association*
J Cancer Res Clin Oncol	*Journal of Cancer Research and Clinical Oncology*
J Cardiopulm Rehabil	*Journal of Cardiopulmonary Rehabilitation*
J Cataract Refract Surg	*Journal of Cataract & Refractive Surgery*
J Cell Biochem	*Journal of Cellular Biochemistry*
J Cell Biol	*Journal of Cell Biology*

Abbreviation	Full Title
J Child Adolesc Group Ther	*Journal of Child and Adolescent Group Therapy*
J Child Lang	*Journal of Child Language*
J Child Psych Psychiatry	*Journal of Child Psychology and Psychiatry*
J Chronic Dis	*Journal of Chronic Diseases* (to 1987). Continued by *Journal of Clinical Epidemiology*
J Clin Anesth	*Journal of Clinical Anesthesia*
J Clin Endocrinol Metab	*Journal of Clinical Endocrinology and Metabolism*
J Clin Epidemiol	*Journal of Clinical Epidemiology*
J Clin Invest	*Journal of Clinical Investigation*
J Clin Microbiol	*Journal of Clinical Microbiology*
J Clin Neurosci	*Journal of Clinical Neuroscience*
J Clin Nurs	*Journal of Clinical Nursing*
J Clin Psychiatry	*Journal of Clinical Psychiatry*
J Clin Virol	*Journal of Clinical Virology*
J Commun Disord	*Journal of Communication Disorders*
J Comp Neurol	*Journal of Comparative Neurology*
J Contemp Psychother	*Journal of Contemporary Psychotherapy*
J Deaf Stud Deaf Educ	*Journal of Deaf Studies and Deaf Education*
J Dent	*Journal of Dentistry*
J Dent Hyg	*Journal of Dental Hygiene*
J Dermatol Sci	*Journal of Dermatological Science*
J Dev Phys Disabil	*Journal of Developmental and Physical Disabilities*
J Diabetes Complications	*Journal of Diabetes and Its Complications*
J Diagn Med Sonography	*Journal of Diagnostic Medical Sonography*
J Emerg Med	*Journal of Emergency Medicine*
J Emerg Nurs	*Journal of Emergency Nursing: JEN*
J Environ Psychol	*Journal of Environmental Psychology*
J Epilepsy	*Journal of Epilepsy*
J Ethnopharmacol	*Journal of Ethnopharmacology*
J Eur Acad Dermatol Venereol	*Journal of the European Academy of Dermatology and Venereology*
J Exp Child Psychol	*Journal of Experimental Child Psychology*
J Exp Med	*Journal of Experimental Medicine*

Abbreviation	Full Title
J Extra Corpor Technol	*Journal of Extra-Corporeal Technology*
J Fam Nurs	*Journal of Family Nursing*
J Fluency Disord	*Journal of Fluency Disorders*
J Gen Physiol	*Journal of General Physiology*
J Gen Virol	*Journal of General Virology*
J Hand Surg Am	*Journal of Hand Surgery (B&E)*
J Head Trauma Rehabil	*Journal of Head Trauma Rehabilitation*
J Health Soc Behav	*Journal of Health and Social Behavior*
J Healthc Manag	*Journal of Healthcare Management*
J Heart Lung Transplant	*Journal of Heart and Lung Transplantation, The*
J Hematother Stem Cell Res	*Journal of Hematotherapy & Stem Cell Research*
J Holist Nurs	*Journal of Holistic Nursing: Official Journal of the American Holistic Nurses' Association*
J Hum Genet	*Journal of Human Genetics*
J Hum Nutr Diet	*Journal of Human Nutrition & Dietetics*
J Immunol	*Journal of Immunology*
J Immunol Methods	*Journal of Immunological Methods*
J Infect Dis	*Journal of Infectious Diseases*
J Intellect Disabil Res	*Journal of Intellectual Disability Research*
J Interferon Cytokine Res	*Journal of Interferon & Cytokine Research*
J Intern Med	*Journal of Internal Medicine*
J Intraven Nurs	*Journal of Intravenous Nursing*
J Invest Dermatol	*Journal of Investigative Dermatology*
J Lab Clin Med	*Journal of Laboratory and Clinical Medicine*
J Laryngol Otol	*Journal of Laryngology and Otology*
J Lipid Res	*Journal of Lipid Research*
J Med Educ	*Journal of Medical Education*
J Med Ethics	*Journal of Medical Ethics*
J Med Humanit	*Journal of Medical Humanities*
J Mem Lang	*Journal of Memory and Language*
J Mol Cell Cardiol	*Journal of Molecular and Cellular Cardiology*
J Nat Prod	*Journal of Natural Products*

Abbreviation	Full Title
J Nerv Ment Dis	Journal of Nervous and Mental Disease
J Neuroimmunol	Journal of Neuroimmunology
J Neurol Neurosurg Psychiatry	Journal of Neurology, Neurosurgery & Psychiatry
J Neurosci	Journal of Neuroscience: The Official Journal of the Society for Neuroscience
J Nucl Med Technol	Journal of Nuclear Medicine Technology
J Nurse Midwifery	Journal of Nurse-Midwifery
J Nurses Staff Dev	Journal for Nurses in Staff Development
J Nutr	Journal of Nutrition
J Nutr Educ	Journal of Nutrition Education
J Nutr Elder	Journal of Nutrition for the Elderly
J Nutr Biochem	Journal of Nutritional Biochemistry
J Obstet Gynecol Neonatal Nurs	Journal of Obstetric, Gynecologic, and Neonatal Nursing: JOGNN
J Orthop Sports Phys Ther	Journal of Orthopaedic and Sports Physical Therapy
J Paediatr Child Health	Journal of Paediatrics and Child Health
J Pain Symptom Manage	Journal of Pain and Symptom Management
J Pediatr	Journal of Pediatrics, The
J Pediatr Psychol	Journal of Pediatric Psychology
J Pharm Sci	Journal of Pharmaceutical Sciences
J Pharmacol Exp Ther	Journal of Pharmacology and Experimental Therapeutics
J Prof Nurs	Journal of Professional Nursing
J Psychiatr Ment Health Nurs	Journal of Psychiatric & Mental Health Nursing
J Psychiatr Res	Journal of Psychiatric Research
J Psychosom Res	Journal of Psychosomatic Research
J Rehabil	Journal of Rehabilitation
J Speech Lang Hear Res	Journal of Speech, Language and Hearing Research
J Stud Alcohol	Journal of Studies on Alcohol
J Subst Abuse Treat	Journal of Substance Abuse Treatment
J Natl Cancer Inst	Journal of the National Cancer Institute
J Neurol Sci	Journal of the Neurological Sciences
J Prosthet Orthot	JPO: Journal of Prosthetics and Orthotics
J R Soc Med	Journal of the Royal Society of Medicine

Abbreviation	Full Title
J Toxicol Clin Toxicol	*Journal of Toxicology—Clinical Toxicology*
J Urol	*Journal of Urology*
J Virol	*Journal of Virology*
J Xray Sci Technol	*Journal of X-Ray Science and Technology*
JAAPA	*JAAPA/Journal of the American Academy of Physician Assistants*
JAMA	*JAMA: Journal of the American Medical Association*
JEMS	*JEMS: Journal of Emergency Medical Services*
JONA	*JONA: The Journal of Nursing Administration*
Lab Med	*Laboratory Medicine*
Lancet	*Lancet*
Lippincotts Prim Care Pract	*Lippincott's Primary Care Practice*
Lung Cancer	*Lung Cancer*
Magn Reson Imaging	*Magnetic Resonance Imaging*
Mark Health Serv	*Marketing Health Services*
Matern Child Health J	*Maternal and Child Health Journal*
MCN Am J Matern Child Nurs	*MCN, American Journal of Maternal Child Nursing*
Med Educ	*Medical Education*
Med J Aust	*Medical Journal of Australia*
Med Sci Sports	*Medicine and Science in Sports*
Medicine	*Medicine*
Methods	*Methods: A Companion to Methods in Enzymology*
Microbiology	*Microbiology*
Midwifery	*Midwifery*
MLO Med Lab Obs	*MLO: Medical Laboratory Observer*
Mod Healthc	*Modern Healthcare*
Mol Aspects Med	*Molecular Aspects of Medicine*
Mol Med Today	*Molecular Medicine Today*
Mol Microbiol	*Molecular Microbiology*
Mol Pharmacol	*Molecular Pharmacology*

Abbreviation	Full Title
N Engl J Med	New England Journal of Medicine
Nat Biotechnol	Nature Biotechnology
Nat Genet	Nature Genetics
Nat Med	Nature Medicine
Nat Neurosci	Nature Neuroscience
Nature	Nature
Neurobiol Aging	Neurobiology of Aging
Neurobiol Dis	Neurobiology of Disease
Neurobiol Learn Mem	Neurobiology of Learning and Memory
Neurogenetics	Neurogenetics
Neurology	Neurology
Neuromuscul Disord	Neuromuscular Disorders
Neuropharmacology	Neuropharmacology
Neuropsychopharmacology	Neuropsychopharmacology
Neurorehabilitation	Neurorehabilitation
Neuroscience	Neuroscience
Neurosurgery	Neurosurgery
Neurotoxicol Teratol	Neurotoxicology and Teratology
Nucl Med Biol	Nuclear Medicine and Biology
Nurs Case Manag	Nursing Case Management
Nurs Forum	Nursing Forum
Nurs Health Care Perspect	Nursing and Health Care Perspectives
Nurs Health Sci	Nursing and Health Sciences
Nurs Outlook	Nursing Outlook
Nurs Res	Nursing Research
Nurs Sci Q	Nursing Science Quarterly
Nurs Times	Nursing Times
Nurse Educ	Nurse Educator
Nurse Pract	Nurse Practitioner, The
Nurse Pract Forum	Nurse Practitioner Forum
Nutr Clin Care	Nutrition in Clinical Care
Nutrition	Nutrition

Abbreviation	Full Title
Obstet Gynecol	Obstetrics and Gynecology
Obstet Gynecol Surv	Obstetrical and Gynecological Survey
Occup Environ Med	Occupational and Environmental Medicine
Occup Ther Health Care	Occupational Therapy in Health Care
Occup Ther J Res	Occupational Therapy Journal of Research
Occup Ther Ment Health	Occupational Therapy in Mental Health
Oncol Nurs Forum	Oncology Nursing Forum
Oncologist	Oncologist, The
Ophthalmic Physiol Opt	Ophthalmic and Physiological Optics
Oral Oncol	Oral Oncology
Oral Surg Oral Med Oral Pathol	Oral Surgery, Oral Medicine, and Oral Pathology (to 1994). Continued by Oral Surgery, Oral Medicine, Oral Pathology, Oral Radiology, and Endodontics
Oral Surg Oral Med Oral Pathol Oral Radiol Endod	Oral Surgery, Oral Medicine, Oral Pathology, Oral Radiology, and Endodontics
Pain	Pain
Pathophysiology	Pathophysiology
Patient Educ Couns	Patient Education and Counseling
Pediatr Intl	Pediatrics International
Pediatr Neurol	Pediatric Neurology
Pediatr Phys Ther	Pediatric Physical Therapy
Pediatrics	Pediatrics
Perfusion	Perfusion
Pharm Sci Technolo Today	Pharmaceutical Science & Technology Today
Pharmacol Ther	Pharmacology and Therapeutics
Phys Occup Ther Geriatr	Physical and Occupational Therapy in Geriatrics
Phys Occup Ther Pediatr	Physical and Occupational Therapy in Pediatrics
Phys Sportsmed	Physician and Sportsmedicine, The
Phys Ther	Physical Therapy
Physician Assist	Physician Assistant
Physiother Can	Physiotherapy Canada
Physiotherapy	Physiotherapy

Abbreviation	Full Title
Plast Reconstr Surg	*Plastic and Reconstructive Surgery*
Postgrad Med	*Postgraduate Medicine*
Postgrad Med J	*Postgraduate Medical Journal*
Practitioner	*Practitioner*
Prev Med	*Preventive Medicine*
Prim Care Update Ob Gyns	*Primary Care Update for OB/GYNS*
Proc Natl Acad Sci U S A	*Proceedings of the National Academy of Sciences*
Prog Retin Eye Res	*Progress in Retinal and Eye Research*
Psychiatr Q	*Psychiatric Quarterly*
Psychiatr Serv	*Psychiatric Services*
Psychiatry	*Psychiatry*
Psychiatry Res	*Psychiatry Research*
Psychoneuroendocrinology	*Psychoneuroendocrinology*
Psychopharmacology	*Psychopharmacology*
Psychosomatics	*Psychosomatics*
Psychother Psychosom	*Psychotherapy and Psychosomatics*
Public Health Nurs	*Public Health Nursing*
Public Health Nutr	*Public Health Nutrition*
Pulm Pharmacol	*Pulmonary Pharmacology*
Pulm Pharmacol Ther	*Pulmonary Pharmacology & Therapeutics*
Radiol Technol	*Radiologic Technology*
Radiology	*Radiology*
Radiother Oncol	*Radiotherapy and Oncology*
Reprod Toxicol	*Reproductive Toxicology*
Res Nurs Health	*Research in Nursing and Health*
Respir Care	*Respiratory Care*
Resuscitation	*Resuscitation*
RN	*RN*
S Afr Med J	*South African Medical Journal*
Scand Audiol	*Scandinavian Audiology*
Scand J Clin Lab Invest	*Scandinavian Journal of Clinical and Laboratory Investigation*

Abbreviation	Full Title
Scand J Clin Lab Invest Suppl	*Scandinavian Journal of Clinical and Laboratory Investigation. Supplement*
Scand J Public Health	*Scandinavian Journal of Public Health*
Science	*Science*
Semin Oncol Nurs	*Seminars in Oncology Nursing*
Soc Psychiatry Psychiatr Epidemiol	*Social Psychiatry and Psychiatric Epidemiology*
Speech Commun	*Speech Communication*
Steroids	*Steroids*
Stroke	*Stroke*
Stud Hist Philos Sci C Stud Hist Philos Biol Biomed Sci	*Studies in History and Philosophy of Science Part C: Studies in History and Philosophy of Biological and Biomedical Sciences*
Surg Gynecol Obstet	*Surgery, Gynecology and Obstetrics* (to 1993). Continued by *Journal of the American College of Surgeons*
Surg Neurol	*Surgical Neurology*
Surg Oncol	*Surgical Oncology*
Surg Technol	*Surgical Technologist*
Surgery	*Surgery*
Surv Ophthalmol	*Survey of Ophthalmology*
Theor Med Bioeth	*Theoretical Medicine & Bioethics*
Top Emerg Med	*Topics in Emergency Medicine*
Top Geriatr Rehabil	*Topics in Geriatric Rehabilitation*
Top Health Inf Manage	*Topics in Health Information Management*
Toxicol Appl Pharmacol	*Toxicology and Applied Pharmacology*
Toxicol Sci	*Toxicological Sciences*
Toxicology	*Toxicology*
Transfusion	*Transfusion*
Transplant Proc	*Transplantation Proceedings*
Trends Biotechnol	*Trends in Biotechnology*
Trends Cardiovasc Med	*Trends in Cardiovascular Medicine*
Trends Cell Biol	*Trends in Cell Biology*
Trends Endocrinol Metab	*Trends in Endocrinology and Metabolism*
Trends Genet	*Trends in Genetics*

Abbreviation	Full Title
Trends Microbiol	*Trends in Microbiology*
Trends Neurosci	*Trends in Neurosciences*
Trends Pharmacol Sci	*Trends in Pharmacological Sciences*
Trop Med Int Health	*Tropical Medicine and International Health*
Ultrason Imaging	*Ultrasonic Imaging*
Ultrasound Med Biol	*Ultrasound in Medicine and Biology*
Urol Oncol	*Urologic Oncology*
Urology	*Urology*
Vaccine	*Vaccine*
Virology	*Virology*
Womens Health Issues	*Women's Health Issues*
World J Microbiol Biotechnol	*World Journal of Microbiology and Biotechnology*

—Compiled by Peter B. Heller, Ph.D.; updated by Connie Pollock

GENERAL BIBLIOGRAPHY

ACQUIRED IMMUNODEFICIENCY SYNDROME (AIDS). *See also* SEXUALLY TRANSMITTED DISEASES (STDs)

Bartlett, John G. *The Johns Hopkins Hospital 2005-6 Guide to Medical Care of Patients with HIV Infection.* 12th ed. Philadelphia: Lippincott Williams & Wilkins, 2005.

Bartlett, John G., and Ann K. Finkbeiner. *The Guide to Living with HIV Infection: Developed at the Johns Hopkins AIDS Clinic.* 6th ed. Baltimore: Johns Hopkins University Press, 2007.

Buckley, R. Michael, and Stephen J. Gluckman, eds. *HIV Infection in Primary Care.* Philadelphia: W. B. Saunders, 2002.

Cichocki, Mark. *Living with HIV: A Patient's Guide.* Jefferson, N.C.: McFarland, 2009.

Clark, Rebecca A., Robert T. Maupin, Jr., and Jill Hayes Hammer. *A Woman's Guide to Living with HIV Infection.* Baltimore: Johns Hopkins University Press, 2004.

Fan, Hung Y., Ross F. Conner, and Luis P. Villarreal. *AIDS: Science and Society.* 5th ed. Sudbury, Mass.: Jones and Bartlett, 2007.

Hubley, John. *The AIDS Handbook: A Guide to the Prevention of AIDS and HIV.* 3d ed. New York: Macmillan, 2002.

Jessen, Heiko, and Hans Jaeger, eds. *Primary HIV Infection: Pathology, Diagnosis, Management.* New York: Georg Thieme, 2005.

Masci, Joseph R. *Outpatient Management of HIV Infection.* 3d ed. Boca Raton, Fla.: CRC Press, 2001.

Matthews, Dawn D., ed. *AIDS Sourcebook.* 3d ed. Detroit: Omnigraphics, 2003.

Princeton, Douglas C. *Manual of HIV/AIDS Therapy.* Rev. ed. Laguna Hills, Calif.: Current Clinical Strategies, 2002.

Shearer, William T., and I. Celine Hansen, eds. *Medical Management of AIDS in Children.* Philadelphia: W. B. Saunders, 2003.

Stine, Gerald J. *AIDS Update 2010.* New York: McGraw-Hill Higher Education, 2010.

World Bank. *Education and HIV/AIDS: A Window of Hope.* Washington, D.C.: Author, 2002.

ALLERGY

Adelman, Daniel C., et al., eds. *Manual of Allergy and Immunology.* 4th ed. Philadelphia: Lippincott Williams & Wilkins, 2002.

Adkinson, N. Franklin, Jr., et al., eds. *Allergy: Principles and Practice.* 6th ed. Philadelphia: Mosby, 2003.

Arshad, S. Hasan. *Allergy.* New York: Churchill Livingstone, 2002.

Brostoff, Jonathan, and Stephen J. Challacombe, eds. *Food Allergy and Intolerance.* 2d ed. New York: W. B. Saunders, 2002.

Decker, Janet M. *Introduction to Immunology.* Hoboken, N.J.: John Wiley & Sons, 2009.

Delves, Peter J., et al. *Roitt's Essential Immunology.* 11th ed. Malden, Mass.: Blackwell, 2006.

Grammer, Leslie C., and Paul A. Greenberger, eds. *Patterson's Allergic Diseases.* 6th ed. Philadelphia: Lippincott Williams & Wilkins, 2002.

Handbook of Allergic Disorders. Philadelphia: Lippincott Williams & Wilkins, 2003.

Kindt, Thomas J., Richard A. Goldsby, and Barbara A. Osborne. *Kuby Immunology.* 6th ed. New York: W. H. Freeman, 2007.

Lieberman, Phil, and John A. Anderson, eds. *Allergic Diseases: Diagnosis and Treatment.* 3d ed. Totowa, N.J.: Humana Press, 2007.

Metcalfe, Dean D., Hugh A. Sampson, and Ronald A. Simon, eds. *Food Allergy: Adverse Reactions to Foods and Food Additives.* 3d ed. Malden, Mass.: Blackwell Science, 2003.

Montanaro, Anthony, ed. *Allergy.* Philadelphia: Saunders/Elsevier, 2006.

Wolf, Raoul L. *Essential Pediatric Allergy, Asthma, and Immunology.* New York: McGraw-Hill, 2004.

ALTERNATIVE/COMPLEMENTARY MEDICINE

Castleman, Michael. *Blended Medicine: How to Integrate the Best Mainstream and Alternative Remedies for Maximum Health and Healing.* Emmaus, Pa.: Rodale Press, 2002.

Ditchek, Stuart, Andrew Weil, and Russell H. Greenfield. *Healthy Child, Whole Child: Integrating the Best of Conventional and Alternative Medicine to Keep Your Kids Healthy.* New York: HarperCollins, 2002.

Freeman, Lyn. *Mosby's Complementary and Alternative Medicine: A Research-Based Approach.* 2d ed. St. Louis, Mo.: Mosby, 2004.

Goldberg, Burton, comp. *Alternative Medicine: The Definitive Guide.* 2d ed. Tiburon, Calif.: Future Medicine, 2002.

Kemper, Kathi J. *The Holistic Pediatrician: A Pediatrician's Comprehensive Guide to Safe and Effective Therapies for the Twenty-five Most Common Ailments of Infants, Children, and Adolescents.* Rev. ed. New York: Quill, 2002.

Mackenzie, Elizabeth R., and Birgit Rakel, eds. *Complementary and Alternative Medicine for Older Adults: A Guide to Holistic Approaches to Healthy Aging.* New York: Springer, 2006.

Micozzi, Marc S., ed. *Fundamentals of Complementary and Integrative Medicine.* 3d ed. St. Louis, Mo.: Saunders/Elsevier, 2006.

Murray, Michael T. *Pill Book Guide to Alternative Medicines.* New York: Bantam, 2002.

Pelletier, Kenneth. *The Best Alternative Medicine.* New York: Fireside, 2002.

Trivieri, Larry, Jr., and John W. Anderson, eds. *Alternative Medicine: The Definitive Guide.* 2d ed. Berkeley, Calif.: Ten Speed Press, 2002.

Weil, Andrew. *Healthy Aging: A Lifelong Guide to Your Physical and Spiritual Well-Being.* New York: Anchor Books, 2007.

White, B. Linda, and Steven Foster. *The Herbal Drugstore.* Emmaus, Pa.: Rodale Press, 2003.

AMBULATORY CARE

Barkin, Roger M., and Peter Rosen, eds. *Emergency Pediatrics: A Guide to Ambulatory Care.* 6th ed. New York: Elsevier, 2003.

Colyar, Margaret R., and Cynthia R. Ehrhardt. *Ambulatory Care Procedures for the Nurse Practitioner.* 2d ed. Philadelphia: F. A. Davis, 2004.

Fiebach, Nicholas H., et al., eds. *Principles of Ambulatory Medicine.* 7th ed. Philadelphia: Lippincott Williams & Wilkins, 2007.

Lewis, Marcia A., and Carol D. Tamparo. *Medical Law, Ethics, and Bioethics for Ambulatory Care.* 5th ed. Philadelphia: F. A. Davis, 2002.

Mengel, Mark B., and L. Peter Schwiebert, eds. *Family Medicine: Ambulatory Care and Medicine.* 4th ed. New York: Lange Medical Books/McGraw-Hill, 2005.

Wachtel, Tom J., and Michael D. Stein, eds. *Practical Guide to the Care of the Ambulatory Patient.* 2d ed. St. Louis, Mo.: Mosby, 2000.

ANATOMY

Abrahams, Peter H., Sandy C. Marks, Jr., and Ralph Hutchings. *McMinn's Color Atlas of Human Anatomy.* 6th ed. St. Louis, Mo.: Mosby/Elsevier, 2008.

Agur, Anne M. R., and Arthur F. Dalley. *Grant's Atlas of Anatomy.* 12th ed. Philadelphia: Wolters Kluwer Health/Lippincott Williams & Wilkins, 2009.

Bo, Walter J., et al. *Basic Atlas of Sectional Anatomy with Correlated Imaging.* 4th ed. Philadelphia: Saunders/Elsevier, 2007.

Eroschenko, Victor P. *Di Fiore's Atlas of Histology with Functional Correlations.* 10th ed. Philadelphia: Lippincott Williams & Wilkins, 2005.

Junqueira, Luis C., et al. *Basic Histology.* 10th ed. New York: McGraw-Hill, 2002.

Marieb, Elaine N. *Essentials of Human Anatomy and Physiology.* 9th ed. San Francisco: Pearson/Benjamin Cummings, 2009.

Moore, Keith L., and Anne M. R. Agur. *Essential Clinical Anatomy.* 4th ed. Philadelphia: Lippincott Williams & Wilkins, 2010.

Moore, Keith L., and T. V. N. Persaud. *The Developing Human.* 8th ed. Philadelphia: Saunders/Elsevier, 2008.

Rohen, Johannes W., Chihiro Yokochi, and Elke Lütjen-Drecoll. *Color Atlas of Anatomy: A Photographic Study of the Human Body.* 6th ed. Philadelphia: Lippincott Williams & Wilkins, 2006.

Scanlon, Valerie, and Tina Sanders. *Essentials of Anatomy and Physiology.* 5th ed. Philadelphia: F. A. Davis, 2007.

Snell, Richard S. *Clinical Neuroanatomy.* 6th ed. Philadelphia: Lippincott Williams & Wilkins, 2006.

Standring, Susan, et al., eds. *Gray's Anatomy.* 40th ed. New York: Churchill Livingstone/Elsevier, 2008.

Tortora, Gerard J., and Bryan Derrickson. *Principles of Anatomy and Physiology.* 12th ed. Hoboken, N.J.: John Wiley & Sons, 2009.

Van De Graaff, Kent M. *Human Anatomy.* 6th ed. Boston: McGraw-Hill, 2002.

ANESTHESIOLOGY

Dunn, Peter F., et al., eds. *Clinical Anesthesia Procedures of the Massachusetts General Hospital.* 7th ed. Philadelphia: Lippincott Williams & Wilkins, 2007.

Fleisher, Lee A., ed. *Anesthesia and Uncommon Diseases.* 5th ed. Philadelphia: Saunders/Elsevier, 2006.

Gregory, George A., ed. *Pediatric Anesthesia.* 4th ed. New York: Churchill Livingstone, 2002.

Kaplan, Joel A., et al., eds. *Kaplan's Cardiac Anesthesia.* 5th ed. Philadelphia: Saunders/Elsevier, 2006.

Lake, Carol L., and Peter D. Booker, eds. *Pediatric Cardiac Anesthesia.* 4th ed. Philadelphia: Lippincott Williams & Wilkins, 2005.

Loeser, John D., ed. *Bonica's Management of Pain.* 4th ed. Philadelphia: Lippincott Williams & Wilkins, 2010.

Miller, Ronald D., ed. *Miller's Anesthesia.* 7th ed. Philadelphia: Churchill Livingstone/Elsevier, 2010.

Motoyama, Etsuro K., and Peter J. Davis, eds. *Smith's Anesthesia for Infants and Children.* 7th ed. Philadelphia: Mosby/Elsevier, 2006.

Palmer, Craig M., Robert D'Angelo, and Michael R. D'Angelo, eds. *Handbook of Obstetric Anesthesia.* 6th ed. New York: Informa Healthcare, 2002.

Sweeny, Frank. *The Anesthesia Fact Book: Everything You Need to Know Before Surgery.* Cambridge, Mass.: Perseus, 2003.

Yao, Fun-Sun F., ed. *Yao and Artusio's Anesthesiology: Problem-Oriented Patient Management.* 5th ed. Philadelphia: Lippincott Williams & Wilkins, 2003.

BIOCHEMISTRY

Alberts, Bruce, et al. *Molecular Biology of the Cell.* 5th ed. New York: Garland, 2008.

Berg, Jeremy M., John L. Tymoczko, and Lubert Stryer. *Biochemistry.* 6th ed. New York: W. H. Freeman, 2007.

Bettleheim, F. A., et al. *Introduction to General, Organic, and Biochemistry.* 8th ed. New York: Brooks/Cole, 2006.

Devlin, Thomas M., ed. *Textbook of Biochemistry: With Clinical Correlations.* 6th ed. Hoboken, N.J.: Wiley-Liss, 2006.

Elliott, William H., and Daphne C. Elliott. *Biochemistry and Molecular Biology.* 3d ed. New York: Oxford University Press, 2005.

Garrett, Reginald H., and Charles M. Grisham. *Biochemistry.* 3d ed. Belmont, Calif.: Thomson Brooks/Cole, 2005.

Murray, Robert K., et al. *Harper's Illustrated Biochemistry.* 27th ed. Stamford, Conn.: Appleton & Lange, 2006.

Nelson, David L., and Michael M. Cox. *Lehninger Principles of Biochemistry.* 4th ed. New York: W. H. Freeman, 2005.

Voet, Donald, and Judith G. Voet. *Biochemistry.* 3d ed. Hoboken, N.J.: John Wiley & Sons, 2004.

CARDIOVASCULAR SYSTEM

Anderson, Robert H., et al., eds. *Paediatric Cardiology.* 3d ed. 2 vols. Philadelphia: Churchill Livingstone/Elsevier, 2010.

Baim, Donald S., ed. *Grossman's Cardiac Catheterization, Angiography, and Intervention.* 7th ed. Philadelphia: Lippincott Williams & Wilkins, 2006.

Crawford, Michael, ed. *Current Diagnosis and Treatment—Cardiology.* 3d ed. New York: McGraw-Hill Medical, 2009.

Eagle, Kim A., and Ragavendra R. Baliga, eds. *Practical Cardiology: Evaluation and Treatment of Common Cardiovascular Disorders.* 2d ed. Philadelphia: Lippincott Williams & Wilkins, 2008.

Ellestad, Myrvin H., and Anila H. Verghese, eds. *Stress Testing: Principles and Practice.* 5th ed. Philadelphia: Davis, 2003.

Fuster, Valentin, et al., eds. *Hurst's The Heart.* 11th ed. 2 vols. New York: McGraw-Hill, 2004.

Fuster, Valentin, Eric J. Topol, and Elizabeth G. Nabel, eds. *Atherosclerosis and Coronary Artery Disease.* 2d ed. Philadelphia: Lippincott Williams & Wilkins, 2005.

Gatzoulis, Michael A., Gary D. Webb, and Piers E. F. Daubeney, eds. *Diagnosis and Management of Adult Congenital Heart Disease.* New York: Churchill Livingstone, 2003.

Gersh, Bernard J., ed. *The Mayo Clinic Heart Book.* 2d ed. New York: William Morrow, 2000.

Goldberger, Ary L. *Clinical Electrocardiography: A Simplified Approach.* 7th ed. Philadelphia: Mosby/Elsevier, 2006.

Goldman, Lee, and Eugene Braunwald, eds. *Primary Cardiology.* 2d ed. New York: Elsevier, 2003.

Koenig, Peter, Ziyad M. Hijazi, and Frank Zimmerman, eds. *Essential Pediatric Cardiology.* New York: McGraw-Hill, 2004.

Park, Myung K. *The Pediatric Cardiology Handbook.* 4th ed. New York: Mosby/Elsevier, 2010.

Von der Lohe, Elizabeth. *Coronary Heart Disease in Women: Prevention, Diagnosis, and Therapy.* New York: Springer, 2003.

Wenger, Nanette Kass, and Peter Collins, eds. *Women and Heart Disease.* 2d ed. New York: Taylor & Francis, 2005.

Zipes, Douglas P., et al., eds. *Braunwald's Heart Disease: A Textbook of Cardiovascular Medicine.* 7th ed. Philadelphia: Saunders/Elsevier, 2005.

CRITICAL CARE

Albert, Richard K., et al., eds. *Clinical Critical Care Medicine.* Philadelphia: Mosby/Elsevier, 2006.

Bongard, Frederick, and Darryl Y. Sue, eds. *Current Critical Care Diagnosis and Treatment.* 3d ed. New York: McGraw-Hill Medical, 2008.

Fink, Mitchell P., et al. *Textbook of Critical Care.* 5th ed. Philadelphia: Saunders/Elsevier, 2005.

Fuhrman, Bradley P., and Jerry J. Zimmerman, eds. *Pediatric Critical Care.* 3d ed. Philadelphia: Mosby/Elsevier, 2006.

Hogan, David E., and Jonathan L. Burstein. *Disaster Medicine.* 2d ed. Philadelphia: Lippincott Williams & Wilkins, 2007.

Irwin, Richard S., et al., eds. *Procedures and Techniques in Intensive Care Medicine.* 3d ed. Philadelphia: Lippincott Williams & Wilkins, 2003.

Irwin, Richard S., and James M. Rippe, eds. *Irwin and Rippe's Intensive Care Medicine.* 5th ed. Philadelphia: Lippincott Williams & Wilkins, 2003.

Lanken, Paul N., et al., eds. *The Intensive Care Unit Manual.* Philadelphia: W. B. Saunders, 2001.

Marini, John J., and Arthur P. Wheeler. *Critical Care Medicine: The Essentials.* 3d ed. Philadelphia: Lippincott Williams & Wilkins, 2006.

Marino, Paul L. *The ICU Book.* 3d ed. Philadelphia: Lippincott Williams & Wilkins, 2007.

Merenstein, Gerald B., and Sandra L. Gardner, eds. *Merenstein and Gardner's Handbook of Neonatal Intensive Care.* 7th ed. Maryland Heights, Mo.: Mosby/Elsevier, 2010.

Murray, Michael J., et al., eds. *Critical Care Medicine: Perioperative Management.* 2d ed. Philadelphia: Lippincott Williams & Wilkins, 2002.

Osborne, Molly L., ed. *Geriatric Critical Care.* Philadelphia: W. B. Saunders, 2003.

Slonim, Anthony D., and Murray M. Pollack, eds. *Pediatric Critical Care Medicine.* Philadelphia: Lippincott Williams & Wilkins, 2006.

Sue, Darryl Y., and Janine R. E. Vintch, eds. *Current Essentials of Critical Care.* New York: Lange Medical Books/McGraw-Hill, 2005.

Udwadia, Farokh Erach. *Principles of Critical Care.* 2d ed. New York: Oxford University Press, 2005.

DENTISTRY

Ash, Major M., Jr., and Stanley J. Nelson. *Wheeler's Dental Anatomy, Physiology, and Occlusion.* 9th ed. St. Louis, Mo.: Saunders/Elsevier, 2010.

Burt, Brian A., and Steven A. Eklund. *Dentistry, Dental Practice, and the Community.* 6th ed. St. Louis, Mo.: Saunders/Elsevier, 2005.

Cohen, Stephen, and Kenneth M. Hargreaves, eds. *Pathways of the Pulp.* 9th ed. St. Louis, Mo.: Mosby/Elsevier, 2006.

Diamond, Richard. *Dental First Aid for Families.* Ravensdale, Wash.: Idyll Arbor, 2000.

Gluck, George M., and William M. Morganstein. *Jong's Community Dental Health.* 5th ed. St. Louis, Mo.: Mosby, 2003.

Langlais, Robert P., and Craig S. Miller. *Color Atlas of Common Oral Diseases.* 4th ed. Philadelphia: Lippincott Williams & Wilkins, 2009.

Mitchell, David A. *An Introduction to Oral and Maxillofacial Surgery.* New York: Oxford University Press, 2006.

Parker, James N., and Philip M. Parker, eds. *The Official Patient Sourcebook on Tooth Decay.* San Diego, Calif.: Icon Health, 2002.

Peterson, Larry J., et al. *Contemporary Oral and Maxillofacial Surgery.* 4th ed. St. Louis, Mo.: Mosby, 2003.

Scully, Crispian, and Athanasios Kalantzis. *Oxford Handbook of Dental Patient Care.* 2d ed. New York: Oxford University Press, 2005.

Weiss, Charles M., and Adam Weiss. *Principles and Practice of Implant Dentistry.* St. Louis, Mo.: Mosby, 2001.

DERMATOLOGY

Arndt, Kenneth A., and Jeffrey T. S. Hsu. *Manual of Dermatologic Therapeutics.* 7th ed. Philadelphia: Lippincott Williams & Wilkins, 2007.

Burns, Tony, et al., eds. *Rook's Textbook of Dermatology.* 7th ed. Malden, Mass.: Blackwell Science, 2004.

Elder, David E., et al., eds. *Lever's Histopathology of the Skin.* 9th ed. Philadelphia: Lippincott Williams & Wilkins, 2005.

Frankel, David H., ed. *Field Guide to Clinical Dermatology.* 2d ed. Philadelphia: Lippincott Williams & Wilkins, 2006.

Freedburg, Irwin M., et al., eds. *Fitzpatrick's Dermatology in General Medicine.* 6th ed. 2 vols. New York: McGraw-Hill, 2003.

Freinkel, Ruth K., and David T. Woodley, eds. *Biology of the Skin.* New York: Parthenon, 2001.

Habif, Thomas P. *Clinical Dermatology: A Color Guide to Diagnosis and Therapy.* 4th ed. New York: Mosby, 2004.

Hall, John C., and Gordon C. Sauer. *Sauer's Manual of*

Skin Diseases. 10th ed. Philadelphia: Lippincott Williams & Wilkins, 2010.

James, William D., Timothy G. Berger, and Dirk M. Elston. *Andrews' Diseases of the Skin: Clinical Dermatology.* 10th ed. Philadelphia: Saunders/Elsevier, 2006.

Mackie, Rona M. *Clinical Dermatology.* 5th ed. New York: Oxford University Press, 2003.

Marks, James G., Jr., and Jeffrey J. Miller. *Lookingbill and Marks' Principles of Dermatology.* 4th ed. Philadelphia: Saunders/Elsevier, 2006.

Parker, James N., and Philip M. Parker, eds. *The Official Patient's Sourcebook on Acne Rosacea.* San Diego, Calif.: Icon Health, 2002.

Spitz, Joel L., ed. *Genodermatoses: A Clinical Guide to Genetic Skin Disorders.* 2d ed. Philadelphia: Lippincott Williams & Wilkins, 2005.

Titman, Penny. *Understanding Childhood Eczema.* New York: Wiley, 2003.

Turkington, Carol, and Jeffrey S. Dover. *The Encyclopedia of Skin and Skin Disorders.* 3d ed. New York: Facts On File, 2007.

Webster, Guy F., and Anthony V. Rawlings, eds. *Acne and Its Therapy.* New York: Informa Healthcare, 2007.

Weedon, David. *Skin Pathology.* 3d ed. Philadelphia: Churchill Livingstone/Elsevier, 2010.

Weston, William L., et al. *Color Textbook of Pediatric Dermatology.* 4th ed. St. Louis, Mo.: Mosby/Elsevier, 2007.

Wolff, Klaus, Richard Allen Johnson, and Dick Suurmond. *Fitzpatrick's Color Atlas and Synopsis of Clinical Dermatology.* 6th ed. New York: McGraw-Hill Medical, 2009.

DIAGNOSIS

Beers, Mark H., et al. *The Merck Manual of Diagnosis and Therapy.* 18th ed. Whitehouse Station, N.J.: Merck Research Laboratories, 2006.

Bickley, Lynn S., and Peter G. Szilagyi. *Bates' Guide to Physical Examination and History Taking.* 9th ed. Philadelphia: Lippincott Williams & Wilkins, 2007.

Bongard, Frederick, and Darryl Y. Sue, eds. *Current Critical Care Diagnosis and Treatment.* 3d ed. New York: McGraw-Hill Medical, 2008.

Collins, R. Douglas. *Differential Diagnosis in Primary Care.* 3d ed. Philadelphia: Lippincott Williams & Wilkins, 2003.

Ferri, Fred F. *Ferri's Differential Diagnosis: A Practical Guide to the Differential Diagnosis of Symptoms, Signs, and Clinical Disorders.* Philadelphia: Mosby/Elsevier, 2006.

Friedman, H. Harold, ed. *Problem-Oriented Medical Diagnosis.* 7th ed. Philadelphia: Lippincott Williams & Wilkins, 2001.

Hay, William W., Jr., et al., eds. *Current Diagnosis and Treatment in Pediatrics.* 18th ed. New York: Lange Medical Books/McGraw-Hill, 2009.

LeBlond, Richard F., Richard L. DeGowin, and Donald D. Brown, eds. *DeGowin's Diagnostic Examination.* 8th ed. New York: McGraw-Hill, 2004.

McPherson, Richard A., and Matthew R. Pincus, eds. *Henry's Clinical Diagnosis and Management by Laboratory Methods.* 21st ed. Philadelphia: Saunders/Elsevier, 2007.

Pagana, Kathleen Deska, and Timothy J. Pagana. *Mosby's Diagnostic and Laboratory Test Reference.* 9th ed. St. Louis, Mo.: Mosby/Elsevier, 2009.

Seidel, Henry M., et al. *Mosby's Guide to Physical Examination.* 6th ed. St. Louis, Mo.: Mosby/Elsevier, 2006.

Seller, Robert H. *Differential Diagnosis of Common Complaints.* 5th ed. Philadelphia: Saunders/Elsevier, 2007.

Silen, William. *Cope's Early Diagnosis of the Acute Abdomen.* 21st ed. New York: Oxford University Press, 2005.

Swartz, Mark H. *Textbook of Physical Diagnosis: History and Examination.* 5th ed. Philadelphia: Saunders/Elsevier, 2006.

Tierney, Lawrence M., Stephen J. McPhee, and Maxine A. Papadakis, eds. *Current Medical Diagnosis and Treatment 2007.* New York: McGraw-Hill Medical, 2006.

DICTIONARIES AND DIRECTORIES

Armitage, Peter, and Theodore Colton, eds. *Encyclopedia of Biostatistics.* 2d ed. Hoboken, N.J.: Wiley Interscience, 2005.

Dorland, W. A. Newman, ed. *Dorland's Illustrated Medical Dictionary.* 31st ed. Philadelphia: Saunders/Elsevier, 2007.

Gilbert, Patricia. *Dictionary of Syndromes and Inherited Disorders.* 3d ed. Chicago: Fitzroy Dearborn, 2000.

Gotto, Antonio M., Jr., ed. *Cornell Illustrated Encyclopedia of Health.* Washington, D.C.: LifeLine Press, 2002.

Leikin, Jerrold B., and Martin S. Lipsky, eds. *American Medical Association Complete Medical Encyclopedia.* New York: Random House Reference, 2003.

McGraw-Hill Encyclopedia of Science and Technology. 10th ed. 20 vols. New York: McGraw-Hill, 2007.

Marcovitch, Harvey, ed. *Black's Medical Dictionary.* 42d ed. Lanham, Md.: Scarecrow Press, 2010.

Miller, Benjamin F., Claire Brackman Keane, and Marie T. O'Toole. *Miller-Keane Encyclopedia and Dictionary of Medicine, Nursing, and Allied Health.* Rev. 7th ed. Philadelphia: Saunders/Elsevier, 2005.

Mosby's Medical Dictionary. 8th ed. St. Louis, Mo.: Mosby/Elsevier, 2009.

PDR for Nonprescription Drugs, Dietary Supplements, and Herbs. 31st ed. Montvale, N.J.: PDR Network, 2010.

Physicians' Desk Reference. 64th ed. Montvale, N.J.: PDR Network, 2009.

Porter, Robert S., et al., eds. *The Merck Manual Home Health Handbook.* Whitehouse Station, N.J.: Merck Research Laboratories, 2009.

Professional Guide to Diseases. 9th ed. Philadelphia: Lippincott Williams & Wilkins, 2008.

Stedman's Medical Dictionary. 28th ed. Philadelphia: Lippincott Williams & Wilkins, 2006.

Venes, Donald, ed. *Taber's Cyclopedic Medical Dictionary.* 21st ed. Philadelphia: F. A. Davis, 2009.

Wagman, Richard J., ed. *The New Complete Medical and Health Encyclopedia.* 4 vols. Chicago: J. G. Ferguson, 2002.

Webster's New World Medical Dictionary. 2d ed. New York: John Wiley & Sons, 2003.

EMERGENCY MEDICINE

American Academy of Orthopaedic Surgeons. *Emergency Care and Transportation of the Sick and Injured.* Edited by Benjamin Gulli, Les Chatelain, and Chris Stratford. 9th ed. Sudbury, Mass.: Jones and Bartlett, 2005.

American College of Emergency Physicians. *Geriatric Emergency Medicine.* Edited by Stephen W. Meldon, O. John Ma, and Robert H. Woolard. New York: McGraw-Hill, 2004.

American Medical Association. *Handbook of First Aid and Emergency Care.* Rev. and updated ed. New York: Random House Reference, 2009.

Caroline, Nancy L. *Nancy Caroline's Emergency Care in the Streets.* 6th ed. Sudbury, Mass.: Jones and Bartlett, 2010.

Fleisher, Gary R., Stephen Ludwig, and Fred M. Henretig, eds. *Textbook of Pediatric Emergency Medicine.* 5th ed. Philadelphia: Lippincott Williams & Wilkins, 2006.

Hamilton, Glenn C., et al. *Emergency Medicine: An Approach to Clinical Problem-Solving.* 2d ed. New York: W. B. Saunders, 2003.

Henry, Mark C., and Edward R. Stapleton. *EMT: Prehospital Care.* 4th ed. St. Louis, Mo.: Mosby/Elsevier, 2010.

Hogan, David E., and Jonathan L. Burstein. *Disaster Medicine.* 2d ed. Philadelphia: Lippincott Williams & Wilkins, 2007.

Knoop, Kevin J., et al., eds. *The Atlas of Emergency Medicine.* 3d ed. New York: McGraw-Hill Medical, 2010.

Krohmer, Jon R., ed. *American College of Emergency Physicians First Aid Manual.* 2d ed. New York: DK, 2004.

Limmer, Daniel, et al. *Emergency Care.* 11th ed. Upper Saddle River, N.J.: Pearson/Prentice Hall Health, 2009.

Marovchick, Vincent J., and Peter T. Pons, eds. *Emergency Medicine Secrets.* 4th ed. Philadelphia: Mosby/Elsevier, 2006.

Marx, John A., et al., eds. *Rosen's Emergency Medicine: Concepts and Clinical Practice.* 7th ed. Philadelphia: Mosby/Elsevier, 2010.

Mistovich, Joseph J., Brent Q. Hafen, and Keith J. Karren. *Prehospital Emergency Care.* 7th ed. Upper Saddle River, N.J.: Brady Prentice Hall Health, 2004.

Roberts, James R., and Jerris R. Hedges, eds. *Clinical Procedures in Emergency Medicine.* 4th ed. Philadelphia: W. B. Saunders, 2004.

Roppolo, Lynn, et al., eds. *Emergency Medicine Handbook: Critical Concepts for Clinical Practice.* Philadelphia: Mosby/Elsevier, 2007.

Scaletta, Thomas A., and Jeffrey J. Schaider. *Emergent Management of Trauma.* 2d ed. Boston: McGraw-Hill, 2001.

Strange, Gary R., et al., eds. *Pediatric Emergency Medicine: A Comprehensive Study Guide.* 2d ed. New York: McGraw-Hill, 2002.

Tintinalli, Judith E., ed. *Emergency Medicine: A Comprehensive Study Guide.* 6th ed. New York: McGraw-Hill, 2004.

ENDOCRINOLOGY AND METABOLISM

Bar, Robert S., ed. *Early Diagnosis and Treatment of Endocrine Disorders.* Totowa, N.J.: Humana Press, 2003.

Becker, Kenneth L., et al., eds. *Principles and Practice of Endocrinology and Metabolism.* 3d ed. Philadelphia: Lippincott Williams & Wilkins, 2001.

DeGroot, Leslie J., and J. Larry Jameson, eds. *Endocrinology.* 5th ed. Philadelphia: Saunders/Elsevier, 2006.

Felig, Philip, and Lawrence A. Frohman. *Endocrinology and Metabolism.* 4th ed. New York: McGraw-Hill, 2001.

Gardner, David G., and Dolores Shoback. eds. *Greenspan's Basic and Clinical Endocrinology.* 8th ed. New York: McGraw-Hill, 2007.

Goodman, H. Maurice. *Basic Medical Endocrinology.* 4th ed. Boston: Academic Press/Elsevier, 2009.

Griffin, James E., and Sergio R. Ojeda, eds. *Textbook of Endocrine Physiology.* 5th ed. New York: Oxford University Press, 2004.

Hadley, Mac E., and Jon E. Levine. *Endocrinology.* 6th ed. Upper Saddle River, N.J.: Pearson/Prentice Hall, 2007.

Henry, Helen L., and Anthony W. Norman, eds. *Encyclopedia of Hormones.* 3 vols. San Diego, Calif.: Academic Press, 2003.

Kronenberg, Henry M., et al., eds. *Williams Textbook of Endocrinology.* 11th ed. Philadelphia: Saunders/Elsevier, 2008.

Lavin, Norman, ed. *Manual of Endocrinology and Metabolism.* 3d ed. Philadelphia: Lippincott Williams & Wilkins, 2002.

Lebovitz, Harold E., ed. *Therapy for Diabetes Mellitus and Related Disorders.* 5th ed. Alexandria, Va.: American Diabetes Association, 2009.

Neal, J. Matthew, ed. *How the Endocrine System Works.* Malden, Mass.: Blackwell Science, 2001.

Porte, Daniel, Jr., Robert S. Sherwin, and Alain Baron, eds. *Ellenberg and Rifkin's Diabetes Mellitus.* 6th ed. New York: McGraw-Hill, 2002.

Ruggieri, Paul, and Scott Isaacs. *A Simple Guide to Thyroid Disorders: From Diagnosis to Treatment.* Omaha, Nebr.: Addicus Books, 2004.

Sperling, Mark A., ed. *Pediatric Endocrinology.* 3d ed. Philadelphia: Saunders/Elsevier, 2008.

ETHICS
American Medical Association. *Code of Medical Ethics: Current Opinions with Annotations, 2006-2007.* Chicago: Author, 2006-2007.

Beauchamp, Tom L., and James F. Childress. *Principles of Biomedical Ethics.* 6th ed. New York: Oxford University Press, 2009.

Beauchamp, Tom L., and LeRoy Walters, eds. *Contemporary Issues in Bioethics.* 7th ed. Belmont, Calif.: Thomson/Wadsworth, 2008.

Campbell, Alistair V., Grant Gillett, and Gareth Jones. *Medical Ethics.* 4th ed. New York: Oxford University Press, 2005.

Devine, Richard J. *Good Care, Painful Choices: Medical Ethics of Ordinary People.* 3d ed. New York: Paulist Press, 2004.

Edge, Raymond S., and John Randall Groves. *Ethics of Health Care: A Guide for Clinical Practice.* 3d ed. Clifton Park, N.Y.: Thomson Delmar Learning, 2006.

Garrett, Thomas M., Harold W. Baillie, and Rosellen M. Garrett. *Health Care Ethics: Principles and Problems.* 5th ed. Upper Saddle River, N.J.: Prentice Hall, 2010.

Jonsen, Albert R., Mark Siegler, and William J. Winslade. *Clinical Ethics: A Practical Approach to Ethical Decisions in Clinical Medicine.* 6th ed. New York: McGraw-Hill, 2006.

Lo, Bernard. *Resolving Ethical Dilemmas: A Guide for Clinicians.* 3d ed. Philadelphia: Lippincott Williams & Wilkins, 2005.

Mappes, Thomas A., and David DeGrazia, eds. *Biomedical Ethics.* 6th ed. Boston: McGraw-Hill, 2006.

Munson, Ronald, comp. *Intervention and Reflection: Basic Issues in Medical Ethics.* 7th ed. Belmont, Calif.: Thomson/Wadsworth, 2004.

Pence, Gregory. *Classic Cases in Medical Ethics: Accounts of Cases That Have Shaped Medical Ethics, with Philosophical, Legal, and Historical Backgrounds.* 4th ed. Boston: McGraw-Hill, 2004.

_____. *Re-creating Medicine: Ethical Issues at the Frontiers of Medicine.* Lanham, Md.: Rowman & Littlefield, 2007.

Rebman, Renée C. *Euthanasia and the Right to Die: Pro/Con Issues.* Berkeley Heights, N.J.: Enslow, 2002.

Torr, James D., ed. *Medical Ethics.* San Diego, Calif.: Greenhaven Press, 2000.

Veatch, Robert M. *The Basics of Bioethics.* 2d ed. Upper Saddle River, N.J.: Prentice Hall, 2003.

EVIDENCE-BASED MEDICINE
Brownson, Ross C., et al., eds. *Evidence-Based Public Health.* New York: Oxford University Press, 2002.

Dawes, Martin, et al. *Evidence-Based Practice: A Primer for Health Care Professionals.* 2d ed. New York: Churchill Livingstone/Elsevier, 2005.

Evans, Michael, ed. *Mosby's Family Practice Sourcebook: An Evidence-Based Approach to Care.* 4th ed. Toronto, Ont.: Mosby/Elsevier, 2006.

Greenhalgh, Trisha. *How to Read a Paper: The Basics*

of Evidence-Based Medicine. 3d ed. Malden, Mass.: BMJ Books/Blackwell, 2006.

Kormos, Bill. *The Massachusetts General Hospital Quick Consult Manual of Evidence-Based Medicine.* 2d ed. Philadelphia: Lippincott Williams & Wilkins, 2007.

Straus, Sharon E., et al. *Evidence-Based Medicine: How to Practice and Teach EBM.* 3d ed. New York: Churchill Livingstone/Elsevier, 2005.

Tierney, Lawrence M., Stephen J. McPhee, and Maxine A. Papadakis, eds. *Current Medical Diagnosis and Treatment 2007.* New York: McGraw-Hill Medical, 2006.

FAMILY MEDICINE

Chan, Paul D., et al. *Family Medicine.* Blue Jay, Calif.: Current Clinical Strategies, 2010.

Chang, Kimberly S. G., et al. *Family Medicine.* 2d ed. Philadelphia: Lippincott Williams & Wilkins, 2007.

Goroll, Allan H., and Albert G. Mulley, eds. *Primary Care Medicine.* 5th ed. Philadelphia: Lippincott Williams & Wilkins, 2006.

Graber, Mark A., Jennifer L. Jones, and Jason K. Wilbur, eds. *University of Iowa: The Family Medicine Handbook.* 5th ed. Philadelphia: Saunders/Elsevier, 2006.

Lipsky, Martin S., and Mitchell S. King. *Blueprints Family Medicine.* 2d ed. Malden, Mass.: Blackwell, 2006.

Rakel, Robert E., ed. *Essential Family Medicine: Fundamentals and Case Studies.* 3d ed. Philadelphia: Saunders/Elsevier, 2006.

_____. *Textbook of Family Practice.* 6th ed. Philadelphia: W. B. Saunders, 2002.

Sloane, Philip D., et al., eds. *Essentials of Family Medicine.* 5th ed. Philadelphia: Lippincott Williams & Wilkins, 2008.

Taylor, Robert B., et al., eds. *Family Medicine: Principles and Practice.* 6th ed. New York: Springer, 2003.

GASTROENTEROLOGY

Boyer, Thomas D., Teresa L. Wright, and Michael P. Manns, eds. *Zakim and Boyer's Hepatology: A Textbook of Liver Disease.* 5th ed. Philadelphia: Saunders/Elsevier, 2006.

Chopra, Sanjiv. *The Liver Book: A Comprehensive Guide to Diagnosis, Treatment, and Recovery.* New York: Simon & Schuster, 2002.

Cunningham, Carin L., and Gerard A. Banez. *Pediatric Gastrointestinal Disorders: Biopsychosocial Assessment and Treatment.* New York: Springer, 2006.

Feldman, Mark, Lawrence S. Friedman, and Lawrence J. Brandt, eds. *Sleisenger and Fordtran's Gastrointestinal and Liver Disease: Pathophysiology, Diagnosis, Management.* New ed. 2 vols. Philadelphia: Saunders/Elsevier, 2010.

Friedman, Scott L., Kenneth R. McQuaid, and James H. Grendell, eds. *Current Diagnosis and Treatment in Gastroenterology.* 2d ed. New York: Lang Medical Books/McGraw-Hill, 2003.

Johnson, Leonard R., ed. *Gastrointestinal Physiology.* 7th ed. Philadelphia: Mosby/Elsevier, 2007.

Kapadia, Cyrus R., James M. Crawford, and Caroline Taylor. *An Atlas of Gastroenterology: A Guide to Diagnosis and Differential Diagnosis.* Boca Raton, Fla.: Pantheon, 2003.

Margolis, Simeon, et al. *Johns Hopkins White Papers 2003: Arthritis, Coronary, Depression and Anxiety, Diabetes, Digestive Disorders, Hypertension and Stroke.* Vol. 1. New York: Rebus, 2002.

Schiff, Eugene R., Michael F. Sorrell, and Willis C. Maddrey, eds. *Schiff's Diseases of the Liver.* 10th ed. Philadelphia: Lippincott Williams & Wilkins, 2007.

Shimberg, Elaine Fantle. *Coping with Chronic Heartburn: What You Need to Know About Acid Reflux and GERD.* New York: St. Martin's Griffin, 2002.

Walker, W. Allan, et al., eds. *Pediatric Gastrointestinal Disease: Pathophysiology, Diagnosis, Management.* 4th ed. Lewiston, N.Y.: B. C. Decker, 2004.

Yamada, Takada, et al., eds. *Textbook of Gastroenterology.* 4th ed. Philadelphia: Lippincott Williams & Wilkins, 2003.

GENETICS AND HEREDITY

Bellenir, Karen, ed. *Genetic Disorders Sourcebook: Basic Consumer Information About Hereditary Diseases and Disorders.* 3d ed. Detroit: Omnigraphics, 2004.

Davis, Dena S. *Genetic Dilemmas: Reproductive Technology, Parental Choices, and Children's Futures.* 2d ed. New York: Routledge, 2010.

Harper, Peter S. *Practical Genetic Counselling.* 6th ed. New York: Oxford University Press, 2004.

Hartwell, Leland, et al. *Genetics: From Genes to Genomes.* 3d ed. Boston: McGraw-Hill, 2008.

Jorde, Lynn B., et al. *Medical Genetics.* Rev. 3d ed. St. Louis, Mo.: Mosby/Elsevier, 2006.

King, Richard A., Jerome I. Rotter, and Arno G. Motulsky, eds. *The Genetic Basis of Common Diseases.* 2d ed. New York: Oxford University Press, 2002.

Korf, Bruce R. *Human Genetics: A Problem-Based Ap-*

proach. 2d ed. Malden, Mass.: Blackwell Science, 2000.

Lewin, Benjamin. *Genes IX.* 9th rev. ed. Sudbury, Mass.: Jones and Bartlett, 2007.

Lewis, Ricki. *Human Genetics: Concepts and Applications.* 9th ed. Dubuque, Iowa: McGraw-Hill, 2009.

McCance, Kathryn L., and Sue M. Huether. *Pathophysiology: The Biologic Basis for Disease in Adults and Children.* 6th ed. St. Louis, Mo.: Mosby/Elsevier, 2010.

Milunsky, Aubrey, ed. *Genetic Disorders of the Fetus: Diagnosis, Prevention, and Treatment.* 6th ed. Hoboken, N.J.: Wiley-Blackwell, 2009.

Nicholl, Desmond S. T. *Introduction to Genetic Engineering.* 3d ed. New York: Cambridge University Press, 2008.

Nussbaum, Robert L., Roderick R. McInnes, and Willard F. Huntington. *Thompson and Thompson Genetics in Medicine.* 7th ed. Philadelphia: Saunders/Elsevier, 2006.

Ridley, Matt. *Nature via Nurture: Genes, Experience, and What Makes Us Human.* New York: HarperCollins, 2003.

Rimoin, David L., et al., eds. *Emery and Rimoin's Principles and Practice of Medical Genetics.* 5th ed. Philadelphia: Churchill Livingstone/Elsevier, 2007.

Scriver, Charles R., et al., eds. *The Metabolic and Molecular Bases of Inherited Disease.* 8th ed. 4 vols. New York: McGraw-Hill, 2001.

Snustad, D. Peter, and Michael J. Simmons. *Principles of Genetics.* 5th ed. Hoboken, N.J.: John Wiley & Sons, 2009.

Turnpenny, Peter, and Sian Ellard. *Emery's Elements of Medical Genetics.* 13th ed. New York: Churchill Livingstone/Elsevier, 2007.

GERIATRICS

Beerman, Susan, and Judith Rappaport-Musson. *Eldercare 911: The Caregiver's Complete Handbook for Making Decisions.* Rev. ed. Amherst, N.Y.: Prometheus Books, 2008.

Beers, Mark H., and Robert Berkow, eds. *The Merck Manual of Geriatrics.* 3d ed. Whitehouse Station, N.J.: Merck Research Laboratories, 2000.

Birren, James E., and K. Warner Schaie, eds. *Handbook of the Psychology of Aging.* 6th ed. Boston: Academic Press/Elsevier, 2007.

Cassel, Christine K., et al., eds. *Geriatric Medicine.* 4th ed. New York: Springer, 2003.

Ferri, Fred F., Marsha Fretwell, and Tom J. Wachtel.

Practical Guide to the Care of the Geriatric Patient. 3d ed. St. Louis, Mo.: Mosby/Elsevier, 2007.

Gauthier, Serge, ed. *Clinical Diagnosis and Management of Alzheimer's Disease.* 3d ed. Abingdon, Oxfordshire, England: Informa Healthcare, 2006.

Ham, Richard, et al., eds. *Primary Care Geriatrics: A Case-Based Approach.* 5th ed. St. Louis, Mo.: Mosby/Elsevier, 2007.

Hazzard, William R., et al., eds. *Principles of Geriatric Medicine and Gerontology.* 5th ed. New York: McGraw-Hill, 2003.

Herdt, Gilbert, and Brian de Vries, eds. *Gay and Lesbian Aging: Research and Future Directions.* New York: Springer, 2004.

Hill, Robert D. *Positive Aging: A Guide for Mental Health Professionals and Consumers.* New York: W. W. Norton, 2006.

Hooyman, Nancy, and H. Asuman Kiyak. *Social Gerontology: A Multidisciplinary Perspective.* New York: Prentice Hall, 2010.

Hoyer, William J., and Paul A. Roodin. *Adult Development and Aging.* 6th ed. Boston: McGraw-Hill, 2009.

Mace, Nancy L., and Peter V. Rabins. *The Thirty-Six-Hour Day: A Family Guide to Caring for Persons with Alzheimer Disease, Related Dementing Illnesses, and Memory Loss in Later Life.* 4th ed. Baltimore: Johns Hopkins University Press, 2006.

Masoro, Edward J., and Steven N. Austad, eds. *Handbook of the Biology of Aging.* 6th ed. Boston: Academic Press/Elsevier, 2007.

Weisstub, David N. *Aging: Caring for Our Elders.* Boston: Kluwer Academic, 2001.

GYNECOLOGY AND OBSTETRICS

Altchek, Albert, Liane Deligdisch, and Nathan Kase, eds. *Diagnosis and Management of Ovarian Disorders.* 2d ed. San Diego, Calif.: Academic Press, 2003.

Ammer, Christine. *The New A to Z of Women's Health: A Concise Encyclopedia.* 6th ed. New York: Checkmark Books, 2009.

Berek, Jonathan S., ed. *Berek and Novak's Gynecology.* 14th ed. Philadelphia: Lippincott Williams & Wilkins, 2007.

Briggs, Gerald G., Roger K. Freeman, and Sumner J. Yaffe. *Drugs in Pregnancy and Lactation: A Reference Guide to Fetal and Neonatal Risk.* 7th ed. Philadelphia: Lippincott Williams & Wilkins, 2005.

Burrow, Gerard N., Thomas P. Duffy, and Joshua A. Copel, eds. *Medical Complications During Pregnancy.* 6th ed. Philadelphia: W. B. Saunders, 2004.

Carey, J. Christopher, and William F. Rayburn. *Obstetrics and Gynecology*. 4th ed. Philadelphia: Lippincott Williams & Wilkins, 2002.

Creasy, Robert K., and Robert Resnik, eds. *Maternal-Fetal Medicine: Principles and Practice*. 5th ed. Philadelphia: W. B. Saunders, 2004.

Cunningham, F. Gary, et al., eds. *Williams Obstetrics*. 23d ed. New York: McGraw-Hill, 2010.

DeCherney, Alan H., and Lauren Nathan, eds. *Current Obstetric and Gynecologic Diagnosis and Treatment*. 9th ed. New York: Lange Medical Books/McGraw-Hill, 2003.

DiSaia, Philip J., and William T. Creasman. *Clinical Gynecologic Oncology*. 6th ed. St. Louis, Mo.: Mosby, 2002.

Emans, S. Jean Herriot, Marc R. Laufer, and Donald P. Goldstein, eds. *Pediatric and Adolescent Gynecology*. 5th ed. Philadelphia: Lippincott Williams & Wilkins, 2005.

Gabbe, Steven G., Jennifer R. Niebyl, and Joe Leigh Simpson, eds. *Obstetrics: Normal and Problem Pregnancies*. 5th ed. Philadelphia: Churchill Livingstone/Elsevier, 2007.

Hacker, Neville F., J. George Moore, and Joseph C. Gambone, eds. *Essentials of Obstetrics and Gynecology*. 4th ed. Philadelphia: W. B. Saunders, 2004.

Katz, Vern L., et al. *Comprehensive Gynecology*. 5th ed. St. Louis, Mo.: Mosby/Elsevier, 2007.

Lowdermilk, Deitra Leonard, and Shannon Perry. *Maternity and Women's Health Care*. 8th ed. St. Louis, Mo.: Mosby, 2003.

Quilligan, Edward J., and Frederick P. Zuspan, eds. *Current Therapy in Obstetrics and Gynecology*. 5th ed. Philadelphia: W. B. Saunders, 2000.

Rock, John A., and Howard W. Jones III, eds. *Te Linde's Operative Gynecology*. 10th ed. Philadelphia: Wolters Kluwer/Lippincott Williams & Wilkins, 2008.

Scott, James R., et al., eds. *Danforth's Obstetrics and Gynecology*. 10th ed. Philadelphia: Lippincott Williams & Wilkins, 2008.

Speroff, Leon, and Marc A. Fritz. *Clinical Gynecologic Endocrinology and Infertility*. 7th ed. Philadelphia: Lippincott Williams & Wilkins, 2005.

Stenchever, Morton A., et al. *Comprehensive Gynecology*. 5th ed. St. Louis, Mo.: Mosby/Elsevier, 2007.

Sweet, Richard L., and Ronald S. Gibbs. *Infectious Diseases of the Female Genital Tract*. 4th ed. Philadelphia: Lippincott Williams & Wilkins, 2002.

HEMATOLOGY

Bick, Roger L. *Disorders of Thrombosis and Hemostasis: Clinical and Laboratory Practice*. 3d ed. Philadelphia: Lippincott Williams & Wilkins, 2002.

Greer, John, et al., eds. *Wintrobe's Clinical Hematology*. 12th ed. Philadelphia: Wolters Kluwer/Lippincott Williams & Wilkins Health, 2009.

Harmening, Denise M., ed. *Clinical Hematology and Fundamentals of Hemostasis*. 5th ed. Philadelphia: F. A. Davis, 2009.

Hillman, Robert S., Kenneth A. Ault, and Henry M. Rinder. *Hematology in Clinical Practice: A Guide to Diagnosis and Management*. 4th ed. New York: McGraw-Hill, 2005.

Hillyer, Christopher D., et al., eds. *Blood Banking and Transfusion Medicine*. 2d ed. Philadelphia: Churchill Livingstone/Elsevier, 2007.

Hoffman, Ronald, et al., eds. *Hematology: Basic Principles and Practice*. 5th ed. Philadelphia: Churchill Livingstone/Elsevier, 2009.

Lichtman, Marshall, et al., eds. *Williams Hematology*. 7th ed. New York: McGraw-Hill, 2006.

Loscalzo, Joseph, and Andrew I. Schafer, eds. *Thrombosis and Hemorrhage*. 3d ed. Philadelphia: Lippincott Williams & Wilkins, 2003.

Nathan, David G., and Stuart H. Orkin, eds. *Nathan and Oski's Hematology of Infancy and Childhood*. 7th ed. Philadelphia: Saunders/Elsevier, 2009.

Rodak, Bernadette, ed. *Hematology: Clinical Principles and Applications*. 2d ed. Philadelphia: W. B. Saunders, 2002.

Spiess, Bruce D., Richard K. Spence, and Aryeh Shander, eds. *Perioperative Transfusion Medicine*. 2d ed. Philadelphia: Lippincott Williams & Wilkins, 2006.

Winslow, Robert M., ed. *Blood Substitutes*. Boston: Academic Press/Elsevier, 2006.

Zucker-Franklin, D., et al. *Atlas of Blood Cells: Function and Pathology*. 3d ed. Philadelphia: Lea & Febiger, 2003.

HOSPITALS AND ADMINISTRATION

American Hospital Association. *Hospital Statistics: The Comprehensive Reference Source for Analysis and Comparison of Hospital Trends*. Chicago: Health Forum, 2008.

Birenbaum, Aaron. *Wounded Profession: American Medicine Enters the Age of Managed Care*. Westport, Conn.: Greenwood Press, 2002.

Bodenheimer, Thomas S., and Kevin Grumbach. *Understanding Health Policy: A Clinical Approach.* 4th ed. New York: McGraw-Hill, 2005.

Cleverley, William O., and Andrew E. Cameron. *Essentials of Health Care Finance.* 6th ed. Sudbury, Mass.: Jones and Bartlett, 2007.

Dranove, David. *The Economic Evolution of American Health Care: From Marcus Welby to Managed Care.* Princeton, N.J.: Princeton University Press, 2002.

Joint Commission on Accreditation of Healthcare Organizations. *2010 Comprehensive Accreditation Manual for Hospitals: The Official Handbook.* Oakbrook Terrace, Ill.: Author, 2009.

Kavaler, Florence, and Allen D. Spiegel. *Risk Management in Health Care Institutions: A Strategic Approach.* 2d ed. Boston: Jones and Bartlett, 2003.

Kovner, Anthony R., and James R. Knickman, eds. *Jonas and Kovner's Health Care Delivery in the United States.* 8th ed. New York: Springer, 2005.

McConnell, Charles R. *The Effective Health Care Supervisor.* 6th ed. Sudbury, Mass.: Jones and Bartlett, 2007.

Shi, Leiyu, and Douglas A. Singh. *Delivering Health Care in America: A Systems Approach.* 3d ed. Boston: Jones and Bartlett, 2004.

Sultz, Harry A., and Kristina M. Young. *Health Care USA: Understanding Its Organization and Delivery.* 5th ed. Sudbury, Mass.: Jones and Bartlett, 2006.

Wolper, Lawrence F., ed. *Health Care Administration: Planning, Implementing, and Managing Organized Delivery Systems.* 4th ed. Boston: Jones and Bartlett, 2004.

IMMUNOLOGY

Abbas, Abul K., and Andrew K. Lichtman. *Basic Immunology: Functions and Disorders of the Immune System.* 2d ed. Philadelphia: Saunders/Elsevier, 2006.

Austen, K. Frank, et al., eds. *Samter's Immunologic Diseases.* 6th ed. Philadelphia: Lippincott Williams & Wilkins, 2001.

Delves, Peter J., et al. *Roitt's Essential Immunology.* 11th ed. Malden, Mass.: Blackwell, 2006.

Detrick, Barbara, Robert G. Hamilton, and James D. Folds, eds. *Manual of Molecular and Clinical Laboratory Immunology.* 7th ed. Washington, D.C.: ASM Press, 2006.

Doughty, Lesley A., and Peter Linden, eds. *Immunology and Infectious Disease.* Norwell, Mass.: Kluwer Academic, 2003.

Frank, Steven A. *Immunology and Evolution of Infectious Disease.* Princeton, N.J.: Princeton University Press, 2002.

Janeway, Charles A., Jr., et al. *Immunobiology: The Immune System in Health and Disease.* 6th ed. New York: Garland Science, 2005.

Kindt, Thomas J., Richard A. Goldsby, and Barbara A. Osborne. *Kuby Immunology.* 6th ed. New York: W. H. Freeman, 2007.

Parkham, Peter. *The Immune System.* 2d ed. New York: Garland Science, 2005.

Parslow, Tristram G., et al., eds. *Medical Immunology.* 10th ed. New York: Lange Medical Books/McGraw-Hill, 2001.

Paul, William E., ed. *Fundamental Immunology.* 5th ed. Philadelphia: Lippincott Williams & Wilkins, 2003.

Playfair, J. H. L., and B. M. Chain. *Immunology at a Glance.* 9th ed. Hoboken, N.J.: Wiley-Blackwell, 2009.

Rose, Noel R., and Ian. R. Mackay, eds. *The Autoimmune Diseases.* 4th ed. St. Louis, Mo.: Academic Press/Elsevier, 2006.

Stiehm, E. Richard, Hans D. Ochs, and Jerry A. Winkelstein, eds. *Immunologic Disorders in Infants and Children.* 5th ed. Philadelphia: W. B. Saunders, 2004.

INFECTIOUS DISEASES

Betts, Robert F., Stanley W. Chapman, and Robert L. Penn, eds. *Reese and Betts' A Practical Approach to Infectious Diseases.* 5th ed. Philadelphia: Lippincott Williams & Wilkins, 2003.

Cohen, Jonathan, and William Powderly, eds. *Infectious Diseases.* 2d ed. St. Louis, Mo.: Mosby, 2004.

Feigin, Ralph D., et al., eds. *Textbook of Pediatric Infectious Diseases.* 5th ed. Philadelphia: W. B. Saunders, 2004.

Frank, Steven A. *Immunology and Evolution of Infectious Disease.* Princeton, N.J.: Princeton University Press, 2002.

Gershon, Anne A., Peter J. Hotez, and Samuel L. Katz, eds. *Krugman's Infectious Diseases of Children.* 11th ed. Philadelphia: Mosby, 2004.

Giesecke, Johan. *Modern Infectious Disease Epidemiology.* 2d ed. New York: Oxford University Press, 2002.

Gorbach, Sherwood L., John G. Bartlett, and Neil R. Blacklow, eds. *Infectious Diseases.* 3d ed. Philadelphia: W. B. Saunders, 2004.

Grace, Christopher, ed. *Medical Management of Infectious Disease.* New York: Marcel Dekker, 2003.

Heymann, David L., ed. *Control of Communicable Diseases Manual*. 19th ed. Washington, D.C.: American Public Health Association, 2008.

Mandell, Gerald L., John E. Bennett, and Raphael Dolin, eds. *Mandell, Douglas, and Bennett's Principles and Practice of Infectious Diseases*. 7th ed. New York: Churchill Livingstone/Elsevier, 2010.

Plotkin, Stanley A., and Walter A. Orenstein, eds. *Vaccines*. 4th ed. Philadelphia: W. B. Saunders, 2004.

Remington, Jack S., et al., eds. *Infectious Diseases of the Fetus and Newborn Infant*. 6th ed. Philadelphia: Saunders/Elsevier, 2006.

INTERNAL MEDICINE

Andreoli, Thomas E., et al., eds. *Andreoli and Carpenter's Cecil Essentials of Medicine*. 8th ed. Philadelphia: Saunders/Elsevier, 2010.

Boon, Nicholas A., et al., eds. *Davidson's Principles and Practice of Medicine*. 20th ed. New York: Churchill Livingstone/Elsevier, 2006.

Cooper, Daniel H., et al., eds. *The Washington Manual of Medical Therapeutics*. 32d ed. Philadelphia: Lippincott Williams & Wilkins, 2007.

Ferri, Fred F., ed. *Practical Guide to the Care of the Medical Patient*. 7th ed. Philadelphia: Mosby/Elsevier, 2007.

Fishman, Mark, et al., eds. *Medicine*. 5th ed. Philadelphia: Lippincott Williams & Wilkins, 2004.

Goldman, Lee, and Dennis Ausiello, eds. *Cecil Textbook of Medicine*. 23d ed. Philadelphia: Saunders/Elsevier, 2007.

Humes, H. David, et al., eds. *Kelley's Textbook of Internal Medicine*. 4th ed. Philadelphia: Lippincott Williams & Wilkins, 2000.

Kasper, Dennis L., et al., eds. *Harrison's Principles of Internal Medicine*. 16th ed. New York: McGraw-Hill, 2005.

Runge, Marschall S., and M. Andrew Gregnati, eds. *Netter's Internal Medicine*. 2d ed. Philadelphia: Saunders/Elsevier, 2009.

Tierney, Lawrence M., Stephen J. McPhee, and Maxine A. Papadakis, eds. *Current Medical Diagnosis and Treatment 2007*. New York: McGraw-Hill Medical, 2006.

LABORATORY METHODS

Diagnostic Tests: A Prescriber's Guide to Test Selection and Interpretation. Philadelphia: Lippincott Williams & Wilkins, 2004.

McClatchey, Kenneth D., ed. *Clinical Laboratory Medicine*. 2d ed. Philadelphia: Lippincott Williams & Wilkins, 2002.

McPherson, Richard A., and Matthew R. Pincus, eds. *Henry's Clinical Diagnosis and Management by Laboratory Methods*. 21st ed. Philadelphia: Saunders/Elsevier, 2007.

Pagana, Kathleen Deska, and Timothy J. Pagana. *Mosby's Diagnostic and Laboratory Test Reference*. 9th ed. St. Louis, Mo.: Mosby/Elsevier, 2009.

Sacher, Ronald A., and Richard A. McPherson. *Widmann's Clinical Interpretation of Laboratory Tests*. 11th ed. Philadelphia: Davis, 2000.

Wallach, Jacques. *Interpretation of Diagnostic Tests*. 8th ed. Philadelphia: Wolters Kluwer Health/Lippincott Williams & Wilkins, 2007.

Wu, Alan H. B., ed. *Tietz Clinical Guide to Laboratory Tests*. 4th ed. St. Louis, Mo.: Saunders/Elsevier, 2006.

LEGAL MEDICINE

American College of Legal Medicine. *Legal Medicine*. 6th ed. Philadelphia: Mosby, 2004.

Boumil, Marcia M., Clifford E. Elias, and Diane Bissonnette Moes. *Medical Liability in a Nutshell*. 2d ed. St. Paul, Minn.: Thomson/West, 2003.

Fremgen, Bonnie F. *Medical Law and Ethics*. 2d ed. Upper Saddle River, N.J.: Pearson/Prentice Hall, 2006.

Furrow, Barry R., et al. *Health Law: Cases, Materials, and Problems*. 5th ed. St. Paul, Minn.: West, 2004.

Garner, Bryan A., ed. *Black's Law Dictionary*. 9th ed. St. Paul, Minn.: Thomson/West, 2008.

Hall, Mark A., Mary Anne Bobinski, and David Orentlicher. *Health Care Law and Ethics*. 6th ed. New York: Aspen, 2003.

Jonsen, Albert R., Mark Siegler, and William J. Winslade. *Clinical Ethics: A Practical Approach to Ethical Decisions in Clinical Medicine*. 6th ed. New York: McGraw-Hill, 2006.

Miller, Robert D. *Problems in Health Care Law*. 9th ed. Sudbury, Mass.: Jones and Bartlett, 2006.

Montgomery, Jonathan. *Health Care Law*. 2d ed. New York: Oxford University Press, 2003.

Pence, Gregory E. *Classic Cases in Medical Ethics: Accounts of Cases That Have Shaped Medical Ethics, with Philosophical, Legal, and Historical Backgrounds*. 4th ed. New York: McGraw-Hill, 2004.

Pozgar, George D. *Legal Aspects of Health Care Administration*. 10th ed. Sudbury, Mass.: Jones and Bartlett, 2006.

MANAGED CARE

Birenbaum, Aaron. *Wounded Profession: American Medicine Enters the Age of Managed Care.* Westport, Conn.: Greenwood Press, 2002.

Bondeson, William B., and James W. Jones, eds. *The Ethics of Managed Care: Professional Integrity and Patient Rights.* Boston: Kluwer Academic, 2002.

Dranove, David. *The Economic Evolution of American Health Care: From Marcus Welby to Managed Care.* Princeton, N.J.: Princeton University Press, 2002.

Fauman, Michael A. *Negotiating Managed Care: A Manual for Clinicians.* Washington, D.C.: American Psychiatric Publishing, 2002.

Freeborn, Donald K., and Clyde R. Pope. *Promise and Performance in Managed Care: The Prepaid Group Practice Model.* Rev. ed. Baltimore: Johns Hopkins University Press, 2000.

Kongstvedt, Peter R. *Managed Care: What It Is and How It Works.* 3d ed. Sudbury, Mass.: Jones and Bartlett, 2009.

_____, ed. *Essentials of Managed Health Care.* 5th ed. Sudbury, Mass.: Jones and Bartlett, 2007.

Marcinko, David Edward, ed. *Dictionary of Health Insurance and Managed Care.* New York: Springer, 2006.

Stanley, Kay B., ed. *Managing Managed Care in the Medical Practice.* 2d ed. Chicago: AMA Press, 2004.

MEDICAL INFORMATICS

Bardram, Jakob E., Alex Mihailidis, and Dadong Wan, eds. *Pervasive Computing in Healthcare.* Boca Raton, Fla.: CRC Press, 2007.

Berman, Jules J. *Biomedical Informatics.* Sudbury, Mass.: Jones and Bartlett, 2007.

Berner, Eta S., ed. *Clinical Decision Support Systems: Theory and Practice.* 2d ed. New York: Springer, 2007.

Davis, James B., ed. *Health and Medicine on the Internet: A Comprehensive Guide to Medical Information on the World Wide Web.* 4th ed. Los Angeles: Practice Management Information, 2003.

Felkey, Bill G., Brent I. Fox, and Margaret R. Thrower. *Health Care Informatics: A Skills-Based Resource.* Washington, D.C.: American Pharmacists Association, 2006.

Friedman, Charles P., and Jeremy C. Wyatt. *Evaluation Methods in Medical Informatics.* 2d ed. New York: Springer, 2006.

Goldstein, Douglas, et al. *Medical Informatics 20/20: Quality and Electronic Health Records Through*

Collaboration, Open Solutions, and Innovation. Sudbury, Mass.: Jones and Bartlett, 2007.

Shortliffe, Edward H., ed. *Biomedical Informatics: Computer Applications in Health Care and Biomedicine.* 3d ed. New York: Springer, 2006.

Smith, Roger P. *The Internet for Physicians.* 3d ed. New York: Springer, 2002.

MICROBIOLOGY

Alcamo, I. Edward. *Microbes and Society: An Introduction to Microbiology.* 2d ed. Sudbury, Mass.: Jones and Bartlett, 2008.

Black, Jacquelyn G. *Microbiology: Principles and Explorations.* 6th ed. Hoboken, N.J.: John Wiley & Sons, 2006.

Brooks, G. F., et al. *Jawetz, Melnick, and Adelberg's Medical Microbiology.* 24th ed. New York: McGraw-Hill, 2007.

Engleberg, N. Cary, Victor DiRita, and Terence S. Dermody, eds. *Schaechter's Mechanisms of Microbial Disease.* 4th ed. Philadelphia: Lippincott Williams & Wilkins, 2007.

Garcia, Lynne Shore. *Diagnostic Medical Parasitology.* 5th ed. Washington, D.C.: ASM Press, 2007.

Gillespie, Stephen, and Kathleen B. Bamford. *Medical Microbiology and Infection at a Glance.* 2d ed. Malden, Mass.: Blackwell, 2003.

Gladwin, Mark, and Bill Trattler. *Clinical Microbiology Made Ridiculously Simple.* 4th ed. Miami: MedMaster, 2009.

Madigan, Michael T., and John M. Martinko. *Brock Biology of Microorganisms.* 12th ed. San Francisco: Pearson/Benjamin Cummings, 2009.

Murray, Patrick R., et al., eds. *Manual of Clinical Microbiology.* 8th ed. Washington, D.C.: ASM Press, 2007.

Murray, Patrick R., Ken S. Rosenthal, and Michael A. Pfaller. *Medical Microbiology.* 6th ed. Philadelphia: Mosby/Elsevier, 2009.

Pommerville, Jeffery C. *Alcamo's Fundamentals of Microbiology.* 9th ed. Sudbury, Mass.: Jones and Bartlett, 2010.

Singleton, Paul, and Diana Sainsbury. *Dictionary of Microbiology and Molecular Biology.* Rev. 3d ed. Hoboken, N.J.: John Wiley & Sons, 2006.

Winn, Washington C., Jr., et al. *Koneman's Color Atlas and Textbook of Diagnostic Microbiology.* 6th ed. Philadelphia: Lippincott Williams & Wilkins, 2006.

NEUROLOGY

Afifi, Adel K., and Ronald A. Bergman. *Functional Neuroanatomy: Text and Atlas*. 2d ed. New York: Lange Medical Books/McGraw-Hill, 2005.

Aminoff, Michael J., David A. Greenberg, and Roger P. Simon. *Clinical Neurology*. 7th ed. New York: McGraw-Hill Medical, 2009.

Bear, Mark F., Barry W. Connors, and Michael A. Paradiso. *Neuroscience: Exploring the Brain*. 3d ed. Philadelphia: Lippincott Williams & Wilkins, 2007.

Bloom, Floyd E., M. Flint Beal, and David J. Kupfer, eds. *The Dana Guide to Brain Health*. New York: Dana Press, 2006.

Carey, Joseph, ed. *Brain Facts: A Primer on the Brain and Nervous System*. 5th ed. Washington, D.C.: Society for Neuroscience, 2006.

Castillo, Mauricio. *Neuroradiology Companion: Methods, Guidelines, and Imaging Fundamentals*. 3d ed. Philadelphia: Lippincott Williams & Wilkins, 2006.

Daube, Jasper R., ed. *Clinical Neurophysiology*. 3d ed. New York: Oxford University Press, 2009.

Evans, Randolph W., ed. *Neurology and Trauma*. 2d ed. New York: Oxford University Press, 2006.

Fenichel, Gerald M. *Clinical Pediatric Neurology: A Signs and Symptoms Approach*. 6th ed. Philadelphia: Saunders/Elsevier, 2009.

Gilman, Sid, and Sarah Winans Newman. *Manter and Gatz's Essentials of Clinical Neuroanatomy and Neurophysiology*. 10th ed. Philadelphia: F. A. Davis, 2003.

Kandel, Eric R., James H. Schwartz, and Thomas M. Jessell, eds. *Principles of Neural Science*. 5th ed. Norwalk, Conn.: Appleton and Lange, 2006.

Kierman, John A. *Barr's The Human Nervous System: An Anatomical Viewpoint*. 9th ed. Philadelphia: Wolters Kluwer/Lippincott Williams & Wilkins, 2009.

Nicholls, John G., A. Robert Martin, and Bruce G. Wallace. *From Neuron to Brain*. 4th ed. Sunderland, Mass.: Sinauer, 2007.

Noback, Charles R., et al. *The Human Nervous System: Structure and Function*. 6th ed. Totowa, N.J.: Humana Press, 2005.

Parsons, Malcolm, and Michael Johnson. *Diagnosis in Color: Neurology*. New York: Mosby, 2001.

Rowland, Lewis P., ed. *Merritt's Textbook of Neurology*. 12th ed. Philadelphia: Lippincott Williams & Wilkins, 2010.

Siegel, George J., et al., eds. *Basic Neurochemistry: Molecular, Cellular, and Medical Aspects*. 7th ed. Burlington, Vt.: Elsevier Academic, 2006.

Swaiman, Kenneth F., Stephen Ashwal, and Donna M. Ferriero, eds. *Pediatric Neurology: Principles and Practice*. 4th ed. Philadelphia: Mosby/Elsevier, 2006.

Victor, Maurice, and Allan H. Ropper. *Adams and Victor's Principles of Neurology*. 9th ed. New York: McGraw-Hill, 2009.

Volpe, Joseph. *Neurology of the Newborn*. 5th ed. Philadelphia: Saunders/Elsevier, 2008.

Waxman, Stephen G. *Correlative Neuroanatomy*. 25th ed. New York: Lange Medical Books/McGraw-Hill, 2002.

NURSING

Berman, Audrey, et al. *Kozier and Erb's Fundamentals of Nursing: Concepts, Process, and Practice*. 8th ed. Upper Saddle River, N.J.: Pearson/Prentice Hall, 2008.

Delaune, Sue C., and Patricia K. Ladner, eds. *Fundamentals of Nursing: Standards and Practices*. 4th ed. Clifton Park, N.Y.: Cengage Learning, 2010.

Ignatavicius, Donna D., and M. Linda Workman, eds. *Medical-Surgical Nursing: Critical Thinking for Collaborative Care*. 5th ed. Philadelphia: Saunders/Elsevier, 2006.

Nettina, Sandra M., ed. *The Lippincott Manual of Nursing Practice*. 8th ed. Philadelphia: Lippincott Williams & Wilkins, 2006.

Wilkinson, Judith M., and Karen Van Leuven. *Fundamentals of Nursing: Theory, Concepts, and Applications*. Philadelphia: F. A. Davis, 2007.

NUTRITION

Bales, Connie Watkins, and Christine Seel Ritchie, eds. *Handbook of Clinical Nutrition and Aging*. Totowa, N.J.: Humana Press, 2004.

Barasi, Mary. *Human Nutrition: A Health Perspective*. 2d ed. New York: Oxford University Press, 2003.

Bendich, Adrianne, and Richard J. Deckelbaum. *Preventive Nutrition: The Comprehensive Guide for Health Professionals*. 3d ed. Totowa, N.J.: Humana Press, 2005.

Clark, Nancy. *Nancy Clark's Sports Nutrition Guidebook*. 4th ed. Champaign, Ill.: Human Kinetics, 2008.

Duyff, Roberta Larson. *American Dietetic Association Complete Food and Nutrition Guide*. 3d ed. Hoboken, N.J.: John Wiley & Sons, 2007.

Garrow, J. S., W. P. T. James, and A. Ralph, eds. *Human Nutrition and Dietetics*. 10th ed. New York: Churchill Livingstone, 2000.

Geissler, Catherine A., and Hilary J. Powers, eds. *Hu-*

man Nutrition. 12th ed. New York: Churchill Livingstone/Elsevier, 2010.

Heimburger, Douglas C., and Jamy D. Ard. *Handbook of Clinical Nutrition.* 4th ed. Philadelphia: Mosby/Elsevier, 2006.

Kleinman, Ronald E., ed. *Pediatric Nutrition Handbook.* 5th ed. Elk Grove Village, Ill.: American Academy of Pediatrics, 2004.

Pennington, Jean A. T., and Judith Spungen Douglass. *Bowes and Church's Food Values of Portions Commonly Used.* 18th ed. Philadelphia: Lippincott Williams & Wilkins, 2005.

Shils, Maurice E., et al., eds. *Modern Nutrition in Health and Disease.* 10th ed. Philadelphia: Lippincott Williams & Wilkins, 2006.

Sizer, Frances Sienkiewicz, and Ellie Whitney. *Nutrition: Concepts and Controversies.* 10th ed. Belmont, Calif.: Thomson Wadsworth, 2006.

Wardlaw, Gordon M., and Anne M. Smith. *Contemporary Nutrition.* 7th ed. New York: McGraw-Hill, 2008.

Whitney, Ellie, and Sharon Rady Rolfes. *Understanding Nutrition.* 12th ed. Belmont, Calif.: Wadsworth, 2009.

ONCOLOGY

Bellenir, Karen, ed. *Cancer Sourcebook: Basic Consumer Health Information About Major Forms and Stages of Cancer.* 5th ed. Detroit: Omnigraphics, 2007.

De Vita, Vincent T., Jr., Samuel Hellman, and Steven A. Rosenberg, eds. *Cancer: Principles and Practice of Oncology.* 7th ed. Philadelphia: Lippincott Williams & Wilkins, 2005.

Dollinger, Malin, et al. *Everyone's Guide to Cancer Therapy.* 5th ed. Kansas City, Mo.: Andrews McMeel, 2008.

Eyre, Harmon J., Dianne Partie Lange, and Lois B. Morris. *Informed Decisions: The Complete Book of Cancer Diagnosis, Treatment, and Recovery.* 2d ed. Atlanta: American Cancer Society, 2002.

Fischer, David S., et al. *The Cancer Chemotherapy Handbook.* 6th ed. St. Louis, Mo.: Mosby, 2003.

Greaves, Mel. *Cancer: The Evolutionary Legacy.* New York: Oxford University Press, 2002.

Greene, Frederick L., et al., eds. *AJCC Cancer Staging Manual.* 6th ed. New York: Springer, 2002.

Hoskins, William J., et al., eds. *Principles and Practice of Gynecologic Oncology.* 4th ed. Philadelphia: Lippincott Williams & Wilkins, 2005.

Kufe, Donald W., et al., eds. *Holland Frei Cancer Medicine.* 7th ed. Hamilton, Ont.: B. C. Decker, 2006.

Pizzo, Philip A., and David G. Poplack, eds. *Principles and Practice of Pediatric Oncology.* 5th ed. Philadelphia: Lippincott Williams & Wilkins, 2006.

Sarg, Michael J., and Ann D. Gross. *The Cancer Dictionary.* 3d ed. New York: Checkmark Books, 2007.

Schottenfeld, David, and Joseph F. Fraumeni, Jr., eds. *Cancer Epidemiology and Prevention.* 3d ed. New York: Oxford University Press, 2006.

Weinberg, Robert. *The Biology of Cancer.* New York: Garland Science, 2007.

OPHTHALMOLOGY

Azar, Dimitri T. *Refractive Surgery.* 2d ed. Philadelphia: Mosby/Elsevier, 2007.

Buettner, Helmut, ed. *Mayo Clinic on Vision and Eye Health: Practical Answers on Glaucoma, Cataracts, Macular Degeneration, and Other Conditions.* Rochester, Minn.: Mayo Foundation for Medical Education and Research, 2002.

Galloway, N. R., et al. *Common Eye Diseases and Their Management.* 3d ed. London: Springer, 2006.

Johnson, Gordon J., et al., eds. *The Epidemiology of Eye Disease.* 2d ed. New York: Oxford University Press, 2003.

Kaufman, Paul L., and Albert Alm. *Adler's Physiology of the Eye: Clinical Application.* 10th ed. St. Louis, Mo.: Mosby, 2003.

Miller, Neil R., et al., eds. *Walsh and Hoyt's Clinical Neuro-ophthalmology.* 6th ed. Philadelphia: Lippincott Williams & Wilkins, 2005.

Nelson, Leonard B., and Scott E. Olitsky, eds. *Harley's Pediatric Ophthalmology.* 5th ed. Philadelphia: Lippincott Williams & Wilkins, 2005.

Palay, David A., and Jay H. Krachmer, eds. *Primary Care Ophthalmology.* 2d ed. Philadelphia: Mosby/Elsevier, 2006.

Riordan-Eva, Paul, and John P. Whitcher. *Vaughan and Asbury's General Ophthalmology.* 17th ed. New York: Lange Medical Books/McGraw-Hill, 2007.

Roy, Frederick Hampton. *Ocular Differential Diagnosis.* 7th ed. Philadelphia: Lippincott Williams & Wilkins, 2002.

Sardegna, Jill, et al. *Encyclopedia of Blindness and Vision Impairment.* 2d ed. New York: Facts On File, 2002.

Spaeth, George L., ed. *Ophthalmic Surgery: Principles and Practice.* 3d ed. Philadelphia: W. B. Saunders, 2003.

Steinert, Roger F., et al., eds. *Cataract Surgery: Techniques, Complications, and Management.* 2d ed. Philadelphia: W. B. Saunders, 2004.

Sutton, Amy L., ed. *Eye Care Sourcebook: Basic Consumer Health Information About Eye Care and Eye Disorders.* 3d ed. Detroit: Omnigraphics, 2008.

Yanoff, Myron, and Ben S. Fine. *Ocular Pathology.* 5th ed. Philadelphia: Mosby, 2002.

ORTHOPEDICS

Borenstein, David G., Sam W. Wiesel, and Scott D. Boden. *Low Back and Neck Pain: Comprehensive Diagnosis and Management.* 3d ed. Philadelphia: W. B. Saunders, 2004.

Bradford, David S., and Thomas A. Zdeblick, eds. *The Spine.* 2d ed. Philadelphia: Lippincott Williams & Wilkins, 2004.

Brotzman, S. Brent, and Kevin E. Wilk. *Clinical Orthopaedic Rehabilitation.* 2d ed. Philadelphia: Mosby, 2003.

Bucholz, Robert W., James D. Heckman, and Charles M. Court-Brown, eds. *Rockwood and Green's Fractures in Adults.* 6th ed. Philadelphia: Lippincott Williams & Wilkins, 2006.

Callaghan, John J., Aaron Rosenberg, and Harry E. Rubash, eds. *The Adult Hip.* 2d ed. Philadelphia: Lippincott Williams & Wilkins, 2007.

Canale, S. Terry, ed. *Campbell's Operative Orthopaedics.* 8th ed. 4 vols. St. Louis, Mo.: Mosby, 2003.

DeLee, Jesse C., and David Drez, Jr. *DeLee and Drez's Orthopaedic Sports Medicine: Principles and Practice.* 2d ed. Philadelphia: W. B. Saunders, 2003.

Delforge, Gary. *Musculoskeletal Trauma: Implications for Sport Injury Management.* Champaign, Ill.: Human Kinetics, 2002.

Magee, David J. *Orthopedic Physical Assessment.* 4th rev. ed. Philadelphia: Saunders/Elsevier, 2007.

Marcus, Robert, David Feldman, and Jennifer Kelsey, eds. *Osteoporosis.* 3d ed. Boston: Academic Press/Elsevier, 2008.

Morrissy, Raymond T., and Stuart L. Weinstein, eds. *Lovell and Winter's Pediatric Orthopaedics.* 6th ed. Philadelphia: Lippincott Williams & Wilkins, 2006.

Neuwirth, Michael, and Kevin Osborn. 2d ed. *The Scoliosis Sourcebook.* New York: McGraw-Hill, 2001.

Rockwood, Charles A., Frederick A. Matsen, and Michael Wirth. *The Shoulder.* 4th ed. 2 vols. St. Louis, Mo.: Saunders/Elsevier, 2009.

OTORHINOLARYNGOLOGY

Bluestone, Charles D., et al., eds. *Pediatric Otolaryngology.* 4th ed. 2 vols. Philadelphia: W. B. Saunders, 2003.

Calhoun, Karen, and David E. Eibling, eds. *Geriatric Otolaryngology.* New York: Taylor & Francis, 2006.

Ferrari, Mario. *PDxMD Ear, Nose, and Throat Disorders.* Philadelphia: PDxMD, 2003.

Hamid, Mohamed, and Aristides Sismanis, eds. *Medical Otology and Neurotology: A Clinical Guide to Auditory and Vestibular Disorders.* New York: Thieme, 2006.

Kennedy, David W., William E. Bolger, and S. James Zinreich, eds. *Diseases of the Sinuses: Diagnosis and Management.* Lewiston, N.Y.: B. C. Decker, 2001.

Lucente, Frank E., and Gady Har-El, eds. *Essentials of Otolaryngology.* 5th ed. Philadelphia: Lippincott Williams & Wilkins, 2004.

Ossoff, Robert H., et al., eds. *The Larynx.* Philadelphia: Lippincott Williams & Wilkins, 2003.

Snow, James B., Jr., and John Jacob Ballenger, eds. *Ballenger's Otorhinolaryngology: Head and Neck Surgery.* 16th ed. Baltimore: Williams & Wilkins, 2003.

Woodson, Gayle E. *Ear, Nose, and Throat Disorders in Primary Care.* Philadelphia: W. B. Saunders, 2001.

PALLIATIVE CARE

Berger, Ann M., John L. Shuster, Jr., and Jamie H. Von Roenn, eds. *Principles and Practice of Palliative Care and Supportive Oncology.* 3d ed. Philadelphia: Lippincott Williams & Wilkins, 2007.

Doyle, Derek, et al., eds. *Oxford Textbook of Palliative Medicine.* 3d ed. New York: Oxford University Press, 2004.

Faull, Christina, Yvonne H. Carter, and Lilian Daniels, eds. *Handbook of Palliative Care.* 2d ed. Malden, Mass.: Blackwell, 2005.

Hallenbeck, James L. *Palliative Care Perspectives.* New York: Oxford University Press, 2003.

Katz, Jeanne, and Sheila Peace, eds. *End of Life in Care Homes: A Palliative Care Approach.* New York: Oxford University Press, 2003.

MacDonald, Neil, et al., eds. *Palliative Medicine: A Case-Based Manual.* 2d ed. New York: Oxford University Press, 2005.

Morrison, R. Sean, and Diane E. Meier, eds. *Geriatric Palliative Care.* New York: Oxford University Press, 2003.

Woodruff, Roger. *Palliative Medicine: Evidence-Based Symptomatic and Supportive Care for Patients with Advanced Cancer.* 4th ed. New York: Oxford University Press, 2004.

PATHOLOGY

Bancroft, John D., and Marilyn Gamble, eds. *Theory and Practice of Histological Techniques.* 6th ed. New York: Churchill Livingstone/Elsevier, 2008.

Corrin, Bryan, and Andrew G. Nicholson. *Pathology of the Lungs.* 2d ed. New York: Churchill Livingstone/Elsevier, 2006.

Crowley, Leonard V. *Introduction to Human Disease: Pathology and Pathophysiology Correlations.* 8th ed. Sudbury, Mass.: Jones and Bartlett, 2010.

Geisinger, Kim R., et al. *Modern Cytopathology.* Philadelphia: Churchill Livingstone, 2004.

Jennette, J. Charles, et al., eds. *Heptinstall's Pathology of the Kidney.* 6th ed. 2 vols. Philadelphia: Lippincott Williams & Wilkins, 2007.

Kilpatrick, Scott E. *Diagnostic Musculoskeletal Surgical Pathology.* Philadelphia: W. B. Saunders, 2004.

Kumar, Vinay, et al., eds. *Robbins Basic Pathology.* 8th ed. Philadelphia: Saunders/Elsevier, 2007.

Kumar, Vinay, Abul K. Abbas, and Nelson Fausto, eds. *Robbins and Cotran Pathologic Basis of Disease.* 8th ed. Philadelphia: Saunders/Elsevier, 2010.

McCance, Kathryn L., and Sue M. Huether. *Pathophysiology: The Biologic Basis for Disease in Adults and Children.* 6th ed. St. Louis, Mo.: Mosby/Elsevier, 2010.

Majno, Guido, and Isabelle Joris. *Cells, Tissues, and Disease: Principles of General Pathology.* 2d ed. New York: Oxford University Press, 2004.

Mills, Stacey E., et al., eds. *Sternberg's Diagnostic Surgical Pathology.* 5th ed. 2 vols. Philadelphia: Wolters Kluwer Health/Lippincott Williams & Wilkins, 2010.

Rosai, Juan. *Rosai and Ackerman's Surgical Pathology.* 9th ed. 2 vols. New York: Mosby, 2004.

Stephens, Alan, James S. Lowe, and Barbara Young, eds. *Wheater's Basic Histopathology: A Color Atlas and Text.* 4th ed. New York: Churchill Livingstone, 2002.

Stocker, J. Thomas, and Louis P. Dehner, eds. *Pediatric Pathology.* 2d ed. Philadelphia: Lippincott Williams & Wilkins, 2001.

Underwood, J. C. E., ed. *General and Systematic Pathology.* 4th ed. New York: Churchill Livingstone, 2004.

PATIENT EDUCATION

American Medical Association. *American Medical Association Family Medical Guide.* 4th rev. ed. Hoboken, N.J.: John Wiley & Sons, 2004.

Bartlett, John G., and Ann K. Finkbeiner. *The Guide to Living with HIV Infection: Developed at the Johns Hopkins AIDS Clinic.* 6th ed. Baltimore: Johns Hopkins University Press, 2007.

Blaivas, Jerry G. *Conquering Bladder and Prostate Problems: The Authoritative Guide for Men and Women.* Rev. ed. Cambridge, Mass.: Da Capo Press, 2001.

Bloom, Floyd E., M. Flint Beal, and David J. Kupfer, eds. *The Dana Guide to Brain Health.* New York: Dana Press, 2006.

Carlson, Karen J., Stephanie A. Eisenstat, and Terra Ziporyn. *The New Harvard Guide to Women's Health.* Cambridge, Mass.: Harvard University Press, 2004.

Conlon, Patrick. *The Essential Hospital Handbook: How to Be an Effective Partner in a Loved One's Care.* New Haven, Conn.: Yale University Press, 2009.

Dollinger, Malin, et al. *Everyone's Guide to Cancer Therapy.* 5th ed. Kansas City, Mo.: Andrews McMeel, 2008.

Duvoisin, Roger C., and Jacob Sage. *Parkinson's Disease: A Guide for Patient and Family.* 5th ed. Philadelphia: Lippincott Williams & Wilkins, 2001.

Foltz-Gray, Dorothy. *The Arthritis Foundation's Guide to Good Living with Rheumatoid Arthritis.* 3d ed. Atlanta: Arthritis Foundation, 2006.

Jackson, Marilynn. *Pocket Guide for Patient Education.* Sudbury, Mass.: Jones and Bartlett, 2009.

Keene, Nancy. *Childhood Leukemia: A Guide for Families, Friends, and Caregivers.* 4th ed. Sebastopol, Calif.: O'Reilly, 2010.

Komaroff, Anthony, ed. *Harvard Medical School Family Health Guide.* New York: Free Press, 2005.

Kushner, Thomasine Kimbrough. *Surviving Healthcare: A Manual for Patients and Their Families.* New York: Cambridge University Press, 2010.

Lorig, Kate, et al. *Patient Education: A Practical Approach.* 3d ed. Thousand Oaks, Calif.: Sage, 2000.

Moore, Stephen W. *Griffith's Instructions for Patients.* 7th ed. Philadelphia: Saunders/Elsevier, 2005.

Porter, Robert S., et al., eds. *The Merck Manual Home Health Handbook.* Whitehouse Station, N.J.: Merck Research Laboratories, 2009.

Saudek, Christopher D., Richard R. Rubin, and Cynthia S. Shump. *The Johns Hopkins Guide to Diabetes: For Today and Tomorrow*. Baltimore: Johns Hopkins University Press, 2001.

Woolf, Alan D., et al., eds. *The Children's Hospital Guide to Your Child's Health and Development*. Cambridge, Mass.: Perseus, 2002.

PEDIATRICS

Behrman, Richard E., Robert M. Kliegman, and Hal B. Jenson, eds. *Nelson Textbook of Pediatrics*. 18th ed. Philadelphia: Saunders/Elsevier, 2007.

Burg, Fredric D., et al. *Gellis and Kagan's Current Pediatric Therapy*. 18th ed. Philadelphia: Saunders/Elsevier, 2006.

Cloherty, John P., Eric C. Eichenwald, and Ann R. Stark, eds. *Manual of Neonatal Care*. 5th ed. Philadelphia: Lippincott Williams & Wilkins, 2004.

Custer, Jason W., and Rachel E. Rau, eds. *The Harriet Lane Handbook: A Manual for Pediatric House Officers*. 18th ed. Philadelphia: Mosby/Elsevier, 2009.

Finberg, Laurence, and Ronald E. Kleinman, eds. *Saunders Manual of Pediatric Practice*. 2d ed. Philadelphia: W. B. Saunders, 2002.

Gomella, Tricia Lacy, et al., eds. *Neonatology: Management, Procedures, On-Call Problems, Diseases, and Drugs*. 5th ed. New York: Lange Medical Books/McGraw-Hill, 2004.

Greydanus, Donald E., Dilip R. Patel, and Helen D. Pratt, eds. *Behavioral Pediatrics*. 3d ed. 2 vols. New York: Nova Biomedical, 2009.

Hay, William W., Jr., et al., eds. *Current Diagnosis and Treatment in Pediatrics*. 18th ed. New York: Lange Medical Books/McGraw-Hill, 2009.

Hoekelman, Robert A., et al., eds. *Primary Pediatric Care*. 4th ed. St. Louis, Mo.: Mosby, 2001.

Kemper, Kathi J. *The Holistic Pediatrician: A Pediatrician's Comprehensive Guide to Safe and Effective Therapies for the Twenty-five Most Common Ailments of Infants, Children, and Adolescents*. Rev. ed. New York: Quill, 2002.

Kimball, Chad T. *Childhood Diseases and Disorders Sourcebook: Basic Consumer Health Information About Medical Problems Often Encountered in Preadolescent Children*. Detroit: Omnigraphics, 2003.

Long, Sarah S., Larry K. Pickering, and Charles G. Prober, eds. *Principles and Practice of Pediatric Infectious Diseases*. 3d ed. Philadelphia: Churchill Livingstone/Elsevier, 2008.

MacDonald, Mhairi G., Mary M. K. Seshia, and Martha D. Mullett, eds. *Avery's Neonatology: Pathophysiology and Management of the Newborn*. 6th ed. Philadelphia: Lippincott Williams & Wilkins, 2005.

McMillan, Julia A., et al., eds. *Oski's Pediatrics: Principles and Practice*. 4th ed. Philadelphia: Lippincott Williams & Wilkins, 2006.

Martin, Richard J., Avroy A. Fanaroff, and Michele C. Walsh, eds. *Fanaroff and Martin's Neonatal-Perinatal Medicine: Diseases of the Fetus and Infant*. 8th ed. 2 vols. Philadelphia: Mosby/Elsevier, 2006.

Merenstein, Gerald B., and Sandra L. Gardner, eds. *Handbook of Neonatal Intensive Care*. 6th ed. St. Louis, Mo.: Mosby/Elsevier, 2006.

Neinstein, Lawrence S. *Adolescent Health Care: A Practical Guide*. 5th ed. Philadelphia: Wolters Kluwer/Lippincott Williams & Wilkins, 2008.

Rudolph, Colin D., and Abraham M. Rudolph, eds. *Rudolph's Pediatrics*. 21st ed. New York: McGraw-Hill, 2003.

Sanghavi, Darshak. *A Map of the Child: A Pediatrician's Tour of the Body*. New York: Henry Holt, 2003.

Taeusch, H. William, Roberta A. Ballard, and Christine A. Gleason, eds. *Avery's Diseases of the Newborn*. 8th ed. Philadelphia: Saunders/Elsevier, 2005.

Tobias, Joseph D., and Jayant K. Deshpande, eds. *Pediatric Pain Management for Primary Care*. 2d ed. Elk Grove Village, Ill.: American Academy of Pediatrics, 2005.

PHARMACOLOGY AND THERAPEUTICS

Allen, Loyd V., Jr., Nicholas G. Popovich, and Howard C. Ansel. *Ansel's Pharmaceutical Dosage Forms and Drug Delivery Systems*. 9th ed. Philadelphia: Lippincott Williams & Wilkins, 2010.

American Pharmaceutical Association. *Handbook of Nonprescription Drugs*. 15th ed. Washington, D.C.: Author, 2006.

Brunton, Laurence L., et al., eds. *Goodman and Gilman's The Pharmacological Basis of Therapeutics*. 11th ed. New York: McGraw-Hill, 2006.

Craig, Charles R., and Robert E. Stitzel, eds. *Modern Pharmacology with Clinical Applications*. 6th ed. Philadelphia: Lippincott Williams & Wilkins, 2004.

Griffith, H. Winter. *Complete Guide to Prescription and Nonprescription Drugs*. Revised and updated by Stephen Moore. New York: Penguin Group, 2010.

Hansten, Philip D., and John R. Horn. *Drug Interactions, Analysis, and Management 2007*. St. Louis, Mo.: Facts and Comparisons, 2007.

Julien, Robert M. *A Primer of Drug Action: A Concise, Nontechnical Guide to the Actions, Uses, and Side Effects of Psychoactive Drugs.* 11th ed. New York: Freeman, 2008.

Katzung, Bertram G., et al., eds. *Basic and Clinical Pharmacology.* 11th ed. New York: McGraw-Hill, 2009.

Keltner, Norman L., and David G. Folks. *Psychotropic Drugs.* 4th ed. St. Louis, Mo.: Mosby/Elsevier, 2005.

Lacy, Charles F., et al. *The Drug Information Handbook.* 17th ed. Hudson, Ohio: Lexi-Comp, 2008.

Liska, Ken. *Drugs and the Human Body, with Implications for Society.* 8th ed. Upper Saddle River, N.J.: Pearson/Prentice Hall, 2009.

McCormack, Rango, et al., eds. *Drug Therapy: Decision Making Guide.* Philadelphia: Saunders/Elsevier, 2007.

PDR for Nonprescription Drugs, Dietary Supplements, and Herbs. 31st ed. Montvale, N.J.: PDR Network, 2010.

PDR Guide to Drug Interactions, Side Effects, and Indications. 63d ed. Montvale, N.J.: PDR, 2008.

Physicians' Desk Reference. 64th ed. Montvale, N.J.: PDR Network, 2009.

Rang, H. P., and Maureen M. Dale. *Rang and Dale's Pharmacology.* 6th ed. New York: Churchill Livingstone/Elsevier, 2007.

Youngkin, Ellis Quinn, et al. *Pharmacotherapeutics: A Primary Care Clinical Guide.* 2d ed. Upper Saddle River, N.J.: Pearson/Prentice Hall, 2005.

Zucchero, Frederic J., et al., eds. *Pocket Guide to Evaluations of Drug Interactions.* 6th ed. Washington, D.C.: American Pharmaceutical Association, 2006.

PHYSICAL MEDICINE AND REHABILITATION

Cameron, Michelle H. *Physical Agents in Rehabilitation: From Research to Practice.* 3d ed. St. Louis, Mo.: Saunders/Elsevier, 2009.

DeLisa, Joel A., et al., eds. *Physical Medicine and Rehabilitation: Principles and Practice.* 4th ed. Philadelphia: Lippincott Williams & Wilkins, 2005.

Garrison, Susan J. *Handbook of Physical Medicine and Rehabilitation Basics.* 2d ed. Philadelphia: Lippincott Williams & Wilkins, 2003.

Kumbhare, Dinesh A., and John V. Basmajian, eds. *Decision Making and Outcomes in Sports Rehabilitation.* New York: Churchill Livingstone, 2000.

Lusardi, Michelle M., and Caroline C. Nielsen. *Orthotics and Prosthetics in Rehabilitation.* 2d ed. St. Louis, Mo.: Saunders/Elsevier, 2007.

Neumann, Donald A. *Kinesiology of the Musculoskeletal System: Foundations for Rehabilitation.* 2d ed. St. Louis, Mo.: Mosby/Elsevier, 2010.

O'Sullivan, Susan, and Thomas J. Schmitz, eds. *Physical Rehabilitation: Assessment and Treatment.* 4th ed. Philadelphia: F. A. Davis, 2001.

Pease, William S., Henry L. Lew, and Ernest W. Johnson, eds. *Johnson's Practical Electromyography.* 4th ed. Philadelphia: Lippincott Williams & Wilkins, 2007.

Tan, Jackson C. *Practical Manual of Physical Medicine and Rehabilitation.* 2d ed. St. Louis, Mo.: Mosby/Elsevier, 2006.

PHYSIOLOGY

Fox, Stuart Ira. *Human Physiology.* 11th ed. Boston: McGraw-Hill, 2010.

Ganong, William F. *Review of Medical Physiology.* 23d ed. New York: Lange Medical Books/McGraw-Hill Medical, 2009.

Guyton, Arthur C., and John E. Hall. *Guyton and Hall Textbook of Medical Physiology.* 12th ed. Philadelphia: Saunders/Elsevier, 2011.

Johnson, Leonard R., ed. *Essential Medical Physiology.* 3d ed. Boston: Academic Press/Elsevier, 2003.

Koeppen, Bruce M., and Bruce A. Stanton, eds. *Berne and Levy Physiology.* 6th ed. St. Louis, Mo.: Mosby/Elsevier, 2010.

Marieb, Elaine N. *Essentials of Human Anatomy and Physiology.* 9th ed. San Francisco: Pearson/Benjamin Cummings, 2009.

Rhoades, Rodney, and Richard Pflanzer. *Human Physiology.* 4th ed. Pacific Grove, Calif.: Brooks/Cole, 2003.

Scanlon, Valerie, and Tina Sanders. *Essentials of Anatomy and Physiology.* 5th ed. Philadelphia: F. A. Davis, 2007.

Seeley, Rod R., Trent D. Stephens, and Philip Tate. *Anatomy and Physiology.* 7th ed. New York: McGraw-Hill, 2006.

Sherwood, Lauralee. *Human Physiology: From Cells to Systems.* 7th ed. Pacific Grove, Calif.: Brooks/Cole/Cengage Learning, 2010.

Shier, David N., Jackie L. Butler, and Ricki Lewis. *Hole's Essentials of Human Anatomy and Physiology.* 10th ed. Boston: McGraw-Hill, 2009.

Thibodeau, Gary A., and Kevin T. Patton. *Anatomy and Physiology.* 7th ed. St. Louis, Mo.: Mosby/Elsevier, 2009.

Tortora, Gerard J., and Bryan Derrickson. *Principles of*

Anatomy and Physiology. 12th ed. Hoboken, N.J.: John Wiley & Sons, 2009.

PREVENTIVE MEDICINE AND PUBLIC HEALTH

Hales, Dianne. *An Invitation to Health Brief.* Updated ed. Belmont, Calif.: Wadsworth/Cengage Learning, 2010.

Koren, Herman. *Illustrated Dictionary and Resource Directory of Environmental and Occupational Health.* 2d ed. Boca Raton, Fla.: CRC Press, 2005.

Lee, Philip R., and Carroll L. Estes, eds. *The Nation's Health.* 7th ed. Sudbury, Mass.: Jones and Bartlett, 2003.

Levy, Barry S., et al., eds. *Occupational Health: Recognizing and Preventing Disease and Injury.* 5th ed. Philadelphia: Lippincott Williams & Wilkins, 2006.

Moeller, Dade W. *Environmental Health.* 3d ed. Cambridge, Mass.: Harvard University Press, 2005.

Rom, William N., ed. *Environmental and Occupational Medicine.* 4th ed. Philadelphia: Wolters Kluwer/Lippincott Williams & Wilkins, 2007.

Wallace, Robert B., ed. *Maxcy-Rosenau-Last Public Health and Preventive Medicine.* 15th ed. New York: McGraw-Hill, 2008.

PRIMARY HEALTH CARE. *See* FAMILY MEDICINE; INTERNAL MEDICINE

PSYCHIATRY

American Psychiatric Association. *Diagnostic and Statistical Manual of Mental Disorders: DSM-IV-TR.* 4th ed. Washington, D.C.: Author, 2000.

Andreasen, Nancy C., and Donald W. Black. *Introductory Textbook of Psychiatry.* 4th ed. Washington, D.C.: American Psychiatric Press, 2006.

Birren, James E., and K. Warner Schaie, eds. *Handbook of the Psychology of Aging.* 6th ed. Boston: Academic Press/Elsevier, 2007.

Blazer, Dan G., David C. Steffens, and Ewald W. Busse, eds. *The American Psychiatric Publishing Textbook of Geriatric Psychiatry.* 4th ed. Washington, D.C.: American Psychiatric Publishing, 2009.

Breedlove, S. Marc, Mark R. Rosenzweig, and Neil V. Watson. *Biological Psychology: An Introduction to Behavioral, Cognitive, and Clinical Neuroscience.* 5th rev. ed. Sunderland, Mass.: Sinauer Associates, 2007.

Davison, Gerald C., and John M. Neale. *Abnormal Psychology.* 9th ed. New York: John Wiley & Sons, 2003.

Goldman, Howard H., ed. *Review of General Psychiatry.* 5th ed. New York: Lange Medical Books/McGraw-Hill, 2000.

Kring, Ann M., et al. *Abnormal Psychology.* 11th ed. Hoboken, N.J.: John Wiley & Sons, 2010.

Lewis, Melvin, ed. *Child and Adolescent Psychiatry: A Comprehensive Textbook.* 4th ed. Philadelphia: Lippincott Williams & Wilkins, 2007.

Oltmanns, Thomas F., et al. *Case Studies in Abnormal Psychology.* 8th ed. Hoboken, N.J.: John Wiley & Sons, 2009.

Rundell, James R., and Michael G. Wise, eds. *The American Psychiatric Press Textbook of Consultation-Liaison Psychiatry.* 2d ed. Washington, D.C.: American Psychiatric Press, 2002.

Sadock, Benjamin J., and Virginia A. Sadock, eds. *Kaplan and Sadock's Comprehensive Textbook of Psychiatry.* 8th ed. Philadelphia: Lippincott Williams & Wilkins, 2005.

Stern, Theodore A., et al., eds. *Massachusetts General Hospital Handbook of General Hospital Psychiatry.* 5th ed. St. Louis, Mo.: Mosby, 2004.

Wiener, Jerry M., and Mina K. Dulcan, eds. *Textbook of Child and Adolescent Psychiatry.* 3d ed. Washington, D.C.: American Psychiatric Publishing, 2004.

Yudofsky, Stuart C., and Robert E. Hales, eds. *The American Psychiatric Publishing Textbook of Neuropsychiatry and Clinical Neurosciences.* 4th ed. Washington, D.C.: American Psychiatric Publishing, 2002.

RADIOLOGY AND IMAGING

Bontrager, Kenneth, and John P. Lampignano. *Textbook of Radiographic Positioning and Related Anatomy.* 7th ed. St. Louis, Mo.: Mosby/Elsevier, 2010.

Bragg, David G., Philip Rubin, and Hedvig Hricak, eds. *Oncologic Imaging.* 2d ed. Philadelphia: W. B. Saunders, 2002.

Cherry, Simon R., James A. Sorenson, and Michael E. Phelps. *Physics in Nuclear Medicine.* 3d ed. Philadelphia: W. B. Saunders, 2003.

Christian, Paul E., Donald Bernier, and James K. Langan, eds. *Nuclear Medicine and PET: Technology and Techniques.* 5th ed. St. Louis, Mo.: Mosby, 2004.

Eisenberg, Ronald L. *Clinical Imaging: An Atlas of Differential Diagnosis.* 4th ed. Philadelphia: Lippincott Williams & Wilkins, 2003.

_____. *Gastrointestinal Radiology: A Pattern Approach.* 4th ed. Philadelphia: Lippincott Williams & Wilkins, 2002.

Halperin, Edward C., et al., eds. *Pediatric Radiation Oncology.* 4th ed. Philadelphia: Lippincott Williams & Wilkins, 2005.

Hendee, William R., Geoffrey S. Ibbott, and Eric G. Hendee. *Radiation Therapy Physics.* 3d ed. Hoboken, N.J.: John Wiley & Sons, 2005.

Kopans, Daniel B. *Breast Imaging.* 3d ed. Baltimore: Lippincott Williams & Wilkins, 2007.

Lee, Joseph K. T., et al., eds. *Computed Body Tomography with MRI Correlation.* 4th ed. Philadelphia: Lippincott Williams & Wilkins, 2006.

Mettler, Fred A., Jr., and Milton J. Guiberteau. *Essentials of Nuclear Medicine Imaging.* 5th ed. Philadelphia: Saunders/Elsevier, 2006.

Novelline, Robert A. *Squire's Fundamentals of Radiology.* 6th ed. Cambridge, Mass.: Harvard University Press, 2004.

Perez, Carlos A., et al., eds. *Principles and Practice of Radiation Oncology.* 4th ed. Philadelphia: Lippincott Williams & Wilkins, 2004.

Reed, James C. *Chest Radiology: Plain Film Patterns and Differential Diagnoses.* 5th ed. Philadelphia: Mosby, 2003.

Resnick, Donald, and Mark J. Kransdorf. *Bone and Joint Imaging.* 3d ed. Philadelphia: Saunders/Elsevier, 2005.

Rumack, Carol M., Stephanie R. Wilson, and J. William Charboneau, eds. *Diagnostic Ultrasound.* 3d ed. St. Louis, Mo.: Mosby/Elsevier, 2005.

Saha, Gopal B. *Physics and Radiobiology of Nuclear Medicine.* 3d ed. New York: Springer, 2006.

Sandler, Martin P., R. Edward Coleman, and James A. Patton, eds. *Diagnostic Nuclear Medicine.* 4th ed. Philadelphia: Lippincott Williams & Wilkins, 2003.

Som, Peter M., and Hugh D. Curtin, eds. *Head and Neck Imaging.* 4th ed. St. Louis, Mo.: Mosby, 2003.

Stoller, David W. *Magnetic Resonance Imaging in Orthopaedic and Sports Medicine.* 3d ed. Philadelphia: Lippincott Williams & Wilkins, 2006.

Weissleder, Ralph, et al. *Primer of Diagnostic Imaging.* 4th ed. Philadelphia: Mosby/Elsevier, 2007.

White, Stuart C., and Michael J. Pharaoh, eds. *Oral Radiology: Principles and Interpretation.* 5th ed. St. Louis, Mo.: Mosby, 2004.

RESPIRATORY SYSTEM

Adams, Francis V. *The Asthma Sourcebook.* 3d ed. New York: McGraw-Hill, 2007.

Barnes, Peter J., and Simon Godfrey. *Asthma.* 2d ed. London: Martin Dunitz, 2000.

Bordow, Richard A., Andrew L. Ries, and Timothy A. Morris, eds. *The Manual of Clinical Problems in Pulmonary Medicine.* 6th ed. Philadelphia: Lippincott Williams & Wilkins, 2005.

Chernick, Victor, et al., eds. *Kendig's Disorders of the Respiratory Tract in Children.* 7th ed. Philadelphia: Saunders/Elsevier, 2006.

Corrin, Bryan, and Andrew G. Nicholson. *Pathology of the Lungs.* 2d ed. New York: Churchill Livingstone/Elsevier, 2006.

Crapo, James D., et al., eds. *Baum's Textbook of Pulmonary Diseases.* 7th ed. Philadelphia: Lippincott Williams & Wilkins, 2004.

Fishman, Alfred P. *Fishman's Manual of Pulmonary Diseases and Disorders.* 3d ed. New York: McGraw-Hill, 2002.

Hagberg, Carin A., ed. *Benumof's Airway Management: Principles and Practice.* 2d ed. Philadelphia: Mosby/Elsevier, 2007.

Hansel, Trevor, and Peter J. Barnes. *An Atlas of Chronic Obstructive Pulmonary Disease.* Boca Raton, Fla.: Pantheon, 2004.

Levitzky, Michael G. *Pulmonary Physiology.* 7th ed. New York: McGraw-Hill Medical, 2007.

Mason, Robert J., et al., eds. *Murray and Nadel's Textbook of Respiratory Medicine.* 5th ed. Philadelphia: Saunders/Elsevier, 2010.

West, John B. *Pulmonary Pathophysiology: The Essentials.* 7th ed. Philadelphia: Wolters Kluwer/Lippincott Williams & Wilkins, 2008.

RHEUMATOLOGY

Clements, Philip J., and Daniel E. Furst, eds. *Systemic Sclerosis.* 2d ed. Philadelphia: Lippincott Williams & Wilkins, 2004.

Harris, Edward D., Jr., et al., eds. *Kelley's Textbook of Rheumatology.* 7th ed. Philadelphia: Saunders/Elsevier, 2005.

Isenberg, David A., et al., eds. *Oxford Textbook of Rheumatology.* 3d ed. New York: Oxford University Press, 2004.

Klippel, John H., ed. *Primer on the Rheumatic Diseases.* 13th ed. New York: Springer, 2008.

Koopman, William J., and Larry W. Moreland, eds. *Arthritis and Allied Conditions: A Textbook of Rheumatology.* 15th ed. Philadelphia: Lippincott Williams & Wilkins, 2005.

Lahita, Robert G. *Rheumatoid Arthritis: Everything You Need to Know.* Rev. ed. New York: Avery, 2004.

Sontheimer, Richard D., and Thomas T. Provost, eds.

Cutaneous Manifestations of Rheumatic Diseases. 2d ed. Philadelphia: Lippincott Williams & Wilkins, 2004.

Wallace, Daniel J., and Bevra Hannahs Hahn, eds. *Dubois' Lupus Erythematosus.* 7th ed. Philadelphia: Lippincott Williams & Wilkins, 2007.

SEXUALLY TRANSMITTED DISEASES (STDs). *See also* ACQUIRED IMMUNODEFICIENCY SYNDROME (AIDS)

Centers for Disease Control and Prevention. *The National Plan to Eliminate Syphilis from the United States.* Atlanta: U.S. Department of Health and Human Services, 2006.

———. *Sexually Transmitted Diseases Treatment Guidelines 2006.* Atlanta: U.S. Department of Health and Human Services, 2006.

Faro, Sebastian. *Sexually Transmitted Diseases in Women.* Philadelphia: Lippincott Williams & Wilkins, 2003.

Larsen, Laura. *Sexually Transmitted Diseases Sourcebook.* Detroit: Omnigraphics, 2009.

McCance, Dennis J., ed. *Human Papilloma Viruses.* New York: Elsevier Science, 2002.

Morse, Stephen A., Ronald C. Ballard, and King K. Holmes. *Atlas of Sexually Transmitted Diseases and AIDS.* 3d ed. New York: Mosby, 2003.

Shoquist, Jennifer, and Diane Stafford. *Encyclopedia of Sexually Transmitted Diseases.* New York: Facts On File, 2003.

Stanberry, Lawrence R., and David I. Bernstein, eds. *Sexually Transmitted Diseases: Vaccines, Prevention, and Control.* San Diego, Calif.: Academic Press, 2000.

Stine, Gerald J. *AIDS Update 2010.* New York: McGraw-Hill Higher Education, 2010.

SPORTS MEDICINE

American College of Sports Medicine. *ACSM's Guidelines for Exercise Testing and Prescription.* 8th ed. Philadelphia: Lippincott Williams & Wilkins, 2010.

Beim, Gloria, and Ruth Winter. *The Female Athlete's Body Book: How to Prevent and Treat Sports Injuries in Women and Girls.* Chicago: Contemporary Books, 2003.

Clark, Nancy. *Nancy Clark's Sports Nutrition Guidebook.* 4th ed. Champaign, Ill.: Human Kinetics, 2008.

Echemendía, Ruben J., ed. *Sports Neuropsychology: Assessment and Management of Traumatic Brain Injury.* New York: Guilford Press, 2006.

Foss, Merle L. *Fox's Physiological Basis for Exercise and Sport.* 6th ed. New York: McGraw-Hill, 2001.

Landry, Gregory L., and David T. Bernhardt. *Essentials of Primary Care Sports Medicine.* Champaign, Ill.: Human Kinetics, 2003.

McArdle, William, Frank I. Katch, and Victor L. Katch. *Exercise Physiology: Energy, Nutrition, and Human Performance.* 7th ed. Boston: Lippincott Williams & Wilkins, 2010.

MacAuley, Domhnall. *Oxford Handbook of Sports and Exercise Medicine.* New York: Oxford University Press, 2007.

Mellion, Morris B., et al., eds. *The Team Physician's Handbook.* 3d ed. New York: Elsevier, 2001.

Noakes, Tim, and Stephen Granger. *Running Injuries: How to Prevent and Overcome Them.* 3d ed. New York: Oxford University Press, 2003.

Norris, Christopher M. *Sports Injuries: Diagnosis and Management.* 3d ed. New York: Butterworth Heinemann, 2004.

Pfeiffer, Ronald P., and Brent C. Mangus. *Concepts of Athletic Training.* 5th ed. Sudbury, Mass.: Jones and Bartlett, 2008.

Plowman, Sharon A., and Denise L. Smith. *Exercise Physiology for Health, Fitness, and Performance.* New York: Wolters Kluwer/Lippincott Williams & Wilkins, 2008.

Powers, Scott K., and Edward T. Howley. *Exercise Physiology: Theory and Application to Fitness and Performance.* 7th ed. New York: McGraw-Hill, 2009.

Scuderi, Giles R., and Peter D. McCann, eds. *Sports Medicine: A Comprehensive Approach.* 2d ed. Philadelphia: Mosby/Elsevier, 2005.

STATISTICS

Chernick, Michael R., and Robert H. Friis. *Introductory Biostatistics for the Health Sciences: Modern Applications Including Bootstrap.* Hoboken, N.J.: Wiley-Interscience, 2003.

D'Agostino, Ralph B., Sr., Lisa M. Sullivan, and Alexa S. Beiser. *Introductory Applied Biostatistics.* Belmont, Calif.: Thomson/Brooks/Cole, 2005.

Daniel, Wayne W. *Biostatistics: A Foundation for Analysis in the Health Sciences.* 9th ed. Hoboken, N.J.: John Wiley & Sons, 2009.

Glantz, Stanton A. *Primer of Biostatistics.* 6th ed. New York: McGraw-Hill, 2005.

Hebel, J. Richard, and Robert J. McCarter. *A Study Guide to Epidemiology and Biostatistics.* 6th ed. Sudbury, Mass.: Jones and Bartlett, 2006.

Le, Chap T. *Health and Numbers: Problems-Based Introduction to Biostatistics.* Malden, Mass.: Blackwell, 2009.

Wassertheil-Smoller, Sylvia. *Biostatistics and Epidemiology: A Primer for Health and Biomedical Professionals.* 3d ed. New York: Springer, 2004.

SUBSTANCE ABUSE

Gahlinger, Paul M. *Illegal Drugs: A Complete Guide to Their History, Chemistry, Use, and Abuse.* Updated and rev. ed. New York: Plume, 2004.

Galanter, Marc, and Herbert D. Kleber, eds. *The American Psychiatric Publishing Textbook of Substance Abuse Treatment.* 3d ed. Washington, D.C.: American Psychiatric Publishing, 2004.

Kuhn, Cynthia, et al. *Buzzed: The Straight Facts About the Most Used and Abused Drugs from Alcohol to Ecstasy.* 3d ed. New York: W. W. Norton, 2008.

Liddle, Howard A., and Cynthia L. Rowe, eds. *Adolescent Substance Abuse: Research and Clinical Advances.* New York: Cambridge University Press, 2006.

Lowinson, Joyce H., et al., eds. *Substance Abuse: A Comprehensive Textbook.* 4th ed. Philadelphia: Lippincott Williams & Wilkins, 2005.

Maisto, Stephen A., Mark Galizio, and Gerard J. Connors. *Drug Use and Abuse.* 4th ed. Belmont, Calif.: Thomson/Wadsworth, 2004.

Rogers, Peter D., and Richard B. Heyman, eds. *Addiction Medicine: Adolescent Substance Abuse.* Philadelphia: W. B. Saunders, 2002.

Weil, Andrew, and Winifred Rosen. *From Chocolate to Morphine: Everything You Need to Know About Mind-Altering Drugs.* Rev. and updated ed. New York: Houghton Mifflin, 2004.

SURGERY

Ashcraft, Keith W., George Whitfield Holcomb, and J. Patrick Murphy, eds. *Pediatric Surgery.* 4th ed. Philadelphia: Saunders/Elsevier, 2005.

Brunicardi, F. Charles, et al., eds. *Schwartz's Principles of Surgery.* 9th ed. New York: McGraw-Hill, 2010.

Callery, Mark P., ed. *Handbook of Reoperative General Surgery.* Malden, Mass.: Blackwell, 2006.

Cameron, John L., ed. *Current Surgical Therapy.* 8th ed. Philadelphia: Mosby/Elsevier, 2004.

Cohn, Lawrence H., and L. Henry Edmunds, Jr., eds. *Cardiac Surgery in the Adult.* 2d ed. New York: McGraw-Hill, 2003.

Corman, Marvin L. *Colon and Rectal Surgery.* 5th ed. Philadelphia: Lippincott Williams & Wilkins, 2005.

Doherty, Gerard M., and Lawrence W. Way, eds. *Current Surgical Diagnosis and Treatment.* 12th ed. New York: Lange Medical Books/McGraw-Hill, 2006.

Fischer, Joseph E., et al., eds. *Mastery of Surgery.* 5th ed. Philadelphia: Wolters Kluwer Health/Lippincott Williams & Wilkins, 2007.

Fuller, Joanna Kotcher. *Surgical Technology: Principles and Practice.* 4th ed. St. Louis, Mo.: Saunders/Elsevier, 2005.

Graham, Sam D., Jr., et al., eds. *Glenn's Urologic Surgery.* 7th ed. Philadelphia: Lippincott Williams & Wilkins, 2009.

Griffith, H. Winter. *Complete Guide to Symptoms, Illness, and Surgery.* Revised and updated by Stephen Moore and Kenneth Yoder. 5th ed. New York: Perigee, 2006.

Khonsari, Siavosh, and Colleen Sintek. *Cardiac Surgery: Safeguards and Pitfalls in Operative Technique.* 3d ed. Philadelphia: Lippincott Williams & Wilkins, 2003.

Lubin, Michael F., ed. *Medical Management of the Surgical Patient: A Textbook of Perioperative Medicine.* 4th ed. New York: Cambridge University Press, 2006.

Moore, Ernest E., David V. Feliciano, and Kenneth L. Mattox. eds. *Trauma.* 5th ed. New York: McGraw-Hill, 2004.

Mulholland, Michael W., et al., eds. *Greenfield's Surgery: Scientific Principles and Practice.* 4th ed. Philadelphia: Lippincott Williams & Wilkins, 2006.

O'Neill, James A., Jr., et al., eds. *Principles of Pediatric Surgery.* 2d ed. St. Louis, Mo.: Mosby, 2004.

Rothrock, Jane C., ed. *Alexander's Care of the Patient in Surgery.* 13th ed. St. Louis, Mo.: Mosby/Elsevier, 2007.

Rutherford, Robert B., ed. *Vascular Surgery.* 6th ed. Philadelphia: Saunders/Elsevier, 2005.

Sellke, Frank W., et al., eds. *Sabiston and Spencer Surgery of the Chest.* 7th ed. Philadelphia: Saunders/Elsevier, 2005.

Townsend, Courtney M., Jr., et al., eds. *Sabiston Textbook of Surgery.* 18th ed. Philadelphia: Saunders/Elsevier, 2008.

Wilmore, Douglas W., et al., eds. *Scientific American Surgery 2006.* New York: Scientific American, 2007.

Yuh, David D., Luca A. Vricella, and William A. Baumgartner, eds. *The Johns Hopkins Manual of*

3360 • GENERAL BIBLIOGRAPHY

Cardiothoracic Surgery. New York: McGraw-Hill, 2007.

Zollinger, Robert M., Jr., and Robert M. Zollinger, Sr. Zollinger's Atlas of Surgical Operations. 8th ed. New York: McGraw-Hill, 2003.

TOXICOLOGY

Baselt, Randall C. Disposition of Toxic Drugs and Chemicals in Man. 8th ed. Foster City, Calif.: Biomedical, 2008.

Dart, Richard C., ed. Medical Toxicology. 3d ed. Philadelphia: Lippincott Williams & Wilkins, 2004.

Flomenbaum, Neal E., et al., eds. Goldfrank's Toxicologic Emergencies. 8th ed. New York: McGraw-Hill, 2006.

Greenberg, Michael I., et al., eds. Occupational, Industrial, and Environmental Toxicology. 2d ed. Philadelphia: Mosby, 2003.

Klaassen, Curtis D., ed. Casarett and Doull's Toxicology: The Basic Science of Poisons. 7th ed. New York: McGraw-Hill, 2008.

Landis, Wayne G., and Ming-ho Yu. Introduction to Environmental Toxicology. 3d ed. Boca Raton, Fla.: Lewis, 2004.

Olson, Kent R., et al., eds. Poisoning and Drug Overdose. 5th ed. New York: Lange Medical Books/ McGraw-Hill, 2007.

Timbrell, John. Introduction to Toxicology. 3d ed. Washington, D.C.: Taylor & Francis, 2003.

TROPICAL MEDICINE

Cook, Gordon C., and Alimuddin I. Zumla, eds. Manson's Tropical Diseases. 22d ed. Philadelphia: Saunders/Elsevier, 2009.

Feldman, Charles, and George A. Sarosi, eds. Tropical and Parasitic Infections in the Intensive Care Unit. New York: Springer, 2005.

Gill, Geoff, and Nick Beeching, eds. Lecture Notes on Tropical Medicine. 5th ed. Malden, Mass: Blackwell, 2004.

Guerrant, Richard L., David H. Walker, and Peter F. Weller, eds. Tropical Infectious Diseases: Principles, Pathogens, and Practice. Philadelphia: Churchill Livingstone/Elsevier, 2006.

Jong, Elaine C., and Russell McMullen, eds. Travel and Tropical Medicine Manual. 4th ed. Philadelphia: Saunders/Elsevier, 2008.

Kwan-Gett, Tao Sheng Clifford, Charles Kemp, and Carrie Kovarik. Infectious and Tropical Diseases: A Handbook for Primary Care. St. Louis, Mo.: Mosby/ Elsevier, 2006.

Lutz, Harald T., and Hassen A. Gharbi, eds. Manual of Diagnostic Ultrasound in Infectious Tropical Diseases. New York: Springer, 2006.

Strickland, G. Thomas, ed. Hunter's Tropical Medicine and Emerging Infectious Diseases. 8th ed. Philadelphia: W. B. Saunders, 2000.

UROLOGY

Alexander, Ivy L., ed. Urinary Tract and Kidney Diseases and Disorders Sourcebook: Basic Consumer Health Information About the Urinary System. 2d ed. Detroit: Omnigraphics, 2005.

Baskin, Laurence S., and Barry A. Kogan, eds. Handbook of Pediatric Urology. 2d ed. Philadelphia: Lippincott Williams & Wilkins, 2005.

Brenner, Barry M., ed. Brenner and Rector's The Kidney. 8th ed. Philadelphia: Saunders/Elsevier, 2008.

Gillenwater, Jay Y., et al., eds. Adult and Pediatric Urology. 4th ed. Philadelphia: Lippincott Williams & Wilkins, 2002.

Graham, Sam D., Jr., et al., eds. Glenn's Urologic Surgery. 7th ed. Philadelphia: Lippincott Williams & Wilkins, 2009.

Greenberg, Arthur, et al., eds. Primer on Kidney Diseases. 4th ed. Philadelphia: Saunders/Elsevier, 2005.

Loughlin, Kevin R., ed. Female Urology. Philadelphia: W. B. Saunders, 2002.

Massry, Shaul G., and Richard J. Glassock, eds. Massry and Glassock's Textbook of Nephrology. 4th ed. Philadelphia: Lippincott Williams & Wilkins, 2001.

Mitch, William E., and Saulo Klahr, eds. Handbook of Nutrition and the Kidney. 6th ed. Philadelphia: Lippincott Williams & Wilkins, 2010.

Schrier, Robert W., ed. Diseases of the Kidney and Urinary Tract. 8th ed. Philadelphia: Wolters Kluwer/ Lippincott Williams & Wilkins, 2007.

_____. Renal and Electrolyte Disorders. 6th ed. Philadelphia: Lippincott Williams & Wilkins, 2003.

Tanagho, Emil A., and Jack W. McAninich, eds. Smith's General Urology. 17th ed. New York: McGraw-Hill, 2008.

Walsh, Patrick C., et al., eds. Campbell-Walsh Urology. 9th ed. 4 vols. Philadelphia: Saunders/Elsevier, 2007.

—Peter B. Heller, Ph.D.; updated by Desiree Dreeuws

RESOURCES

ABORTION. *See* REPRODUCTIVE ISSUES

ACQUIRED IMMUNODEFICIENCY SYNDROME
   (AIDS)
AIDS Info
   P.O. Box 6303
   Rockville, MD 20849-6303
   800-HIV-0440
   TTY: 888-480-3739
   Fax: 301-315-2818
   E-mail: ContactUs@aidsinfo.nih.gov
   Web site: http://www.aidsinfo.nih.gov
   This federal Public Health Service project maintains
a database on AIDS clinical trials. Provides informa-
tion on the location of AIDS trials, criteria for inclusion
or exclusion, and related assistance.

Centers for Disease Control and Prevention
   (CDC)
   HIV/AIDS
   800-CDC-INFO
   TTY: 888-232-6348
   E-mail: cdcinfo@cdc.gov
   Web site: http://www.cdc.gov/hiv
   This federal program offers information on AIDS
and AIDS-related issues. Provides referrals to physi-
cians, support groups, self-help groups, legal organiza-
tions, housing agencies, hospices, and home care
services.

Gay Men's Health Crisis
   The Tisch Building
   119 W. 24th Street
   New York, NY 10011
   800-AIDS-NYC
   212-367-1000
   Web site: http://www.gmhc.org
   Provides support and therapy groups for persons
with AIDS and their families. Offers volunteer crisis
counselors, a buddy program for assistance with tasks,
and an HIV-AIDS prevention program.

Good Samaritan Project
   3030 Walnut
   Kansas City, MO 64108
   816-561-8784

   Fax: 816-531-7199
   Web site: http://www.gsp-kc.org
   The mission of this organization is to provide supportive and responsive care for a diverse community of
individuals affected by HIV-AIDS and to raise awareness through education and advocacy.

Project Inform
   1375 Mission Street
   San Francisco, CA 94103-2621
   800-822-7422
   415-558-8669
   Fax: 415-558-0684
   Web site: http://www.projinf.org
   This clearinghouse and hotline provides AIDS and
HIV treatment information and advocacy as well as information on current drugs and where they can be
obtained.

WORLD: An Information and Support Network by,
   for, and About Women with HIV-AIDS
   414 13th Street
   2d Floor
   Oakland, CA 94612
   510-986-0340
   Fax: 510-986-0341
   Web site: http://www.womenhiv.org
   Offers support and information for women infected
with or affected by AIDS or HIV. Sponsors retreats and
classes.

ADDICTION—ALCOHOL, DRUGS, AND SMOKING
Al-Anon/Alateen
   1600 Corporate Landing Parkway
   Virginia Beach, VA 23454-5617
   888-4AL-ANON
   757-563-1600
   Fax: 757-563-1655
   E-mail: wso@al-anon.org
   Web site: http://www.al-anon.org
   Provides a free self-help program of recovery from
the family disease of alcoholism, based on the Twelve
Steps and Twelve Traditions of Alcoholics Anony-
mous. Includes Alateen, a program for younger family
members affected by another person's drinking.

Alcoholics Anonymous (AA)
P.O. Box 459
New York, NY 10163
212-870-3400
Web site: http://www.aa.org
This is a free self-help program for recovery from alcoholism. Members work to recover from alcoholism and help others to achieve sobriety through a Twelve-Step program, in which members share experiences, strength, and hope with one another. Web site provides information on local chapters of AA in the United States and Canada.

Cocaine Anonymous World Services
P.O. Box 492000
Los Angeles, CA 90049-8000
800-347-8998 (referral service)
310-559-5833
Fax: 310-559-2554
E-mail: cawso@ca.org
Web site: http://www.ca.org
Refers callers to local self-help Twelve-Step groups for persons addicted to cocaine and other mind-altering drugs.

Dual Recovery Anonymous
P.O. Box 8107
Prairie Village, KS 66208
913-991-2703
E-mail: draws@draonline.org
Web site: http://www.draonline.org
This self-help support group is based on the Twelve-Step program; for persons who have alcohol or drug addictions along with mental or emotional disorders.

Families Anonymous
P.O. Box 3475
Culver City, CA 90231-3475
800-736-9805
Fax: 310-815-9682
E-mail: famanon@FamiliesAnonymous.org
Web site: http://www.familiesanonymous.org
This Twelve-Step support group is for persons dealing with drug abuse or related behavior problems of a family member or friend. Refers callers to the nearest meetings, which are held throughout the world. Also provides referrals to other Twelve-Step programs and other resources and organizations.

Jewish Alcoholics, Chemically Dependent Persons, and Significant Others (JACS)
120 West 57th Street
New York, NY 10019
212-397-4197
Fax: 212-399-3525
E-mail: jacs@jacsweb.org
Web site: http://www.jacsweb.org
Promotes and assists recovery from chemical dependency for Jewish alcoholics and addicts, their families, and their friends.

National Center for Chronic Disease Prevention and Health Promotion
Office on Smoking and Health
800-CDC-INFO
TTY: 888-232-6348
E-mail: tobaccoinfo@cdc.gov
Web site: http://www.cdc.gov/tobacco
This site from the Centers for Disease Control and Prevention provides information on smoking cessation, smoking and teens, smoking during pregnancy, and passive smoking, among other resources. Also offers a comprehensive collection of Web links.

National Institute on Alcohol Abuse and Alcoholism (NIAAA)
5635 Fishers Lane, MSC 9304
Bethesda, MD 20892-9304
301-443-3860
E-mail: niaaaweb-r@exchange.nih.gov
Web site: http://www.niaaa.nih.gov
Provides information on clinical trials, intramural research, and publications and answers frequently asked questions, among other services.

Phoenix Center on Addiction and the Family
164 West 74th Street
New York, NY 10023
646-505-2060
Fax: 212-595-2553
E-mail: coaf@phoenixhouse.org
Web site: http://www.coaf.org
Provides information on the effects of parental abuse of alcohol and other substances on children. Looks for solutions to the problems of children of alcoholics.

Pride Institute
800-54-PRIDE
E-mail: support@pride-institute.com

Web site: http://www.pride-institute.com

Helps lesbian, gay, and bisexual individuals with chemical dependency and mental health problems.

Rational Recovery
  P.O. Box 800
  Lotus, CA 95651
  530-621-2667, 530-621-4374
  Web site: http://www.rational.org
  Nonspiritual self-help program for recovery from substance addictions and overeating.

Women for Sobriety, Inc.
  P.O. Box 618
  Quakertown, PA 18951-0618
  215-536-8026
  Fax: 215-538-9026
  Web site: http://www.womenforsobriety.org
  Self-help group specifically for female alcoholics based on the Thirteen Acceptance Statements.

AGENT ORANGE
National Veterans Service Fund, Inc.
  P.O. Box 2465
  Darien, CT 06820-0465
  800-521-0198
  E-mail: NatVetSvc@optonline.net
  Web site: http://www.angelfire.com/ct2/natvetsvc
  Offers case-managed social services and limited medical assistance to Vietnam and Persian Gulf War veterans. Provides information on Agent Orange and works to see that affected veterans receive proper treatment. Helps veterans' children with birth defects.

AGING AND ELDER CARE
Children of Aging Parents
  P.O. Box 167
  Richboro, PA 18954
  800-227-7294
  E-mail: info@caps4caregivers.org
  Web site: http://www.caps4caregivers.org
  This national information and referral service is for caregivers of elderly persons. Organizes and promotes caregivers' support groups, workshops, seminars, and conferences.

Eldercare Locator
  800-677-1116
  E-mail: eldercarelocator@spherix.com
  Web site: http://www.eldercare.gov

A federal service that provides information on state and local resources for community-based services for the elderly.

Little Brothers-Friends of the Elderly
  255 North Ashland Avenue
  Chicago, IL 60607-1019
  312-455-1000
  Fax: 312-455-9674
  E-mail: general@littlebrotherschicago.org
  Web site: http://www.littlebrothers.org
  Provides friendship and assistance to persons over seventy years of age who live alone and do not have emotional and physical help from families. Sponsors visitation programs and provides transportation, information, and referrals.

National Council on the Aging (NCOA)
  1901 L Street NW
  4th Floor
  Washington, DC 20036
  202-479-1200
  TDD: 202-479-6674
  Fax: 202-479-0735
  Web site: http://www.ncoa.org
  Answers questions on services available to seniors. Sponsors groups relating to such topics as employment for seniors, rural aging, adult day care, senior housing, and volunteer programs for seniors.

ALBINISM
National Organization for Albinism and
  Hypopigmentation (NOAH)
  P.O. Box 959
  East Hampstead, NH 03826-0959
  800-473-2310
  603-887-2310
  Fax: 800-648-2310
  Web site: http://www.albinism.org
  Provides information on albinism and coordinates and promotes support groups for persons with albinism.

ALLERGIES
American Academy of Allergy, Asthma, and
  Immunology
  555 East Wells Street
  Suite 1100
  Milwaukee, WI 53202-3823
  800-822-2762
  414-272-6071

E-mail: info@aaaai.org
Web site: http://www.aaaai.org

An organization that provides consumers, professionals, and media with comprehensive information on allergies and related conditions and diseases.

ALZHEIMER'S DISEASE

Alzheimer's Association
225 North Michigan Avenue
Suite 1700
Chicago, IL 60601-7633
800-272-3900
312-335-8700
TDD: 312-403-3073
Fax: 866-699-1246
E-mail: info@alz.org
Web site: http://www.alz.org

Promotes family support systems for relatives of persons with Alzheimer's disease.

Alzheimer's Disease Education and Referral Center
P.O. Box 8250
Silver Spring, MD 20907-8250
800-438-4380
Fax: 301-495-3334
Web site: http://www.nia.nih.gov/alzheimers

Federal service through the National Institute on Aging that provides information on Alzheimer's disease, including symptoms and current research, and makes referrals to other organizations.

AMPUTATION

National Amputation Foundation
40 Church Street
Malverne, NY 11565
516-887-3600
Fax: 516-887-3667
E-mail: amps76@aol.com
Web site: http://www.nationalamputation.org

Assists veterans and other amputees in employment and social and mental rehabilitation. Sponsors a program in which amputees who have returned to normal life visit new amputees.

AMYOTROPHIC LATERAL SCLEROSIS (ALS)

ALS Association
27001 Agoura Road
Suite 250
Calabasas Hills, CA 91301-5104
888-949-2577

818-880-9007
Fax: 818-880-9006
Web site: http://www.alsa.org

Provides research and information on ALS and patient care.

ANOREXIA NERVOSA. *See* EATING DISORDERS

APNEA

American Sleep Apnea Association
6856 Eastern Avenue NW
Suite 203
Washington, DC 20012
202-293-3650
Fax: 202-293-3656
Web site: http://www.sleepapnea.org

Offers educational programs and support groups through the Awake Network.

ARTHRITIS

Arthritis Foundation
P.O. Box 7669
Atlanta, GA 30357-0669
800-283-7800
404-872-7100
Web site: http://www.arthritis.org

Provides information on arthritis support groups, exercise classes, and other resources for persons with arthritis. Also offers information, education, and publications specific to juvenile arthritis.

ASTHMA. *See* LUNG DISORDERS

ATAXIA

National Ataxia Foundation
2600 Fernbrook Lane
Suite 119
Minneapolis, MN 55447-4752
763-553-0020
Fax: 763-553-0167
E-mail: naf@ataxia.org
Web site: http://www.ataxia.org

Provides services and information to victims of ataxia and their families.

ATTENTION-DEFICIT DISORDER (ADD)

Attention Deficit Disorder Association
P.O. Box 7557
Wilmington, DE 19803-9997
800-939-1019

E-mail: info@add.org

Web site: http://www.add.org

Offers support to persons with attention-deficit disorder and their families. Maintains a database of support groups.

Children and Adults with Attention Deficit/
  Hyperactivity Disorder
  8181 Professional Place
  Suite 150
  Landover, MD 20785
  800-233-4050
  301-306-7070
  Fax: 301-306-7090
  Web site: http://www.chadd.org

Local groups provide information and support for families affected by ADD.

AUTISM

Autism Society of America
  4330 East-West Highway
  Suite 350
  Bethesda, MD 20814
  800-3-AUTISM
  301-657-0881
  Web site: http://www.autism-society.org

Provides information, education, and publications about autism, as well as online services and referrals.

AUTOIMMUNE DISORDERS

American Autoimmune Related Diseases
  Association
  22100 Gratiot Avenue
  East Detroit, MI 48021
  586-776-3900
  Fax: 586-776-3903
  Web site: http://www.aarda.org

Provides education and information on autoimmunity, which causes several serious chronic diseases.

BATTEN'S DISEASE

Batten Disease Support and Research Association
  166 Humphries Drive
  Suite 2
  Reynoldsburg, OH 43068
  800-448-4570
  740-927-4298
  E-mail: bdsra1@bdsra.org
  Web site: http://www.bdsra.org

Provides support group activities, referrals, and information for families of children with Batten's disease.

BED-WETTING. *See* **INCONTINENCE**

BIRTH DEFECTS. *See also* **SPECIFIC DEFECTS**

Birth Defect Research for Children, Inc.
  800 Celebration Avenue
  Suite 225
  Celebration, FL 34747
  407-566-8403
  E-mail: staff@birthdefects.org
  Web site: http://www.birthdefects.org

A nonprofit organization that provides parents and expectant parents with information about birth defects and support services for their children.

March of Dimes
  1275 Mamaroneck Avenue
  White Plains, NY 10605
  914-997-4488
  Web site: http://www.marchofdimes.com

An organization that supports research into the prevention of birth defects and offers consumers a range of excellent information on myriad birth defects, prenatal testing, and pregnancy health.

BLINDNESS. *See* **VISION DISORDERS**

BRAIN DISORDERS

American Brain Tumor Association
  2720 River Road
  Des Plaines, IL 60018
  800-886-2282
  847-827-9910
  Fax: 847-827-9918
  E-mail: info@abta.org
  Web site: http://hope.abta.org

Provides educational materials and resource information to patients, families, and medical professionals. Mentors support group leaders and offers a database of support groups and a pen-pal program.

Brain Injury Association of America
  1608 Spring Hill Road
  Suite 110
  Vienna, VA 22182
  800-444-6443
  703-761-0750

Fax: 703-761-0755
Web site: http://www.biausa.org
Provides services to persons with brain injuries and their families as well as information about traumatic brain injury. Links callers with support groups and local resources.

Brain Tumor Society
   124 Watertown Street
   Suite 2D
   Watertown, MA 02472
   800-770-8287
   617-924-9997
   Fax: 617-924-9998
   E-mail: info@braintumor.org
   Web site: http://www.braintumor.org
   Support for brain tumor patients and their families.

BULIMIA. *See* **EATING DISORDERS**

BURNS
Phoenix Society for Burn Survivors, Inc.
   1835 R W Berends Drive SW
   Grand Rapids, MI 49519-4955
   800-888-2876
   616-458-2773
   Fax: 616-458-2831
   E-mail: info@phoenixsociety.org
   Web site: http://www.phoenix-society.org
   This is a self-help service organization for burn survivors and their families. Offers seminars and school and job reentry programs.

CANADIAN ORGANIZATIONS
Canadian Centre for Occupational Health and
   Safety (CCOHS)/Le Centre canadien d'hygiène
   et de sécurité au travail (CCHST)
   135 Hunter Street East
   Hamilton, Ontario, Canada L8N 1M5
   905-572-2981
   Fax: 905-572-2206
   Web site: http://www.ccohs.ca (English);
     http://www.cchst.ca (French)
   A not-for-profit federal department corporation that seeks the elimination of work-related illnesses and injuries.

Canadian Public Health Association (CPHA)
   400-1565 Carling Avenue
   Ottawa, Ontario, Canada K1Z 8R1

   613-725-3769
   Fax: 613-725-9826
   E-mail: info@cpha.ca
   Web site: http://www.cpha.ca/en/default.aspx
   A national, independent, not-for-profit, and voluntary association representing public health in Canada, with links to the international public health community.

Health Canada/Santé Canada
   Address Locator 0900C2
   Ottawa, Ontario, Canada K1A 0K9
   866-225-0709
   613-957-2991
   TTY: 800-267-1245
   Fax: 613-941-5366
   E-mail: Info@hc-sc.gc.ca
   Web site: http://www.hc-sc.gc.ca/index-eng.php
     (English); http://www.hc-sc.gc.ca/index-fra.php
     (French)
   The federal department responsible for helping Canadians maintain and improve their health. Offers consumer safety information and information about First Nations, Inuit, and Aboriginal health.

Public Health Agency of Canada (PHAC)/L'Agence
   de la santé publique du Canada (ASPC)
   Ontario office:
   130 Colonnade Road
   Address Locator 6501H
   Ottawa, Ontario, Canada K1A 0K9
   Manitoba office:
   1015 Arlington Street
   Winnipeg, Manitoba, Canada R3E 3R2
   204-789-2000
   Fax: 204-789-7878
   Web site: http://www.phac-aspc.gc.ca/index-eng
     .php (English); http://www.phac-aspc.gc.ca/
     index-fra.php (French)
   This government agency, formed in 2004, was created in response to growing concerns about the capacity of Canada's public health system to anticipate and respond effectively to public health threats.

CANCER
American Cancer Society
   250 Williams Street
   Atlanta, GA 30303
   800-ACS-2345
   TTY: 866-228-4327
   Web site: http://www.cancer.org

Provides general information on cancer and information on the group's programs and services. Offers Look Good, Feel Better, a free, nonmedical program to help women overcome the appearance-related side effects of radiation and chemotherapy treatment.

Candlelighters Childhood Cancer Foundation
    10400 Connecticut Avenue
    Suite 205
    Kensington, MD 20895
    800-366-CCCF
    301-962-3520
    Fax: 301-962-3521
    E-mail: staff@candlelighters.org
    Web site: http://www.candlelighters.org
    Provides information, support, and advocacy to families of children and adolescents with cancer, survivors of childhood cancer, and professionals who work with them.

National Cancer Institute
    NCI Public Inquiries Office
    6116 Executive Boulevard
    Suite 3036A
    Bethesda, MD 20892-8322
    800-4-CANCER
    TTY: 800-332-8615
    E-mail: cancergovstaff@mail.nih.gov
    Web site: http://www.cancer.gov
    A component of the National Institutes of Health (NIH), the NCI is the federal government's principal agency for cancer research and training. Offers information on cancer treatment and diagnosis, clinical trials, rehabilitation, home care, financial aid, palliative care, supportive care for the side effects of treatment, quitting smoking, and cancer prevention.

National Coalition for Cancer Survivorship
    1010 Wayne Avenue
    Suite 770
    Silver Spring, MD 20910
    301-650-9127
    Fax: 301-565-9670
    E-mail: info@canceradvocacy.org
    Web site: http://www.canceradvocacy.org
    Provides support to cancer survivors and their families and friends. Facilitates peer support and maintains a list of organizations that are concerned with survivorship.

R. A. Bloch Cancer Foundation, Inc.
    1 H&R Block Way
    Kansas City, MO 64105
    800-433-0464
    816-854-5050
    Fax: 816-854-8024
    E-mail: hotline@blochcancer.org
    Web site: http://www.blochcancer.org
    Matches patients with volunteers who have had the same type of cancer. Provides resources, information, and free "Fighting Cancer" booklet.

Susan G. Komen for the Cure
    5005 LBJ Freeway
    Suite 250
    Dallas, TX 75244
    800-GO-KOMEN
    972-855-1600
    Fax: 972-855-1605
    Web site: http://www.komen.org
    Trained volunteers provide information and resources to individuals concerned about breast health or breast cancer.

Y-ME National Breast Cancer Organization
    135 South LaSalle Street
    Suite 2000
    Chicago, IL 60603
    800-221-2141
    312-986-8338
    Fax: 312-294-8597
    Web site: http://www.y-me.org
    Provides information, referrals, and emotional support to women concerned about or diagnosed with breast cancer. National toll-free hotline is staffed by trained personnel and volunteers who have experienced breast cancer. Publications include information tailored for single women with breast cancer, teens, and partners of women with breast cancer.

CAREGIVERS. *See* AGING AND ELDER CARE;
    CHRONIC ILLNESSES

CELIAC SPRUE
Celiac Sprue Association (CSA)
    P.O. Box 31700
    Omaha, NE 68131-0700
    877-CSA-4CSA
    402-558-0600
    Fax: 402-558-1347

E-mail: celiacs@csaceliacs.org
Web site: http://www.csaceliacs.org

Support and information on maintaining a gluten-free diet for persons affected by celiac sprue. Publications include a cookbook for gluten-free cooking.

CEREBRAL PALSY

United Cerebral Palsy
  1660 L Street NW
  Suite 700
  Washington, DC 20036
  800-872-5827
  202-776-0406
  Fax: 202-776-0414
  E-mail: info@ucp.org
  Web site: http://www.ucp.org

Provides information and referrals. Local affiliates provide family and individual support, early intervention programs, personal assistance and assistive technology services, and community-integrated living arrangements.

CHILDBIRTH. *See* REPRODUCTIVE ISSUES

CHRONIC FATIGUE SYNDROME AND
  FIBROMYALGIA

National Chronic Fatigue Syndrome and
  Fibromyalgia Association (NCFSFA)
  P.O. Box 18426
  Kansas City, MO 64133
  816-737-1343
  E-mail: information@ncfsfa.org
  Web site: http://www.ncfsfa.org

Provides information, support, and local groups for sufferers of chronic fatigue and fibromyalgia.

CHRONIC ILLNESSES

MUMS National Parent-to-Parent Network
  150 Custer Court
  Green Bay, WI 54301-1243
  877-336-5333 (parents only)
  920-336-5333
  Fax: 920-339-0995
  E-mail: mums@netnet.net
  Web site: http://www.netnet.net/mums

For parents or caregivers of a child with a disability, rare disorder, chromosomal abnormality, or serious health condition. Matches parents whose children have similar conditions so they can offer support for one another.

Parents Helping Parents
  1400 Parkmoor Avenue
  Suite 100
  San Jose, CA 95126
  408-727-5775
  Fax: 408-286-1116
  Web site: http://www.php.com

Offer support for parents of children with special needs, including those with chronic or terminal illnesses. Assists new and ongoing parent support groups and resource centers.

Well Spouse Foundation
  63 West Main Street
  Suite H
  Freehold, NJ 07728
  800-838-0879
  732-577-8899
  Fax: 732-577-8644
  Web site: http://www.wellspouse.org

Provides emotional support network for the spouse or partner of a chronically ill patient. Establishes local groups and provides information and materials.

CLEFT LIP AND PALATE

Children's Craniofacial Association (CAA)
  13140 Coit Road
  Suite 517
  Dallas, TX 75240
  800-535-3643
  214-570-9099
  Fax: 214-570-8811
  E-mail: contactCCA@ccakids.com
  Web site: http://www.ccakids.org

Refers callers to support groups for persons and families affected by craniofacial anomalies. Provides referrals to doctors and explains how to get financial assistance for food, travel, and lodging related to these conditions.

Cleft Palate Foundation
  1504 East Franklin Street
  Suite 102
  Chapel Hill, NC 27514-2820
  800-24-CLEFT
  919-933-9044
  Fax: 919-933-9604
  Web site: http://www.cleftline.org

Provides general information on cleft lip, cleft palate, and craniofacial anomalies to affected persons and their families as well as information about health care teams and support groups for these conditions.

FACES: The National Craniofacial Association
    P.O. Box 11082
    Chattanooga, TN 37401
    800-3FACES3
    E-mail: faces@faces-cranio.org
    Web site: http://www.faces-cranio.org
    Provides information on related support groups and financial assistance for expenses while traveling for reconstructive surgery, based on financial and medical need. Provides referrals to other resources and organizations, support networks, and a speakers' bureau.

National Foundation for Facial Reconstruction
    317 East 34th Street
    Room 901
    New York, NY 10016
    212-263-6656
    Fax: 212-263-7534
    Web site: http://www.nffr.org
    Works to help children and others with craniofacial conditions to lead productive lives.

COLITIS. *See* CROHN'S DISEASE

COLOSTOMY. *See* ILEOSTOMY AND COLOSTOMY

CORNELIA DE LANGE SYNDROME
Cornelia de Lange Syndrome-USA Foundation
    302 West Main Street
    Suite 100
    Avon, CT 06001
    800-223-8355, 800-753-2357
    860-676-8166, 860-676-8255
    Fax: 860-676-8337
    E-mail: info@cdlsusa.org
    Web site: http://www.cdlsusa.org
    Provides information and support for families, friends, and professionals dealing with Cornelia de Lange syndrome.

CROHN'S DISEASE
Crohn's and Colitis Foundation of America
    (CCFA)
    386 Park Avenue South
    17th Floor
    New York, NY 10016
    800-932-2423

E-mail: info@ccfa.org
Web site: http://www.ccfa.org
Provides support groups, educational publications, and programs on Crohn's disease and ulcerative colitis.

CYSTIC FIBROSIS
Cystic Fibrosis Foundation
    6931 Arlington Road
    Bethesda, MD 20814
    800-FIGHT-CF
    301-951-4422
    Fax: 301-951-6378
    E-mail: info@cff.org
    Web site: http://www.cff.org
    Supports more than one hundred specialized care centers for people with cystic fibrosis.

DEATH AND DYING
American Association of Retired Persons (AARP)
    Grief and Loss Program
    601 E Street NW
    Washington, DC 20049
    888-OUR-AARP
    Web site: http://www.aarp.org/families/grief_loss
    This national outreach group consists of widowed volunteers who visit, support, and offer referrals to new widows and widowers. Includes a link to information in Spanish.

Center for Loss in Multiple Birth (CLIMB)
    P.O. Box 91377
    Anchorage, AK 99509
    907-222-5321
    E-mail: climb@pobox.alaska.net
    Web site: http://www.climb-support.org
    Provides peer support for parents who have lost a multiple birth child during pregnancy or after birth. Newsletter includes resources for dealing with multiple birth loss and names of parents willing to share experiences. Includes a link to information in Spanish.

Children's Hospice International
    1101 King Street
    Suite 360
    Alexandria, VA 22314
    800-24-CHILD
    703-684-0330
    E-mail: info@chionline.org
    Web site: http://www.chionline.org
    Provides information on children's hospices, refer-

rals to local hospices, and education for affected children and their families.

Compassionate Friends
  P.O. Box 3696
  Oak Brook, IL 60522-3696
  877-969-0010
  630-990-0010
  Fax: 630-990-0246
  Web site: http://www.compassionatefriends.org
  This is a self-help organization for parents and siblings of a child who has died, with chapters throughout the United States. Includes a link to information in Spanish.

Helping Other Parents in Normal Grieving
  (HOPING)
  P.O. Box 27452
  Lansing, MI 48909-7452
  888-288-0967
  E-mail: info@lansingbabyloss.org
  Web site: lansingbabyloss.org
  Provides support for parents who have lost an infant to miscarriage, stillbirth, or infant death, from trained parents who have had a similar experience.

National Hospice and Palliative Care Organization
  (NHPCO)
  1731 King Street
  Suite 100
  Alexandria, VA 22314
  800-658-8898
  703-837-1500
  Fax: 703-837-1233
  E-mail: nhpco_info@nhpco.org
  Web site: http://www.nhpco.org
  Provides information on caring for terminally ill patients and their families. Gives referrals to hospices throughout the United States. Includes a link to information in Spanish.

Parents of Murdered Children, Inc.
  100 East Eighth Street
  Suite 202
  Cincinnati, OH 45202
  888-818-POMC
  513-721-5683
  Fax: 513-345-4489
  E-mail: natlpomc@aol.com
  Web site: http://www.pomc.org

This self-help organization offers support for anyone who has had a family member or friend murdered. Provides information about grief and the criminal justice system. Establishes self-help groups that meet regularly. Works on violence prevention programs.

SHARE: Pregnancy and Infant Loss Support
  402 Jackson Street
  St. Charles, MO 63301
  800-821-6819
  636-947-6164
  Fax: 636-947-7486
  Web site: http://www.nationalshareoffice.com
  Provides support, information, and referrals for parents who have suffered miscarriage, stillbirth, or infant death. Assists local groups in organizing.

DEPRESSION. *See* **MENTAL HEALTH**

DIABETES
American Diabetes Association
  ATTN: National Call Center
  1701 North Beauregard Street
  Alexandria, VA 22311
  800-DIABETES
  E-mail: AskADA@diabetes.org
  Web site: http://www.diabetes.org
  Provides training, guidance, and education on diabetes. Includes a link to information in Spanish.

Juvenile Diabetes Research Foundation
  International
  26 Broadway
  14th Floor
  New York, NY 10004
  800-533-CURE
  Fax: 212-785-9595
  E-mail: info@jdrf.org
  Web site: http://www.jdrf.org
  Regional groups offer support and activities for families affected by diabetes. Provides information on specific diabetes needs. Includes a link to information in Spanish.

National Diabetes Information Clearinghouse
  (NDIC)
  1 Information Way
  Bethesda, MD 20892-3560
  800-860-8747

TTY: 866-569-1162
Fax: 703-738-4929
E-mail: ndic@info.niddk.nih.gov
Web site: http://diabetes.niddk.nih.gov
This clearinghouse offers information and publications on diabetes. Gives referrals to support groups and other relevant organizations. Includes a link to information in Spanish.

DIGESTIVE DISORDERS
National Digestive Diseases Information
  Clearinghouse (NDDIC)
  2 Information Way
  Bethesda, MD 20892-3570
  800-891-5389
  TTY: 866-569-1162
  Fax: 703-738-4929
  E-mail: nddic@info.niddk.nih.gov
  Web site: http://digestive.niddk.nih.gov
  Provides information on the prevention and management of digestive diseases and referrals to relevant support groups and other organizations. Offers publications on many digestive disorders.

DISABILITIES, GENERAL
American Network of Community Options and
  Resources (ANCOR)
  101 King Street
  Suite 380
  Alexandria, VA 22314
  703-535-7850
  Fax: 703-535-7860
  E-mail: ancor@ancor.org
  Web site: http://www.ancor.org
  This umbrella group for several hundred agencies provides services and support to persons with disabilities.

Americans with Disabilities Act
  U.S. Department of Justice
  950 Pennsylvania Avenue NW
  Civil Rights Division
  Disability Rights Section-NYA
  Washington, DC 20530
  800-514-0301
  TTY: 800-514-0383
  Fax: 202-307-1198
  Web site: http://www.usdoj.gov/crt/ada
  This government service provides information on Titles II and III of the Americans with Disabilities Act.

Information is available over the phone from specialists, or documents may be ordered by fax or mail.

Association for the Help of Retarded Children
  AHRC New York City
  83 Maiden Lane
  New York, NY 10038
  212-780-2500
  TTY: 800-662-1220
  Web site: http://www.ahrcnyc.org
  Provides support, training, clinics, and residential facilities for the mentally retarded and disabled and their families.

Easter Seals
  233 South Wacker Drive
  Suite 2400
  Chicago, IL 60606
  800-221-6827
  312-726-6200
  TTY: 312-726-4258
  Fax: 312-726-1494
  E-mail: info@easterseals.org
  Web site: http://www.easterseals.com
  Provides information and referrals for people with disabilities and special needs, and their families. Includes a link to information in Spanish.

Federation for Children with Special Needs
  1135 Tremont Street
  Suite 420
  Boston, MA 02120
  800-331-0688 (in Mass.)
  617-236-7210
  Fax: 617-572-2094
  E-mail: fcsninfo@fcsn.org
  Web site: http://www.fcsn.org
  Coalition of groups concerned with children and adults with disabilities. Provides information on resources, basic rights, and obtaining services. Works for parent involvement in the care of children with disabilities and chronic illnesses and supports parent training and information. Includes a link to information in Spanish.

HEATH Resource Center
  George Washington University
  2134 G Street NW
  Washington, DC 20052-0001
  800-449-7343

202-994-6160'
Fax: 202-994-8613
E-mail: askheath@gwu.edu
Web site: http://www.heath.gwu.edu

This national clearinghouse for people with disabilities who are seeking education or training after high school provides information about access, accommodations, program modifications, and national organizations. Gives referrals to local resources.

National Dissemination Center for Children with
  Disabilities (NICHCY)
  1825 Connecticut Avenue NW
  Suite 700
  Washington, DC 20009
  800-695-0285
  202-884-8200
  Fax: 202-884-8441
  E-mail: nichcy@aed.org
  Web site: http://www.nichcy.org

Provides information packets and resources regarding special education and disability related issues. Offers technical assistance to parents and groups.

DISEASES, RARE. *See* **RARE DISEASES**

DONORS, MARROW AND ORGANS
Center for Organ Recovery and Education (CORE)
  204 Sigma Drive
  RIDC Park
  Pittsburgh, PA 15238
  800-DONORS-7
  Fax: 412-963-3563
  E-mail: hbulvony@core.org
  Web site: http://www.core.org

Provides general information on becoming an organ donor. Accepts referrals for potential donors.

Living Bank
  P.O. Box 6725
  Houston, TX 77265-6725
  800-528-2971
  Fax: 713-961-0979
  E-mail: info@livingbank.org
  Web site: http://www.livingbank.org

Maintains a registry of organ donors. Provides educational materials and registration forms for organ donation.

National Marrow Donor Program
  3001 Broadway Street Northeast
  Suite 100
  Minneapolis, MN 55413-1753
  800-MARROW-2
  612-627-5800 (outside the United States)
  E-mail: patientinfo@nmdp.org
  Web site: http://www.marrow.org

This central registry of unrelated potential volunteer marrow donors provides transplant information for patients with leukemia, aplastic anemia, and other life-threatening diseases.

DOWN SYNDROME
ACDS
  4 Fern Place
  Plainview, NY 11803
  516-933-4700
  Fax: 516-933-9524
  Web site: http://www.acds.org

This is a resource and information source for parents of children with Down syndrome. Provides referrals and offers programs in New York State for preschool-age children and their siblings and recreational programs and support groups for older children.

National Down Syndrome Congress
  1370 Center Drive
  Suite 102
  Atlanta, GA 30338
  800-232-NDSC
  770-604-9500
  Fax: 770-604-9898
  E-mail: info@ndsccenter.org
  Web site: http://www.ndsccenter.org

Assists parents in finding ways to meet children's needs, coordinates local parents' groups, and provides a clearinghouse for information on Down syndrome. Includes a link to information in Spanish.

National Down Syndrome Society
  666 Broadway
  New York, NY 10012
  800-221-4602
  Fax: 212-979-2873
  E-mail: info@ndss.org
  Web site: http://www.ndss.org

Provides information and referral services to families, local support groups, and community programs. Includes a link to information in Spanish.

DWARFISM
Little People of America, Inc.
  250 El Camino Real
  Suite 201
  Tustin, CA 92780
  888-LPA-2001
  714-368-3689
  Fax: 714-368-3367
  E-mail: info@lpaonline.org
  Web site: http://www.lpaonline.org
  Provides support, publications, and information for dwarfs and other persons of short stature.

DYSLEXIA
International Dyslexia Association
  40 York Road
  4th Floor
  Baltimore, MD 21204-5202
  800-ABCD-123
  410-296-0232
  Fax: 410-321-5069
  Web site: http://www.interdys.org
  .Provides information, publications, and a computer database on dyslexia. Makes referrals for diagnosis and treatment.

EATING DISORDERS
National Eating Disorders Organization
  603 Stewart Street
  Suite 803
  Seattle, WA 98101
  800-931-2237
  206-382-3587
  Fax: 206-829-8501
  E-mail: info@NationalEatingDisorders.org
  Web site: http://www.nationaleatingdisorders.org
  Offers a referral service, support group packet, prevention video, and general information on eating disorders. Includes a link to information in Spanish.

ELDER CARE. *See* AGING AND ELDER CARE

ENDOMETRIOSIS. *See* WOMEN'S HEALTH

EPILEPSY
Epilepsy Foundation
  8301 Professional Place
  Landover, MD 20785
  800-332-1000
  Web site: http://www.epilepsyfoundation.org

Provides referrals and basic information on epilepsy for patients, families, physicians, and others. Includes a link to information in Spanish.

FATTY ACID OXIDATION DISORDERS
FOD: All in This Together
  P.O. Box 54
  Okemos, MI 48805-0054
  517-381-1940
  Fax: 866-290-5206
  E-mail: deb@fodsupport.org
  Web site: http://www.fodsupport.org
  Provides information to families affected by fatty oxidation disorders.

FIBROMYALGIA. *See* CHRONIC FATIGUE SYNDROME AND FIBROMYALGIA

FRAGILE X SYNDROME
National Fragile X Foundation
  P.O. Box 190488
  San Francisco, CA 94119
  800-688-8765
  925-938-9300
  Fax: 925-938-9315
  Web site: http://www.fragilex.org
  Provides information about fragile X syndrome and gives referrals to specialists and support groups. Includes a link to information in Spanish.

GALACTOSEMIA
Parents of Galactosemic Children, Inc.
  P.O. Box 2401
  Mandeville, LA 70470-2401
  866-900-PGC1
  Web site: http://www.galactosemia.org
  Provides support and information for parents of children with galactosemia.

GAUCHER'S DISEASE
National Gaucher Foundation
  2227 Idlewood Road
  Suite 6
  Tucker, GA 30084
  800-504-3189
  Fax: 770-934-2911
  E-mail: ngf@gaucherdisease.org
  Web site: http://www.gaucherdisease.org
  Provides support and information for persons with Gaucher's disease.

GENDER REASSIGNMENT SURGERY

Renaissance Transgender Association, Inc.
  987 Old Eagle School Road
  Suite 719
  Wayne, PA 19087
  610-975-9119
  E-mail: info@ren.org
  Web site: http://www.ren.org
  Offers support and resources for transgender persons, including those who have had or wish to have gender reassignment surgery.

GENERAL

Angel Flight America
  1515 East 71st Street
  Suite 312
  Tulsa, OK 74136
  918-749-8992
  Fax: 918-745-0879
  E-mail: angel@angelflight.com
  Web site: http://www.angelflight.com
  Offers free air transportation to ambulatory patients who are traveling to and from specialized medical treatment and are in financial need.

Centers for Disease Control and Prevention (CDC)
  National Center for Injury Prevention and Control
    (NCIPC)
  Mailstop K-65
  4770 Buford Highway NE
  Atlanta, GA 30341-3717
  800-CDC-INFO
  TTY: 888-232-6348
  Fax: 770-488-4760
  E-mail: cdcinfo@cdc.gov
  Web site: http://www.cdc.gov/injury
  Offers a number of documents related to injury prevention and control. Both nontechnical information for patients and technical information for health care providers can be obtained.

MedicAlert Foundation International
  2323 Colorado Avenue
  Turlock, CA 95382
  888-633-4298
  209-668-3333 (from outside the United States)
  Fax: 209-669-2450
  Web site: http://www.medicalert.org
  Provides medical facts pertaining to the MedicAlert emblem worn on bracelets or neck chains, with an emergency hotline number for medical professionals to call for further details. Operators available in many languages. Also gives information on obtaining a Medic-Alert emblem.

National Patient Travel Center
  c/o Mercy Medical Airlift
  4620 Haygood Road
  Suite 1
  Virginia Beach, VA 23455
  800-296-1217
  757-318-9174
  Fax: 757-318-9107
  E-mail: info@mercymedical.org
  Web site: http://www.mercymedical.org
  Provides information on and referral to airline, charitable, and commercial service options for patients needing transport to specialized treatment facilities or places of continuing care.

National Rehabilitation Information Center
  8201 Corporate Drive
  Suite 600
  Landover, MD 20785
  800-346-2742
  301-459-5900
  TTY: 301-459-5984
  E-mail: naricinfo@heitechservices.com
  Web site: http://www.naric.com
  This is a national disability and rehabilitation library and information center. Provides information on assistive devices and products. Also does document searches and takes orders for publications.

Office of Minority Health Resource Center
  P.O. Box 37337
  Washington, DC 20013-7337
  800-444-6472
  E-mail: info@omhrc.gov
  Web site: http://www.minorityhealth.hhs.gov
  This government agency is primarily for health professionals but gives information and referrals on minority health-related topics to the general public. Also offers resource lists and publications. Provides information to Latinos and Asians in their native languages.

Research! America
  1101 King Street
  Suite 520
  Alexandria, VA 22314-2960

800-366-CURE
703-739-2577
Fax: 703-739-2372
E-mail: info@researchamerica.org
Web site: http://www.researchamerica.org
Offers resource referrals, data, and contact names for organizations nationwide that offer support and information on a wide range of diseases and disorders.

St. Jude Children's Research Hospital
262 Danny Thomas Place
Memphis, TN 38105
901-595-3300
Web site: http://www.stjude.org
Provides information on referrals to St. Jude Children's Research Hospital, which serves children who have not received extensive treatment for a disease being studied. Includes a link to information in Spanish.

Visiting Nurse Associations of America (VNAA)
900 19th Street NW
Suite 200
Washington, DC 20006
202-384-1420
Fax: 202-384-1444
E-mail: vnaa@vnaa.org
Web site: http://www.vnaa.org
Gives referrals to callers' nearest Visiting Nurse Association. Services include general nursing; physical, occupational, and speech therapy; medical social services; case management; personal care; advanced therapies; adult day care; parent aid; care for the dying; nutritional counseling; friendly visit services; AIDS education and treatment; Meals on Wheels; and specialized nursing services.

GENETIC DISEASES. *See also* **SPECIFIC DISEASES**
Genetic Alliance
4301 Connecticut Avenue NW
Suite 404
Washington, DC 20008-2369
202-966-5557
Fax: 202-966-8553
E-mail: info@geneticalliance.org
Web site: http://www.geneticalliance.org
Provides information and support to persons and families affected by genetic disorders. Offers referrals to appropriate genetic support groups and professionals.

GLYCOGEN STORAGE DISEASES
Association for Glycogen Storage Disease
P.O. Box 896
Durant, IA 52747
563-514-4022
E-mail: maryc@agsdus.org
Web site: http://www.agsdus.org
Facilitates communication between patients and families of patients with glycogen storage diseases (GSDs) and provides information to families, patients, and health care professionals. Provides referrals for treatment and helps members get equipment needed to care for GSD patients.

GRIEF. *See* **DEATH AND DYING**

GROWTH DISORDERS
Human Growth Foundation
997 Glen Cove Avenue
Suite 5
Glen Head, NY 11545
800-451-6434
Fax: 516-671-4055
E-mail: hgf1@hgfound.org
Web site: http://www.hgfound.org
Provides information and support for individuals suffering from physical growth problems and their families. Includes a link to information in Spanish.

GUILLAIN-BARRÉ SYNDROME
GBS/CIDP Foundation International
The Holly Building
104½ Forrest Avenue
Narberth, PA 19072
866-224-3301
610-667-0131
Fax: 610-667-7036
E-mail: info@gbsfi-cidp.com
Web site: http://www.gbsfi-cidp.org
Develops support groups for persons suffering from Guillain-Barré syndrome (GBS) and chronic inflammatory demyelinating polyneuropathy (CIDP), as well as their families.

HANSEN'S DISEASE. *See* **LEPROSY**

HEADACHE

National Headache Foundation
820 N. Orleans
Suite 217
Chicago, IL 60610
888-NHF-5552
312-274-2650
E-mail: info@headaches.org
Web site: http://www.headaches.org

Operates local support groups and provides information for headache sufferers, their families, and physicians.

HEARING LOSS

International Hearing Dog, Inc. (IHDI)
5901 E. 89th Avenue
Henderson, CO 80640
303-287-3277
Fax: 303-287-3425
E-mail: IHDI@aol.com
Web site: http://www.ihdi.org

Trains and places hearing dogs, who alert their hearing-impaired owners to doorbells, crying children, smoke alarms, ringing telephones, and other sounds that require attention or could indicate danger.

Starkey Hearing Foundation
6700 Washington Avenue South
Eden Prairie, MN 55344
800-328-8602
Fax: 952-828-6946
Web site: http://www.sotheworldmayhear.org

This foundation gives away hearing instruments and batteries, promotes hearing health awareness, and conducts research and education.

HEART ATTACK, DISEASE, AND FAILURE

Mended Hearts, Inc.
7272 Greenville Avenue
Dallas, TX 75231-4596
888-HEART-99
214-360-6149
Fax: 214-360-6145
E-mail: info@mendedhearts.org
Web site: http://www.mendedhearts.org

Local groups offer advice, encouragement, and support for patients and families affected by heart disease.

HEMOCHROMATOSIS

Iron Overload Diseases Association
525 Mayflower Road
West Palm Beach, FL 33405
866-768-8629
561-586-8246
E-mail: iod@ironoverload.org
Web site: http://www.ironoverload.org

Works with patients, families, and doctors. Offers patient referrals by phone.

HEMOPHILIA

National Hemophilia Foundation
116 West 32d Street
11th Floor
New York, NY 10001
212-328-3700
Fax: 212-328-3777
E-mail: handi@hemophilia.org
Web site: http://www.hemophilia.org

Support, education, and information for families affected by hemophilia.

HEPATITIS

Hepatitis Foundation International
504 Blick Drive
Silver Spring, MD 20904
800-891-0707
301-622-4200
Fax: 301-622-4702
E-mail: info@hepatitisfoundation.org
Web site: http://www.hepfi.org

Provides education and information about viral hepatitis. Maintains a database of support groups.

HERPES

American Social Health Association (ASHA)
Herpes Resource Center
P.O. Box 13827
Research Triangle Park, NC 27709
800-227-8922
919-361-8400
Fax: 919-361-8425
Web site: http://www.ashastd.org/herpes/
herpes_overview.cfm

Provides support and information for persons with recurring genital herpes infections and referrals to self-help groups in the United States and Canada.

HISTIOCYTOSIS
Histiocytosis Association of America
332 North Broadway
Pitman, NJ 08071
800-548-2758
856-589-6606
Fax: 856-589-6614
E-mail: association@histio.org
Web site: http://www.histio.org
Provides peer counseling, information, physician referrals, and parent/patient networking.

HIV. *See* **ACQUIRED IMMUNODEFICIENCY SYNDROME (AIDS)**

HOSPICE. *See* **DEATH AND DYING**

HUNTINGTON'S DISEASE
Huntington's Disease Society of America
505 Eighth Avenue
Suite 902
New York, NY 10018
800-345-HDSA
212-242-1968
Fax: 212-239-3430
E-mail: hdsainfo@hdsa.org
Web site: http://www.hdsa.org
Provides information and referrals to local support groups, chapter social workers, physicians, nursing homes, and other resources. Crisis intervention and other support available.

HYDROCEPHALUS
Guardians of Hydrocephalus Research Foundation
2618 Avenue Z
Brooklyn, NY 11235
718-743-4473
Fax: 718-743-1171
E-mail: ghrf2618@aol.com
Web site: http://ghrforg.org
Provides information on hydrocephalus.

Hydrocephalus Association
870 Market Street
Suite 705
San Francisco, CA 94102
888-598-3789
415-732-7040
Fax: 415-732-7044
E-mail: info@hydroassoc.org

Web site: http://www.hydroassoc.org
Facilitates networking among families affected by hydrocephalus, creates training for families, and sponsors social gatherings. Provides information in English and Spanish.

ILEOSTOMY AND COLOSTOMY
United Ostomy Associations of America, Inc.
P.O. Box 66
Fairview, TN 37062-0066
800-826-0826
E-mail: info@uoaa.org
Web site: http://www.uoaa.org
Provides information and referrals to support groups for persons who have had a colostomy, ileostomy, or similar surgical operation.

ILLNESSES, CHRONIC. *See* **CHRONIC ILLNESSES**

IMMUNIZATION
Centers for Disease Control and Prevention (CDC)
National Immunization Program (NIP)
NIP Public Inquiries
Mailstop E-05
1600 Clifton Road, NE
Atlanta, GA 30333
800-CDC-INFO
TTY: 888-232-6348
Fax: 888-232-3299
E-mail: cdcinfo@cdc.gov
Web site: http://www.cdc.gov/vaccines
Offers a number of documents related to immunization. Includes information on immunization schedules and general information on vaccines, information on specific vaccines, and how to report adverse reactions to vaccines. Provides nontechnical information for patients and technical information for health care providers.

IMMUNODEFICIENCY DISORDERS
Immune Deficiency Foundation (IDF)
40 West Chesapeake Avenue
Suite 308
Towson, MD 21204
800-296-4433
E-mail: idf@primaryimmune.org
Web site: http://www.primaryimmune.org
Provides information for patients with inherited immunodeficiency diseases and their families and for medical professionals.

IMPOTENCE. *See* SEXUAL DISORDERS AND
   DYSFUNCTION

INCONTINENCE
National Association for Continence (NAFC)
   P.O. Box 1019
   Charleston, SC 29402-1019
   800-BLADDER
   843-377-0900
   Fax: 843-377-0905
   E-mail: memberservices@nafc.org
   Web site: http://www.nafc.org
   This is a clearinghouse for information and services
related to incontinence and assistive devices. Provides
education, advocacy, and support on the causes, prevention, diagnosis, treatment, and management alternatives for persons with incontinence. Includes a link
to information in Spanish.

Simon Foundation for Continence
   P.O. Box 815
   Wilmette, IL 60091
   800-23-SIMON
   847-864-3913
   Fax: 847-864-9758
   Web site: http://www.simonfoundation.org
   Provides peer support and a speaker's bureau. Man-
ages educational and self-help support groups on urinary and bowel incontinence and organizes self-help
groups.

INFERTILITY. *See* REPRODUCTIVE ISSUES

INTRAVENTRICULAR HEMORRHAGE
IVH Parents
   P.O. Box 56-1111
   Miami, FL 33256-1111
   305-232-0381
   Fax: 305-223-9890
   Provides support and information for parents of chil-
dren with intraventricular hemorrhage.

KIDNEY DISORDERS
American Association of Kidney Patients (AAKP)
   3505 East Frontage Road
   Suite 315
   Tampa, FL 33607
   800-749-2257
   Fax: 813-636-8122
   E-mail: info@aakp.org

   Web site: http://www.aakp.org
   This is an advocacy organization for kidney patients,
persons on dialysis, and those with kidney transplants.
Includes a link to information in Spanish.

American Kidney Fund (AKF)
   6110 Executive Boulevard
   Suite 1010
   Rockville, MD 20852
   800-638-8299
   E-mail: helpline@kidneyfund.org
   Web site: http://www.kidneyfund.org
   Provides financial assistance for individuals with
chronic kidney failure.

Cystinosis Research Network
   302 Whytegate Court
   Lake Forest, IL 60045
   866-276-3669
   847-735-0471
   Fax: 847-235-2773
   E-mail: info@cystinosis.org
   Web site: http://www.cystinosis.org
   A volunteer, nonprofit organization dedicated to
supporting and advocating research, providing family
assistance, and educating the public and medical communities about cystinosis.

National Kidney Foundation
   30 East 33d Street
   New York, NY 10016
   800-622-9010
   212-889-2210
   Fax: 212-689-9261
   Web site: http://www.kidney.org
   Makes referrals to local agencies. Supports patient
services such as transportation, drug banks, and educational projects.

KLINEFELTER SYNDROME
KS&A: Knowledge Support & Action
   P.O. Box 461047
   Aurora, CO 80046-1047
   888-999-9428
   Fax: 303-400-3454
   E-mail: info@genetic.org
   Web site: http://www.genetic.org
   Offers support and information for persons and fam-
ilies affected by Klinefelter syndrome, trisomy X, mo-
saicism, and other conditions caused by an uncommon

number of X and/or Y chromosomes. Facilitates networking and the exchange of information.

LEAD POISONING

U.S. Environmental Protection Agency (EPA)
National Lead Information Center
422 South Clinton Avenue
Rochester, NY 14620
800-424-LEAD
Fax: 585-232-3111
Web site: http://www.epa.gov/lead
This is a government program providing information about lead poisoning and its prevention. Includes a link to information in Spanish.

LEARNING DISABILITIES

Learning Disabilities Association of America
(LDA)
4156 Library Road
Pittsburgh, PA 15234-1349
412-341-1515
Fax: 412-344-0224
Web site: http://www.ldanatl.org
Information, publications, and referral service concerning learning disabilities. State and local groups provide services to families, including camps and recreation programs.

LEPROSY

American Leprosy Missions (ALM)
1 ALM Way
Greenville, SC 29601
800-543-3135
864-271-7040
Fax: 864-271-7062
E-mail: amlep@leprosy.org
Web site: http://leprosy.org
Provides medical, rehabilitation, and social care, as well as information about leprosy. Refers callers to treatment centers.

LEUKEMIA

Leukemia and Lymphoma Society
1311 Mamaroneck Avenue
White Plains, NY 10605
800-955-4LSA
Web site: http://www.leukemia.org
Provides callers with referrals in their area and offers educational materials and financial aid. Includes a link to information in Spanish.

LEUKODYSTROPHY

United Leukodystrophy Foundation (ULF)
2304 Highland Drive
Sycamore, IL 60178
800-728-5483
Fax: 815-895-2432
E-mail: office@ulf.org
Web site: http://www.ulf.org
Offers information and support to persons suffering from leukodystrophy and their families. Coordinates communication among families.

LIVER DISORDERS

American Liver Foundation
75 Maiden Lane
Suite 603
New York, NY 10038
212-668-1000
Fax: 212-483-8179
Web site: http://www.liverfoundation.org
Provides physician referrals and information on support groups for persons with liver disease and their families.

LUNG DISORDERS

American Lung Association
1301 Pennsylvania Avenue NW
Washington, DC 20004
800-LUNG-USA, 800-548-8252
202-785-3355, 202-452-1805
Web site: http://www.lungusa.org
This organization seeks to prevent lung disease and promote lung health. The Web site includes in-depth information and recent research findings, a guide to local events and programs, and a section to share personal stories. Includes a link to information in Spanish.

Lung Line
National Jewish Medical and Research Center
1400 Jackson Street
Denver, CO 80206
800-222-5864, 800-423-8891
Web site: http://www.nationaljewish.org
Registered nurses provide information on the detection, treatment, and prevention of lung and immunological diseases and allergies, and give referrals to local doctors.

LUPUS
Lupus Foundation of America
  2000 L Street NW
  Suite 710
  Washington, DC 20036
  800-558-0121
  202-349-1155
  Fax: 202-349-1156
  Web site: http://www.lupus.org
  Provides information on lupus. Refers callers to local chapters, which provide support group details and physician referrals. Includes a link to information in Spanish.

LYME DISEASE
American Lyme Disease Foundation (ALDF)
  P.O. Box 466
  Lyme, CT 06371
  E-mail: inquire@aldf.com
  Web site: http://www.aldf.com
  Provides educational materials and information regarding Lyme disease and maintains a physician referral service. Includes a link to information in Spanish.

MAPLE SYRUP URINE DISEASE (MSUD)
MSUD Research Foundation
  P.O. Box 2512
  Gilbert, AZ 85299
  480-710-1144, 480-813-8209
  Fax: 480-219-8216
  E-mail: azmsud@cox.net
  Web site: http://www.msudresearchfoundation.org
  Provides information on MSUD. Works for better communication between affected families and health care professionals.

MARFAN SYNDROME
National Marfan Foundation
  22 Manhasset Avenue
  Port Washington, NY 11050
  800-8-MARFAN
  516-883-8712
  Fax: 516-883-8040
  E-mail: staff@marfan.org
  Web site: http://www.marfan.org
  Provides information on Marfan syndrome and a support network for patients and families.

MARROW DONORS. *See* DONORS, MARROW AND ORGANS

MÉNIÈRE'S DISEASE
Vestibular Disorders Association (VEDA)
  P.O. Box 13305
  Portland, OR 97213-0305
  800-837-8428
  503-229-7705
  Fax: 503-229-8064
  Web site: http://www.vestibular.org
  A nonprofit organization that provides information to the public and health professionals about inner-ear balance disorders such as Ménière's disease, benign paroxysmal positional vertigo, and labyrinthitis. Includes a link to information in Spanish.

MENOPAUSE. *See* WOMEN'S HEALTH

MENTAL HEALTH
Depression and Bipolar Support Alliance (DBSA)
  730 N. Franklin Street
  Suite 501
  Chicago, IL 60654-7225
  800-826-3632
  Fax: 312-642-7243
  Web site: http://www.dbsalliance.org
  Provides information on depressive and bipolar illnesses as medical diseases and promotes self-help for affected persons and their families.

Emotions Anonymous International
  P.O. Box 4245
  St. Paul, MN 55104-0245
  651-647-9712
  Fax: 651-647-1593
  E-mail: info3498fjsd@emotionsanonymous.org
  Web site: http://www.emotionsanonymous.org
  This is a self-help group using a 12-step program for recovery from emotional illnesses. Provides publications, information, and referrals to local groups. Includes a link to information in Spanish.

International Foundation for Research and
  Education on Depression (iFred)
  P.O. Box 17598
  Baltimore, MD 12197-1598
  410-268-0044
  Fax: 443-782-0739
  E-mail: info@ifred.org
  Web site: http://www.ifred.org
  Provides referrals to doctors who specialize in treating depression and a list of local support groups.

Mental Health America
  2000 North Beauregard Street
  6th Floor
  Alexandria, VA 22311
  800-969-6642
  703-684-7722
  TTY: 800-433-5959
  Fax: 703-684-5968
  E-mail: infoctr@mentalhealthamerica.net
  Web site: http://www.nmha.org
  Offers regional support groups, information and referral programs, and other patient advocacy services.

National Alliance on Mental Illness (NAMI)
  3803 North Fairfax Drive
  Suite 100
  Arlington, VA 22203
  800-950-NAMI
  703-524-7600
  Web site: http://www.nami.org
  Provides emotional support and practical guidance for the mentally ill and their families. Offers referrals to local groups. Includes a link to information in Spanish.

National Institute of Mental Health (NIMH)
  6001 Executive Boulevard
  Room 8184, MSC 9663
  Bethesda, MD 20892-9663
  866-615-6464
  301-443-4513
  TTY: 301-443-8431
  Fax: 301-443-4279
  E-mail: nimhinfo@nih.gov
  Web site: http://www.nimh.nih.gov
  This government organization tries to help people better understand mental health and mental disorders. Provides the fax-on-demand service Mental Health FAX4U, with four hundred documents on mental illnesses such as Alzheimer's disease, bipolar disorder, depression, and seasonal affective disorder.

National Mental Health Consumers' Self-Help
  Clearinghouse
  1211 Chestnut Street
  Suite 1207
  Philadelphia, PA 19107
  800-553-4539
  215-751-1810
  Fax: 215-636-6312
  E-mail: info@mhselfhelp.org

  Web site: http://www.mhselfhelp.org
  Provides technical assistance in the development of self-help projects, information referrals, publications, and consulting services.

National Resource and Training Center on
  Homelessness and Mental Illness
  *E-mail:*generalinquiry@center4si.com
  Web site: http://www.nrchmi.samhsa.gov
  Provides technical assistance and comprehensive information on the treatment, services, and housing needs of homeless persons with severe mental illnesses.

Pride Institute
  800-54-PRIDE
  E-mail: support@pride-institute.com
  Web site: http://www.pride-institute.com
  Helps lesbian, gay, and bisexual individuals with chemical dependency and mental health problems.

MENTAL RETARDATION
Best Buddies
  100 SE Second Street
  Suite 2200
  Miami, FL 33131
  800-89-BUDDY
  305-374-2233
  Fax: 305-374-5305
  Web site: http://www.bestbuddies.org
  Facilitates friendships between people with mental retardation and others in the community.

MISCARRIAGE. *See* **DEATH AND DYING;**
  REPRODUCTIVE ISSUES

MUCOPOLYSACCHARIDOSIS (MPS)
National MPS Society
  P.O. Box 14686
  Durham, NC 27709-4686
  877-MPS-1001
  919-806-0101
  Fax: 919-806-2055
  E-mail: info@mpssociety.org
  Web site: http://www.mpssociety.org
  Refers parents whose children have been diagnosed with MPS or mucolipidosis (ML) to other families dealing with these diseases.

MULTIPLE BIRTHS. *See also* **REPRODUCTIVE ISSUES**
National Organization of Mothers of Twins
  Clubs, Inc.
  2000 Mallory Lane
  Suite 130-600
  Franklin, TE 37067-8231
  248-231-4480
  E-mail: info@nomotc.org
  Web site: http://www.nomotc.org
  Local groups provide information on multiples and their care.

Triplet Connection
  P.O. Box 429
  Spring City, UT 84662
  435-851-1105
  Fax: 435-462-7466
  Web site: http://www.tripletconnection.org
  Helps parents of triplets and larger multiple births prepare for and deal with high-risk multiple births. Provides supports and facilitates networking. Offers information on such topics as breast-feeding, medical services, preventing premature births, and clothing and equipment exchanges. Also provides support for mothers who have lost one or more babies of a multiple birth.

Twinless Twins Support Group International
  P.O. Box 980481
  Ypsilanti, MI 48198-0481
  888-205-8962
  E-mail: contact@twinlesstwins.org
  Web site: http://www.twinlesstwins.org
  Provides support to persons who have lost a multiple-birth sibling through death or disappearance and others dealing with multiple-birth losses. Also works to reunite multiple-birth siblings who were separated through adoption or for other reasons.

MULTIPLE SCLEROSIS
National Multiple Sclerosis Society
  733 Third Avenue
  New York, NY 10017
  800-FIGHT-MS
  Web site: http://www.nationalmssociety.org
  Provides services to persons with multiple sclerosis through local chapters.

MUSCULAR DYSTROPHY
Muscular Dystrophy Association (MDA)
  National Headquarters
  3300 E. Sunrise Drive
  Tucson, AZ 85718
  800-F572-1717
  Web site: http://www.mdausa.org
  Combats neuromuscular diseases through research programs, medical and community services, and professional and public health education. Provides referrals to local groups for information about support groups, clinics, and summer camps. Includes a link to information in Spanish.

MYASTHENIA GRAVIS
Myasthenia Gravis Foundation of America, Inc.
  355 Lexington Avenue
  15th Floor
  New York, NY 10017
  800-541-5454
  212-297-2156
  Fax: 212-3700-9047
  E-mail: mgfa@myasthenia.org
  Web site: http://www.myasthenia.org
  Provides publications and information on myasthenia gravis.

NARCOLEPSY
Narcolepsy Network, Inc.
  P.O. Box 294
  Pleasantville, NY 10570
  888-292-6522
  401-667-2523
  Fax: 401-633-6567
  Web site: http://www.narcolepsynetwork.org
  Provides referral service, support group meetings, and communication among members.

NEUROFIBROMATOSIS
Children's Tumor Foundation
  95 Pine Street
  16th Floor
  New York, NY 10005
  800-323-7938
  212-344-6633
  Fax: 212-747-0004
  E-mail: info@ctf.org
  Web site: http://www.ctf.org
  Provides information, peer counseling, and referral services.

Neurofibromatosis, Inc.
   P.O. Box 66884
   Chicago, IL 60666
   800-942-6825
   630-627-1115
   Fax: 630-627-1117
   Web site: http://www.nfinc.org
Offers support, peer counseling, and information for patients and families affected by neurofibromatosis. Provides referrals to medical resources.

NIEMANN-PICK DISEASE
National Niemann-Pick Disease Foundation
   P.O. Box 49
   401 Madison Avenue, Suite B
   Ft. Atkinson, WI 53538
   877-287-3672
   920-563-0930
   Fax: 920-563-0931
   E-mail: nnpdf@nnpdf.org
   Web site: http://www.nnpdf.org
Support and phone referrals for parents of children with Niemann-Pick disease. Provides information on genetic counseling.

NUTRITION
American Dietetic Association (ADA)
   120 South Riverside Plaza
   Suite 2000
   Chicago, IL 60606-6995
   800-877-1600
   Web site: http://www.eatright.org
The largest organization of food and nutrition professionals in the United States. Provides referrals to local registered dieticians and answers questions on food and nutrition.

OBESITY AND WEIGHT LOSS
Overeaters Anonymous (OA)
   World Service Office
   P.O. Box 44020
   Rio Rancho, NM 87174-4020
   505-891-2664
   Fax: 505-891-4320
   Web site: http://www.oa.org
This is a Twelve-Step support group for persons who want to stop their compulsive overeating.

Take Off Pounds Sensibly (TOPS)
   4575 South Fifth Street
   Milwaukee, WI 53207-0360
   414-482-4620
   E-mail: topsinteractive@tops.org
   Web site: http://www.tops.org
This is a self-help weight loss support group using group dynamics, competition, and recognition. Participants are required to consult with a doctor about weight loss goals and diets. Includes a link to information in Spanish.

OBSESSIVE-COMPULSIVE DISORDER. *See* MENTAL HEALTH

ORGAN DONORS. *See* DONORS, MARROW AND ORGANS

OSTEOPOROSIS
National Osteoporosis Foundation (NOF)
   1150 17th Street NW
   Washington, DC 20036
   800-231-4222
   202-223-2226
   Web site: http://www.nof.org
Provides information about osteoporosis.

PAGET'S DISEASE
Paget Foundation
   120 Wall Street
   Suite 1602
   New York, NY 10005-4001
   800-23-PAGET
   212-509-5335
   Fax: 212-509-8492
   E-mail: PagetFdn@aol.com
   Web site: http://www.paget.org
Provides information, patient assistance, and referrals to medical specialists for persons with Paget's disease, primary hyperparathyroidism, fibrous dysplasia, and osteopetrosis.

PAIN MANAGEMENT
American Chronic Pain Association (ACPA)
   P.O. Box 850
   Rocklin, CA 95677
   800-533-3231
   Fax: 916-632-3208
   E-mail: acpa@pacbell.net
   Web site: http://www.theacpa.org

Offers mutual support groups for sufferers of pain lasting more than six months. Provides information on pain management. Includes a link to information in Spanish.

PARALYSIS

National Spinal Cord Injury Association (NSCIA)
 1 Church Street
 Suite 600
 Rockville, MD 20850
 800-962-9629, 866-387-2196
 E-mail: info@spinalcord.org
 Web site: http://www.spinalcord.org
 Assists persons with spinal cord injuries or diseases. Facilitates networking for parents of children with spinal cord injuries or related diseases.

PARKINSON'S DISEASE

American Parkinson Disease Association, Inc.
 (ADPA)
 135 Parkinson Avenue
 Staten Island, NY 10305
 800-223-2732
 718-981-8001
 Fax: 1-718-981-4399
 E-mail: apda@apdaparkinson.org
 Web site: http://www.apdaparkinson.org
 Maintains information and referral centers and more than eight hundred support groups for patients and families.

National Parkinson Foundation, Inc.
 1501 NW 9th Avenue
 Miami, FL 33136-1494
 800-327-4545
 305-243-6666
 Fax: 305-243-6073
 E-mail: contact@parkinson.org
 Web site: http://www.parkinson.org
 Provides information and referrals to local medical facilities. Offers evaluations at the National Parkinson Foundation Center and sponsors regional support groups.

Parkinson's Disease Foundation (PDF)
 1359 Broadway
 Suite 1509
 New York, NY 10018

 800-457-6676
 212-923-4700
 Fax: 212-923-4778
 E-mail: info@pdf.org
 Web site: http://www.pdf.org
 Provides information about Parkinson's disease and referrals to physicians and hospitals.

PHENYLKETONURIA (PKU)

Children's PKU Network
 3790 Via De La Valle
 Suite 120
 Del Mar, CA 92014
 800-377-6677
 858-509-0767
 Fax: 858-509-0768
 E-mail: pkunetwork@aol.com
 Web site: http://www.pkunetwork.org
 Provides support groups, crisis intervention, financial assistance, and discount dietary aids for families affected by PKU.

PHOBIAS. *See* MENTAL HEALTH

POLIOMYELITIS

Post-Polio Health International (PHI)
 4207 Lindell Boulevard
 Suite 110
 St. Louis, MO 63108-2915
 314-534-0475
 Fax: 314-534-5070
 E-mail: info@post-polio.org
 Web site: http://www.post-polio.org
 Facilitates networking among persons who have had polio. Provides information and encourages research into the long-term effects of polio.

PORPHYRIA

American Porphyria Foundation
 4900 Woodway
 Suite 780
 Houston, TX 77056-1837
 866-APF-3635
 713-266-9617
 Fax: 713-840-9552
 Web site: http://www.porphyriafoundation.com
 Provides information on porphyria to affected persons, parents, and physicians.

PRADER-WILLI SYNDROME

Prader-Willi Syndrome Association (USA)
   8588 Potter Park Drive
   Suite 500
   Sarasota, FL 34238
   800-926-4797
   941-312-0400
   Fax: 941-312-0142
   Web site: http://www.pwsausa.org
   Provides information, referrals, and publications on Prader-Willi syndrome.

PREGNANCY. *See* REPRODUCTIVE ISSUES

PREMATURE BIRTH. *See also* MULTIPLE BIRTHS; REPRODUCTIVE ISSUES

Premature Baby-Premature Child
   E-mail: 5martin@bellsouth.net
   Web site: http://www.prematurity.org
   Offers advice and support for premature children with special needs and their parents.

PURINE METABOLIC DISORDERS

Purine Research Society
   5424 Beech Avenue
   Bethesda, MD 20814-1730
   301-530-0354
   Fax: 301-564-9597
   E-mail: purine@erols.com
   Web site: http://www.purineresearchsociety.org
   Provides information on purine metabolic disorders, including gout, purine autism, Lesch-Nyban syndrome, and ADA deficiency.

RARE DISEASES

National Organization for Rare Disorders (NORD)
   55 Kenosia Avenue
   P.O. Box 1968
   Danbury, CT 06813-1968
   800-999-6673
   203-744-0100
   TDD: 203-797-9590
   Fax: 203-798-2291
   E-mail: orphan@rarediseases.org
   Web site: http://www.rarediseases.org
   Gathers and disseminates information on more than three thousand rare diseases. Facilitates networking between patients with the same disorder.

REPRODUCTIVE ISSUES. *See also* SURROGATE PARENTING

American Academy of Husband-Coached Childbirth
   P.O. Box 5224
   Sherman Oaks, CA 91413-5224
   818-788-6662
   800-4-A-BIRTH
   Web site: http://www.bradleybirth.com
   Refers callers to local teachers of the Bradley method of natural childbirth.

Couple to Couple League International, Inc.
   P.O. Box 111184
   Cincinnati, OH 45211-1184
   800-745-8252
   513-471-2000
   Web site: http://www.ccli.org
   Sponsors local groups for couples who wish to space pregnancies by timing intercourse in accordance with a woman's natural cycle of fertility, rather than by using contraceptives. Educational publications available in English, Polish, and Spanish.

La Leche League International
   P.O. Box 4079
   Schaumburg, IL 60168-4079
   800-LA-LECHE
   847-519-7730
   Fax: 847-519-0035
   Web site: http://www.lalecheleague.org
   Provides help, education, and encouragement for mothers who want to breast-feed or who are breast-feeding. Offers informal discussion groups, telephone support, and publications. Includes a link to information in Spanish.

Lamaze International
   2025 M Street NW
   Suite 800
   Washington, DC 20036-3309
   800-368-4404
   202-367-1128
   Fax: 202-367-2128
   Web site: http://www.lamaze.org
   Provides information about the Lamaze method of prepared childbirth and how to locate a local certified childbirth educator.

Liberty Godparent Foundation
P.O. Box 4199
Lynchburg, VA 24502
800-542-4453
434-845-3466
Fax: 434-845-1751
Web site: http://www.godparent.org
A Christian maternity home that provides housing, education, medical care, and counseling for single, pregnant young women who wish to keep their child or place their child up for adoption. Offers a twenty-four-hour help line.

National Abortion Federation (NAF)
1660 L Street NW
Suite 450
Washington, DC 20036
800-772-9100
202-667-5881
Fax: 202-667-5890
E-mail: naf@prochoice.org
Web site: http://www.prochoice.org
Provides information and referrals to local abortion providers and information on pregnancy and abortion procedures.

National Infertility Network Exchange (NINE)
P.O. Box 204
East Meadow, NY 11554
516-794-5772
Fax: 516-794-0008
E-mail: info@nine-infertility.org
Web site: http://www.nine-infertility.org
Provides peer support group, education, and referrals for persons who are infertile.

National Life Center
686 North Broad Street
Woodbury, NJ 08096
800-848-LOVE
856-848-1819
Fax: 856-848-2380
Web site: http://www.nationallifecenter.com
Provides free pregnancy tests and medical, legal, and professional counseling referrals. Shelter, adoption, maternity care, and baby clothing are available through local affiliates. The toll-free number directs callers to the nearest pro-life pregnancy service.

Planned Parenthood Federation of America
434 West 33d Street
New York, NY 10001
800-230-PLAN
212-541-7800
Fax: 212-245-1845
Web site: http://www.plannedparenthood.org
Offers information on human sexuality and reproductive health. The toll-free number automatically connects callers to a local Planned Parenthood health center.

Postpartum Support International (PSI)
P.O. Box 60931
Santa Barbara, CA 93160
800-944-4PPD
805-967-7636
Fax: 323-204-0635
E-mail: PSIOffice@postpartum.net
Web site: http://www.postpartum.net
Clearinghouse for information on postpartum depression, providing referrals, educational materials, and support for affected women and their families. Includes a link to information in Spanish.

REYE'S SYNDROME
National Reye's Syndrome Foundation, Inc.
P.O. Box 829
Bryan, OH 43506
800-233-7393
419-924-9000
Fax: 419-924-9999
E-mail: nrsf@reyessyndrome.org
Web site: http://www.reyessyndrome.org
Provides a resource clearinghouse and support groups for patients with Reye's syndrome and their families. Gives referrals to treatment centers across the United States.

RUBINSTEIN-TAYBI SYNDROME
Rubinstein-Taybi Parent Group
P.O. Box 146
Smith Center, KS 66967
888-447-2989
Web site: http://www.rubinstein-taybi.org
Provides support and information for parents of children with Rubinstein-Taybi syndrome.

SCHIZOPHRENIA. *See* **MENTAL HEALTH**

SCLERODERMA
Scleroderma Foundation
  300 Rosewood Drive
  Suite 105
  Danvers, MA 01923
  800-722-HOPE
  978-463-5843
  Fax: 978-463-5809
  E-mail: sfinfo@scleroderma.org
  Web site: http://www.scleroderma.org
  Provides education and emotional support for persons and families affected by scleroderma.

Scleroderma Research Foundation
  220 Montgomery Street
  Suite 1411
  San Francisco, CA 94104
  800-441-CURE
  415-834-9444
  Fax: 415-834-9177
  Web site: http://www.srfcure.org
  Provides support for parents and families and offers doctor referrals on scleroderma, a rare autoimmune disorder in which the body's immune system attacks its own tissues.

SCOLIOSIS
Scoliosis Association, Inc.
  P.O. Box 811705
  Boca Raton, FL 33481-1705
  800-800-0669
  561-994-4435
  Fax: 561-994-2455
  E-mail: normlipin@aol.com
  Web site: http://www.scoliosis-assoc.org
  Provides support for persons suffering from curvature of the spine and related problems.

SELF-HELP ORGANIZATIONS, GENERAL
American Self-Help Clearinghouse
  St. Clare's Health Services
  25 Pocono Road
  Denville, NJ 07834-2995
  973-989-1122
  Web site: http://www.mentalhelp.net/selfhelp
  Publishes *The Self-Help Sourcebook*, which lists several hundred state and local self-help groups and self-help clearinghouses and gives information on how to start a self-help group. The publication is inexpensive and updated every other year.

National Mental Health Consumers' Self-Help
  Clearinghouse
  1211 Chestnut Street
  Suite 1207
  Philadelphia, PA 19107
  800-553-4539
  215-751-1810
  Fax: 215-636-6312
  E-mail: info@mhselfhelp.org
  Web site: http://www.mhselfhelp.org
  Provides technical assistance in the development of self-help projects, information referrals, publications, and consulting services.

SEXUAL DISORDERS AND DYSFUNCTION
American Urological Association Foundation
  1000 Corporate Boulevard
  Linthicum, MD 21090
  866-RING-AUA
  410-689-3700
  Fax: 410-689-3800
  E-mail: auafoundation@auafoundation.org
  Web site: http://www.auafoundation.org/
    auafhome.asp
  Educates patients, the public, and health care providers on sexual health issues, including erectile dysfunction. Includes a link to information in Spanish.

Sex Addicts Anonymous
  P.O. Box 70949
  Houston, TX 77270
  800-477-8191
  713-869-4902
  E-mail: info@saa-recovery.org
  Web site: http://www.saa-recovery.org
  This is a Twelve-Step support group for persons who compulsively repeat sexual behavior that is detrimental to their lives.

Sexaholics Anonymous
  P.O. Box 3565
  Brentwood, TN 37024
  866-424-8777
  615-370-6062
  Fax: 615-370-0882

E-mail: saico@sa.org
Web site: http://www.sa.org
This Twelve-Step self-help group is for persons who want to stop self-destructive thinking and behavior, such as the use of pornography, adultery, incest, or criminal sexual activity.

Survivors of Incest Anonymous
    World Service Office
    P.O. Box 190
    Benson, MD 21018-9998
    410-893-3322
    Web site: http://www.siawso.org
This nonprofit organization for victims of incest and other sexual abuse is based on the Twelve Steps and Twelve Traditions of Alcoholics Anonymous.

SEXUALLY TRANSMITTED DISEASES (STDs).
    See also **ACQUIRED IMMUNODEFICIENCY**
    SYNDROME (AIDS); HERPES
Centers for Disease Control and Prevention (CDC)
    STD Prevention Fax Information Service
    Fax: 888-CDC-FAXX
A number of documents related to STDs and other health issues are available from the CDC Fax Information Service as well as from its Web site. Both nontechnical information for patients and technical information for health care providers can be obtained.

SICKLE CELL DISEASE
Sickle Cell Disease Association of America
    231 East Baltimore Street
    Suite 800
    Baltimore, MD 21202
    800-421-8453
    410-528-1555
    Fax: 410-528-1495
    E-mail: scdaa@sicklecelldisease.org
    Web site: http://www.sicklecelldisease.org
Provides referrals to local chapters for educational materials and medical help.

SJÖGREN'S SYNDROME
Sjögren's Syndrome Foundation, Inc.
    6707 Democracy Boulevard
    Suite 325
    Bethesda, MD 20817
    800-475-6473
    301-530-4420
    Fax: 301-530-4415

E-mail: tms@sjogrens.org
Web site: http://www.sjogrens.org
This is a clearinghouse for information about Sjögren's syndrome.

SLEEP DISORDERS. *See also* **APNEA**
National Sleep Foundation
    1522 K Street NW
    Suite 500
    Washington, DC 20005
    202-347-3471
    Fax: 202-347-3472
    E-mail: nsf@sleepfoundation.org
    Web site: http://www.sleepfoundation.org
A nonprofit organization dedicated to improving public health and safety by achieving understanding of sleep and sleep disorders and by supporting education, sleep-related research, and advocacy.

SMOKING. *See* **ADDICTION—ALCOHOL, DRUGS, AND SMOKING**

SPINA BIFIDA
Spina Bifida Association
    4590 MacArthur Boulevard NW
    Suite 250
    Washington, DC 20007-4226
    800-621-3141
    202-944-3285
    Fax: 202-944-3295
    E-mail: sbaa@sbaa.org
    Web site: http://www.sbaa.org
Provides support and information for families affected by spina bifida. Refers callers to local chapters. Includes a link to information in Spanish.

SPONDYLITIS
Spondylitis Association of America
    P.O. Box 5872
    Sherman Oaks, CA 91413
    800-777-8189
    818-981-1616
    E-mail: info@spondylitis.org
    Web site: http://www.spondylitis.org
Provides information and support for persons and families of persons suffering from ankylosing spondylitis, psoriatic arthritis, and Reiter's syndrome.

STRESS. *See* **MENTAL HEALTH**

STROKES
American Stroke Association
    National Center
    7272 Greenville Avenue
    Dallas, TX 75231-4596
    888-4-STROKE
    Web site: http://www.strokeassociation.org
    A division of the American Heart Association that focuses on reducing disability and death from stroke through research, education, fund-raising, and advocacy.

National Institute of Neurological Disorders and
    Stroke (NINDS)
    NIH Neurological Institute
    P.O. Box 5801
    Bethesda, MD 20824
    800-352-9424
    301-496-5751
    TTY: 301-468-5981
    Web site: http://www.ninds.nih.gov
    A government agency that conducts, fosters, coordinates, and guides research on the causes, prevention, diagnosis, and treatment of strokes and other neurological disorders. Includes a link to information in Spanish.

National Stroke Association
    9707 East Easter Lane
    Building B
    Centennial, CO 80112
    800-STROKES
    Fax: 303-649-1328
    E-mail: info@stroke.org
    Web site: http://www.stroke.org
    An organization committed to fighting strokes in the United States. Provides education, services, and community-based activities in prevention, treatment, rehabilitation, and recovery. Includes a link to information in Spanish.

Stroke Clubs International
    805 12th Street
    Galveston, TX 77550
    409-762-1022
    E-mail: strokeclubs@earthlink.net
    Support and information for stroke victims, families, and caregivers. Has a list of more than nine hundred clubs in the United States.

STURGE-WEBER SYNDROME
Sturge-Weber Foundation
    P.O. Box 418
    Mount Freedom, NJ 07970-0418
    800-627-5482
    973-895-4445
    Fax: 973-895-4846
    Web site: http://www.sturge-weber.org
    Provides information and support for persons suffering from Sturge-Weber syndrome, Klippel-Trenaunay syndrome, and port-wine stains, as well as for their families.

STUTTERING
Stuttering Foundation of America
    3100 Walnut Grove Road
    Suite 603
    P.O. Box 11749
    Memphis, TN 38111-0749
    800-992-9392
    901-452-7343
    Fax: 901-452-3931
    E-mail: info@stutteringhelp.org
    Web site: http://www.stuttersfa.org
    Provides referrals to speech pathologists, a nationwide resource list, and free brochures.

SUDDEN INFANT DEATH SYNDROME (SIDS)
First Candle/SIDS Alliance
    1314 Bedford Avenue
    Suite 210
    Baltimore, MD 21208
    800-221-7437
    410-653-8226
    E-mail: info@firstcandle.org
    Web site: http://www.firstcandle.org
    This organization seeks to advance infant health and survival in the fight against infant mortality resulting from SIDS, stillbirth, and miscarriage. Offers support and information for affected families.

SUICIDE. *See* **DEATH AND DYING**

SURROGATE PARENTING. *See also*
    REPRODUCTIVE ISSUES
Center for Surrogate Parenting, Inc. (CSP)
    9 State Circle
    Suite 302
    Annapolis, MD 21401

410-990-9860
Fax: 410-990-9862
Web site: http://www.creatingfamilies.com
Provide support for surrogate parents, enabling them to share experiences and information. Offer information about egg donation.

Organization of Parents Through Surrogacy (OPTS)
P.O. Box 611
Gurnee, IL 60031
847-782-0224
E-mail: bzager@msn.com
Web site: http://www.opts.com
Provides support for families created through surrogate parenting, including phone and e-mail support for members. Also provides information and referrals to infertile couples.

TAY-SACHS DISEASE
National Tay-Sachs and Allied Diseases
Association, Inc.
2001 Beacon Street
Suite 204
Boston, MA 02135
800-906-8723
Fax: 617-277-0134
E-mail: info@ntsad.org
Web site: http://www.ntsad.org
Offers support groups for parents of children with Tay-Sachs and related diseases. Also acts as a clearinghouse of information for families and professionals.

TERMINAL ILLNESSES. *See* **AGING AND ELDER CARE; DEATH AND DYING**

TERMINAL ILLNESSES, WISHES FOR CHILDREN WITH
Children's Wish Foundation International, Inc.
8615 Roswell Road
Atlanta, GA 30350-7526
800-323-WISH
770-393-WISH
Fax: 770-393-0683
Web site: http://www.childrenswish.org
Seeks to fulfill the wishes of terminally ill children.

Dream Factory, Inc.
National Headquarters
200 West Broadway
Suite 504

Louisville, KY 40202
800-456-7556
502-561-3001
Fax: 502-561-3004
Web site: http://www.dreamfactoryinc.org
Seeks to fulfill the wishes of chronically or critically ill children and works to promote a more positive family atmosphere in the face of a prolonged illness.

Make-a-Wish Foundation of America
4742 North 24th Street
Suite 400
Phoenix, AZ 85016-4862
800-722-WISH
602-279-WISH
Fax: 602-279-0855
Web site: http://www.wish.org
Seeks to fulfill the wishes of children with terminal illnesses or other life-threatening conditions.

TORTICOLLIS
National Spasmodic Torticollis Association (NTSA)
Orange Coast Memorial Medical Center
9920 Talbert Avenue
Fountain Valley, CA 92708
800-487-8385
E-mail: NSTAmail@aol.com
Web site: http://www.torticollis.org
Provides support for persons with spasmodic torticollis.

TOURETTE'S SYNDROME
Tourette's Syndrome Association (TSA), Inc.
42-40 Bell Boulevard
Suite 205
Bayside, NY 11361
718-224-2999
Fax: 718-279-9596
Web site: http://tsa-usa.org
Offers physician referrals and provides access to support groups and other services for persons with Tourette's syndrome and their families. Helps people identify and understand Tourette's syndrome. Includes a link to information in Spanish.

TUBERCULOSIS. *See* **LUNG DISORDERS**

TURNER SYNDROME
Turner Syndrome Society of the United States
10960 Millridge North Drive

Suite 214A
Houston, TX 77014
800-365-9944
Fax: 832-912-6446
Web site: http://www.turnersyndrome.org
Provides support and information for families affected by Turner syndrome.

URINARY DISORDERS. *See* **INCONTINENCE;**
 KIDNEY DISORDERS

VISION DISORDERS
American Council of the Blind
2200 Wilson Boulevard
Suite 650
Arlington, VA 22201
800-424-8666
202-467-5081
Fax: 703-465-5085
Web site: http://www.acb.org
Promotes the independence and dignity of blind and visually impaired persons. Includes the Council of Citizens with Low Vision International, which offers outreach programs, advocacy, and educational services for partially sighted and low-vision persons.

American Foundation for the Blind
2 Penn Plaza
Suite 1102
New York, NY 10121
800-AFB-LINE
212-502-7600
Fax: 212-502-7777
E-mail: afbinfo@afb.net
Web site: http://www.afb.org
This is an information and referral service for organizations for the blind. Includes a reference directory of services in the United States.

Blind Children's Fund
201 S. University Street
Mt. Pleasant, MI 48858
989-779-9966
Fax: 989-779-0015
E-mail: BCF@blindchildrensfund.org
Web site: http://www.blindchildrensfund.org
Promotes the health, education, and welfare of blind and visually impaired infants and preschoolers.

Blinded Veterans Association
477 H Street NW
Washington, DC 20001-2694
800-669-7079
202-371-8880
Fax: 202-371-8258
E-mail: bva@bva.org
Web site: http://www.bva.org
Provides information on benefits and services for blinded veterans.

Guide Dog Foundation for the Blind
371 East Jericho Turnpike
Smithtown, NY 11787-2976
800-548-4337
631-930-9000
Fax: 631-930-9009
E-mail: info@guidedog.org
Web site: http://www.guidedog.org
Provides trained guide dogs to the visually impaired. Provides a training program, a dog, all necessary equipment, and airfare within the United States at no charge to students accepted by the program.

Lighthouse International
The Sol and Lillian Goldman Building
111 East 59th Street
New York, NY 10022-1202
800-829-0500
212-821-9200
TTY: 212-821-9713
Fax: 212-821-9707
E-mail: info@lighthouse.org
Web site: http://www.lighthouse.org
Provides educational material on vision and childhood development, vision and aging, and low vision. Gives referrals to vision rehabilitation agencies, low-vision resources, and support groups nationwide. Includes a link to information in Spanish.

National Association for Parents of Children with
Visual Impairments (NAPVI)
P.O. Box 317
Watertown, MA 02471
800-562-6265
617-972-7441
Fax: 617-972-7444
E-mail: napvi@perkins.org

Web site: http://www.spedex.com/napvi

Database provides support group of parents of visually impaired persons. Includes a link to information in Spanish.

National Library Service for the Blind and
Physically Handicapped (NLS)
Library of Congress
1291 Taylor Street NW
Washington, DC 20542
888-NLS-READ
202-707-5100
TDD: 202-707-0744
Fax: 202-707-0712
E-mail: nls@loc.gov
Web site: http://www.loc.gov/nls

Provides Braille and audio books and free loans to persons with vision problems or other physical disabilities that prevent the person from reading. Makes referrals to state and local libraries.

WILSON'S DISEASE

Wilson's Disease Association International
1802 Brookside Drive
Wooster, OH 44691
888-264-1450
330-264-1450
Fax: 330-264-0974
E-mail: info@wilsonsdisease.org
Web site: http://www.wilsonsdisease.org

Provides support and financial aid to needy families, information, and coordination among members and related organizations.

WOMEN'S HEALTH

Endometriosis Association
8585 N. 76th Place
Milwaukee, WI 53223

800-992-3636 (United States), 800-426-2END
(Canada)
414-355-2200
Fax: 414-355-6065
Web site: http://www.endometriosisassn.org

Sponsors self-help support and informational meetings. Provides brochures in twenty-three languages and publications specifically for teens. Includes a link to information in Spanish.

North American Menopause Society (NAMS)
5900 Landerbrooke Drive
Suite 390
Mayfield Heights, OH 44124
440-442-7550
Fax: 440-442-2660
E-mail: info@menopause.org
Web site: http://www.menopause.org

Provides information on midlife medical issues. Maintains a database of menopause care providers and support groups.

Older Women's League (OWL)
National Office
1828 L Street NW
Suite 801
Washington, DC 20036
800-825-3695
Fax: 202-332-2949
E-mail: owl@owl-national.org
Web site: http://www.owl-national.org

Information on and support for issues affecting middle-aged and older women, such as health care and insurance, maintaining independence, and support for family caregivers.

—Irene Struthers Rush;
updated by Connie Pollock

WEB SITE DIRECTORY

GENERAL

The following Web sites offer a broad range of clinical and consumer health information, research news, and features such as interactive tools, searchable databases, and discussion boards.

A.D.A.M. Medical Encyclopedia
http://www.nlm.nih.gov/medlineplus/
   encyclopedia.html

Aging in the Know
http://www.healthinaging.org/agingintheknow

American Academy of Pediatrics
http://www.aap.org

American Dental Association
http://www.ada.org

American Geriatrics Society
http://www.americangeriatrics.org

American Medical Association
http://www.ama-assn.org

Anatomy Atlases
http://www.anatomyatlases.org

Centers for Disease Control and Prevention
http://www.cdc.gov

Consumer Health: Cushing/Whitney Medical
   Library
http://www.med.yale.edu/library/portals/
   consumer.html

Dictionary.com: Medical Dictionaries
http://www.dictionary.reference.com/medical

Digital Book Index
http://www.digitalbookindex.org

Dirline: Directory of Health Organizations
http://dirline.nlm.nih.gov

Drug Information Portal
http://druginfo.nlm.nih.gov/drugportal

FreeBooks4Doctors
http://www.freebooks4doctors.com

Genetics Home Reference
http://ghr.nlm.nih.gov

Global Library of Women's Medicine
http://www.glowm.com

Hospital Compare
http://www.hospitalcompare.hhs.gov

Household Products Database
http://householdproducts.nlm.nih.gov

Human Anatomy Online
http://www.innerbody.com

International Classification of Diseases
http://www.who.int/classifications/icd/en

Kids Health
http://www.kidshealth.org

Lab Tests Online
http://www.labstestsonline.org

MayoClinic.com
http://www.mayoclinic.com

MedicalStudent.com
http://www.medicalstudent.com

Medicine Net
http://www.medicinenet.com

MedlinePlus
http://medlineplus.gov

Medscape
http://www.medscape.com

Men's Health Network
http://www.menshealthnetwork.org

National Academies Press
http://www.nap.edu

National Cancer Institute
http://cancer.gov

National Center for Biotechnology Information
  Bookshelf
http://www.ncbi.nlm.nih.gov/books

National Center for Complementary and Alternative
  Medicine
http://nccam.nih.gov

National Eye Institute
http://www.nei.nih.gov

National Human Genome Research Institute
http://www.genome.gov

National Institute on Drug Abuse
http://www.nida.nih.gov

National Institutes of Health
http://nih.gov

National Library of Medicine
http://www.nlm.nih.gov

National Mental Health Information Center
http://mentalhealth.samhsa.gov

National Women's Health Resource Center
http://www.healthywomen.org

NIHSeniorHealth
http://nihseniorhealth.gov

Office of Minority Health Resource Center
http://minorityhealth.hhs.gov

Online Books Page
http://onlinebooks.library.upenn.edu

PubMed Central
http://www.pubmedcentral.nih.gov

Recalls, Market Withdrawals, and Safety Alerts
http://www.fda.gov/Safety/Recalls

RxList: The Internet Drug Index
http://www.rxlist.com

Stanford Health Library
http://healthlibrary.stanford.edu

Tox Town (Toxic Substances)
http://toxtown.nlm.nih.gov

U.S. Department of Health and Human Services
http://www.hhs.gov

U.S. Food and Drug Administration
http://www.fda.gov

User's Guide to Finding and Evaluating Health
  Information on the Web
http://mlanet.org/resources/userguide

WebMD
http://www.webmd.com

Who Named It? A Dictionary of Medical Eponyms
http://www.whonamedit.com

Womenshealth.gov
http://4women.gov

World Health News
http://www.worldhealthnews.harvard.edu

World Health Organization
http://www.who.int

ABORTION
National Right to Life Organization
http://www.nrlc.org
    Site offers sources of information on pro-life issues
in relation to abortion, organization support, euthanasia, and federal legislation.

Planned Parenthood
http://www.plannedparenthood.org
    Site of a leading sexual and reproductive health care
provider and advocate. Emphases on protecting access
to abortion, providing affordable birth control, and sex
education.

ACCIDENTS

National Center for Emergency Medicine
   Informatics
http://ncemi.org
   Site provides Web links, answers frequently asked
questions, and offers automatic e-mail list subscrip-
tions, bibliographies, and articles.

ACQUIRED IMMUNODEFICIENCY SYNDROME
   (AIDS)

AIDSinfo
http://www.aidsinfo.nih.gov
   HIV- and AIDS-related information from the U.S.
Department of Health and Human Services.

AIDS.org
http://www.aids.org
   Provides fact sheets, answers frequently asked questions, and offers AIDS treatment news, a newsletter,
and a bookstore.

National Pediatric AIDS Network
http://www.npan.org
   Site provides education, advocacy, and emotional
support to those with HIV/AIDS; promotes research
into prevention and treatment; helps remove the stigma
associated with the disease; and promotes the prevention of HIV transmission.

ALCOHOLISM

Alcoholics Anonymous
http://www.aa.org
   A group whose primary purpose is to help members
stay sober and help other alcoholics to achieve sobriety.

National Clearinghouse for Alcohol and Drug
   Information
http://ncadi.samhsa.gov
   A consumer Web site of the Substance Abuse and
Mental Health Services Administration. Provides access to publications on alcoholism, provides a treatment facility locator, lists statistics, and lists other information and resources.

ALZHEIMER'S DISEASE

Alzheimer's Association
http://www.alz.org
   An organization dedicated to researching the prevention and treatment of Alzheimer's disease. The
Benjamin B. Green-Field Library and Resource Center

collects a wide range of materials on Alzheimer's disease and related disorders and provides services to family members, educators and students, health professionals, social service agencies, and the general public.

AMPUTATION

Amputation Prevention Global Resource Center
http://www.diabetesresource.com
   Site offers clinical, educational, and research information on amputation.

AMYOTROPHIC LATERAL SCLEROSIS

ALS Association
http://www.alsa.org
   Site describes the mission and service of this national nonprofit voluntary health organization dedicated solely to the fight against amyotrophic lateral
sclerosis, also known as Lou Gehrig's disease.

ANEMIA

Anemia.com
http://www.anemia.com
   A group formed as a collaborative effort with the National Kidney Foundation, the Wellness Community,
and the National Anemia Action Council, Anemia
Lifeline works to increase awareness of the signs and
symptoms of anemia associated with serious diseases,
provide educational materials about anemia, and promote the understanding that treating anemia can help
patients with serious diseases live healthier and more
productive lives.

ANOREXIA NERVOSA

National Association of Anorexia Nervosa and
   Associated Disorders
http://www.anad.org
   A site that provides hotline counseling, a national
network of free support groups, referrals to health care
professionals, and education and prevention programs
to promote self-acceptance and healthy lifestyles.

ARTHRITIS

Arthritis Foundation
http://www.arthritis.org
   The site of the Arthritis Foundation, whose mission
is to support research to find the cure for and prevention
of arthritis and to improve the quality of life for those
affected by arthritis.

ASTHMA

American Lung Association

http://www.lungusa.org

Includes detailed information and updated research findings, a guide to local events and programs, and a section to share personal stories.

Asthma and Allergy Foundation of America

http://www.aafa.org

Site describes the mission of this nonprofit organization dedicated to finding a cure for and controlling asthma and allergic diseases.

ATTENTION-DEFICIT DISORDER

Children and Adults with Attention Deficit/
   Hyperactivity Disorder

http://www.chadd.org

Site describes this parent-based organization formed to better the lives of individuals with attention-deficit disorders and their families.

AUTISM

Autism Society of America

http://www.autism-society.org

Site provides information for parents with newly diagnosed children, general information about the society, and information about local chapters.

AUTOIMMUNE DISORDERS

American Autoimmune Related Diseases
   Association

http://www.aarda.org

A site that provides information on a range of autoimmune disorders, a section on women and autoimmunity, a newsletter, and links to resources, among other features.

BIOLOGICAL SUBSTANCES

U.S. Army Medical Research Institute of Infectious
   Diseases

http://www.usamriid.army.mil

This site includes information on how to recognize and treat illness caused by biological substances.

BIPOLAR DISORDERS

Depression and Bipolar Support Alliance

http://www.ndmda.org

Offers information on mood disorders, support groups, referrals for mental health professionals, research links, and discussion forums.

BIRTH DEFECTS

March of Dimes

http://www.marchofdimes.org

Web site offers a range of excellent fact sheets on myriad birth defects and disorders, information about prenatal testing, and special sections for pregnant women and for researchers and professionals.

BITES AND STINGS

Spiders and Other Arachnids

http://spiders.ucr.edu

Site provides links to information about the spider, scorpion, bee, wasp, and ant species worldwide whose bites cause morbidity and mortality.

BLINDNESS

American Foundation for the Blind

http://www.afb.org

Site of the American Foundation for the Blind (AFB), which publishes materials about blindness for professionals and consumers and maintains and preserves the Helen Keller Archives, one of the world's largest collections of print materials on blindness. AFB also maintains the Careers Technology Information Bank, a network of North American individuals who are blind.

National Federation of the Blind

http://www.nfb.org

The site of the National Federation of the Blind, which provides public education about blindness, information and referral services, scholarships, literature and publications about blindness, aids and appliances and other adaptive equipment, advocacy services and protection of civil rights, job opportunities, development and evaluation of technology, and support for blind persons and their families.

Prevent Blindness America

http://www.preventblindness.org

Founded in 1908, this group is dedicated to fighting blindness and saving eyesight. Its efforts are focused on promoting a continuum of vision care, public and professional education, certified vision screening training, and community and patient service programs and research.

BONE DISORDERS

National Institutes of Health, Osteoporosis and
   Related Bone Diseases National Resource Center

http://www.niams.nih.gov/bone

Comprehensive site with newsletters, research bibliographies, and fact sheets, among other features.

BONE MARROW TRANSPLANTATION
Blood and Marrow Transplant Information Network
http://www.bmtinfonet.org

Site contains a resource directory, information on transplant centers in the United States and Canada, a drug database, and a news bulletin, among other features.

BRAIN DISORDERS
Dana.org
http://www.dana.org

A nonprofit organization of neuroscientists that was formed to provide information about the personal and public benefits of brain research. The Web site is research oriented and gives excellent information and links on current brain studies, new diagnosis and treatment technology, and brain-related news stories.

BREAST CANCER
National Alliance of Breast Cancer Organizations
http://www.nabco.org

Site describes this nonprofit resource for information about breast cancer, providing current research information, treatment options, support referrals, and links.

Sisters Network
http://www.sistersnetworkinc.org

A national breast cancer network that provides on-line health information, support, and referrals to African American women who have had or who have breast cancer.

BURPING
National Digestive Disease Information
  Clearinghouse
http://digestive.niddk.nih.gov/ddiseases/pubs/gas

This section, "Gas in the Digestive Tract," provides information on burping and the possible signs and symptoms that it represents.

CANADIAN SITES
Canadian Centre for Occupational Health and
  Safety (CCOHS)/Le Centre canadien d'hygiène
  et de sécurité au travail (CCHST)
http://www.ccohs.ca (English)
http://www.cchst.ca (French)

A not-for-profit federal department corporation that seeks the elimination of work-related illnesses and injuries.

Canadian Public Health Association (CPHA)
http://www.cpha.ca/en/default.aspx

A national, independent, not-for-profit, and voluntary association representing public health in Canada, with links to the international public health community.

Health Canada/Santé Canada
http://www.hc-sc.gc.ca/index-eng.php (English)
http://www.hc-sc.gc.ca/index-fra.php (French)

The federal department responsible for helping Canadians maintain and improve their health. Offers consumer safety information and information about First Nations, Inuit, and Aboriginal health.

Public Health Agency of Canada (PHAC)/L'Agence
  de la santé publique du Canada (ASPC)
http://www.phac-aspc.gc.ca/index-eng.php (English)
http://www.phac-aspc.gc.ca/index-fra.php (French)

This government agency, formed in 2004, was created in response to growing concerns about the capacity of Canada's public health system to anticipate and respond effectively to public health threats.

CANCER
American Cancer Society
http://www.cancer.org

Site describes the mission of this organization, dedicated to helping everyone who faces cancer through research, patient services, early detection, treatment, and education.

Cancer Care
http://www.cancercare.org

Site provides information, including links and resources, to help people who have cancer, and their families and friends, cope with the disease.

CARPAL TUNNEL SYNDROME
Carpal Tunnel Syndrome Place
http://www.ctsplace.com

Web page offers information about the disorder, ergonomic products for sale, message boards, and myriad research links.

CEREBRAL PALSY

United Cerebral Palsy

http://www.ucp.org

A leading source of information on cerebral palsy, acting as a pivotal advocate for the rights of persons with any disability. One of the largest health charities in the United States, United Cerebral Palsy helps advance the independence, productivity, and full citizenship of people with cerebral palsy and other disabilities.

CERVICAL, OVARIAN, AND UTERINE CANCERS

National Cervical Cancer Coalition

http://www.nccc-online.org

Site describes this grassroots advocacy coalition for issues concerning cervical cancer screening and the traditional Pap test.

Ovarian Cancer National Alliance

http://www.ovariancancer.org

This group was formed in 1997 by leaders from seven ovarian cancer groups. Its primary goal is to establish a coordinated national effort to place ovarian cancer education, policy, and research issues prominently on the agendas of national policy makers and women's health care leaders.

CHILDBIRTH

Baby Center

http://www.babycenter.com/pregnancy

An excellent site that offers comprehensive information on all topics related to pregnancy and childbirth.

Childbirth.org

http://www.childbirth.org

A site that helps users learn about childbirth options and how to find the best possible care during pregnancy. Includes many links of an educational, informational, and personal nature.

CHOLESTEROL

HealthCentral.com

http://www.healthcentral.com/cholesterol

Site provides information on lowering cholesterol levels and on cholesterol and the heart, as well as the opportunity to join a cholesterol discussion group.

CHRONIC FATIGUE SYNDROME

CFIDS Association of America

http://www.cfids.org

A group dedicated to understanding and eliminating chronic fatigue and immune dysfunction syndrome (CFIDS). Focuses on increasing the pace of CFIDS research, achieving public policy victories for people with CFIDS, and directing mainstream attention on the disease.

CLEFT PALATE

Cleft Palate Foundation

http://www.cleftline.org

Web site is divided into two sections, one for patients and families and one for professionals. The group offers publications, information and support, and annual research grants.

CLINICAL TRIALS

CenterWatch Clinical Trials Listing Service

http://www.centerwatch.com

Site provides national and international listings of clinical trials in all therapeutic areas.

ClinicalTrials.gov

http://www.clinicaltrials.gov

Site sponsored by the National Institutes of Health provides patients, family members, health care professionals, and members of the public access to information on clinical trials for a wide range of diseases and conditions.

COLITIS

Crohn's and Colitis Foundation of America

http://www.ccfa.org

Provides support groups and a wide range of educational publications and programs on Crohn's disease and ulcerative colitis.

COLON CANCER

Colon Cancer Alliance

http://www.ccalliance.org

A national patient advocacy organization dedicated to ending the suffering caused by colorectal cancer. The Colon Cancer Alliance is the official patient support partner of the National Colorectal Cancer Research Alliance.

CONGENITAL HEART DISEASE

American Heart Association

http://www.americanheart.org

A group dedicated to reducing disability and death from cardiovascular diseases and stroke. Offers thorough information on a wide range of cardiovascular diseases, referrals to emergency cardiovascular care classes, and research statistics and articles.

CONTRACEPTION
Planned Parenthood
http://www.plannedparenthood.org
Site describes the philosophy of Planned Parenthood: that knowledge empowers people to make better choices about their health and sexuality. Offers a wide range of information resources including pamphlets, books, newsletters, and a list of helpful Web sites.

CORNEAL TRANSPLANTATION
Tissue Banks International
http://www.tbionline.org
Site describes an international network of eye and tissue banks that recovers and provides ocular and other human tissue for use in transplants and other surgeries.

CORNELIA DE LANGE SYNDROME
Cornelia de Lange Syndrome-USA Foundation
http://www.cdlsusa.org
A family support organization that promotes the early and accurate diagnosis of Cornelia de Lange syndrome (CLS) and research into the causes and manifestations of the syndrome. It helps people with a diagnosis of CLS and others with similar characteristics.

CREUTZFELDT-JAKOB DISEASE
Creutzfeldt-Jakob Disease Foundation
http://cjdfoundation.org
Site describes resources to promote research, education, and awareness of the disease, as well as to provide support services for persons affected by Creutzfeldt-Jakob disease.

Dana.org
http://www.dana.org
A nonprofit organization of neuroscientists that was formed to provide information about the personal and public benefits of brain research. The Web site is research oriented and gives excellent information and links on current brain studies, new diagnosis and treatment technology, and brain-related news stories.

CROHN'S DISEASE
Crohn's and Colitis Foundation of America
http://www.ccfa.org

Provides support groups and a wide range of educational publications and programs on Crohn's disease and ulcerative colitis.

CYSTIC FIBROSIS
Cystic Fibrosis Foundation
http://www.cff.org
Web site offers comprehensive information about the disease, locations of local Cystic Fibrosis Foundation chapters and care centers, information about research and clinical trials, and advice on living with the disease.

DEMENTIAS
Dana.org
http://www.dana.org
A nonprofit organization of neuroscientists that was formed to provide information about the personal and public benefits of brain research. The Web site is research oriented and gives excellent information and links on current brain studies, new diagnosis and treatment technology, and brain-related news stories.

Psychiatry24x7.com
http://www.psychiatry24x7.com
Provides information for caregivers and health care professionals about the latest developments in research and caregiving for dementia.

DEPRESSION
Depression and Bipolar Support Alliance
http://www.dbsalliance.org
Offers information on mood disorders, support groups, referrals for mental health professionals, research links, and discussion forums.

DERMATITIS
American Academy of Dermatology
http://www.aad.org
The site's public resources section offers good information about dermatitis, as well as coverage of other dermatological disorders.

DIABETES
American Diabetes Association
http://www.diabetes.org
Gives comprehensive information on type 1 and type 2 diabetes and updated research and scientific findings, provides community forums and news stories, and helps decipher health insurance issues, among other features.

Children with Diabetes
http://www.childrenwithdiabetes.com
Site provides information that helps children with diabetes and their families learn about the disease and meet other diabetics.

Diabetes Monitor
http://www.diabetesmonitor.com
Site monitors diabetes-related happenings on the Web.

Diabetes.com
http://www.diabetes.com
Site provides an information resource and online community for diabetics. Includes sections on diet and exercise, intimacy, risk factors and prevention, and information on symptoms.

DOMESTIC VIOLENCE
National Coalition Against Domestic Violence
http://www.ncadv.org
A site that defines domestic violence and offers information on community responses, getting help, and public policy.

DOWN SYNDROME
National Down Syndrome Society
http://www.ndss.org
An excellent organization that focuses on research, advocacy, and education. The Web site promotes virtual communities and provides updated information about events.

DRUG USE
ClubDrugs.gov
http://clubdrugs.gov
Information from the U.S. National Institutes of Health and National Institute on Drug Abuse.

National Clearinghouse for Alcohol and Drug
    Information
http://ncadi.samhsa.gov
A consumer Web site of the Substance Abuse and Mental Health Services Administration. Provides access to publications on drug abuse, provides a treatment facility locator, lists statistics, and lists other information and resources.

DWARFISM
Little People of America
http://www.lpaonline.org
A nonprofit organization that provides support and information to people of short stature and their families. Web site offers a research library, answers frequently asked questions, and provides information on local chapters.

DYSLEXIA
International Dyslexia Association
http://www.interdys.org
Web site includes a bookstore and information on new assistive technologies. Divided into sections for children, teenagers, college students, adults, educators, and parents.

EATING DISORDERS
National Association of Anorexia Nervosa and
    Associated Disorders
http://www.anad.org
A site that provides hotline counseling, a national network of free support groups, referrals to health care professionals, and education and prevention programs to promote self-acceptance and healthy lifestyles.

National Eating Disorders Association
http://www.nationaleatingdisorders.org
This nonprofit organization works to prevent eating disorders and to provide treatment referrals to those suffering from anorexia nervosa, bulimia, and binge eating disorder and those concerned with body image and weight issues.

ECZEMA
National Eczema Society
http://www.eczema.org
Site about one of the most established organizations worldwide dedicated to the needs of people with eczema, dermatitis, and sensitive skin. Offers medical information and links.

EMPHYSEMA
American Lung Association
http://www.lungusa.org
Includes detailed information and updated research findings, a guide to local events and programs, and a section to share personal stories.

National Emphysema Foundation

http://www.emphysemafoundation.org

Site offers tips on exercises, inhaler uses, and other helpful items for those with emphysema.

ENCEPHALITIS

Dana.org

http://www.dana.org

A nonprofit organization of neuroscientists that was formed to provide information about the personal and public benefits of brain research. The Web site is research oriented and gives excellent information and links on current brain studies, new diagnosis and treatment technology, and brain-related news stories.

ENDOCARDITIS

American Heart Association

http://www.americanheart.org

A group dedicated to reducing disability and death from cardiovascular diseases and stroke. Offers thorough information on a wide range of cardiovascular diseases, referrals to emergency cardiovascular care classes, and research statistics and articles.

ENDOMETRIOSIS

Endometriosis.org

http://www.endometriosis.org

A Web site that answers frequently asked questions about the disease and offers research articles, case histories, information about local support groups, diagnosis and treatment facts, and a glossary.

ENVIRONMENTAL HEALTH

Environmental Diseases from A to Z

http://www.niehs.nih.gov/health/topics/atoz

Site provides information from the National Institute of Environmental Health Sciences, National Institutes of Health.

Scorecard

http://www.scorecard.org

Site provides a database allowing users to see chemical pollution on street maps of their own communities.

EPILEPSY

Epilepsy Foundation

http://www.epilepsyfoundation.org

A national organization dedicated to education, research, and advocacy. Web site offers information on careers and employment, parent support groups and children's programs, and online interest groups, among many other features.

FETAL ALCOHOL SYNDROME

National Organization on Fetal Alcohol Syndrome

http://www.nofas.org

A group committed to raising public awareness of fetal alcohol syndrome and to developing and implementing plans for prevention, intervention, education, and advocacy.

FIBROMYALGIA

Fibromyalgia Network

http://www.fmnetnews.com

An organization that provides updated information about fibromyalgia and chronic fatigue syndrome. Its goal is to enrich the lives of patients by providing education, improving awareness, and promoting research.

National Fibromyalgia Association

http://www.fmaware.org

An excellent resource for those living with fibromyalgia. Offers updated information on the disease, resource links, and a magazine.

FOOD POISONING

U.S. Food and Drug Administration Center for Food Safety and Applied Nutrition

http://fda.gov/food

Site provides information on food safety, nutrition, and wholesomeness, as well as the notices on food recalls.

USDA/FDA Food Safety Information Center

http://foodsafety.nal.usda.gov

Site provides information about foodborne illness prevention to educators, trainers, and organizations developing education and training materials for food workers and consumers.

FOOT DISORDERS

American Podiatric Medical Association

http://www.apma.org

Provides information on many types of foot disorders, such as bunions, athlete's foot, foot and ankle injuries, hammertoe, heel pain, leg cramps, nail problems, neuromas, and warts.

FRAGILE X SYNDROME
FRAXA Research Foundation
http://www.fraxa.org
A group that works to support scientific research aimed at finding a treatment and cure for fragile X syndrome.

GENETIC DISEASES
Alliance of Genetic Support Groups
http://www.geneticalliance.org
Site provides information on an international coalition of individuals, professionals, and genetic support organizations working together to enhance the lives of everyone affected by genetic conditions.

Hereditary Disease Foundation
http://www.hdfoundation.org
Site describes the mission of this nonprofit, basic science organization dedicated to the cure of genetic disease.

GLAUCOMA
Glaucoma Research Foundation
http://www.glaucoma.org
A group that strives toward restoring the sight and independence of individuals with glaucoma through research and education, with the ultimate goal of finding a cure.

GRIEF AND GUILT
GriefNet.org
http://griefnet.org
A Web community of persons dealing with grief, death, and major loss. Offers e-mail-based support groups for adults and children.

GUILLAIN-BARRÉ SYNDROME
GBS/CIDP Foundation International
http://www.gbsfi-cidp.com
A Web site focused on providing informative support and increasing the opportunities for patients, family, and friends to create networks and communicate.

GULF WAR SYNDROME
Gulf War Veteran Resource Pages
http://www.gulfweb.org
Considers the health effects created by the 1991 Persian Gulf War. Additionally, the site is a community center for veterans of the conflict that gives them opportunities to locate fellow soldiers, discuss issues, and tell their stories.

HEADACHES
National Headache Foundation
http://www.headaches.org
Operates local support groups and provides information for headache sufferers, their families, and physicians.

HEARING LOSS AND TESTS
Hearing Exchange
http://www.hearingexchange.com
An online community designed to foster the exchange of information and to provide support for the hearing impaired.

HEART ATTACK AND DISEASE
American Heart Association
http://www.americanheart.org
Site provides comprehensive information on heart disease and conditions, healthy lifestyles, and resources and offers interactive health tools.

HEMOPHILIA
National Hemophilia Foundation
http://www.hemophilia.org
A Web site that promotes education, research, and advocacy on behalf of people with bleeding disorders.

HEPATITIS
Hepatitis Foundation International
http://www.hepfi.org
A foundation that teaches the public and hepatitis patients how to prevent, diagnose, and treat viral hepatitis and supports research into the prevention, treatment, and cure of the disease.

HERNIA
Hernia Resource Center
http://www.herniainfo.com
Answers frequently asked questions about hernias and provides the latest medical news and research, information on surgical treatment options, and tools for finding a doctor who specializes in hernias.

HERPES
American Social Health Association: Herpes
    Resource Center
http://www.ashastd.org/herpes/herpes_overview.cfm
A group that focuses on increasing education, public awareness, and support to anyone concerned about herpes.

HISTIOCYTOSIS
Histiocytosis Association of America
http://www.histio.org
Established in 1986 to connect patients and families dealing with histiocytic disorders. In addition to outreach and educational efforts, the group funds clinical trials and scientific research projects to identify better treatments and ultimately cure these diseases.

HODGKIN'S DISEASE
Lymphoma Information Network
http://www.lymphomainfo.net/hodgkins
Offers information on the diagnosis and treatment options for adult and childhood Hodgkin's disease and resources for further research.

HOLISTIC MEDICINE
American Holistic Health Association
http://www.ahha.org
A Web site dedicated to honoring the whole person and encouraging people to participate actively in their own health and health care.

HOMEOPATHY
National Center for Homeopathy
http://www.homeopathic.org
Offers resources on research, training, and how to find a homeopathic practitioner.

HOSPICE
National Hospice and Palliative Care Organization
http://www.nhpco.org
A group that advocates for the terminally ill and their families, develops public and professional educational programs and materials to enhance understanding and availability of hospice and palliative care, and conducts research, among other activities.

HYDROCEPHALUS
Hydrocephalus Association
http://www.hydroassoc.org
A Web site that provides information and resources, support, and educational help to patients with hydrocephalus and their parents.

HYPERTENSION
American Society of Hypertension
http://www.ash-us.org
A group dedicated to promoting and encouraging the development, advancement, and exchange of scientific information in all aspects of the research, diagnosis, and treatment of hypertension and related cardiovascular diseases.

HYPOGLYCEMIA
Hypoglycemia Support Foundation
http://www.hypoglycemia.org
Provides diet information, self-tests for the disease, and helpful Web links.

HYSTERECTOMY
Hysterectomy Association
http://www.hysterectomy-association.org.uk
A group based in the United Kingdom dedicated to providing impartial information to women who have had, or who are contemplating, a hysterectomy and to enable them to make appropriate decisions for their long-term health.

Hystersisters.com
http://www.hystersisters.com
An online community of women who give and receive support for hysterectomy decisions and recovery. Offers resources that allow visitors to explore options and make decisions for themselves.

ILEOSTOMY AND COLOSTOMY
United Ostomy Association
http://www.uoa.org
A support group for ostomy patients that stresses education, information, support, and advocacy.

IMMUNE DISORDERS
Immune Web
http://www.immuneweb.org
A mailing list and resource center for people with chronic fatigue syndrome, multiple chemical sensitivities, lupus, allergies, environmental illness, fibromyalgia, candidiasis, and other immune system disorders. Offers good articles on several immunodeficiency disorders, "safe" product lists, and annotated links to other Web sites.

IMMUNIZATION AND VACCINATION
Vaccine Place
http://www.vaccineplace.com
Site provides access to current news about vaccines and an annotated database of vaccine resources on the Web.

Red Book Online

http://aapredbook.aappublications.org

Site provides information about vaccinations and infectious diseases involving children. Lists recommended immunization schedule for children up to age eighteen.

INCONTINENCE

National Association for Continence

http://www.nafc.org

A clearinghouse for information and services related to incontinence and assistive devices. Provides education, advocacy, and support on the causes, prevention, diagnosis, treatment, and management options for persons with incontinence.

INFERTILITY

International Council on Infertility Information Dissemination

http://www.inciid.org

An online resource of comprehensive, consumer-targeted infertility information that covers cutting-edge technologies and treatments. Provides fact sheets of treatments, an interactive area for member participation, a library and glossary, and a comprehensive professional directory of clinics and doctors who specialize in infertility treatment.

INFLUENZA

Centers for Disease Control and Prevention

http://www.cdc.gov/flu

Gives updates on current areas of infection, provides resources for prevention and control, and answers frequently asked questions.

INTERNET MEDICINE

Office for the Advancement of Telehealth

http://www.hrsa.gov/telehealth

An organization devoted to advancing the use of telehealth and Internet-based medicine to facilitate improvement in the state of public health and research on public health.

IRRITABLE BOWEL SYNDROME

Irritable Bowel Syndrome Self Help and Support Group

http://www.ibsgroup.org

Provides support to those who suffer from irritable bowel syndrome (IBS) and their family members and information for medical professionals who want to learn more about IBS. Works to educate those who are living with IBS and to increase awareness about this and other functional gastrointestinal disorders.

National Digestive Diseases Information Clearinghouse

http://digestive.niddk.nih.gov

Site offers an overview of irritable bowel syndrome; its causes, effects, and treatments; and suggestions for further reading.

JUVENILE RHEUMATOID ARTHRITIS

Arthritis Foundation

http://www.arthritis.org

Provides information on arthritis support groups, exercise classes, and other resources for persons with arthritis. Also offers information, education, and publications specific to juvenile arthritis.

KIDNEY DISORDERS

National Kidney Foundation

http://www.kidney.org

Offers thorough information on myriad kidney problems and diseases; supports patient services such as transplantation, drug banks, and educational projects; and makes referrals to local agencies.

KIDNEY TRANSPLANTATION

American Kidney Fund

http://www.akfinc.org

Provides financial assistance for individuals with chronic kidney failure.

KLINEFELTER SYNDROME

Klinefelter Syndrome and Associates

http://www.genetic.org

Offers support and information for persons and families affected by Klinefelter syndrome. Facilitates networking and the exchange of information.

LACTOSE INTOLERANCE

Lactose.co.uk

http://www.lactose.co.uk

A site based in the United Kingdom that provides excellent information about lactose intolerance, irritable bowel syndrome, allergens, and food allergies.

National Digestive Diseases Information
Clearinghouse: Lactose Intolerance
http://digestive.niddk.nih.gov/ddiseases/pubs/
lactoseintolerance
A U.S. government site offering detailed information on lactose intolerance.

LEARNING DISABILITIES
Learning Disabilities Association of America
http://www.ldanatl.org
Information, publications, and referral service concerning learning disabilities. State and local groups provide services to families, including camps and recreation programs.

LEUKEMIA
Leukemia and Lymphoma Society of America
http://www.leukemia.org
A group dedicated to funding blood cancer research, education, and patient services for patients with leukemia and other lymphatic diseases.

LIVER CANCER
Liver Cancer Network
http://www.livercancer.com
A group whose mission is to provide liver cancer patients and their families with the basic knowledge needed to communicate better with their physicians. Gives excellent information about the anatomy of the liver and the diagnosis and treatment of liver cancer.

LIVER DISORDERS
American Liver Foundation
http://www.liverfoundation.org
Provides physician referrals and information on support groups for persons with liver disease and their families.

LUNG CANCER
Lung Cancer Online Foundation
http://www.lungcanceronline.org
A Web site that strives to improve the quality of care and quality of life for people with lung cancer by funding lung cancer research and providing information to patients and families.

LUPUS
Lupus Foundation of America
http://www.lupus.org
A group dedicated to improving the diagnosis and treatment of lupus, supporting individuals and families

affected by the disease, increasing awareness of lupus among health professionals and the public, and finding a cure.

LYME DISEASE
American Lyme Disease Foundation
http://www.aldf.com
Provides educational materials and information regarding Lyme disease and maintains a physician referral service.

Lyme Disease Association
http://www.lymediseaseassociation.org
An organization dedicated to Lyme disease education and prevention and to raising money for research projects.

LYMPHADENOPATHY AND LYMPHOMA
Leukemia and Lymphoma Society of America
http://www.leukemia.org
A group dedicated to funding blood cancer research, education, and patient services for patients with leukemia and other lymphatic diseases.

Lymphoma Focus
http://www.lymphomafocus.org
This site is divided into two areas: one for lymphoma patients, caregivers, and the public; the other for physicians, nurses, and other health care professionals. Features include streaming video Webcasts, text transcripts, and articles.

Lymphoma Information Network
http://www.lymphomainfo.net/hodgkins
Offers information on the diagnosis and treatment options for adult and childhood Hodgkin's disease and resources for further research.

MACULAR DEGENERATION
American Macular Degeneration Foundation
http://www.macular.org
Provides information to clinicians and patients regarding the latest in research regarding macular degeneration. Offers an award-winning video for helping patients cope with this debilitating illness.

Macular Degeneration Foundation
http://www.eyesight.org
Site describes this charitable educational and research foundation dedicated to discovering the cause of and developing cures for macular degeneration.

MALARIA

Malaria Foundation International
http://www.malaria.org

A site that serves as a gateway for the Malaria Foundation International, a group that funds global outreach projects designed to fight malaria and that raises public awareness and provides education about the disease.

MARFAN SYNDROME

National Marfan Foundation
http://www.marfan.org

A group that seeks to disseminate accurate information about this condition to patients, family members, and the health care community; to provide a communication network for patients and their relatives; and to support and foster research.

MASSAGE

American Massage Therapy Association
http://www.amtamassage.org

Site provides information and references about massage, methods and techniques, alternative and holistic care, and general information related to massage therapy.

MEDICARE

Medicare: The Official Government Site for People with Medicare
http://www.medicare.gov

Provides information on the quality of care provided by health care facilities approved by Medicare.

MELANOMA

Melanoma Patients' Information Page
http://www.melanoma.org/community/bulletin-board

Provides support and information to patients with melanoma; allows them to be proactive participants in their treatment decisions.

MENINGITIS

Meningitis Research Foundation
http://www.meningitis.org

Provides information about symptoms and different types of the disease, the latest news, and research links, among other features.

MENOPAUSE

North American Menopause Society
http://www.menopause.org

A site run by a scientific research organization that includes an excellent section covering the range of menopause symptoms and treatment and providing referral lists and resource links, among other features.

MENTAL RETARDATION

American Association on Intellectual and Developmental Disabilities
http://www.aamr.org

A group for professionals in the mental health field that promotes progressive policies, research, effective practices, and universal human rights for people with mental retardation.

Best Buddies International
http://www.bestbuddies.org

Facilitates friendships among people with mental retardation and others in the community.

MULTIPLE SCLEROSIS

National Multiple Sclerosis Society
http://www.nationalmssociety.org

Provides services to persons with multiple sclerosis through local chapters and promotes research, educates, advocates on critical issues, and organizes a wide range of programs.

NARCOLEPSY

Narcolepsy Network
http://www.narcolepsynetwork.org

Provides referral services, support group meetings, and communication among members.

Stanford School of Medicine Center for Narcolepsy
http://med.stanford.edu/school/Psychiatry/narcolepsy

Site describes the Stanford University center, providing an outline of the disorder, details of current research, and information about publications.

NEURALGIA, NEURITIS, AND NEUROPATHY

Facial Neuralgia Resources
http://facial-neuralgia.org

Covers a range of information about facial neuralgias, other cranial neuralgias, and neuralgia-like disorders.

Trigeminal Neuralgia Association
http://www.tna-support.org

A group that serves as an advocate for patients suffering from trigeminal neuralgia and related facial pain conditions by providing information, encouraging research, and offering support.

NEUROFIBROMATOSIS
Children's Tumor Foundation
http://www.ctf.org

Site of a nonprofit foundation dedicated to improving the health and well-being of individuals and families affected by neurofibromatoses.

NIEMANN-PICK DISEASE
National Niemann-Pick Disease Foundation
http://www.nnpdf.org

A group that promotes advocacy, research, support, and awareness.

NUTRITION
U.S. Department of Agriculture
http://www.MyPyramid.gov

Government site that offers information about nutrition, including personalized guidelines.

OBESITY
American Obesity Association
http://www.obesity.org

A comprehensive Web site with information on the disease, research resources, advocacy, disability issues, community action, and personal stories, among many other topics.

OBSESSIVE-COMPULSIVE DISORDER
Obsessive-Compulsive Foundation
http://www.ocfoundation.org

A group that educates the public and professional communities about obsessive-compulsive disorder (OCD) and related disorders, provides assistance to individuals with OCD and their families and friends, and funds research into causes and effective treatments.

OSTEONECROSIS
National Osteonecrosis Foundation
http://www.nonf.org

The goal of this organization is to provide funding for medical research and education of patients, physicians, and other health professionals about osteonecrosis and Perthes' disease.

OSTEOPOROSIS
National Osteoporosis Foundation
http://www.nof.org

A leading resource for people seeking updated, medically sound information on the causes, prevention, detection, and treatment of osteoporosis.

Osteoporosis and Related Bone Diseases National Resource Center
http://www.niams.nih.gov/health_info/bone

This center at the National Institutes of Health offers fact sheets, research bibliographies, newsletters, and links.

PAIN MANAGEMENT
American Pain Foundation
http://www.painfoundation.org

Web site of one of the major advocacy and support organizations for persons in pain and for health professionals and caregivers. Provides links to helpful resources, including academic journals, and links to information on "pain law and ethics" and finding care.

PANCREATITIS
Pancreatitis Supporters' Network
http://www.pancreatitis.org.uk

A group based in the United Kingdom that provides medical information and support. Offers valuable information on drugs, advances in medical research, and book and Web resources.

PANIC ATTACKS
AnxietyPanic.com
http://www.anxietypanic.com

A good portal site that provides resources for understanding of anxiety disorders and their research and treatment.

PARALYSIS
Christopher and Dana Reeve Foundation
http://www.christopherreeve.org

Site describes this advocacy organization that supports research into spinal cord injuries and nervous system disorders that cause paralysis.

Cure Paralysis Now
http://www.cureparalysisnow.org

Site offers information for professionals and patients on advancing progress to cure spinal cord paralysis.

PARKINSON'S DISEASE
National Parkinson Foundation
http://www.parkinson.org

Site provides the latest news and developments in Parkinson's disease research and includes a list of publications and events.

Parkinson's Disease Foundation
http://www.pdf.org
A national group devoted to education, advocacy, and the funding of research for the disease.

PHENYLKETONURIA
National PKU News
http://www.pkunews.org
A site that focuses on news and information about the disease. Includes personal stories, research links, and diet-related information, among other features.

PHOBIAS
AnxietyPanic.com
http://www.anxietypanic.com
A good portal site that provides resources for support, understanding anxiety disorders, treatment, and research. Phobias are specifically covered in one section.

POLIOMYELITIS
Post-Polio Health International
http://www.post-polio.org
A site that offers research and educational materials about polio and postpolio syndrome as well as networking opportunities and advocacy for patients.

PORPHYRIA
American Porphyria Foundation
http://www.porphyriafoundation.com
Seeks to enhance public awareness about the disease, develop educational programs and distribute educational literature for patients and physicians, and support research to improve treatment and ultimately lead to a cure.

POSTPARTUM DEPRESSION
Postpartum Support International
http://www.postpartum.net
Offers resources for mothers and their families, a bookstore, information on support groups, and forums.

POST-TRAUMATIC STRESS DISORDER
National Center for Posttraumatic Stress Disorder
http://www.ncptsd.va.gov
A program of the U.S. Department of Veterans Affairs that seeks to advance the clinical care and social welfare of veterans through research, education, and training in the science, diagnosis, and treatment of post-traumatic stress disorder and other stress-related disorders.

PTSD Alliance
http://www.ptsdalliance.org
A group of professional and advocacy organizations that provide educational resources to individuals diagnosed with post-traumatic stress disorder (PTSD) and their loved ones, those at risk for developing PTSD, and health care professionals.

PRADER-WILLI SYNDROME
Prader-Willi Syndrome Association
http://www.pwsausa.org
A group dedicated to serving individuals affected by Prader-Willi syndrome, their families, and health care professionals. Provides information, education, and support services to its members.

PROSTATE CANCER
National Prostate Cancer Coalition
http://www.fightprostatecancer.org
A network of survivors, doctors, researchers, activists, and partnering advocate organizations that serves as a source for prostate cancer information and education.

PSORIASIS
National Psoriasis Foundation
http://www.psoriasis.org
A national nonprofit organization whose mission is to help improve the quality of life of people who have psoriasis and psoriatic arthritis. Gives comprehensive information on research, treatment, and community resources.

PSYCHIATRIC DISORDERS
AllPsych Online
http://allpsych.com/disorders
A site that covers adult psychiatric disorders and personality disorders, including etiology, symptoms, treatment options, and prognosis.

PULMONARY DISEASES
American Lung Association
http://www.lungusa.org
Includes detailed information and updated research findings, a guide to local events and programs, and a section to share personal stories.

RESUSCITATION

American Heart Association CPR and Emergency Cardiovascular Care

http://www.americanheart.org

Site offers updated cardiopulmonary resuscitation guidelines.

ROSACEA

Rosacea.org

http://www.rosacea.org

A nonprofit organization whose mission is to improve the lives of people with rosacea by raising awareness, providing public health information, and supporting research on this widespread but little-known disorder. Web site provides information for patients and physicians, a newsletter, and a glossary.

RUBINSTEIN-TAYBI SYNDROME

RTS: Rubinstein-Taybi Syndrome

http://www.rubinstein-taybi.org

A site devoted to people diagnosed with Rubinstein-Taybi syndrome and their families. Provides medical information, links to resources, and a forum.

SCHIZOPHRENIA

National Allegiance for Research on Schizophrenia and Depression

http://www.narsad.org

This site provides excellent information on a range of mental health disorders, including schizophrenia. Also covers updated research and provides personal stories.

SCOLIOSIS

National Scoliosis Foundation

http://www.scoliosis.org

Provides updated medical research information, physician referrals, and community support.

SKIN CANCER

Skin Cancer Foundation

http://www.skincancer.org

Promotes public education about skin cancer through campaigns against Sun exposure and early detection. Supports research into new diagnostic techniques and therapies.

SLEEP DISORDERS

National Sleep Foundation

http://www.sleepfoundation.org

Along with good information about the range of sleep disorders, the site also provides information on sleeping tips, children and sleep, and sleep services, among other features.

SMOKING

National Center for Chronic Disease Prevention and Health Promotion, Office on Smoking and Health

http://www.cdc.gov/tobacco

This site from the Centers for Disease Control and Prevention provides information on smoking cessation, smoking and teens, smoking during pregnancy, and passive smoking, among other resources. Also offers a comprehensive collection of Web links.

SPINA BIFIDA

Spina Bifida Association

http://www.sbaa.org

Promotes the prevention of spina bifida and strives to enhance the lives of all affected. Offers a newsletter, physician referrals, and scholarship funds, among other services.

SPINAL CORD DISORDERS

NINDS Spinal Cord Injury Information Page

http://www.ninds.nih.gov/disorders/sci

Site from the National Institute of Neurological Disorders and Stroke contains good information about spinal cord injuries, current research, and support organizations.

STEROIDS

Anabolic Steroid Abuse

http://www.steroidabuse.gov

The National Institutes of Health and the National Institute on Drug Abuse provide information about steroid abuse.

STROKES

American Stroke Association

http://www.strokeassociation.org

Gives information on warning signs, stroke care, and stroke programs. Offers newsletters and scientific and professional research links, among other features.

STURGE-WEBER SYNDROME

Sturge-Weber Foundation

http://www.sturge-weber.com

A comprehensive resource for all individuals interested in birthmarks and Sturge-Weber and Klippel-Trenaunay syndromes. Provides education and referrals and promotes research and awareness.

STUTTERING

Stuttering Foundation of America

http://www.stuttersfa.org

Provides free online resources, services, and support to those who stutter and their families, as well as support for research into the causes of stuttering.

SUDDEN INFANT DEATH SYNDROME

SIDS Network

http://sids-network.org

Provides news about current research, answers frequently asked questions about sudden infant death syndrome, and offers fact sheets on such topics as sleep, smoking, and apnea.

SUICIDE

Suicide Awareness Voices of Education

http://www.save.org

Offers resources for suicide prevention, suicide survivors, and families coping with a suicide loss.

TAY-SACHS DISEASE

National Tay-Sachs and Allied Diseases Association

http://www.ntsad.org

A group dedicated to the treatment and prevention of Tay-Sachs and related diseases and to information and support services for individuals and families affected by these diseases.

THALASSEMIA

Cooley's Anemia Foundation

http://www.cooleysanemia.org

Provides information for patients and their families, medical personnel, donors, and anyone interested in learning about Cooley's anemia and other forms of thalassemia.

Northern California Comprehensive Thalassemia Center

http://www.thalassemia.com

This center's program is designed to provide medical care, education, outreach, genetic counseling, and psychosocial care to patients, their families, and those at risk for carrying the disease.

THYROID DISORDERS

EndocrineWeb.com

http://www.endocrineweb.com

A site that provides a good overview of thyroid and related complications and disorders.

TOURETTE'S SYNDROME

Tourette Syndrome Association

http://www.tsa-usa.org

A group supporting advocacy, education, and research about this disorder.

TOXICOLOGY

Agency for Toxic Substances and Disease Registry

http://www.atsdr.cdc.gov

A public health agency under the U.S. Department of Health and Human Services that is an excellent resource for current information on risks associated with toxic substances, for specialists and for the public.

TRANSPLANTATION

OrganDonor.gov

http://www.organdonor.gov

Site provides advice on how to become an organ and tissue donor and answers questions about the many myths and facts surrounding donation.

TRAVEL

Centers for Disease Control, Traveler's Health

http://wwwnc.cdc.gov/travel

Site provides updated information on health precautions for U.S. citizens traveling internationally.

Tissue Banks International

http://www.tbionline.org

Site describes an international network that recovers and provides human tissue for use in transplants and other surgeries.

United Network for Organ Sharing
http://www.unos.org

A site that provides detailed information for patients and family members about the transplantation procedure, living with a transplant, current transplant research, and how to donate organs.

TREMORS
International Essential Tremor Foundation
http://www.essentialtremor.org

An organization created to provide information, services, and support to individuals and families affected by essential tremor. Encourages and promotes research in an effort to determine causes, treatment, and ultimately a cure.

TUBERCULOSIS
American Lung Association
http://www.lungusa.org

A group initially founded to fight tuberculosis, it now targets its efforts toward asthma, tobacco control, and environmental health in addition to the global rise of tuberculosis. The Web site offers a comprehensive fact sheet about the disease, as well as resources for advocacy, research, and relevant news stories.

TURNER SYNDROME
Turner Syndrome Society of the United States
http://www.turnersyndrome.org

A group that encourages medical research, the dissemination of updated medical research information, and social support services to individuals, families, physicians, and the general public.

VISION DISORDERS
National Foundation for Eye Research
http://www.nfer.org

Site provides consumers and professionals with access to developing technology for treating impaired vision.

WOUNDS
Wound Care Institute
http://www.woundcare.org

Users can search this site for a variety of articles on the care of wounds resulting from diabetes.

—Mary Allen Carey, Ph.D.;
updated by Desiree Dreeuws

SALEM HEALTH

MAGILL'S MEDICAL GUIDE

ENTRIES BY ANATOMY OR SYSTEM AFFECTED

Motor skill development
Necrosis
Neurofibromatosis
Niemann-Pick disease
Nuclear medicine
Nuclear radiology
Orthopedic surgery
Orthopedics
Orthopedics, pediatric
Osgood-Schlatter disease
Osteochondritis juvenilis
Osteogenesis imperfecta
Osteomyelitis
Osteonecrosis
Osteopathic medicine
Osteoporosis
Paget's disease
Periodontitis
Physical rehabilitation
Pigeon toes
Podiatry
Polydactyly and syndactyly
Prader-Willi syndrome
Rheumatology
Rickets
Rubinstein-Taybi syndrome
Sarcoma
Scoliosis
Slipped disk
Spinal cord disorders
Spine, vertebrae, and disks
Sports medicine
Teeth
Temporomandibular joint (TMJ) syndrome
Tendon disorders
Tendon repair
Upper extremities

BRAIN
Abscess drainage
Abscesses
Acidosis
Addiction
Adrenal glands
Adrenoleukodystrophy
Agnosia
Alcoholism
Altitude sickness
Alzheimer's disease
Amnesia
Anesthesia
Anesthesiology
Aneurysmectomy

Aneurysms
Angiography
Anosmia
Antianxiety drugs
Antidepressants
Aphasia and dysphasia
Aromatherapy
Attention-deficit disorder (ADD)
Auras
Batten's disease
Biofeedback
Body dysmorphic disorder
Brain
Brain damage
Brain disorders
Brain tumors
Caffeine
Carbohydrates
Carotid arteries
Chiari malformations
Chronic wasting disease (CWD)
Cluster headaches
Cognitive development
Coma
Computed tomography (CT) scanning
Concussion
Cornelia de Lange syndrome
Corticosteroids
Craniotomy
Creutzfeldt-Jakob disease (CJD)
Cytomegalovirus (CMV)
Defibrillation
Dehydration
Dementias
Developmental stages
Dizziness and fainting
Down syndrome
Drowning
Dyskinesia
Dyslexia
Electroencephalography (EEG)
Embolism
Embolization
Emotions: Biomedical causes and effects
Encephalitis
Endocrine glands
Endocrinology
Endocrinology, pediatric
Enteroviruses
Epilepsy
Failure to thrive
Fetal alcohol syndrome

Fetal surgery
Fetal tissue transplantation
Fibromyalgia
Fragile X syndrome
Frontotemporal dementia (FTD)
Galactosemia
Gigantism
Gulf War syndrome
Hallucinations
Head and neck disorders
Headaches
Hearing
Huntington's disease
Hydrocephalus
Hypertension
Hypnosis
Hypotension
Hypothalamus
Infarction
Intraventricular hemorrhage
Jaundice
Kinesiology
Kluver-Bucy syndrome
Lead poisoning
Learning disabilities
Leukodystrophy
Light therapy
Listeria infections
Malaria
Marijuana
Melatonin
Memory loss
Meningitis
Mental retardation
Migraine headaches
Narcolepsy
Narcotics
Nausea and vomiting
Neuroimaging
Neurology
Neurology, pediatric
Neurosurgery
Nicotine
Niemann-Pick disease
Nuclear radiology
Parkinson's disease
Pharmacology
Pharmacy
Phenylketonuria (PKU)
Pick's disease
Pituitary gland
Poliomyelitis
Polycystic kidney disease

Positron emission tomography
   (PET) scanning
Prader-Willi syndrome
Prion diseases
Psychiatric disorders
Psychiatry
Psychiatry, child and adolescent
Psychiatry, geriatric
Rabies
Restless legs syndrome
Reye's syndrome
Rocky Mountain spotted fever
Sarcoidosis
Schizophrenia
Seizures
Shock therapy
Shunts
Sleep
Sleep disorders
Sleeping sickness
Sleepwalking
Stammering
Strokes
Sturge-Weber syndrome
Subdural hematoma
Synesthesia
Syphilis
Tetanus
Thrombolytic therapy and TPA
Thrombosis and thrombus
Tics
Tinnitus
Tourette's syndrome
Toxicology
Toxoplasmosis
Transient ischemic attacks (TIAs)
Trembling and shaking
Tumor removal
Tumors
Unconsciousness
Vagus nerve
Vertigo
Weight loss medications
Wilson's disease
Yellow fever

BREASTS
Abscess drainage
Abscesses
Breast biopsy
Breast cancer
Breast disorders
Breast-feeding
Breast surgery

Breasts, female
Cyst removal
Cysts
Fibrocystic breast condition
Gender reassignment surgery
Glands
Gynecology
Gynecomastia
Klinefelter syndrome
Mammography
Mastectomy and lumpectomy
Mastitis
Tumor removal
Tumors

CELLS
Acid-base chemistry
Antibodies
Bacteriology
Batten's disease
Biological therapies
Biopsy
Cells
Cholesterol
Conception
Cytology
Cytomegalovirus (CMV)
Cytopathology
Dehydration
DNA and RNA
E. coli infection
Enzymes
Fluids and electrolytes
Food biochemistry
Gaucher's disease
Genetic counseling
Genetic engineering
Glycolysis
Gram staining
Gulf War syndrome
Host-defense mechanisms
Immunization and vaccination
Immunology
In vitro fertilization
Karyotyping
Kinesiology
Laboratory tests
Lipids
Magnetic field therapy
Microbiology
Microscopy
Mutation
Pharmacology
Pharmacy

Phlebotomy
Plasma
Pus
Toxicology

CHEST
Anatomy
Antihistamines
Asthma
Bacillus Calmette-Guérin (BCG)
Bones and the skeleton
Breasts, female
Bronchiolitis
Bronchitis
Bypass surgery
Cardiac rehabilitation
Cardiology
Cardiology, pediatric
Chest
Choking
Common cold
Congenital heart disease
Coughing
Croup
Cystic fibrosis
Defibrillation
Diaphragm
Electrocardiography (ECG or EKG)
Embolism
Emphysema
Gulf War syndrome
Heart
Heart transplantation
Heart valve replacement
Heartburn
Heimlich maneuver
Hiccups
Interstitial pulmonary fibrosis (IPF)
Legionnaires' disease
Lung cancer
Lungs
Pacemaker implantation
Pityriasis rosea
Pleurisy
Pneumonia
Pneumothorax
Pulmonary diseases
Pulmonary medicine
Pulmonary medicine, pediatric
Respiration
Respiratory distress syndrome
Resuscitation
Sarcoidosis
Sneezing

Thoracic surgery
Trachea
Tuberculosis
Wheezing
Whooping cough

CIRCULATORY SYSTEM
Aneurysmectomy
Aneurysms
Angina
Angiography
Angioplasty
Antibodies
Antihistamines
Apgar score
Arrhythmias
Arteriosclerosis
Atrial fibrillation
Biofeedback
Bleeding
Blood and blood disorders
Blood pressure
Blood testing
Blood vessels
Blue baby syndrome
Bypass surgery
Cardiac arrest
Cardiac rehabilitation
Cardiac surgery
Cardiology
Cardiology, pediatric
Cardiopulmonary resuscitation
   (CPR)
Carotid arteries
Catheterization
Chest
Cholesterol
Circulation
Claudication
Congenital heart disease
Coronary artery bypass graft
Decongestants
Deep vein thrombosis
Defibrillation
Dehydration
Diabetes mellitus
Dialysis
Disseminated intravascular
   coagulation (DIC)
Diuretics
Dizziness and fainting
Ebola virus
Echocardiography
Edema

Electrocardiography (ECG or EKG)
Electrocauterization
Embolism
End-stage renal disease
Endarterectomy
Endocarditis
Ergogenic aids
Exercise physiology
Facial transplantation
Food allergies
Heart
Heart attack
Heart disease
Heart failure
Heart transplantation
Heart valve replacement
Heat exhaustion and heatstroke
Hematology
Hematology, pediatric
Hemorrhoid banding and removal
Hemorrhoids
Hormones
Hyperbaric oxygen therapy
Hypercholesterolemia
Hypertension
Hypotension
Intravenous (IV) therapy
Ischemia
Juvenile rheumatoid arthritis
Kidneys
Kinesiology
Klippel-Trenaunay syndrome
Liver
Lymph
Lymphatic system
Marburg virus
Marijuana
Mitral valve prolapse
Motor skill development
Nosebleeds
Obesity
Obesity, childhood
Osteochondritis juvenilis
Pacemaker implantation
Palpitations
Phlebitis
Phlebotomy
Placenta
Plaque, arterial
Plasma
Preeclampsia and eclampsia
Pulmonary edema
Pulse rate
Resuscitation

Reye's syndrome
Rheumatic fever
Sarcoidosis
Scleroderma
Septicemia
Shock
Shunts
Smoking
Sports medicine
Stenosis
Stents
Steroid abuse
Strokes
Sturge-Weber syndrome
Systems and organs
Testicular torsion
Thrombocytopenia
Thrombolytic therapy and TPA
Thrombosis and thrombus
Transfusion
Transient ischemic attacks (TIAs)
Transplantation
Typhus
Uremia
Varicose vein removal
Varicose veins
Vascular medicine
Vascular system
Vasculitis
Venous insufficiency

EARS
Adenoids
Adrenoleukodystrophy
Agnosia
Altitude sickness
Antihistamines
Audiology
Auras
Biophysics
Cartilage
Cornelia de Lange syndrome
Cytomegalovirus (CMV)
Deafness
Decongestants
Dyslexia
Ear infections and disorders
Ear surgery
Ears
Earwax
Fragile X syndrome
Hearing
Hearing aids
Hearing loss

Hearing tests
Histiocytosis
Leukodystrophy
Ménière's disease
Motion sickness
Myringotomy
Nervous system
Neurology
Neurology, pediatric
Osteogenesis imperfecta
Otoplasty
Otorhinolaryngology
Pharynx
Plastic surgery
Quinsy
Rubinstein-Taybi syndrome
Sense organs
Speech disorders
Tinnitus
Vasculitis
Vertigo
Wiskott-Aldrich syndrome

ENDOCRINE SYSTEM
Addison's disease
Adrenal glands
Adrenalectomy
Adrenoleukodystrophy
Assisted reproductive technologies
Bariatric surgery
Biofeedback
Breasts, female
Carbohydrates
Congenital adrenal hyperplasia
Congenital hypothyroidism
Contraception
Corticosteroids
Diabetes mellitus
Dwarfism
Eating disorders
Emotions: Biomedical causes and
    effects
End-stage renal disease
Endocrine disorders
Endocrine glands
Endocrinology
Endocrinology, pediatric
Ergogenic aids
Failure to thrive
Fibrocystic breast condition
Gender reassignment surgery
Gestational diabetes
Gigantism
Glands

Goiter
Hashimoto's thyroiditis
Hormone therapy
Hormones
Hot flashes
Hyperhidrosis
Hyperparathyroidism and
    hypoparathyroidism
Hypoglycemia
Hypothalamus
Klinefelter syndrome
Liver
Melatonin
Nonalcoholic steatohepatitis (NASH)
Obesity
Obesity, childhood
Overtraining syndrome
Pancreas
Pancreatitis
Parathyroidectomy
Pituitary gland
Placenta
Plasma
Polycystic ovary syndrome
Postpartum depression
Prader-Willi syndrome
Prostate enlargement
Prostate gland
Prostate gland removal
Sexual differentiation
Small intestine
Steroid abuse
Steroids
Sweating
Systems and organs
Testicular cancer
Testicular surgery
Thymus gland
Thyroid disorders
Thyroid gland
Thyroidectomy
Turner syndrome
Weight loss medications

EYES
Adenoviruses
Adrenoleukodystrophy
Agnosia
Albinos
Antihistamines
Astigmatism
Auras
Batten's disease
Behçet's disease

Blindness
Blurred vision
Botox
Cataract surgery
Cataracts
Chlamydia
Color blindness
Conjunctivitis
Corneal transplantation
Cornelia de Lange syndrome
Cytomegalovirus (CMV)
Dengue fever
Diabetes mellitus
Dyslexia
Enteroviruses
Eye infections and disorders
Eye surgery
Eyes
Face lift and blepharoplasty
Galactosemia
Glaucoma
Gonorrhea
Gulf War syndrome
Jaundice
Juvenile rheumatoid arthritis
Keratitis
Kluver-Bucy syndrome
Laser use in surgery
Leukodystrophy
Macular degeneration
Marfan syndrome
Marijuana
Microscopy, slitlamp
Motor skill development
Multiple chemical sensitivity
    syndrome
Myopia
Ophthalmology
Optometry
Optometry, pediatric
Pigmentation
Ptosis
Refractive eye surgery
Reiter's syndrome
Rubinstein-Taybi syndrome
Sarcoidosis
Sense organs
Sjögren's syndrome
Strabismus
Sturge-Weber syndrome
Styes
Tears and tear ducts
Toxoplasmosis
Trachoma

Klippel-Trenaunay syndrome
Kwashiorkor
Lactose intolerance
Laparoscopy
Lipids
Liver
Malabsorption
Malnutrition
Marburg virus
Marijuana
Metabolism
Motion sickness
Muscles
Nausea and vomiting
Nonalcoholic steatohepatitis
 (NASH)
Noroviruses
Nutrition
Obesity
Obesity, childhood
Obstruction
Pancreas
Pancreatitis
Peristalsis
Pharynx
Pinworm
Poisoning
Poisonous plants
Polycystic kidney disease
Polyps
Premenstrual syndrome (PMS)
Proctology
Protozoan diseases
Pyloric stenosis
Radiation sickness
Rectum
Reiter's syndrome
Rotavirus
Roundworm
Salmonella infection
Scleroderma
Sense organs
Shigellosis
Shunts
Small intestine
Soiling
Stenosis
Stomach, intestinal, and pancreatic
 cancers
Systems and organs
Tapeworm
Taste
Teeth
Toilet training

Trichinosis
Tumor removal
Tumors
Typhoid fever
Ulcer surgery
Ulcers
Vagotomy
Vasculitis
Vitamins and minerals
Weaning
Weight loss and gain
Worms

GENITALS
Adrenoleukodystrophy
Aphrodisiacs
Assisted reproductive technologies
Behçet's disease
Candidiasis
Catheterization
Cervical, ovarian, and uterine
 cancers
Cervical procedures
Chlamydia
Circumcision, female, and genital
 mutilation
Circumcision, male
Congenital adrenal hyperplasia
Contraception
Culdocentesis
Cyst removal
Cysts
Electrocauterization
Embolization
Endometrial biopsy
Episiotomy
Erectile dysfunction
Fragile X syndrome
Gender identity disorder
Gender reassignment surgery
Genital disorders, female
Genital disorders, male
Glands
Gonorrhea
Gynecology
Hemochromatosis
Hermaphroditism and
 pseudohermaphroditism
Herpes
Human papillomavirus (HPV)
Hydroceles
Hyperplasia
Hypospadias repair and
 urethroplasty

Infertility, female
Infertility, male
Klinefelter syndrome
Kluver-Bucy syndrome
Masturbation
Orchiectomy
Orchitis
Pap test
Pelvic inflammatory disease (PID)
Penile implant surgery
Prader-Willi syndrome
Rape and sexual assault
Reproductive system
Rubinstein-Taybi syndrome
Semen
Sexual differentiation
Sexual dysfunction
Sexuality
Sexually transmitted diseases
 (STDs)
Sperm banks
Sterilization
Syphilis
Testicles, undescended
Testicular cancer
Testicular surgery
Testicular torsion
Toilet training
Trichomoniasis
Urology
Urology, pediatric
Uterus
Vas deferens
Vasectomy
Warts

GLANDS
Abscess drainage
Abscesses
Addison's disease
Adrenal glands
Adrenalectomy
Adrenoleukodystrophy
Assisted reproductive technologies
Biofeedback
Breasts, female
Contraception
Cyst removal
Cysts
Dengue fever
Diabetes mellitus
DiGeorge syndrome
Dwarfism
Eating disorders

Dyskinesia
Electroencephalography (EEG)
Embolism
Epilepsy
Esophagus
Facial transplantation
Fetal tissue transplantation
Fibromyalgia
Hair loss and baldness
Hair transplantation
Head and neck disorders
Headaches
Hydrocephalus
Lice, mites, and ticks
Meningitis
Migraine headaches
Nasal polyp removal
Nasopharyngeal disorders
Neuroimaging
Neurology
Neurology, pediatric
Neurosurgery
Oral and maxillofacial surgery
Pharynx
Polyps
Rhinoplasty and submucous
    resection
Rubinstein-Taybi syndrome
Seizures
Shunts
Sports medicine
Strokes
Sturge-Weber syndrome
Subdural hematoma
Tears and tear ducts
Temporomandibular joint (TMJ)
    syndrome
Thrombosis and thrombus
Tinnitus
Unconsciousness
Whiplash

HEART
Acidosis
Aneurysmectomy
Aneurysms
Angina
Angiography
Angioplasty
Anxiety
Apgar score
Arrhythmias
Arteriosclerosis
Atrial fibrillation

Biofeedback
Bites and stings
Blood pressure
Blood vessels
Blue baby syndrome
Bypass surgery
Caffeine
Cardiac arrest
Cardiac rehabilitation
Cardiac surgery
Cardiology
Cardiology, pediatric
Cardiopulmonary resuscitation
    (CPR)
Carotid arteries
Catheterization
Circulation
Congenital heart disease
Cornelia de Lange syndrome
Coronary artery bypass graft
Defibrillation
DiGeorge syndrome
Diuretics
Echocardiography
Electrical shock
Electrocardiography (ECG or EKG)
Embolism
End-stage renal disease
Endocarditis
Enteroviruses
Exercise physiology
Fatty acid oxidation disorders
Glycogen storage diseases
Heart
Heart attack
Heart disease
Heart failure
Heart transplantation
Heart valve replacement
Hemochromatosis
Hypertension
Hypotension
Infarction
Internal medicine
Intravenous (IV) therapy
Juvenile rheumatoid arthritis
Kinesiology
Lyme disease
Marfan syndrome
Marijuana
Methicillin-resistant *Staphylococcus*
    aureus (MRSA) infections
Mitral valve prolapse
Nicotine

Obesity
Obesity, childhood
Pacemaker implantation
Palpitations
Plaque, arterial
Plasma
Prader-Willi syndrome
Pulmonary edema
Pulse rate
Respiratory distress syndrome
Resuscitation
Reye's syndrome
Rheumatic fever
Rubinstein-Taybi syndrome
Sarcoidosis
Scleroderma
Shock
Sports medicine
Stenosis
Stents
Steroid abuse
Strokes
Thoracic surgery
Thrombolytic therapy and TPA
Thrombosis and thrombus
Toxoplasmosis
Transplantation
Ultrasonography
Uremia
Yellow fever

HIPS
Aging
Arthritis
Arthroplasty
Arthroscopy
Bone disorders
Bones and the skeleton
Chiropractic
Dwarfism
Fracture and dislocation
Fracture repair
Hip fracture repair
Hip replacement
Liposuction
Lower extremities
Orthopedic surgery
Orthopedics
Orthopedics, pediatric
Osteoarthritis
Osteochondritis juvenilis
Osteonecrosis
Osteoporosis
Physical rehabilitation

Pityriasis rosea
Rheumatoid arthritis
Rheumatology
Sciatica

IMMUNE SYSTEM
Acquired immunodeficiency
  syndrome (AIDS)
Adenoids
Adenoviruses
Allergies
Antibiotics
Antibodies
Antihistamines
Arthritis
Asthma
Autoimmune disorders
Bacillus Calmette-Guérin (BCG)
Bacterial infections
Bacteriology
Bedsores
Bile
Biological therapies
Bites and stings
Blood and blood disorders
Bone grafting
Bone marrow transplantation
Candidiasis
Cells
Chagas' disease
Childhood infectious diseases
Chronic fatigue syndrome
Cornelia de Lange syndrome
Coronaviruses
Corticosteroids
Cytology
Cytomegalovirus (CMV)
Cytopathology
Dermatology
Dermatopathology
DiGeorge syndrome
Disseminated intravascular
  coagulation (DIC)
E. coli infection
Ebola virus
Ehrlichiosis
Emotions: Biomedical causes and
  effects
Endocrinology
Endocrinology, pediatric
Enzyme therapy
Enzymes
Epstein-Barr virus
Facial transplantation

Food allergies
Fungal infections
Gluten intolerance
Grafts and grafting
Gram staining
Guillain-Barré syndrome
Gulf War syndrome
Hashimoto's thyroiditis
Healing
Hematology
Hematology, pediatric
Histiocytosis
Hives
Homeopathy
Host-defense mechanisms
Human immunodeficiency virus
  (HIV)
Immune system
Immunization and vaccination
Immunodeficiency disorders
Immunology
Immunopathology
Juvenile rheumatoid arthritis
Kawasaki disease
Leprosy
Lymph
Lymphatic system
Magnetic field therapy
Marburg virus
Measles
Microbiology
Monkeypox
Multiple chemical sensitivity
  syndrome
Mumps
Mutation
Myasthenia gravis
Nicotine
Noroviruses
Oncology
Pancreas
Pharmacology
Pharynx
Plasma
Poisoning
Poisonous plants
Pulmonary diseases
Pulmonary medicine
Pulmonary medicine, pediatric
Pus
Rh factor
Rheumatology
Rubella
Sarcoidosis

Sarcoma
Scarlet fever
Scleroderma
Serology
Severe acute respiratory syndrome
  (SARS)
Severe combined immunodeficiency
  syndrome (SCID)
Sjögren's syndrome
Small intestine
Smallpox
Sneezing
Stevens-Johnson syndrome
Stress
Stress reduction
Systemic lupus erythematosus
  (SLE)
Systems and organs
Thalidomide
Thymus gland
Tonsils
Toxicology
Transfusion
Transplantation
Vasculitis
Vitiligo
Wiskott-Aldrich syndrome

INTESTINES
Abdomen
Abdominal disorders
Acidosis
Adenoviruses
Amebiasis
Anal cancer
Anus
Appendectomy
Appendicitis
Appetite loss
Bacterial infections
Bariatric surgery
Bypass surgery
Campylobacter infections
Carbohydrates
Celiac sprue
Chyme
Clostridium difficle infections
Colic
Colitis
Colon
Colon therapy
Colonoscopy and sigmoidoscopy
Colorectal cancer
Colorectal polyp removal

Colorectal surgery
Constipation
Crohn's disease
Diarrhea and dysentery
Digestion
Diverticulitis and diverticulosis
E. coli infection
Eating disorders
Endoscopy
Enemas
Enterocolitis
Fiber
Fistula repair
Food poisoning
Gastroenteritis
Gastroenterology
Gastroenterology, pediatric
Gastrointestinal disorders
Gastrointestinal system
Gluten intolerance
Hemorrhoid banding and removal
Hemorrhoids
Hernia
Hernia repair
Hirschsprung's disease
Ileostomy and colostomy
Indigestion
Infarction
Internal medicine
Intestinal disorders
Intestines
Irritable bowel syndrome (IBS)
Kaposi's sarcoma
Kwashiorkor
Lactose intolerance
Laparoscopy
Malabsorption
Malnutrition
Metabolism
Nutrition
Obesity
Obesity, childhood
Obstruction
Peristalsis
Pinworm
Polyps
Proctology
Rectum
Rotavirus
Roundworm
Salmonella infection
Small intestine
Soiling
Sphincterectomy

Stomach, intestinal, and pancreatic
  cancers
Tapeworm
Toilet training
Trichinosis
Tumor removal
Tumors
Typhoid fever
Ulcer surgery
Ulcers
Vasculitis
Worms

JOINTS
Amputation
Arthritis
Arthroplasty
Arthroscopy
Braces, orthopedic
Bursitis
Carpal tunnel syndrome
Cartilage
Casts and splints
Chlamydia
Collagen
Corticosteroids
Cyst removal
Cysts
Endoscopy
Exercise physiology
Fracture and dislocation
Fragile X syndrome
Gout
Gulf War syndrome
Hammertoe correction
Hammertoes
Hip fracture repair
Juvenile rheumatoid arthritis
Klippel-Trenaunay syndrome
Kneecap removal
Ligaments
Lyme disease
Methicillin-resistant *Staphylococcus*
  aureus (MRSA) infections
Motor skill development
Orthopedic surgery
Orthopedics
Orthopedics, pediatric
Osteoarthritis
Osteochondritis juvenilis
Osteomyelitis
Osteonecrosis
Physical rehabilitation
Reiter's syndrome

Rheumatoid arthritis
Rheumatology
Rotator cuff surgery
Sarcoidosis
Scleroderma
Spondylitis
Sports medicine
Systemic lupus erythematosus
  (SLE)
Temporomandibular joint (TMJ)
  syndrome
Tendinitis
Tendon disorders
Tendon repair
Von Willebrand's disease

KIDNEYS
Abdomen
Abscess drainage
Abscesses
Adrenal glands
Adrenalectomy
Babesiosis
Carbohydrates
Corticosteroids
Cysts
Dialysis
Diuretics
End-stage renal disease
Galactosemia
Hantavirus
Hematuria
Hemolytic uremic syndrome
Hypertension
Hypotension
Infarction
Internal medicine
Intravenous (IV) therapy
Kidney cancer
Kidney disorders
Kidney transplantation
Kidneys
Laparoscopy
Lithotripsy
Metabolism
Methicillin-resistant *Staphylococcus*
  aureus (MRSA) infections
Nephrectomy
Nephritis
Nephrology
Nephrology, pediatric
Nuclear medicine
Nuclear radiology
Polycystic kidney disease

Preeclampsia and eclampsia
Proteinuria
Pyelonephritis
Renal failure
Reye's syndrome
Rocky Mountain spotted fever
Sarcoidosis
Scleroderma
Stone removal
Stones
Toilet training
Transplantation
Ultrasonography
Uremia
Urinalysis
Urinary disorders
Urinary system
Urology
Urology, pediatric
Vasculitis

KNEES
Amputation
Arthritis
Arthroplasty
Arthroscopy
Bone disorders
Bones and the skeleton
Bowlegs
Braces, orthopedic
Bursitis
Cartilage
Casts and splints
Endoscopy
Exercise physiology
Fracture and dislocation
Joints
Kneecap removal
Knock-knees
Liposuction
Lower extremities
Orthopedic surgery
Orthopedics
Orthopedics, pediatric
Osgood-Schlatter disease
Osteoarthritis
Osteonecrosis
Physical rehabilitation
Rheumatoid arthritis
Rheumatology
Sports medicine
Tendinitis
Tendon disorders
Tendon repair

LEGS
Amputation
Arthritis
Arthroplasty
Arthroscopy
Bone disorders
Bones and the skeleton
Bowlegs
Bursitis
Casts and splints
Cerebral palsy
Cornelia de Lange syndrome
Deep vein thrombosis
Dwarfism
Dyskinesia
Fracture and dislocation
Fracture repair
Gigantism
Hemiplegia
Hip fracture repair
Kneecap removal
Knock-knees
Liposuction
Lower extremities
Methicillin-resistant *Staphylococcus aureus* (MRSA) infections
Muscle sprains, spasms, and disorders
Muscles
Muscular dystrophy
Numbness and tingling
Orthopedic surgery
Orthopedics
Orthopedics, pediatric
Osteoarthritis
Osteoporosis
Paralysis
Paraplegia
Physical rehabilitation
Pigeon toes
Pityriasis rosea
Poliomyelitis
Quadriplegia
Rheumatoid arthritis
Rheumatology
Rickets
Sciatica
Sports medicine
Tendinitis
Tendon disorders
Tendon repair
Thalidomide
Varicose vein removal
Varicose veins

Vasculitis
Venous insufficiency

LIGAMENTS
Bones and the skeleton
Casts and splints
Collagen
Connective tissue
Flat feet
Joints
Kidneys
Ligaments
Muscle sprains, spasms, and disorders
Muscles
Orthopedic surgery
Orthopedics
Orthopedics, pediatric
Osteogenesis imperfecta
Physical rehabilitation
Slipped disk
Spleen
Sports medicine
Tendon disorders
Tendon repair
Whiplash

LIVER
Abdomen
Abdominal disorders
Abscess drainage
Abscesses
Alcoholism
Amebiasis
Babesiosis
Bile
Blood and blood disorders
Chyme
Circulation
Cirrhosis
Corticosteroids
Cytomegalovirus (CMV)
Edema
Embolization
Endoscopic retrograde cholangiopancreatography (ERCP)
Fatty acid oxidation disorders
Fetal surgery
Galactosemia
Gastroenterology
Gastroenterology, pediatric
Gastrointestinal disorders
Gastrointestinal system
Gaucher's disease

Glycogen storage diseases
Hematology
Hematology, pediatric
Hemochromatosis
Hemolytic disease of the newborn
Hepatitis
Histiocytosis
Internal medicine
Jaundice
Jaundice, neonatal
Kaposi's sarcoma
Liver
Liver cancer
Liver disorders
Liver transplantation
Malabsorption
Malaria
Metabolism
Methicillin-resistant *Staphylococcus aureus* (MRSA) infections
Niemann-Pick disease
Nonalcoholic steatohepatitis (NASH)
Polycystic kidney disease
Reye's syndrome
Schistosomiasis
Shunts
Thrombocytopenia
Transplantation
Wilson's disease
Yellow fever

LUNGS
Abscess drainage
Abscesses
Acute respiratory distress syndrome (ARDS)
Adenoviruses
Allergies
Altitude sickness
Anthrax
Antihistamines
Apgar score
Apnea
Asbestos exposure
Aspergillosis
Asphyxiation
Asthma
Bacterial infections
Bronchi
Bronchiolitis
Bronchitis
Cardiopulmonary resuscitation (CPR)

Chest
Childhood infectious diseases
Choking
Chronic obstructive pulmonary disease (COPD)
Coccidioidomycosis
Common cold
Coronaviruses
Corticosteroids
Coughing
Croup
Cystic fibrosis
Cytomegalovirus (CMV)
Diaphragm
Diphtheria
Drowning
Edema
Embolism
Emphysema
Endoscopy
Exercise physiology
Fetal surgery
Hantavirus
Heart transplantation
Heimlich maneuver
Hiccups
Histiocytosis
H1N1 influenza
Hyperbaric oxygen therapy
Hyperventilation
Hypoxia
Infarction
Influenza
Internal medicine
Interstitial pulmonary fibrosis (IPF)
Intravenous (IV) therapy
Kaposi's sarcoma
Kinesiology
Legionnaires' disease
Lung cancer
Lung surgery
Lungs
Marijuana
Measles
Mesothelioma
Multiple chemical sensitivity syndrome
Nicotine
Niemann-Pick disease
Oxygen therapy
Plague
Pleurisy
Pneumonia

Pneumothorax
Pulmonary diseases
Pulmonary edema
Pulmonary hypertension
Pulmonary medicine
Pulmonary medicine, pediatric
Respiration
Respiratory distress syndrome
Resuscitation
Rhinoviruses
Sarcoidosis
Scleroderma
Severe acute respiratory syndrome (SARS)
Smoking
Sneezing
Thoracic surgery
Thrombolytic therapy and TPA
Thrombosis and thrombus
Toxoplasmosis
Transplantation
Tuberculosis
Tularemia
Tumor removal
Tumors
Vasculitis
Wheezing
Whooping cough
Wiskott-Aldrich syndrome

LYMPHATIC SYSTEM
Adenoids
Angiography
Antibodies
Bacillus Calmette-Guérin (BCG)
Bacterial infections
Biological therapies
Blood and blood disorders
Blood vessels
Breast cancer
Breast disorders
Breasts, female
Bruises
Burkitt's lymphoma
Cancer
Cervical, ovarian, and uterine cancers
Chemotherapy
Circulation
Colon cancer
Coronaviruses
Corticosteroids
DiGeorge syndrome
Edema

Elephantiasis
Gaucher's disease
Histology
Hodgkin's disease
Immune system
Immunology
Immunopathology
Kawasaki disease
Klippel-Trenaunay syndrome
Liver cancer
Lower extremities
Lung cancer
Lymph
Lymphadenopathy and lymphoma
Lymphatic system
Malignancy and metastasis
Mononucleosis
Oncology
Overtraining syndrome
Prostate cancer
Sarcoidosis
Skin cancer
Sleeping sickness
Small intestine
Splenectomy
Stomach, intestinal, and pancreatic
  cancers
Systems and organs
Thymus gland
Tonsillectomy and adenoid
  removal
Tonsillitis
Tonsils
Tularemia
Tumor removal
Tumors
Upper extremities
Vascular medicine
Vascular system

MOUTH
Acid reflux disease
Adenoids
Behçet's disease
Braces, orthodontic
Candidiasis
Canker sores
Cavities
Cleft lip and palate
Cleft lip and palate repair
Cold sores
Cornelia de Lange syndrome
Crowns and bridges
Dengue fever

Dental diseases
Dentistry
Dentistry, pediatric
Dentures
DiGeorge syndrome
Dyskinesia
Endodontic disease
Esophagus
Facial transplantation
Fluoride treatments
Gingivitis
Gum disease
Halitosis
Hand-foot-and-mouth disease
Heimlich maneuver
Herpes
Jaw wiring
Kawasaki disease
Lesions
Lisping
Mouth and throat cancer
Nicotine
Nutrition
Oral and maxillofacial surgery
Orthodontics
Periodontal surgery
Periodontitis
Pharynx
Plaque, dental
Rape and sexual assault
Reiter's syndrome
Root canal treatment
Rubinstein-Taybi syndrome
Sense organs
Sjögren's syndrome
Smoking
Taste
Teeth
Teething
Temporomandibular joint (TMJ)
  syndrome
Thumb sucking
Tooth extraction
Toothache
Ulcers
Wisdom teeth

MUSCLES
Acidosis
Acupressure
Amputation
Amyotrophic lateral sclerosis
Anesthesia
Anesthesiology

Apgar score
Ataxia
Back pain
Bed-wetting
Bedsores
Bell's palsy
Beriberi
Bile
Biofeedback
Botox
Botulism
Breasts, female
Carbohydrates
Cerebral palsy
Chest
Chiari malformations
Childhood infectious diseases
Chronic fatigue syndrome
Claudication
Creutzfeldt-Jakob disease (CJD)
Cysts
Diaphragm
Ebola virus
Electromyography
Emotions: Biomedical causes and
  effects
Ergogenic aids
Exercise physiology
Facial transplantation
Fatty acid oxidation disorders
Feet
Fibromyalgia
Flat feet
Foot disorders
Glycogen storage diseases
Glycolysis
Guillain-Barré syndrome
Gulf War syndrome
Head and neck disorders
Hemiplegia
Hiccups
Joints
Kinesiology
Leukodystrophy
Ligaments
Lower extremities
Marburg virus
Mastectomy and lumpectomy
Methicillin-resistant *Staphylococcus
  aureus* (MRSA) infections
Motor neuron diseases
Motor skill development
Multiple chemical sensitivity
  syndrome

Multiple sclerosis
Muscle sprains, spasms, and
    disorders
Muscles
Muscular dystrophy
Necrotizing fasciitis
Neurology
Neurology, pediatric
Numbness and tingling
Orthopedic surgery
Orthopedics
Orthopedics, pediatric
Osgood-Schlatter disease
Osteopathic medicine
Overtraining syndrome
Palsy
Paralysis
Paraplegia
Parkinson's disease
Physical rehabilitation
Poisoning
Poliomyelitis
Ptosis
Quadriplegia
Rabies
Respiration
Restless legs syndrome
Rheumatoid arthritis
Rotator cuff surgery
Seizures
Speech disorders
Sphincterectomy
Sports medicine
Steroid abuse
Strabismus
Tattoos and body piercing
Temporomandibular joint (TMJ)
    syndrome
Tendon disorders
Tendon repair
Tetanus
Tics
Torticollis
Tourette's syndrome
Trembling and shaking
Trichinosis
Upper extremities
Weight loss and gain
Yellow fever

MUSCULOSKELETAL SYSTEM
Acupressure
Amputation
Amyotrophic lateral sclerosis

Anatomy
Anesthesia
Anesthesiology
Arthritis
Ataxia
Atrophy
Back pain
Bed-wetting
Bell's palsy
Beriberi
Biofeedback
Bone cancer
Bone disorders
Bone grafting
Bone marrow transplantation
Bones and the skeleton
Botulism
Bowlegs
Braces, orthopedic
Breasts, female
Cartilage
Casts and splints
Cells
Cerebral palsy
Chest
Childhood infectious diseases
Chiropractic
Chronic fatigue syndrome
Claudication
Cleft lip and palate
Cleft lip and palate repair
Collagen
Congenital hypothyroidism
Connective tissue
Craniosynostosis
Cysts
Dengue fever
Depression
Diaphragm
Dwarfism
Ear surgery
Ears
Ehrlichiosis
Electromyography
Emotions: Biomedical causes
    and effects
Ergogenic aids
Ewing's sarcoma
Exercise physiology
Feet
Fetal alcohol syndrome
Fibromyalgia
Flat feet
Foot disorders

Fracture and dislocation
Fracture repair
Gigantism
Glycolysis
Guillain-Barré syndrome
Hammertoe correction
Hammertoes
Head and neck disorders
Heel spur removal
Hematology
Hematology, pediatric
Hematomas
Hemiplegia
Hip fracture repair
Hip replacement
Hyperparathyroidism and
    hypoparathyroidism
Jaw wiring
Joints
Juvenile rheumatoid arthritis
Kinesiology
Kneecap removal
Knock-knees
Kyphosis
Ligaments
Lower extremities
Marfan syndrome
Marijuana
Mastectomy and lumpectomy
Methicillin-resistant *Staphylococcus
    aureus* (MRSA) infections
Motor neuron diseases
Motor skill development
Multiple sclerosis
Muscle sprains, spasms, and
    disorders
Muscles
Muscular dystrophy
Myasthenia gravis
Neurology
Neurology, pediatric
Nuclear medicine
Nuclear radiology
Numbness and tingling
Orthopedic surgery
Orthopedics
Orthopedics, pediatric
Osteochondritis juvenilis
Osteogenesis imperfecta
Osteomyelitis
Osteonecrosis
Osteopathic medicine
Osteoporosis
Paget's disease

NERVOUS SYSTEM

Abscess drainage
Abscesses
Acupressure
Addiction
Adenoviruses
Adrenoleukodystrophy
Agnosia
Alcoholism
Altitude sickness
Alzheimer's disease
Amnesia
Amputation
Amyotrophic lateral sclerosis
Anesthesia
Anesthesiology
Aneurysmectomy
Aneurysms
Anosmia
Antidepressants
Anxiety
Apgar score
Aphasia and dysphasia
Apnea
Aromatherapy
Ataxia
Atrophy
Attention-deficit disorder (ADD)
Auras
Autism
Back pain
Balance disorders
Batten's disease
Behçet's disease
Bell's palsy
Beriberi
Biofeedback
Botulism
Brain
Brain damage
Brain disorders
Brain tumors
Caffeine
Carpal tunnel syndrome
Cells
Cerebral palsy
Chagas' disease
Chiari malformations
Chiropractic
Chronic wasting disease (CWD)
Claudication
Cluster headaches
Cognitive development
Coma

Computed tomography (CT)
  scanning
Concussion
Congenital hypothyroidism
Craniotomy
Creutzfeldt-Jakob disease (CJD)
Cysts
Deafness
Defibrillation
Dementias
Developmental disorders
Developmental stages
Diabetes mellitus
Diphtheria
Disk removal
Dizziness and fainting
Down syndrome
Dwarfism
Dyskinesia
Dyslexia
E. coli infection
Ear surgery
Ears
Ehrlichiosis
Electrical shock
Electroencephalography (EEG)
Electromyography
Emotions: Biomedical causes and
  effects
Encephalitis
Endocrinology
Endocrinology, pediatric
Enteroviruses
Epilepsy
Eye infections and disorders
Eyes
Facial transplantation
Fetal alcohol syndrome
Fetal tissue transplantation
Fibromyalgia
Frontotemporal dementia (FTD)
Gigantism
Glands
Guillain-Barré syndrome
Hallucinations
Hammertoe correction
Head and neck disorders
Headaches
Hearing aids
Hearing loss
Hearing tests
Heart transplantation
Hemiplegia
Histiocytosis

Huntington's disease
Hydrocephalus
Hypnosis
Hypothalamus
Insect-borne diseases
Intraventricular hemorrhage
Irritable bowel syndrome (IBS)
Kinesiology
Lead poisoning
Learning disabilities
Leprosy
Light therapy
Listeria infections
Local anesthesia
Lower extremities
Lyme disease
Malaria
Maple syrup urine disease
  (MSUD)
Marijuana
Memory loss
Meningitis
Mental retardation
Mercury poisoning
Migraine headaches
Motor neuron diseases
Motor skill development
Multiple chemical sensitivity
  syndrome
Multiple sclerosis
Myasthenia gravis
Narcolepsy
Narcotics
Nausea and vomiting
Nervous system
Neuralgia, neuritis, and neuropathy
Neurofibromatosis
Neuroimaging
Neurology
Neurology, pediatric
Neurosurgery
Niemann-Pick disease
Nuclear radiology
Numbness and tingling
Orthopedic surgery
Orthopedics
Orthopedics, pediatric
Overtraining syndrome
Paget's disease
Palsy
Paralysis
Paraplegia
Parkinson's disease
Pharmacology

Appetite loss
Aromatherapy
Asperger's syndrome
Attention-deficit disorder (ADD)
Auras
Autism
Bariatric surgery
Biofeedback
Bipolar disorders
Body dysmorphic disorder
Bonding
Brain
Brain disorders
Bulimia
Chronic fatigue syndrome
Club drugs
Cluster headaches
Cognitive development
Colic
Coma
Concussion
Corticosteroids
Death and dying
Delusions
Dementias
Depression
Developmental disorders
Developmental stages
Dizziness and fainting
Domestic violence
Down syndrome
Dyskinesia
Dyslexia
Eating disorders
Electroencephalography (EEG)
Emotions: Biomedical causes and
    effects
Endocrinology
Endocrinology, pediatric
Facial transplantation
Factitious disorders
Failure to thrive
Fibromyalgia
Frontotemporal dementia (FTD)
Gender identity disorder
Grief and guilt
Gulf War syndrome
Hallucinations
Headaches
Hormone therapy
Hormones
Hydrocephalus
Hypnosis
Hypochondriasis

Hypothalamus
Kinesiology
Klinefelter syndrome
Learning disabilities
Light therapy
Marijuana
Memory loss
Menopause
Mental retardation
Midlife crisis
Migraine headaches
Miscarriage
Morgellons disease
Motor skill development
Narcolepsy
Narcotics
Neurology
Neurology, pediatric
Neurosis
Neurosurgery
Nicotine
Nightmares
Obesity
Obesity, childhood
Obsessive-compulsive disorder
Overtraining syndrome
Palpitations
Panic attacks
Paranoia
Pharmacology
Pharmacy
Phobias
Pick's disease
Postpartum depression
Post-traumatic stress disorder
Prader-Willi syndrome
Precocious puberty
Prescription drug abuse
Psychiatric disorders
Psychiatry
Psychiatry, child and adolescent
Psychiatry, geriatric
Psychoanalysis
Psychosis
Psychosomatic disorders
Puberty and adolescence
Rabies
Rape and sexual assault
Restless legs syndrome
Schizophrenia
Seasonal affective disorder
Separation anxiety
Sexual dysfunction
Sexuality

Shock therapy
Sibling rivalry
Sleep
Sleep disorders
Sleepwalking
Soiling
Speech disorders
Sperm banks
Stammering
Steroid abuse
Stillbirth
Stress
Strokes
Stuttering
Substance abuse
Suicide
Synesthesia
Tics
Tinnitus
Toilet training
Tourette's syndrome
Weight loss and gain
Wilson's disease

REPRODUCTIVE SYSTEM
Abdomen
Abdominal disorders
Abortion
Acquired immunodeficiency
    syndrome (AIDS)
Adrenoleukodystrophy
Amenorrhea
Amniocentesis
Anatomy
Anorexia nervosa
Assisted reproductive technologies
Breast-feeding
Breasts, female
Candidiasis
Catheterization
Cervical, ovarian, and uterine
    cancers
Cervical procedures
Cesarean section
Childbirth
Childbirth complications
Chlamydia
Chorionic villus sampling
Circumcision, female, and genital
    mutilation
Circumcision, male
Conception
Congenital adrenal hyperplasia
Contraception

Intravenous (IV) therapy
Itching
Jaundice
Kaposi's sarcoma
Kawasaki disease
Laceration repair
Laser use in surgery
Leishmaniasis
Leprosy
Lesions
Lice, mites, and ticks
Light therapy
Lower extremities
Lyme disease
Marburg virus
Measles
Melanoma
Methicillin-resistant *Staphylococcus aureus* (MRSA) infections
Moles
Monkeypox
Morgellons disease
Multiple chemical sensitivity syndrome
Nails
Necrosis
Necrotizing fasciitis
Neurofibromatosis
Nicotine
Numbness and tingling
Obesity
Obesity, childhood
Otoplasty
Pigmentation
Pinworm
Pityriasis alba
Pityriasis rosea
Plastic surgery
Poisonous plants
Polycystic ovary syndrome
Polydactyly and syndactyly
Porphyria
Psoriasis
Radiation sickness
Rashes
Reiter's syndrome
Ringworm
Rocky Mountain spotted fever
Rosacea
Roseola
Rubella
Sarcoidosis
Scabies
Scarlet fever

Scurvy
Sense organs
Shingles
Skin
Skin cancer
Skin disorders
Skin lesion removal
Smallpox
Stretch marks
Sturge-Weber syndrome
Sunburn
Sweating
Systemic lupus erythematosus (SLE)
Tattoo removal
Tattoos and body piercing
Touch
Tularemia
Typhus
Umbilical cord
Upper extremities
Vasculitis
Vitiligo
Von Willebrand's disease
Warts
Wiskott-Aldrich syndrome
Wrinkles

SPINE
Anesthesia
Anesthesiology
Atrophy
Back pain
Bone cancer
Bone disorders
Bones and the skeleton
Cerebral palsy
Chiari malformations
Chiropractic
Diaphragm
Disk removal
Fracture and dislocation
Head and neck disorders
Kinesiology
Laminectomy and spinal fusion
Lumbar puncture
Marfan syndrome
Meningitis
Motor neuron diseases
Multiple sclerosis
Muscle sprains, spasms, and disorders
Muscles
Muscular dystrophy

Nervous system
Neuralgia, neuritis, and neuropathy
Neurology
Neurology, pediatric
Neurosurgery
Numbness and tingling
Orthopedic surgery
Orthopedics
Orthopedics, pediatric
Osteoarthritis
Osteogenesis imperfecta
Osteoporosis
Paget's disease
Paralysis
Paraplegia
Physical rehabilitation
Poliomyelitis
Quadriplegia
Radiculopathy
Sciatica
Scoliosis
Slipped disk
Spina bifida
Spinal cord disorders
Spine, vertebrae, and disks
Spondylitis
Sports medicine
Stenosis
Sympathectomy
Whiplash

SPLEEN
Abdomen
Abdominal disorders
Abscess drainage
Abscesses
Anemia
Bleeding
Gaucher's disease
Hematology
Hematology, pediatric
Immune system
Internal medicine
Jaundice, neonatal
Lymph
Lymphatic system
Metabolism
Methicillin-resistant *Staphylococcus aureus* (MRSA) infections
Niemann-Pick disease
Sarcoidosis
Splenectomy
Thrombocytopenia
Transplantation

STOMACH

Abdomen
Abdominal disorders
Abscess drainage
Abscesses
Acid reflux disease
Adenoviruses
Allergies
Bariatric surgery
Botulism
Bulimia
Burping
Bypass surgery
Campylobacter infections
Chyme
Clostridium difficile infection
Coccidioidomycosis
Colitis
Crohn's disease
Digestion
Eating disorders
Endoscopic retrograde
    cholangiopancreatography (ERCP)
Endoscopy
Esophagus
Food biochemistry
Food poisoning
Gastrectomy
Gastroenteritis
Gastroenterology
Gastroenterology, pediatric
Gastrointestinal disorders
Gastrointestinal system
Gastrostomy
Gluten intolerance
Halitosis
Heartburn
Hernia
Hernia repair
Indigestion
Influenza
Internal medicine
Kwashiorkor
Lactose intolerance
Malabsorption
Malnutrition
Metabolism
Motion sickness
Nausea and vomiting
Nutrition
Obesity
Obesity, childhood
Peristalsis
Poisoning

Poisonous plants
Pyloric stenosis
Radiation sickness
Rotavirus
Roundworm
Salmonella infection
Small intestine
Stomach, intestinal, and pancreatic
    cancers
Ulcer surgery
Ulcers
Vagotomy
Vitamins and minerals
Weaning
Weight loss and gain

TEETH

Braces, orthodontic
Cavities
Cornelia de Lange syndrome
Crowns and bridges
Dental diseases
Dentistry
Dentistry, pediatric
Dentures
Endodontic disease
Fluoride treatments
Forensic pathology
Fracture repair
Gastrointestinal system
Gingivitis
Gum disease
Jaw wiring
Lisping
Nicotine
Nutrition
Oral and maxillofacial surgery
Orthodontics
Osteogenesis imperfecta
Periodontal surgery
Periodontitis
Plaque, dental
Prader-Willi syndrome
Root canal treatment
Rubinstein-Taybi syndrome
Teeth
Teething
Temporomandibular joint (TMJ)
    syndrome
Thumb sucking
Tooth extraction
Toothache
Veterinary medicine
Wisdom teeth

TENDONS

Carpal tunnel syndrome
Casts and splints
Collagen
Connective tissue
Cysts
Exercise physiology
Ganglion removal
Hammertoe correction
Joints
Kneecap removal
Orthopedic surgery
Orthopedics
Orthopedics, pediatric
Osgood-Schlatter disease
Physical rehabilitation
Sports medicine
Tendinitis
Tendon disorders
Tendon repair

THROAT

Acid reflux disease
Adenoids
Antihistamines
Asbestos exposure
Auras
Bulimia
Catheterization
Choking
Croup
Decongestants
Drowning
Epiglottitis
Epstein-Barr virus
Esophagus
Fifth disease
Gastroenterology
Gastroenterology, pediatric
Gastrointestinal disorders
Gastrointestinal system
Goiter
Head and neck disorders
Heimlich maneuver
Hiccups
Histiocytosis
H1N1 influenza
Laryngectomy
Laryngitis
Mouth and throat cancer
Nasopharyngeal disorders
Nicotine
Nosebleeds
Otorhinolaryngology

Pharyngitis
Pharynx
Pulmonary medicine
Pulmonary medicine, pediatric
Quinsy
Respiration
Rhinitis
Rhinoviruses
Smoking
Sore throat
Strep throat
Tonsillectomy and adenoid
    removal
Tonsillitis
Tonsils
Tracheostomy
Voice and vocal cord disorders

URINARY SYSTEM
Abdomen
Abdominal disorders
Abscess drainage
Abscesses
Adenoviruses
Adrenalectomy
Bed-wetting
Bladder cancer
Bladder removal
Candidiasis
Catheterization
Circumcision, male
Cystitis
Cystoscopy
Cysts
Dialysis
Diuretics
E. coli infection
End-stage renal disease
Endoscopy
Fetal surgery
Fistula repair
Fluids and electrolytes
Geriatrics and gerontology
Hematuria
Hemolytic uremic syndrome
Hermaphroditism and
    pseudohermaphroditism
Host-defense mechanisms
Hyperplasia

Hypertension
Incontinence
Internal medicine
Kidney cancer
Kidney disorders
Kidney transplantation
Kidneys
Laparoscopy
Lithotripsy
Nephrectomy
Nephritis
Nephrology
Nephrology, pediatric
Pediatrics
Penile implant surgery
Plasma
Proteinuria
Pyelonephritis
Reiter's syndrome
Renal failure
Reye's syndrome
Schistosomiasis
Stone removal
Stones
Systems and organs
Testicular cancer
Toilet training
Transplantation
Trichomoniasis
Ultrasonography
Uremia
Urethritis
Urinalysis
Urinary disorders
Urinary system
Urology
Urology, pediatric

UTERUS
Abdomen
Abdominal disorders
Abortion
Amenorrhea
Amniocentesis
Assisted reproductive technologies
Cervical, ovarian, and uterine
    cancers
Cervical procedures
Cesarean section

Childbirth
Childbirth complications
Chorionic villus sampling
Conception
Contraception
Culdocentesis
Dysmenorrhea
Ectopic pregnancy
Electrocauterization
Embolization
Endocrinology
Endometrial biopsy
Endometriosis
Fistula repair
Gender reassignment surgery
Genetic counseling
Genital disorders, female
Gynecology
Hermaphroditism and
    pseudohermaphroditism
Hyperplasia
Hysterectomy
In vitro fertilization
Infertility, female
Internal medicine
Laparoscopy
Menopause
Menorrhagia
Menstruation
Miscarriage
Multiple births
Myomectomy
Obstetrics
Pap test
Pelvic inflammatory disease
    (PID)
Placenta
Pregnancy and gestation
Premature birth
Premenstrual syndrome (PMS)
Prostate enlargement
Reproductive system
Sexual differentiation
Sperm banks
Sterilization
Stillbirth
Tubal ligation
Ultrasonography
Uterus

ENTRIES BY SPECIALTIES AND RELATED FIELDS

E. coli infection
Emerging infectious diseases
Endocarditis
Epidemics and pandemics
Fluoride treatments
Gangrene
Gastroenteritis
Genomics
Gonorrhea
Gram staining
Impetigo
Infection
Laboratory tests
Legionnaires' disease
Leprosy
Listeria infections
Lyme disease
Mastitis
Methicillin-resistant Staphylococcus
  aureus (MRSA) infections
Microbiology
Microscopy
Necrotizing fasciitis
Nephritis
Opportunistic infections
Osteomyelitis
Pelvic inflammatory disease (PID)
Plague
Pneumonia
Pus
Salmonella infection
Sarcoidosis
Scarlet fever
Serology
Shigellosis
Staphylococcal infections
Strep throat
Streptococcal infections
Syphilis
Tetanus
Tonsillitis
Tropical medicine
Tuberculosis
Tularemia
Typhoid fever
Typhus
Whooping cough

BIOCHEMISTRY
Acid-base chemistry
Acidosis
Adrenal glands
Antibodies
Antidepressants

Autopsy
Bacteriology
Caffeine
Carbohydrates
Cholesterol
Collagen
Colon
Connective tissue
Corticosteroids
Digestion
Endocrine glands
Endocrinology
Endocrinology, pediatric
Enzyme therapy
Enzymes
Ergogenic aids
Fatty acid oxidation disorders
Fluids and electrolytes
Fluoride treatments
Food biochemistry
Food Guide Pyramid
Fructosemia
Gaucher's disease
Genetic engineering
Genomics
Glands
Glycogen storage diseases
Glycolysis
Gram staining
Histology
Hormones
Hypothalamus
Leptin
Leukodystrophy
Lipids
Macronutrients
Malabsorption
Metabolism
Nephrology
Nephrology, pediatric
Niemann-Pick disease
Nutrition
Ovaries
Pathology
Pharmacology
Pharmacy
Pituitary gland
Plasma
Protein
Respiration
Retroviruses
Rhinoviruses
Small intestine
Stem cells

Steroids
Thymus gland
Toxicology
Urinalysis
Wilson's disease

BIOTECHNOLOGY
Antibodies
Assisted reproductive technologies
Biological therapies
Bionics and biotechnology
Biophysics
Cloning
Computed tomography (CT)
  scanning
Defibrillation
Dialysis
Echocardiography
Electrocardiography (ECG or EKG)
Electroencephalography (EEG)
Fatty acid oxidation disorders
Gene therapy
Genetic engineering
Genomics
Glycogen storage diseases
Huntington's disease
Hyperbaric oxygen therapy
In vitro fertilization
Magnetic resonance imaging (MRI)
Pacemaker implantation
Positron emission tomography
  (PET)scanning
Prostheses
Severe combined immunodeficiency
  syndrome (SCID)
Single photon emission computed
  tomography (SPECT)
Sperm banks
Stem cells
Xenotransplantation

CARDIOLOGY
Acute respiratory distress syndrome
  (ARDS)
Aging
Aging: Extended care
Aneurysmectomy
Aneurysms
Angina
Angiography
Angioplasty
Anxiety
Arrhythmias
Arteriosclerosis

Atrial fibrillation
Biofeedback
Blood pressure
Blood vessels
Blue baby syndrome
Bypass surgery
Cardiac arrest
Cardiac rehabilitation
Cardiac surgery
Cardiology
Cardiology, pediatric
Cardiopulmonary resuscitation
   (CPR)
Carotid arteries
Catheterization
Chest
Cholesterol
Circulation
Congenital heart disease
Coronary artery bypass graft
Critical care
Critical care, pediatric
Defibrillation
DiGeorge syndrome
Diuretics
Dizziness and fainting
Echocardiography
Electrocardiography (ECG or EKG)
Emergency medicine
End-stage renal disease
Endocarditis
Enteroviruses
Exercise physiology
Fetal surgery
Food Guide Pyramid
Geriatrics and gerontology
Heart
Heart attack
Heart disease
Heart failure
Heart transplantation
Heart valve replacement
Hematology
Hemochromatosis
Hypercholesterolemia
Hypertension
Hypotension
Infarction
Internal medicine
Ischemia
Kinesiology
Leptin
Lesions
Marfan syndrome

Metabolic syndrome
Mitral valve prolapse
Mucopolysaccharidosis (MPS)
Muscles
Neonatology
Nicotine
Noninvasive tests
Nuclear medicine
Pacemaker implantation
Palliative medicine
Palpitations
Paramedics
Physical examination
Plaque, arterial
Plasma
Polycystic kidney disease
Prader-Willi syndrome
Progeria
Prostheses
Pulmonary edema
Pulmonary hypertension
Pulse rate
Rheumatic fever
Rubinstein-Taybi syndrome
Sarcoidosis
Sports medicine
Stenosis
Stents
Thoracic surgery
Thrombolytic therapy and TPA
Thrombosis and thrombus
Transplantation
Ultrasonography
Uremia
Vascular medicine
Vascular system
Vasculitis
Venous insufficiency

CRITICAL CARE
Accidents
Acidosis
Aging: Extended care
Amputation
Anesthesia
Anesthesiology
Apgar score
Atrial fibrillation
Brain damage
Burns and scalds
Carotid arteries
Catheterization
Club drugs
Coma

Critical care
Critical care, pediatric
Defibrillation
Diuretics
Drowning
Echocardiography
Electrical shock
Electrocardiography (ECG or EKG)
Electroencephalography (EEG)
Embolization
Emergency medicine
Emergency medicine, pediatric
Emergency rooms
Emerging infectious diseases
Epidemics and pandemics
First aid
Geriatrics and gerontology
Grafts and grafting
Hantavirus
Heart attack
Heart transplantation
Heat exhaustion and heatstroke
Hospitals
Hyperbaric oxygen therapy
Hyperthermia and hypothermia
Hypotension
Hypoxia
Infarction
Intensive care unit (ICU)
Intravenous (IV) therapy
Methicillin-resistant *Staphylococcus*
   aureus (MRSA) infections
Necrotizing fasciitis
Neonatology
Nursing
Oncology
Osteopathic medicine
Pain management
Palliative medicine
Paramedics
Psychiatry
Psychiatry, child and adolescent
Psychiatry, geriatric
Pulmonary medicine
Pulmonary medicine, pediatric
Pulse rate
Radiation sickness
Resuscitation
Safety issues for children
Safety issues for the elderly
Severe acute respiratory syndrome
   (SARS)
Shock
Stevens-Johnson syndrome

Thrombolytic therapy and TPA
Toxic shock syndrome
Tracheostomy
Transfusion
Tropical medicine
Wounds ·

CYTOLOGY
Acid-base chemistry
Bionics and biotechnology
Biopsy
Blood testing
Cancer
Carcinoma
Cells
Cholesterol
Cytology
Cytopathology
Dermatology
Dermatopathology
E. coli infection
Enzymes
Fluids and electrolytes
Food biochemistry
Gaucher's disease
Genetic counseling
Genetic engineering
Genomics
Glycolysis
Gram staining
Healing
Hematology
Hematology, pediatric
Histology
Hyperplasia
Immune system
Immunology
Karyotyping
Laboratory tests
Lipids
Melanoma
Metabolism
Microscopy
Mutation
Oncology
Pathology
Pharmacology
Pharmacy
Plasma
Pus
Rhinoviruses
Sarcoma
Serology
Side effects

Stem cells
Toxicology

DENTISTRY
Abscess drainage
Abscesses
Aging: Extended care
Anesthesia
Anesthesiology
Braces, orthodontic
Canker sores
Cavities
Crowns and bridges
Dental diseases
Dentistry
Dentistry, pediatric
Dentures
Endodontic disease
Fluoride treatments
Forensic pathology
Fracture and dislocation
Fracture repair
Gastrointestinal system
Gingivitis
Gum disease
Halitosis
Head and neck disorders
Jaw wiring
Lisping
Local anesthesia
Mouth and throat cancer
Nicotine
Oral and maxillofacial surgery
Orthodontics
Osteogenesis imperfecta
Periodontal surgery
Periodontitis
Plaque, dental
Plastic surgery
Prader-Willi syndrome
Prostheses
Root canal treatment
Rubinstein-Taybi syndrome
Sense organs
Sjögren's syndrome
Teeth
Teething
Temporomandibular joint (TMJ)
   syndrome
Thumb sucking
Tooth extraction
Toothache
Von Willebrand's disease
Wisdom teeth

DERMATOLOGY
Abscess drainage
Abscesses
Acne
Adrenoleukodystrophy
Age spots
Albinos
Anthrax
Anti-inflammatory drugs
Athlete's foot
Bedsores
Bile
Biopsy
Birthmarks
Blisters
Body dysmorphic disorder
Boils
Burns and scalds
Carcinoma
Chickenpox
Coccidioidomycosis
Corns and calluses
Corticosteroids
Cryotherapy and cryosurgery
Cyst removal
Cysts
Dermatitis
Dermatology
Dermatology, pediatric
Dermatopathology
Eczema
Electrocauterization
Enteroviruses
Facial transplantation
Fungal infections
Ganglion removal
Glands
Gluten intolerance
Grafts and grafting
Gray hair
Hair
Hair loss and baldness
Hair transplantation
Hand-foot-and-mouth disease
Healing
Histology
Hives
Hyperhidrosis
Impetigo
Itching
Laser use in surgery
Lesions
Lice, mites, and ticks
Light therapy

Local anesthesia
Melanoma
Methicillin-resistant *Staphylococcus aureus* (MRSA) infections
Moles
Monkeypox
Morgellons disease
Multiple chemical sensitivity syndrome
Nail removal
Nails
Necrotizing fasciitis
Neurofibromatosis
Pigmentation
Pinworm
Pityriasis alba
Pityriasis rosea
Plastic surgery
Podiatry
Poisonous plants
Polycystic ovary syndrome
Prostheses
Psoriasis
Puberty and adolescence
Rashes
Reiter's syndrome
Ringworm
Rocky Mountain spotted fever
Rosacea
Sarcoidosis
Scabies
Scleroderma
Sense organs
Side effects
Skin
Skin cancer
Skin disorders
Skin lesion removal
Stevens-Johnson syndrome
Stretch marks
Sturge-Weber syndrome
Sunburn
Sweating
Systemic lupus erythematosus (SLE)
Tattoo removal
Tattoos and body piercing
Touch
Vasculitis
Vitiligo
Von Willebrand's disease
Warts
Wiskott-Aldrich syndrome
Wrinkles

EMBRYOLOGY
Abortion
Amniocentesis
Assisted reproductive technologies
Birth defects
Blue baby syndrome
Brain damage
Brain disorders
Cerebral palsy
Chorionic villus sampling
Cloning
Conception
Down syndrome
Embryology
Fetal alcohol syndrome
Gamete intrafallopian transfer (GIFT)
Genetic counseling
Genetic diseases
Genetics and inheritance
Genomics
Growth
Hermaphroditism and pseudohermaphroditism
In vitro fertilization
Karyotyping
Klinefelter syndrome
Miscarriage
Mucopolysaccharidosis (MPS)
Multiple births
Nicotine
Obstetrics
Ovaries
Placenta
Pregnancy and gestation
Reproductive system
Rh factor
Rubella
Sexual differentiation
Spina bifida
Stem cells
Teratogens
Toxoplasmosis
Ultrasonography
Uterus

EMERGENCY MEDICINE
Abdominal disorders
Abscess drainage
Accidents
Acidosis
Adrenoleukodystrophy
Aging
Altitude sickness

Amputation
Anesthesia
Anesthesiology
Aneurysms
Angiography
Appendectomy
Appendicitis
Asphyxiation
Atrial fibrillation
Biological and chemical weapons
Bites and stings
Bleeding
Blurred vision
Botulism
Brain damage
Bruises
Burns and scalds
Cardiac arrest
Cardiology
Cardiology, pediatric
Cardiopulmonary resuscitation (CPR)
Carotid arteries
Casts and splints
Catheterization
Cesarean section
Choking
Club drugs
Coma
Computed tomography (CT) scanning
Concussion
Critical care
Critical care, pediatric
Croup
Defibrillation
Diphtheria
Dizziness and fainting
Domestic violence
Drowning
Echocardiography
Electrical shock
Electrocardiography (ECG or EKG)
Electroencephalography (EEG)
Embolization
Emergency medicine
Emergency medicine, pediatric
Emergency rooms
Epiglottitis
First aid
Food poisoning
Fracture and dislocation
Frostbite
Grafts and grafting

Head and neck disorders
Heart attack
Heart transplantation
Heat exhaustion and heatstroke
Heimlich maneuver
Hemorrhage
H1N1 influenza
Hospitals
Hyperbaric oxygen therapy
Hyperthermia and hypothermia
Hyperventilation
Hypotension
Hypoxia
Infarction
Intensive care unit (ICU)
Intoxication
Intravenous (IV) therapy
Jaw wiring
Laceration repair
Local anesthesia
Lumbar puncture
Lung surgery
Meningitis
Monkeypox
Necrotizing fasciitis
Noninvasive tests
Nosebleeds
Nursing
Osteopathic medicine
Oxygen therapy
Pain management
Paramedics
Peritonitis
Physician assistants
Plague
Plastic surgery
Pneumonia
Pneumothorax
Poisoning
Pulmonary diseases
Pulmonary medicine
Pulmonary medicine, pediatric
Pulse rate
Pyelonephritis
Radiation sickness
Resuscitation
Reye's syndrome
Rocky Mountain spotted fever
Safety issues for children
Safety issues for the elderly
Salmonella infection
Severe acute respiratory syndrome
  (SARS)
Shock

Side effects
Snakebites
Spinal cord disorders
Splenectomy
Sports medicine
Staphylococcal infections
Stevens-Johnson syndrome
Streptococcal infections
Strokes
Sunburn
Surgical technologists
Thrombolytic therapy and TPA
Toxic shock syndrome
Tracheostomy
Transfusion
Transplantation
Unconsciousness
Wheezing
Wounds

ENDOCRINOLOGY
Addison's disease
Adrenal glands
Adrenalectomy
Adrenoleukodystrophy
Anti-inflammatory drugs
Assisted reproductive technologies
Bariatric surgery
Breasts, female
Carbohydrates
Chronobiology
Congenital adrenal hyperplasia
Congenital hypothyroidism
Corticosteroids
Cushing's syndrome
Diabetes mellitus
Dwarfism
End-stage renal disease
Endocrine disorders
Endocrine glands
Endocrinology
Endocrinology, pediatric
Enzymes
Ergogenic aids
Failure to thrive
Food Guide Pyramid
Galactosemia
Gamete intrafallopian transfer
  (GIFT)
Gender identity disorder
Gender reassignment surgery
Geriatrics and gerontology
Gestational diabetes
Gigantism

Glands
Goiter
Growth
Gynecology
Gynecomastia
Hair loss and baldness
Hashimoto's thyroiditis
Hemochromatosis
Hermaphroditism and
  pseudohermaphroditism
Hormone therapy
Hormones
Hot flashes
Hyperadiposis
Hyperparathyroidism and
  hypoparathyroidism
Hyperplasia
Hypertrophy
Hypoglycemia
Hypothalamus
Hysterectomy
Infertility, female
Infertility, male
Internal medicine
Klinefelter syndrome
Laboratory tests
Laparoscopy
Leptin
Liver
Melatonin
Menopause
Menstruation
Metabolic disorders
Metabolic syndrome
Nephrology
Nephrology, pediatric
Neurology
Neurology, pediatric
Niemann-Pick disease
Nonalcoholic steatohepatitis (NASH)
Nuclear medicine
Obesity
Obesity, childhood
Ovaries
Pancreas
Pancreatitis
Parathyroidectomy
Pharmacology
Pharmacy
Pituitary gland
Plasma
Polycystic ovary syndrome
Precocious puberty
Prostate enlargement

ETHICS
Abortion
Animal rights vs. research
Assisted reproductive technologies
Circumcision, female, and genital
    mutilation
Circumcision, male
Cloning
Defibrillation
Ergogenic aids
Ethics
Euthanasia
Fetal surgery
Fetal tissue transplantation
Gender identity disorder
Gene therapy
Genetic engineering
Genomics
Gulf War syndrome
Health Canada
Health care reform
Hippocratic oath
Law and medicine
Living will
Malpractice
Marijuana
Münchausen syndrome by proxy
Palliative medicine
Sperm banks
Stem cells
Xenotransplantation

EXERCISE PHYSIOLOGY
Acidosis
Back pain
Biofeedback
Blood pressure
Bone disorders
Bones and the skeleton
Cardiac rehabilitation
Cardiology
Carotid arteries
Circulation
Defibrillation
Dehydration
Echocardiography
Electrocardiography (ECG or EKG)
Ergogenic aids
Exercise physiology
Fascia
Glycolysis
Heart
Heat exhaustion and heatstroke
Hypoxia

Kinesiology
Ligaments
Lungs
Massage
Metabolism
Motor skill development
Muscle sprains, spasms, and
    disorders
Muscles
Nutrition
Orthopedic surgery
Orthopedics
Orthopedics, pediatric
Overtraining syndrome
Oxygen therapy
Physical rehabilitation
Physiology
Pulmonary diseases
Pulmonary medicine
Pulmonary medicine, pediatric
Pulse rate
Respiration
Sports medicine
Stenosis
Steroid abuse
Sweating
Tendinitis
Vascular system

FAMILY MEDICINE
Abdominal disorders
Abscess drainage
Abscesses
Acne
Acquired immunodeficiency
    syndrome (AIDS)
Alcoholism
Allergies
Alzheimer's disease
Amyotrophic lateral sclerosis
Anemia
Angina
Anosmia
Antianxiety drugs
Antidepressants
Antihistamines
Anti-inflammatory drugs
Antioxidants
Arthritis
Athlete's foot
Atrophy
Attention-deficit disorder (ADD)
Bacterial infections
Bed-wetting

Bell's palsy
Beriberi
Biofeedback
Birthmarks
Bleeding
Blisters
Blood pressure
Blurred vision
Body dysmorphic disorder
Boils
Bronchiolitis
Bronchitis
Bunions
Burkitt's lymphoma
Burping
Caffeine
Candidiasis
Canker sores
Carotid arteries
Casts and splints
Chagas' disease
Chickenpox
Childhood infectious diseases
Chlamydia
Cholecystitis
Cholesterol
Chronic fatigue syndrome
Cirrhosis
Clinics
Clostridium difficile infection
Cluster headaches
Coccidioidomycosis
Cold sores
Common cold
Constipation
Contraception
Corticosteroids
Coughing
Cryotherapy and cryosurgery
Cytomegalovirus (CMV)
Death and dying
Decongestants
Deep vein thrombosis
Defibrillation
Dehydration
Dengue fever
Depression
Diabetes mellitus
Diaper rash
Diarrhea and dysentery
Digestion
Dizziness and fainting
Domestic violence
Earwax

FORENSIC MEDICINE
Autopsy
Blood and blood disorders
Blood testing
Bones and the skeleton
Cytopathology
Dermatopathology
DNA and RNA
Forensic pathology
Genetics and inheritance
Genomics
Hematology
Histology
Immunopathology
Laboratory tests
Law and medicine
Pathology

GASTROENTEROLOGY
Abdomen
Abdominal disorders
Acid reflux disease
Acidosis
Adenoviruses
Amebiasis
Amyotrophic lateral sclerosis
Anal cancer
Anthrax
Anus
Appendectomy
Appendicitis
Bariatric surgery
Bile
Bulimia
Bypass surgery
Campylobacter infections
Celiac sprue
Cholecystectomy
Cholecystitis
Cholera
Chyme
Clostridium difficile infection
Colic
Colitis
Colon
Colonoscopy and sigmoidoscopy
Colorectal cancer
Colorectal polyp removal
Colorectal surgery
Computed tomography (CT)
    scanning
Constipation
Critical care
Critical care, pediatric

Crohn's disease
Cytomegalovirus (CMV)
Diarrhea and dysentery
Digestion
Diverticulitis and diverticulosis
E. coli infection
Emergency medicine
Endoscopic retrograde
    cholangiopancreatography (ERCP)
Endoscopy
Enemas
Enterocolitis
Enzymes
Epidemics and pandemics
Esophagus
Failure to thrive
Fiber
Fistula repair
Food allergies
Food biochemistry
Food poisoning
Gallbladder
Gallbladder cancer
Gallbladder diseases
Gastrectomy
Gastroenteritis
Gastroenterology
Gastroenterology, pediatric
Gastrointestinal disorders
Gastrointestinal system
Gastrostomy
Giardiasis
Glands
Gluten intolerance
Heartburn
Hemochromatosis
Hemolytic uremic syndrome
Hemorrhoid banding and removal
Hemorrhoids
Hernia
Hernia repair
Hirschsprung's disease
Ileostomy and colostomy
Indigestion
Infarction
Internal medicine
Intestinal disorders
Intestines
Irritable bowel syndrome (IBS)
Lactose intolerance
Laparoscopy
Lesions
Liver
Liver cancer

Liver disorders
Liver transplantation
Malabsorption
Malnutrition
Metabolism
Nausea and vomiting
Nonalcoholic steatohepatitis (NASH)
Noroviruses
Nutrition
Obstruction
Pancreas
Pancreatitis
Peristalsis
Poisonous plants
Polycystic kidney disease
Polyps
Proctology
Pyloric stenosis
Rectum
Rotavirus
Roundworm
Salmonella infection
Scleroderma
Shigellosis
Small intestine
Soiling
Stenosis
Stevens-Johnson syndrome
Stomach, intestinal, and pancreatic
    cancers
Stone removal
Stones
Tapeworm
Taste
Toilet training
Trichinosis
Ulcer surgery
Ulcers
Vagotomy
Vagus nerve
Vasculitis
Von Willebrand's disease
Weight loss and gain
Wilson's disease
Worms

GENERAL SURGERY
Abscess drainage
Adenoids
Adrenalectomy
Amputation
Anesthesia
Anesthesiology
Aneurysmectomy

Appendectomy
Bariatric surgery
Biopsy
Bladder removal
Bone marrow transplantation
Breast biopsy
Breast surgery
Bunions
Bypass surgery
Casts and splints
Cataract surgery
Catheterization
Cervical procedures
Cesarean section
Cholecystectomy
Circumcision, female, and genital
    mutilation
Circumcision, male
Cleft lip and palate repair
Coccidioidomycosis
Colon
Colorectal polyp removal
Colorectal surgery
Corneal transplantation
Coronary artery bypass graft
Craniotomy
Cryotherapy and cryosurgery
Cyst removal
Defibrillation
Disk removal
Ear surgery
Electrocauterization
Endarterectomy
Endometrial biopsy
Eye surgery
Face lift and blepharoplasty
Fistula repair
Ganglion removal
Gastrectomy
Gender identity disorder
Gender reassignment surgery
Grafts and grafting
Hair transplantation
Hammertoe correction
Heart transplantation
Heart valve replacement
Heel spur removal
Hemorrhoid banding and removal
Hernia repair
Hip replacement
Hydroceles
Hypospadias repair and
    urethroplasty
Hypoxia

Hysterectomy
Infarction
Intravenous (IV) therapy
Kidney transplantation
Kneecap removal
Laceration repair
Laminectomy and spinal fusion
Laparoscopy
Laryngectomy
Laser use in surgery
Lesions
Liposuction
Liver transplantation
Lung surgery
Mastectomy and lumpectomy
Mesothelioma
Myomectomy
Nail removal
Nasal polyp removal
Nephrectomy
Neurosurgery
Oncology
Ophthalmology
Orthopedic surgery
Otoplasty
Parathyroidectomy
Penile implant surgery
Periodontal surgery
Phlebitis
Plasma
Plastic surgery
Polydactyly and syndactyly
Polyps
Prostate gland removal
Prostheses
Pulse rate
Rhinoplasty and submucous
    resection
Rotator cuff surgery
Shunts
Skin lesion removal
Small intestine
Sphincterectomy
Splenectomy
Sterilization
Stone removal
Surgery, general
Surgery, pediatric
Surgical procedures
Surgical technologists
Sympathectomy
Tattoo removal
Tendon repair
Testicular surgery

Thoracic surgery
Thyroidectomy
Tonsillectomy and adenoid removal
Toxic shock syndrome
Trachea
Tracheostomy
Transfusion
Transplantation
Tumor removal
Ulcer surgery
Vagotomy
Varicose vein removal
Vasectomy
Xenotransplantation

GENETICS
Adrenal glands
Adrenoleukodystrophy
Aging
Agnosia
Albinos
Alzheimer's disease
Amniocentesis
Assisted reproductive technologies
Attention-deficit disorder (ADD)
Autoimmune disorders
Batten's disease
Bioinformatics
Biological therapies
Bionics and biotechnology
Birth defects
Bone marrow transplantation
Breast cancer
Breast disorders
Chorionic villus sampling
Cloning
Cognitive development
Color blindness
Colorectal cancer
Congenital adrenal hyperplasia
Congenital disorders
Cornelia de Lange syndrome
Cystic fibrosis
Diabetes mellitus
DiGeorge syndrome
DNA and RNA
Down syndrome
Dwarfism
Embryology
Endocrinology
Endocrinology, pediatric
Enzyme therapy
Enzymes
Failure to thrive

Fetal surgery
Fragile X syndrome
Fructosemia
Galactosemia
Gaucher's disease
Gender identity disorder
Gene therapy
Genetic counseling
Genetic diseases
Genetic engineering
Genetics and inheritance
Genomics
Grafts and grafting
Hematology
Hematology, pediatric
Hemophilia
Hermaphroditism and
    pseudohermaphroditism
Huntington's disease
Hyperadiposis
Immunodeficiency disorders
In vitro fertilization
Karyotyping
Klinefelter syndrome
Klippel-Trenaunay syndrome
Laboratory tests
Leptin
Leukodystrophy
Malabsorption
Maple syrup urine disease (MSUD)
Marfan syndrome
Mental retardation
Metabolic disorders
Motor skill development
Mucopolysaccharidosis (MPS)
Muscular dystrophy
Mutation
Neonatology
Nephrology
Nephrology, pediatric
Neurofibromatosis
Neurology
Neurology, pediatric
Niemann-Pick disease
Obstetrics
Oncology
Osteogenesis imperfecta
Ovaries
Pediatrics
Phenylketonuria (PKU)
Polycystic kidney disease
Polydactyly and syndactyly
Polyps
Porphyria

Prader-Willi syndrome
Precocious puberty
Reproductive system
Retroviruses
Rh factor
Rhinoviruses
Rubinstein-Taybi syndrome
Sarcoidosis
Screening
Severe combined immunodeficiency
    syndrome (SCID)
Sexual differentiation
Sexuality
Sperm banks
Stem cells
Synesthesia
Tay-Sachs disease
Tourette's syndrome
Transplantation
Turner syndrome
Wiskott-Aldrich syndrome

**GERIATRICS AND
    GERONTOLOGY**
Age spots
Aging
Aging: Extended care
Alzheimer's disease
Arthritis
Assisted living facilities
Atrophy
Bed-wetting
Blindness
Blood pressure
Blurred vision
Bone disorders
Bones and the skeleton
Brain
Brain disorders
Cartilage
Cataract surgery
Cataracts
Chronic obstructive pulmonary
    disease (COPD)
Corns and calluses
Critical care
Crowns and bridges
Deafness
Death and dying
Dementias
Dentures
Depression
Domestic violence
Dyskinesia

Emergency medicine
End-stage renal disease
Endocrinology
Euthanasia
Family medicine
Fatigue
Fiber
Fracture and dislocation
Fracture repair
Gray hair
Hearing aids
Hearing loss
Hip fracture repair
Hip replacement
Hormone therapy
Hormones
Hospitals
Incontinence
Joints
Memory loss
Nursing
Nutrition
Ophthalmology
Orthopedics
Osteoporosis
Pain management
Palliative medicine
Paramedics
Parkinson's disease
Pharmacology
Pick's disease
Psychiatry
Psychiatry, geriatric
Radiculopathy
Rheumatology
Safety issues for the elderly
Sleep disorders
Spinal cord disorders
Spine, vertebrae, and disks
Suicide
Vision disorders
Wrinkles

GYNECOLOGY
Abortion
Amenorrhea
Amniocentesis
Assisted reproductive technologies
Biopsy
Bladder removal
Breast biopsy
Breast cancer
Breast disorders
Breast-feeding

Breasts, female
Cervical, ovarian, and uterine
    cancers
Cervical procedures
Cesarean section
Childbirth
Childbirth complications
Chlamydia
Circumcision, female, and genital
    mutilation
Conception
Contraception
Culdocentesis
Cyst removal
Cystitis
Cysts
Dysmenorrhea
Electrocauterization
Embolization
Endocrinology
Endometrial biopsy
Endometriosis
Endoscopy
Episiotomy
Fibrocystic breast condition
Gender reassignment surgery
Genital disorders, female
Glands
Gonorrhea
Gynecology
Hermaphroditism and
    pseudohermaphroditism
Herpes
Hormone therapy
Hormones
Hot flashes
Human papillomavirus (HPV)
Hyperplasia
Hysterectomy
In vitro fertilization
Incontinence
Infertility, female
Internal medicine
Laparoscopy
Leptin
Lesions
Mammography
Mastectomy and lumpectomy
Mastitis
Menopause
Menorrhagia
Menstruation
Myomectomy
Nutrition

Obstetrics
Ovarian cysts
Ovaries
Pap test
Pelvic inflammatory disease (PID)
Peritonitis
Polycystic ovary syndrome
Polyps
Postpartum depression
Preeclampsia and eclampsia
Pregnancy and gestation
Premenstrual syndrome (PMS)
Rape and sexual assault
Reiter's syndrome
Reproductive system
Sexual differentiation
Sexual dysfunction
Sexuality
Sexually transmitted diseases
    (STDs)
Sterilization
Syphilis
Toxemia
Toxic shock syndrome
Trichomoniasis
Tubal ligation
Turner syndrome
Ultrasonography
Urethritis
Urinary disorders
Urology
Uterus
Von Willebrand's disease
Warts

HEMATOLOGY
Acid-base chemistry
Acidosis
Acquired immunodeficiency
    syndrome (AIDS)
Anemia
Babesiosis
Biological therapies
Bleeding
Blood and blood disorders
Blood testing
Blood vessels
Bone grafting
Bone marrow transplantation
Bruises
Burkitt's lymphoma
Cholesterol
Circulation
Connective tissue

Cyanosis
Cytology
Cytomegalovirus (CMV)
Cytopathology
Deep vein thrombosis
Dialysis
Disseminated intravascular
    coagulation (DIC)
Epidemics and pandemics
Ergogenic aids
Fluids and electrolytes
Forensic pathology
Healing
Hematology
Hematology, pediatric
Hemolytic disease of the newborn
Hemolytic uremic syndrome
Hemophilia
Hemorrhage
Histiocytosis
Histology
Hodgkin's disease
Host-defense mechanisms
Hypercholesterolemia
Hyperlipidemia
Hypoglycemia
Immune system
Immunology
Infection
Ischemia
Jaundice
Jaundice, neonatal
Kidneys
Laboratory tests
Leukemia
Liver
Lymph
Lymphadenopathy and lymphoma
Lymphatic system
Malaria
Nephrology
Nephrology, pediatric
Niemann-Pick disease
Nosebleeds
Palliative medicine
Phlebotomy
Plasma
Rh factor
Septicemia
Serology
Sickle cell disease
Stem cells
Subdural hematoma
Thalassemia

Anxiety
Appetite loss
Arrhythmias
Arteriosclerosis
Aspergillosis
Autoimmune disorders
Babesiosis
Bacillus Calmette-Guérin (BCG)
Bacterial infections
Bariatric surgery
Bedsores
Behçet's disease
Beriberi
Bile
Biofeedback
Bleeding
Blood vessels
Body dysmorphic disorder
Bronchiolitis
Bronchitis
Burkitt's lymphoma
Burping
Bursitis
Campylobacter infections
Candidiasis
Cardiac surgery
Carotid arteries
Casts and splints
Chickenpox
Childhood infectious diseases
Cholecystitis
Cholesterol
Chronic fatigue syndrome
Chyme
Cirrhosis
Claudication
Cluster headaches
Coccidioidomycosis
Colitis
Colon
Colonoscopy and sigmoidoscopy
Common cold
Congenital hypothyroidism
Constipation
Corticosteroids
Coughing
Crohn's disease
Cyanosis
Defibrillation
Dengue fever
Diabetes mellitus
Dialysis
Diaphragm
Diarrhea and dysentery

Digestion
Disseminated intravascular
   coagulation (DIC)
Diuretics
Diverticulitis and diverticulosis
Dizziness and fainting
Domestic violence
E. coli infection
Edema
Embolism
Emphysema
End-stage renal disease
Endocarditis
Endocrine glands
Endoscopic retrograde
   cholangiopancreatography (ERCP)
Endoscopy
Enteroviruses
Epidemics and pandemics
Factitious disorders
Family medicine
Fatigue
Fever
Fiber
Fungal infections
Gallbladder
Gallbladder diseases
Gangrene
Gastroenteritis
Gastroenterology
Gastroenterology, pediatric
Gastrointestinal disorders
Gastrointestinal system
Gaucher's disease
Genetic diseases
Geriatrics and gerontology
Goiter
Gout
Guillain-Barré syndrome
Hantavirus
Headaches
Heart
Heart attack
Heart disease
Heart failure
Heartburn
Heat exhaustion and heatstroke
Hematuria
Hemochromatosis
Hepatitis
Hernia
Histology
Hodgkin's disease
H1N1 influenza

Human immunodeficiency virus
   (HIV)
Hypercholesterolemia
Hyperlipidemia
Hypertension
Hyperthermia and hypothermia
Hypertrophy
Hypoglycemia
Hypotension
Hypoxia
Incontinence
Indigestion
Infarction
Infection
Inflammation
Influenza
Internal medicine
Intestinal disorders
Intestines
Ischemia
Itching
Jaundice
Kaposi's sarcoma
Kidney disorders
Kidneys
Klippel-Trenaunay syndrome
Legionnaires' disease
Leprosy
Lesions
Leukemia
Liver
Liver disorders
Lyme disease
Lymph
Lymphadenopathy and lymphoma
Malignancy and metastasis
Metabolic syndrome
Methicillin-resistant Staphylococcus
   aureus (MRSA) infections
Mitral valve prolapse
Monkeypox
Mononucleosis
Motion sickness
Multiple sclerosis
Nephritis
Nephrology
Nephrology, pediatric
Niemann-Pick disease
Nonalcoholic steatohepatitis (NASH)
Nosebleeds
Nuclear medicine
Nutrition
Obesity
Obesity, childhood

Occupational health
Opportunistic infections
Osteopathic medicine
Paget's disease
Pain
Palliative medicine
Palpitations
Pancreas
Pancreatitis
Parasitic diseases
Parkinson's disease
Peristalsis
Peritonitis
Pharyngitis
Pharynx
Phlebitis
Physical examination
Physician assistants
Physiology
Plaque, arterial
Plasma
Pneumonia
Polyps
Proctology
Psoriasis
Puberty and adolescence
Pulmonary edema
Pulmonary medicine
Pulmonary medicine, pediatric
Pulse rate
Pyelonephritis
Radiopharmaceuticals
Rashes
Rectum
Renal failure
Reye's syndrome
Rheumatic fever
Rheumatoid arthritis
Roundworm
Rubella
Sarcoidosis
Scarlet fever
Schistosomiasis
Sciatica
Scurvy
Septicemia
Severe acute respiratory syndrome
   (SARS)
Sexuality
Sexually transmitted diseases
   (STDs)
Shingles
Shock
Sickle cell disease

Small intestine
Sneezing
Sports medicine
Staphylococcal infections
Stevens-Johnson syndrome
Stone removal
Stones
Streptococcal infections
Stress
Supplements
Systemic lupus erythematosus
   (SLE)
Tapeworm
Tetanus
Thrombosis and thrombus
Toxic shock syndrome
Tumor removal
Tumors
Ulcer surgery
Ulcers
Ultrasonography
Viral infections
Vitamins and minerals
Weight loss medications
Whooping cough
Wilson's disease
Worms
Wounds

MICROBIOLOGY
Abscesses
Amebiasis
Anthrax
Antibiotics
Antibodies
Aspergillosis
Autopsy
Bacillus Calmette-Guérin (BCG)
Bacterial infections
Bacteriology
Bionics and biotechnology
Campylobacter infections
Clostridium difficile infection
Coccidioidomycosis
Dengue fever
Drug resistance
E. coli infection
Enteroviruses
Epidemics and pandemics
Epidemiology
Fluoride treatments
Fungal infections
Gangrene
Gastroenteritis

Gastroenterology
Gastroenterology, pediatric
Gastrointestinal disorders
Gastrointestinal system
Genetic engineering
Genomics
Gram staining
Hematuria
Immune system
Immunization and vaccination
Immunology
Impetigo
Laboratory tests
Listeria infections
Methicillin-resistant *Staphylococcus
   aureus* (MRSA) infections
Microbiology
Microscopy
Opportunistic infections
Pathology
Pharmacology
Pharmacy
Plasma
Protozoan diseases
Pus
Serology
Severe acute respiratory syndrome
   (SARS)
Smallpox
Toxic shock syndrome
Toxicology
Tropical medicine
Tuberculosis
Urinalysis
Urology
Urology, pediatric
Viral infections

NEONATOLOGY
Apgar score
Birth defects
Blue baby syndrome
Bonding
Cardiology, pediatric
Cesarean section
Childbirth
Childbirth complications
Chlamydia
Cleft lip and palate
Cleft lip and palate repair
Congenital disorders
Congenital heart disease
Critical care, pediatric
Cystic fibrosis

Disseminated intravascular
  coagulation (DIC)
Down syndrome
E. coli infection
Endocrinology, pediatric
Failure to thrive
Fetal alcohol syndrome
Fetal surgery
Gastroenterology, pediatric
Genetic diseases
Genetics and inheritance
Hematology, pediatric
Hemolytic disease of the newborn
Hydrocephalus
Intraventricular hemorrhage
Jaundice
Jaundice, neonatal
Karyotyping
Malabsorption
Maple syrup urine disease (MSUD)
Motor skill development
Multiple births
Neonatology
Nephrology, pediatric
Neurology, pediatric
Nicotine
Nursing
Obstetrics
Orthopedics, pediatric
Pediatrics
Perinatology
Phenylketonuria (PKU)
Physician assistants
Premature birth
Pulmonary medicine, pediatric
Pulse rate
Respiratory distress syndrome
Rh factor
Shunts
Sudden infant death syndrome
  (SIDS)
Surgery, pediatric
Tay-Sachs disease
Toxoplasmosis
Transfusion
Trichomoniasis
Tropical medicine
Umbilical cord
Urology, pediatric
Well-baby examinations

NEPHROLOGY
Abdomen
Cysts

Diabetes mellitus
Dialysis
Diuretics
E. coli infection
Edema
End-stage renal disease
Hematuria
Hemolytic uremic syndrome
Internal medicine
Kidney cancer
Kidney disorders
Kidney transplantation
Kidneys
Lesions
Lithotripsy
Nephrectomy
Nephritis
Nephrology
Nephrology, pediatric
Palliative medicine
Polycystic kidney disease
Polyps
Preeclampsia and eclampsia
Proteinuria
Pyelonephritis
Renal failure
Sarcoidosis
Stenosis
Stone removal
Stones
Transplantation
Uremia
Urinalysis
Urinary disorders
Urinary system
Urology
Urology, pediatric
Vasculitis

NEUROLOGY
Adrenoleukodystrophy
Agnosia
Altitude sickness
Alzheimer's disease
Amnesia
Amyotrophic lateral sclerosis
Anesthesia
Anesthesiology
Aneurysmectomy
Aneurysms
Anosmia
Aphasia and dysphasia
Apnea
Ataxia

Atrophy
Attention-deficit disorder (ADD)
Audiology
Auras
Back pain
Balance disorders
Batten's disease
Bell's palsy
Biofeedback
Biophysics
Botox
Brain
Brain damage
Brain disorders
Brain tumors
Caffeine
Carotid arteries
Carpal tunnel syndrome
Cerebral palsy
Chiari malformations
Chiropractic
Chronic wasting disease (CWD)
Chronobiology
Claudication
Cluster headaches
Concussion
Cornelia de Lange syndrome
Craniotomy
Creutzfeldt-Jakob disease (CJD)
Critical care
Critical care, pediatric
Cysts
Deafness
Dementias
Developmental stages
Disk removal
Dizziness and fainting
Dyskinesia
Dyslexia
Ear infections and disorders
Ears
Electrical shock
Electroencephalography (EEG)
Electromyography
Emergency medicine
Emotions: Biomedical causes and
  effects
Encephalitis
Enteroviruses
Epilepsy
Fascia
Fetal tissue transplantation
Frontotemporal dementia (FTD)
Grafts and grafting

Guillain-Barré syndrome
Hallucinations
Head and neck disorders
Headaches
Hearing
Hearing aids
Hearing loss
Hearing tests
Hematomas
Hemiplegia
Hiccups
Huntington's disease
Hyperhidrosis
Hypothalamus
Hypoxia
Infarction
Intraventricular hemorrhage
Jaundice, neonatal
Learning disabilities
Lesions
Leukodystrophy
Lower extremities
Lumbar puncture
Marijuana
Melatonin
Memory loss
Ménière's disease
Meningitis
Mercury poisoning
Migraine headaches
Morgellons disease
Motor neuron diseases
Motor skill development
Multiple chemical sensitivity
    syndrome
Multiple sclerosis
Myasthenia gravis
Narcolepsy
Nervous system
Neuralgia, neuritis, and neuropathy
Neurofibromatosis
Neurology
Neurology, pediatric
Neurosurgery
Niemann-Pick disease
Numbness and tingling
Optometry, pediatric
Otorhinolaryngology
Pain
Palliative medicine
Palsy
Paralysis
Paraplegia
Parkinson's disease

Phenylketonuria (PKU)
Physical examination
Pick's disease
Poliomyelitis
Porphyria
Prader-Willi syndrome
Preeclampsia and eclampsia
Prion diseases
Psychiatry
Psychiatry, child and adolescent
Psychiatry, geriatric
Quadriplegia
Rabies
Radiculopathy
Restless legs syndrome
Reye's syndrome
Rubinstein-Taybi syndrome
Sarcoidosis
Sciatica
Seizures
Sense organs
Shock therapy
Skin
Sleep
Sleep disorders
Sleepwalking
Smell
Snakebites
Spina bifida
Spinal cord disorders
Spine, vertebrae, and disks
Stem cells
Stenosis
Strokes
Sturge-Weber syndrome
Stuttering
Subdural hematoma
Sympathectomy
Synesthesia
Taste
Tay-Sachs disease
Tetanus
Tics
Tinnitus
Torticollis
Touch
Tourette's syndrome
Transient ischemic attacks
    (TIAs)
Trembling and shaking
Unconsciousness
Upper extremities
Vagotomy
Vagus nerve

Vasculitis
Vertigo
Vision
Wilson's disease

NUCLEAR MEDICINE
Biophysics
Imaging and radiology
Invasive tests
Magnetic resonance imaging
    (MRI)
Noninvasive tests
Nuclear medicine
Nuclear radiology
Positron emission tomography
    (PET) scanning
Radiation therapy
Radiopharmaceuticals
Single photon emission computed
    tomography (SPECT)

NURSING
Acidosis
Aging: Extended care
Allied health
Anesthesiology
Atrophy
Bedsores
Cardiac rehabilitation
Carotid arteries
Casts and splints
Critical care
Critical care, pediatric
Defibrillation
Diuretics
Emergency medicine
Emergency medicine, pediatric
Epidemics and pandemics
Fiber
Geriatrics and gerontology
Holistic medicine
Home care
H1N1 influenza
Hospitals
Hypoxia
Immunization and vaccination
Infarction
Intravenous (IV) therapy
Neonatology
Noninvasive tests
Nursing
Nutrition
Palliative medicine
Pediatrics

Physical examination
Physician assistants
Polycystic ovary syndrome
Pulse rate
Radiculopathy
Surgery, general
Surgery, pediatric
Surgical procedures
Surgical technologists
Well-baby examinations

NUTRITION
Aging: Extended care
Anorexia nervosa
Antioxidants
Appetite loss
Bariatric surgery
Bedsores
Beriberi
Bile
Breast-feeding
Bulimia
Carbohydrates
Cardiac rehabilitation
Cholesterol
Colon
Dietary reference intakes (DRIs)
Digestion
Eating disorders
Exercise physiology
Fatty acid oxidation disorders
Fiber
Food allergies
Food biochemistry
Food Guide Pyramid
Fructosemia
Galactosemia
Gastroenterology
Gastroenterology, pediatric
Gastrointestinal disorders
Gastrointestinal system
Geriatrics and gerontology
Gestational diabetes
Gluten intolerance
Glycogen storage diseases
Hyperadiposis
Hypercholesterolemia
Irritable bowel syndrome (IBS)
Jaw wiring
Kwashiorkor
Lactose intolerance
Leptin
Leukodystrophy
Lipids

Macronutrients
Malabsorption
Malnutrition
Metabolic disorders
Metabolic syndrome
Metabolism
Nursing
Nutrition
Obesity
Obesity, childhood
Osteoporosis
Phytochemicals
Pituitary gland
Plasma
Polycystic ovary syndrome
Protein
Scurvy
Small intestine
Sports medicine
Supplements
Taste
Tropical medicine
Ulcers
Vagotomy
Vitamins and minerals
Weaning
Weight loss and gain
Weight loss medications

OBSTETRICS
Amniocentesis
Apgar score
Assisted reproductive technologies
Birth defects
Breast-feeding
Breasts, female
Cervical, ovarian, and uterine
  cancers
Cesarean section
Childbirth
Childbirth complications
Chorionic villus sampling
Conception
Congenital disorders
Cytomegalovirus (CMV)
Disseminated intravascular
  coagulation (DIC)
Down syndrome
Ectopic pregnancy
Embryology
Emergency medicine
Episiotomy
Family medicine
Fetal alcohol syndrome

Fetal surgery
Gamete intrafallopian transfer
  (GIFT)
Genetic counseling
Genetic diseases
Genetics and inheritance
Genital disorders, female
Gestational diabetes
Gonorrhea
Growth
Gynecology
Hemolytic disease of the newborn
In vitro fertilization
Incontinence
Intravenous (IV) therapy
Invasive tests
Karyotyping
Listeria infections
Miscarriage
Multiple births
Neonatology
Nicotine
Noninvasive tests
Obstetrics
Ovaries
Perinatology
Pituitary gland
Placenta
Polycystic ovary syndrome
Postpartum depression
Preeclampsia and eclampsia
Pregnancy and gestation
Premature birth
Pyelonephritis
Reproductive system
Rh factor
Rubella
Sexuality
Sperm banks
Spina bifida
Stillbirth
Teratogens
Toxemia
Toxoplasmosis
Trichomoniasis
Ultrasonography
Urology
Uterus

OCCUPATIONAL HEALTH
Acidosis
Agnosia
Altitude sickness
Asbestos exposure

Asphyxiation
Bacillus Calmette-Guérin (BCG)
Back pain
Biofeedback
Blurred vision
Carcinogens
Cardiac rehabilitation
Carpal tunnel syndrome
Defibrillation
Environmental diseases
Environmental health
Gulf War syndrome
Hearing aids
Hearing loss
Home care
Interstitial pulmonary fibrosis
    (IPF)
Lead poisoning
Leukodystrophy
Lung cancer
Lungs
Mercury poisoning
Mesothelioma
Multiple chemical sensitivity
    syndrome
Nasopharyngeal disorders
Occupational health
Pneumonia
Prostheses
Pulmonary diseases
Pulmonary medicine
Pulmonary medicine, pediatric
Radiation sickness
Skin cancer
Skin disorders
Stress
Stress reduction
Tendinitis
Tendon disorders
Tendon repair
Toxicology

ONCOLOGY
Aging
Aging: Extended care
Amputation
Anal cancer
Antibodies
Antioxidants
Anus
Asbestos exposure
Biological therapies
Biopsy
Bladder cancer

Bladder removal
Blood testing
Bone cancer
Bone disorders
Bone grafting
Bone marrow transplantation
Bones and the skeleton
Brain tumors
Breast biopsy
Breast cancer
Breasts, female
Burkitt's lymphoma
Cancer
Carcinogens
Carcinoma
Cells
Cervical, ovarian, and uterine
    cancers
Chemotherapy
Colon
Colorectal cancer
Colorectal polyp removal
Cryotherapy and cryosurgery
Cytology
Cytopathology
Dermatology
Dermatopathology
Disseminated intravascular
    coagulation (DIC)
Embolization
Endometrial biopsy
Epstein-Barr virus
Ewing's sarcoma
Fibrocystic breast condition
Gallbladder cancer
Gastrectomy
Gastroenterology
Gastrointestinal disorders
Gastrointestinal system
Gastrostomy
Gene therapy
Genital disorders, female
Genital disorders, male
Gynecology
Hematology
Histology
Hodgkin's disease
Human papillomavirus (HPV)
Hysterectomy
Imaging and radiology
Immunology
Immunopathology
Intravenous (IV) therapy
Kaposi's sarcoma

Karyotyping
Kidney cancer
Laboratory tests
Laryngectomy
Laser use in surgery
Lesions
Liver cancer
Lung cancer
Lung surgery
Lungs
Lymph
Lymphadenopathy and lymphoma
Malignancy and metastasis
Mammography
Massage
Mastectomy and lumpectomy
Melanoma
Mesothelioma
Mouth and throat cancer
Necrosis
Nephrectomy
Nicotine
Oncology
Oral and maxillofacial surgery
Pain management
Palliative medicine
Pap test
Pathology
Pharmacology
Pharmacy
Plastic surgery
Proctology
Prostate cancer
Prostate gland
Prostate gland removal
Prostheses
Pulmonary diseases
Pulmonary medicine
Radiation sickness
Radiation therapy
Radiopharmaceuticals
Rectum
Retroviruses
Sarcoma
Serology
Skin
Skin cancer
Skin lesion removal
Small intestine
Smoking
Stem cells
Stenosis
Stomach, intestinal, and pancreatic
    cancers

Cytology
Cytopathology
Dermatopathology
Disease
Electroencephalography (EEG)
Embolization
Emerging infectious diseases
Epidemics and pandemics
Epidemiology
Forensic pathology
Frontotemporal dementia (FTD)
Hematology
Hematology, pediatric
Histology
Homeopathy
Immunopathology
Inflammation
Karyotyping
Laboratory tests
Ligaments
Malignancy and metastasis
Mesothelioma
Microbiology
Microscopy
Motor skill development
Mutation
Nicotine
Niemann-Pick disease
Noninvasive tests
Oncology
Pathology
Polycystic ovary syndrome
Prion diseases
Radiculopathy
Retroviruses
Rhinoviruses
Serology
Toxicology

PEDIATRICS
Acne
Adrenoleukodystrophy
Amenorrhea
Appendectomy
Appendicitis
Attention-deficit disorder (ADD)
Batten's disease
Bed-wetting
Birth defects
Birthmarks
Blurred vision
Bronchiolitis
Bulimia
Burkitt's lymphoma

Cardiology, pediatric
Casts and splints
Chickenpox
Childhood infectious diseases
Cholera
Circumcision, female, and genital
  mutilation
Circumcision, male
Cleft lip and palate
Cleft lip and palate repair
Cognitive development
Colic
Congenital disorders
Congenital heart disease
Cornelia de Lange syndrome
Critical care, pediatric
Croup
Cystic fibrosis
Cytomegalovirus (CMV)
Dentistry, pediatric
Dermatology, pediatric
Diabetes mellitus
Diaper rash
Diarrhea and dysentery
DiGeorge syndrome
Domestic violence
Down syndrome
Dwarfism
Ehrlichiosis
Emergency medicine, pediatric
Endocrinology, pediatric
Enterocolitis
Epiglottitis
Ewing's sarcoma
Failure to thrive
Family medicine
Fatty acid oxidation disorders
Fetal surgery
Fever
Fifth disease
Fistula repair
Food Guide Pyramid
Fructosemia
Gastroenterology, pediatric
Gaucher's disease
Gender identity disorder
Genetic diseases
Genetics and inheritance
Giardiasis
Gigantism
Glycogen storage diseases
Growth
Gynecomastia
Hand-foot-and-mouth disease

Hematology, pediatric
Hemolytic uremic syndrome
Hirschsprung's disease
Hives
H1N1 influenza
Hormones
Hydrocephalus
Hypospadias repair and
  urethroplasty
Intravenous (IV) therapy
Juvenile rheumatoid arthritis
Kawasaki disease
Klippel-Trenaunay syndrome
Kluver-Bucy syndrome
Kwashiorkor
Learning disabilities
Leukodystrophy
Listeria infections
Malabsorption
Malnutrition
Maple syrup urine disease
  (MSUD)
Massage
Measles
Menstruation
Metabolic disorders
Motor skill development
Mucopolysaccharidosis (MPS)
Multiple births
Multiple sclerosis
Mumps
Münchausen syndrome by proxy
Muscular dystrophy
Neonatology
Nephrology, pediatric
Neurology, pediatric
Niemann-Pick disease
Nightmares
Nosebleeds
Nursing
Nutrition
Obesity, childhood
Optometry, pediatric
Orthopedics, pediatric
Osgood-Schlatter disease
Osteogenesis imperfecta
Otoplasty
Otorhinolaryngology
Pediatrics
Perinatology
Phenylketonuria (PKU)
Pigeon toes
Pinworm
Pituitary gland

Poliomyelitis
Polydactyly and syndactyly
Porphyria
Prader-Willi syndrome
Precocious puberty
Premature birth
Progeria
Psychiatry, child and adolescent
Puberty and adolescence
Pulmonary medicine, pediatric
Pulse rate
Pyloric stenosis
Rashes
Reflexes, primitive
Respiratory distress syndrome
Reye's syndrome
Rheumatic fever
Rhinitis
Rickets
Roseola
Rotavirus
Roundworm
Rubella
Rubinstein-Taybi syndrome
Safety issues for children
Scarlet fever
Seizures
Severe combined immunodeficiency
  syndrome (SCID)
Sexuality
Sibling rivalry
Soiling
Sore throat
Steroids
Stevens-Johnson syndrome
Strep throat
Streptococcal infections
Sturge-Weber syndrome
Styes
Sudden infant death syndrome
  (SIDS)
Surgery, pediatric
Tapeworm
Tay-Sachs disease
Teething
Testicles, undescended
Testicular torsion
Thumb sucking
Toilet training
Tonsillectomy and adenoid removal
Tonsillitis
Tonsils
Trachoma
Tropical medicine

Urology, pediatric
Weaning
Well-baby examinations
Whooping cough
Wiskott-Aldrich syndrome
Worms

PERINATOLOGY
Amniocentesis
Assisted reproductive technologies
Birth defects
Breast-feeding
Cesarean section
Childbirth
Childbirth complications
Chorionic villus sampling
Congenital hypothyroidism
Critical care, pediatric
Embryology
Fatty acid oxidation disorders
Fetal alcohol syndrome
Glycogen storage diseases
Hematology, pediatric
Hydrocephalus
Karyotyping
Metabolic disorders
Motor skill development
Neonatology
Neurology, pediatric
Nursing
Obstetrics
Pediatrics
Perinatology
Pregnancy and gestation
Premature birth
Reflexes, primitive
Shunts
Stillbirth
Sudden infant death syndrome
  (SIDS)
Trichomoniasis
Umbilical cord
Uterus
Well-baby examinations

PHARMACOLOGY
Acid-base chemistry
Acidosis
Aging: Extended care
Anesthesia
Anesthesiology
Antianxiety drugs
Antibiotics
Antibodies

Antidepressants
Antihistamines
Anti-inflammatory drugs
Bacteriology
Blurred vision
Chemotherapy
Club drugs
Corticosteroids
Critical care
Critical care, pediatric
Decongestants
Digestion
Diuretics
Drug resistance
Dyskinesia
Emergency medicine
Emergency medicine, pediatric
Enzymes
Epidemics and pandemics
Ergogenic aids
Fluids and electrolytes
Food biochemistry
Genetic engineering
Genomics
Geriatrics and gerontology
Glycolysis
Herbal medicine
Homeopathy
Hormones
Laboratory tests
Marijuana
Melatonin
Mesothelioma
Metabolism
Narcotics
Nicotine
Oncology
Over-the-counter medications
Pain management
Pharmacology
Pharmacy
Poisoning
Polycystic ovary syndrome
Prader-Willi syndrome
Prescription drug abuse
Psychiatry
Psychiatry, child and adolescent
Psychiatry, geriatric
Rheumatology
Self-medication
Side effects
Sports medicine
Steroid abuse
Steroids

Substance abuse
Thrombolytic therapy and TPA
Toxicology
Tropical medicine

PHYSICAL THERAPY
Aging: Extended care
Amputation
Amyotrophic lateral sclerosis
Arthritis
Atrophy
Back pain
Bell's palsy
Biofeedback
Bowlegs
Burns and scalds
Cardiac rehabilitation
Casts and splints
Cerebral palsy
Cornelia de Lange syndrome
Disk removal
Dyskinesia
Electromyography
Exercise physiology
Fascia
Grafts and grafting
Hemiplegia
Hip fracture repair
Hip replacement
Home care
Hydrotherapy
Kinesiology
Knock-knees
Leukodystrophy
Ligaments
Lower extremities
Massage
Motor skill development
Muscle sprains, spasms, and
    disorders
Muscles
Muscular dystrophy
Neurology
Neurology, pediatric
Numbness and tingling
Orthopedic surgery
Orthopedics
Orthopedics, pediatric
Osteopathic medicine
Osteoporosis
Pain management
Palsy
Paralysis
Paraplegia

Parkinson's disease
Physical examination
Physical rehabilitation
Plastic surgery
Prostheses
Pulse rate
Quadriplegia
Radiculopathy
Rickets
Scoliosis
Slipped disk
Spina bifida
Spinal cord disorders
Spine, vertebrae, and disks
Sports medicine
Tendinitis
Tendon disorders
Torticollis
Upper extremities
Whiplash

PLASTIC SURGERY
Aging
Amputation
Bariatric surgery
Birthmarks
Body dysmorphic disorder
Botox
Breast cancer
Breast disorders
Breast surgery
Breasts, female
Burns and scalds
Cancer
Carcinoma
Circumcision, female, and genital
    mutilation
Circumcision, male
Cleft lip and palate
Cleft lip and palate repair
Craniosynostosis
Cyst removal
Cysts
Dermatology
Dermatology, pediatric
DiGeorge syndrome
Face lift and blepharoplasty
Facial transplantation
Gender reassignment surgery
Grafts and grafting
Hair loss and baldness
Hair transplantation
Healing
Jaw wiring

Laceration repair
Liposuction
Malignancy and metastasis
Moles
Necrotizing fasciitis
Neurofibromatosis
Obesity
Obesity, childhood
Oral and maxillofacial surgery
Otoplasty
Otorhinolaryngology
Plastic surgery
Prostheses
Ptosis
Rhinoplasty and submucous
    resection
Skin
Skin lesion removal
Sturge-Weber syndrome
Surgical procedures
Tattoo removal
Tattoos and body piercing
Varicose vein removal
Varicose veins
Vision
Wrinkles

PODIATRY
Athlete's foot
Bone disorders
Bones and the skeleton
Bunions
Cartilage
Corns and calluses
Feet
Flat feet
Foot disorders
Fungal infections
Hammertoe correction
Hammertoes
Heel spur removal
Joints
Lesions
Lower extremities
Nail removal
Orthopedic surgery
Orthopedics
Physical examination
Pigeon toes
Podiatry
Polydactyly and syndactyly
Tendon disorders
Tendon repair
Warts

PREVENTIVE MEDICINE
Acidosis
Acupressure
Acupuncture
Aging: Extended care
Alternative medicine
Antibodies
Aromatherapy
Assisted living facilities
Bacillus Calmette-Guérin (BCG)
Biofeedback
Braces, orthopedic
Caffeine
Cardiac surgery
Cardiology
Chiropractic
Cholesterol
Chronobiology
Disease
Echocardiography
Electrocardiography (ECG or EKG)
Environmental health
Exercise physiology
Family medicine
Fiber
Genetic counseling
Geriatrics and gerontology
Holistic medicine
Host-defense mechanisms
Hypercholesterolemia
Immune system
Immunization and vaccination
Immunology
Mammography
Massage
Meditation
Melatonin
Mesothelioma
Noninvasive tests
Nursing
Nutrition
Occupational health
Osteopathic medicine
Over-the-counter medications
Pharmacology
Pharmacy
Physical examination
Phytochemicals
Polycystic ovary syndrome
Preventive medicine
Psychiatry
Psychiatry, child and adolescent
Psychiatry, geriatric
Rhinoviruses

Screening
Serology
Spine, vertebrae, and disks
Sports medicine
Stress
Stress reduction
Tendinitis
Tropical medicine
Yoga

PROCTOLOGY
Anal cancer
Anus
Bladder removal
Colon
Colonoscopy and sigmoidoscopy
Colorectal cancer
Colorectal polyp removal
Colorectal surgery
Crohn's disease
Diverticulitis and diverticulosis
Endoscopy
Fistula repair
Gastroenterology
Gastrointestinal disorders
Gastrointestinal system
Genital disorders, male
Geriatrics and gerontology
Hemorrhoid banding and removal
Hemorrhoids
Hirschsprung's disease
Internal medicine
Intestinal disorders
Intestines
Irritable bowel syndrome (IBS)
Palliative medicine
Physical examination
Proctology
Prostate cancer
Prostate gland
Prostate gland removal
Rectum
Reproductive system
Urology
Polyps

PSYCHIATRY
Addiction
Adrenoleukodystrophy
Aging
Aging: Extended care
Alcoholism
Alzheimer's disease
Amnesia

Amyotrophic lateral sclerosis
Anorexia nervosa
Antianxiety drugs
Antidepressants
Anxiety
Appetite loss
Asperger's syndrome
Attention-deficit disorder (ADD)
Auras
Autism
Bariatric surgery
Bipolar disorders
Body dysmorphic disorder
Bonding
Brain
Brain damage
Brain disorders
Breast surgery
Bulimia
Chronic fatigue syndrome
Circumcision, female, and genital
  mutilation
Club drugs
Corticosteroids
Delusions
Dementias
Depression
Developmental disorders
Developmental stages
Domestic violence
Dyskinesia
Eating disorders
Electroencephalography (EEG)
Emergency medicine
Emotions: Biomedical causes
  and effects
Factitious disorders
Failure to thrive
Family medicine
Fatigue
Frontotemporal dementia
  (FTD)
Gender identity disorder
Gender reassignment surgery
Grief and guilt
Gynecology
Hallucinations
Huntington's disease
Hypnosis
Hypochondriasis
Hypothalamus
Incontinence
Intoxication
Kluver-Bucy syndrome

Light therapy
Marijuana
Masturbation
Memory loss
Mental retardation
Midlife crisis
Morgellons disease
Münchausen syndrome by proxy
Neurosis
Neurosurgery
Nicotine
Nightmares
Obesity
Obesity, childhood
Obsessive-compulsive disorder
Pain
Pain management
Palliative medicine
Panic attacks
Paranoia
Penile implant surgery
Phobias
Pick's disease
Postpartum depression
Post-traumatic stress disorder
Prader-Willi syndrome
Prescription drug abuse
Psychiatric disorders
Psychiatry
Psychiatry, child and adolescent
Psychiatry, geriatric
Psychoanalysis
Psychosis
Psychosomatic disorders
Rape and sexual assault
Restless legs syndrome
Schizophrenia
Seasonal affective disorder
Separation anxiety
Sexual dysfunction
Sexuality
Shock therapy
Single photon emission computed
    tomography (SPECT)
Sleep
Sleep disorders
Speech disorders
Steroid abuse
Stress
Stress reduction
Substance abuse
Sudden infant death syndrome
    (SIDS)
Suicide

Synesthesia
Tinnitus
Toilet training
Tourette's syndrome

PSYCHOLOGY
Addiction
Aging
Aging: Extended care
Alcoholism
Amnesia
Amyotrophic lateral sclerosis
Anorexia nervosa
Anxiety
Appetite loss
Aromatherapy
Asperger's syndrome
Attention-deficit disorder (ADD)
Auras
Bariatric surgery
Bed-wetting
Biofeedback
Bipolar disorders
Bonding
Brain
Brain damage
Brain disorders
Bulimia
Cardiac rehabilitation
Cirrhosis
Club drugs
Cognitive development
Death and dying
Delusions
Depression
Developmental disorders
Developmental stages
Domestic violence
Dyslexia
Eating disorders
Electroencephalography (EEG)
Emotions: Biomedical causes
    and effects
Environmental health
Factitious disorders
Failure to thrive
Family medicine
Forensic pathology
Gender identity disorder
Gender reassignment surgery
Genetic counseling
Grief and guilt
Gulf War syndrome
Gynecology

Hallucinations
Holistic medicine
Hormone therapy
Huntington's disease
Hypnosis
Hypochondriasis
Hypothalamus
Juvenile rheumatoid arthritis
Kinesiology
Klinefelter syndrome
Kluver-Bucy syndrome
Learning disabilities
Light therapy
Marijuana
Meditation
Memory loss
Mental retardation
Midlife crisis
Motor skill development
Münchausen syndrome by proxy
Neurosis
Nightmares
Nutrition
Obesity
Obesity, childhood
Obsessive-compulsive disorder
Occupational health
Overtraining syndrome
Pain management
Palliative medicine
Panic attacks
Paranoia
Phobias
Pick's disease
Plastic surgery
Polycystic ovary syndrome
Postpartum depression
Post-traumatic stress disorder
Prescription drug abuse
Psychosomatic disorders
Puberty and adolescence
Restless legs syndrome
Separation anxiety
Sexual dysfunction
Sexuality
Sibling rivalry
Sleep
Sleep disorders
Sleepwalking
Speech disorders
Sports medicine
Steroid abuse
Stillbirth
Stress

Stress reduction
Sturge-Weber syndrome
Stuttering
Substance abuse
Sudden infant death syndrome (SIDS)
Suicide
Synesthesia
Temporomandibular joint (TMJ) syndrome
Tics
Toilet training
Tourette's syndrome
Weight loss and gain
Yoga

PUBLIC HEALTH
Acquired immunodeficiency syndrome (AIDS)
Acute respiratory distress syndrome (ARDS)
Adenoviruses
Aging: Extended care
Allied health
Alternative medicine
Amebiasis
Anthrax
Antibodies
Asbestos exposure
Assisted living facilities
Babesiosis
Bacillus Calmette-Guérin (BCG)
Bacteriology
Beriberi
Biological and chemical weapons
Biostatistics
Blood banks
Blood testing
Botulism
Carcinogens
Chagas' disease
Chickenpox
Childhood infectious diseases
Chlamydia
Cholera
Chronic obstructive pulmonary disease (COPD)
Clinics
Club drugs
Common cold
Coronaviruses
Corticosteroids
Creutzfeldt-Jakob disease (CJD)
Dengue fever

Department of Health and Human Services
Dermatology
Diarrhea and dysentery
Diphtheria
Domestic violence
Drug resistance
E. coli infection
Ebola virus
Elephantiasis
Emergency medicine
Environmental diseases
Epidemics and pandemics
Epidemiology
Fetal alcohol syndrome
Food poisoning
Forensic pathology
Gonorrhea
Gulf War syndrome
Hantavirus
Health Canada
Health care reform
Hepatitis
H1N1 influenza
Hospitals
Human immunodeficiency virus (HIV)
Immunization and vaccination
Influenza
Insect-borne diseases
Kwashiorkor
Lead poisoning
Legionnaires' disease
Leishmaniasis
Leprosy
Lice, mites, and ticks
Lyme disease
Macronutrients
Malaria
Malnutrition
Managed care
Marburg virus
Marijuana
Measles
Medicare
Meningitis
Methicillin-resistant *Staphylococcus aureus* (MRSA) infections
Microbiology
Monkeypox
Multiple chemical sensitivity syndrome
Mumps
Necrotizing fasciitis

Nicotine
Niemann-Pick disease
Nursing
Nutrition
Occupational health
Osteopathic medicine
Parasitic diseases
Pharmacology
Pharmacy
Physical examination
Physician assistants
Pinworm
Plague
Pneumonia
Poliomyelitis
Polycystic ovary syndrome
Prion diseases
Protozoan diseases
Psychiatry
Psychiatry, child and adolescent
Psychiatry, geriatric
Rabies
Radiation sickness
Rape and sexual assault
Retroviruses
Rhinoviruses
Roundworm
Rubella
Salmonella infection
Schistosomiasis
Screening
Serology
Severe acute respiratory syndrome (SARS)
Sexually transmitted diseases (STDs)
Shigellosis
Sleeping sickness
Smallpox
Syphilis
Tapeworm
Tattoos and body piercing
Tetanus
Toxicology
Toxoplasmosis
Trichinosis
Trichomoniasis
Tropical medicine
Tuberculosis
Tularemia
Typhoid fever
Typhus
Whooping cough
World Health Organization

Geriatrics and gerontology
Gout
Hip replacement
Hydrotherapy
Inflammation
Joints
Ligaments
Lyme disease
Orthopedic surgery
Orthopedics
Orthopedics, pediatric
Osteoarthritis
Osteonecrosis
Palliative medicine
Physical examination
Radiculopathy
Rheumatic fever
Rheumatoid arthritis
Rheumatology
Rotator cuff surgery
Sarcoidosis
Scleroderma
Sjögren's syndrome
Spondylitis
Sports medicine
Vasculitis

SEROLOGY
Anemia
Babesiosis
Blood and blood disorders
Blood testing
Cholesterol
Cytology
Cytopathology
Dialysis
Epidemics and pandemics
Fluids and electrolytes
Forensic pathology
Hematology
Hematology, pediatric
Hemophilia
Hodgkin's disease
Host-defense mechanisms
Hyperbaric oxygen therapy
Hypercholesterolemia
Hyperlipidemia
Hypoglycemia
Immune system
Immunology
Immunopathology
Jaundice
Laboratory tests
Leukemia

Lymph
Malaria
Pathology
Plasma
Rh factor
Rhinoviruses
Sarcoidosis
Septicemia
Serology
Sickle cell disease
Thalassemia
Transfusion

SPEECH PATHOLOGY
Adenoids
Agnosia
Alzheimer's disease
Amyotrophic lateral sclerosis
Aphasia and dysphasia
Audiology
Autism
Cerebral palsy
Cleft lip and palate
Cleft lip and palate repair
Deafness
Dyslexia
Ear infections and disorders
Ear surgery
Ears
Electroencephalography (EEG)
Hearing loss
Hearing tests
Home care
Jaw wiring
Laryngitis
Learning disabilities
Lisping
Paralysis
Pharynx
Rubinstein-Taybi syndrome
Speech disorders
Strokes
Stuttering
Subdural hematoma
Thumb sucking
Voice and vocal cord disorders

SPORTS MEDICINE
Acidosis
Acupressure
Anorexia nervosa
Arthroplasty
Arthroscopy
Athlete's foot

Atrophy
Biofeedback
Blurred vision
Bones and the skeleton
Braces, orthopedic
Cardiology
Cartilage
Casts and splints
Critical care
Defibrillation
Dehydration
Eating disorders
Emergency medicine
Ergogenic aids
Exercise physiology
Fiber
Fracture and dislocation
Fracture repair
Glycolysis
Head and neck disorders
Heat exhaustion and heatstroke
Hematomas
Hydrotherapy
Joints
Kinesiology
Ligaments
Macronutrients
Massage
Motor skill development
Muscle sprains, spasms, and
    disorders
Muscles
Nutrition
Orthopedic surgery
Orthopedics
Orthopedics, pediatric
Overtraining syndrome
Oxygen therapy
Physical examination
Physical rehabilitation
Physiology
Psychiatry
Psychiatry, child and adolescent
Pulse rate
Radiculopathy
Rotator cuff surgery
Safety issues for children
Spine, vertebrae, and disks
Sports medicine
Steroid abuse
Steroids
Tendinitis
Tendon disorders
Tendon repair

TOXICOLOGY
Acidosis
Biological and chemical weapons
Bites and stings
Blood testing
Botulism
Club drugs
Critical care
Critical care, pediatric
Cyanosis
Defibrillation
Dermatitis
Eczema
Emergency medicine
Environmental diseases
Environmental health
Food poisoning
Forensic pathology
Gaucher's disease
Hepatitis
Herbal medicine
Homeopathy
Intoxication
Itching
Laboratory tests
Lead poisoning
Liver
Mold and mildew
Multiple chemical sensitivity
  syndrome
Nicotine
Occupational health
Pathology
Pharmacology
Pharmacy
Poisoning
Poisonous plants
Rashes
Sarcoidosis
Side effects
Snakebites
Toxicology
Toxoplasmosis
Urinalysis

UROLOGY
Abdomen
Abdominal disorders
Adenoviruses
Bed-wetting
Bladder cancer
Bladder removal
Catheterization
Chlamydia

Circumcision, male
Congenital adrenal hyperplasia
Cystitis
Cystoscopy
Dialysis
Diuretics
E. coli infection
Endoscopy
Erectile dysfunction
Fetal surgery
Fluids and electrolytes
Gender reassignment surgery
Genital disorders, female
Genital disorders, male
Geriatrics and gerontology
Gonorrhea
Hemolytic uremic syndrome
Hermaphroditism and
  pseudohermaphroditism
Hydroceles
Hyperplasia
Hypospadias repair and
  urethroplasty
Incontinence
Infertility, male
Kidney cancer
Kidney disorders
Kidney transplantation
Kidneys
Lesions
Lithotripsy
Nephrectomy
Nephritis
Nephrology
Nephrology, pediatric
Orchiectomy
Palliative medicine
Pediatrics
Pelvic inflammatory disease (PID)
Penile implant surgery
Polycystic kidney disease
Polyps
Prostate cancer
Prostate enlargement
Prostate gland
Prostate gland removal
Proteinuria
Pyelonephritis
Reiter's syndrome
Reproductive system
Schistosomiasis
Semen
Sexual differentiation
Sexual dysfunction

Sexually transmitted diseases
  (STDs)
Sterilization
Stevens-Johnson syndrome
Stone removal
Stones
Syphilis
Testicles, undescended
Testicular cancer
Testicular surgery
Testicular torsion
Toilet training
Transplantation
Trichomoniasis
Ultrasonography
Uremia
Urethritis
Urinalysis
Urinary disorders
Urinary system
Urology
Urology, pediatric
Vas deferens
Vasectomy

VASCULAR MEDICINE
Acidosis
Amputation
Aneurysmectomy
Aneurysms
Angiography
Angioplasty
Anti-inflammatory drugs
Arteriosclerosis
Biofeedback
Bleeding
Blood and blood disorders
Blood pressure
Blood vessels
Bruises
Bypass surgery
Cardiac surgery
Carotid arteries
Catheterization
Cholesterol
Circulation
Claudication
Defibrillation
Dehydration
Diabetes mellitus
Dialysis
Embolism
Embolization
End-stage renal disease

Endarterectomy
Exercise physiology
Glands
Healing
Hematology
Hematology, pediatric
Hemorrhoid banding and removal
Hemorrhoids
Histology
Hypercholesterolemia
Hyperlipidemia
Infarction
Ischemia
Klippel-Trenaunay syndrome
Lesions
Lipids
Lymphatic system
Mitral valve prolapse
Necrotizing fasciitis
Nicotine
Osteochondritis juvenilis
Phlebitis
Plaque, arterial
Plasma
Podiatry
Preeclampsia and eclampsia
Progeria
Pulse rate
Shunts
Smoking
Stents
Strokes
Sturge-Weber syndrome
Thrombolytic therapy and TPA
Thrombosis and thrombus
Toxemia
Transfusion
Transient ischemic attacks (TIAs)

Varicose vein removal
Varicose veins
Vascular medicine
Vascular system
Venous insufficiency
Von Willebrand's disease

VIROLOGY
Acquired immunodeficiency
    syndrome (AIDS)
Biological and chemical weapons
Chickenpox
Childhood infectious diseases
Chlamydia
Chronic fatigue syndrome
Common cold
Coronaviruses
Creutzfeldt-Jakob disease (CJD)
Croup
Cytomegalovirus (CMV)
Dengue fever
Drug resistance
Ebola virus
Encephalitis
Enteroviruses
Epidemics and pandemics
Epstein-Barr virus
Fever
Gastroenteritis
Hantavirus
Hepatitis
Herpes
H1N1 influenza
Human immunodeficiency virus
    (HIV)
Human papillomavirus (HPV)
Infection
Influenza

Laboratory tests
Marburg virus
Measles
Microbiology
Microscopy
Monkeypox
Mononucleosis
Mumps
Noroviruses
Opportunistic infections
Parasitic diseases
Pelvic inflammatory disease (PID)
Poliomyelitis
Pulmonary diseases
Rabies
Retroviruses
Rheumatic fever
Rhinitis
Rhinoviruses
Roseola
Rotavirus
Rubella
Sarcoidosis
Serology
Severe acute respiratory syndrome
    (SARS)
Sexually transmitted diseases
    (STDs)
Shingles
Smallpox
Tonsillitis
Tropical medicine
Viral hemorrhagic fevers
Viral infections
Warts
Yellow fever
Zoonoses

PERSONAGES INDEX

INDEX

A page number or range in boldface type indicates that an entire entry devoted to that topic appears in the Guide.

Artificial limbs. *See* Prostheses

Artificial nutrition and hydration, 3203

Artificial respiration, 496

Artificial respirator, 2519

Artificial skin, 456

Artificial teeth. *See* Dentures

Asanas, 3191

Asbestos, 3203

Asbestos exposure, **217-219**, 1024, 1936-1937

Asbestosis, 217

Ascaris lumbricoides, 2617

Ascites, 610, 935, 1212, 1804, 1807, 2074, 2322, 3061

Ascites praecox, 3272

Ascorbic acid, 2659

Aseptic fever, 3272

Aseptic techniques, 2879, 3203

Asherman's syndrome, 113, 3272

Ashkenazi Jews, 1223, 2916

Asian American health, **219-222**

Asparaginase, 1029

Asperger, Hans, 260, 809

Asperger's syndrome, **222-224**, 260, 808-809, 2892, 3203

Aspergillosis, **224-226**, 1187, 1971, 3272

Asphyxia neonatorum, 3272

Asphyxiants, 19

Asphyxiation, **226**, 884, 1420, 2945, 3203, 3272; fetal, 2831

Aspiration, 46, 328, 423, 744, 747, 884, 1199, 1680-1681, 2471, 3041, 3203

Aspiration pneumonia, 3272

Aspirin, 181, 543, 1610, 2233, 2401, 2589, 2726, 2856, 2954-2955, 3053, 3056

Asplenia, 3272

Assessment, 823, 3203

Assisted living facilities, **227-231**

Assisted reproductive technologies, **231-235**, 1197, 1616, 1968, 3203; ethics and, 1060

Association of American Medical Colleges (AAMC), 1894

Astereognosis, 3272

Asthenia, 3272

Asthenopia, 3272

Asthma, 90, 224, **235-242**, 446, 595, 793, 1556, 1661, 1828, 1918, 1921, 2237, 2517-2518, 2525-2526, 2528, 2575, 3162, 3204,

3272; African Americans and, 67; first aid, 1133; mold and, 1971

Asthmatic eosinophilia, 3272

Astigmatism, **242-243**, 510, 1075, 1077, 1086, 2564, 2671, 3131, 3133, 3204, 3272

Astroblastoma, 3272

Astrocytes, 414

Astrocytoma, 3272

Astrocytosis, 3272

Asymptomatic, 3204

Ataxia, **243-244**, 3204, 3272

Ataxia-telangiectasia, 3272

Ataxic dysarthria, 3272

Ateliosis, 3272

Atelorachidia, 3272

Atherectomy, 1397, 2818

Atherosclerosis, 3204. *See also* Arteriosclerosis

Athetosis, 3272

Athletes, 1053, 2236, 2823

Athlete's foot, **245**, 1110, 1185, 1954, 2035, 3204, 3272

Athlete's heart, 3272

Athletic injuries. *See* Sports injuries

Atom, 3204

Atopic dermatitis, 793-796, 931, 2375

ATP. *See* Adenosine triphosphate (ATP)

Atresia, 3272

Atria, 1390

Atrial fibrillation, 203, **245-246**, 485, 488, 769, 945, 1393, 1401, 2955, 3204, 3272

Atrial septic defect, 3272

Atrial standstill, 3272

Atrial tachycardia, 3272

Atrioventricular (A-V) node, 488, 1391, 2013, 2238, 3204

Atrioventricular defects, 683

Atrioventricular dissociation, 3272

Atrium, 3204

Atrophic rhinitis, 2604

Atrophoderma, 3272

Atrophy, **246-248**, 1551, 1818, 1980, 2013, 2259, 3070, 3204, 3272; vaginal, 1911

Atropine, 1454

Attention-deficit disorder (ADD), **248-251**, 2491, 2974, 3273

Attention-deficit hyperactivity disorder. *See* Attention-deficit disorder (ADD)

Attenuation, 3204

Audiology, 160, **251-256**, 3204

Audiometer, 3204

Auditory brainstem potential (ABR) test, 1387

Auditory dyslexia, 899

Auditory nerve, 3204

Auditory system, 3204

Aural rehabilitation, 255, 3204

Auras, **256-257**, 1360, 1964, 3204, 3273

Auscultation, 2344, 3204

Autism, 222-223, **257-261**, 807-808, 2785, 3204, 3273; mercury and, 1935

Autoantibody, 2897, 3204

Autografts, 456, 1306, 1308, 3204

Autoimmune disorders, 176, **261-265**, 587, 589, 848, 1325-1326, 1449, 1608, 1612, 1698, 2026, 2298, 2596, 2733, 2896, 3204, 3273; endometriosis and, 1011

Autologous, 3204

Autologous transplants, 3020

Automated external defibrillators (AEDs), 478, 763, 2586, 3204

Automated quantitative cytometry (AQC), 1823

Automation, 1729

Automobile accidents, 3163

Autonomic nervous system, 302, 1392, 1541, 2085, 2325, 2361, 2890, 3204; yoga and, 3191

Autonomy, 811

Autopsy, **266-271**, 1166, 2300, 3204

Autosomal dominant diseases, 1238

Autosomal dominant gene, 3204

Autosomal recessive diseases, 1238

Autosomal recessive gene, 3204

Autosomes, 3204

Autotransplantation, 3204

A-V node. *See* Atrioventricular (A-V) node

Avian influenza, **271-275**, 1602, 2681

Avoidance, 2426

Avulsions, 1368

Axons, 977, 1477, 2084, 2098, 2272, 3204

Azathiaprine, 3018

Azithromycin, 1762

Azotemia, 2050, 3071

AZT. *See* Zidovudine

Blood thinners. *See* Anticoagulants

Blood transfusion, 2709. *See also* Transfusion

Blood transfusion reactions, 90, 372, 1613, 3014

Blood typing, 366, 377, 1730, 2590, 2677, 3009, 3206

Blood vessels, **379-381**, 448, 645, 1427, 1816, 3061, 3068, 3103; growth, 3105; inflammation, 3107

Blood withdrawal. *See* Phlebotomy

Bloom's disease, 3274

Blount's disease, 406

Blue baby syndrome, **381-382**, 730, 3274

Blue Gene project, 306

Blue skin, 381, 729

Blundell, James, 370

Blurred vision, **382-383**, 1846, 2029, 3274

Blushing, 2890

BMI. *See* Body mass index (BMI)

Bodamer, Joachim, 80

Body composition, 2774

Body dysmorphic disorder, **383-384**, 3206, 3274

Body mass index (BMI), 1094, 2144, 3207

Body piercing, **2914-2916**

Body temperature, 1417, 1545, 1547, 2890; sleep and, 2747. *See also* Fever

Boils, **385**, 1951, 2531, 3274

Bolus, 598, 1056, 3207

Bonding, **385-387**, 435

Bone cancer, **388-392**, 1067, 2195, 3274

Bone cells. *See* Osteocytes

Bone densitometry, 2220

Bone disorders, 388-389, 391, **392-395**, 400, 450, 706, 1163, 1466, 1727, 2094, 2206, 2209, 2212, 2217, 2219, 2244, 2597, 2608-2609

Bone fractures. *See* Fractures

Bone grafting, **395**, 2212, 3207

Bone marrow, 357, 389, 396, 466, 1422, 1425, 1592, 1605, 1773, 1775, 2815, 2953, 3207

Bone marrow transplantation, **395-398**, 400, 1309, 1483-1484, 1605-1606, 1775, 2543, 2683, 2724, 3207

Bone matrix, 398

Bone scan, 389, 3207

Bones, 391, 395, **398-403**, 690, 707, 1067, 1108, 1141, 1173, 1367, 1476, 1693, 1696, 2011, 2195, 2197, 2384, 2552, 2599, 3066, 3207; broken, 503, 1367, 1465

Bordeu, Théophile, 1282

Botox, **403-404**, 1431, 1532, 1966, 2386, 3207; prostate enlargement and, 2467

Botulism, 19, 282, 403, **404-405**, 1159, 1954, 2386, 3207, 3274

Bouchard's nodes, 2206

Bovine growth hormone, 1245, 1247

Bovine spongiform encephalopathy, 593, 710, 3274. *See also* Mad cow disease

Bowel movements, 1474

Bowlegs, **405-406**, 894, 1724, 2195

Bowman's capsule, 1715, 3207

Bowman's glands, 2770, 3207

BPH. *See* Benign prostatic hyperplasia (BPH)

Braces, orthodontic, **406-408**, 780, 784, 2193

Braces, orthopedic, **408-410**, 1784, 2652

Brachmann-de Lange syndrome, 698

Brachytherapy, 427

Bradycardia, 194, 201, 884, 1401, 2530, 3207, 3274

Bradyesthesia, 3274

Bradykinesia, 2292-2293

Bradykinin, 1644

Bradypnea, 3274

Braille, 362

Brain, 137, **410-416**, 632, 948, 978, 1477, 1524, 2100, 2107, 2552, 2685, 2901, 3207; aging and, 70; anatomy of the, 410, 2901; bleeding in, 1680, 1819; hemispheres, 978, 2109; implants, 317; inflammation, 986; mapping of, 2096; sleep and, 2747

Brain, water on the. *See* Hydrocephalus

Brain damage, 17, 80, **416-417**, 478, 658, 660, 885, 899, 978, 1044, 1930, 2991

Brain death, 419, 660, 3207, 3274

Brain disorders, 106, 244, 412, **417-421**, 551, 668, 899, 949, 986, 1176, 1907-1908, 2662

Brain hemorrhage, 1680, 1819

Brain stem, 3207

Brain tumors, 192, **422-423**, 950, 2087, 2274, 2662-2663

Brain waves, 948-949, 2748

Branched-chain alpha-ketoacid dehydrogenase (BCKD), 1878

BRCA1 gene, 425, 429, 530, 542, 1885, 1887

BRCA2 gene, 425, 429, 530, 542

Breast augmentation, 437, 2386

Breast biopsy, 326, **423-424**, 437, 3207

Breast cancer, 220, 423, **424-430**, 437, 443, 596, 1236, 1874, 2120, 2545, 3171, 3207, 3274; screening and, 2656

Breast cysts, 732, 744, 1885

Breast disorders, **430-432**, 442, 549, 1128, 1888

Breast-feeding, **432-437**, 1866, 1888, 3151

Breast implants, 438-439, 1873, 2386

Breast milk, 433-434, 1889, 3152

Breast reduction, 438, 2385

Breast self-examination, 2656

Breast surgery, **437-440**, 2385

Breasts, 549, 1872; female, 423, 425, 438, **440-445**, 1128, 1280, 2348, 2385, 2569, 3207; male, 1338

Breathing, 194, 496, 706, 721, 1420, 1554, 2388, 3162. *See also* Respiration

Breathing difficulty. *See* Dyspnea; Pulmonary diseases; Respiration; Respiratory distress syndrome

Breathing exercises, 3191

Breech birth, 536, 558, 561-562

Breech position, 3207

Bridges, **723-724**, 785

Briggs, Robert, 624

Bright, Richard, 2480

Bright's disease, 2076

Broca's area, 191

Broken bones, 1367, 1465

Bronchi, **445-446**, 1827, 3003, 3207

Bronchiectasis, 1825

Bronchioles, 236, 445-446, 1827, 3207

Cleft lip, **611-616**, 3211, 3276; repair, **616-617**, 2385
Cleft palate, **611-616**, 617, 2335, 2785, 3142, 3211, 3276; repair, **616-617**, 2385
Clinical examination, 3211
Clinical laboratory, 3211
Clinical trials, **617-619**, 1148, 3211
Clinics, **619-621**, 3211
Clitoridectomy, 603, 2571
Clitoris, 603, 2569
Clomiphene, 1617
Cloning, 234, **621-625**, 3211; hair, 1345
Closed head injury, 3276
Clostridia, 1200, 1954, 2943, 2945
Clostridium difficile infection, **625-626**
Clot, 3211, 3276
Clotting factors, 2382, 3211. *See also* Coagulation factors
Club drugs, **626-628**
Clubbing, 2035
Clubfoot, 1110, 1163
Cluster headaches, **628-630**, 1361, 1363, 3211, 3276
CME. *See* Continuing medical education
CMV. *See* Cytomegalovirus (CMV)
Coagulation, 761, 3211. *See also* Blood clotting
Coagulation factors, 356, 358, 1436, 3144
Cobalamin, 141
Cobb angle measurement, 2651
Cocaine, 49-50, 53, 150, 187, 511, 679, 963, 1103, 1453; anesthesia, 1813
Cocci, 1312-1313
Coccidioidomycosis, **630-632**, 3211, 3276
Cochlea, 753, 914, 1378, 2670, 3211
Cochlear implants, 316, 754, 1379-1380
Cockayne syndrome, 894
Cocktail therapy, 37, 1519
Code situation, 1504
Codeine, 1453
Cognitive, 3211
Cognitive development, 72, **632-637**, 810, 1323
Cognitive functioning, 3211
Cognitive therapy, 52, 2270

Cohort studies, 1041
Colchicine, 1304, 1454
Cold, therapeutic use of, 724, 2352
Cold agglutinin disease, 3276
Cold-blooded organisms, 1122, 1545
Cold sores, **637**, 1463, 3211, 3276
Colectomy, 656
Coley, William B., 314, 1549
Colic, **638-640**, 3276
Colitis, 626, **640-645**, 649, 656, 834, 836, 1127, 1207, 1213, 1219, 1582, 1670, 2458, 3211, 3276
Collagen, 501, **645-646**, 689, 1367, 1476, 1784, 2369, 2386, 2647, 2851, 3185, 3211
Collagen vascular disease, 3276
Collapsed lung. *See* Pneumothorax
Collaterals, 3211
Collecting duct, 3211
Collection kits, 1731
Collimator, 3211
Colombo, Realdo, 369
Colon, 2, 101, **646-648**, 655, 691, 842, 856, 1017, 1206, 1213, 1218, 1473, 1580-1581, 1669, 1673, 2319, 2456, 2561, 3211; irrigation of, 647
Colon cancer, 648-649, **651-654**, 656, 1213-1214, 1444, 1582-1583, 1671, 1674, 1916, 1920, 2141, 2458, 2561, 2657; women and, 3174
Colon polyp removal, 649, **654-655**, 2458
Colon polyps, 2420
Colon surgery, **655-657**, 2456
Colon therapy, 102, **647-648**, 3211
Colonoscopy, **648-650**, 652, 654, 858, 1017, 1208, 1681, 2457, 2657, 3211
Color blindness, **650-651**, 679, 1087, 1239, 2671, 3129, 3211, 3276
Color synesthesia, 2893
Colorado tick fever, 1780
Colorectal cancer, 3276. *See also* Colon cancer; Rectal cancer
Colorectal polyp removal. *See* Colon polyp removal; Rectal polyp removal
Colorectal surgery. *See* Colon surgery; Rectal surgery

Colostomy, 656, 859, **1580-1585**, 3211
Colostrum, 433, 1514, 3211
Colposcopy, 534
Coma, 419, **657-661**, 2400, 2402, 2405, 2539, 3064, 3211, 3276
Combat neurosis, 2428
Commissurotomy, 2109, 3211
Common cold, 447, **661-666**, 2047, 2049, 2227, 2390, 2524, 2607, 2682, 2770, 2911, 3211, 3276
Communication, 3211
Comparative genomics, 306, 1263
Compartment syndrome, 504, 1428
Competition, 2717
Complement, 1604, 1613, 3212
Complement system, 1513, 1644, 2079
Complications, 2726, 3212
Compounding, 2328, 3212
Compression, breast, 1872
Compulsions, 186, 259, 2152, 3212, 3276
Computed tomography (CT) scanning, **667-669**, 1002, 1220, 1588-1589, 1807, 1823, 2096, 2118, 2169, 2545, 2856, 3212
Conception, **669-674**, 1616, 1634, 1638, 2434, 3212
Concordance, 3212
Concrete operations stage, 634, 812
Concussion, 17, **674-676**, 1358, 3212, 3276
Conditioning, 49, 2269, 2343
Condom, 692-693, 1922; female, 692
Conductive hearing loss, 753, 914, 1379, 1383, 3212
Cone biopsy, 534
Conenose bug, 538
Cones, 650, 1084, 3130, 3212
Confidential, 3212
Confidentiality, 1060
Conflict resolution, 2720
Congenital, 3212
Congenital adrenal hyperplasia, 60, **676-678**, 1538, 3212, 3276
Congenital disorders, **678-681**, 3212, 3276. *See also* Birth defects
Congenital heart disease, 381, 489, **681-686**, 893, 3212, 3276
Congenital hypothyroidism, 400, **686-688**, 892, 1864, 2968. *See also* Cretinism

Eating habits, 199
Eating while asleep, 2756
Eaton-Lambert's syndrome, 3279
Ebola virus, **924-927**, 1035, 1879, 3122, 3279
Ebstein's anomaly, 3279
Ecchymoma, 3279
Ecchymoses, 354, 852, 3217, 3279
ECG or EKG. *See* Electrocardiography (ECG or EKG)
ECG waves, 3217
Echocardiogram, 3217
Echocardiography, 490, **927-929**, 1402, 2119, 2255, 3061, 3217
Echoviruses, 1020
Eclampsia, **2432-2433**, 2438, 2995, 3217, 3279. *See also* Preeclampsia
Ecology, 3217
Ecosystem, 3217
Ecstasy, 627
-ectomy, 3217
Ectopic pregnancy, **929-930**, 2309, 2437, 2821, 3217, 3279
Ectropion, 1075, 1077
Eczema, 793, 796, **931**, 2743, 3169, 3217, 3279
ED. *See* Erectile dysfunction
Edema, 104, 805, 828, **932-936**, 1355, 1401, 1406, 1478, 1628, 1863, 2074, 2274, 3114, 3217, 3279
Edema, pulmonary. *See* Pulmonary edema
Education; dental, 777; medical, 96-97, 118, 568, **936-941**, 1097, 1494, 1895, 2214, 2330, 2396, 2925; special, 1931, 2786
Edwards, Robert, 1619
Edwards syndrome, 679, 3279
EEG. *See* Electroencephalography (EEG)
Effector, 3217
Efficacy, 3217
Effusions, 1680
Eflornithine, 2759
Egg. *See* Ovum
Ego, 2502
Ehlers-Danlos syndrome, 645, 1784
Ehrlich, Paul, 314, 370, 539, 1516
Ehrlichiosis, **942-943**, 3217, 3279
Ejaculation, 669, 2568, 3217
EKG. *See* Electrocardiography (ECG or EKG)

Elastic cartilage, 502
Elastin, 501, 689, 983, 1784, 3217
Elbow, 3217
Elder abuse, 874, 876
Elderly, 75, 1266, 1384, 1465, 2331, 2350, 2358, 2499; bedsores and, 296; eating disorders and, 919
Electric anesthesia, 151, 3217
Electrical burns, 455
Electrical shock, 456, **943-944**, 3217, 3279
Electrocardiography (ECG or EKG), 323, 478, 490, 684, **945-947**, 1397, 1402, 2119, 2238, 2584, 3217
Electrocauterization, 534, **947-948**, 3217
Electroconvulsive therapy, 2711, 3217
Electrodermal response, 302
Electrodermal response biofeedback, 3217
Electroencephalography (EEG), 302, 412, **948-950**, 2096, 2664, 2748, 3217
Electrolysis, 1341
Electrolyte imbalance, 1104, 1141, 2567
Electrolytes, 764, **1139-1143**, 1730, 1839, 2140, 2382, 3083, 3217. *See also* Fluids
Electromagnetic fields, 322
Electromyograph, 302, 3217
Electromyography, 131, **950-952**, 2014, 2351, 2850, 3217
Electron volt, 3218
Electrons, 1588, 3218
Elephantiasis, **952-957**, 1832, 1841, 2289, 2618, 3028, 3182, 3218, 3279
ELISA. *See* Enzyme-linked immunosorbent assay (ELISA)
Embolism, 203, 418, 761, 934, **957**, 990, 1172, 1575, 2339, 2853, 2955-2956, 2959, 3099, 3106, 3218; pulmonary, 2730
Embolization, **958-959**
Embolus, 3218, 3279
Embryo, 960, 1618, 2158, 2434, 2685, 3218
Embryo transfer, 1617
Embryology, **959-964**, 3218
Embryonic development, 340, 612, 671, 681-682, 892, 960, 1083,

1320, 2100, 2436, 2685, 2794, 2800
Embryonic stem cells, 2813
EMDR. *See* Eye movement desensitization and reprocessing (EMDR)
E-medicine, 1664. *See also* Telemedicine
Emergency contraceptive pills, 694
Emergency medical services, 3218
Emergency medical technicians (EMTs), 966, 2277, 2584
Emergency medicine, 491, **964-970**, 972, 1582, 2277, 2584, 3218; informed consent and, 1058; pediatric, **970-972**
Emergency room, 619, 965, **972-974**, 1510, 3218
Emerging diseases, 3218, 3279
Emerging infectious diseases, **974-977**
Emery-Dreifuss syndrome, 3279
Emetic, 3218
EMG. *See* Electromyography
Emotional development, 810
Emotions, biomedical causes and effects, **977-981**, 1556, 2748
Emphysema, 227, 591, **981-985**, 1033, 1478, 1744, 1828, 1918, 1921, 2237, 2517-2518, 2526-2527, 2575, 2774, 3162, 3218, 3279; senile, 70
EMTs. *See* Emergency medical technicians (EMTs)
Enamel, 514, 2919, 3218
Encephalitis, 192, 553, 772, **986-988**, 1020, 2086, 3194, 3218, 3279; West Nile, 3160
Encephalocele, 680
Encephalopathy, 1805, 1807, 3218
Encephelotrigeminal angiomatosis, 2858
Encoscopy, 2457
End-stage renal disease, **988-990**, 1896, 2413, 3218, 3280; African Americans and, 66
Endarterectomy, 206, **990-991**, 1921, 2856, 3218
Endemic disease, 3218
Endocarditis, 160, 472, 490, 928, **991-993**, 1397, 1413, 2922, 3218, 3280; bacterial, 992
Endocrine, 3218

Endocrine disorders, 137, **993-997**,
1001, 1004, 1299, 1621, 1730,
3280
Endocrine glands, 136, **997-999**,
1004, 1278, 1476, 1502, 2261,
2967, 3218
Endocrine pancreas, 3218
Endocrine system, 997, 1004, 2903,
3218; anatomy of, 993, 999;
changes in aging, 1267
Endocrinology, 997, **999-1002**,
1282, 3218; pediatric, **1003-1005**
Endodontic disease, **1005-1006**,
3218, 3280
Endodontics, 780, 2612, 3218
Endogenous, 3218
Endogenous viruses, 3187
Endolymph, 3218
Endometrial biopsy, **1006-1007**,
3218
Endometrial cancer, 530-532, 1006,
1255-1256, 3091
Endometrial hyperplasia, 1538
Endometriosis, 902, 929, **1008-1014**,
1254-1255, 1336, 1616, 1634,
1737, 1927, 2570, 3091, 3218,
3280
Endometrium, 2569, 3091
Endoplasmic reticulum, 645, 3218
Endorphins, 39, 99, 2247, 2443
Endoscope, 3218
Endoscopic retrograde
cholangiopancreatography
(ERCP), **1014-1015**, 1190, 1192,
3218
Endoscopy, 216, 328, 654, 835,
858, **1015-1018**, 1196, 1207,
1211, 1680-1681, 1737, 1795,
2163, 2226, 2879, 2884, 3057,
3219
Endospores, 2943, 3219
Endosteum, 398
Endothelium, 3219
Endotoxins, 1123
Endotracheal tube, 150-151, 2280,
3219
Enemas, 101, 920, **1018-1019**, 3219
Energy, 3219
Energy medicine, 102
Energy production, 1294
Engorgement, 1889
Enkephalins, 2443
Enlarged prostate. *See* Prostate
enlargement

ENT (ear, nose, and throat)
medicine. *See*
Otorhinolaryngology
Entacapone, 2295
Entamoeba histolytica, 112
Enterococcus, 888
Enterocolitis, **1019-1020**, 1474
Enterostomal therapists, 1583
Enteroviruses, 987, **1020-1021**,
1354, 3219, 3280
Entropion, 1075, 1077
Enuresis, 3205, 3280. *See also* Bed-
wetting
Environment, 1039, 3219
Environmental disasters, 716
Environmental diseases, 217, 341,
1021-1027, 3219, 3280
Environmental health, 382, 1022,
1027-1028, 2999, 3219
Environmental medicine, 3219
Environmental toxicology, 1246,
3219
Enzyme-linked immunosorbent
assay (ELISA), 38
Enzyme therapy, 102, **1029**, 1107,
1224, 1230, 1292, 1941, 2113,
3219
Enzymes, 2, 22, 102, 733, 735, 842,
1029-1035, 1107, 1155, 1218,
1291, 1735, 1797, 1938, 1946,
1989, 2262, 2916, 3219
EOAE test. *See* Evoked otoacoustic
emissions (EOAE) test
Eosinophils, 1513, 1592
Ephedra, 2876, 3156
Ephedrine, 1055
Epidemics, 848, 926, 975, **1035-
1038**, 1041, 1600, 1646, 1759,
1763, 2407, 2410, 2519, 3176,
3219, 3280. *See also* Pandemics
Epidemiology, 1022, **1038-1042**,
2410, 2452, 3219; genetic, 2481
Epidermis, 2033, 2369, 2735, 2737,
2742, 3219
Epididymis, 2568, 3098, 3112, 3219
Epididymitis, 1919, 1922, 2190,
3112
Epididymoorchitis, 2190
Epidural anesthesia, 146, 536, 558,
3219
Epidural hematomas, 18
Epiglottis, 1042
Epiglottitis, 722, **1042**, 2048, 2051,
2334, 3003

Epilepsy, 257, 412, 419-420, 949,
978, **1043-1047**, 2086, 2128,
2257, 2662-2663, 2772, 3219,
3280
Epinephrine, 60, 1146, 1281, 3219.
See also Adrenaline
Epi-Pen, 1146, 3219
Epiphora, 1081
Epiphyses, 1171
Episiotomy, 557, 1010, **1048-1049**,
3219
Epistaxis, 356, 358, 2123, 2210
Epithelial cells, 745
Epithelial tissue, 135, 1307, 1476,
3044, 3219
Epley, John, 289
Epstein-Barr virus, 264, 452, **1049-
1051**, 1463, 1955, 1974, 2953,
3127
ER. *See* Emergency room
Erb's palsy, 2259
ERCP. *See* Endoscopic retrograde
cholangiopancreatography (ERCP)
Erectile dysfunction, **1051-1053**,
3219, 3280. *See also* Sexual
dysfunction
Erection, 1051, 1259, 2310, 2568,
2690, 3219
Ergogenic aids, **1053-1055**
Ergonomics, 951, 2929, 3219
Ergot, 1971
Ergotamines, 1966
Ergotism, 1185
Erikson, Erik, 635, 810, 1960
Erythema, 3280
Erythema multiforme, 3219
Erythema nodosum, 297, 3219
Erythematous, 3219
Erythralgia, 3280
Erythremia, 3280
Erythroblastosis, 3280
Erythroblastosis fetalis. *See*
Hemolytic disease of the newborn
Erythrocytes, 364, 1422, 1426,
1716, 1773, 2078, 2382, 3219
Erythromycin, 1762, 2639
Erythropoietin, 1054, 1503, 1716,
2078
Escherich, Theodore, 905
Escherichia coli. See *E. coli*
infection
Esophageal cancer, 1056, 1213;
heartburn and, 1416
Esophageal spasm, 2320

Food, 199, 462, 1152, 1216, 1221, 1565-1566, 1673, 2145-2146, 2911; genetic engineering of, 1245
Food additives, 1149
Food allergies, 89, 92, **1144-1147**, 1480, 3222, 3281
Food and Drug Administration (FDA), 618, 787, **1147-1151**, 1161, 1491, 2327, 2876, 2999, 3138
Food biochemistry, **1151-1156**, 1673, 1787, 3222
Food group, 3222
Food Guide Pyramid, **1156-1158**
Food poisoning, 19, 284, 405, 836-837, **1158-1162**, 1204, 1219, 1435, 1954, 2810, 3049, 3222, 3281
Foot disorders, 450-451, 700, 1110, 1138, **1163-1165**, 2367, 2397
Foramen magnum, 3222
Forceps, 557
Forearm, 3222
Foremilk, 433, 3222
Forensic, 3222
Forensic autopsy, 3222
Forensic medicine, 1165, 1746, 2922, 2999
Forensic pathology, 269, **1165-1167**, 1246, 2300, 3222
Forensic toxicology, 3222
Foreskin, 606
Forgetfulness, 2631
Formal operations stage, 634, 812
Formula feeding, 436
Forteo, 2221
Fosamax, 2212, 2221
Foscarnet, 750
Fourier-transform, 3222
Fovea, 1084, 3130
Fracture repair, 19, 503, **1173-1175**, 1465, 1692, 2807
Fractures, 19, 391-392, 409, 503, **1167-1173**, 1174, 1692, 2195, 2199, 2203, 2218, 2279, 2384, 2807, 3222, 3281; facial, 1692; nonunion of, 1171
Fragile X syndrome, **1175-1176**, 3281
Framingham Heart Study, 1041, 1408
Fraternal twins, 1991
Freckles, 2369, 2743
Free association, 2503

Free radical theory of aging, 71, 3222
Free radicals, 71, 182, 2740, 2876
Freezing, 725
Frequency, 3223
Fresh-frozen plasma, 3013
Freud, Sigmund, 186, 188, 635, 810, 813, 1558, 2153, 2493, 2501, 2720, 2979
Frölich, Alfred, 1282
Frontal lobe, 3223
Frontotemporal dementia (FTD), **1176-1178**, 2365, 3223, 3281
Frostbite, 730, **1178-1182**, 1546, 2352, 3223, 3281
Frozen section biopsy, 328, 3223
Fructose, 1183
Fructosemia, **1182-1183**, 1799, 3281
FSH. See Follicle-stimulating hormone (FSH)
FTD. See Frontotemporal dementia (FTD)
Full-term, 3223
Functional disease, 846, 1214, 3223
Functional genomics, 306, 1263
Functional magnetic resonance imaging (fMRI), 3223
Fungal infections, 224, 245, 470, 630, **1183-1188**, 2035, 2176, 2609, 3223, 3281
Fungi, 172, 1184-1185, 1953-1954, 1970
Fungiform papillae, 2909, 3223
Fungus, 3223
Furuncle, 385
Fusion inhibitors, 37
Future of Family Medicine (FMM) Project, 1099

GABA. See Gamma-aminobutyric acid (GABA)
Gag reflex, 3093
Galactoceles, 431
Galactorrhea, 113, 1338
Galactose, 1189
Galactosemia, 1154, **1189**, 1240, 1568, 1799
Galen of Pergamum, 338, 369, 417, 502, 1061, 1829, 2772
Gallbladder, 300, 574-575, **1189-1191**, 1193, 1206, 1214, 1797, 2161, 2163, 2825, 2840, 3060; imaging, 1014
Gallbladder cancer, 115, **1191-1193**, 1195

Gallbladder diseases, 7, 575-576, **1193-1197**, 3281
Gallbladder removal. See Cholecystectomy
Gallo, Robert, 2178, 2588
Gallstone removal. See Gallstones; Stone removal
Gallstones, 300, 574, 576, 1014, 1136, 1190, 1192, 1689, 1738, 2162-2163, 2266, 2825, 2837-2840, 3223, 3281. See also Gallbladder diseases; Stone removal; Stones
Gamete intrafallopian transfer (GIFT), 233, **1197-1199**, 1635, 3223
Gametes, 3223
Gametogenesis, 2231
Gamma-aminobutyric acid (GABA), 168, 2443, 2748
Gamma camera, 2551, 2730, 3223
Gamma globulin, 1593, 1704
Gamma-hydroxybutyrate, 627
Gamma rays, 322, 1587, 2551, 2729, 3223
Ganciclovir, 750
Ganglion, 744, 3223
Ganglion removal, 744, **1199-1200**
Gangliosides, 2916
Gangrene, 282, 818, 848, 1180, **1200-1201**, 1546, 1954, 2064, 2352, 2744, 2890, 3223, 3281; dry, 1200
Gardasil, 531, 1521, 1602
Garlic, 1455
Gas, 458
Gas-bloat syndrome, 458
Gas exchange, 1826-1827, 3223
Gas gangrene, 1200, 3183
Gasser syndrome, 1434
Gastrectomy, **1201-1202**, 3052, 3223
Gastric, 3223
Gastric banding, 290
Gastric bypass, 290
Gastric juice, 2, 841, 1674-1675, 1728
Gastric lavage, 3000
Gastritis, 8, 1219, 3223, 3281. See also Abdominal disorders; Gastroenteritis; Gastrointestinal disorders
Gastroenteritis, **1203-1205**, 1219, 1435, 2121, 2616, 2633, 3223, 3281

HPSAs. *See* Health professions shortage areas (HPSAs)
HPV. *See* Human papillomavirus (HPV)
Hullihen, Simon P., 2188
Human chorionic gonadotropin, 1967, 2158, 2377
Human genome, 306, 1230, 1262, 1265
Human Genome Project, 316, 1262, 1264, 2020, 2481. *See also* Genomics
Human immunodeficiency virus (HIV), 34, 373, 414, 607, 679, 769, 975, 1104, 1187, 1437, 1515, **1518-1520**, 1605, 1732, 2178, 2588, 2700, 3009, 3124, 3178, 3228
Human leukocyte antigen (HLA), 1713, 3228
Human papillomavirus (HPV), 133, 312, 531, **1520-1522**, 1602, 3228
Human Proteome Organization, 2482
Humerus, 3066, 3228
Humor, 634
Humoral response, 176
Humors, theory of, 269, 338, 367, 1191, 1563
Hunter, William, 502
Hunter syndrome, 1989
Huntington's disease, 413, 419, 678, 1119, 1233, 1238, 1250, **1522-1523**, 2994, 3069, 3228, 3283
Hurler's syndrome, 1120, 1989, 3283
Hurthle cell carcinoma, 3283
Hutchinson-Gilford syndrome, 72, 2459
Hutchinson's disease, 3283
Hyaline cartilage, 501
Hyaline membrane disease, 3284
Hyaluronic acid, 2207, 3185
Hydatid disease, 2289
Hydatidosis, 3284
Hydradenitis, 3284
Hydramnios, 3284
Hydrating solutions, 1678
Hydro-, 3228
Hydrocarbon, 3228
Hydrocelectomy, 1523, 3228
Hydroceles, 1260, **1523**, 2938, 3228, 3284
Hydrocephalus, 419-420, 768, 1234,

1524-1525, 1680, 1820, 1930, 2304, 2306, 2716, 2794, 3228, 3284; fetal surgery and, 1114
Hydrochloric acid, 841, 843, 1219, 3055, 3092, 3138
Hydrocortisone, 1453, 3228
Hydrogenation, 1786
Hydronephrosis, 3071
Hydrophilic, 3228
Hydrophobic, 3228
Hydrops fetalis, 2948
Hydrostatic pressure, 932, 934, 1841
Hydrotherapy, 100, **1526-1527**, 2353, 3228; colon, 647
Hydroxymethylglutaryl coenzyme A, 580
Hygiene, 3228
Hygiene hypothesis, 240, 1145
Hygienic Laboratory, 2055
Hyper-, 3228
Hyperactivity, 248, 2974. *See also* Attention-deficit disorder (ADD)
Hyperadiposis, **1527-1528**, 3284
Hyperalimentation, 3228
Hyperandrogenism, 2414, 3228
Hyperbaric oxygen therapy, **1528-1530**
Hyperbarism, 3284
Hyper-beta-alaninemia, 3284
Hyperbetalipoproteinemia, 3284
Hyperbilirubinemia, 3284
Hypercalcemia, 1141, 2838
Hypercholesterolemia, **1530-1531**, 1918, 2828; familial, 1252
Hypercoagulation, 762
Hyperglycemia, 1944, 3228
Hyperhidrosis, 404, **1531-1532**, 2890
Hyperinsulinemia, 2414, 3228
Hyperlipidemia, 204, 816, 1238, **1532-1534**, 1918, 2141, 2266, 3228, 3284
Hypernatremia, 3228, 3284
Hyperopia, 382, 1075, 1077, 1086, 2564, 2671, 3131, 3133, 3228, 3284
Hyperparathyroidism, **1534-1538**, 2291, 2838, 3229, 3284
Hyperplasia, 1006, **1538**, 1550, 1802, 2462, 2470, 3229, 3284
Hypersensitivity, 89, 1613, 3229
Hypersplenism, 2803
Hypertension, 153, 205, 302, 375, 420, 769, 1040, 1392, 1401,

1539-1544, 1552, 1662, 1918, 1944, 2145, 2313, 2690, 2857, 3100, 3229, 3284; African Americans and, 66; Asian Americans and, 221; kidney disease and, 989; portal, 610, 2716; pregnancy and, 2432, 2995; renal failure and, 2566; renovascular, 3100; screening and, 2655
Hyperthermia, **1544-1550**, 2867, 3229, 3284
Hyperthyroidism, 998, 1532, 2966. *See also* Graves' disease
Hypertonia, 3284
Hypertrophy, 442, 1413, **1550-1553**, 2016, 2018, 3229
Hyperuricemia, 1303
Hyperventilation, **1554-1555**, 2269, 3229
Hyphae, 1185, 3229
Hypnosis, 120, **1555-1559**, 2850, 3229
Hypo-, 3229
Hypoadrenocorticism, 54
Hypocalcemia, 1141, 3229
Hypochondriasis, **1559-1564**, 3229, 3284
Hypocretins, 2040
Hypodermis, 3229
Hypogammaglobulinemia, 1604-1605
Hypoglycemia, 864, **1564-1569**, 2662, 2834, 3229, 3284; newborns and, 1272
Hypogonadism, 1919, 1922
Hypogonadotropic hypogonadism, 2513
Hypokalemic paralysis, 2275
Hypomania, 335
Hyponychium, 2033
Hypoparathyroidism, **1534-1538**, 3229, 3284. *See also* Hyperparathyroidism
Hypophysectomy, 2107
Hypopituitarism, 1475, 2374
Hypopnea, 2751
Hypospadias, 1569, 2569, 3229, 3284
Hypospadias repair, **1569-1570**
Hypotension, 376, **1570-1571**, 3229
Hypothalamus, 60, 412, 994, 997, 999, 1281, 1417, **1571-1572**, 2145, 2373, 2770, 2965, 3229

Influenza, 273, 975, 1037, 1158, 1495, 1600, **1645-1649**, 1661, 1919, 1921, 2093, 2520, 3125, 3127, 3230, 3285; avian, **271-275**, 1602, 2681; H1N1, 975, **1495-1498**, 1602, 3228, 3282; viral, 566
Influenza B, 564-565, 1599
Informed consent, 968, 1057, 3230
Infrared light, 2352
Ingrown nails, 2032
Ingrown toenails, 1164, 2034
Inguinal hernias, 1101, 1458-1459, 1461, 2570, 3230
Inhalant, 3230
Inhalers, 239
Inheritance, 870, **1248-1253**, 3230
Inhibitions, 2975
Injection, 3230
Injuries, 17, 408, 448, 2246; brain, 416; children and, 2623; elderly and, 2629. *See also* Wounds
Inner ear, 289, 3115, 3230
Inoculate, 3230
Inotropic drugs, 1407, 3230
Inpatient care, 3230
Insane, 3230
Insect-borne diseases, 953, **1649-1655**, 1853. *See also* Arthropod-borne diseases; Bites; Stings
Insecticides, 1653
Insemination, 3231
Insomnia, 1911, 2749, 2755, 3231, 3285. *See also* Sleep disorders
Inspiration, 3231
Instincts, 2502
Instinctual drives, 3231
Institute for Genome Research, 1264
Institute of Medicine (IOM), 3174
Institutional Review Board, 618, 968
Insulin, 2, 66, 475, 815-818, 822, 994-995, 1001, 1154, 1244, 1271, 1280, 1297, 1503, 1505, 1565-1567, 2025, 2263, 2414, 2438, 2834, 2902, 2904, 3231; fetal, 1272
Insulin growth factor, 1131
Insulin resistance, 1944
Insulin resistance syndrome, 3285
Insurance, 1372
Integra, 456
Integrase, 3231
Intelligence, 72
Intelligence quotient (IQ), 259, 1929

Intense pulsed light therapy, 3095
Intensive care, 3231. *See also* Critical care, Critical care, pediatric
Intensive care unit (ICU), 712-713, 717, **1655-1658**, 2066
Intercourse, 669, 672, 692, 739-741, 2568, 2690, 3076
Intercourse, painful. *See* Dyspareunia
Interferometry, 1703
Interferon, 313, 3127, 3231
Intergenic regions, 1263
Interleukin receptors, 2683
Interleukins, 313
Intermittent care, 3231
Intermittent claudication, 380, 610, 3231
Internal medicine, **1659-1662**, 3231
International Classification of Diseases, 823
Internet medicine, **1663-1667**, 2925. *See also* Telemedicine
Internship, 938, 3231
Interstitial, 3231
Interstitial compartment, 932
Interstitial cystitis, 277
Interstitial fluid, 1832
Interstitial nephritis, 1708
Interstitial pulmonary fibrosis (IPF), **1667-1668**, 3231, 3285
Intertrigo, 471, 796
Intervertebral disks, 3231
Intervertebral foramina, 3231
Intestinal cancer, **2832-2836**
Intestinal disorders, 641, 691, 720, 832, 1019, 1457, **1668-1672**
Intestinal lumen, 3231
Intestines, 2, 646, 1580, **1672-1676**, 3231
In-toeing, 2367
Intoxication, **1676-1677**, 3231
Intracellular fluid, 1139, 3231
Intracytoplasmic sperm injection, 234, 1198, 1617
Intraocular pressure, 1284, 1287, 3231
Intraperitoneal therapy, 531
Intrauterine devices (IUDs), 693, 694, 929
Intrauterine growth retardation, 2377
Intravascular fluid, 3231
Intravenous (IV) therapy, **1677-1679**, 2279, 3231

Intravenous pyelogram (IVP), 1588, 1706
Intraventricular hemorrhage, **1679-1680**, 3231, 3285
Intrinsic factor, 1203
Intubation, 3003, 3231
Invasive, 3231
Invasive tests, **1680-1682**
Investigational new drugs, 1148
Involuntary muscle contractions, 3231
Iodine, 687, 995, 1001, 1299, 1587, 1864, 1866, 2553, 2965, 2969-2970
Iodine deficiency, 687, 1864, 2965
IOM. *See* Institute of Medicine (IOM)
Ionization, 3231
Ions, 322, 1139, 2262, 3231
Iontophoresis, 1532
Ipecac, 3231
IPF. *See* Interstitial pulmonary fibrosis (IPF)
IQ. *See* Intelligence quotient (IQ)
Iraq War, 1024
Iridectomy, 1286
Iris, 507, 1074, 2172, 3130, 3231
Iritis, 1074, 1077, 2565
Iron, 1423, 1431, 1797, 1941, 2140
Iron-deficiency anemia, 3231, 3285. *See also* Anemia, iron-deficiency
Iron lung, 2408
Irritable bowel syndrome (IBS), 639, 833, 835, 1206, 1214, 1625, **1682-1686**, 2321, 2458, 3285; fibromyalgia and, 1130
Irritants, 19
Ischemia, 126, 203, 205, 418, 460, 488, 701, 848, 1400, 1529, 1626, **1686-1687**, 2063, 2352, 2380, 2853, 2955, 3099, 3231, 3285
Islets of Langerhans, 997, 1280, 2261, 3232
Isoflavones, 2364
Isoimmunization, 124, 2158, 2831
Isokinetic, 3232
Isoleucine, 1878
Isotonic, 3232
Isotopes, 1587
Isotypes, 3232
Itching, 553, 794-796, 1480, **1687-1688**, 1779, 2372, 2404, 2609, 2638, 3232, 3285
-itis, 3232

Lipopigment, 292
Lipopolysaccharide (LPS), 3234
Lipoproteins, 579, 1426, 1845, 3234
Liposarcoma, 2637
Liposomes, 1229
Liposuction, 1528, **1790-1793**, 3234
Lips, 616, 1216, 1988
Liquid X, 627
Lisping, **1793-1794**, 2784, 3286
Lister, Joseph, 2395
Listeria infections, 1159, **1794-1795**, 3286
Lithium, 336, 791, 2491, 3234
Lithotripsy, 1196, 1717, **1795-1796**, 2837-2838, 3087, 3234
Liver, 2, 7, 300, 609, 1206, 1211, 1214, 1447, 1592, **1796-1800**, 1804, 1809, 2112, 2116, 2553, 2716, 3019, 3234; glycogen storage diseases, 1291
Liver cancer, 7, 1214, 1799, **1800-1803**, 1806-1807, 3286
Liver disorders, 7, 84, 589, 609, 658, 935, 1447-1448, 1567, 1689, 1798, 1800-1801, **1803-1809**, 1919, 2116, 2690, 2716, 3167
Liver failure, 454, 1211, 1809, 2050
Liver spots, 68
Liver transplantation, 1211, 1800, 1808, **1809-1811**, 2117, 3019, 3234
Living will, 1065, 1472, **1811-1812**, 2586, 3234
Lobectomy, 3234
Lobotomy, 2109, 3234
Lobular carcinoma in situ, 426
Lobule, 3234
Local anesthesia, 144, 150, **1812-1814**, 3110, 3234
Local block, 144
Lockjaw. *See* Tetanus
Long-term care, 3234
Longitudinal studies, 1041
Lordosis, 2800
Lorenzo's oil, 63, 1778
Loss-of-control syndrome, 3234
Lotronex, 1684-1685
Lou Gehrig's disease. *See* Amyotrophic lateral sclerosis
Lovaas, O. Ivar, 223, 259
Lovastatin, 1778
Low blood pressure. *See* Hypotension

Low-density lipoproteins (LDLs), 579, 1530, 1788, 2828, 3234
Lower, Richard, 370
Lower esophageal sphincter (LES), 26, 1415
Lower extremities, 127, **1814-1819**, 3094, 3100, 3234; prostheses for, 2475
LPS. *See* Lipopolysaccharide (LPS)
LSD, 627
Lubricants, 692
Lujo fever, 3122
Lumbar puncture, 145, 1680-1681, 1728, **1819-1820**, 1908, 2285, 3234
Lumbar vertebrae, 3234
Lumen, 3234
Lumpectomy, 427, 437, **1884-1888**, 3041, 3172, 3234. *See also* Mastectomy
Lumps, breast. *See* Breast cancer; Breast disorders; Breasts, female; Fibrocystic breast condition
Lung, collapsed. *See* Pneumothorax
Lung cancer, **1821-1824**, 1828, 1916, 1920, 1936, 2517, 2526, 2773, 3286; women and, 3171
Lung disease, 1667, 1918, 2774. *See also* Pulmonary diseases
Lung disorders, 2521
Lung reduction, 592
Lung surgery, **1824-1826**
Lung toxicants, 310
Lung transplantation, 592
Lungs, 445, 547, 982-983, 1017, 1824, **1826-1830**, 2388, 2394, 2516, 2524, 2552, 2573, 2902, 3234; acidosis and, 28; fetal, 124
Lunula, 2033, 3234
Lupus, 138, 264, 848, 1164, 1478, 3234, 3286; endometriosis and, 1011. *See also* Systemic lupus erythematosus (SLE)
Luteal phase defect, 1007
Lutein, 2364
Luteinizing hormone (LH), 232, 672, 1000, 1281, 2373
Lyme disease, 347, 1780, **1830-1832**, 2626, 3194, 3234, 3286
Lymph, 1476, 1592, **1832-1833**, 1839, 3234
Lymph nodes, 1481-1483, 1592, 1832-1833, 1839, 1974, 3234
Lymphadenectomy, 3234

Lymphadenitis, 954
Lymphadenopathy, **1833-1838**, 3234, 3286
Lymphangitis, 954
Lymphatic disorders. *See* Lymphadenopathy; Lymphoma
Lymphatic system, 56, 953, 1592, 1832, **1838-1843**, 2983, 3234; anatomy of, 1481, 1592, 1833-1834, 1838
Lymphedema, 1832, 1841
Lymphocytes, 365, 470, 816, 1145, 1481, 1513, 1592, 1604, 1773, 1833, 1839, 1842, 2677, 2964, 3018, 3235
Lymphogranuloma venereum, 572, 3286
Lymphoid interstitial pneumonia, 3286
Lymphoma, 452, 1463, 1481, **1833-1838**, 1841, 2832, 2952, 3235, 3286
Lyric Hearing Aid, 1382
Lysosomal storage diseases, 1223, 1789, 2916
Lysosomes, 518-519, 1291, 1512, 3235
Lysosyme, 2917, 3235

McCune-Albright syndrome, 2430-2431
McDowell, Ephraim, 1576
McKenzie method, 279
Macronutrients, **1844-1846**, 2139
Macrophages, 176, 1475, 1592, 1628-1629, 1827, 2635, 3235
Macrosomia, 1272
Macula, 3130
Macular degeneration, 360-361, 1075, 1077, **1846-1849**, 2774, 3131, 3133, 3235, 3286
Mad cow disease, 593, 710, 2453, 3286
Maduromycosis, 1186
Magnesium, 2140, 3138
Magnetic field therapy, 102, **1849-1850**, 3235
Magnetic resonance imaging (MRI), 131, 207, 324, 388, 1002, 1220, 1586, 1807, **1850-1852**, 2096, 2118, 2546, 2856, 3235
Magnetoencephalography (MEG), 2096
Magnets, 1557, 1849, 1851

Monosaccharides, 1152
Monosodium glutamate (MSG), 2891
Monosomy, 3287
Monozygotes, 3237
Montagnier, Luc, 2178
Mood disorders, 75, 789, 979, 2711
Morbid obesity, 3237
Morbidity, 3237
Morbidity and Mortality Weekly Report, 522
Mordant, 3237
Morgellons disease, **1976-1977**, 3237, 3287
Morgue, 3238
Morning-after pills, 694
Morning sickness, 2060-2061
Moro reflex, 2562
Morphea, 2647
Morphine, 730, 1453, 2042, 2469
Morphologic changes, 267
Morquio syndrome, 1989
Morselli, Enrique, 384
Mortality, 3238
Morton, William T. G., 149
Morton's neuroma, 1164
Mosaicism, 879, 881
Mosquitoes, 772, 953, 955, 987, 1650, 1853, 3160, 3189, 3194
Moss, F. A., 1895
Mother-infant attachment, 635, 811
Motility, 3238
Motion sickness, **1977-1979**, 2059-2060, 2671, 3238, 3287
Motor, 3238
Motor disabilities, 526
Motor neuron, 3238
Motor neuron diseases, 131, **1979-1983**, 3238, 3287
Motor seizure, 3287
Motor skill development, **1983-1987**
Motor weakness, 3238, 3287
Mouth, 1216, 1512, 1988; dry, 2733
Mouth cancer, **1988-1989**
MPS. *See* Mucopolysaccharidosis (MPS)
MRI. *See* Magnetic resonance imaging (MRI)
mRNA. *See* Messenger ribonucleic acid (mRNA)
MRSA infections. *See* Methicillin-resistant *Staphylococcus aureus* (MRSA) infections

MSUD. *See* Maple syrup urine disease (MSUD)
Mucoepidermoid carcinoma, 3287
Mucolipidosis, 3287
Mucopolysaccharidosis (MPS), **1989-1990**, 3238, 3287
Mucosa, 3238
Mucous glands, 1279
Mucous membrane, 3238
Mucus, 1279, 1512, 1827, 2770, 3238
Müllerian ducts, 2685, 3238
Multiple births, 233, 1618, **1990-1996**
Multiple chemical sensitivity syndrome, **1996-1997**, 3288
Multiple infarct dementia, 768, 1904
Multiple myeloma, 3288
Multiple sclerosis, 264, 1327, 1479, **1998-2003**, 2087, 2274, 2690, 2727, 2795, 3238, 3288; endometriosis and, 1011
Multipotent, 3238
Mumps, 563, 1218, **2003-2006**, 2190, 3238, 3288
Münchausen syndrome, 834, 1093, 2399
Münchausen syndrome by proxy, **2006-2007**, 2399, 3288
Murmur, 3238, 3288. *See also* Heart murmurs
Muscle cells, 745, 1295, 1307
Muscle contraction, 3238
Muscle cramps, 2009
Muscle fibers, 3238
Muscle pain, 1130, 2008
Muscle relaxant, 3238
Muscle sprains, spasms, and disorders, 1325, 1818, 1980, **2007-2011**, 2013, 2016, 2945, 2972, 3164
Muscle weakness, 2026
Muscles, 136, 409, 831, 1069, 1109, 1296, 1551, 1980, 2007, **2011-2016**, 2026, 2197, 2273, 2353, 2668, 2929, 2944, 3238; aging and, 70; atrophy, 247; chest, 547; glycogen storage diseases, 1291; lower extremities, 1815; upper extremities, 3067
Muscular dystrophy, 138, 1239, 1241, 1552, 1818, 2008, 2013, 2015, **2016-2021**, 2275, 3070,

3238, 3288; Duchenne, 1251, 1818, 2013, 2016, 2018-2019, 3070
Musculature, 3238
Musculoskeletal, 3238
Mushrooms, 2405
Mustard gas, 310
Mutagen, 3238
Mutation, 341, 465, 519, 733, 735-736, 868, 879, 883, 892, 962, 1032, 1233, **2021-2026**, 2168, 2298, 2833, 3044, 3238, 3288; recessive, 735
Mutism, 3288
Myasthenia gravis, 265, 952, 1479, 1608, 1610, 2008-2009, 2014, **2026-2028**, 2275, 2964, 3238, 3288
Mycetoma, 3238
Myco-, 3238
Mycobacteria, 278, 3035
Mycobacterium, 3238
Mycobacterium avium complex, 2176
Mycosis, 3238
Mycosis fungoides, 2740
Mycotoxins, 1185, 1971
Myelin, 62, 1326-1327, 1477, 1998, 2001, 2086-2087, 2091
Myelin sheath, 1778
Myelography, 1820
Myenteric plexus, 2317
Myocardial infarction. *See* Heart attack
Myocardium, 489, 3238
Myoclonus, 2749, 3238
Myomas, 3045
Myomectomy, 1336, 1573, 1915, **2028-2029**, 3238
Myopathy, 2008
Myopia, 382, 1076-1077, 1086, **2029-2030**, 2564, 2671, 3131, 3133, 3238, 3288
Myosarcoma, 3045
Myostatin, 1245
MyPyramid, 1156. *See also* Food Guide Pyramid
Myringotomy, 911, 916, **2030-2031**, 3238

NAD. *See* Nicotinamide adenine dinucleotide (NAD)
Nail bed, 2033
Nail plate, 2033

Phrenic reflex, 294
Phylogenetics, 3246
Physiatry, 2350, 3246
Physical deconditioning, 1105, 3246
Physical examination, 1659, **2344-2349**, 2806, 3246
Physical fitness, 1073, 1111
Physical modalities, 3246
Physical rehabilitation, 128, 2015, **2349-2354**, 2805, 3246
Physical sciences, 3246
Physical therapy, 95, 128, 527, 620, 1467, 1488, 1526, 1699, 1719, 2010, 2018, 2350, 2805
Physician assistants, **2355-2359**, 3246
Physiological, 3246
Physiology, **2359-2364**, 3246
Phytochemicals, **2364**, 2875, 3246
Piaget, Jean, 632, 636, 810, 1323
Pica, 259
Pick, Arnold, 1177
Pick's disease, 768, **2365-2367**
PID. *See* Pelvic inflammatory disease (PID)
Piebaldism, 2743
Piercings. *See* Body piercing
Pigeon toes, **2367-2368**
Pigmentation, 81, 1900, **2368-2372**, 2743, 3246; disorders, 3141
Pigs, 3187
Piles, 3246. *See also* Hemorrhoids
Pilocarpine, 1286
Pilosebaceous, 3246
Pimples, 29, 799, 2531, 2860, 3246. *See also* Acne
Pinched nerve, 278
Pineal gland, 994-995, 997, 1281, 1902, 2747
Pinel, Philippe, 2492
Pinkeye. *See* Conjunctivitis
Pinworms, 2289, **2372-2373**, 2618, 3290
Pitocin, 1504, 2159
Pituitary gland, 401, 891-892, 993-994, 997, 999, 1002, 1274, 1281, 1323, 1924, 2107, **2373-2375**, 2771, 2903, 3246
Pituitary tumors, 728, 1274
Pityriasis, 2744
Pityriasis alba, **2375**
Pityriasis rosea, **2376-2377**
P-K test, 93

PKU. *See* Phenylketonuria (PKU)
Placebo, 332, 2249, 3246
Placenta, 556-557, 584, 960, 1992, 2158, 2313, **2377-2378**, 2433-2434, 3246
Placenta abruptio, 560, 2313, 2377, 2441, 2831
Placenta previa, 536, 2313, 2377, 2441
Placental insufficiency, 2377
Plague, 308, 975, 1037, 1652, **2378-2380**, 3194, 3246, 3290; bubonic, 2378, 3028, 3195; pneumonic, 2379, 2519
Plaintiff, 3246
Plantar, 3246
Plantar fasciitis, 1101
Plantar warts, 1110, 1164, 3146, 3148, 3246
Plants, 1452, 2364
Plaque, 514, 701, 3246; arterial, 202, 203, 488, 601, 990, 1392, 1395, 1400, 1533, 1540, **2380-2381**, 2818, 2828, 2853, 2955, 3099, 3290; dental, 24, 774-775, 779, 1276, 1331, 2315, **2381-2382**, 2920, 2986, 3290
Plasma, 366, 370, 1421, 1437, 1610, 1832, **2382-2383**, 2902, 3013, 3246
Plasma coagulation system, 356
Plasma exchange, 2001, 2027, 2953
Plasma proteins, 3246
Plasmapheresis, 1327, 1437, 1610, 2009, 3108
Plasmids, 622, 886, 904, 1229
Plasmin, 2954, 3246
Plasminogen, 2954
Plastic surgery, 68, 384, 1089, 1791, 2227, **2383-2388**, 3186, 3247. *See also* Cosmetic surgery; Reconstructive surgery
Plasticity, 3247
Platelets, 356-357, 359, 365, 370, 1422, 1436, 1773, 2382, 2952, 2954, 2958, 3012, 3144, 3169, 3247
Pleura, 547, 1825, 1827, 2388, 3247
Pleurisy, **2388-2389**, 2390, 3247, 3290
Pluripotent, 3247
PMDD. *See* Premenstrual dysphoric disorder (PMDD)

PML. *See* Progressive multifocal leukoencephalopathy (PML)
PMS. *See* Premenstrual syndrome (PMS)
Pneumococcal infections, 888
Pneumocystis pneumonia, 36, 2177, 2391, 3247, 3290
Pneumonia, 47, 282, 447, 631, 661, 663, 1187, 1600, 1661, 1726, 1759, 1822, 1828, 1919, 2379, **2389-2393**, 2516, 2526, 2803, 3162, 3247, 3290
Pneumonic plague, 2379, 2519
Pneumothorax, 1825, 1827, **2393-2395**, 3247, 3290
PNP. *See* Purine nucleoside phosphorylase (PNP)
Podiatry, 1111, **2395-2398**, 3247
Point-of-service plans, 1376, 1876
Poison control centers, 1134
Poison ivy, 2404
Poison oak, 2404
Poison sumac, 2404
Poisoning, 18, 20, 269, 659, 715, 848, 1150, 1530, **2398-2404**, 2627, 2670, 3000, 3247, 3290; first aid, 1134
Poisonous plants, **2404-2406**, 3247, 3290
Poisons, 18, 269, 347, 746, 1039, 2299, 2402, 2671, 2998, 3000
Poliomyelitis, 564-565, 1020-1021, 1479, 1596, 1598, **2406-2412**, 2795, 3124, 3126, 3247
Pollen, 1357
Pollution, 706, 1027, 1039, 1828
Polyarteritis, 3109
Polychondritis, 502
Polycystic kidney disease, 1250, 1716, **2412-2413**, 3247, 3290
Polycystic ovary syndrome, 114, 744, 2231, **2413-2415**, 2570, 3247, 3290
Polycythemia, 730, 3247
Polydactyly, 341, **2415-2417**, 3247, 3290
Polydipsea, 3290
Polyesthesia, 3290
Polygraph, 979
Polyhydramnios, 123
Polymerase chain reaction, 327, 374, 377, 1244, 1505, 1647, 1990, 3247
Polymethylmethacrylate, 2386, 3247

Taste buds, 2669, 2908, 2910, 3259
Taste cell, 3259
Taste disorders, 2911
Tattoo removal, **2913-2914**
Tattoos, **2914-2916**
Taussig-Bing syndrome, 3295
Taxanes, 466
Taxol, 427, 542, 1454
Tay-Sachs disease, 678, 736, 1233, 1250, 1789, 1939, 1941, **2916-2917**, 3295
Tear ducts, 1081, **2917-2918**
Tear gas, 310
Tears, 1278, 2733, **2917-2918**, 3131
Technetium, 1587
TEE. *See* Transesophageal echocardiography (TEE)
Teeth, 406, 513, 723, 779, 783-784, 1216, 1321, 1332, 2187, 2191, 2193, 2315, 2381, 2612, **2918-2923**, 2985, 3168, 3259
Teething, **2923-2925**
Telangiectases, 356
Telangiectasia, 3295
Telehealth, 2925
Telemedicine, 1664, **2925-2926**
Telomeres, 468, 624
Temin, Howard, 2588
Temperature. *See* Body temperature; Fever
Temporal lobe seizure, 1044
Temporal lobectomy, 1047
Temporal lobes, 3259
Temporomandibular joint, 3259
Temporomandibular joint (TMJ) syndrome, 2186, **2926-2927**, 3295
Tend-and-befriend response, 2847
Tender points, 1130
Tendinitis, 1101, 2009-2010, 2615, 2807, **2927-2929**, 2931, 3259, 3295
Tendinosis, 2928
Tendon disorders, 2204, **2929-2931**
Tendon repair, **2931-2932**
Tendons, 645, 690, 1100, 1109, 1199, 1816, 2198, 2204, 2668, 2807, 2928-2929, 2931, 3067, 3259
Tennis elbow, 2009-2010, 2808, 2928, 2930, 3070
Tenosynovitis, 2009-2010, 2930
TENS. *See* Transcutaneous electrical nerve stimulation (TENS)

Tensile strength, 3259
Tension-type headaches, 1361, 1363
Tentorial herniation, 3295
Teratogenesis, 3295
Teratogens, 341, 961, 1112, 2436, **2932-2933**, 3259
Teratology, 3259
Teriparatide, 2221
Terminal illness, 755, 1506, 2869, 2872
Terminally ill, extended care for the, 1063, 2252, **2933-2937**
Termites, 2286
Terrorism, 307, 310
Test kits, 1731
Testes, 1258, 1281, 1523, 2567, 2685, 2940, 3259
Testicle removal. *See* Orchiectomy
Testicles, 1919, 2190, 2942; undescended, **2937-2938**, 3295
Testicular cancer, 1260, 1916, 2189, **2938-2939**, 2941
Testicular surgery, 1523, **2940-2941**
Testicular torsion, 1919, 1922, **2942**, 3259, 3295
Testosterone, 1053, 1227, 1258, 1281, 1552, 2465, 2685, 2690, 2696, 2826, 3259
Tests. *See* Invasive tests; Laboratory tests; Noninvasive tests
Tetanospasmin, 2944
Tetanus, 282, 564, 1181, 1201, 1597, 1954, **2942-2947**, 2965, 3183, 3259, 3295; acellular pertussis, 565
Tetany, 1536-1537, 2945, 3295
Tetracycline, 3006
Tetrahydrocannabinol (THC), 1882
Tetralogy of Fallot, 381, 683
Thalamus, 412, 2748
Thalassemia, 140, 1250, 2722, **2947-2948**, 3259, 3295
Thalidomide, 297, 313, 343, 962, 1150, 2932, **2948-2949**, 3259
Thanatology, 3259
Thanotophoric dwarfism, 894
THC. *See* Tetrahydrocannabinol (THC)
Theophylline, 595, 984
Therapeutic index, 541
Therapeutics, 3259
Thermogenesis, 3259
Thermometers, 1125
Thermometry, 1126

Thermoregulation, 1517, 1545-1546, 2743, 2890
Thermoregulatory set point, 3259
Thiamine, 299, 1153, 1864, 1878, 2366, 3137
Thigh, 3259
Thimerosal, 1935
Third-degree burn, 456, 2991
Thoracentesis, 1681
Thoracic, 3259
Thoracic duct, 3259
Thoracic surgery, 485, 549, **2949-2951**
Thoracotomy, 2950
Thorax, 3259. *See also* Chest
Threadworms, 2372
Throat, 1739, 1827, 1988, 2224, 3004-3005
Throat, sore. *See* Sore throat
Throat cancer, **1988-1989**, 2335
Thrombin, 2954, 3259
Thrombocytes, 3260. *See also* Platelets
Thrombocytopenia, 357, **2951-2953**, 3013, 3169, 3260
Thromboembolism, 3260, 3295
Thrombolytic drugs, 3260
Thrombolytic therapy, 957, **2953-2958**
Thrombophlebitis, 3114
Thrombosis, 203, 601, 934, 2337, 2380, 2853, **2958-2962**, 3106, 3260, 3295; deep vein, 761-762
Thrombotic thrombocytopenia purpura, 2952
Thrombus, 602, 761, 934, 957, 2237, 2337, 2853, 2955, **2958-2962**, 3114, 3260, 3295
Thrush, 471
Thumb sucking, 2192, **2962-2964**
Thymectomy, 2027
Thymus gland, 839, 994, 1592, 1610, 2009, 2026, 2683, **2964-2965**, 3260; removal, 2027
Thyroglossal cysts, 732
Thyroid disorders, 264, 998, 1001, 1281, 1299, 1356, 1503, **2965-2967**, 2968
Thyroid gland, 686, 994, 997, 1000-1001, 1280, 1298, 1356, 1864, 2128, 2553, 2903, 2965, **2967-2971**, 3260; imaging of, 1587
Thyroid hormone, 2971

Thyroid hormone-releasing hormone (TRH), 2374
Thyroid-stimulating hormone (TSH), 1281, 2373
Thyroidectomy, 1001, **2971-2972**, 3260
Thyroxine, 1280, 1299, 1356, 2846, 2965-2966, 2968, 3260
TIAs. *See* Transient ischemic attacks (TIAs)
Tibia, 1815-1816, 2204, 3260
Tibia vara, 406
Tic douloureux, 2108, 2973
Ticks, 276, 942, 987, **1779-1783**, 1830, 2611, 3194. *See also* Lice
Tics, 897, 2785, **2972-2976**, 2994, 3295
Timolol maleate, 1286
Tincture, 1492, 3260
Tinea nigra, 1185
Tinea pedis, 245
Tinea versicolor, 1185, 2375
Tingling, 257, 1180, 1326, 1911, **2132-2133**, 2991. *See also* Numbness
Tinnitus, 908-909, 1384, 2671, **2977-2978**, 3115, 3260, 3295
Tiredness. *See* Fatigue
Tissue culture, 3260
Tissue death. *See* Necrosis
Tissue plasminogen activator (TPA or tPA), 1029-1030, 2585, **2953-2958**, 3260
Tissue typing, 3260
Tissues, 135, 326, 2363, 2668, 3260; damage, 1772
TMJ syndrome. *See* Temporomandibular joint (TMJ) syndrome
Tobacco, 50, 1025, 1988, 2111, 2316, 2450, 2517; American Indians and, 115
Toddlers, 811
Todd's paralysis, 2275
Toenail removal. *See* Nail removal
Toenails, 2032, 2034; ingrown, 1164, 2034
Toes, 1108, 1815-1816, 2033, 2367
Toes, extra. *See* Polydactyly
Toes, fused. *See* Syndactyly
Toilet training, 811, 1622, **2978-2980**
Tolerance, 48, 3260

Toman, Walter, 2721
Tomograms, 667
Tomography, 3260
Tongue, 1216, 1988, 2669, 2908-2909
Tongue thrusting, 2192
Tonic-clonic seizure. *See* Grand mal seizure
Tonometer, 1288, 3260
Tonsillectomy, 57, 353, 917, 2334, 2536, 2782, **2980-2982**, 2984, 3260
Tonsillitis, 1840, 2048, 2051, 2334, 2536, 2980, **2982-2983**, 2984, 3260, 3295
Tonsils, 1840, 2334, 2980, 2982, **2983-2984**, 3260; nasopharyngeal, 56
Tooth decay, 514, 1005, 1143, 2381, 2986, 3260, 3295. *See also* Cavities
Tooth extraction, 780, 2921, **2985**, 3168, 3260
Tooth loss, 784, 2316; smoking and, 2773
Tooth pulp, 3260
Toothache, 774, 776, **2986**, 3260, 3295
Tophi, 1303
Tophus, 3260
Topical, 3260
Topical anesthesia, 144
Torsion, 2940
Tort, 3260
Torticollis, 404, **2987**, 3295
Totipotence, 3260
Touch, 2668, **2987-2993**, 3260
Tourette's syndrome, 2154, 2974-2975, **2993-2995**, 3295
Tourniquet, 2341
Toxemia, 2441, **2995-2996**, 3260, 3295
Toxic epidermal necrolysis, 2829
Toxic shock syndrome, 282, 1926, 2810, 2844, 2891, **2996-2998**, 3261, 3295
Toxicity, selective, 539
Toxicokinetics, 3261
Toxicology, 269, 1022, 1491, **2998-3001**, 3261
Toxins, 102, 347, 403-404, 679, 1755, 1799-1800, 2299, 2324, 2399, 2674, 2943, 2998, 3261; metal, 1023

Toxoid, 3261
Toxoplasmosis, 161, 1159, 2176, 2289, 2483, **3001-3003**, 3194-3195, 3261, 3295
TPA. *See* Tissue plasminogen activator (TPA or tPA)
Trabeculectomy, 1287
Trabeculoplasty, 1080
Trace elements, 3261
Trace evidence, 3261
Tracer, 3261
Trachea, 445, 1017, 1824, 1827, 2573, **3003-3004**, 3005, 3261
Tracheal transplantation, 3004
Tracheomalacia, 3003
Tracheostomy, 713, 1420, 1658, 2946, **3004-3006**, 3261
Trachoma, 361, 696, 1074, 1076, **3006**, 3028, 3261, 3295
Tracking, 1665
Tract, 3261
Traction, 503, 1170-1171, 1173
Traffic accidents, 2630. *See also* Accidents
Trance, 1555
Tranquilizers, 2155, 2750
Transcription, 3261
Transcutaneous electrical nerve stimulation (TENS), 2251
TransCyte, 456
Transducer (probe), 3261
Transduction, 622
Transesophageal echocardiography (TEE), 928
Transfats, 2140
Transference, 3261
Transfusion, 142, 370-372, 1575, 1730, 2592, 2709, **3007-3016**, 3261
Transgender, 3261
Transgenic organisms, 625
Transient ischemic attacks (TIAs), 192, 204, 205, 418, 420, 2853, **3016-3017**, 3105, 3261, 3295
Transitional cell carcinoma, 3261
Translation, 3261
Translocation, 879, 883, 2637
Transmission, 3261
Transplantation, 160, 396, 750, 1249, 1411, 1593, 1711-1712, 2815, 2885, **3017-3023**, 3261; bone marrow, **395-398**, 400, 1309, 1483-1484, 1605-1606, 1775, 2543, 2683, 2724; cloning

for, 625; corneal, **696-698**, 1077, 1080; ethics and, 1060; facial, **1090-1092**, 2188; hair, 1341, 1346, **1348-1350**; heart, 1393, 1407, **1409-1412**, 2951; kidney, 989, 1710, **1711-1713**, 2073, 2076, 2083; liver, 1800, 1808, **1809-1811**, 2117, 3019; lung, 592; tracheal, 3004

Transposition of the great arteries, 683-684

Transposon, 887

Transsexualism, 1227, 2688

Transsexuals, 3261

Transthoracic echocardiography (TTE), 928

Transverse processes, 3261

Transvestism, 3261

Trauma, 120, 715, 848, 1358, 1465, 2279, 2299, 2350, 2794, 3261, 3295

Trauma, emotional, 120, 2426

Trauma centers, 974, 3261

Travelers' diarrhea, 113, 833, 836, 1219, 3295

Treacher Collins syndrome, 3295

Treatment, 3261

Trembling, 3023

Tremors, 2293, 3023-3024

Trench fever, 1652

Trench mouth, 1276, 3295. *See also* Vincent's infection

Trephination, 2109, 3261

Trephine, 3261

Tretinoin, 2851

Triage, 967, 971, 973, 1509, 3261

Triangle model in epidemiology, 1039

Trichiasis, 3006

Trichinellosis, 3024

Trichinosis, 2289, 2618, **3024-3025**, 3182

Trichomonas vaginalis, 1254

Trichomoniasis, 1255-1256, 2700, 2703, **3025-3027**, 3261

Tricyclic antidepressants, 169, 177, 979, 1966, 3262

Trigeminal nerve, 628, 2187, 2858

Triglycerides, 1152, 1673, 1786, 1788, 1797, 1844, 1918, 2656

Triiodothyronine, 1280

Trimester, 3262

Triple test, 3262

Triplets, 1993, 1995

Triptans, 1966

Trismus, 2536, 3168

Trisomy, 3262, 3295

Trisomy C syndrome, 3295

Trisomy 21. *See* Down syndrome

Tropical diseases, 956, 1853, 2288, 3027, 3189

Tropical medicine, 2640, **3027-3033**, 3262

Trousseau's sign, 3295

Trudeau, Edward Livingston, 3038

Trunk, 3262

Trust, 811, 813

Trypanosomes, 538, 2759

Trypanosomiasis, 2178, 2759, 3296

TSH. *See* Thyroid-stimulating hormone (TSH)

TTE. *See* Transthoracic echocardiography (TTE)

Tubal ligation, 695, 1738, 2820, **3033-3034**, 3112, 3262

Tubal pregnancy, 929

Tubercles, 3034

Tuberculin skin test, 3036

Tuberculosis, 224, 277, 282, 523, 769, 887, 975, 1596, 1828, 2517, 2524, 2526, **3034-3039**, 3194, 3262, 3296; Asian Americans and, 221

Tuberculous laryngitis, 1740

Tubular reabsorption, 3262

Tubular secretion, 3262

Tubulointerstitial nephritis, 2074

Tularemia, 1780, **3039-3040**

Tumor removal, 652, 1840, **3040-3043**

Tumor suppressor genes, 1252, 1859

Tumor vaccines, 1707

Tumors, 349, 422, 465, 651, 653, 748, 1002, 1067, 1566, 1671, 1739, 1801, 1858, 2126, 2168, 2226, 2264, 2470, 2570, 3040, **3043-3048**, 3061, 3262, 3296; nerve, 2094

Tunnel vision, 1078

Turbidity, 3074

Turbulence, 601

Turgor, 3262

Turner syndrome, 113, 550, 679, 892, 962, 1004, 1703, 1994, 2685, **3048-3049**, 3296

Twin-twin transfusion syndrome, 1115, 1993

Twins, 623, 1115, 1234, 1991, 3262. *See also* Multiple births; Vanishing twin syndrome

Tympanic membrane, 753, 911, 1378, 2669, 3262

Tympanoplasty, 911, 916, 3262

Type A individuals, 2848

Type B individuals, 2848

Typhoid fever, 2632, **3049-3050**, 3262, 3296

Typhus, 1652, 1780, **3050-3051**, 3262, 3296

Tyramine, 1965

Tyrosine, 1965, 2368

Tyrosine kinase inhibitors, 313

Ulcer surgery, **3052-3054**

Ulcerative colitis, 647, 3262, 3296. *See also* Colitis

Ulcers, 8, 297, 598, 1136, 1202, 1207, 1213, 1219, 1662, 1674, 1744, 3052, **3054-3058**, 3092, 3114, 3262, 3296; corneal, 2173; decubitus, 295; mouth, 297, 474

Ulna, 3066, 3262

Ulnar, 3262

Ultrasonic, 3262

Ultrasonography, 426, 1207, 1220, 1234, 1586, 1795, 2119, 2158, 2312, 2838, **3058-3063**, 3262

Ultrasound, 206-207, 342, 928, 1194, 1586, 1807, 2159, 2855, 2857

Ultraviolet light, 2369, 2487, 2740

Ultraviolet radiation, 2369-2370, 3262

Umbilical cord, 2158, 2377, 2436, 2943, **3063-3064**; entanglement, 2831

Umbilical hernias, 1461

Umbilicus, 3262

Unconsciousness, 674, 2037, 2400, **3064-3065**, 3262, 3296

Underbite, 407

Universal coverage, 1370, 3262

Upper arm, 3262

Upper extremities, 128, **3065-3070**, 3262; prostheses for, 2475

Uprima, 2692

Urban, Jerome, 1887

Urea, 2076, 3071, 3262

Uremia, 989, **3071-3072**, 3262, 3296

Venipuncture, 1426, 2341, 3264
Venography, 2339
Venom, 347, 2776
Venous admixture, 730
Venous insufficiency, **3114-3115**, 3264, 3296
Venous thrombosis, 934, 957, 2339, 3106, 3264, 3296
Venter, Craig, 1264
Ventilator, 47
Ventricles, 1390, 3264
Ventricular fibrillation, 201, 488, 762, 943, 945, 1393, 1401, 2242, 2584
Ventricular remodeling, 486
Ventricular tachycardia, 762
Ventriculoperitoneal shunts, 2716, 3264
Venules, 379
Vermiform appendix. *See* Appendix
Vertebrae, 279, 545, 567, 569, 1726, 2108, 2762, **2797-2802**, 3264
Vertigo, 289, 863, 908, 2670, 2854, **3115-3116**, 3264, 3296
Very long chain fatty acids, 62, 1778
Vesalius, Andreas, 502, 1784
Vesicants, 310
Vesicle, 3264
Vestibular, 3264
Veterans, 1329, 2428
Veterinary medicine, 159, **3117-3121**, 3264
Viability, 1748
Viagra, 1052-1053
Vicodin, 2251, 2445
Videoconferencing, 2925
Vierordt, Karl, 368
Villi, 3264
Vinca alkaloids, 542
Vincent's infection, 774, 776
Vioxx, 181, 1149
Viral hemorrhagic fevers, **3121-3123**, 3296
Viral infections, 6, 8, 57, 272, 552, 564, 662, 750, 887, 924, 1020, 1050, 1132, 1204, 1354-1355, 1448, 1463, 1518, 1628, 1630, 1645, 1660, 1798, 1879, 1973, 2003, 2524, 2587, 2589, 2607, 2616, 3122, **3123-3129**, 3189; arthropod-borne, 3027
Virchow, Rudolf, 749, 2064
Virilization, 3264

Virions, 3124, 3264
Virulence, 3264
Virulence factors, 904
Viruses, 57, 172, 662-663, 666, 848, 887, 925, 1020, 1645, 1890, 1953, 1955, 1975, 2524, 2538, 2587, 2607, 3046, 3122-3123, 3264; endogenous, 3187; use as vectors, 1229
Vision, 322, 1084, 2180, 2669, 3115, **3129-3132**; blurred, 382-383, 1846, 2029; color, 650
Vision correction, 243, 1081, 3133
Vision disorders, 242, 243, 360, 382, 507, 509, 1074, 1079-1081, 1267, 1285, 1846, 1848, 2029, 2184, 2564, 2671, 2842, **3132-3136**
Visual acuity, 3264
Visual dyslexia, 899
Visual reinforcement audiometry (VRA), 1388
Vital organs, 3264
Vital signs, 2727
Vitamin A, 2140, 3136
Vitamin A acid, 32
Vitamin A deficiency, 1705, 1864, 1866
Vitamin B deficiency, 141, 1203, 1864, 1866, 2907, 3137
Vitamin C, 183, 690, 2140, 2658, 3137
Vitamin C deficiency, 2658. *See also* Scurvy
Vitamin D, 2141, 2222, 2736, 3137, 3172, 3174
Vitamin D deficiency, 1864, 1866, 2143, 2608, 3137
Vitamin E, 183, 2141, 2444, 3137
Vitamin K, 598, 2954
Vitamin K deficiency, 353, 3013, 3137
Vitamins, 183, 300, 353, 848, 1153, 1797, 1844, 1863, 1865, 2140, 2299, 2658, 2875, **3136-3140**, 3264
Vitiligo, 2375, 2743, **3140-3142**, 3264, 3296
Vitravene, 319
Vitrectomy, 1077, 3264
Vitreous, 3130
Vitreous humor, 3264
Vitrification, 1640
Vocal cord disorders, **3142-3144**

Vocal cord polyps, 2420
Vocal cords, 1740
Voice box. *See* Larynx
Voice disorders, 1740, 2785, **3142-3144**
Voltage, 3264
Voluntary euthanasia, 3264
Vomiting, 20, 920, 1219, **2058-2063**, 2121, 2319, 2533, 2671, 3264, 3296. *See also* Nausea
Vomiting, self-induced. *See* Bulimia; Purging
Von Behring, Emil, 176, 1516
Von Neumann machine, 3264
Von Recklinghausen's tumor, 3296
Von Willebrand's disease, 353, 357-358, 1436, 1438, **3144-3145**, 3264, 3296
VRA. *See* Visual reinforcement audiometry (VRA)
Vulva, 732, 1334, 2569
Vygotsky, Lev, 634, 636

Wagner-Jauregg, Julius, 1125
Waksman, Selman, 543, 3038
Wald, Lillian, 1489
Waldemeyer's ring, 2980
Walking, 288, 1466
Wandering, 2631
Warburg effect, 1297
Warfare, 307
Warfarin, 2955
Warm-blooded organisms, 1122, 1545
Warts, 799, 1164, 1520, 1739, 1858, 3046, **3146-3150**, 3264, 3296; genital, 726, 1255-1256, 1520-1521, 2700-2701, 3147, 3149; plantar, 1110, 1164, 3146, 3148
Wasting, 3264
Watchful waiting, 2466
Water, 1139, 1714; therapy in, 1526. *See also* Hydrotherapy
Water loss, 764
Water on the brain. *See* Hydrocephalus
Watery eyes, 1075, 1077
Wavelength, 3264
Waxes, 1786
Weaning, **3150-3153**
Web sites, 1664
Wedge argument, 3264
Wegener's granulomatosis, 3109
Weight gain, 2145, 2150, **3153-3156**